STRUCTURE AND MECHANISM IN ORGANIC CHEMISTRY

SECOND EDITION

BY C. K. INGOLD

Structure and Mechanism in Organic Chemistry

Second Edition

BY C. K. INGOLD

Professor of Chemistry, University College
University of London

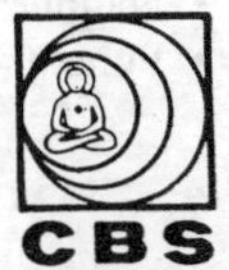

CBS Publishers & Distributors Pvt. Ltd.

New Delhi • Bengaluru • Chennai • Kochi • Kolkata • Mumbai
Hyderabad • Nagpur • Patna • Pune • Vijayawada

ISBN: 81-239-0975-6

First Indian Reprint: 1994

This edition has been published in India by arrangement with Cornell University, USA

Published by **Satish Kumar Jain** and produced by **Varun Jain** for
CBS Publishers & Distributors Pvt. Ltd.,
4819/XI Prahlad Street, 24 Ansari Road, Daryaganj, New Delhi - 110002
delhi@cbspd.com, cbspubs@airtelmail.in • www.cbspd.com
Ph.: 23289259, 23266861, 23266867 • Fax: 011-23243014

Corporate Office: 204 FIE, Industrial Area, Patparganj, Delhi - 110 092
Ph: 49344934 • Fax: 011-49344935
E-mail: publishing@cbspd.com • publicity@cbspd.com

Branches:

- ***Bengaluru:*** 2975, 17th Cross, K.R. Road, Bansankari 2nd Stage, Bengaluru - 70 • Ph: +91-80-26771678/79 • Fax: +91-80-26771680 E-mail: cbsbng@gmail.com, bangalore@cbspd.com
- ***Chennai:*** No. 7, Subbaraya Street, Shenoy Nagar, Chennai - 600030 Ph: +91-44-26681266, 26680620 • Fax: +91-44-42032115 E-mail: chennai@cbspd.com
- ***Kochi:*** Ashana House, 39/1904, A.M. Thomas Road, Valanjambalam, Ernakulum, Kochi • Ph: +91-484-4059061-65 Fax: +91-484-4059065 • E-mail: cochin@cbspd.com
- ***Kolkata:*** 6-B, Ground Floor, Rameshwar Shaw Road, Kolkata - 700014 Ph: +91-33-22891126/7/8 • E-mail: kolkata@cbspd.com
- ***Mumbai:*** 83-C, Dr. E. Moses Road, Worli, Mumbai - 400018 Ph: +91-9833017933, 022-24902340/41 • E-mail: mumbai@cbspd.com

Representatives:

- Hyderabad: 0-9885175004
- Patna: 0-9334159340
- Vijayawada: 0-9000660880
- Nagpur: 0-9021734563
- Pune: 0-9623451994

Printed at:
Neekunj Print Process, Delhi (India)

Preface to the Second Edition

THE first edition of *Structure and Mechanism in Organic Chemistry* was written in 1950–51, when the formation of the subject had been accomplished, and the work of consolidation and development, by a vastly increased number of workers, was only just beginning. This work has so flourished since then as to constitute a large part of the story now to be told. In this edition, about two-thirds of the text of the previous one has been retained, with only minor emendations, and more than that amount of new writing has been added.

Three times only have I been withdrawn long enough from daily duties to undertake comprehensive writing—writing intended to help the pulling together of organic chemistry. The first time was in 1932, when, during a period at Stanford University, I produced a review article published in 1934. In 1950 came a second opportunity, when, as Baker Lecturer at Cornell University, I wrote the first edition of this book. The invitation to be National Science Foundation Fellow at Vanderbilt University in 1964 made possible the undertaking of this edition, amidst congenial and relaxed surroundings. Thus, to Academic America, acting always with the co-operation of University College, London, I owe my three long interludes for quiet reflexion.

I am very grateful for all the personal help I have received. I had some most valuable lessons on homolytic organic reactions from my son, who also gave me hundreds of original references, and revised, sometimes changing extensively, my own first attempts at writing in this area. These parts of the book could appropriately have appeared under joint authorship, as I would myself have preferred. Other parts of the text have benefited greatly from the help I have had from colleagues, in particular Dr. D. V. Banthorpe, Dr. H. M. R. Hoffmann,

Dr. M. D. Johnson, Professor A. Maccoll, Dr. J. H. Ridd, Professor C. A. Vernon, and Dr. A. Wassermann. I am especially grateful to my wife, who has checked many references and corrected many small mistakes. And the whole typescript, based on my almost illegible hand-copy, is her work.

C. K. INGOLD

April, 1967

POSTSCRIPT (April, 1969).—My wife has also taken the major part in "author's" proofreading.

Preface to the First Edition

THIS book records, and in its later chapters extends, a course of lectures which, as George Fisher Baker Non-resident Lecturer in Chemistry, I gave in the Baker Laboratory, Cornell University, during the Fall Term of 1950–51.

I should like to express my sincere gratitude to Professor F. A. Long for all the trouble he took to make my duties easy and my visit enjoyable. I am deeply grateful to him and to all the staff of the Baker Laboratory for the generosity of their welcome and the great kindness they extended to me throughout my stay. I wish to thank their colleagues and students also for their acceptance of me into their congenial society.

I am much indebted to a number of friends, most of them on this side of the water, who have in various ways shared with me the task of preparing the present manuscript. Professor E. D. Hughes gave me his private notes on a number of subjects: the substance of Chapter XI in particular is due essentially to him. That of Chapter XV is similarly due to Professor J. F. Bunnett of Reed College, Portland, Oregon, whose co-operation I enjoyed during his tenure of a Fulbright Fellowship in London. Dr. A. Wassermann gave me the same kind of aid in the composition of part of Chapter XII. Dr. R. A. Buckingham helped me with part of Chapter II. Among those, not of my own College nor of Cornell University, who were kind enough to give me important new information in advance of its publication were Dr. J. W. Baker of the University of Leeds, Dr. H. M. E. Cardwell of the University of Oxford, Dr. M. Magat of the University of Paris, Dr. A. K. Mills of Guinness's Brewery, Dublin, Dr. J. D. Roberts of the Massachusetts Institute of Technology, and Professor F. H. Westheimer of the University of Chicago. It seems hardly necessary to say that my friends of the Baker Laboratory, and my colleagues here, have contributed largely to my education in many matters which have affected this book. I am grateful for the permission which several investigators have given me to reproduce diagrams from their original papers, as is indicated by the references under the reproductions. I feel much indebted to the writers of the books and reviews to which reference is given in the text on the numerous occasions on which I have made use of them.

When this manuscript was written, Professor E. D. Hughes read the whole of it, Dr. A. Maccoll most of it, Dr. D. P. Craig and Dr. A. Wassermann large portions of it, and Dr. J. N. E. Day, Dr. P. B. D. de la Mare, and Dr. J. F. J. Dippy selected chapters. I thank these good friends for the time they have devoted to this work. They have given me much expert criticism and many valuable suggestions, of which I have been glad to take advantage. I thank my wife, who has done most of the heavy routine work involved in the composition. I believe that, had I not accepted her doctrine that it is better to finish an imperfect book than never to finish a perfect one, this particular book would never have appeared.

As its title indicates, it deals with the structure of molecules and the mechanism of reactions in organic chemistry. However, the wide scope of this subject has necessitated the imposition of limitations. As to structure, attention has concentrated on molecules in their normal states. As to reactions, discussion has been restricted substantially to those classes of homogeneous molecular reactions on which the present broad pattern of organic chemistry mainly depends. Thus a very appreciable fraction of the field indicated by the title remains uncovered. But I have been writing chiefly for the university student, and, rightly or wrongly, I have adopted the policy of limitation by selection.

University College, London C. K. INGOLD
December, 1951

POSTSCRIPT (February, 1953).—During the passage of this book through processes of publication, Dr. John R. Johnson has very kindly co-operated with the staff of the Cornell University Press in solving the numerous problems that have arisen. I am sincerely grateful both to him and to them.—C. K. I.

Contents

STRUCTURE AND MECHANISM IN ORGANIC CHEMISTRY

CHAPTER I

Valency and Molecular Structure

(1) DEVELOPMENT OF THE THEORY OF MOLECULAR STRUCTURE

IN 1808 Dalton published his atomic theory; and in 1812 Berzelius advanced the earliest theory of chemical combination. This so-called dualistic theory of combination was based on the study of inorganic substances, and envisaged binding as an electrostatic attraction between oppositely charged atoms. About 1840 the dualistic theory was overthrown as a result of the work of Dumas and others, who showed it to be incompatible with the accumulating facts of organic chemistry. Much later, following the announcement of Arrhenius's theory of electrolytic dissociation in 1887, the idea of electrostatic binding was revived, but now only in relation to ionising compounds.

In the meantime, mainly between 1840 and 1860, the work of Gerhardt, Laurent, Cannizzaro, Frankland, Williamson, Kekulé, and many others had clarified the numerical aspect of valency. Largely as part of the same work, the unitary theory of molecular constitution was developed, through its transitional forms, the radical and type theories, into the structural theory. This made no attempt to specify the physical nature of the forces holding atoms. It assumed binding power as an intrinsic property of atoms, the number of bonds formed by an atom, its valency, being characteristic for each kind of atom.

The idea that chemical binding must also have a geometrical aspect was not at once accepted as axiomatic; but it became accepted as a result of van't Hoff and Le Bel's recognition in 1874 of the specific geometrical arrangement of carbon bonds.

At the close of the last century the single term valency was used to mean both the charge on an element in its ionic form and the number of bonds by which an atom holds others in a structure. The circumstance that these numbers are often identical facilitated the dual usage. However, there was considerable confusion, structural bonds being frequently assumed where none had been shown to exist. In this period Werner was foremost in maintaining a clear distinction between an electrically neutral assembly of kinetically separable ions, and a kinetically individual molecular or ionic structure; and therefore between the charge number of an ion, and the co-ordination number, as he called it, of an atom, that is, the number of atoms bound by it structurally.

Regularities concerning the valency numbers of elements had attracted attention from an early time. Mendeléjeff, when formulating his periodic law in 1869, pointed out that valency is closely related to the numbers of the periodic groups, and normally changes by one unit from one group to the next. After the discovery of the electron by Thomson and Wiechert in 1897, several attempts were made to express the connexion between valency and group number in electronic terms. Thus Abegg assigned to each element a positive valency, equal to the group number, and a negative valency, such that the sum of the two, neglecting signs, was always eight; and he designated as the normal valency of an element, whichever, apart from signs, was the smaller. His interpretation was that all atoms have eight places for electrons, the positive valency, that is, the periodic group number, being the number of such places actually occupied in the neutral atom.[1] As Drude expressed the matter, Abegg's normal valency, when positive, represented the number of easily detached electrons, and, when negative, the number of easily added electrons.[2] The theory of octet stability could hardly have been rendered in a clearer form than this before 1913, when, as a result of the work of Fajans and Soddy, and especially of Moseley, the numbers of electrons in the atoms became known.

Already in 1911, Rutherford had established the nuclear theory of the atom. In 1916 the celebrated papers by Kossel[3] and by Lewis[4] appeared, which outlined the grouping of atomic electrons in concentric *shells*, the first a shell of two electrons, a *duplet*, the second a shell of eight, the third of eight, and the higher shells of less regular character, but always ending in a shell of eight, an *octet*, in the atoms of the inert gases. These assignments have since proved correct, though they were made before the rules of quantisation were understood. The specific geometrical ideas with which they were associated in the two theories were different, but inessential. It was essential in both theories that the electron shells reach their highest degree of stability and completeness in the inert gases, helium with its shell of two, neon with its shells of two and eight, and so on; and also that atoms having a few electrons more or less than in an inert gas would tend to lose or acquire electrons, in such a way as to produce the electronic structure of the inert gas. The formation of many stable ions, those of potassium, calcium, sulphide, and chloride, for example, could thus be understood.

[1] R. Abegg, *Z. anorg. Chem.*, 1904, **39**, 330.

[2] P. Drude, *Ann. Physik*, 1904, **14**, 722.

[3] W. Kossel, *Ann. Physik*, 1916, **49**, 229.

[4] G. N. Lewis, *J. Am. Chem. Soc.*, 1916, **38**, 762.

Lewis's theory involved a further step of quite fundamental importance, inasmuch as he recognised the *sharing* of electrons as a second process by which stable electron groups could be produced. Thus he achieved an electronic interpretation of the structural bond of chemistry. His hypothesis was that the bond consisted of a pair of electrons belonging jointly to two atoms and contributing to the completion of the electron shells of each. Sharing economises electrons, so that atoms, which, when free, had insufficient, could, when combined, have sufficient electrons to complete their shells. A bond satisfied one unit of combining power, normally represented by one electron, of each of two atoms, and therefore the content of a bond was two electrons, which themselves constituted a stable group. Lewis regarded the electron *pair*, or duplet, as the most fundamental of electron groups, and considered valency octets to consist of four duplets, whether all the electrons are shared or not. This idea has also proved correct, although it was advanced a decade before the discovery of electron spin and of Pauli's principle.

The bond of two shared electrons is much the most important type of bond on which molecular structure depends: it is the bond of the classical structural theory of chemistry. Langmuir gave it the name *covalent bond*. A weaker form of bond is known which depends on the sharing of a single electron. Binding by the sharing of electrons generally is called *covalent binding*. In case the sharing is equal, the binding is called *homopolar binding*.

The electrostatic attraction between ions was termed *electrovalency* by Langmuir. It constitutes a strong force; yet it very often fails to hold ions together in solution, because of the similarly strong, competing electrostatic attraction between the ions and the solvent. In general, electrostatic attraction may arise between oppositely charged ions, between ions and permanent or induced dipoles, and between two dipoles. Electrostatic attraction is a factor of considerable importance for molecular structure; and a measure of such *electrostatic binding* is often associated with covalent binding.

(2) ELECTRONIC CHARACTER OF COVALENCY[5]

(2a) Atomic Binding.—Lewis assumed that when two hydrogen atoms, a hydrogen and a fluorine atom, or two fluorine atoms combined, each atom, being one electron short of the number needed to complete its valency shell, supplies one electron to the shared duplet constituting the bond, each hydrogen atom thus completing its duplet, and each

[5] G. N. Lewis, "Valence and the Structure of Atoms and Molecules," Chemical Catalog Co., New York, 1923.

fluorine atom its octet; and that other atoms would similarly combine to complete their stable valency shells; so that carbon, for example, would form four bonds with hydrogen or fluorine. He expressed these ideas in formulae in which the electrons of the valency shells are represented by dots, while the literal symbols for the elements are allowed to stand, not as previously for neutral atoms, but for the positively charged kernels of atoms, that is, the atomic nuclei together with any completed inner shells of electrons:

$$H\cdot + H\cdot \rightarrow H{:}H$$

$$:\underset{\cdot\cdot}{\ddot{F}}\cdot + :\underset{\cdot\cdot}{\ddot{F}}\cdot \rightarrow :\underset{\cdot\cdot}{\ddot{F}}{:}\underset{\cdot\cdot}{\ddot{F}}:$$

$$H\cdot + :\underset{\cdot\cdot}{\ddot{F}}\cdot \rightarrow H{:}\underset{\cdot\cdot}{\ddot{F}}:$$

$$\cdot\underset{\cdot}{\dot{C}}\cdot + 4H\cdot \rightarrow \begin{array}{c} H \\ \cdot\cdot \\ H{:}C{:}H \\ \cdot\cdot \\ H \end{array}$$

$$\cdot\underset{\cdot}{\dot{C}}\cdot + 4{:}\underset{\cdot\cdot}{\ddot{F}}\cdot \rightarrow \begin{array}{c} \cdot\cdot \\ :F: \\ \cdot\cdot\ \ \cdot\cdot\ \ \cdot\cdot \\ :F{:}C{:}F: \\ \cdot\cdot\ \ \cdot\cdot\ \ \cdot\cdot \\ :F: \\ \cdot\cdot \end{array}$$

The process of forming a covalent bond by means of one electron of each of the combining atoms will be called *colligation*: the atoms may be said to colligate with each other. It is to be distinguished from the alternative way of forming a two-electron bond, co-ordination, which is to be discussed in the next Section. It must be emphasized that the distinction is in the process by which the bond is formed, not in the bond itself.

In the word "colligation" the prefix "co-" signifies, as in "covalency," a qualitative similarity of behaviour of each combining atom toward the other in the act of combination. Specifically, "colligation" means that, with such a mutuality of interaction, each atom acquires the other as a "ligand."[6]

By reversing equations such as the foregoing, we obtain a picture of one way in which the covalent bond can be broken, namely, so

[6] The terms "ligand," "ligancy," "quadriligant," and so on are today frequently used in place of the older words, "valency" and its congeners, because the former refer only to what is bound, and cannot have read into them unintended theories about the constitutions of the bonds involved.

that one of the electrons which constituted the bond is retained by each of the atoms which had formed the bond. This mode of bond fission is called *homolysis*.

(2b) Co-ordination.—Although the above-written formulae completely correspond in the number and arrangement of their bonds to the formulae of the classical structural theory, such correspondence, as Lewis pointed out, is not universal: the theory of the electron-pair bond and of the valency octet leads to a number of structures which differ significantly from those previously accepted. Moreover, the new formulae abolish some unsatisfactory features of the old, including a number to which Werner had directed attention.[7] Indeed, the electronic theory includes and interprets Werner's theory, also going beyond it by eliminating some unreal distinctions which it had retained. Thus, Werner discussed the formation and structure of ammonium salts, and of fluoroborates: according to him, nitrogen used its three principal valencies in ammonia, and employed a subsidiary valency, which was in some way qualitatively different, to hold the fourth hydrogen atom of ammonium salts: a similar description was applied to the formation of fluoroborates. Lewis admitted no distinction between the bonds holding the four hydrogen atoms, or the four fluorine atoms: he expressed the formation of the ammonium and fluoroborate ions as follows:

$$H^+ + \begin{matrix} & H & \\ & \ddot{} & \\ : & N & :H \\ & \ddot{} & \\ & H & \end{matrix} \rightarrow \left[\begin{matrix} & H & \\ & \ddot{} & \\ H: & N & :H \\ & \ddot{} & \\ & H & \end{matrix} \right]^+$$

$$\begin{matrix} & \ddot{F} & \\ :\ddot{F}: & B & \\ & \ddot{F} & \end{matrix} + :\ddot{F}:^- \rightarrow \left[\begin{matrix} & \ddot{F} & \\ :\ddot{F}: & \ddot{B} & :\ddot{F}: \\ & \ddot{F} & \end{matrix} \right]^-$$

Werner called the process of binding by the use of a subsidiary valency *co-ordination*. In its electronic interpretation, this process evidently constitutes another general method of producing a two-electron bond, namely, through the acceptance by one atom, which must have room for two additional electrons in its valency shell, of a share of a pair of unshared electrons of another atom. All the reactions by which Werner illustrated binding by subsidiary valencies retain this feature in their electronic interpretation. No distinction being now

[7] A. Werner, "Neuere Anschauungen auf den Gebiete der Anorganischen Chemie," Vieweg, Braunschweig, 1905.

admitted between Werner's two kinds of valency, it is natural that even bonds which he would have classified as principal valencies can be formed in the same way. Thus the hydrogen molecule might be formed, not only from two hydrogen atoms, but also from a proton and a hydride ion; just as a hydrogen fluoride molecule may be, and commonly is, formed from a proton and a fluoride ion:

$$H^+ + H:^- \rightarrow H:H$$

$$H^+ + :\ddot{\underset{\cdot\cdot}{F}}:^- \rightarrow H:\ddot{\underset{\cdot\cdot}{F}}:$$

Following Sidgwick, it is customary to summarise all such processes of bond-formation under the term co-ordination. Even though, etymologically, the word is not aimed quite exactly to this developed objective, the historical reasons for retaining Werner's word are very strong.

Colligation and co-ordination are two ways of forming a bond; but the bond is the same, once it is formed. Some authors use different signs for a bond according to how they suppose it to have been formed, but this is allowing the description of a non-unique hypothetical process to confuse the representation of a product, whose constitution is independent of any such process.

By reversing the last four equations, we obtain illustrations of the second method by which a covalent bond can be broken, namely, so that both the electrons of the bond are retained by one of the separating atoms. This process is termed *heterolysis*.

(2c) Multiple Bonds.—The electronic interpretation of a number of the double and triple bonds of classical structural formulae is completely straightforward. The double bond of ethylene and of carbonyl compounds is represented as containing two shared pairs of electrons, and the triple bond of acetylene and of cyanides, three shared pairs:

```
H.   .H     H.   .
 :C::C:      :C::O:     H:C:::C:H     H:C:::N:
H·   ·H     H·   ·
```

(2d) Dipolar Bonds.—Two examples will serve to demonstrate the character of these bonds. Consider first the compound of ammonia with trimethylboron. It was formerly classified as a "molecular" compound. Werner considered the nitrogen and boron atoms to be linked with a subsidiary valency, and he wrote the compound $H_3N \cdots BMe_3$. The electronic theory regards this ligancy as a covalent bond, and the formation of the compound as a process of co-ordination:

$$\begin{array}{ccccccc} & \mathrm{H} & & \mathrm{R} & & \mathrm{H} & \mathrm{R} \\ \mathrm{H}: & \ddot{\underset{\cdot\cdot}{\mathrm{N}}}: & + & \ddot{\underset{\cdot\cdot}{\mathrm{B}}}:\mathrm{R} & \rightarrow \mathrm{H}: & \ddot{\underset{\cdot\cdot}{\mathrm{N}}}: & \ddot{\underset{\cdot\cdot}{\mathrm{B}}}:\mathrm{R} \\ & \mathrm{H} & & \mathrm{R} & & \mathrm{H} & \mathrm{R}\end{array}$$

The electronic formula shows, however, that the nitrogen atom is in the quadricovalent condition characteristic of an ammonium ion: so far as concerns the nitrogen atom, the compound is indeed a substituted ammonium ion. Again, the boron atom is in the quadricovalent condition obtaining, for instance, in the fluoroborate ion: so far as concerns this atom, the compound is a substituted borate ion. In order to signalise these analogies, it is convenient to attach sign-labels to the nitrogen and boron atoms, the compound being regarded as a dipolar ion, $H_3N^+B^-R_3$.

As the second example, consider trimethylamine-oxide, which was formerly written with a double bond, $Me_3N{=}O$. However, the electronic theory formulates this bond as a single covalent bond. It could be formed by co-ordination between the trimethylamine molecule and an atom of oxygen:

$$\begin{array}{cccccc} & \mathrm{R} & & & & \mathrm{R} \\ \mathrm{R}: & \ddot{\underset{\cdot\cdot}{\mathrm{N}}}: & + & \ddot{\underset{\cdot\cdot}{\mathrm{O}}}: & \rightarrow \mathrm{R}: & \ddot{\underset{\cdot\cdot}{\mathrm{N}}}:\ddot{\underset{\cdot\cdot}{\mathrm{O}}}: \\ & \mathrm{R} & & & & \mathrm{R}\end{array}$$

Here the nitrogen atom is again bound as in ammonium ions. The oxygen atom is in the unicovalent condition characteristic of hydroxide, phenoxide, or other 'oxide ions. Again it is convenient to signalise these conditions by the use of sign labels, the compound being considered as a dipolar ion, $R_3N^+O^-$.

The kind of bond illustrated, that is, a single covalent bond between atoms constituting a formal dipole, may be called a *dipolar bond*. The theory of the shared duplet and the valency octet places many such bonds in simple inorganic molecules, including most of the oxy-acids, together with their halides, anhydrides, and other derivatives. The theory places one such bond in the nitro-group, one in the azoxy-group, one in sulphoxides, and two in sulphones. It places what may be called a *dipolar double bond*, that is, a covalent double bond between atoms constituting a formal dipole, in the diazo-group, and in the azido-group:[8]

[8] The bond here called a *dipolar bond* has previously been termed a *semipolar double bond* and a *co-ordinate bond*. The name used in the text is preferred, because some of the bonds concerned have never been regarded as double, and because co-ordination by no means always produces charges. Lewis considered that the bond should not receive a distinctive name, but it seems not to have proved convenient to do without one.

```
  +  ..-          +  ..-                         :O:-
R:N:O:          R:N:O:         ..+..-         .. ..
  ..  ..          ..  ..       R:S :O:        R:S :O:-
  ..              ..            .. ..           +.. ..
 :O:             :N:R           R             +  R

           R.  +  -              ..  +  -
            .C::N::N:          R:N::N::N:
           R.      ..                   .
```

During the growth of the physical theory of binding, the concepts underlying these structures have been modified, largely, however, in ways that can best be treated by reading added significance into the structures, which remain the correct starting point from which to pursue these developments.

(2e) Polarity of Bonds.—Polarity enters into molecular constitution in more subtle ways than those which depend on formal charges. Consider again the covalent bond between formally uncharged atoms. As Lewis was careful to point out, the hypothesis of sharing does not imply a general equality of possession of the shared electrons by the atoms concerned. In the hydrogen molecule, or the fluorine molecule, the electrons must, for obvious reasons, be equally shared between the atoms. But in hydrogen fluoride, the shared electrons should be considered to belong much more to the fluorine atom than to the hydrogen atom. Therefore the molecule should possess a dipole moment, with hydrogen at the positive and fluorine at the negative end of the dipole. Furthermore, such electrical dissymmetry should reduce the energy needed to split the molecule into hydrogen and fluoride ions.

The following *isoelectronic* series will serve as the basis for a more detailed discussion:

```
   H         H        H
   ..        ..       ..        ..        ..
 H:C:H      :N:H     :O:H      :F:H      :Ne:
   ..        ..       ..        ..        ..
   H         H
```

In all these molecules, the total nuclear charge, to the combined field of which all the electrons must be subject, is the same, namely, ten units. However, on passing towards the right, successive units of positive charge are removed from their peripheral situations to the central position, from which they must be expected to exert a firmer general control over the octet of electrons. Therefore, comparing in several molecules a particular shared pair, say, that binding the hydrogen atom written on the right in each of the first four formulae, it can be deduced that this pair will belong progressively more to the central atom, and less to hydrogen, along the series CH_4, NH_3, OH_2, FH. The hydrogen atom should become increasingly positive; and this should affect physical properties, such as dipole moments, and chemical reactions, such as the ionic dissociation of the compounds as acids. If the electron-pair under consideration were in each case binding some other common atom, say, carbon, instead of hydrogen, then, increasingly along the series, electrons should be withdrawn from carbon. This likewise should influence the physical properties of the compounds, and also their chemical reactions, as we shall have occasion later to illustrate.

The above series may also be used for comparisons with respect to an unshared electron-pair, say, that written on the left in each of the last four formulae. This electron-pair should be progressively more strongly bound along the series NH_3, OH_2, FH, Ne. The effect of this should likewise be apparent in physical properties, such as polarisability, and chemical properties, such as basicity.

The terms *electronegative* and *electropositive* have been applied to atoms and atomic groups throughout the whole history of chemical molecular theory. On account of a chain of ideas originating with Berzelius, atoms and groups have been classified as electronegative if they conferred or enhanced acidic properties, and electropositive if they behaved in the opposite way. The groups $—CH_3$, $—NH_2$, —OH, —F, or, if we prefer, the central atoms of those groups, form a series in order of increasing electronegativity. The preceding explanation shows that the term *electronegativity* summarises those properties which result from the power of an atom to *attract* electrons from attached atoms, that is, from the strength of the *positive* electrical field of the atom. Conversely, *electropositivity* implies the *repulsion* of electrons, and a dominating *negative* electrical field.

It is to be expected that electronegativity will, quite generally, increase as an atom, or the central atom of a group, is displaced, in successive units of atomic number, towards the right-hand side of Mendeléjeff's periodic table. This applies so long as the atoms compared are all formally neutral, or at least possess the same formal charge. It should be noted that atoms and groups carrying a *positive* ionic charge are, by virtue of that fact, *electronegative*: they are among the most strongly electronegative groups known. Thus, the group $—NH_3^+$ is much more strongly electronegative than $—NH_2$, or, indeed, than any group of the series $—CH_3$, $—NH_2$, —OH, —F. Similarly, atoms and groups bearing a *negative* ionic charge are *electropositive*. Thus the group $—O^-$ is much more strongly electropositive than —OH, or than any of the series of neutral groups.

(2f) The Binding of Hydrogen.—As the hydrogen atom is small compared to other bound atoms, its nucleus can be approached especially closely by the unshared electron-pairs of other atoms, with the consequence that electrostatic attraction plays a particularly large part in determining the behaviour of bound hydrogen. Two effects of this are of outstanding importance.

The first relates to the great *mobility, as proton*, of hydrogen bound to electronegative atoms, which also possess unshared electrons, particularly atoms of the nitrogen, oxygen, and fluorine families. In bonds with such atoms, the proton is so little screened that the close approach, thereby permitted, of an active unshared electron-pair of another atom, can lead to the development of an electrostatic attraction for the proton strong enough to be competitive with the original bond. Thus only a very small energy barrier resists proton-transfers between electronegative atoms in such an example as the following:

$$:\ddot{\underset{\cdot\cdot}{F}}:H + :\ddot{\underset{\cdot\cdot}{F}}:^- \rightarrow :\ddot{\underset{\cdot\cdot}{F}}:^- + H:\ddot{\underset{\cdot\cdot}{F}}:$$

It is for this reason that isomerism depending on differences in the position of attachment of protons to electronegative atoms, for instance, among the inorganic oxy-acids, is unknown.

The second effect arises from the circumstance that, during the period in which two molecules are close enough together to permit facile proton-transfer, the proton is strongly attracted, by one kind of force or another, to *both* the atoms between which it can be transferred: the bond may switch, and even switch repeatedly, but *forces* in both directions remain; and they will tend to hold the species together. This form of association of two atoms through hydrogen is called a *hydrogen bond*. Three types of phenomena depending on hydrogen bonds may be mentioned. (1) The hydrogen bonding may be strong enough to maintain the combination of species as a kinetically individual particle of long life in solution. Thus the hydrogen difluoride ion $(FHF)^-$ is a kinetically stable entity. (2) Weaker forms of hydrogen bonding can produce striking effects in condensed systems, in which hydrogen bonds can be formed with such frequency that, despite a short individual life, the number of such bonds present is always large. This is the interpretation given to the association, manifested by reduced volatility, raised viscosity, and other altered physical properties, which is recognised in many pure liquids, notably, ammonia, water, hydrogen fluoride, primary and secondary amines, alcohols, phenols, and inorganic and organic acids. (3) When the components of a hydrogen bond are present in the same molecule, and are suitably articulated by the structure, intramolecular hydrogen bonds of considerable permanence may be established. Such bonds affect physical properties by repressing the intermolecular hydrogen bonding in which the groups concerned would otherwise have engaged. So volatility is raised, and viscosity lowered. They also affect chemical properties by resisting the normal functional behaviour of the groups, for example, the acidic ionisation of the proton. To cite but one of the many available examples of these effects, salicylaldehyde is notably more volatile than *p*-hydroxybenzaldehyde.

(3) PHYSICAL INTERPRETATION OF COVALENCY

Lewis discovered the material constitution of the covalent bond. But he could not describe the forces involved, because they were of a nature unknown in classical physics. Their discovery was one of the achievements of quantum mechanics.

(3a) Quantum Mechanics.[9]—In 1900 Planck introduced the quantum of action, h; in 1905 Einstein suggested the wave-particle duality of radiation; in 1913 Bohr employed the quantum to construct the first successful theory of atomic phenomena; in 1923 de Broglie applied the idea of wave-particle duality to the electron; and in 1925 quantum mechanics was discovered, in one form by Heisenberg, and in another by Schrödinger, whose method is the more directly related to the duality concept.

In this method, the behaviour of an elementary particle, in particular an electron, is expressed by that of a function, usually called Ψ, of the co-ordinates and the time, under the action of an operator correlated with the kinetic and potential energy. The operator gives to Ψ the properties of a wave, whose frequency ν is linked with the energy E through Planck's relation $E=h\nu$, while $|\Psi|^2$ becomes the probability distribution function of the particle. If several electrons are considered the *wave-function* Ψ is a function of *all* their co-ordinates, as well as of the time.

Quantum mechanics does not calculate precise trajectories, but *probabilities* of the position and momentum of particles. This is quite fundamental; for, as Heisenberg has pointed out, it is inconceivable that the position and momentum of a particle could both be exactly known. His *uncertainty principle* requires that the product of the ranges of uncertainty of a co-ordinate and of the corresponding momentum cannot be less than Planck's constant h; and that any pair of dynamical variables whose product has the dimensions of action—energy and time constitute another such pair—will have this property: the more precisely one is defined the more the other must become blurred. This is the essential meaning of the quantum of action.

[9] V. Rojansky, "Introductory Quantum Mechanics," Prentice-Hall, New York, 1946.

(3b) Atomic States and Orbitals.[10]—A general property of mechanical waves in any bounded system is that of becoming *stationary waves* having certain allowed forms and frequencies, as determined by the characteristics of the system. In like manner, the Ψ function for electrons restricted by the attractive potential of an atomic nucleus can assume stationary wave forms, having discrete frequencies. This is the wave property in terms of which Schrödinger described the *stationary states of atoms.*

In the description of an atomic state, the time is left indefinite; and thus the energy may be exactly defined. The concept of a state therefore pictures electrons as moving in undefined trajectories, but with a calculable probability distribution in the space about the nucleus. For many purposes, this distribution can be considered as one of averaged density of electronic charge. With this idea in mind, it is called a *charge-density distribution.*

The basic problem in the quantum mechanics of atomic states is that of the stationary states of hydrogen. It has been fully solved. The manifold of stationary states discloses the orbital quantum numbers, n, l, and m_l, and the rules of development of their values, as indicated in Table 3-1. It reveals their significance in relation to the symmetry and orientation of the wave functions Ψ, and of the electronic charge-density functions $|\Psi|^2$, and in relation to the number and type of nodal surfaces that these functions contain.

Table 3-1.—Rules of Development of Atomic Quantum Numbers.
(Shown for first three n. The series continues indefinitely.)

n	1	2				3								
l	0	0	1			0	1			2				
m_l	0	0	−1	0	+1	0	−1	0	+1	−2	−1	0	+1	+2
Symbol	1*s*	2*s*	2*p*			3*s*	3*p*			3*d*				

The forms of the electronic density functions for the 1-quantum and the four 2-quantum states of the hydrogen atom are illustrated in Fig. 3-1. The 1*s* state, the normal state of the atom, has a spherically symmetrical charge density, which fades radially in an exponential way. The 2-quantum states, which are first-excited states of equal energy, have one nodal surface each; the 2*s* state is spherical, its

[10] G. Herzberg, "Atomic Spectra and Atomic Structure," Blackie, London and Glasgow, 1937.

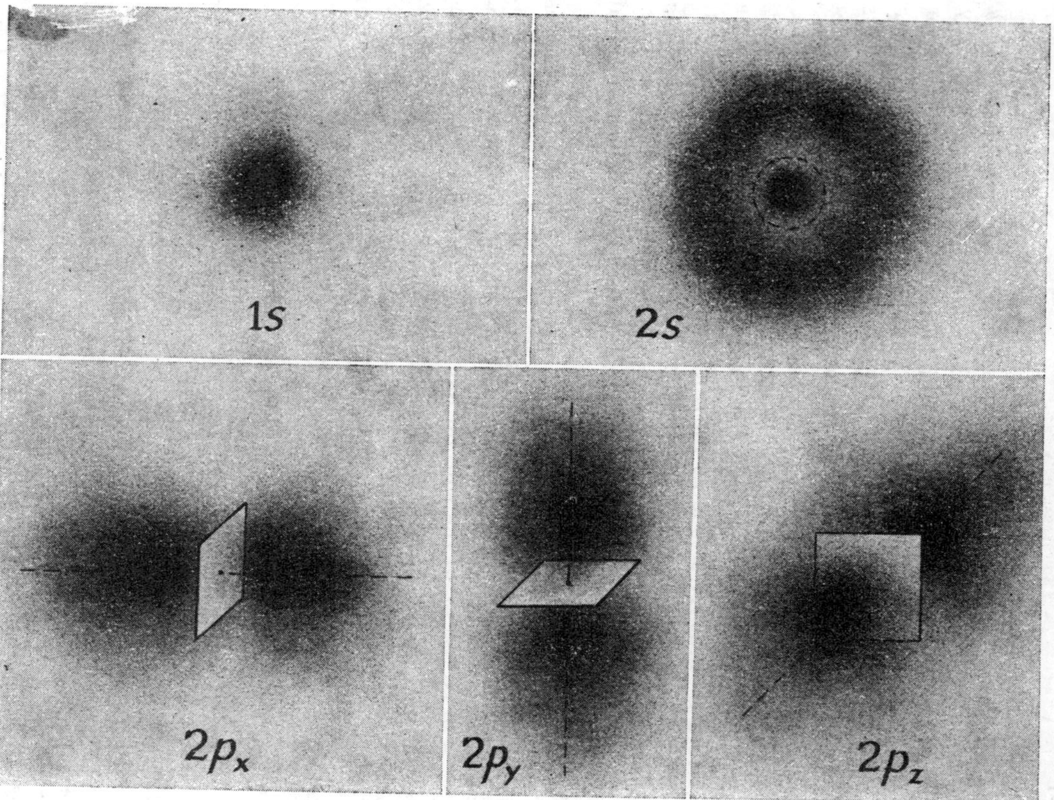

Fig. 3-1.—Illustrating the electronic charge-density distribution in the lower states of the hydrogen atom. The interior spherical node in the 2s state is represented by the broken circle. The plane nodes of the 2p states are indicated by the squares (represented as opaque to aid perspective).

node being a spherical surface; while the three $2p$ states, which differ from each other only in their mutually perpendicular orientations, are axially symmetrical, their nodes being planes. The nine 3-quantum states are second-excited states of equal energy, and have two nodal surfaces each; the single $3s$ and the three $3p$ states are like the $2s$ and $2p$ states, but possess each an extra spherical node; while the five $3d$ states have somewhat more complicated forms.

That the lowest energy state of the hydrogen atom does not contain an electron in stationary contact with the attracting nucleus is consistent with the uncertainty principle. If an electron could be held against the nucleus, then, its position being closely defined, an enormous uncertainty of momentum would result, and an enormous total energy would be required to accommodate the allowed variation of momentum. By permitting to the electron an increasing range of movement about the nucleus, this minimal required energy will be made to fall, while the actual electrostatic energy due to the separation will be caused to rise. Clearly there will be an optimal size of atom, namely, that which gives the atom the smallest energy that both electrostatics and quantum mechanics allow. The generalisation follows that any bound particle, in its most stable state, must move with an energy, called *zero-point energy*, which decreases if the range of motion can be increased. We shall refer to this principle on several later occasions.

Single-electron wave functions, such as describe the states of the hydrogen atom, are called *orbitals*, and electrons in such states are said to "occupy" the orbitals. It is convenient to think of the orbitals, occupied or not, as pre-existing, and as mapping out the space about a nucleus, much as one formerly thought of Bohr's orbits.

Part of the importance of the problem of hydrogen atom is that the normal and excited states of hydrogen suggest a model for an approximate treatment of the normal states of all atoms. To an adjustable nuclear charge, furnished with a series of orbitals having the quantum numbers, and therefore the symmetry and nodes, of those of hydrogen, electrons are successively supplied, and are assumed to enter the energetically lowest orbitals up to the limit of capacity of each.

The limit of capacity of an orbital is two electrons. For in 1925 Uhlenbeck and Goudsmit discovered that an electron has a property called *spin*, which gives it an angular momentum and a magnetic moment; and that, in a magnetic field, this moment can be oriented in only two ways, namely, with or against the field. This is expressed by saying that an electron has, besides its three spatial quantum numbers, n, l, and m_l, a spin quantum number, m_s, with the unit-spaced pair of values $+\frac{1}{2}$ and $-\frac{1}{2}$.

In the same year Pauli announced his *exclusion principle*, which requires that no more than two electrons can occupy a stable orbital, and that, when two do so, their spins, and the associated angular momenta and magnetic moments, must be oriented in opposition, or, as it is sometimes expressed, *paired*. The exclusion principle requires that no two electrons can be alike in both orbital motion and spin. In particular, electrons with the same n and l, *equivalent electrons*, as they are called, must be distinct in either m_l or m_s. So, if they are alike in m_l, and thus belong to the same orbital, they must be unlike in m_s, that is, paired.

The energy sequence of the orbitals in polyelectronic atoms differs qualitatively from that of hydrogen. For in polyelectronic atoms, the source of the potential acting on any one electron is not localised in the nucleus, but is distributed through the atom. On this account, the energy of the orbital now depends, not only on n, but also on l (though still not on m_l). Thus sets of orbitals with the same principal quantum number n become energetically separated into sub-sets: p orbitals are raised above the s orbital, d orbitals above the p orbitals, and so on. The stability sequence of the orbitals in the normal atoms of lower atomic number is qualitatively indicated[11] in Fig. 3-2.

The rule, given by Hund, for the order of filling of *equivalent orbitals*, that is, orbitals of the same n and l, in normal atoms—for instance, the three $2p$ orbitals—is that each such orbital accepts one electron, all such electrons having parallel spins, before any of the orbitals accepts a second electron, necessarily one with a spin opposed to the other spins. This rule of *maximum multiplicity*, as it is called, derives from the generalised exclusion principle. Electrons with like spins will not only go into different orbitals, but also, when there, will so move in correlation with one another as to keep maximally apart in space. This will minimise their electrostatic repulsion energy, and so will make the polyelectronic system more stable than if the electrons, in their different orbitals, had had unlike spins, and therefore had not had their motions brought into spatial correlation by the exclusion principle. Quite generally, for normal and excited atoms, and even outside the limitation to equivalent orbitals, states having single electrons with parallel spins in different orbitals will lie lower in energy than states of the same distribution of electrons among the orbitals, that is, the same *electron configuration*, but with the single electrons having opposed spins.

[11] L. Pauling, "Nature of the Chemical Bond," Cornell University Press, Ithaca, New York, 3rd Edn., 1960, p. 49.

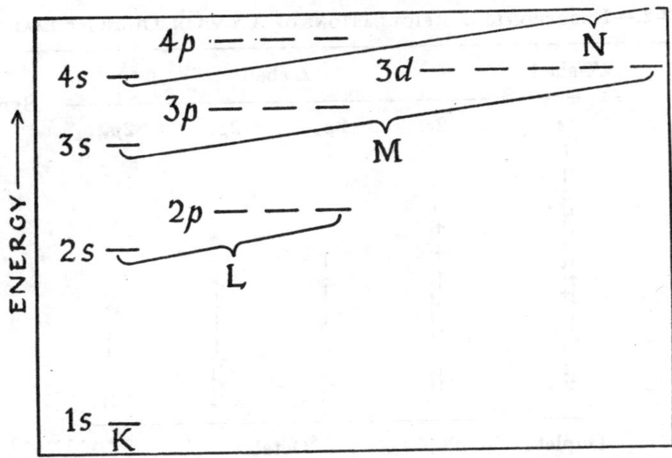

FIG. 3-2.—Approximate stability sequence for atomic orbitals.

As an example, one applying to normal atoms, and within the limitation of equivalent orbitals, we may refer to the electron configurations of the atoms of the elements of the first period. This is illustrated in Table 3-2, which shows the mode of development in normal atoms of the *K* and *L* shells, that is, of the first duplet and octet: the electrons are represented by arrows, pairs of opposed arrows indicating paired spins.

As a matter of terminology, an atom with all spins paired is said to be in a *singlet* state. The normal helium and neon atoms are singlet. An atom with one unpaired spin is said to be in a *doublet* state. The hydrogen and normal boron and fluorine atoms are doublet. An atom with two parallel spins is said to be in a *triplet* state. The normal (free) carbon and oxygen atoms are triplet, in accordance with Hund's rule. For the same reason, the normal nitrogen atom is in a *quartet* state. An atom with n parallel spins is said to be in an $(n+1)$-*let* state; and $n+1$ is called the *multiplicity*. The same terminology is applied to molecules. An odd-electron molecule, such as nitric oxide, is normally in a doublet state. Nearly all even-electron molecules have all spins paired, and so are normally in singlet states. But the normal oxygen molecule is exceptional, in that it has two parallel spins, and thus is in a triplet state.

An interesting geometrical property of orbitals is that, when *equivalent* orbitals are *all equally* occupied, as are the $2p$ orbitals in the normal nitrogen and neon atoms, then the total charge distribution (given by $\Sigma|\Psi|^2$) attains spherical symmetry. It follows that, when all but one of the orbitals of an equivalent set are equally occupied, the total

TABLE 3-2.—ELECTRONIC CONFIGURATIONS OF ATOMS IN THEIR NORMAL STATES.

	K shell	*L* shell				Symmetry
	$1s$	$2s$	$2p_x$	$2p_y$	$2p_z$	
H	↑					*S*
He	↑↓					*S*
Li	↑↓	↑				*S*
Be	↑↓	↑↓				*S*
B	↑↓	↑↓	↑			*P*
C	↑↓	↑↓	↑	↑		*P*
N	↑↓	↑↓	↑	↑	↑	*S*
O	↑↓	↑↓	↑↓	↑	↑	*P*
F	↑↓	↑↓	↑↓	↑↓	↑	*P*
Ne	↑↓	↑↓	↑↓	↑↓	↑↓	*S*
	Duplet	Octet				

charge distribution will have the axial symmetry of that of a single orbital of the set. Thus, while the atoms marked *S* in the right-hand column of Table 3-2 have full spherical symmetry, those marked *P* only have the axial symmetry of a spheroid.

(3c) Bond Orbitals.—Just as the stationary-wave property is fundamental for the discussion of the atom, so another general wave property, called *resonance*, is fundamental for the discussion of atomic binding. In mechanics, the phenomenon termed resonance occurs when two systems, capable of sustaining similar stationary waves, are connected or allowed to merge to some degree: then, a stationary wave actually present in one original system will disturb the other system, thereby becoming itself non-stationary: and there will become established in the united system two new stationary waves, one having a reduced and the other an increased frequency. The analogous property of Ψ waves, and its effect in altering the energies of states, were discovered by Heisenberg in 1926. It was shown to be the main source of the strength of the covalent bond by Heitler and London in 1927.

It is convenient to consider first the simpler case of binding by a single shared electron, as in the hydrogen molecule ion, H_2^+. Let us suppose that two protons A and B are held at various fixed distances apart, and that an electron is supplied to A to produce a normal hydrogen atom. At the outset, the distance is assumed to be great enough to preclude interaction. Then it is reduced sufficiently to secure that the occupied orbital about A will overlap slightly with the similar but unoccupied orbital about B. The electron will now be able to pass between the equivalent orbitals, which on this account will cease to represent stationary states: there will be resonance, the two original atomic orbitals becoming replaced by *molecular orbitals*, which, spreading symmetrically over the two protons, take account of movement of the electron between them. There will be two such orbitals, one with a reduced, and the other with an increased energy; the former, designated by its symmetry as $1s\sigma$, and classified as a *bonding orbital*, will have no nodal surface; and the latter, designated as $2p\sigma$, and classified as an *antibonding orbital*, will have a nodal plane, perpendicular to the internuclear line, half-way between the nuclei. We shall be interested mainly in the more stable state of the system, that in which the former orbital is occupied. Now let the internuclear distance be shortened somewhat further, so that resonance is increased. Then the energy of the more stable orbital will be further depressed, and that of the less stable will be further increased. However, as the internuclear distance continues to be shortened, the reduction in the energy of the more stable orbital cannot continue, because at really small distances internuclear repulsion must increase the energy steeply. Therefore there must be an optimal separation, which minimises the energy; and this is the equilibrium bond length in the normal state of the molecular ion.

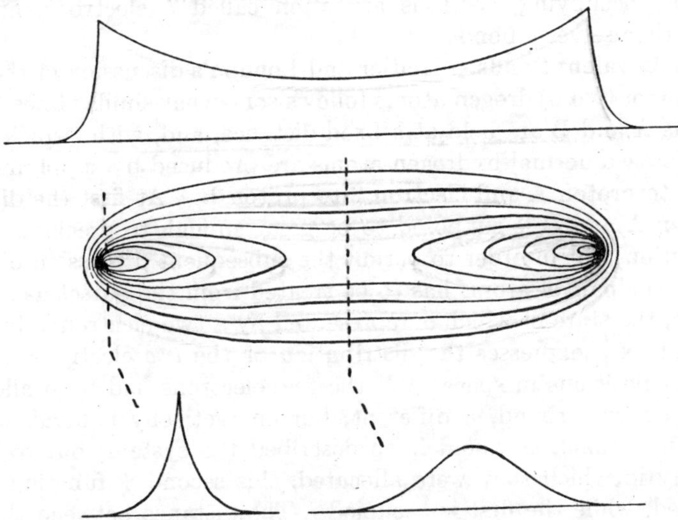

FIG. 3-3.—Electron distribution function of the hydrogen molecule-ion (after Burrau). The upper diagram represents the function along a line through the nuclei, and the centre one the contours of the function over a plane through the nuclei, while the lower diagrams show the function along lines perpendicular to the internuclear line, through a nucleus (left), and through the point mid-way between the nuclei (right).

Calculations have shown, in agreement with spectroscopic determinations, that the bond length of the ion is 1.06 *A*, while the bond energy is 61 kcal./mole.[12] The resonance accounts for about 80% of this energy. The remaining 20% arises from so-called deformation, that is, the circumstance that, even in the absence of resonance, a proton and a hydrogen atom would attract each other owing to the ability of the proton to polarise the atom. The calculated electron distribution function is represented in Fig. 3-3. It shows the electron to be contained mainly between the nuclei in the space around the internuclear line, the nuclei being very little shielded on the side of either remote from the other. From the value and width of the function over a central section perpendicular to the internuclear line, one sees that the electron is present in this half-way position to a greater extent than over a parallel section through either nucleus. This warns us that we must not regard the resonance as a switching of the electron between the alternative atoms, but rather as a form of motion which becomes mixed inseparably with the original atomic motion, thereby changing it into a homogeneous molecular motion. As the occupation of this molecular orbital constitutes a bond, the orbital may be called a *bond orbital*. Bond orbitals which, like this one, are circularly symmetrical about the internuclear line are termed σ orbitals, and the occupying electrons are often called σ electrons, and the bonds themselves σ bonds.

(3d) Covalent Bonds.—Heitler and London's discussion of the combination of two hydrogen atoms follows somewhat similar lines. Two protons A and B are held at a fixed distance, and, with two electrons 1 and 2, two normal hydrogen atoms are produced by supplying electron 1 to proton A and electron 2 to proton B. At first the distance between A and B is supposed to be great enough to preclude atomic interaction; but in order to permit the subsequent discussion of interaction, the pair of atoms has to be treated from the outset as a single system, the state of which is represented by a two-electron Ψ function (so that $|\Psi|^2$ expresses the distribution of the *two* electrons over all *pairs* of positions in space). If the two electrons had been allocated the other way round, a different, but energetically equivalent two-electron Ψ function would have described the system; but owing to the way in which they were allocated, this second Ψ function is unoccupied, while the first is occupied. The distance between the protons is now shortened sufficiently to allow either electron a limited

[12] O. Burrau, *Kgl. Danske Videnskab. Sclskab*, **1927**, **7**, 1; L. Pauling, *Chem. Revs.*, 1928, **5**, 173; B. N. Finkelstein and G. E. Horowitz, *Z. Physik*, 1928, **48**, 118; E. A. Hylleraas, *ibid.*, 1931, **71**, 739; B. N. Dickinson, *J. Chem. Phys.*, 1933, **1**, 317; G. Jaffé, *Z. Physik*, 1934, **87**, 535.

possibility of being captured by the proton to which it was not originally assigned. There will then be resonance: for the electrons can now spontaneously change atoms, passing over from the distribution of the occupied to that of the originally unoccupied Ψ function. Thus the originally occupied function will no longer represent a stationary state; nor will the originally unoccupied Ψ function, because the electrons can exchange both ways. These Ψ functions will become replaced by molecular two-electron Ψ functions, each of which will treat the alternative allocations of electrons symmetrically, thus taking account of the reversible exchange. There will be two such two-electron functions, one, when occupied, representing a state of reduced, and the other one of increased, energy. When the protons are brought progressively closer together, the energy of the more stable of these states becomes further reduced owing to the increased resonance, then passes through a minimum, and finally increases, essentially on account of internuclear repulsion. Simultaneously, the energy of the less stable state increases continuously. The former state represents the formation of the normal molecule, and the latter repulsion between atoms. These energy relations are illustrated in Fig. 3-4.

The spectroscopic value of the bond length of the hydrogen molecule

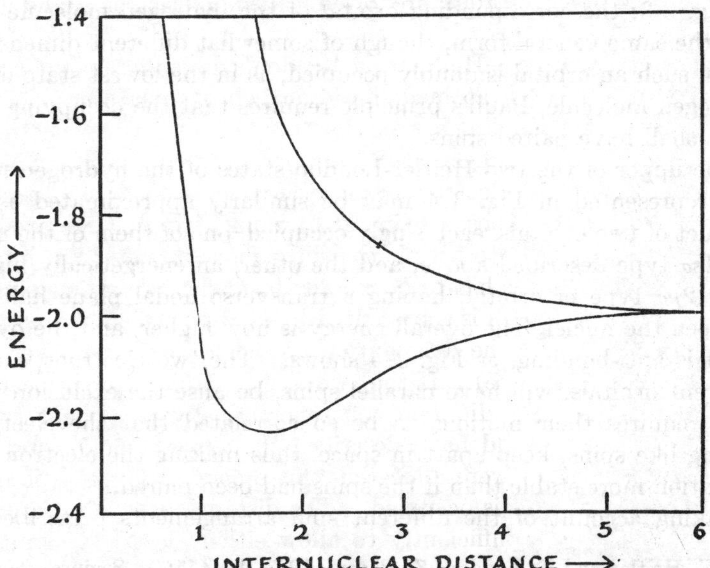

FIG. 3-4.—Energy of two interacting normal hydrogen atoms as a function of the internuclear distance (after Segiura). The units are atomic units: energy unit = 13.53 electron-volts = 312 kcal./mole; length unit = 0.528 *A*.

is 0.740 *A*, and that of the bond energy is 102.6 kcal./mole. The calculations of Heitler and London, after some extension and refinement by Segiura, and by Wang, yielded 80% of this energy as resonance energy of electron exchange. Weinbaum showed that a further 5% is accounted for by removing the implicit assumption that the two electrons are never present together in the same atom. The remaining 15% is to be attributed to forms of interaction summarised as deformation, of which complete account is taken in the calculations of James and Coolidge, which exactly reproduce the bond energy, as well as other known physical constants of the molecule.[13]

As with atoms, so with molecules, it is convenient, though it is an approximation, to describe polyelectronic systems in terms of one-electron wave-functions, that is, orbitals. In each such orbital, the occupying electron is taken to be moving in the field of the nucleus and the smoothed-out field of the other electron or electrons. Thus, the two-electron wave-function of the lower of the two Heitler-London states of the hydrogen molecule represented in Fig. 3–4 may be approximated as the product of two co-incident and identical one-electron wave-functions, or orbitals, and may accordingly be described as a "doubly occupied" orbital. This orbital is of the nodeless bonding type, $1s\sigma$, already illustrated for the hydrogen molecule ion in Fig. 3-3: the corresponding orbital of the hydrogen molecule is of just the same general form, though of somewhat different dimensions. When such an orbital is doubly occupied, as in the lowest state of the hydrogen molecule, Pauli's principle requires that the occupying electrons shall have paired spins.

The upper of the two Heitler-London states of the hydrogen molecule represented in Fig. 3–4 may be similarly approximated as the product of two orbitals, each singly occupied, one of them of the nodeless $1s\sigma$ type described above, and the other, an energetically higher-lying $2p\sigma$ type of orbital, having a transverse nodal plane half-way between the nuclei. The overall energy is now higher, and the overall effect is anti-bonding, as Fig. 3–4 shows. The two electrons, now in different orbitals, will have parallel spins, because the exclusion principle requires their motions to be so correlated that the electrons, having like spins, keep apart in space, thus making the electron configuration more stable than if the spins had been paired.

Taking account of the different spin arrangements prescribed by

[13] W. Heitler and F. London, *Z. Physik*, 1927, **44**, 455; Y. Segiura, *ibid.*, **45**, 484; S. C. Wang, *Phys. Rev.*, 1928, **31**, 579; N. Rosen, *ibid.*, 1931, **38**, 2099; S. Weinbaum, *J. Chem. Phys.*, 1933, **1**, 593; H. M. James and A. S. Coolidge, *ibid.*, 1933, **1**, 825.

Pauli's principle in the two hydrogen-molecule states of Fig. 3–4, Heitler and London explained that their theory of the interaction of two hydrogen atoms is in principle a general theory of covalency formation, as well as of the steric resistance of non-combining atoms to mutual compression. Thus, while two hydrogen atoms may either combine or repel in consequence of electron exchange, a hydrogen atom and a helium atom, or two helium atoms, can only repel. The reason is that Pauli's principle is preserved in the helium atoms only if electrons with parallel spins are exchanged, and this leads to interaction states of the type of that represented by the upper curve in Fig. 3-4. The conclusion follows that, at distances short enough to permit electron exchange, unpaired electrons by exchange repel electron duplets with paired spins, while all such duplets by exchange repel each other. On the other hand, two unpaired electrons have the possibility to form a covalent bond. More generally, two atomic orbitals, which two electrons in all are available to occupy, may form a bond orbital, which by double occupation becomes a covalent bond.

Bond formation by exchange is consistent with the uncertainty principle, according to which bound particles in their most stable states possess a zero-point energy related to the range of motion. Exchange provides additional opportunities of electron motion, thereby reducing the electronic zero-point energy. Thus a more stable system will result, unless the zero-point state is rendered inaccessible by Pauli's principle.

(4) INTERPRETATION OF STEREOCHEMICAL FORM

(4a) Directed Single Bonds.—The development of Heitler and London's interpretation of the covalent bond, in relation to the formation of molecules from polyelectronic atoms, and especially with reference to the directional properties of bonds, is due mainly to Pauling and to Slater.[14] Pauling has evolved from the formal theory certain general rules concerning bond formation. He points out that the atomic orbitals of two electrons engaged in forming a bond will tend to overlap with each other, and to avoid overlapping with the orbitals of other electrons: the reason is that overlapping facilitates electron exchange, which is the main source of the stability of bonds, and of the instability of interpenetrated non-bonding electron-pairs. From this it is deduced that a non-spherical orbital will tend to form a bond in the direction of greatest concentration of the orbital; and that, while

[14] L. Pauling, *Proc. Nat. Acad. Sci.* (U. S.), 1928, **14**, 359; *J. Am. Chem. Soc.*, 1931, **53**, 1367; "Nature of the Chemical Bond," 3rd Edn., 1960, p. 108; J. C. Slater, *Phys. Rev.*, 1931, **37**, 481.

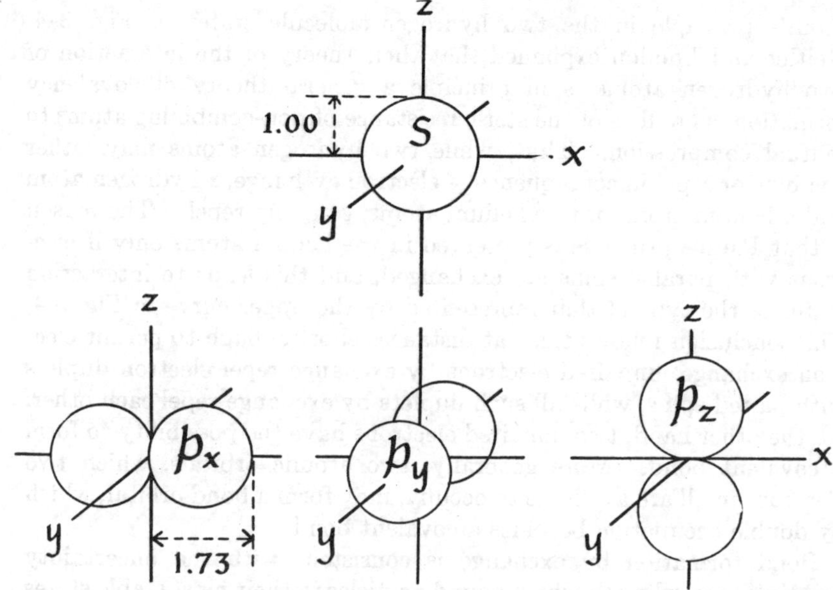

FIG. 4-1.—Polar graphs of *s* and *p* orbitals (the magnitudes-in-angle are indicated).

in general stable orbitals form stable bonds, an orbital concentrated in one direction will tend to form stronger bonds than another orbital of similar stability but less locally concentrated.

An approximate idea of the relative concentration and distribution-in-direction of atomic orbitals of the same principal quantum number is afforded by the polar graphs of their angular dependence: that factor, contained in Ψ, which depends on angle is plotted as a radius-vector, and a surface is thereby described, whose distance from the origin in any direction gives the magnitude of Ψ in its dependence on direction. The polar graph of an *s* orbital is a spherical surface, and that of a *p* orbital is a pair of equal spherical surfaces in contact at the nucleus (Fig. 4-1). Taking the magnitude in dependence upon angle of an *s* orbital to be 1 for all directions, then that of a *p* orbital for the direction in which it is maximal is $\sqrt{3} = 1.73$. Pauling, with the overlapping principle in mind, regards these figures as indicating the strengths of the bonds formed by the orbitals, and he calls the figures the "strengths" of the orbitals, although, for a reason mentioned later, we shall term them simply the *magnitudes-in-angle*, thereby avoiding the implication that they are accurate measures of bonding strength. Pauling deduces that a *p* orbital will form stronger bonds than will an *s* orbital of the same principal quantum number; and also that two *p* orbitals in the same atom will tend to form bonds at right angles.

There is some experimental support for these conclusions. The normal oxygen atom has two singly occupied *p* orbitals, and no redistribution of electrons in the *L* shell can give it any more (Table 3-2, p. 18). Therefore oxygen, and other atoms with a like electronic configuration, such as sulphur, can form two covalent bonds with atoms, such as hydrogen or fluorine, each of which has one singly occupied orbital. It is known that molecules produced from such atoms are always angular, although the angles are nearly always appreciably greater than a right angle. Thus in water the angle is 105.0°, in fluorine monoxide 101.5°, and in hydrogen sulphide 92.3°. There are several causes which might lead the angle to exceed 90°. One would be electrostatic repulsion between the bonds of like polarity. Another would be steric repulsion between the bonds, supposing that the fully formed bond orbitals concentrate between the atoms, leaving only reduced portions on the remote sides of the divalent atom. A third cause would be steric repulsion between the bound atoms, if they are large enough. A fourth possible cause is that a widened angle leads, through the process of hybridisation discussed below, to more stable bonds but less stable unshared duplets, and that the balance of these effects might favour some degree of widening.

The normal nitrogen atom has all three *p* orbitals singly occupied (Table 3-2), and therefore can, equally with other atoms of like configuration, form three covalent bonds with univalent atoms. It is known that the molecules thus formed are invariably pyramidal, although again the bond angles are greater than a right angle, being, for example, 106.8° in ammonia, 102.5° in nitrogen trifluoride, and within the range 96–104° in the trihalides of phosphorus, arsenic, and antimony.

Beryllium, boron, and carbon atoms can form with univalent atoms, such as hydrogen or fluorine, larger numbers of bonds than their normal electronic configurations would suggest (Table 3-2, p. 18). The reason is that these atoms have both unoccupied and doubly occupied orbitals in their *L* shells. This permits a redistribution of *L* electrons, to produce excited atomic states of the configurations indicated in Table 4-1. Such excitations must be regarded as accompanying bond formation, when the excitation energy is less than the extra energy liberated by the increased bond formation. In these examples, the bonding energy is additionally augmented by the process called *hybridisation,* now to be considered.

In analogy with degenerate vibrations and waves in mechanical

TABLE 4-1.—ELECTRONIC CONFIGURATIONS OF ATOMS IN EXCITED STATES.

	K shell	L shell				Symmetry
	$1s$	$2s$	$2p_x$	$2p_y$	$2p_z$	
Be*	↑↓	↑	↑			P
B*	↑↓	↑	↑	↑		P
C*	↑↓	↑	↑	↑	↑	S

systems, a number of orbitals of exactly equal energy are always equivalent to the same number of independent mixtures of them. Thus if the three equivalent *p* orbitals are mixed to give three independent new orbitals, these are completely similar, the effect of the mixing being only that of a rotation of the co-ordinate axes. By an extension of this principle, if some energy process involving orbitals is under consideration, then orbitals whose energies approximate to one another to within the energy of the process can become mixed during the process; and they will then become mixed in just that way which leads to the most stable end-product.

For example, the excited carbon atom, C* in Table 4-1, can form four bonds. But it will not use its *s* and *p* orbitals directly for this purpose, because the mixing of *s* with *p* orbitals yields hybrid orbitals, which are more locally concentrated, and can therefore produce stronger bonds. The *s* and *p* orbitals have the important geometrical property that, when they are so mixed as to fulfil the condition of producing *one* hybrid orbital having the greatest magnitude-in-angle (which, on the scale used for *s* and *p* orbitals, is 2.00) of any orbital that could be formed from these components, then the mixing will in fact produce *four* orbitals of that magnitude-in-angle; and these orbitals are equivalent; and their bonding directions are mutually inclined at the tetrahedral angle 109°28′. The polar graph of such a *tetrahedral orbital* is shown in Fig. 4-2.

The result is, of course, basic for the stereochemistry of carbon. It must apply equally to silicon, and to other atoms with like bonding orbitals, including nitrogen, phosphorus, etc., on the one hand, and boron, aluminium, etc., on the other, when these atoms are rendered quadricovalent by co-ordination. It applies quite generally to quadricovalency depending only on *s* and *p* orbitals.

The boron atom, as well as other atoms with similar outer electronic structure, can analogously form three equivalent hybrid orbitals. Their bonding directions lie in a plane, at angles of 120°. The magnitude-in-angle of such a *plane-trigonal orbital*, 1.99, is practically the same as that of a tetrahedral orbital (Fig. 4-2). A number of tervalent

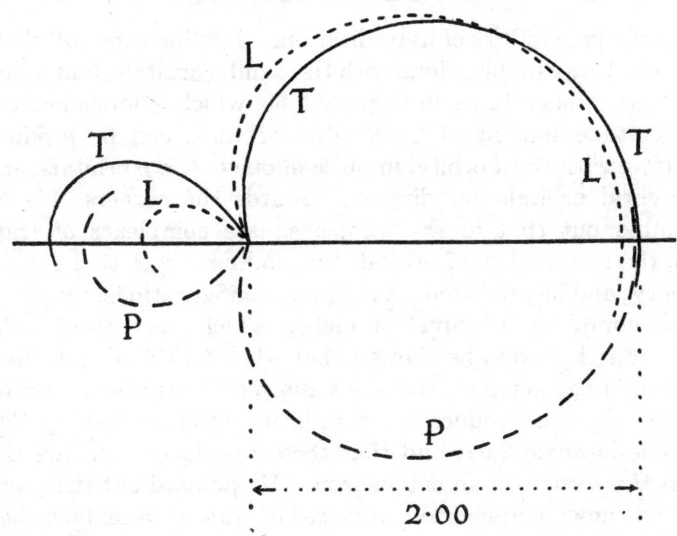

FIG. 4-2.—Polar graphs of *s-p* hybrid orbitals: L—linear (magnitude-in-angle 1.93); P—plane-trigonal (magnitude-in-angle 1.99); T—tetrahedral (magnitude-in-angle 2.00).

boron compounds (BF_3, BCl_3, BBr_3, BMe_3) have been shown to have the plane-trigonal configuration.

The beryllium atom, and atoms having a similar valency shell, can form two equivalent hybrid orbitals. Their bonding directions make an angle of 180°, and so they lead to linear structures. The magnitude-in-angle of such a *linear orbital*, 1.93, is near enough to those of the other hybrid orbitals (Fig. 4-2) to indicate that this orbital will be comparable to them in its ability to form strong bonds, in particular, stronger bonds than could be formed by a *p* orbital. The proved cases of linear covalent bonding are among compounds of the heavier elements, such as mercury ($HgCl_2$, $HgBr_2$, HgI_2, Hg_2Cl_2, etc.).

A tetrahedral orbital, which is a mixture of $\frac{1}{4}$ of an *s* orbital with $\frac{3}{4}$ of a *p* orbital, is often designated sp^3; similarly, a trigonal orbital, consisting of $\frac{1}{3}$ of an *s* and $\frac{2}{3}$ of a *p* orbital, is described as sp^2; and a linear orbital, composed of $\frac{1}{2}$ of an *s* and $\frac{1}{2}$ of a *p* orbital, is described as an *sp* orbital.

Some of the most striking successes of the orbital theory of binding, as developed by Pauling, relate to the compounds of the transition metals, which have available for binding, not only the *s* and *p* orbitals of their highest principal quantum number, but also such *d* orbitals of the next lower principal quantum number (which are of about the same energy) as are not occupied by unshared electrons. This greatly enriches the possibilities of hybridisation. Pauling showed[15] that when one *d* orbital is available, along with the *s* and *p* orbitals, four equivalent orbitals, with magnitudes-in-angle of 2.69, which is much greater than the magnitude-in-angle of tetrahedral orbitals, can be produced by hybridising with the *d* orbital in place of one of the *p* orbitals; and that these hybrid orbitals are directed towards the corners of a square. He pointed out that in the known square complexes of transition metals, the availability of orbitals for binding is just that required by the theory; and he predicted some square configurations, *e.g.*, in quadricovalent complexes of bivalent nickel, which were afterwards confirmed. Furthermore, he showed that when two *d* orbitals are available for binding, together with the *s* and *p* orbitals, then hybridisation of all the six can produce six equivalent orbitals, having the high magnitude-in-angle 2.92; and that these hybrid orbitals are directed towards the corners of an octahedron. He pointed out that, again, in the many known octahedral complexes of transition metals, the availability of orbitals is as required by theory. When four or five *d* orbitals could be used for bond formation, then other geometrical arrangements of bonds become possible,[16] some of which are known.[17]

Pauling has suggested[14] that the magnitudes-in-angle, and hence the bonding properties, of the *s*-*p* hybrid orbitals can in higher approximation be improved by including small proportions of *d* and *f* orbitals in the hybridisation. These additional component orbitals must often have higher principal quantum numbers, and, if occupied, relatively high energies, circumstances that would resist their participation in more than small proportions; but, as R. S. Mulliken has said in other connexions, a little hybridisation can go a long way; and the improved resultant bonding will certainly cause some inclusion of the additional orbitals. Pauling calculates that a maximum improvement to the bond-forming properties of a tetrahedral orbital, an improvement measured by an increase of magnitude-in-angle from 2.00 to 2.76, would be produced by the inclusion of 4% of a *d* orbital and 20% of an *f* orbital. This is indeed a maximum; but a certain proportion, though it is hard to say how much, of it is bound to be realised in bond-forming orbitals, on account of the energetic benefit to the resulting bonds. This effect would not arise in unshared-electron orbitals.

(4b) Double and Triple Bonds.—Two models have been suggested for double bonds, such, for example, as that present in ethylene. One model, originally proposed by Pauling and Slater,[14] and recently

[15] L. Pauling, *J. Am. Chem. Soc.*, 1931, **53**, 1367.

[16] R. Hultgren, *Phys. Rev.*, 1932, **40**, 891.

[17] L. Pauling, "Nature of the Chemical Bond," 3rd Edn., 1960, Chap. V, p. 145.

further developed by Pauling,[17] treats the two shared duplets in an equivalent manner, essentially as two bent single bonds formed from tetrahedral orbitals by bonding in directions considerably inclined to the best bonding directions. In the other model, proposed by Hückel and supported by Penney,[18] one shared duplet is regarded as composing a single bond of the usual σ type, whilst the other duplet, which constitutes the chemically reactive part of the double bond, is considered to be formed by lateral bonding between atomic p orbitals. These two models are not as widely different from each other as might appear. In an approximate treatment of molecules, known as the molecular orbital method, the two models lead to the same overall electron distribution.[19] To this extent, the manner of division into doubly occupied bond orbitals is an arbitrary choice. In other approximations this is not so, and the best model to use may depend on the purpose in view. But for general purposes, the Hückel-Penney model has a great advantage, as Hückel obviously intended, in the almost automatic ease with which it interprets "conjugation," a phenomenon with which we shall be dealing in Chapter II. It does this not only for open-chain polyunsaturated systems, such as that of buta-1,3-diene (for which, indeed, it may quantitatively overempha-

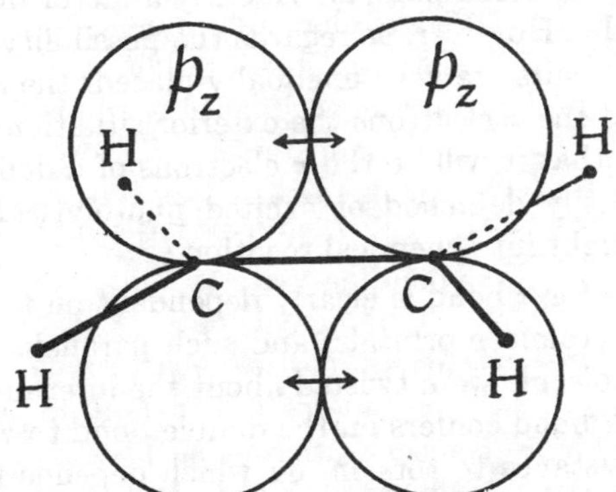

Fig. 4-3.—Interaction of p orbitals (represented by their polar graphs) to form a π orbital, which by double occupation becomes the π component of the double bond in ethylene. (The σ electron-pairs are represented only by their symmetry axes, namely, the relevant internuclear lines.)

[18] E. Hückel, *Z. Physik*, 1930, **60**, 423; W. G. Penney, *Proc. Roy. Soc.* (London), 1934, **A, 144**, 166; **A, 146**, 223.

[19] G. G. Hall and J. E. Lennard-Jones, *Proc. Roy. Soc.* (London), 1951, **A, 205**, 357.

size the importance of conjugation), but also, and quite realistically, for aromatic systems, such as that of benzene.

In this model (to describe it for the example of ethylene), the *s* orbital and two *p* orbitals of each carbon atom are assumed to hybridise to give three plane-trigonal orbitals, two of which form the bonds with hydrogen, while the third forms a bond between the carbon atoms of the usual σ type. All these bonds lie in a plane. Each carbon atom is now left with a singly occupied *p* orbital, having its symmetry axis normal to the plane of the atoms; and lateral interaction between these p_z orbitals is assumed to produce the second component of the double bond (Fig. 4-3). Pauli's principle is satisfied if, in each component of the double bond, electron spins are paired.

Just as for the original p_z orbitals, so for the bond orbital which they yield by lateral interaction, the plane of the nuclei is a nodal plane. Such bond orbitals are termed π orbitals, and the electrons occupying them π electrons, while the bond component formed by such occupation is called a π bond. The charge distribution in a π bond thus forms two layers, one on either side of the molecular plane (Fig. 4-4). In particular, a π bond has zero charge along, and only a small charge density near, the internuclear line, along and immediately about which the electronic charge of the σ bond is concentrated. This degree of separation of the electron pairs is evidently a factor in the stability of the double bond. However, as regards the possibility of disturbance, the two electron pairs are very unequally placed: the σ electrons have the interior, and the π electrons the exterior situation; and hence one can understand that it will be the π electrons of a double bond which are the more easily detached or excited photolytically and are the more easily brought into chemical reaction.

The strength of a π bond is clearly dependent on the parallelism of the axes of the atomic *p* orbitals; and such parallelism would be destroyed if the molecule were twisted about the internuclear line. For this reason the π bond confers on the double bond to which it belongs that marked resistance to torsion, on which depends the geometrical isomerism, which is observed among double-bonded carbon and nitrogen compounds.

There is a certain dubiety about the hybridisation in the Hückel-Penney model: it could be plane-trigonal, as originally assumed, or it could proceed so as to give two tetrahedral and one linear orbital, or in any intermediate way that still leaves one *p* orbital for the formation of the π bond. The chief geometrical distinction would be found in the external single-bond angle, which would be reduced from 120° under plane-trigonal hybridisation, to 109°28′ between the bonds of tetrahedral orbitals. External single-bond angles are known that are

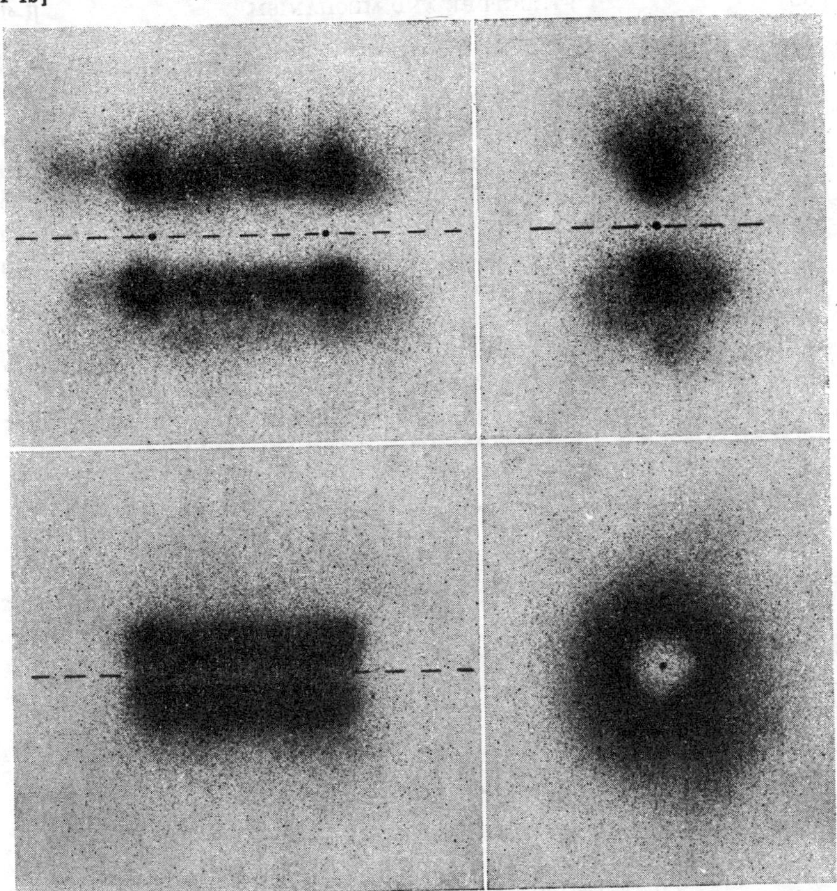

FIG. 4–4.—Illustrating the density distribution of π electrons in the double bond (above), and in the triple bond (below). A side-view and an end-view are given in each case.

close to either of these values, or lie in the range between them. For ethylene the $\widehat{HCH}$ angle is 117.6°,[20] and for formaldehyde 115.8°.[21] For 1,1-difluoroethylene the $\widehat{FCF}$ angle is 109.6°[22] and for 1,1-dichloroethylene the $\widehat{ClCCl}$ angle is 113.6°.[23] For *iso*butylene and tetramethyl-

[20] From infra-red spectrum: H. C. Allen and E. K. Plyler, *J. Am. Chem. Soc.*, 1958, **80**, 2673. From Raman spectrum: J. M. Dowlong and B. P. Stoicheff, *Canadian J. Phys.*, 1959, **37**, 703.

[21] From micro-wave spectrum: T. Oka, *J. Phys. Soc. Japan*, 1960, **12**, 2274.

[22] From micro-wave spectrum: W. F. Edgell, P. A. Kinsley, and J. W. Amy, *J. Am. Chem. Soc.*, 1957, **79**, 2691.

[23] From micro-wave spectrum: S. Sekino and T. Nishikawa, *J. Phys. Soc., Japan*, 1957, **12**, 43.

ethylene the external $\widehat{CCC}$ angles are less accurately known, but are about 111°.[24]

The corresponding theory of the triple bond requires (to employ acetylene as the example) that the *s* orbital and one *p* orbital of each carbon atom shall produce two linear hybridised orbitals, one of which forms the bond with hydrogen, while the other forms a σ bond between the carbon atoms. All the atoms now lie along a straight line. Each carbon atom is left with two *p* orbitals, whose symmetry axes are perpendicular to each other and to the internuclear line. These *p* orbitals of either carbon atom interact laterally with those of the other, each with each, to form two π orbitals. Each π orbital is occupied by two electrons with paired spins. These four electrons constitute what may be called the π shell of the triple bond (Fig. 4-5).

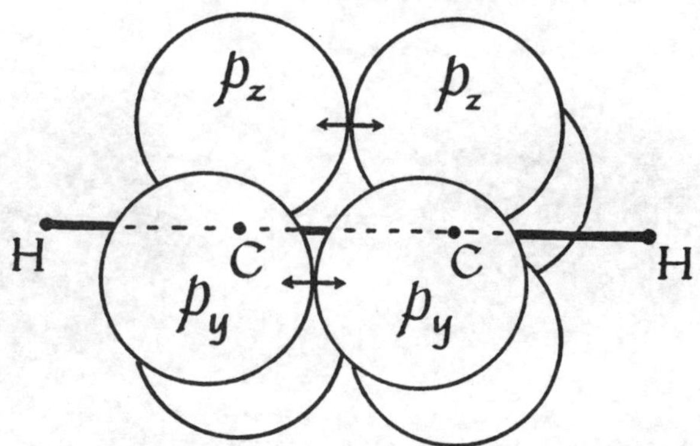

FIG. 4-5.—Interaction of *p* orbitals (represented by their polar graphs) to form the π orbitals of the triple bond of acetylene.

Owing to the orthogonal arrangement of the atomic *p* orbitals, the formed π orbitals must evidently have their nodal planes intersecting at right angles along the internuclear line. This implies that the maxima of electronic density of either electron pair will lie in the plane of zero electronic density of the other pair. But, furthermore, the geometrical property (Section **3b**), through which two equally occupied *p* orbitals together build up a total charge-density distribution with full circular symmetry about the axis of the third *p* orbital, secures that two equally occupied π orbitals will produce a total electron distribu-

[24] By electron diffraction: L. Pauling and L. O. Brockway, *J. Am. Chem. Soc.*, 1937, 59, 1223.

tion, which is circularly symmetrical about the internuclear line. It follows that the π shell of a triple bond has the general form of a cylindrical sheath, the axial interior of which is relatively empty of π electrons (Fig. 4-4). However, the electrons of the σ component of the bond will have their main concentration along this axial region.

As with the double bond, it is the externally situated π electrons of the triple bond that are the more easily removed or disturbed, photolytically or chemically. On the other hand, whilst the π component of a double bond might be uncoupled by torsion, such disruption in the π shell of a triple bond is evidently impossible, a circumstance doubtless of significance in relation to the great thermal stability of some simple triple-bonded compounds.

There is evidence that CH bonds become more polar, the hydrogen end becoming more positive, along the series, methane, ethylene, acetylene, the most striking fact being the ability of acetylene to form metallic compounds. Walsh has related this to the increase in the proportions ($\frac{1}{4}$, $\frac{1}{3}$, and $\frac{1}{2}$) in which the s component is contained in the s-p hybrid orbitals of carbon along the above series.[25] An s orbital, more than a p orbital, and therefore an s component, more than a p component of a hybrid orbital tend to keep the electrons near the carbon nucleus, and consequently away from the hydrogen nucleus.[26]

[25] A. D. Walsh, *Disc. Faraday Soc.*, 1947, 2, 18.

[26] This can be deduced from Fig. 3-2, which shows the s levels lying lower than corresponding p levels. It is, of course, consistent with the pictures in Fig. 3-1, which show s orbitals with a maximum of electron density at the nucleus, and p orbitals with zero electron density at the nucleus.

CHAPTER II

Interactions between and within Molecules*

* The material of this chapter, and of the three next following, is drawn largely from the writer's paper "Principles of an Electronic Theory of Organic Reactions" (*Chem. Revs.*, 1934, 15, 225). Detailed references to this paper are omitted from the text.

(5) ELECTRONIC INTERACTIONS BETWEEN NON-REACTING MOLECULES

IT WILL be useful, in preparation for the study of electronic interactions between the parts of a molecule, to classify the known types of interaction between separate, non-reacting molecules. All those types of interaction which arise between molecules are expected to contribute to the interactions between suitably disposed parts of the same molecule; although within molecules there are also, as we shall note later, certain characteristically internal types of interaction, which are fundamentally dependent on the mode of binding. But it is convenient to consider intermolecular interactions first: they may be classified broadly as electrostatic, electrokinetic, and exchange interactions.

(5a) Electrostatic Interactions.—Almost all molecules possess a series of electrostatic characteristics, which are summarised in the general term *polarisation*. This implies that a molecule has an external electrostatic field. In general, such fields are most simply regarded as a series of superposed fields, each with a characteristic spatial distribution. Fields of long range are produced only when the molecule is an ion.[1] The electrostatic potential arising on account of the nett ionic charge $\pm Ze$ is everywhere proportional to the charge; it varies with distance as the inverse-first power, r^{-1}, and is independent of direction. If the molecule has no nett charge, but has a dipole moment, it will produce a field of medium range. The potential of this field will be everywhere proportional to the dipole moment μ, will vary with distance as r^{-2}, and will depend on direction (since μ is a vector), being, for instance, positive near the hydrogen atom, and negative near the fluorine atom of a hydrogen fluoride molecule. If the molecule has not a dipole moment, but is not too highly symmetrical, it may possess a quadrupole moment, which will give it a field of short range. The potential of this field will be everywhere proportional to the quadrupole moment θ, will vary with distance as r^{-3}, and will depend on direction (since θ is a tensor) being, for example, positive near each end, and negative near the sides of a hydrogen molecule. Any electric charge or system of charges, when placed within the effective range of any of these potential fields, will experience a force. The

[1] We generalise the term "molecule" to include any kinetically independent particle, atom, neutral molecule, or monatomic or polyatomic ion.

force derived from any potential, acting on a single electric charge—on a "pole," as we may say—will be proportional to the gradient of the potential; and the force acting on a dipole will be proportional to the spatial rate of change of the gradient; and so on.

All molecules possess the electrostatic property of *polarisability*. This depends on the readiness of the distributions of nuclear and electronic charges to undergo displacement in opposite directions in an electrostatic field, thereby creating an induced dipole moment. The induced moment is proportional to the polarisability α of the polarisable molecule, and to the potential gradient of the inducing electric field; and it is a function of orientation (α being a tensor). If the electric field originates in another molecule, then a force will arise between the source of the field and the induced dipole moment. Like the force acting on a permanent dipole, the force on this induced dipole will be proportional to the spatial rate of change of the gradient of the potential; it will also be proportional to the induced moment.

All the above-mentioned forces, whether arising from the polarisation of molecules alone, or from their polarisation and polarisability jointly, are considered to contribute significantly to the *electrostatic forces*, which participate in molecular cohesion.

(5b) Electrokinetic Interactions.—These are short-range forces, which the above discussion does not disclose, because it treats the electrons in a molecule as sufficiently represented by a static distribution of electronic charge, and neglects otherwise the actual motion of the electrons. The electrokinetic forces depend fundamentally on this motion; and they are invariably forces of attraction. Their nature was recognised by London especially.[2] As he showed, they are universally present forces, and are often the strongest of the forces of attraction, collectively known as van der Waals forces, on which the condensation of matter depends.

The nature of *electrokinetic forces*[3] can be understood by considering two helium atoms, situated too far apart to permit an important amount of electron exchange. These atoms will then attract each other, even though they have no permanent dipole or quadrupole moments. For the nucleus and each electron of one atom will exert individual forces on the nucleus and each electron of the other; and

[2] R. Eisenschitz and F. London, *Z. Physik*, 1930, 60, 491; F. London, *ibid.*, 1930, 63, 245; *Z. physik. Chem.*, 1930, B, 11, 222.

[3] They are commonly called *dispersion forces*, for the reason that London showed how they could be approximately calculated from data for optical dispersion. They are also called *London forces*, and would probably be universally so called, but for the fact that London also discovered the even more important forces of electron exchange.

the electrons will tend to adapt their motion so as to minimise the overall interaction energy. Thus, if we think of the atoms as situated to the right and left of each other, then, when the electrons of one atom are predominantly towards the right-hand side of that atom, the electrons of the other atom will have a greater probability of being found towards the right than towards the left; and when the electrons of one atom are towards the left, those of the other will tend towards the left. Thus there will always be attraction. As described, it is an attraction of fluctuating dipole-induced dipoles. The interaction energy will vary with distance as r^{-6}, though this is only the leading term of a series of electrokinetic interactions of still shorter range, terms in r^{-8}, r^{-10}, etc.

As London pointed out, electrokinetic forces are non-saturative; that is, they possess the property that the existence of an attraction between two atoms does not interfere appreciably with the attraction of either for a third atom. This is evidently a necessary property for the interpretation of condensation. It contrasts strongly with the behaviour of the forces of electron exchange that lead to covalency formation.

(5c) Exchange Interactions.—At very short distances (*e.g.*, below 2.8 *A* for two neon atoms, or 3.4 *A* for two argon atoms) exchange forces dominate all others. Their physical nature has been discussed in Chapter I. Where Pauli's principle allows, they lead to covalency formation. If we are dealing with molecules in which all possible bonds have been formed, they lead to repulsion.

This repulsion increases very sharply with diminishing distance, as is illustrated by the curves in Fig. 5-1 for the interaction energy of two argon atoms: the steep left-hand branch of either curve shows the predominating repulsion due to exchange at short distances, and the much less steep right-hand branch represents the relatively weak electrokinetic attraction, which dominates at greater distances. Between these branches lies the energy minimum, the position of which gives the equilibrium distance between the atoms in the condensed state, and (after correction for zero-point and thermal energy) the heat of evaporation.

Theoretically, exchange energy should, for distances not too small, obey an expression of the type $R(r)e^{-r/\rho}$, where $R(r)$ is a polynomial in r and ρ is a constant. It is usual in numerical calculations to replace $R(r)$ by a constant b, hoping to absorb most of the error by mutual adjustment of the constants. The electrokinetic energy being represented by its leading term, that in r^{-6}, the total interaction energy U is expressed by the equation,

$$U = be^{-r/\rho} - cr^{-6}$$

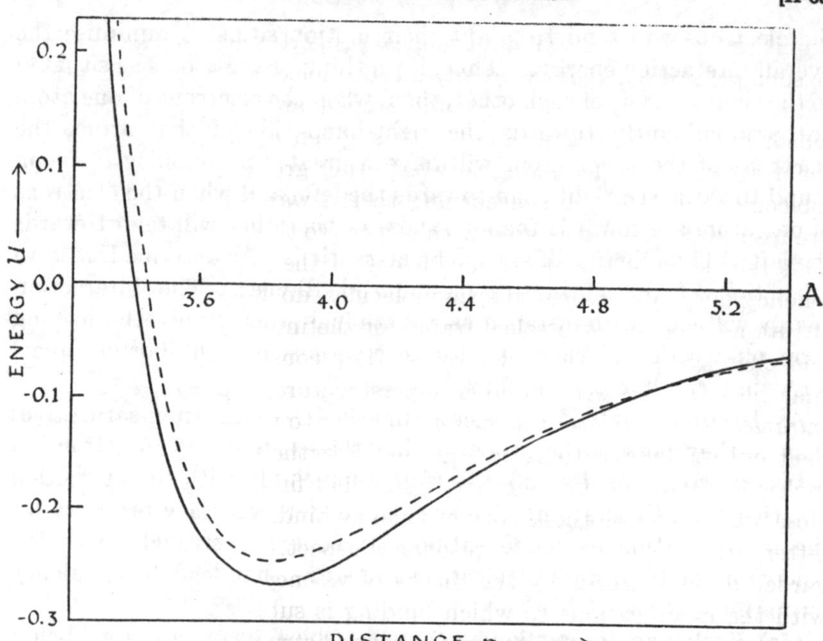

FIG. 5-1.—Energy of interaction of two argon atoms, calculated from the equation $U = be^{-r/\rho} - cr^{-6}$. The full-line curve uses Buckingham's constants, and the broken-line curve revised constants given by Corner. The energy for an atom-pair is multiplied by Avogadro's number, and then expressed in kilocalories in order to facilitate comparison with values given elsewhere for other interaction energies.

where the constants b, c, and ρ are to be evaluated empirically. This equation has proved very successful for the representation of equations of state, transport properties, and crystal properties of the inert gas atoms, and of some other non-polar molecules. The curves in Fig. 5-1 are drawn from this equation with constants given by Buckingham and by Corner.[4]

(6) EXISTENCE AND SIGNIFICANCE OF ELECTRONIC INTERACTION WITHIN MOLECULES

(6a) Existence of Intramolecular Interaction.—Chemistry would be a much simpler science than it is, if every combined atom or group of

[4] J. E. Lennard-Jones in R. H. Fowler's "Statistical Mechanics," Cambridge Univ. Press, 1935, Chap. 10; R. H. Fowler and E. A. Guggenheim, "Statistical Thermodynamics," Cambridge Univ. Press, 1939, Chap. 7; R. A. Buckingham, *Proc. Roy. Soc.* (London), 1938, A, **168**, 264; J. Corner, *Trans. Faraday Soc.*, 1948, **44**, 914. The writer is indebted to Dr. Buckingham for assistance in preparing this Section.

atoms carried its physical and chemical properties, or its contributions to such properties, unchanged into all the molecules in which it participates. We know that this does not happen, and that those properties which are especially associated with a given atom or group usually differ appreciably, according to what other groups are present in the molecular structure, and according to the way in which such other groups are bound and located with respect to the given atom or group. This tells us that the electronic theory of the atom, and that of the valency binding of atoms to form molecules, do not by themselves constitute a sufficient theoretical frame for the interpretation of physical and chemical properties. However, they constitute a basis; and on that basis we have to build a superstructure, namely, a theory of *intramolecular electronic interaction*, in order to take account of the evident effects which atoms and groups, together present in the same molecule, have on one another. We shall find that this theory has close analogies with the theory of valency binding, possessing, like the latter, an electrostatic and a resonance aspect. It can, indeed, be regarded as an extension of the theory of valency, inasmuch as it deals with the modifications to which binding is subject, owing to mutual interactions between the parts of a bonded structure.

(6b) Intramolecular Interaction and Physical Properties.—One of the obvious fields in which to look for manifestations of intramolecular interaction is that of molecular physical properties. For example, we have noted that molecules possess a class of electrostatic properties, collectively termed "polarisation," and that for neutral molecules its most important measure is the molecular dipole moment. One may enquire how far the term polarisation can be given precise meaning when applied, not only to complete molecules, but also to atoms and atomic groups in combination; and how far, in particular, molecular dipole moments can be analysed into characteristic contributions attributable to atoms and atomic groups. The matter has a history. After the principles underlying the determination of molecular dipole moments had been set forth by Debye,[5] but before many dipole moments had actually been measured, Thomson suggested[6] that such moments should be calculable by vector summation of characteristic atomic and group contributions. Soon afterwards dipole moments began to be measured more extensively, and it quickly became clear that a rough relationship of the suggested kind exists. Then followed a succession of attempts to establish an accurately additive principle, and to construct tables of group moments from which molecular mo-

[5] P. Debye, *Physik. Z.*, 1912, **13**, 97; "Polare Molekeln," Hirzel, Leipzig, 1929.
[6] J. J. Thomson, *Phil. Mag.*, 1923, **46**, 513.

ments could be computed by vector addition. Naturally, these attempts could not succeed, first, for the reason that, since molecules have the property of polarisability, as well as their polarisation, internal induction must produce new moments; and secondly, because exact additivity would imply the absence of intramolecular electrical interaction, which is an essential basis for the interpretation of general chemical properties.[7] As measurements became more numerous and more accurate, it became increasingly clear that the deviations from additivity were very general, and much too large to be neglected. The next phase in the development of the subject, namely, the correlation of the deviations with structure, and with other phenomena dependent on internal interaction, will be considered in Chapter III. However, although accurate additivity could not be established, the rough additive principle remains; and hence it is qualitatively valid to regard groups as possessing polarisation, even though the magnitudes which measure it are not accurately constant and characteristic.

A somewhat similar situation prevails with respect to the analysis of molecular polarisability into atomic and group components. The mean polarisability of a molecule (average of the tensor) is given, apart from a constant numerical factor, by the molecular refraction of the gaseous or liquid substance; and it has long been known that molecular refraction exhibits an approximation to an additive principle. There are deviations; but large deviations are less widespread than with dipole moments, arising, as we shall note in Chapter III, mainly in the presence of high polarisation, and of all types of unsaturation, including unshared valency electrons, incomplete valency-electron shells, and multiple bonds. It can thus be understood that, throughout the earlier development of the study of molecular refraction, the adopted procedure was to admit large deviations as constitutive effects, leaving only the small ones to be smoothed over by the averaging processes involved in the calculations of atomic and group contributions. Here again then, deviations from additivity are found, which demonstrate intramolecular electronic effects; and yet it remains true as an approximation that bound atoms and groups have their own polarisabilities, although the measuring magnitudes cannot be regarded as strictly constant and characteristic.

(6c) Intramolecular Interaction and Equilibria in Chemical Reactions.—In some of the following chapters, we shall be occupied with effects of intramolecular electrical interaction on various chemical

[7] C. K. Ingold, *Ann. Repts. on Progress Chem.* (Chem. Soc. London), 1926, 23, 144

reactions. Two aspects of such a study have to be sharply distinguished, namely, the thermodynamic and the kinetic aspects.

We here introduce the thermodynamic aspect with the remark that it has no concern with the rate of reaction, which depends on reaction mechanism: it has no concern with mechanism. The thermodynamic aspect of a reaction relates to the ultimate extent to which the factors can, by any mechanism, be converted into the products, or could be so converted in the absence of any limitation whatsoever with respect to time. This equilibrium degree of conversion is independent of mechanism, and depends only on the factors and the products, and on the physical conditions, such as pressure and temperature.

The equilibrium degree of conversion in a reaction

$$A + B + \cdots = X + Y + \cdots$$

may be expressed by an *equilibrium constant*, K, usually so defined that it is zero when there is no conversion, and infinity when there is complete conversion at equilibrium:

$$K = \frac{[X][Y]\cdots}{[A][B]\cdots}$$

Here the quantities $[X]\cdots$ are, strictly, activities; but they are often replaced by some measure of the concentrations (gaseous partial pressures, mole-fractions, molalities, molarities, etc.), when these are considered to be approximately proportional to the activities. This equilibrium constant[8] depends, differentially, on each of two thermodynamic functions of the collectively considered factors, and the collectively considered products of the reaction. First, it depends on the difference, ΔH, in the *enthalpy* of the factors and products: this, if not the same, is usually very nearly the same as the difference, ΔE, in their internal *energies*, the distinction amounting only to an allowance ($p\Delta v$) for any external work that is done, if the reaction is not conducted at constant volume. Secondly, the equilibrium constant depends on the difference, ΔS, in the *entropies* of the factors and products: entropy is the thermodynamic measure of the statistical probability of a system. The two differences are often expressed in combination as a single difference, ΔG, of *free energy*, the relation with

[8] It is not necessary here to go further into the ways in which K may be specified, or into the manner in which the related thermodynamic functions of the factors and products are defined to suit the specification chosen (the "standard state" conventions). These are described in G. N. Lewis and M. Randall's "Thermodynamics," McGraw-Hill, New York, 1923, Chap. 22.

the equilibrium constant therefore having several alternative forms:

$$\Delta G = \Delta H - T\Delta S = \Delta E + p\Delta v - T\Delta S = -RT \ln K$$

If we rewrite the essence of these equations in the form,

$$K = e^{\Delta S/R} \cdot e^{-\Delta H/RT}$$

we see at once that the products will be more completely formed the greater their entropy, and the smaller their enthalpy, relatively to the corresponding properties of the factors.

In order to understand how, for instance, the enthalpy or free energy might be differently influenced in the factors and products of a reaction by intramolecular electrical effects, consider a factor molecule A—B and a product molecule A—B′ of the reaction,

$$\text{A—B} + \cdots \rightleftarrows \text{A—B}' + \cdots$$

assuming that B′ is more electropositive than B, that is, that B′ repels electrons more strongly than does B, towards and within the common molecular residue A. Side by side with this system, consider a second similar system in which A has been constitutionally modified to A_1,

$$\text{A}_1\text{—B} + \cdots \rightleftarrows \text{A}_1\text{—B}' + \cdots$$

it being assumed that A_1 is more electronegative than A, that is, that A_1 has a greater affinity for electrons than A has. Then the extra polarisation of B′ as compared with B, and the extra polarisation of A_1 as compared with A, will co-operate in the new product molecule A_1—B′, producing a negative energy of interaction. That is, the new product molecule will be more stable relatively to its factor A_1—B, than the old product molecule A—B′ was relatively to its factor A—B. Therefore, as we pass from the first reaction to the second, the position of equilibrium should be shifted in the direction favouring products. This conclusion is based on a consideration of an expected difference of energy differences, when we pass from the first reaction to the second. It should hold provided that, as seems very often to be the case, the analogous difference of entropy differences can be neglected.

The nature of this last assumption can be appreciated with the help of an example. Suppose that $A = C_6H_5$, $B = CO_2H$, $B' = CO_2^-$, and $A_1 = p\text{-}NO_2 \cdot C_6H_4$, the first reaction being the aqueous ionisation of benzoic acid, and the second that of *p*-nitrobenzoic acid:

$$C_6H_5 \cdot CO_2H \rightleftarrows C_6H_5 \cdot CO_2^- + H^+ \text{ (in water)}$$

$$NO_2 \cdot C_6H_4 \cdot CO_2H \rightleftarrows NO_2 \cdot C_6H_4 \cdot CO_2^- + H^+ \text{ (in water)}$$

Then the extra polarisation of B′, as compared with B, will consist essentially in the negative ionic charge of the carboxylate ion. This will produce large overall energy effects, first, by orienting and attracting the permanent water dipoles, and secondly, by inducing extra dipoles in the organic residue, and in the nearer water molecules. It will also produce a large entropy effect, chiefly through the restrictions placed on the positions of the nearer water molecules, restrictions which diminish the statistical probability of the solvated state of the ion. Our assumption is that these effects on energy, and on entropy, are carried over without substantial change from the first reaction to the second. We assume, for example, that the dipolar field of the nitro-group will not much affect the strength of the attraction, or the fixity of position of those water molecules which are closest to the carboxylate ion group, and are therefore of chief importance for the energy and entropy of the solvated ion. The matter can as easily be argued with reference to the energy and entropy effects arising from the interactions of the nitro-group with its near surroundings. Our assumption would then take the equivalent form that these effects of the substituent can be considered as carried, without substantial change, from the factors into the products of the reactions. But outside all these effects, which are assumed approximately to cancel in the difference of differences of energy, and in the difference of differences of entropy, stands uncompensated the internal interaction of the two extra polarisations[9] together present in the *p*-nitrobenzoate ion. This must produce a residual energy effect. In a molecule such as that considered, in which the interacting centres are fairly well separated, and there is little possibility of stereochemical deformation, the interaction can produce no large residual entropy effect.

For these reasons we must expect a greater equilibrium degree of ionisation of *p*-nitrobenzoic acid than of benzoic acid, and this is in accordance with observations. It is usual (see Chapter XIV) to measure the equilibrium degree of ionisation by means of the *acidity constant*,

$$K_a = [H_3\overset{+}{O}][\overset{-}{B}]/[HB]$$

alternatively called *strength* of the acid HB in water, and often expressed in the logarithmic form,

$$pK_a = -\log_{10} K_a$$

The observed values[9] for benzoic and *p*-nitrobenzoic acids are as follows:

$C_6H_5 \cdot CO_2H$ (pK_a 4.20) $\quad$ *p*-$NO_2 \cdot C_6H_4 \cdot CO_2H$ (pK_a 3.42)

The above description of the electrical interactions which influence

[9] J. F. J. Dippy, *Chem. Revs.*, 1939, 25, 151; H. B. Watson, "Modern Theories of Organic Chemistry," Clarendon Press, Oxford, 2nd Edn., 1941, Chap. 2.

equilibria was oversimplified, and must be extended. It was oversimplified inasmuch as *group polarisations* were treated as though they could be carried unaltered from one compound into another: it was implied that the extra polarisation of A_1, compared with A, was carried unaltered from A_1—B into A_1—B′, while the extra polarisation of B′ compared with B, was carried unchanged from A—B′ to A_1—B′, so that one had only to consider the interaction of these unaltered extra polarisations in A_1—B′. This cannot be correct; for, as we saw in Section **6b**, group polarisations are not constant, but become modified by mutual interaction; and the modifications involved in our problem, that is, the *interaction polarisations*, must be taken into account. The group polarisation of A will be altered when A—B is converted into A—B′; and the interaction producing the alterations will produce an energy effect, and perhaps an entropy effect. The group A_1 will not be equally prone to interaction, so that its group polarisation will be differently altered when A_1—B is converted into A_1—B′; and therefore this interaction will produce a different energy effect, and possibly its own entropy effect. We are interested in the difference between these energy effects, and in the difference if any, in the entropy effects. They measure the part played by interaction polarisation in determining the effect of a constitutional modification on equilibria. It is sometimes an important part.

For example, on the basis of the discussion which neglected interaction polarisation, we might have expected, on account of the electronegativity of the methoxyl oxygen atom, that *p*-anisic acid, $MeO\cdot C_6H_4\cdot CO_2H$, would be a stronger acid than benzoic acid, that is, that it would have a higher K_a, and a lower pK_a. In fact, *p*-anisic acid is a weaker acid than benzoic acid, as is shown by the following values:[10]

$C_6H_5\cdot CO_2H$ (pK_a 4.20) *p*-$MeO\cdot C_6H_4\cdot CO_2H$ (pK_a 4.47)

This is attributed to interaction polarisation (essentially a "mesomeric effect," as we shall describe it later), which is expected to be present in both *p*-anisic acid and its anion, but to be stronger in, and thus selectively to stabilise, the undissociated acid.[11]

(6d) Intramolecular Interaction and Rates of Chemical Reactions.— The kinetic aspect of reactions is concerned fundamentally with mechanism: the reactants come together, and the atoms regroup themselves, breaking old bonds and forming new ones: reaction rate is determined by the details of this process, not merely by the final result.

Our interest will be concentrated on thermal reactions, and in these

[10] J. F. J. Dippy, *loc. cit.*; H. B. Watson, *loc. cit.*

[11] C. K. Ingold, *J. Chem. Soc.*, **1933**, 1124.

there are two features of the regrouping process which are so general that they guide all consideration of the details. The first is that it is scarcely ever necessary to supply sufficient energy to break the old bonds completely before the new bonds can begin to be formed: the bond-breaking and bond-forming processes are synchronous. This assumption was first clearly stated by Lewis,[12] and it was developed as part of a general theory by London.[13] For many gas reactions the principle is interpreted as referring to the breaking and formation of covalency bonds. For many reactions in solution, it bears a similar interpretation. But for many other reactions in solution, a broader interpretation is required, because of the occurrence of strong electrostatic binding, as in the solvation of ions.[14] Thus covalency fission may occur synchronously with ion solvation, without the simultaneous formation of a new covalency; and again, covalency formation may synchronise with ion desolvation.

The second general principle, stated by London,[13] is that almost all thermal reactions are "adiabatic." This means that they do not involve an electronic excitation, and that, therefore, as the atoms regroup themselves, the potential energy of the system will vary in a continuous manner, in accord with the Franck-Condon principle.

The significance of these principles may be illustrated by the simple model of a gas reaction between an atom and a diatomic molecule:

$$X + Y—Z = X—Y + Z$$

As X is brought up to Y—Z, interaction between the bonding electron of X and the bond electrons of Y—Z will cause Y and Z progressively to separate. At first the potential energy will rise, but not by so much as would correspond to the separation of Y and Z in the absence of the interaction, essentially because an electron of Y can now pair in two ways, and this form of resonance reduces the energy of the system. A similar description applies, if we suppose Z to be brought up to X—Y. Between these initial and final states there will be a configuration X · · · Y · · · Z, called the *transition state*, having the greatest energy of any intermediate configuration through which the system is bound to pass. But this maximal energy is, because of the resonance, less than would be needed to dissociate either diatomic molecule.[15] In the transition state, Y is bound by partial covalencies to both X and Z.

[12] G. N. Lewis, "Valence and the Structure of Atoms and Molecules," Chemical Catalog Co., New York, 1923, p. 113.

[13] F. London, *Z. Elektrochem.*, 1929, 35, 552.

[14] E. D. Hughes and C. K. Ingold, *J. Chem. Soc.*, 1935, 244.

[15] For X = Y = Z = H the rise in energy at the transition state is 9 kcal./mole, as against a dissociation energy of 103 kcal./mole.

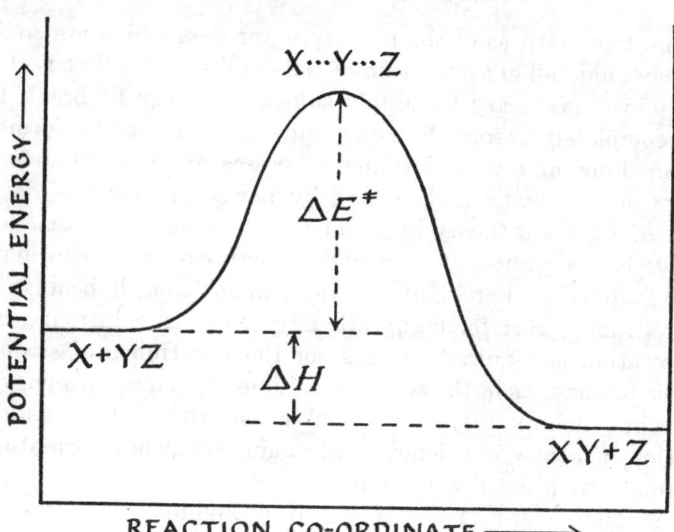

FIG. 6-1.—Variation of potential energy accompanying the reaction X+YZ =XY+Z. The heat of reaction ΔH, and the energy of activation $\Delta E^{\neq}$ are uncorrected for the zero-point and thermal energies of the relevant species.

If a coordinate is defined to measure the progress of the atomic regrouping, the variation of potential energy during the process will be represented by a continuous curve of the general form shown in Fig. 6-1.

The difference ΔE of potential energy between the initial and transition states is the uncorrected *energy of activation* of the reaction. It requires correction, first, for the difference in the zero-point energies of vibration of the initial and transition states, and secondly, for the difference in their thermal energies at the temperature of reaction.

In order to understand more completely what is meant by the term "reaction co-ordinate," it is necessary to consider the potential energy as a function of all the internal co-ordinates of the system, $3n-6$ co-ordinates for an n-atomic system. In the three-atom system there are three internal co-ordinates, but a simplified description can be based on the consideration that, in all configurations approaching that of the transition state, the atoms X and Z repel each other, so that the transition state is certain to be included in an abridged description in which only linear configurations of the three atoms are explicitly taken into account. Under this restriction, there remain two internal co-ordinates, and these can conveniently be taken as the distances XY and YZ. In this co-ordinate system, the potential energy can be represented by a surface, which consists, as the contour diagram in Fig. 6-2 shows, of

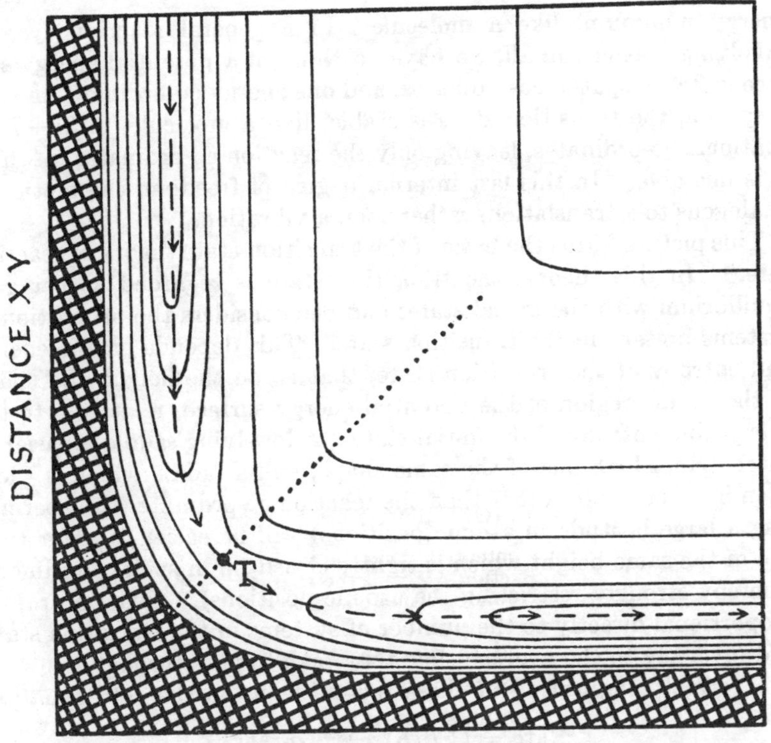

FIG. 6-2.—Variation of potential energy with linear configurations of the reaction system X+YZ=XY+Z. The form of the energy surface is indicated by energy contours: two valleys, representing initial and final states, meet in a saddle-point, which represents the transition state (T). The reaction co-ordinate, indicated by the broken line, passes through an energy maximum at the transition state. But the orthogonal co-ordinate, indicated by the dotted line, passes through an energy minimum at the transition state.

two valleys meeting in a saddle-point, which represents the transition state. The *reaction co-ordinate* passes along the floor of either valley and over the saddle-point, always following the lowest possible path from one valley floor to the other. The curve in Fig. 6-1 is the profile of a section of this surface, taken along the reaction co-ordinate.

In the transition state, the reaction co-ordinate corresponds to what would be the vibrational co-ordinate, $\overrightarrow{X}$—Y—$\overrightarrow{Z}$, if XYZ were a stable molecule. However, the transition state is at an energy maximum, not, like a molecule, at a minimum, in *this* particular co-ordinate. But in the orthogonal co-ordinate, $\overleftrightarrow{X}$—Y—$\overrightarrow{Z}$, the transition state is at an energy minimum, like a molecule. In a general reaction system, involving n atoms in all, we have to think of a potential energy surface in $3n-6$ spatial co-ordinates, and one energy co-ordinate. In such a system, the transition state is stable, like a molecule, in $3n-7$ vibrational co-ordinates, leaving only the reaction co-ordinates in which it is unstable. In this last internal degree of freedom, the motion is analogous to a translation, rather than a vibration.

This picture forms the basis of the transition-state theory of reaction rate.[16] In this theory, the transition state is regarded as being in equilibrium with the initial state; and one considers the proportion of systems present in the transition state. This depends on the energy and entropy of the transition state, that is, on the height and shape of the saddle region of the potential energy surface, relatively to the energy and entropy of the initial state. A low-lying saddle is easier to enter than a high one of the same shape, and a saddle which is wide-open in co-ordinates other than the reaction co-ordinate (thus permitting a large latitude in atomic positions) will be easier to enter than one of the same height which is tightly closed-up in such co-ordinates (thereby strongly restricting the atomic positions). Reaction rate is proportional directly to the number of systems in the transition state, and inversely to the average time they take to pass through it.

A formal composition of these factors leads to the rate equation,

$$\text{Rate} = (kT/h)\cdot e^{\Delta S^{\neq}/R}\cdot e^{-\Delta H^{\neq}/RT}$$

The rate is measured by k, the *rate constant* in the kinetic equation

$$\text{Rate} = k[\text{A}]^a[\text{B}]^b \cdots$$

for a reaction of *order a* in factor A, b in factor B, the *total order* being $a+b+\cdots$; and k is Boltzmann's constant; and h is Planck's constant; while $\Delta H^{\neq}$, the *heat of activation*, and $\Delta S^{\neq}$, the *entropy of activation*, are differences between the relevant thermodynamic functions of the transition and initial states. In reckoning the entropy of the transition state, it is convenient to omit the part dependent on motion in the reaction co-ordinate. The factor kT/h takes care of this part, as well as of the dependence of rate on time of passage through the transition state. The heat of activation is an approximation to the *energy of activation*, the difference consisting only in a small adjustment in respect of kinetic energy, and one for external work, if any:

[16] H. Pelzer and E. Wigner, *Z. physik. Chem.*, 1932, **B**, 15, 445; H. Eyring, *J. Chem. Phys.*, 1935, **3**, 107; M. G. Evans and M. Polanyi, *Trans. Faraday, Soc.* 1935, **31**, 875; W. F. K. Wynne-Jones and H. Eyring, *J. Chem. Phys.*, 1935, **3**, 492; S. Glasstone, K. J. Laidler, and H. Eyring, "Theory of Rate Processes," McGraw-Hill, New York, 1941.

$$\Delta E^{\neq} = \Delta H^{\neq} + kT - p\Delta v^{\neq}$$

In the elementary form in which the mass-law is normally applied in reaction kinetics, the brackets [ ] in the above rate equation are taken to be concentrations. However, the theory that reaction rate is proportional to the fraction of systems maintained in the transition state, obviously involves a correction in terms of activities or activity coefficients, when the latter differ significantly from unity. The thermodynamic activity, $a^{\neq} = c^{\neq}f^{\neq}$, of the transition state should be proportional to the product of the activities, $a_A = c_A f_A$, etc., of all the reactant molecules; and therefore the concentration of systems in the transition state $c^{\neq}$, to which reaction rate should be proportional, should be equal to this activity product divided by the activity coefficient of the transition state. Thus we arrive at the rate equation

$$\text{Rate} = kc_A{}^a c_B{}^b \cdots \frac{f_A{}^a f_B{}^b \cdots}{f^{\neq}}$$

where the c's are concentrations, and the f's activity coefficients, $f^{\neq}$ being the activity coefficient of the transition state. For reactions in solution, the activity coefficient factor should take care of all departures from ideality. This rate equation was advanced by Brönsted in 1922, who thereby anticipated some of the ideas of the transition state theory.[17]

It must be admitted that it is seldom possible to use the explicit equation of the transition-state theory in unambiguous numerical calculations of reaction rate, for lack of sufficiently detailed information about the energy surfaces of reactions. Nevertheless, we can often profitably apply the ideas of the theory in qualitative discussions of effects of molecular structure, or of solvent, on the heat and entropy of activation, and therefore on rate of reaction.

The quantities which are usually computed from measurements of the temperature dependence of reaction rate are the parameters A and E_A of the Arrhenius equation,

$$k = Ae^{-E_A/RT}$$

Comparison with the transition-state equation for reaction rate shows that the Arrhenius equation is only an approximation, inasmuch as it represents by the constant A a number of quantities which actually depend on temperature. However, in general, these quantities vary much more slowly with temperature than does the factor $e^{-E_A/RT}$, so that a quite small adjustment in the value of E_A can almost completely

[17] J. N. Brönsted, *Z. physik. Chem.*, 1922, **102**, 169.

absorb the slow variation, over the ranges of temperature used in practice. For this reason, it is usual to accept the *Arrhenius activation energy* E_A as an approximation to the energy of activation, and to take the logarithm of the *Arrhenius frequency factor A* as an approximate measure (a nearly linear function) of the entropy of activation; and to regard both these quantities as reflecting in a semi-quantitative way, the variations in the energy and entropy of activation over a series of reactions, or for a reaction in a series of solvents.

With this picture of the general nature of the factors determining reaction rate, let us take up the question of how electrical effects might influence energy or entropy of activation, and therefore reaction rate. It may be assumed that very many reagents act primarily either on the valency electrons, or on the positive atomic kernel of the atom attacked, and that therefore the development in the first case, of a high, or in the second, of a low, electronic density in that atom will facilitate the formation of the transition state. An equivalent statement is that, in the transition state, the site of reaction becomes a highly polar centre, which either requires electrons to be drawn away from, or requires them to be driven back into, the rest of the molecule. Whichever of these requirements actually obtains for some particular reaction, polar substituents cannot fail either to assist, or to impede, its fulfilment.

Consider the case of a reaction between A—B and C, in which C attacks a positive atomic kernel in B, forming a transition state [A—B$^{\neq}$ · · · C], wherein electrons are driven back into the radical A to a greater extent than they were in the initial molecule A—B:

$$\text{A—B} + \text{C} \text{—}[\text{A—B}^{\neq} \cdots \text{C}] \rightarrow \text{A—B}' + \text{C}'$$

Consider, side by side with this, a similar reaction in which A has been structurally modified to A_1, where A_1 has a greater affinity for electrons than A has:

$$\text{A}_1\text{—B} + \text{C} \text{—}[\text{A}_1\text{—B}^{\neq} \cdots \text{C}] \rightarrow \text{A}_1\text{—B}' + \text{C}'$$

Then, by an argument closely similar to that used in Section **6c** in connexion with constitutional polar effects on chemical equilibria, it follows that the energy of activation of the second reaction will be the smaller. Accordingly, the rate of the second reaction will be the greater, provided that, as is very often true, the effect of the structural change in producing a difference in the entropies of activation can be neglected. If A should be structurally modified in a different way to give A_2, where A_2 has a smaller affinity for electrons than has A, then the effect of the modification on the energy of activation, and on the rate of the reaction, should be the opposite of that described. If the reaction is of the opposite polar kind, the reagent C attacking the valency electrons of B, to form a transition state in which electrons are attracted from the radical A more than they were in the original molecule, then, the kinetic effect of changing A either into A_1, or into A_2, will in each case be the opposite of that already mentioned.

As an example, let $A = C_6H_5$, $B = H$, $C = NO_2^+$, $A_1 = p\text{-}NO_2 \cdot C_6H_4$, $B' = NO_2$, and $C' = H^+$. The reactions compared are the nitration of benzene in any one position, and of nitrobenzene in, say, the para-position, the substituting agent in both cases being the nitronium ion:

$$C_6H_5 \cdot H + NO_2^+ — \left[C_6H_5^+ \begin{matrix} \diagup H \\ \\ \diagdown NO_2 \end{matrix} \right] \rightarrow C_6H_5 \cdot NO_2 + H^+$$

$$NO_2 \cdot C_6H_4 \cdot H + NO_2^+ — \left[NO_2 \cdot C_6H_4^+ \begin{matrix} \diagup H \\ \\ \diagdown NO_2 \end{matrix} \right] \rightarrow NO_2 \cdot C_6H_4 \cdot NO_2 + H^+$$

In these reactions the nitronium ion attacks the electrons of the benzenoid carbon atom to form a transition state (shown in brackets), in which positive polarity is acquired by the reaction centre. The prior presence of a nitro-group with its formal dipole should lead to an interaction in the transition state, which increases the energy of activation of nitration of the nitrobenzene in comparison with that of unsubstituted benzene. Experimentally, the rate of nitration of nitrobenzene is so much smaller than that of benzene that the two rates cannot be measured under identical conditions. It can be estimated from known data that the rates of the reactions compared must differ by a factor of about 10^8. On theoretical grounds one would expect that almost the whole of this difference arises from a difference in the energy of activation. As the molecules are fairly rigid, and as the modification of structure is made at some distance from the reaction centre, no marked change in the entropy of activation is to be anticipated. However, a constitutional change in close proximity to the site of reaction (as in an ortho-substitution), or an alteration in the solvent in which the reaction is carried out, would change the shape of the energy surface at the saddle-point, and we should then have to expect a difference in the entropy as well as in the energy of activation.

The preceding description of electrical kinetic effects requires to be extended, much in the same way as that in which the initially given description of electrical thermodynamic effects was extended in Section 6c. The above discussion of kinetic effects was limited to what may be called *polarisation effects*, inasmuch as the extra polarisation introduced into a molecule by a constitutional modification was considered as a constant attribute of the modification, a *group polarisation*, assumed to be carried unchanged from the initial state of the system into the transition state, there to interact with the special polarity acquired in that state by the site of reaction, thus influencing the energy, and possibly the entropy, of activation. However, this can only be a partial description of electrical kinetic effects: there remain what may be called *polarisability effects*. For the special polarity of the reaction centre in the transition state must deform the total electronic system, producing a temporary interaction polarisation; and this will be altered by any constitutional modification which alters the polarisability of the electronic system, or, as we may express it, introduces a new polarisability, with respect to the deforming field. Thus the constitutional modification will be associated with a *temporary interaction polarisation*, not present in the initial state, but present in the transition state, where it must interact with the special polarisation acquired by the reaction centre, thereby influencing the energy, and perhaps the entropy, of activation of the reaction.

For example, if we were to take account only of polarisation effects, we should expect that, on account of the electronegativity of the methoxyl group, anisole would be nitrated in the para-position more slowly, and with larger energy of activation, than benzene would be nitrated in any one position. In fact, anisole is nitrated much more rapidly than benzene, the difference being so great that the two rates have never been directly compared in identical experimental conditions. The rate ratio is probably[18] greater than 10^4. This striking reversal of what should be expected on the basis of the polarisation of anisole is attributed to a polarisability effect: the positive polarity acquired in the transition state causes the methoxyl group temporarily to supply electrons to the reaction site in that state, even though an electron displacement in this direction is contrary to the normal polarity of the methoxyl group.

Comparing this discussion with that of Section 6c, we see that the parts played by group polarisation and interaction polarisation in the control of reaction equilibria are paralleled respectively by polarisation effects and polarisability effects in the control of reaction rates.

[18] P. B. D. de la Mare and C. A. Vernon have estimated the ratio to be 1.2×10^9 for bromination (*J. Chem. Soc.*, **1951**, 1764).

But, of course, there is a difference in time-dependence: group polarisation and interaction polarisation are both properties of normal molecular states: a polarisation effect arises from polarity in a normal state; but a polarisability effect is a temporary interaction, not referable to polarity in a normal state. Kinetic polarisability effects are of great importance, as we shall have later occasion to observe.

(6e) Intramolecular Interaction and Stereochemical Form.—As was noted in Chapter I, the single bond has, according to theory, full circular symmetry about its internuclear axis. It follows that rotation about single bonds, such as the CC bond in ethane, should be completely free, except in so far as this conclusion might be modified by effects of internal interaction. That such rotation is not free was shown by Kemp and Pitzer,[19] and by Kistiakowsky, Lacher, and Stitt,[20] by reference to the entropy and low-temperature heat-capacity of ethane. At the temperature of liquid air, the contributions to the specific heat of all vibrations, excepting torsional oscillation, are negligible because of the large magnitudes of the vibrational quanta. The excess of the specific heat over the part ($3R$) due to molecular translation and rotation arises from torsional oscillation. If relative rotation of the methyl groups were completely free, this contribution would be that of a rotation ($0.5R$). If such movement were very slightly resisted, the contribution could be larger (because of the potential energy). If the movement were strongly resisted, so that the torsional frequency was high, then the contribution would be negligible (because of the large size of the quantum). In fact, it is about $0.3R$. The same conclusion was reached at about the same time by Howard[21] from an analysis of the rotational structures of infra-red absorption bands of ethane. He estimated the torsional oscillation frequency at 230 cm.$^{-1}$. From the thermal data the frequency 280 cm.$^{-1}$ had been calculated. A later analysis by G. L. Smith of infra-red fine structure has given 290 cm.$^{-1}$; and finally direct observation by Weiss and Leroi[22] of the very weak infra-red twisting bands, symmetry-forbidden, but allowed by a Coriolis interaction, has shown the fundamental frequency to be 289 cm.$^{-1}$. It is thus much lower than the twisting frequency of ethylene (1027 cm.$^{-1}$).[23] The height of the

[19] J. D. Kemp and K. S. Pitzer, *J. Chem. Phys.*, 1936, **4**, 749; *J. Am. Chem. Soc.*, 1937, **59**, 276.

[20] G. B. Kistiakowsky, J. R. Lacher, and F. Stitt, *J. Chem. Phys.*, 1938, **6**, 407; 1939, **7**, 289.

[21] J. B. Howard, *J. Chem. Phys.*, 1937, **5**, 451.

[22] L. G. Smith, *J. Chem. Phys.*, 1949, **17**, 139; S. Weiss and G. E. Leroi, *ibid.*, 1968, **48**, 262.

[23] R. L. Arnett and B. L. Crawford jr., *J. Chem. Phys.*, 1950, **18**, 118.

energy barrier resisting internal rotation has been estimated with good consistency to be 2.93 kcal./mole. (Thus the zero-point level is 0.41 kcal./mole above the minimum potential energy.) This is sufficiently large, relatively to the equipartition value at ordinary temperature (0.6 kcal./mole), to ensure that nearly all the molecules are in the favoured conformation; but it is too small, considered as an activation energy, to suggest that one could isolate geometrical isomers of ethane derivatives having barriers of a similar height.

Molecular models that differ only as after relative rotation round one or more single bonds (or, as we ought to say, "formal" single bonds) are called *conformations.* The symmetry of ethane requires that its stable conformation be one of two alternatives. Either it is what is called *eclipsed*, that is, with pairs of methyl hydrogen atoms coinciding in projection on a transverse plane; or it is *staggered*, that is, with one methyl group so rotated that its bonds lie symmetrically between those of the other methyl group in the projection. In 1949, L. G. Smith showed, by a detailed rotational analysis of infra-red bands, that the stable conformation of ethane is the staggered one.[22]

Actually, the same conclusion had been less directly reached a little earlier, by a study of the stabilities of *cyclo*alkanes. A stable eclipsed model for ethane would imply an attraction of the CH bonds of either carbon atom for those of the other. Such an attraction would produce stability in *cyclo*pentane, in the almost strainless planar form of which all C_2-units are in the eclipsed conformation, relatively to *cyclo*hexane, which cannot simultaneously achieve strainlessness and eclipsed conformations in all its C_2-units. On the contrary, a stable staggered model for ethane would imply repulsion between the CH bonds of each carbon atom and those of the other. Such repulsion would lead to instability in *cyclo*pentane, the CH bonds in which cannot assume staggered positions, relatively to *cyclo*hexane, one of the out-of-plane strainless forms of which, the trigonal, so-called "chair" form, has all its C_2-units in the staggered conformation. The heats of combustion of a number of *cyclo*alkanes were measured by Spitzer and Huffman, who concluded that *cyclo*hexane, the only one that can simultaneously have its ring completely strainless and all its C_2-units exactly staggered, is the most stable of the series:[24]

n in $(CH_2)_n$	5	6	7	8
$-\Delta^{25°}_{gas}/n$ (kcal./mole)	158.7	157.4	158.3	158.8

Hassel demonstrated by X-ray, electron diffraction, and dipole-moment measurements that simple *cyclo*hexane compounds remain

[24] R. Spitzer and H. M. Huffman, *J. Am. Chem. Soc.*, 1947, **69**, 211.

firmly in the "chair" conformation, shown below, in all phases of matter, even the gas phase. The other strainless, though less stable, conformation of *cyclo*hexane, the so-called "boat" form, is really a manifold of conformations, so mutually convertible by coordinated strainless rotations around the ring bonds, that each in turn of the three pairs of most remote carbon atoms constitute the "prow" and "stern" of the "boat," *i.e.*, lie on a plane of symmetry. However, each of these conformations has two C_2-units, the "sides" of the "boat," in eclipsed form; and there is a general belief that the stable conformations within the manifold will lie between those described, so avoiding all such eclipsing. They will have no plane of symmetry, but will have a 2-fold rotational axis of symmetry, as shown below.

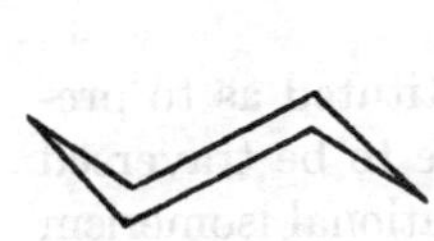

"Chair" conformation of *cyclo*hexane. (Has a 3-fold rotational and a 6-fold alternating axis of symmetry.)

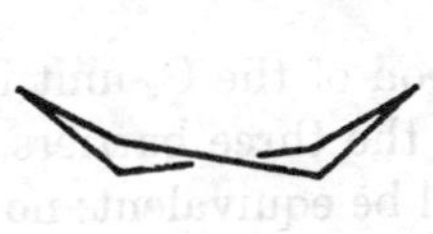

"Boat" conformation of *cyclo*hexane (metastable). (Has a 2-fold rotational axis of symmetry.)

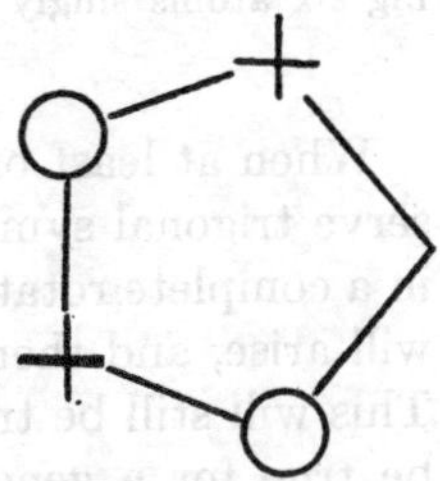

Proposed[27] equilibrium conformation of *cyclo*pentane: + = above, and O = below, median plane by 0.32 *A*.

The *cyclo*pentane ring avoids eclipsed C_2-units by not being flat, although the most nearly strainless conformation would be flat. This has been shown by thermal measurements[25] and supported by analyses of infra-red and microwave spectra[26] and by measurements on electric double refraction.[27] The geometry of the stable conformation is not known with precision but may approximate to that represented above.[27]

A number of simple open-chain derivatives and analogues of ethane have been investigated by thermal, spectral, and other physical methods in order to determine their stable conformations and also the heights of the energy barriers that resist rotation around their single bonds. When a derivative of ethane has six single-bonded substituent atoms, the staggered conformation is always favoured. But when the

[25] J. G. Aston, S. C. Schumann, H. L. Fink, and P. M. Doty, *J. Am. Chem. Soc.*, 1941, **63**, 2029; 1943, **65**, 541; K. S. Pitzer and W. D. Gwinn, *ibid.*, 1941, **63**, 3313; J. E. Kilpatrick, K. S. Pitzer, and R. Spitzer, *ibid.*, 1947, **69**, 2483.

[26] F. A. Miller and R. G. Inskeep, *J. Chem. Phys.*, 1950, **18**, 1510; G. W. Rathjens jr., *J. Chem. Phys.*, 1962, **36**, 2401.

[27] C. G. LeFèvre and R. J. W. LeFèvre, *J. Chem. Soc.*, 1956, 3549.

number of substituent atoms is reduced to five, one being doubly bonded, then one single bond becomes eclipsed with the double bond. These stable conformations are shown in Newman projections below.

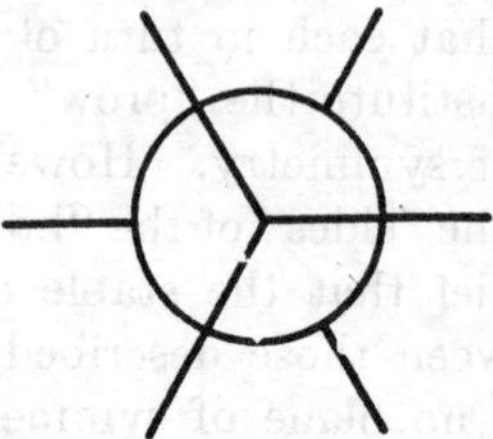

Stable conformation of a C_2-unit bearing six atoms singly bound.

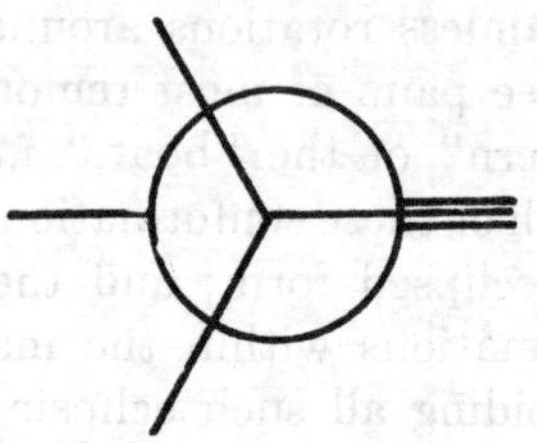

Stable conformation of a C_2-unit bearing five atoms singly and one doubly bound.

When at least one carbon of the C_2-unit is so substituted as to preserve trigonal symmetry, the three barriers that have to be traversed in a complete rotation will be equivalent: no conformational isomerism will arise, and there will be just one barrier height for the compound. This will still be true when one carbon carries a double bond. It will be true for a generalised XY-unit of octet-forming atoms, provided that either X, or Y, or both, have trigonal symmetry. It will still be true if one of these atoms has the number of its other bonds reduced to two. A number of barrier heights in molecules that do not show conformational isomerism are contained in Table 6-1.[28]

It is noteworthy that for C_2-units with six flanking atoms the barrier height is 3 kcal./mole, independently of the nature of the flanking atoms, provided that these are small enough collectively. There appears to be a threshold of collective size, above which the barrier rises, as in $CF_3 \cdot CCl_3$ and $CCl_3 \cdot CCl_3$. The barrier is reduced when the central C_2-unit is changed to a CX- or an XY-unit, with a longer and weaker torsion bond; and it is reduced in CX-units in which the number of bonds of X that must simultaneously cross eclipsed positions during rotation is diminished from three to two, and to one. Again, the barrier is diminished when a double bond to carbon is introduced; and it is diminished still more if the double bond is to an oxygen atom. As we shall see later, the π electrons in a carbonyl group are strongly

[28] Nearly all the figures in this table are from D. J. Millen's Chapter IV in P. B. D. de la Mare and W. Klyne's "Progress in Stereochemistry," Butterworths, London, 1962, Vol. 3, p. 138; the article gives full references to the original literature. The figures for C_2Cl_6, $CCl_3 \cdot SiCl_3$, and Si_2Cl_6 come from an electron-diffraction study by Y. Morino and E. Hirota, *J. Chem. Phys.*, 1958, 28, 185.

TABLE 6-1.—ENERGETIC HEIGHTS OF BARRIERS RESTRICTING ROTATION ROUND SINGLE BONDS.

Bond	Barrier height kcal./mole	Bond	Barrier height kcal./mole
CH_3—CH_3	2.90	CH_3—SiH_3	1.70
CH_3—CH_2F	3.33	CH_3—SiH_2F	1.56
CH_3—CH_2Cl	3.56	CH_3—$SiHF_2$	1.24
CH_3—CH_2Br	3.57	CH_3—SiF_3	1.20
CH_3—CH_2I	3.22		
CH_3—$CH_2{\cdot}CN$	3.05	CH_3—GeH_3	1.20
CH_3—CHF_2	3.18		
CH_3—CF_3	3.04	CCl_3—$SiCl_3$	4.3
CH_3—CCl_3	2.91	$SiCl_3$—$SiCl_3$	1.0
CF_3—CF_3	3.02		
CF_3—CCl_3	6.00	CH_3—$CH{:}CH_2$	1.98
CCl_3—CCl_3	10.8		
		CH_3—$CH{:}O$	1.16
CH_3—NH_2	1.96	CH_3—$CF{:}O$	1.04
CH_3—OH	1.07	CH_3—$CCl{:}O$	1.30
CH_3—SH	1.27	CH_3—$C(CN){:}O$	1.21

concentrated towards the oxygen atom, and hence in our examples are drawn away from the torsion-sustaining bond and so from the theatre of the interactions that create the resistance to torsion.

It seems evident that the forces that restrict rotation in ethane, and in its substitution products with small-atom substituents, are repulsions between the bonds flanking the C_2-unit, repulsions which are maximised when the flanking bonds are in eclipsed positions. The repulsions must occur mainly between those parts of the flanking bonds which are nearer the carbon nuclei of the central C_2-unit and hence are nearer to each other. Or we may say, the repulsions must be mainly between those parts of the flanking bonds which are within the carbon radii of the C_2-unit. The reason for thinking so is that the resulting energy barriers are so nearly independent of the nature of the flanking atoms, as long as these are small enough. It is generally thought that the repulsive forces are mainly those of electron exchange, although quadrupole-quadrupole repulsions, and possibly other electrostatic interactions, may contribute.

Now if the flanking bonds were, within the carbon radii of the C_2-unit, no different from equally occupied sp^3 carbon orbitals, there would be no barrier to rotation; for three such orbitals of a tetrahedral atom build up an electron distribution with full circular symmetry about the axis of the fourth orbital. Therefore we must admit a difference between such orbitals and the bonds they form—a difference applying even to those parts of the bonds which are within the carbon radii. This difference reduces the full circular symmetry of the assembly of three atomic orbitals to trigonal symmetry in the assembly of three bonds, giving trefoil character to the electron distribution over a section through the three bonds, perpendicular to the line of the torsion-sustaining bond. In filling in this idea, we might follow Pauling in assuming that the atomic orbitals sp^3, in higher approximation, become concentrated more closely about their individual symmetry axes, by the inclusion of small proportions of *d* and *f* orbitals. Or, if we do not wish to follow the description of atomic orbitals to so high an approximation, because these orbitals will in any case be greatly changed on conversion to bond orbitals, we may reflect simply that the bond orbitals of the flanking bonds must become concentrated, relatively to their parent, carbon-atomic, sp^3 orbitals, by the nuclei of the flanking atoms that the bond orbitals bind. This itself will give trefoil cross sections of electron density to the sets of flanking bonds, and so lead to an oscillating interaction energy during rotation round the central C_2-bond.

It is easily understood that, when one of the flanking bonds is a double bond, a single bond will be eclipsed with it; for the single bond will then lie on the nodal plane of the π bond orbital, *i.e.*, in a plane of zero π-electron density.

When neither substituted methyl group in the C_2-unit has trigonal symmetry, conformational (*i. e.* rotational) isomerism arises: the three rotational energy hollows are no longer all equivalent. We may describe the isomers belonging to the several hollows by specifying for each the smallest angle with which unique or other fiducial groups, belonging one to each of the substituted methyl groups, can be connected by a helix about the C_2-bond as axis.[29] The helical angle is designated + or −, or, according to a newer suggestion, *P* or *M* (for "plus" and "minus"),[30] according as the helix is right- or left-handed. All isomers having helical angles other than 0° and 180° have chirality (handedness) and would, if separately isolated, exhibit optical activity: the labels *P* and *M* distinguish the enantiomers. When the magnitude of the helical angle is only approximately known (and often also when it is exactly known), semi-quantitative terms, or their abbreviations, namely, synperiplanar (*sp*), synclinal (*sc*), anticlinal (*ac*), and antiperiplanar (*ap*), are employed in order to describe helical

[29] W. Klyne and V. Prelog, *Experientia*, 1960, **16**, 521.

[30] R. S. Cahn, C. K. Ingold, and V. Prelog, *Angew. Chem., internat. Edit.*, 1966, **5**, 383.

angles believed to be within ±30° of the idealised angles, 0°, ±60°, ±120°, and 180°, respectively.

The simplest systems of conformational isomers are those which arise, in a substituted ethane, when each substituted methyl group carries two identical atoms or groups, and one unique one. The unique substituents in the two substituted methyl groups then become fiducial. If we describe each isomer by the helical inter-relation of its two fiducial substituents, the isomer system comprises one antiperiplanar isomer, and two enantiomeric synclinal isomers, that is, the *ap*, *P-sc*, and *M-sc* isomers, represented below. In a plot of energy *versus* torsion angle, the hollow containing the antiperiplanar isomer would lie between the equivalent hollows containing synclinal enantiomers; but the antiperiplanar hollow might lie either lower or higher in energy than the pair of synclinal hollows:

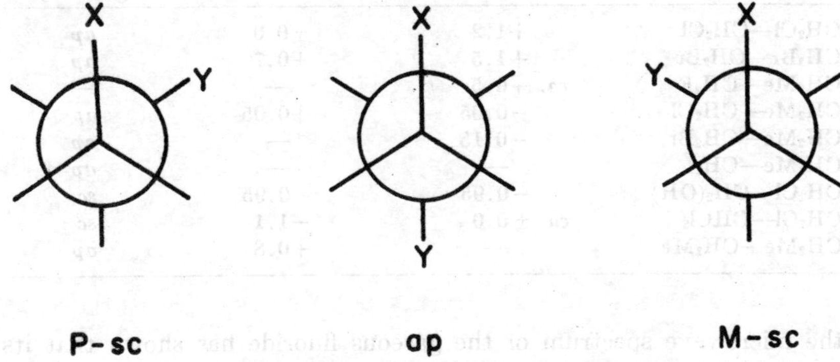

The existence of such isomers is shown,[31] in the first place, by the Raman and infra-red spectra of ethylene dichloride and ethylene dibromide. Each spectrum consists of two superposed spectra, one of which fades at low temperatures, thus indicating isomers of different stabilities in equilibrium. The low-temperature spectra show that, in these particular molecules, the more stable rotational isomers have the antiperiplanar conformation (centro-symmetric). This conclusion is supported by the dipole moments, which fall considerably as the temperature is reduced. The antiperiplanar isomers can be isolated in a pure form by merely cooling; for the solid substances consist of these pure isomers. From the effects of temperature on the spectra of the vapours, it is concluded that the synclinal isomers of

[31] The evidence is summarised by S. Mizushima in his "Structure of Molecules and Internal Rotation," Academic Press, New York, 1954, where full references to the original literature are given.

ethylene dichloride and dibromide are less stable by 1.2 and 1.5 kcal./mole, respectively, than their antiperiplanar isomers. The heights of the barriers separating the isomers are not known, but they must amount to several kcal./mole, or the bands in the spectra would be broader than they are.

Some relative stabilities in a number of sets of isomers are given in Table 6-2.[32] The relative stabilities are not always in the direction illustrated by the ethylene dihalides. In the *n*-propyl halides, whether as gases or liquids, the balance of stability between the synclinal and antiperiplanar isomers is in the opposite sense. An investigation of

TABLE 6-2.—RELATIVE STABILITIES OF ROTATIONAL ISOMERS.

	$E_{sc}-E_{ap}$ (kcal./mole)		Isomers constituting solid
	Gas	Liquid	
$CH_2Cl—CH_2Cl$	+1.2	±0.0	*ap*
$CH_2Br—CH_2Br$	+1.5	+0.7	*ap*
$CH_2Me—CH_2F$	*ca.* +0.5	—	—
$CH_2Me—CH_2Cl$	−0.05	+0.05	*ap*
$CH_2Me—CH_2Br$	−0.15	—	*ap*
$CH_2Me—CH_2I$	—	—	*ap*
$CH_2Cl—CH_2(OH)$	−0.95	−0.95	*sc*
$CH_2Cl—CHCl_2$	*ca.* ±0.0	−1.1	*sc*
$CH_2Me—CH_2Me$	—	+0.8	*ap*

the microwave spectrum of the gaseous fluoride has shown that its synclinal isomers, with helical angles of ±63° about the C_1C_2-bond, are more stable than the antiperiplanar isomer by 0.47±0.31 kcal./mole. Anticlinal barriers of about 4 kcal./mole separate the synclinal enantiomers from the antiperiplanar isomer, whilst the synclinal enantiomers themselves are separated by a synperiplanar barrier of about 10 kcal./mole. The rotation spectrum shows also that all isomers have barriers restricting methyl rotation about the C_2C_3-bond: it amounts to 2.9 kcal./mole in the synclinal isomers and to 2.7 kcal./mole in the antiperiplanar isomer. In gaseous and liquid *n*-propyl chloride, and in gaseous *n*-propyl bromide, the synclinal isomers are

[32] Nearly all the data in the table are from D. J. Millen's article in de la Mare and Klyne's "Progress in Stereochemistry," Vol. **3**, p. 138, where references to the original literature will be found. The figures in the table and the text referring to *n*-propyl fluoride are from a study by E. Hirota of the microwave spectrum of that substance, *J. Chem. Phys.*, 1962, **37**, 283.

again slightly more stable than the antiperiplanar. However, the solid chloride and the solid bromide are both pure antiperiplanar forms, presumably because, despite their lesser molecular stabilities, they have higher lattice energies. The synclinal form of ethylene chlorohydrin is more stable by 1.0 kcal./mole than the antiperiplanar form, in the gaseous and liquid states; and now the solid substance consists entirely of the synclinal racemate, though whether the *P*- and *M*-enantiomers pack together into the same racemic crystal, or whether they separately constitute enantiomeric crystals, which could be picked out, has not yet been reported. 1,1,2-Trichloroethane is in a similar case. In Table 6-2 a plus sign means that the antiperiplanar isomer is the most stable, and a minus sign that the synclinal isomers are the more stable.

In propane, and in *iso*butane, each methyl group lies in staggered conformation with respect to the non-terminal carbon atom. The simplest alkane that can exhibit conformational isomerism is *n*-butane (Table 6-2, last line). Its synclinal and antiperiplanar forms are both present in the liquid, the latter form predominating. The solid material consists of the pure antiperiplanar isomer, in which the carbon chain is a plane zig-zag, and the whole molecule is centro-symmetric. All the higher normal alkanes, in the solid state, are in their planar zig-zag conformations, the even-carbon members of the series being centro-symmetric. In the stable conformation of *cyclo*hexane, all the ring-bonds are synclinal, having, alternately, *P* and *M* helical angles between the flanking ring-bonds. In the stable conformation of *cyclo*decane,[33] two ring-bonds are antiperiplanar, whilst the remaining eight ring-bonds form a balanced assembly of *P* and *M* synclinal bonds. In the following representations of these substances, *P* and *M* are written for *P-sc* and *M-sc*, respectively.

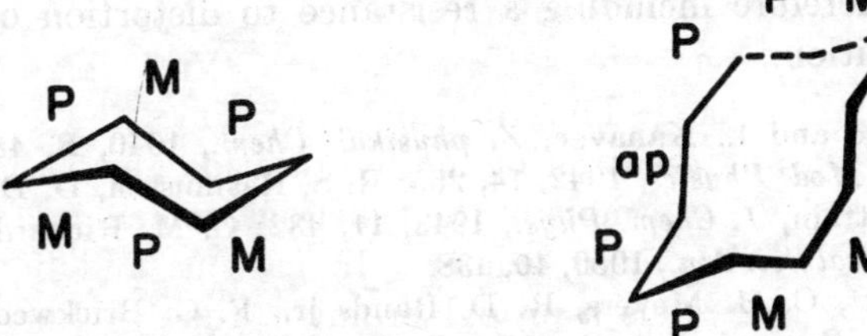

Rotational isomerism depending on internal interactions of quite a different type has been demonstrated, for example, in buta-1,3-diene, in which rotation round the central, formally single, bond is restricted.

[33] J. D. Dunitz and V. Prelog, *Angew. Chem.*, 1960, **72**, 896.

This molecule has been examined by spectral[34] and thermal[35] methods, and the conclusions agree, those given by the latter method being the more detailed. The isomers are not those which would result from repulsions between the atoms and groups attached to the two interior carbon atoms: such isomers would be out-of-plane, enantiomeric, and energetically equivalent to each other. Actually there are two isomers, both of planar type and energetically non-equivalent, that having like atoms antiperiplanar to each other being the more stable. The synperiplanar isomer lies 2.3 kcal./mole higher in energy. A barrier of 4.9 kcal./mole resists conversion of the antiperiplanar to the synperiplanar form. Other such cases have been established. Acrolein has been examined by both microwave[36] and ultrasonic[37] methods, and the conclusions agree, those of the latter method being the more detailed. For this unsaturated aldehyde, and for a number of its derivatives, the antiperiplanar isomer is the more stable; the synperiplanar isomer has about 2 kcal./mole more energy, and a barrier of at least 7 kcal./mole restricts conversion of the former isomer into the latter. The infra-red spectrum of glyoxal[38] shows that this molecule exists almost entirely in the antiperiplanar form. Presumably the synperiplanar isomer is less stable by rather more than 2 kcal./mole. The barrier height is not known. These and other such situations are summarised in Table 6-3.

It is considered that, when a formally single bond occurs between two double bonds, the factor called conjugation, about which more will be said in Section 7, plays a dominant part. In this form of interaction, the unsaturation of the double bonds spreads over the intervening bond, giving it, even though it is formally single, some part of the character of a double bond, including a strong tendency towards a planar disposition of its atoms and all the atoms directly attached to them, and therefore including a resistance to distortion out of that planar disposition.

[34] K. Bradaco and L. Kahavec, *Z. physikal. Chem.*, 1940, **B, 48,** 63; R. S. Mulliken, *Rev. Mod. Physics*, 1942, **14,** 265; R. S. Rasmussen, D. D. Tunnicliff, and R. R. Brettain, *J. Chem. Phys.*, 1943, **11,** 432; C. M. Richards and J. R. Nielsen, *J. Optical Sci. Am.*, 1950, **40,** 438.

[35] R. B. Scott, C. H. Meyers, R. D. Rands jr., F. G. Brickwedde, and N. Bekkendahl, *J. Research Nat. Bur. Standards*, 1945, **35,** 39; J. G. Aston, G. J. Szasz, W. H. Wooley, and F. G. Brickwedde, *J. Chem. Phys.*, 1946, **14,** 87.

[36] R. Wagner, J. Fine, J. W. Simmons, and J. H. Goldstein, *J. Chem. Phys.*, 1957, **26,** 634.

[37] M. S. de Groot and J. Lamb, *Proc. Roy. Soc.*, 1957, **A, 242,** 36.

[38] A. R. H. Cole and H. W. Thompson, *Proc. Roy. Soc.*, 1949, **A, 200,** 10.

TABLE 6-3.—RELATIVE STABILITIES AND HEIGHTS OF ENERGY BARRIERS PROTECTING PLANAR ROTATIONAL ISOMERS.

	Energy (kcal./mole)			
Antiperiplanar		Barrier		Synperiplanar
H(CH=CH₂)C–C(=CH₂)H	0.0	4.9	2.3	H(CH=CH₂)C–C(=CH₂)H
H(H₂C=)C–C(=O)H	0.0	7.0	2.1	H(H₂C=)C–C(=O)H
H(O=)C–C(=O)H	0.0	—	>2	H(O=)C–C(=O)H
H(O=)C–O–H	2.2	11	0.0	H(O=)C–O–H
O=N–O–H	0.0	9	0.5	O=N–O–H
O=N–O–Me	0.0	10	0.5	O=N–O–Me
O=N–O–Et	0.5	9	0.0	O=N–O–Et

This concept can be extended. As we shall see in Section 7, the unsaturation that an atom, such as oxygen or nitrogen, may possess by virtue of its unshared valency electrons, can also interact conjugatively with the unsaturation of a double bond, through an intervening formally single bond. This effect also will give to the single bond some of the character of a double bond, including a ten-

dency towards a planar arrangement of all its flanking bonds, and therefore including a resistance to torsion out of the planar arrangement.

The simplest oxy-olefinic example would be vinyl alcohol; but that is unavailable. The simplest oxy-carbonyl example is formic acid. An investigation of its infra-red spectrum has shown[39] that it consists of two isomers, which are both planar. The more stable has the hydroxyl hydrogen atom and the carbonyl oxygen atom in synperiplanar relation to each other. The antiperiplanar isomer is less stable by 2.2 kcal./mole. The barrier resisting conversion of the more stable isomer to the less stable has the somewhat high value of 11 kcal./mole. Nitrous acid and its esters form a group of examples of this type of effect, as summarised in Table 6-3. Nitrous acid itself has been investigated by a microwave method.[40] Methyl nitrite has been examined by a thermodynamic method,[41] and both methyl and ethyl nitrite have been studied by a nuclear-magnetic-resonance technique.[42] In these examples the balance of stability between the isomers is quite small, and not always in the same direction. But all the barrier heights are again of the order of 10 kcal./mole.

If two-fold symmetry is introduced at one end or the other of the formally single bond, or, for that matter, at both ends, conformational isomerism disappears, but the barrier to rotation remains. The phenyl group in phenol has two-fold symmetry, because, as we shall see in Section 7, the double-bond unsaturation of the benzene ring is spread symmetrically round the ring. A microwave investigation of phenol has shown[43] that the hydroxyl hydrogen atom lies in the plane of the phenyl ring, and that a barrier of 3.1 kcal./mole resists its rotation around the oxygen-phenyl bond. The nitro-group has two-fold symmetry, for, as we shall see also in Section 7, its double-bond unsaturation is symmetrically spread between its NO-bonds. An investigation of the infra-red spectrum of nitric acid has shown[44] that it is a planar molecule, and that a barrier of 9 kcal./mole resists rotation of the hydroxyl hydrogen atom out of the plane of the other atoms. A microwave investigation of methyl nitrate has shown[45] that this

[39] T. Miyazawa and K. S. Pitzer, *J. Chem. Phys.*, 1959, **30**, 1076.

[40] L. H. Jones, K. M. Badger, and G. E. Moore, *J. Chem. Phys.*, 1951, **19**, 599.

[41] P. Gray and M. W. Pratt, *J. Chem. Soc.*, 1958, 3403.

[42] L. H. Piette and W. A. Anderson, *J. Chem. Phys.*, 1959, **30**, 899; P. Gray and L. W. Reeves, *ibid.*, 1960, **32**, 1878.

[43] T. Kojima, *J. Phys. Soc. Japan*, 1960, **15**, 284.

[44] H. Cohn, C. K. Ingold, and H. G. Poole, *J. Chem. Soc.*, 1952, 4272.

[45] W. B. Dixon and E. B. Wilson, *J. Chem. Phys.*, 1961, **35**, 191.

TABLE 6-4.—BARRIERS RESTRICTING ROTATION ROUND FORMALLY SINGLE BONDS IN PLANAR SINGLE-ISOMER MOLECULES.

Molecule	Barrier height kcal./mole	Molecule	Barrier height kcal./mole
C_6H_5—O—H	3.1	H(O=)C—N(Me)$_2$	7
O_2N—O—H	9	Me(O=)C—N(Me)$_2$	12
O_2N—O—Me	9	O_2N—NO_2	2.9

molecule is in just the same case, as will be seen from the figures in Table 6-4.

We should achieve two-fold symmetry at the unshared-electron end of the formally single bond, if, in a molecule such as aniline or formamide, the forces of conjugation were strong enough completely to overcome the intrinsic tendency of a terligant nitrogen atom to pyramidal bonding, and so completely to flatten these molecules. We do not know whether or not the forces of conjugation do completely succeed in doing this in aniline; but it has been shown in a microwave study[46] of formamide, that the stereochemical dominance of conjugation is not complete, and that its NH-bonds are turned out of the NCO-plane by about 10°. However, a nuclear-magnetic-resonance study of dimethylformamide, and of dimethylacetamide, has shown[47] that these molecules, apart from their methyl hydrogen atoms, are flat, and that a moderate energy barrier resists rotation round the CN-bond of the amide group. The figures are in Table 6-4.

Dinitrogen tetroxide has two-fold symmetry at each end of the NN-bond. It is a planar molecule. Its small barrier to internal rotation[48] has to be considered in relation to the small dissociation energy of the bond, 13.7 kcal./mole.

These and all other attractive forces which might produce rotational isomerism of the planar type illustrated can at short distances be com-

[46] C. C. Costain and J. W. Dowling, *J. Chem. Phys.*, **1960**, *32*, 158.
[47] H. S. Gutowsky and C. H. Holn, *J. Chem. Phys.*, **1956**, *25*, 1228.
[48] H. G. Snyder and I. C. Hisatsune, *J. Mol. Spect.*, **1957**, *1*, 139.

pletely overcome by the strong repulsive forces of electron exchange, which may thereby produce a much more stable isomerism of the out-of-plane type. Probably these forces are beginning to operate, and to lead to an enhanced resistance to rotation, in simple ethane derivatives in which the collective size of the substituents rises above a certain threshold, as it appears to do in $CF_3 \cdot CCl_3$ and $CCl_3 \cdot CCl_3$ (Table 6-1). However, the best filled-in field of examples is that of the biaryl series.

In 1922, Christie and Kenner,[49] while examining what proved to be an untenable hypothesis concerning the stereochemical form of biphenyl, optically resolved 6,6′-dinitrodiphenic acid. In 1926 the correct explanation was given almost simultaneously by Turner and LeFèvre,[50] by Bell and Kenyon,[51] and by Mills,[52] and it is that, in the course of rotation round the internuclear bond, the ortho-groups of one ring so closely approach those of the other as to create a steric repulsion, which inhibits planar forms, and indeed, raises such high energy barriers between the enantiomeric out-of-plane forms that they do not undergo interconversion in ordinary conditions.[53]

NO_2 HO_2C O_2N CO_2H CO_2H HO_2C O_2N NO_2

Enantiomeric forms of 6,6′-dinitrodiphenic acid

A similar type of rotational isomerism, depending on the restriction of rotation round a CN single bond, was discovered by Mills and Elliot[54] in the example of N-benzenesulphonyl-N(8-nitro-1-naphthyl)-glycine:

$C_6H_5 \cdot SO_2—N—CH_2 \cdot CO_2H$ NO_2 $CO_2H \cdot CH_2—N—SO_2 \cdot C_6H_5$ NO_2

Enantiomeric forms of N-benzenesulphonyl-
-N(8-nitro-1-naphthyl)-glycine

[49] G. H. Christie and J. Kenner, *J. Chem. Soc.*, 1922, **121**, 614.

[50] E. E. Turner and R. J. W. LeFèvre, *Chemistry & Industry*, 1926, **45**, 831, 883.

[51] F. Bell and J. Kenyon, *Chemistry & Industry*, 1926, **45**, 864.

[52] W. H. Mills, *Chemistry & Industry*, 1926, **45**, 884, 905.

[53] R. Kuhn and O. Albrecht could observe no appreciable racemisation when a solution of 6,6′-dinitrodiphenic acid in 2*N* aqueous sodium hydroxide was heated at 160° for several hours (*Ann.*, 1927, **455**, 272).

[54] W. H. Mills and K. A. C. Elliot, *J. Chem. Soc.*, 1928, **130**, 1291.

Subsequent work on this type of isomerism has consisted largely in the detailed study of the effect of different combinations of rotation-restricting groups on optical stability. In the biphenyl series, optical isomerides have been separately obtained with three, with two, and even with one substituent, ortho- to the internuclear bond, though with fewer ortho-substituents it is the more necessary that they should be large ones.[55] The height of the rotation-restricting barrier is given approximately by the experimental activation energy of racemisation, as determined from the temperature coefficient of the rate by means of the Arrhenius equation. Successful attempts have been made by Westheimer and others to calculate barrier heights from what is known about the repulsive potentials between the rotation-restricting atoms and groups, and about the force constants of those bonds by whose stretching or bending the interatomic compressions of the planar configuration could be relieved. One of the calculated results was experimentally confirmed at a later time and by another group of workers. Some of these observed and calculated energy values are listed in Table 6-5.

There are several classes of aromatic compounds, notably nitro-compounds and amines, for which it is inferred that an internal interaction, similar to that illustrated for buta-1,3-diene, orients the atoms of the substituent in, or as nearly as possible in, the plane of the benzene ring. The evidence is that the physical and chemical properties normally associated with the nitro- or amino-substituent, become significantly changed when ortho-groups are present, which by a repulsive interaction, such as produces isomerism in biphenyl compounds, would inhibit a planar or approximately planar orientation of the substituent. Effects of this kind will be considered later; and we also leave for later discussion those more detailed effects of intramolecular interaction on stereochemical form which reveal themselves by measurements of bond length, or bond angle, or by refined spectroscopic tests for molecular symmetry (Chapters III and IV).

(6f) External Transmission of Intramolecular Interaction.—It is to be expected that, in general, interaction between any group in a molecule and some other part of the molecule, where an effect of the interaction might be observed, will be transmitted in two broadly different ways, namely, through the intervening atoms and bonds, that is, the intervening electronic system, of the molecule itself, and through the space immediately outside the molecule. Transmission

[55] The only known case of optical activity depending on one ortho-group in a biphenyl is that of M. S. Lesslie and E. E. Turner, who resolved 3′-bromobiphenyl-2-trimethylarsonium salts. They were unable to resolve the corresponding 2-trimethylammonium salts (*J. Chem. Soc.*, **1933**, 1588).

TABLE 6-5.—ARRHENIUS ACTIVATION ENERGIES OF RACEMISATION AND CALCULATED ENERGY BARRIERS RESTRICTING ROTATION AROUND SINGLE BONDS IN DIPHENYL AND ARYLAMINE DERIVATIVES.

Compound	Medium	E_A (observed) kcal./mole	ΔE (calcd.) kcal./mole	Reference
2,2'-diamino-6,6'-dimethyldiphenyl (NH_2, CH_3; CH_3, NH_2)	As gas, or in Ph_2O	45.1	—	1
6-nitrodiphenic acid (NO_2, CO_2H; CO_2H)	In $2N$-aq. Na_2CO_3	22.6	—	2
(NO_2, CO_2H; NO_2, NO_2; CO_2H)	In $2N$-aq. Na_2CO_3	22.6	—	3
(NO_2, OMe; CO_2H)	EtOH	~20	—	4
(HO_2C, I; CO_2H, I I)	Na salt in water	28.0	29–33	5
(HO_2C, I; CO_2H, I)	Na salt in water	21.6	21–23	5
(HO_2C, Br; CO_2H, Br)	—	19±0.5	18	5, 6
($CH_3\cdot CO\cdot NMe$, SO_3^-, Me)	Na salt in water	22.6	—	7

[1] G. B. Kistiakowsky and W. R. Smith, *J. Am. Chem. Soc.*, 1936, **58**, 1043.
[2] R. Kuhn and O. Albrecht, *Ann.*, 1927, **455**, 272.
[3] *Idem, ibid.*, 1927, **458**, 221.
[4] C. C. Li and R. Adams, *J. Am. Chem. Soc.*, 1935, **57**, 1565.
[5] M. Reiger and F. H. Westheimer, *ibid.*, 1950, **72**, 19. (The greater energy value for the tetra-iodo- than for the di-iodo-acid is attributed to the "buttressing effect" of the exterior iodine atoms in the former compound on the interior iodine atoms.) Cf. C. C. K. Ling and M. M. Harris, *J. Chem. Soc.*, 1964, 1825.
[6] F. H. Westheimer and J. E. Mayer, *J. Chem. Phys.*, 1946, **14**, 733; F. H. Westheimer, *ibid.*, 1947, **15**, 252. The experimental result is by M. M. Harris, *Proc. Chem. Soc.*, 1959, 367; M. M. Harris and R. K. Mitchell, *J. Chem. Soc.*, 1960, 1905.
[7] W. H. Mills and R. M. Kelham, *J. Chem. Soc.*, 1937, 274.

through the atoms and bonds, *internal transmission*, as we may call it, is dependent in a sensitive and rather complicated way on the intervening electronic structure: this dependence will be our concern in Section 7. Transmission through the space outside the molecule, *external transmission*, will operate much as for interactions between different molecules, as discussed in Section 5. The space immediately outside the molecule may be the empty space outside a gas molecule, or the solvent-filled space outside a solute molecule. And solvent molecules that are polar and can turn, or that are polarisable and so can become polar, in response to the forces that they are transmitting, will strongly influence what forces arrive at the receiving end of the transmission.

According to the model, considered in Section 5, of interactions between different molecules, three kinds of force are expected to be conveyed from an origin in a molecule to other parts of the same molecule by external transmission. The first consists in the long-range electrostatic forces emanating from poles and dipoles. Their observed effects are described as *field effects*. The second kind of force comprises the shorter-range electrokinetic forces, which depend on electron correlation between non-exchanging electron pairs. They are weak forces, and their intramolecular effects, which have only occasionally been distinguished, have been termed *electrokinetic effects*. The third kind of force consists in the strong, short-range forces of electron exchange between electron-pairs. The effects of these forces, long known in the phenomena of steric hindrance, are called *steric effects*, or sometimes, in order to make a distinction explained below, *primary steric effects*.

With the addition of the following schematic summary of this breakdown of externally transmitted intramolecular interactions, we leave their effects on physical properties and chemical reactions to be illustrated in the later Chapters:

External Transmission of {
- electrostatic forces produces *Field Effects*
- electrokinetic forces produces *Electrokinetic Effects*
- exchange forces produces *Steric Effects*.

Of course, there is often interplay between externally and internally transmitted interactions. One well-studied situation is that in which steric repulsions so change the geometrical forms of molecules that they considerably modify the internally transmitted interactions. We shall refer to this phenomenon as the *secondary steric effect*.

(7) INTERNAL TRANSMISSION OF INTRAMOLECULAR INTERACTION

When an interaction is transmitted through, and by means of, an electronic system, it alters the positions and motions of the intervening electrons. Thus theories of transmitted interactions are essentially theories of electron displacement.

(7a) Modes of Electron Displacement in the Theory of Intramolecular Interaction.—All theories of electron displacement start from the electronic theory of the atom and of valency, the basic importance of which is that, by its insistence on the stability of certain electron groups, notably the duplet and the octet, it limits the modes of electron displacement that may be assumed as mechanisms for the internal transmission of electrical effects. The electronic theory requires that electron displacements will preserve the pairing of electrons, and the octets or other stable electron groups in the atoms, as completely as is possible.

Two modes of electron displacement have been found, which preserve these electron groups. The first is characterised by the circumstance that all the displaced electron duplets remain bound in their original atomic octets. Displacements of this form were first assumed by Lewis,[56] who showed how the electrical dissymmetry, arising from the unequal sharing of electrons between unlike atoms, that is, from electropositivity or electronegativity, could be propagated along a chain of bound atoms (like or unlike) in a mode resembling electrostatic induction. This is called the *inductive mode* of electron displacement, and it is often represented by attaching to the bond signs, arrowheads indicating the direction towards which the electrons are concentrated. Thus the symbol

$$Cl \leftarrow C \leftarrow C \leftarrow C$$

indicates that the electronegativity of chlorine, and the resulting electrical dissymmetry in the carbon-chlorine bond, has caused the electrons of the carbon-carbon bonds to concentrate in the general direction of the chlorine atom. It is not to be thought, however, that the electron displacements represented by the arrow-signs are all equal: the carbon-chlorine dipole will induce a smaller dipole in the adjacent carbon-carbon bond, because the electrons there are otherwise constrained: and these dipoles will induce a still smaller dipole in the next carbon-carbon bond. Thus the effect will decrease with each successive stage of relay. Each carbon atom, losing electrons in greater proportion than it receives them, will become the seat of a small positive charge. The situation might be represented by the following expression,

[56] G. N. Lewis, "Valence and the Structure of Atoms and Molecules," p. 139.

$$\overset{\delta-}{Cl}\leftarrow\overset{\delta+}{C}\leftarrow\overset{\delta\delta+}{C}\leftarrow\overset{\delta\delta\delta+}{C}$$

where $\delta-$ and $\delta+$ denote small fractions of a unit of charge, and the added δ's indicate successive orders of smallness, resulting from the attenuation caused by relay.

Lewis regarded the inductive mode of electron displacement as describing a permanent molecular condition, such as could influence physical properties and chemical equilibria. He discussed, as an example, the difference in the acid strengths of chloroacetic acid and acetic acid, supposing that the electrons of every bond in the former molecule, relatively to those of the corresponding bond in the latter, would be displaced towards the chlorine atom; and that this effect, on reaching the ionisable proton, would cause it to be dissociated more easily from the former molecule than from the latter:

$$Cl\leftarrow CH_2\leftarrow CO\leftarrow O\leftarrow H$$

$$H—CH_2—CO—O—H$$

In so far as the inductive mode of electron displacement enters into the description of the normal states of molecules, it is called the *inductive effect.* Its quantal re-description will be set forth later. We shall also note later that the same mode of electron displacement becomes involved in activation processes, that is, in the formation of the transition states of chemical reactions.

The second mode of electron displacement that preserves duplets and octets is characterised by the substitution of one duplet for another in the same atomic octet. Displacements of this type were first assumed by Lowry,[57] who showed how the entrance into an octet of an unshared duplet possessed by a neighbouring atom could cause the ejection of another duplet, which would then either become unshared, or initiate a similar exchange further along the molecule. This displacement by substitution is especially characteristic of unsaturated molecules, and may be called the *conjugative mode* of displacement, since, as we shall see, it can be regarded as a development of the early concept of conjugation in unsaturated systems. It is usually indicated by curved arrows pointing from the duplets, or from the positions which the chemical formula assumes the duplets to occupy, towards the situations in the directions of which the displacements are considered to occur. Thus the arrows contained in the symbol

$$R_2N—C═C—C═O$$

connote duplet displacements which could convert the non-dipolar

[57] T. M. Lowry, *J. Chem. Soc.*, 1923, 123, 822, 1886; *Nature*, 1925, 114, 376.

structure towards and possibly into the dipolar structure thus:

$$R_2N{-}C{=}C{-}C{=}O \rightarrow R_2\overset{+}{N}{=}C{-}C{=}C{-}\overset{-}{O}$$

Lowry himself did not regard his mechanism of electron displacement as describing a permanent molecular condition: to him, it was a mode of chemical transformation, the mechanism of a molecular activation occurring in the course of a chemical reaction. The assumption that the conjugative mechanism enters into the description of the normal states of molecules was made by Hilda Ingold and the writer.[58] This implies that duplets in a structure such as that written above may at the same time be partly shared and partly unshared, or may belong simultaneously to two bonds. This assumption brings the discussion of physical properties and chemical equilibria into the scope of the theory. To the extent that the conjugative mode of electron displacement applies to the normal states of molecules, it is called the *mesomeric effect* (or *mesomerism*). Its quantal re-description will be set forth later.

These are the two general modes of electron displacement recognised in molecules with completed electron shells. Two others are known, which become permitted in the presence of incomplete shells. But these mechanisms are much more specialised in application, and need not be introduced here.

The inductive effect and the mesomeric effect, being time-independent effects of electron displacement, that is, factors controlling the permanent distribution of electrons in the ground states of molecules, are together summarised in the single term *polarisation effects.*

Most of the commonly measured physical properties of molecules, such as their dimensions, elastic constants, and dipole moments, though not their electronic absorption spectra, are properties only of the ground states of the molecules. In the study of such properties, therefore, the only internally transmitted polar effects of which we should need to take account are the two summarised as polarisation effects.

Chemical equilibria depend differentially on the energy and entropy of the ground states of the factors and products of the reversible reaction. In the study of chemical equilibria, therefore, the only internally transmitted polar effects of which we should need to take account are the polarisation effects.

In problems of reaction rate, on the other hand, we have to deal differentially with the initial and transition states of reaction. The

[58] **C. K. Ingold and E. H. Ingold, *J. Chem. Soc.*, 1926, 1310.**

initial state of reaction is composed of the ground states of the factors of reaction; and on their account, we must take the polarisation effects into consideration. In describing the transition state of reaction, we may, as a first formal step, consider the polarisation effects to be carried unchanged from the initial state into the transition state. But after that, we must allow for the extra polarisation that arises during activation, and hence has arisen in the transition state, in consequence of the electrical demands of the reaction centre on the surrounding polarisable structure. This extra polarisation, which, as was first pointed out by Florence Shaw and the writer,[59] can be highly important for reaction rates, is fleeting, and could not be studied like polarisation in any permanent state. It can be assessed only from the electronic requirements of the reaction and the polarisability of the structure. For that reason, the two modes of electron displacement that we have distinguished already, when operating during reaction in this time-dependent way, are collectively called *polarisability effects.*

A polarisability effect by the inductive mode of electron displacement is called an *inductomeric effect.* Its recognition came later[60] than that of the corresponding but time-independent inductive effect. A polarisability effect by the conjugative mode of electron displacement is called the *electromeric effect.* As we have seen, it was postulated by Lowry[57] before its time-independent counterpart, the mesomeric effect, was recognised. The inductomeric effect is generally less important than the electromeric effect, because the σ electrons mainly involved with the former are more strongly bound, and hence are less polarisable, than are the π electrons concerned with the latter.

The electric polarisability of a molecule, that is, the mobility of its electrons under a deforming electric field, can be studied in appropriate physical properties, notably dielectric and optical properties of the ground state. Thus the factors of polarisability, the inductomeric and electromeric effects, can to some extent be studied physically. Polarisability depends on the accessibility, to electrons of the ground state, of unoccupied, quantally allowed, excited states. Thus the factors of polarisability have a certain connexion with excited electronic states, and hence with spectral properties.

Let us now put together the pieces of this framework of the theory of the internal transmission of electronic interaction, noting, as is done in Table 7–1, its dependence on two modes of electron displacement, and the separation of effects due to each mode into time-independent

[59] C. K. Ingold and F. R. Shaw, *J. Chem. Soc.*, **1927**, 2918.

[60] C. K. Ingold, *J. Chem. Soc.*, **1933**, 1120.

TABLE 7-1.—INTERNAL TRANSMISSION OF ELECTRONIC INTERACTION. BREAKDOWN OF EFFECTS, AND THEIR APPLICATION TO PHENOMENA.

Electronic modes	Electronic effects	
	Polarisation effect	Polarisability effect
Inductive (→) (I)	Inductive (I_s)	Inductomeric (I_d)
Conjugative (⤵) (K)	Mesomeric (M)	Electromeric (E)
Applicability	Many physical properties	Optical properties
	Reaction equilibria	—
	Reaction rate	Reaction rate

and time-dependent parts. We note also the classes of observational phenomena to which the various effects apply.

This table contains some symbols—the arrow symbols introduced already, and also some letter symbols. The latter are unnecessary in simple situations, but in more or less complicated ones they are a convenience. They lend themselves to summary statements of the direction and mode of electron shifts: prefixed by plus or minus signs, they refer to electropositive or electronegative shifts. Most of the letters used have an obvious origin and are well-established, but K, for the conjugative mode of electron displacement, was introduced by Olah relatively recently.[61] The symbols I_s and I_d, where the subscripts stand for "static" and "dynamic," were introduced by Johnson, and used by Remick.[62]

(7b) Pre-electronic Background of the Theory of Intramolecular Electronic Interaction.—Our ideas about electron displacement have an extensive background in the pre-electronic theories of organic chemistry. On account of its great place in the history of chemical thought, this subject deserves a book to itself. Here, however, we can represent it only by a very bare outline.

The dualistic theory, promulgated by Berzelius in 1812, never com-

[61] G. A. Olah, "Einführung in der Theoretische Organische Chemie," Akademie-Verlag, Berlin, 1960, pp. 180–181. The old symbol T for "tautomeric" had only historical associations, and, as a change to C for "conjugative" has obvious inconveniences in organic chemistry, Olah, writing in German, went over to the German initial letter, K, as we now do. Such substitution has been made familiar in English texts through the use of k or K, as well as of C, for "constant" in mathematics.

[62] J. R. Johnson in H. Gilman's "Organic Chemistry," Wiley, New York, 1938, p. 1015; A. E. Remick, "Electronic Interpretations of Organic Chemistry," Wiley, New York, 1st Edn., 1943.

pletely lost its hold on chemistry, though it seemed to do so after 1840, when Dumas and his associates showed that it did not fit the pattern of organic chemistry. But in the 1870's we see dualism being re-introduced in a vestigial way in order to correlate the data, which were then beginning to accumulate, about the orientation of aromatic substitution. Some first substituents in the benzene molecule oriented second substituents to the meta-positions, whilst other first substituents oriented second to the ortho- and para-positions. Koerner,[63] Hübner,[64] and Noelting[65] all considered that the meta-orienting groups were those which normally conferred acidic properties on, or enhanced pre-existing acidic properties in, the molecules that contained these groups; and, since the time of Berzelius, acidic properties had been associated with the idea of electrical negativity. Ortho- and para-orienting substituents included those which normally conferred or enhanced basic properties; and such properties had been linked by Berzelius with the idea of electrical positivity (cf. Chapter VI). In the 1890's, Michael[66] was sign-labelling aliphatic atoms in ketones and esters, in order to schematize metal-uptake by these compounds, and their alkylation, and in order to represent the directions in which molecules, which can thus be sign-labelled, will add to unsaturated ketones and esters (cf. Chapters XIII and XV). Michael had the idea of electropolar quality, propagated by contact, and thus of electropolarity able to spread from an atom possessing it to adjacent parts of the molecule. Thus, by the end of the century this revived but milder form of dualism was essentially ready for re-expression, by means of the electronic theory of valency, which after 1916 became available as an embryonic form of the theory of electron displacement by the inductive mode.

Thiele's famous twelve papers, printed together in 1898,[67] constituted a major break-through in chemical theory. He demonstrated, in many examples, how two double bonds separated by a single bond act as if "yoked together"—as if "conjugated"—giving 1,4-addition, as of bromine to buta-1,3 diene (Chapter XIII). He assumed that the unsaturation of the double bonds spread over the intervening single bond, leaving relatively isolated centres of unsaturated reactivity at the ends of the "conjugated system." He interpreted the apparently reduced unsaturation of benzene on the ground that it was

[63] W. Koerner, *Gazz. chim. ital.*, 1874, **4**, 305, 446.

[64] H. Hübner, *Ber.*, 1875, **8**, 878.

[65] E. Noelting, *Ber.*, 1876, **9**, 1797.

[66] A. Michael, *J. prak. Chem.*, 1892, **46**, 204; *et seq.*; *ibid.*, 1899, **60**, 286; *et seq.*

[67] J. Thiele, *Ann.*, 1898, **306**, 87.

a conjugated system without any ends (Chapter IV). One has only to restate all this on the basis that a bond is two electrons in order to see in it a pre-electronic foundation-statement of the conjugative mode of electron displacement. Moreover, as Thiele regarded his redistributions of bonded affinity as permanently present in his conjugated unsaturated molecules, his theory belongs particularly to the foundations of the theory of the mesomeric effect.

Thiele's theory lacked generality in only one important respect: it made no allowance for the unsaturation of latent valencies, such as we would today represent by unshared valency electrons, or incomplete valency shells; and hence it made no allowance for the participation of latent valencies in conjugation. However, this deficiency was supplied in a theory by Flurscheim, first promulgated in 1902,[68] in explanation of the dependence on group-structure of orientation in aromatic substitution (Chapter VI). Flurscheim gave an important place in his theory to potential valencies, as of terligant nitrogen, allowing their binding power to spread by conjugation, just as Thiele would have done if he had recognised latent valencies as units of unsaturation, capable of conjugation with other units, such as double bonds. Flurscheim's theory was also one of permanent affinity redistribution, as he established very clearly by applying it to a problem of chemical equilibrium,[69] that of the dependence on constitution of the strengths of acids and bases (Chapter XIV). All this was most important preparation for the theory of the mesomeric effect.

As the years went by, ideas of electropolarity gradually entered this group of theories. Thiele's theory was non-electropolar. Flurscheim did employ the idea of electropolar quality, but rather by superposing Michael's concepts on his own, than by associating polarity in an essential way with conjugative valency redistributions. Coming to considerably later times, Arndt's theory, in 1924, of intermediate stages between the formally dipolar aromatic, and the non-dipolar unsaturated, structures of a pyrone, employed redistributions of partial valencies similar to those assumed in Flurscheim's theory, but went further than the latter in the definiteness with which it associated polarity changes with valency redistributions.[70] So Arndt's theory was particularly closely related to the theory of mesomerism, which was to succeed it two years later. Arndt's theory was not developed broadly; indeed, it was hardly developed at all outside the field of pyrones and thiopyrones, which it correctly treated as oxonium and

[68] B. Flurscheim, *J. prak. Chem.*, 1902, **66**, 321.

[69] B. Flurscheim, *J. Chem. Soc.*, 1909, **95**, 722; 1910, **97**, 91; *J. Soc. Chem. Ind.* (London). 1925, **44**, 246.

[70] F. Arndt, E. Scholz, and F. Nachtway, *Ber.*, 1924, **57**, 1903.

sulphonium anhydro-bases (Chapter XI). Robinson expounded the same theory in 1925 for other aromatic oxonium and ammonium anhydro-bases, using electronic terminology, but with a classification of aromatic electrons that would not now be accepted;[71] and again the application was only to anhydro-bases (Chapter XI).

Going back, once more, to the turn of the century, we find, in Lapworth's theory of polar molecular activations during reaction, a pre-electronic foundation-statement of the theory of the electromeric effect.[72] Lapworth assumed partial valencies to arise, on activation, from incipient ionisations; and the necessarily polar partial valencies thus created, he redistributed according to the pattern that had been proposed by Thiele. In a later restatement, he represented the temporarily produced partial valencies by the model of Faraday tubes of force,[73] but the theory was essentially the same. It was a distinguishing merit of Lapworth's theory that from the outset he integrated the idea of polarity with valency. That he was thus led to the incorrect theory of alternate polarities (Chapter VI) was due, not to the integration, but to its form. However, Lapworth was clear, at least from 1901 onwards, that chemical reactions are electrical transactions, necessarily involving polar selectivity (Chapters VI, XIII, and XV).

An important late phase in the development of the theory of electron displacement was the synthesis of the various polar effects into a single theoretical picture, as set out in Table 7-1. The first step in this direction was taken by Lucas and his collaborators, who, in 1924, brought together the previously only separately employed inductive and electromeric effects.[74] They showed how the former effect might be supposed to assist and give direction to the latter, as, for example, in the activation of olefins during their addition reactions:

$$CH_3—CH\overset{\frown}{=}CH$$

Here, the methyl group is assumed to exert an inductive effect, which promotes an electromeric activation of the double bond as shown, so leading to the uptake of a proton from an adding hydrogen bromide molecule at the terminal carbon atom, with the production, therefore, of *iso*propyl bromide (Chapter XIII). Similar combinations of in-

[71] J. W. Armit and R. Robinson, *J. Chem. Soc.*, 1925, **127**, 1604. Characteristically aromatic electrons were assumed to be in multiples of 6, naphthalene, for example, having 12.

[72] A. Lapworth, *J. Chem. Soc.*, 1898, **73**, 445; 1901, **79**, 1265.

[73] A. Lapworth, *Proc. Manchester Lit. Phil. Soc.*, 1920, **64**, No. 3; *J. Chem. Soc.*, 1922, 121, 416; *Nature*, 1925, **115**, 625.

[74] H. J. Lucas and A. Y. Jameson, *J. Am. Chem. Soc.*, 1924, **46**, 2475; H. J. Lucas and H. W. Moyse, *ibid.*, 1925, **47**, 1459; H. J. Lucas, T. P. Simpson, and J. M. Carter, *ibid.*, p. 1462.

ductive and electromeric effects were assumed in 1926 by Robinson and his associates,[75] particularly in explanation of orientation in aromatic substitution. In 1926 the writer with Hilda Ingold introduced the mesomeric effect,[58] and in 1927 with Florence Shaw employed combinations of the inductive, mesomeric, and electromeric effects,[59] in an interpretation, jointly, of orientation and reactivity in aromatic substitution (Chapter VI). Even though the concept of the inductomeric effect was introduced only some years later,[60] the theory of electron displacement was complete enough at that stage to be applied over all the phenomenological fields set out in Table 7-1.

In the next four Sections we shall discuss in order the four component polar effects, but here only from the standpoint of general principle, not that of phenomenological illustration; for it is to the latter aspect that most of the rest of this book is devoted.

(7c) Inductive Effects of Bound Atoms and Groups.—Electron repulsions and attractions within molecules are most usefully treated on a relative basis; and, by convention, the standard of reference is hydrogen. A group may be said to be electropositive, or to repel electrons, if it does so more than hydrogen would in the same molecular situation. Thus a group X is described as electropositive, or electron-repelling, in a compound X—CR_3, if the electron content in the residue CR_3 is greater than in the compound H—CR_3. It is not a serious difficulty that there is no physically indicated point along the bond X—C or H—C at which X or H ends and C begins: it is known that the single-bond radius of the carbon atom is a nearly constant quantity (0.77 *A*), which it would be fair to accept as providing a conventional atomic boundary for the purposes of comparison. Again, a group Y may be described as electronegative, or electron-attracting, in Y—CR_3, if here the electron content of CR_3 is less than in H—CR_3. Using the already defined symbols, these ideas can be represented as follows:

$X \rightarrow CR_3$	H—CR_3	$Y \leftarrow CR_3$
$+I$ effect	Standard	$-I$ effect

It has been mentioned several times that group polarisations are not accurately constant and characteristic, but are affected by interaction polarisation arising from the molecular environment. It is convenient to set up the problem of classifying groups by their polarisation in a form in which this disturbance is minimised; and we shall do so, if we

[75] J. Allan, A. E. Oxford, R. Robinson, and J. C. Smith, *J. Chem. Soc.*, 1926, 401.

suppose that the groups considered are singly present as substituents in derivatives of alkanes.

A major electrostatic distinction must be drawn between formally charged and formally neutral groups. Anionic substituents, for example,

$$\leftarrow\bar{O} \qquad \leftarrow\bar{S}$$

are expected, as a whole, to repel electrons strongly in comparison with neutral groups, considered as a whole. Cationic groups, as a class, for example,

$$\rightarrow\overset{+}{N}R_3 \qquad \rightarrow\overset{+}{S}R_2$$

should strongly attract electrons relatively to neutral groups, as a class. Groups with formal dipolar bonds, for example

$$\rightarrow\overset{+-}{NO_2} \qquad \rightarrow\underset{+-}{\overset{+-}{SO_2}}R \qquad \rightarrow\overset{+-}{SO}R$$

are always bound through their cationic centres to the remainder of the molecule to which they belong, and therefore they should attract electrons relatively to neutral groups. These, of course, are broad relationships, taking no account of individual variations, which may lead to some overlapping between the various series.

Individual variations depending on chemical type become apparent on considering a series of different groups in the same state of formal charge. This may be illustrated by reference to neutral groups, although the arguments would be equally applicable to anionic, cationic, or dipolar groups with identical formal charges. Along the isoelectronic series,

$$\rightarrow CH_3, \qquad \rightarrow NH_2, \qquad \rightarrow OH, \qquad \rightarrow F$$

the total nuclear charge becomes progressively centralised; and thus, as was noted in Section **2e**, the groups attract electrons progressively more strongly. This relationship may be expected to repeat itself among similar groups whose central atoms belong to the other periods which, in Mendeléjeff's periodic table, end in a halogen.

The electrical dissymmetry of the bound fluorine atom is expected to be reduced in similarly bound chlorine by a compensating polarisation of the core electrons of the latter. The compensation should increase with the size of the core in the heavier halogens; and thus we should expect the electron attraction of halogens to increase with diminishing atomic number, that is, to increase along the series

$$\rightarrow I, \qquad \rightarrow Br, \qquad \rightarrow Cl, \qquad \rightarrow F$$

A similar relationship should appear among groups with central atoms belonging to the oxygen and nitrogen families in the periodic classification.

Thus, a regular connection between the inductive effect of an atom and its position in the periodic table of the elements is indicated. If R is a non-polar or feebly polar group (such as hydrogen or alkyl), then all groups, such as $—NR_2$, —OR, —SR, —Hal, =NR, =O, ≡N, should attract electrons relatively to the methyl group. The extent of the attraction should increase with the number of the periodic group, and decrease with increasing period number. On account of the greater opportunities for electron displacement which are furnished by the additional electrons in multiple bonds, the electron attraction of a multiply bound atom should be greater than that of the corresponding singly bound atom.

Deuterium is slightly electropositive relative to light hydrogen. This was discovered experimentally by Halevi in 1956, by examination of effects of deuterium substitution on acid strengths; and it has been confirmed by others in a variety of such studies since (Chapter XIV), as well as in observed dipole moments (Chapter III). The CD bond has a slightly smaller average length than the CH bond,[76] and the contraction may press the bond electrons towards the electrons in the rest of the molecule, so creating an effect of electropositivity.

It is a consequence of the premises stated that the inductive effect of all alkyl groups is zero. This follows for the methyl group from the symmetry and non-polar character of ethane and methane, and for other alkyl groups from a succession of such comparisons. However, the inference depends on the circumstance that the alkane molecular framework has been selected for the purpose of standardising and minimising the effects of interaction polarisation. The real conclusion concerning alkyl groups is that, unlike the groups already considered, the intrinsic polarity of which renders their classification qualitatively insensitive to the disturbance of interaction polarisation, alkyl groups will exert essentially those polar effects which are impressed on them by the other polar groups present in the molecule: that is, the

[76] This is a consequence of the normal (Morse-curve) anharmonicity of binding, which makes bond-stretching increasingly easier than bond-contraction, and hence makes time-average bond lengths increasingly greater, as the amplitude of vibration becomes increased. On passing from C—H to C—D, the zero-point amplitude becomes decreased, because of the increased mass moving in the same force-field; and hence, over a time average, the bond is shortened. For a discussion of these and related matters, see E. Halevi, *Prog. Phys. Chem.*, 1963, 1, 109.

inductive polarisation of alkyl groups is mainly interaction polarisation. In this connexion, the important property of alkyl groups is that they are more polarisable than hydrogen; and thus $-CH_3$ becomes weakly electron-repelling when the comparison is between $CH_3{\rightarrow}CO_2H$ and $H{-}CO_2H$, or between $CH_3{\rightarrow}CH_2Cl$ and $H{-}CH_2Cl$. Since the majority of commonly encountered substituents are attractors of electrons, alkyl groups usually function as weakly electron-repelling groups.

As a substratum to these somewhat weak polar effects of methyl, and hence of all alkyl, groups in substituted alkanes, methyl groups are not strictly neutral, but are very weakly electronegative, in alkanes themselves. The writer deduced this some time ago from the fact that alkane absorption spectra are not independent of homology. This shows that the electrons are not completely located in the bonds, but can in some degree move from bond to bond, with the consequence that molecular orbitals can be constructed which, by taking this migratory movement into account, become energetically non-equivalent to the composing bond orbitals. This granted, it follows that, increasingly with homology, the electrons will concentrate towards the ends of an alkane chain, so that a methyl group, replacing hydrogen, withdraws electrons slightly from the rest of the alkane molecule. One suspects, by analogy with hyperconjugation (Section 7i), that most of this mobility resides in the CH bond electrons. Today, we have some relatively direct evidence that this expected polarity is real: some of this evidence will be summarised in Chapter III (Section 8d).

The unsaturated hydrocarbon radicals, such as vinyl, phenyl, and ethynyl, have next to be considered. It has been observed experimentally in several ways, as we shall have occasion later to notice, that alkyl groups behave as if they repel electrons when bound to such unsaturated systems:

$$CH_3{\rightarrow}CH{=}CH_2 \qquad CH_3{\rightarrow}C_6H_5 \qquad CH_3{\rightarrow}C{\equiv}CH$$

A completely equivalent statement is that the radicals vinyl, phenyl, and ethynyl act as attractors of electrons when present as substituents in an alkane. The electron attraction by vinyl and phenyl groups seems to be of the same order of intensity, while that of the ethynyl groups is considerably stronger. Moreover the ethynyl group definitely attracts electrons from the phenyl group, and it probably does so from the vinyl group:

$$HC{\equiv}C{\leftarrow}CH{=}CH_2 \qquad HC{\equiv}C{\leftarrow}C_6H_5$$

Walsh's explanation of such relationships is as described in Section **4b**: vinyl and phenyl carbon atoms form their single bonds using plane-trigonal, or some approximation to plane-trigonal orbitals, while the ethynyl carbon atom forms its single bond with a linear orbital: the former hybrid orbitals have somewhat larger proportions, and the linear orbital a considerably larger proportion of *s* component, than has the ordinary tetrahedral orbital of carbon: and these increased proportions of *s* component, by tending to concentrate the electrons more towards the carbon nucleus, confer increased electronegativity on the carbon atom.

It is possible that this effect enhances the electro-negativity of other groups containing doubly and triply bound carbon, for example, the carbonyl and cyano-groups.

The conclusions so far set forth in this Section are summarised in Table 7-2.

In making this qualitative and relative assessment of the inductive effects of groups, we have treated the driving forces of inductive electron displacement as electrostatic in a more or less classical sense. But, of course, electrostatics must act under the quantum restrictions of stationary states. Suppose that we combine neutral CH_3 with neutral F by pure colligation, to form, at first, strictly homopolar CH_3—F; and suppose that then we "let the electrons go." The homopolar molecule is not in a stationary state, and the electrons, when released, will indeed "go," building up a dipole, yet continuing to move against the electrostatic field that their displacement will be creating, until the stationary state is reached. This step in the formation of the normal molecule, $CH_3 \rightarrow F$, with its dipole, will, as a natural process, be associated with a decrease of energy. Starting again, let us now suppose that we combine CH_3^+ with F^- by pure co-ordination, to form, at first, the electrovalent or ion-pair molecule $CH_3^+F^-$; and that then we "let the electrons go." Again they will "go," and we shall obtain the normal polar but essentially covalent molecule $CH_3 \rightarrow F$ with a larger reduction of energy.

All this can be re-described in terms of quantal resonance. To say so is a platitude, because quantal resonance is involved in all chemical binding, from that in the hydrogen molecule-ion upward; and just what resonance is involved in a given case is not determined by any natural circumstance of the case, but is a pure artifact of the approximation from which we choose to start the description of the binding.

If we conceptually first build homopolar methyl fluoride, or first build ion-pair methyl fluoride, then quantal resonance between these

TABLE 7-2.—INDUCTIVE EFFECTS OF GROUPS.

Electron Repulsion $(+I)$						
$-D$	>	$-H$				
$-\bar{N}R$	>	$-\bar{O}$				
$-\bar{S}e$	>	$-\bar{S}$	>	$-\bar{O}$		
$-C(CH_3)_3$	>	$-CH(CH_3)_2$	>	$-CH_2(CH_3)$	>	$-CH_3$
Electron Attraction $(-I)$						
$-\overset{+}{O}R_2$	>	$-\overset{+}{N}R_3$				
$-\overset{+}{N}R_3$	>	$-\overset{+}{P}R_3$	>	$-\overset{+}{As}R_3$	>	$-\overset{+}{Sb}R_3$
$-\overset{+}{O}R_2$	>	$-\overset{+}{S}R_2$	>	$-\overset{+}{Se}R_2$	>	$-\overset{+}{Te}R_2$
$-\overset{+}{O}R_2$	>	$-OR$				
$=\overset{+}{N}R_2$	>	$-\overset{+}{N}R_3$	>	$-\overset{+-}{NO_2}$	>	$-NR_2$
$-\overset{+-}{\overset{+-}{S}}O_2R$	>	$-\overset{-}{\overset{+-}{\overset{+}{S}}}O_3$	>	$-\overset{+-}{S}OR$	>	$-SR$
$-\overset{+}{S}R_2$	>	$-\overset{+-}{S}OR$				
$-F$	>	$-OR$	>	$-NR_2$	[>	$-CR_3$]
$-F$	>	$-Cl$	>	$-Br$	>	$-I$
$-OR$	>	$-SR$	>	$-SeR$		
$-SiR_3$	>	$-GeR_3$				
$=O$	>	$=NR$	[>	$=CR_2$]		
$=O$	>	$-OR$				
$\equiv N$	>	$=NR$	>	$-NR_2$		
$-C\equiv CR$	>	$-CR=CR_2$	[>	$-CR_2\cdot CR_3$]		
$-CH_3$	>	$-H$				

structures will be necessary to pass from either to the normal molecule. Pauling has illustrated the energy effect, associated with the resonance step in such an approach to the description of a polar covalency, by means of the formation heats of diatomic molecules.[77] He shows, for example, that the formation heats of the hydrogen halides are all greater than the arithmetic means, or, what is theoretically more relevant, the geometric means, of the formation heats of hydrogen and of the appropriate halogens.

[77] L. Pauling, "Nature of the Chemical Bond," 3rd Edn., 1960, Chap. III, p. 64.

For simplicity, let us consider the formation of the bond dipole in methyl fluoride as a two-electron problem, neglecting the effect of the electron shift on the other electrons. Suppose that the two electrons of concern are first put into the bond orbital of the homopolar structure A. Then their two-electron wave function Ψ_A (which, when squared, gives the probability distribution of the two electrons over all pairs of positions in space) will be rendered non-stationary by the existence of an unshared-electron orbital on fluorine in the ionic structure B, into which the bond-electrons of A could "leak" to form the ionic structure B:

$$\text{(A)} \qquad CH_3\text{—}F \qquad\qquad \overset{+}{C}H_3 \quad \overset{-}{F} \qquad \text{(B)}$$

Thus, electrons, originally placed in the bond orbital of A, and having the wave function Ψ_A, can be spontaneously captured by the fluorine-atomic orbital of B, when they would have the wave-function Ψ_B; and so, as the capture can be reversed, neither Ψ_A nor Ψ_B is a stationary state. The stationary state must include the motions between Ψ_A and Ψ_B; and, in first approximation, they can be represented by normalised mixtures of Ψ_A and Ψ_B, the ground stationary state being of the form $a\Psi_A+b\Psi_B$, where a is the larger of the two positive mixing coefficients a and b. From the non-stationary non-polar structure Ψ_A to the stationary polar state $a\Psi_A+b\Psi_B$, there will be a decrease of energy, the resonance energy of the bond polarity. It is to be associated with the greater latitude of electron motion allowed in the mixed wave-function, and with the consequential reduction, prescribed by the uncertainty principle, in the electronic zero-point energy of the electropolar ground state.

Thus the energy of the inductive effect, as of every factor in chemical combination, is resonance energy. In the example of the acidity of chloroacetic acid, by which G. N. Lewis originally illustrated the inductive effect, we start from one non-polar and a series of polar structures, as follows:

$$Cl\text{—}CH_2\text{—}CO\text{—}O\text{—}H \qquad\qquad \overset{-}{Cl} \;\; \overset{+}{C}H_2\text{—}CO\text{—}O\text{—}H$$

$$Cl\text{—}\overset{-}{C}H_2 \;\; \overset{+}{C}O\text{—}O\text{—}H \qquad\qquad Cl\text{—}CH_2\text{—}\overset{-}{CO} \;\; \overset{+}{O}\text{—}H$$

$$Cl\text{—}CH_2\text{—}CO\text{—}\overset{-}{O} \;\; \overset{+}{H}$$

The wave-function of the normal, inductively polarised state will be a mixture of the wave-functions of all these structures. The energy of the normal state will lie lower than the energies of any of the structures, even the non-polar one.

(7d) Inductomeric Effects of Bound Atoms and Groups.—Polarisability effects result from the action of those electric forces which arise at the reaction centre in the transition state of a reaction on the polarisable residues in the molecular system. The sign of a polarisability effect will depend on the electronic requirements of the reaction; and always it will be such as to facilitate reaction. The magnitude of a polarisability effect will depend jointly on the strength of the electronic requirements of the reaction, and on the polarisability of the systems which the reaction centre deforms.

By inductomeric polarisability is understood the polarisability which atoms and groups in saturated combination exhibit along the lines of their bonds. Such polarisability must depend generally on the strength of binding of the valency electrons: the more strongly they are bound, the less they are polarisable. For isoelectronic atoms with completed valency shells, inductomeric polarisability thus depends on electronegativity: the more electronegative an atom, the less will it be polarisable. First, then, we must expect the inductomeric polarisability of an atom to be strongly decreased by a positive ionic charge, and, of course, strongly increased by a negative charge:

$$-\bar{O} > -OR > -\overset{+}{O}R_2$$

Secondly, we should expect the inductomeric polarisability of isoelectronic atoms having the same formal charge to decrease towards the right-hand side of a Mendeléjeff period:

$$-CR_3 > -NR_2 > -OR > -F$$

Then, we know from optical data (Chapter III) that atomic valency shells having a higher principal quantum number are more polarisable than similar shells with a lower quantum number: it appears that, in atoms of higher atomic number, the effect on polarisability of the greater distance of the valency electrons from the nucleus outweighs that of the greater imperfections of screening by the core electrons. Since optical data show also that bonds are more polarisable along their length than transversely (Chapter III), we may expect inductomeric polarisability to follow the trend of overall polarisability in similar valency shells. Thus, on empirical grounds, we have to expect that inductomeric polarisability will diminish with decreasing atomic number in the same Mendeléjeff group:

$$-I > -Br > -Cl > -F$$

Finally, additional inductomeric polarisability will be furnished by additional electrons of multiple bonds, apart from any electromeric polarisability that may arise through the participation of the multiple bonds in conjugative electron displacements.

The hydrogen atom is, naturally, less polarisable than any neutral group containing hydrogen. As Halevi has pointed out, deuterium is slightly less polarisable than protium.[76] This follows from measurements of optical refraction, and should be expected theoretically, because the CD bond is slightly shorter than the CH bond, so that the nuclei come slightly closer to their bond electrons.[76]

The conclusions of this Section are summarised in Table 7-3.

TABLE 7-3.—THE ± INDUCTOMERIC POLARISABILITIES OF GROUPS.

—H	>	—D						
$—\bar{O}$	>	—OR	>	$—\overset{+}{O}R_2$; etc.				
$—CR_3$	>	$—NR_2$	>	—OR	>	—F; etc.		
—I	>	—Br	>	—Cl	>	—F; etc.		
≡N	>	=NR	>	$—NR_2$; etc.				
$—CR_3$	>	$—CHR_2$	>	$—CH_2R$	>	$—CH_3$	>	H

For very small electron displacements, inductomeric polarisability must be the same in both directions. But for large displacements, this symmetry is expected to break down, the electrons being shifted more easily one way than the other. As to where the dissymmetry enters, and how important it becomes, we have at present no reliable information.

Even for small displacement, polarisability does not work classically. An electric field does not displace electrons necessarily in the direction of the field. A molecule is subject to quantum restrictions, and an electric field, acting on its ground state, can only change the positions and motions of the electrons in that state by mixing-in a certain fraction, proportional for small fields to the field intensity, of the positions and motions of the electrons as they would be in one or more of the quantally allowed excited states. Thus, the polarisability of a ground state depends on the manifold of excited states, and depends especially on the more easily accessible excited states. Inductomeric polarisability will depend, in particular, on polar excited states, to which polar structures, such as those written above for methyl fluoride and for chloroacetic acid, may often be treated as first approximations. The greater the accessibility of these polar states, or of some of them, that is, the lower they lie in energy, and the more their orbitals overlap spatially with the orbitals of the ground state, so as to facilitate electron capture, the greater the inductomeric polarisability of the ground state will be.

(7e) Mesomeric Effects in Unsaturated Systems.—Suppose that we have an imaginary molecule containing a formally non-polar, conjugated unsaturated system, such as

$$R_2N{-}C{=}C{-}C{=}O$$

in which there is as yet no mesomeric effect: the distribution of electron pairs among the atoms is assumed to be exactly as the theory of valency would represent it. Now suppose that conjugative electron displacements are allowed to proceed freely, until the real molecule is produced, that is, until the internal energy of the system is minimised:

$$(\delta+) \quad R_2\overset{\curvearrowright}{N{-}}C{=}\overset{\curvearrowright}{C{-}}C{=}\overset{\curvearrowright}{O} \quad (\delta-)$$

According to the theory of the mesomeric effect, the distribution of electron-pairs in the mesomeric molecule will be intermediate between that which the theory of valency would require for the original non-dipolar structure, and for the alternative dipolar structure,

$$R_2\overset{+}{N}{=}C{-}C{=}C{-}\overset{-}{O}$$

The conjugative electron displacements, which we allowed to occur in the original non-polar structure, must therefore have built up charges at the ends of the mesomeric system (as is indicated by the signs $\delta+$ and $\delta-$). Moreover, during the conversion of the non-polar structure into the mesomeric state, the electrons must have been moving against the electrostatic forces which they were progressively creating: when they could do this no longer, the mesomeric state was fully formed.

For the purpose of discussing the extent of mesomeric displacements in different systems, the simplest point of view from which to start is to regard the extent of displacement as determined by an equilibrium between certain non-electrostatic displacement-promoting forces, the nature of which we have still to consider, and the electrostatic resisting forces. At the outset, we take the displacement-promoting forces for granted; and, carefully choosing systems for comparison which will make them as closely similar as may be, we consider the relative intensities with which electrostatic resistance to displacement may be expected to develop in different cases. Later, we shall consider the displacement-promoting forces, and how they would be expected to vary from one system to another.

It will have been noted that, in the system represented above, one of the terminal atoms increases its covalency, becoming positively charged, while the other decreases its covalency, becoming negatively charged. Evidently, in dealing with the electrostatic resistance to mesomeric displacement, it is necessary to consider the factors which confer on a bound atom, with a complete valency shell of electrons, a tendency to increase or decrease its covalency.

Increases of covalency depend on the possession of unshared electron pairs, and on their power of interaction with an adjacent atomic nucleus. The affinity of the unshared electrons for the nucleus of another atom in turn depends on the strength of their binding, that is, on the electronegativity of the atom to which they belong. Accordingly, a major distinction must be expected between charged and formally neutral groups: negatively charged groups, as a whole, will tend to increase their covalency, becoming more nearly neutral, to a greater extent than will neutral groups, which on increasing their covalency become positively charged; and neutral groups, as a class, will tend to increase their covalency more than will positively charged groups:

$$—\bar{O} > —OR > —\overset{+}{O}R_2$$

For groups in any one state of formal charge, for instance, neutral groups, one must expect a connexion between tendency to increase covalency and the position of the central atom in the periodic table of the elements. As was noted in Section **2e**, the affinity of unshared electrons for the nucleus of another atom decreases with increasing electronegativity along an isoelectronic series. Therefore, tendency to increase covalency must diminish along a Mendeléjeff period:

$$—NR_2 > —OR > —F$$

When comparing elements in the same Mendeléjeff group, another factor has to be taken into account, namely, the stereochemical consequences of any difference of principal quantum number between the valency shells of the atoms concerned and of carbon. The increase of covalency involved in the mesomeric effect is partial double-bond formation, and, because of the overlap principle, double bonds are the more easily formed when the atoms concerned, in particular, the p orbitals of their valency shells, are of about the same size. Therefore one can understand that, as is established by the evidence of dipole moments (Chapter III) and chemical equilibria (Chapters XIII and

XIV), the halogens stand in the following order with respect to their capacity to increase covalency in the mesomeric effect,

$$—F > —Cl > —Br > —I$$

while elements of the oxygen family yield the analogous order,

$$—OR > —SR > —SeR$$

When any of these groups, X, is attached to an unsaturated residue, for example, vinyl or phenyl, the conjugative mode of electron displacement will always operate in such a way as to decrease the electron content of X, and increase that of the unsaturated residue. With respect to this electron displacement, the group X is acting electropositively, and so we label the resulting mesomeric effect $+M$:

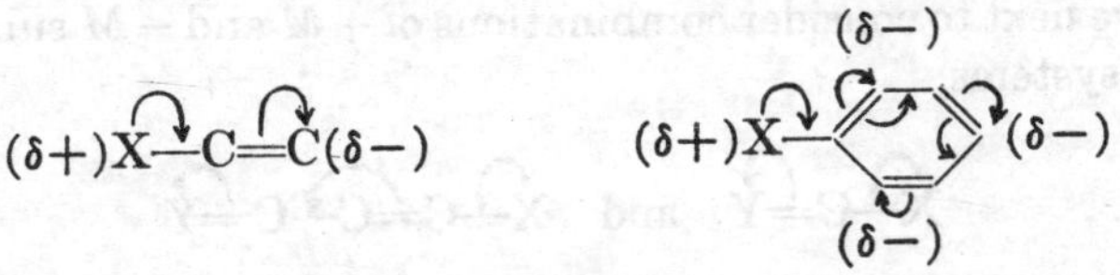

$$(\delta+)X—C=C(\delta-) \qquad (\delta+)X—C_6H_5\ (\delta-)\ (\delta-)\ (\delta-)$$

$+M$ effect

If those groups which exert a $+M$ effect are severally bound to *the same* unsaturated system, then the relative intensities of the mesomeric effects should correspond to the relative tendencies of the substituents to increase their covalency.

The decreases of covalency with which we are concerned in this discussion involve loss of multiplicity in a multiple bond. By means of electrostatic and stereochemical arguments quite similar to those already used, it may be deduced that a positive ionic charge, a high group number in the Mendeléjeff table, and a high period number in the table, will be the main factors that should enhance the tendency of a multiply bound atom towards a reduction of its covalency. Thus we may expect the inequality

$$=\overset{+}{N}R_2 > =NR$$

on account of the difference of charge,

$$=O > =NR$$

because of the difference of group number in the periodic table, and

$$=S > =O$$

owing to the difference in the Mendeléjeff period number.

When any of these substituents, Y, terminates an unsaturated system, the group Y will act electronegatively, withdrawing electrons from the system: we label the resulting mesomeric effect $-M$:

$$(\delta-)\overset{\frown}{Y}=C-C=C(\delta+) \qquad (\delta-)\overset{\frown}{Y}=C-C_6H_5\ (\delta+)\ (\delta+)\ (\delta+)$$

$-M$ effect

If the groups Y are severally associated with *the same* unsaturated system, then the mesomeric polarisations should correspond to the relative tendencies of the substituents to reduce their covalency.

The above conclusions are summarised in Table 7-4.

We have next to consider combinations of $+M$ and $-M$ substituents, as in the systems,

$$X-C=Y \quad \text{and} \quad X-C=C-C=Y$$

The carboxyl group, and its various derived forms, furnish an interesting series of examples of the simpler system. Let us consider how the electronic structure of these forms should vary when X and Y are varied independently. By keeping Y the same, and allowing X to become any of a succession of groups having progressively reduced

TABLE 7-4.—MESOMERIC EFFECTS OF GROUPS.

Electron Repulsion Dependent on Covalency Increase ($+M$)

$-\bar{O} > -OR > -\overset{+}{O}R_2$

$-\bar{S} > -SR > -\overset{+}{S}R_2$

$-I > -\overset{+}{I}R$

$-NR_2 > -OR > -F$

$-OR > -SR > -SeR$

$-F > -Cl > -Br > -I$

Electron Attraction Dependent on Covalency Decrease ($-M$)

$=\overset{+}{N}R_2 > =NR$

$=O > =NR > =CR_2$

$=S > =O$

$\equiv N > \equiv CR$

$+M$ effects, a series may be constructed along which the internal mesomeric electron displacement should diminish. Such a series is the following:

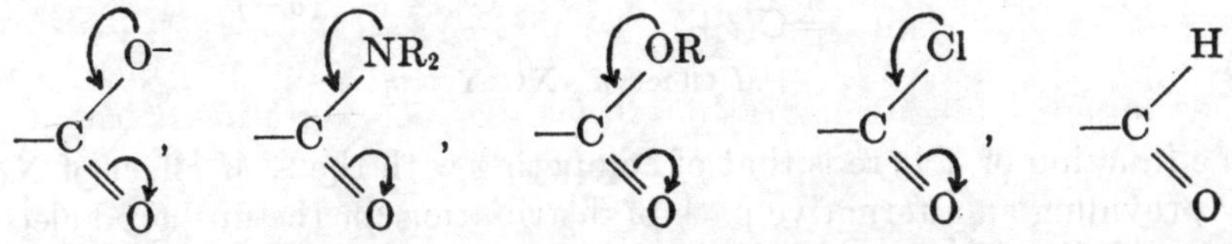

$$\text{—C(O}^-\text{)=O},\quad \text{—C(NR}_2\text{)=O},\quad \text{—C(OR)=O},\quad \text{—C(Cl)=O},\quad \text{—C(H)=O}$$

At the head stands the carboxylate ion group, the symmetry of which shows that the mesomeric displacement here has its maximum value, equivalent to the transfer of 0.5 electron from one oxygen atom to the other. At the other end is the aldehyde group, in which the internal mesomeric charge-transfer is zero. Now when any of these groups is bound through its carbon atom to an unsaturated residue, such as vinyl or phenyl, the group as a whole must act electronegatively, that is, must withdraw electrons, for the structural reason that the group Y (the doubly-bound oxygen atom) is conjugated with the unsaturated residue, whereas the group X is not thus conjugated, being separated from the unsaturated residue by two single bonds:

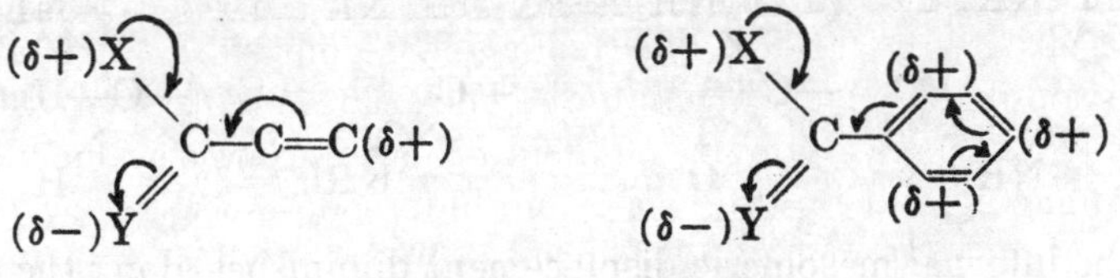

$$(\delta+)\text{X}\!-\!\text{C}(=\text{Y}(\delta-))\!-\!\text{C}\!=\!\text{C}(\delta+)\qquad (\delta+)\text{X}\!-\!\text{C}(=\text{Y}(\delta-))\!-\!\text{C}_6\text{H}_5\ (\delta+)(\delta+)(\delta+)$$

$-M$ effect of $\cdot$CX:Y

What X does is to compete with this $-M$ effect of the whole group by providing an alternative source of electrons for absorption by the doubly-bound oxygen atom. Thus the relative $-M$ effects of the complete groups will be given by inverting the series representing the relative mesomeric displacements within the groups:

$$\text{—CHO} > \text{—CO·Cl} > \text{—CO}_2\text{R} > \text{—CO·NR}_2 > \text{—CO}_2^-$$

$-M$ effects

It is worth noticing that when these groups are bound to the unsaturated residue, not through the carbon atom, but through X, then the groups exert $+M$ effects, that is, they act electropositively. For now it is X which is conjugated with the unsaturated residue and Y which is not:

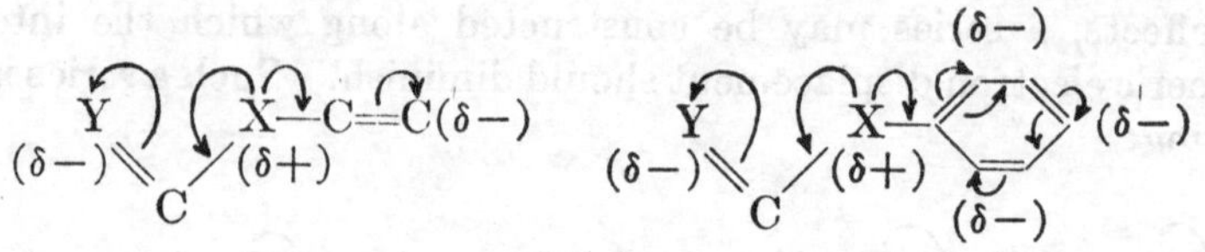

$+M$ effect of $\cdot XC:Y$

The function of Y here is that of competing with the $+M$ effect of X, by providing an alternative path of distribution for the unshared electrons of X. Thus acylation always diminishes the $+M$ effects of amino- and hydroxyl groups. But as between amides and esters, the order of the intensities of the effects will be the opposite of that already given:

$$RCO\cdot NR\text{—} > RCO\cdot O\text{—}$$

$+M$ effects

Series of another type may be constructed by keeping X the same and allowing Y to become any of a succession of groups having progressively reduced $-M$ effects, as in the following illustration:

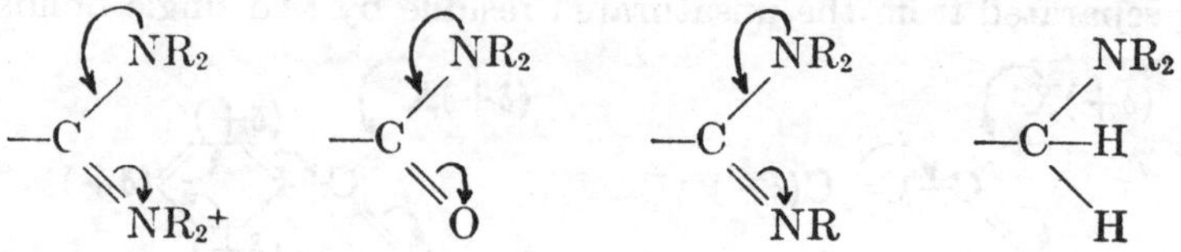

Here the internal mesomeric displacement diminishes along the series: in the first example, it is maximal, amounting to the transport of 0.5 electron from one nitrogen atom to the other: in the last example it is zero. If these groups are bound through their carbon atoms to an unsaturated residue, then, for a reason already given, the complete groups will exert $-M$ effects. This they will do with an intensity which diminishes with the $-M$ effect of Y, because X, which gives rise to the competing effect, is constant throughout the series:

$$\text{—}C(:\overset{+}{N}R_2)\cdot NR_2 > \text{—}CO\cdot NR_2 > \text{—}C(:NR)\cdot NR_2$$

$-M$ effects

If the groups are bound to the unsaturated residue, not through carbon, but through the atom X, which in these examples is the singly-bound nitrogen atom, then, for a reason given above, the complete groups will exert $+M$ effects. These effects will be reduced by competition with the mesomeric effects within the groups; but such competition becomes progressively weaker with the successive changes in Y along the series. Therefore the intensities of the $+M$ effects of the complete groups will stand in the following order:

$$RCH_2 \cdot NR— > RC(:NR) \cdot NR— > RCO \cdot NR— > R(:\overset{+}{N}R_2) \cdot NR—$$

$+M$ effects

The mesomeric effects in the simple systems X·C:Y should be found again in the more extended systems X·C:C·C:Y. Thus the properties of the carboxyl group ought to reappear in the β-keto-enol group:

$$H—O—C{=}O \qquad H—O—C{=}C—C{=}O$$

One's general impression of β-keto-enols, such as acetylacetone (which is mainly enolic under ordinary conditions), is that they are not strikingly like carboxylic acids: in particular their aqueous acid strengths are much smaller than are those of carboxylic acids. However, it has to be observed that the formation of an internal hydrogen bond (Section **2f**) is stereochemically feasible in β-keto-enols. It is certain that such bonds are formed in the simpler aliphatic β-keto-enols, which are much too volatile to be ordinary hydroxy-compounds, and are even more volatile than the isomeric β-diketones. Such hydrogen bonding will necessarily interfere with the normal functions of the terminal groups of the mesomeric system:

$$CH_3—C{=}CH—C—CH_3 \quad (\text{O—H}\cdots\text{O}) \qquad (pK_a \sim 8)$$

But when this kind of hydrogen bonding is impeded, or wholly prevented, for example, by including the β-keto-enolic system in a carbon ring, as in dimethyldihydroresorcinal, or "crystalline dimeric methylketen" (which are also mono-enols, having the formulae given below), then the properties become much more like those of a carboxylic acid. Dimethyldihydroresorcinol was originally mistaken for a carboxylic acid. Its aqueous acid strength[78] is not very much smaller than that of acetic acid, while that of the dimeric methylketen is larger than that of acetic acid, and that of the dibasic acid *cyclo*-butenedioldione (so-called "squaric acid," obtained, *e.g.*, by hydrolysis of the dimer of $CF_2:CCl_2$) is larger in both steps of ionisation.[79] The figures are below (acetic acid has pK_a 4.20):

[78] V. von Schilling, *Ann.*, 1900, **308**, 193. Some degree of internal hydrogen bonding may be permitted in dimethyldihydroresorcinol by the flexibility of the six-membered carbon ring.

[79] R. B. Woodward and G. Small, *J. Am. Chem. Soc.*, 1950, **72**, 1297; G. Monks and P. Hegenberg, *Angew. Chem. Internat. Edit.*, 1966, **5**, 888.

$$\text{(p}K_a\ 5.15)\quad (CH_3)_2C\begin{matrix} CH_2-C(=O)- \\ CH_2-C(OH)= \end{matrix}CH$$

$$CH_3-CH\begin{matrix} C(=O) \\ C(OH) \end{matrix}C-CH_3 \quad (\text{p}K_a\ 2.8) \qquad \begin{matrix} O=C-C\cdot OH \\ O=C-C\cdot OH \end{matrix} \quad \begin{matrix} (\text{p}K_{a1}\ \sim 1) \\ (\text{p}K_{a2}\ \ 2.2) \end{matrix}$$

Tropolone illustrates a still more expanded carboxyl-type system' X·C:C·C:C·C:C·C:Y, though only in a form permitting hydrogen bonding, as is clear from the pK_a value:[80]

$$\text{Tropolone (CH=CH, CH, CH—CH ring; C=O}\cdots\text{H—O—C)} \quad (\text{p}K_a\ 6.7)$$

That chemical functions are normally not much altered when an additional unit ·C=C· is included in a conjugated system was first recognised and illustrated by Angeli, and was stated as a general principle by him in 1924.[81]

Systems similar to the $+M$ mesomeric systems X—C=Y, but with a central nitrogen atom, are present in the nitro-, azoxy-, nitrite, nitrosamine, diazo-oxy, and diazo-amino-groups, as well as in several more complex groups:

$$\overset{-}{O}-\overset{+}{N}(-)=O \qquad \overset{-}{O}-\overset{+}{N}(-)=NR$$

$$-O-N=O \qquad >N-N=O \qquad -O-N=NR \qquad >N-N=NR$$

[80] W. von E. Doering and L. H. Knox, *J. Am. Chem. Soc.*, 1951, **73**, 828.
[81] A. Angeli, *Atti. R. Acad. Lincei*, 1924 [v], **33**, 109.

In the nitro-group the mesomeric displacements are maximal, corresponding to the transport of 0.5 electron from one oxygen atom to the other.

The carboxylate ion, the amidinium ion, the nitro-group, and the anions of β-keto-enols are examples of systems into which mesomerism brings a symmetry that is not represented in any valency structure. Such symmetry is sometimes indicated by the use of a *curved bond sign* for a pair of electrons which is either partly shared and partly unshared, or is shared simultaneously in two bonds:

$$[O—C—O]^- \qquad [R_2N—C—NR_2]^+ \qquad O—N—O$$

$$[O—C—C—C—O]^-$$

There is nothing in the theory of the mesomerism, either of the simple $+M$ systems, X—C=C, etc., or of the self-compensating $\pm M$ systems, X—C=Y, etc., or of systems analogous to either but with a central nitrogen atom, which prevents the atom X from being doubly bound to the central atom in the valency structure, provided that X has unshared electrons and could be triply bound. Ketens and diazo-compounds furnish examples of a $+M$ effect operating by increased covalency in an original double bond:

$$O=C=CR_2 \qquad \bar{N}=\overset{+}{N}=CR_2$$

This, without doubt, is why ketens and diazo-compounds accept a proton on the terminal carbon atom so easily in their reactions. In the case of keten, it has been established (Chapter III) that the mesomeric displacement of electrons is considerable, even though, from the outset, they have to move against the dipole field in the carbonyl group. Cyanates and azides provide examples of the $\pm M$ effect in systems with contiguous double bonds. Here the mesomeric displacements can evidently occur in either direction, the less important being that indicated by the arrows underneath the following formulae:

$$RN=C=O \qquad \bar{N}=\overset{+}{N}=NR$$

In carbon dioxide, the nitronium ion, and the azide ion, the two directions of displacement are equally important for reasons of symmetry; and thus mesomerism cannot produce a new dipole, though it can produce a new quadrupole. It will make detailed differences to the electron distribution, by causing the electron pairs of the terminal atoms to become less sharply differentiated as shared and unshared, and less localised, than would be represented by the usual valency formulae:

$O{=}C{=}O$ $\qquad$ $O{=}\overset{+}{N}{=}O$ $\qquad$ $\overset{-}{N}{=}\overset{+}{N}{=}\overset{-}{N}$

A most important type of balanced conjugation is that of the unsaturated hydrocarbons: buta-1:3-diene is the simplest example:

$CH_2{=}CH{-}CH{=}CH_2$

Again no dipole can be produced: but the two-way displacements will produce a new quadrupole, and will delocalise the electron pairs, destroying the sharp differentiation in their assignment, in the valency formula, to individual bonds; and the displacements will therefore tend to even-up the average electron contents of the bonds along the carbon chain, much as Thiele's theory described with reference to the affinity contents of the bonds.

The strong limitation imposed on mesomeric displacements in neutral conjugated systems by the formation of terminal charges, especially charges on carbon, does not apply to a closed conjugated system. In such a system, the electron displacements are free, so far as electrostatic factors are concerned, to proceed until, if the symmetry so allows, there is complete equality in the electron contents of the bonds. The fundamental example is benzene, and the statement just made can be considered as an electronic version of both Kekulé's oscillation hypothesis and Thiele's partial-valency formula for benzene, as we shall observe in more detail in Chapter IV:

→ ←

We have now to consider the nature of the forces which promote the mesomeric displacement of electrons. As in every approximation to the description of chemical combination, and as illustrated already for inductive electron displacement, these forces are those of electron delocalisation, which leads, in accordance with the uncertainty principle, to a reduced electronic zero-point energy, the reduction being described as resonance energy.

The fundamental model was provided in 1927 by Heitler and London's theory of the formation of a covalency by exchange resonance. In 1929 Burton and the writer[82] suggested that the forces of mesomer-

[82] H. Burton and C. K. Ingold, *Proc. Leeds Phil. Lit. Soc.*, Sci. Sect., 1929, 1, 421.

ism arise from the delocalisation of electrons permitted by the existence of alternative valency structures: they thus explained the stability of aromatic free radicals and the related ions. In 1931–32 Hückel[83] discussed the case of benzene very thoroughly, applying an existing, and developing a new, quantum mechanical formalism for the purpose. In 1932 Pauling[84] discussed a number of typically mesomeric molecules, including carbon dioxide, benzene, the macromolecule of graphite, and the carbonate and nitrate ions, attributing their form and stability to quantal resonance. In 1933 the writer indicated[85] how such ideas were to be incorporated in the general theory of mesomerism, as developed up to that time. In 1933 also Pauling and Wheland[86] extended Hückel's work on benzene, developing a simpler mathematical method, which they were able to apply to other aromatic hydrocarbons, including free radicals. Some further developments in the quantitative treatment of such problems are mentioned in Chapter IV.

In order to explain these concepts, let us consider the example of the carboxylate ion. We shall suppose that all the electrons, except four, are localised in atomic or bond orbitals, thus constituting a molecular frame or core, leaving over only the two pairs of electrons, the effect of whose opportunities for changing orbitals is to be investigated. At first suppose that these electrons are assigned, one pair to an oxygen-atomic p orbital, and the other to a double-bond π orbital, as required by the valency structure A:

$$\text{(A)}\quad \bar{\text{O}}\text{—}\underset{|}{\text{C}}\text{=O} \qquad\qquad \text{O=}\underset{|}{\text{C}}\text{—}\bar{\text{O}}\quad \text{(B)}$$

Assuming these electrons to remain as assigned, their motion can be described by a four-electron wave-function, Ψ_A (meaning that $|\Psi_A|^2$ gives the probability distribution of the four electrons over all possible combinations of four positions in space). There is another energetically equivalent four-electron wave-function Ψ_B, corresponding in an analogous way to the valency structure B; but, as the problem is set up, Ψ_A is the occupied function, while Ψ_B is unoccupied.[87] However, the electronic motion admitted in Ψ_A allows the electrons such

[83] E. Hückel, *Z. Physik*, 1931, **70**, 204; **72**, 310; 1932, **76**, 628.

[84] L. Pauling, *Proc. Nat. Acad. Sci.* (U. S.), 1932, **18**, 293.

[85] C. K. Ingold, *J. Chem. Soc.*, **1933**, 1120.

[86] L. Pauling and G. W. Wheland, *J. Chem. Phys.*, 1933, **1**, 322.

[87] In comparing the pattern of the theory with that of the formation of the covalent bond of hydrogen (Section **3d**), it is to be noted that one *valency structure* corresponds to one *assignment* of electrons to the two hydrogen atoms (not to one *atom*).

excursions as provide them with opportunities to be captured into, or lost from the carbon bond-orbitals; that is, the electrons can pass spontaneously from the occupied function Ψ_A to the originally unoccupied function Ψ_B. Thus there will be resonance: the originally occupied Ψ function will no longer represent a stationary state; nor will the originally unoccupied Ψ function. These functions will become replaced by two new four-electron wave-functions for the system, each of which will treat the alternative assignments of electrons to atomic and bond orbitals in a symmetrical manner, thus blending into the electronic motion the extra motion admitted by the resonance. There will be two such four-electron functions, one, when occupied, representing a state of reduced, and the other a state of increased, energy. The former is the normal mesomeric state. The defect in its energy, relatively to the energy of a valency structure, is known as resonance energy, or, more specifically, the *mesomeric energy*. The state of increased energy is an excited mesomeric state: it is mainly interesting in relation to optical properties.

Thus it is electron delocalisation which, limited by electrostatic restrictions, provides the driving force of mesomerism, producing more stable systems, and often establishing new dipoles, sometimes against the permanent electrostatic dipoles. In symmetrical systems such as carbon dioxide and buta-1:3-diene, mesomerism produces no permanent dipoles; but the formal neutrality of the terminal atoms represents an average of instantaneous states of charge, which fluctuate over a wider range than they would have done otherwise. In benzene, the electron contents of the six bonds, rendered equivalent by mesomerism, are likewise means of somewhat widely fluctuating electron contents (Chapter IV).

In an example, such as the carbonate or nitrate ion, which has three equivalent valency structures, mesomerism will produce a normal state and two excited states. The Ψ functions of each of these states will be related symmetrically to those of the three covalent structures; and thus the molecule will have trigonal symmetry, as is indicated below for the carbonate ion by curved bond-signs, the ionic charge being symmetrically divided among the oxygen atoms:

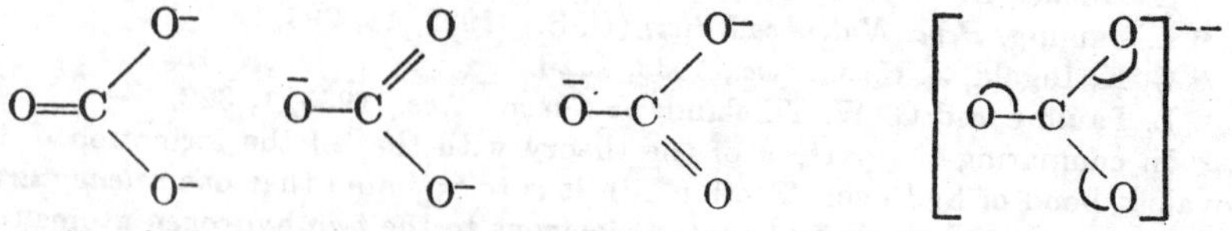

Covalent structures of the carbonate ion

Mesomeric state

When the covalent structures of a mesomeric molecule are not energetically equivalent, as in the undissociated carboxyl group, the carboxylic ester group, or amide group, in cyanates, or azides, or in vinyl chloride, aniline, or benzaldehyde—this, indeed, is the general case—then mesomerism will be less effective in producing an electron distribution more stable than that expressed by the most stable of the covalent structures. But provided that the atomic and bond orbitals of the less stable covalent structures are *accessible* in any degree to electrons placed originally in the orbitals of the most stable structure, mesomerism will occur, with the production of a normal state which is to some extent more stable than the most stable covalent structure. In such a case, mesomeric energy is conventionally reckoned with reference to the most stable of the valency structures.

Carbon dioxide and buta-1,3-diene illustrate partial specialisations of the general case, as do nitroamines and nitric esters: in these examples more than two covalent structures are associated in the conjugation, but only some of them are equivalent. The energy relations between the valency structures and mesomeric states for a number of general and specialised systems are qualitatively schematised in Fig. 7-1. The rules are that the states spread themselves over a range of energies, which extends both above and below the range covered by the structures; and that the mesomeric energy will be the larger the greater the number of structures which are low-lying relatively to the most stable (the reference) structure. We may infer that a more extended conjugated system will be stabilised by more mesomeric energy than a similar, but less extended, one. Thus, the β-keto-enolate ion will have more mesomeric energy than the carboxylate ion, and hexa-1,3,5-triene more than buta-1,3-diene:

$$\text{X—C=C—C=C} > \text{X—C=C}$$
$$\text{C=C—C=C—C=Y} > \text{C=C—C=Y}$$
$$\text{X—C=C—C=Y} > \text{X—C=Y}$$
$$\text{C=C—C=C—C=C} > \text{C=C—C=C}$$

(7f) Mesomerism and Stereochemical Form.—The stereochemical consequences of mesomerism are brought out most simply—sometimes even in an oversimplified form—by the Hückel-Penney picture of the double bond, designed as this picture is to achieve easy extension to conjugated systems (Section 4b). Conjugation is considered to arise through lateral overlap between atomic *p* orbitals or between π orbitals derived from *p* orbitals. It follows that the normal mesomeric state will achieve maximum stability when such orbital overlap is maxi-

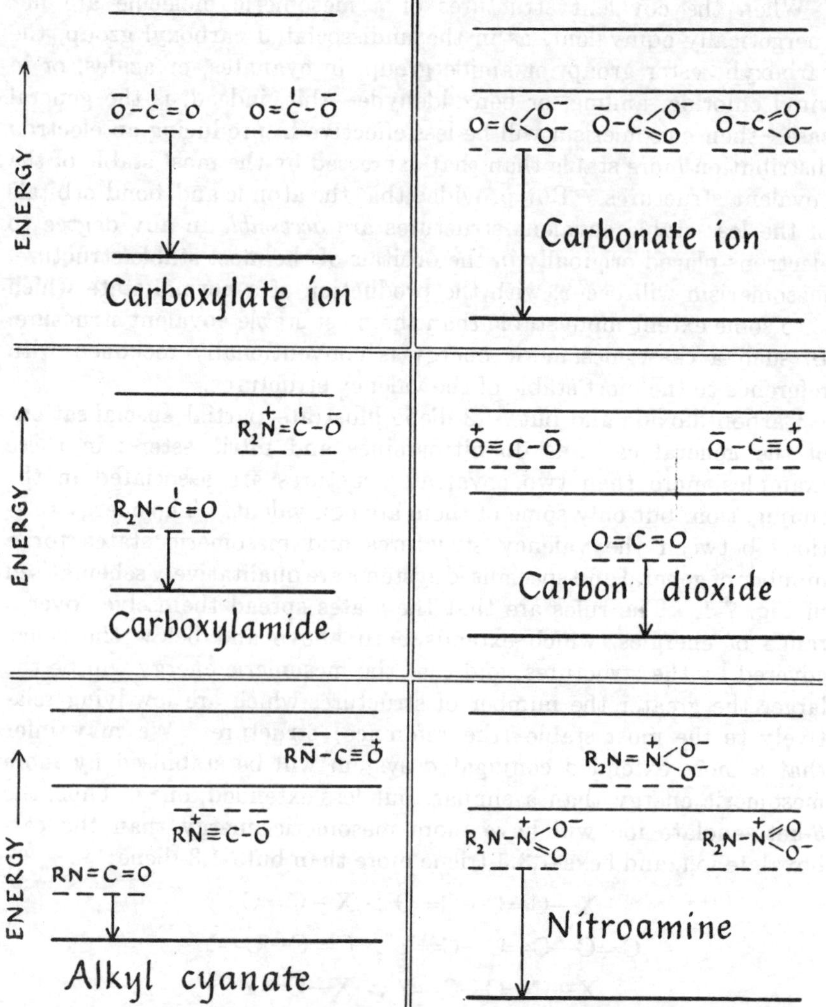

FIG. 7-1.—Schematic energy levels of mesomeric molecules. Energies of covalent structures (which exist only imaginatively as initial approximations) are represented by broken lines, and energies of mesomeric states by full lines. The arrows indicate the conventional mesomeric energies.

mised, that is, when the p and π orbitals concerned have a common nodal plane, or, in other words, when all the atoms of the conjugated system, and all the σ bonds attached to them, lie in a plane. This is illustrated for buta-1,3-diene, and for the carboxylamide group, in Fig. 7-2.

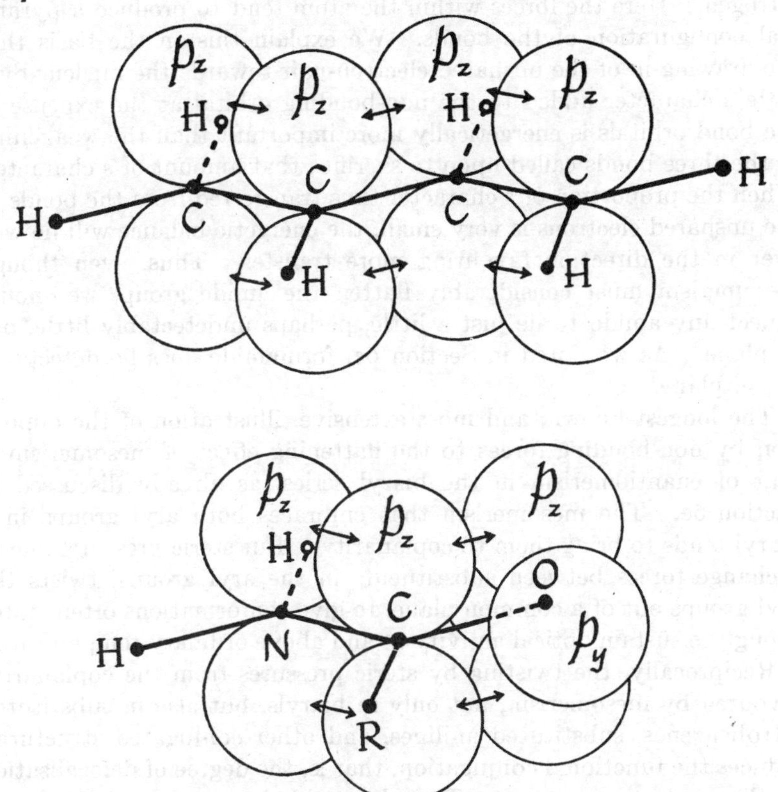

FIG. 7-2.—Illustrating the stability of the planar arrangement of the atoms and their σ bonds in a conjugated system: above, buta-1,3-diene; below, the carboxylamide group. The interacting atomic p_z orbitals are represented by their polar graphs: the interactions are not independent, because Pauli's principle must be satisfied at each atom. The σ bonds are represented by their symmetry axes, the internuclear lines. The oxygen atom of the carboxylamide group has a non-conjugated p_y orbital (shown), and an s (or perhaps, an s-p hybrid) orbital (not shown), both occupied by unshared electrons.

This simple theory explains the lack of free rotation, and the stability of planar or near-planar conformations, about the central, formally single, bond in a number of conjugated systems discussed in Section **6e**, for example, buta-1,3-diene, formic acid, various amides, nitric acid, esters of nitrous and nitric acids, and phenol. On the other hand, both bonding and non-bonding forces may oppose, with varying degrees of success, the flattening influence of mesomerism.

As an illustration of the effect of bonding forces we refer to terligant nitrogen. Here the forces within the atom tend to produce a pyramidal configuration of the bonds. We explain this on the basis that the drawing-in of the unshared electron-pair towards the nucleus by a little *s* character added to the non-bonding orbital at the expense of the bond orbitals is energetically more important than the weakening of the three bonds called upon to sacrifice that amount of *s* character. When the proportion of *s* character thus transferred from the bonds to the unshared electrons is very small, the energetic balance will lie well over in the direction favouring more transfer. Thus, even though mesomerism must considerably flatten the amide group, we should expect any amide to lie just a little, perhaps undetectably little, out of plane. As we noted in Section **6e**, formamide does lie detectably out of plane.

The longest known, and most extensive, illustration of the opposition by non-bonding forces to the flattening effect of mesomerism is that of enantiomerism in the biaryl series, as already discussed in Section **6e**. The mesomerism that embraces both aryl groups in a biaryl tends to bring them to coplanarity. But steric pressure, due to exchange forces between substituents in the aryl groups, twists the aryl groups out of a common plane, to give conformations often stable enough to sustain optical activity at and above ordinary temperatures.

Reciprocally, the twisting by steric pressures from the coplanarity favoured by mesomerism, not only in biaryls, but also in substituted nitrobenzenes, substituted anilines, and other conjugated structures, reduces the functional conjugation, that is, the degree of delocalisation in the π electron system. The observable consequences in altered physical properties, such as dipole moments, and altered chemical reactivity, as in acid-base equilibria, or aromatic substitution rates, are summarised under the term "secondary steric effects," and will be illustrated in Chapters III, VI, and XIV.

(7g) Electromeric Effects in Unsaturated Systems.—By an electromeric effect is meant the conjugative electron displacement produced in a mesomeric system by the action of the forces which arise at the reaction centre in the transition state of reaction. The electromeric effect being a polarisability effect, its direction is always such as to facilitate reaction.

When a mesomeric system is produced by the conjugation of a single $+M$ group X, or a single $-M$ group Y (or a $\pm M$ group), with an unsaturated hydrocarbon residue, for example, in

$$X{-}C{=}C \quad \text{or} \quad C{=}C{-}C{=}Y$$

then the amount of conjugative electron displacement, which converts the reference structure into the normal mesomeric state, is never more than a small fraction (nearly always under 10%) of what would be involved in a complete conversion to the dipolar structure,

$$\overset{+}{X}{=}C{-}\overset{-}{C} \quad \text{or} \quad \overset{+}{C}{-}C{=}C{-}\overset{-}{Y}$$

This is clear from the evidence of dipole moments (Chapter III). It is, of course, implied that the mesomeric energy is somewhat small. In such cases, the main possibility of additional conjugative displacements is towards the dipolar structure; and therefore strong electromeric effects are *strongly unidirectional*, $+M$ groups giving strong $+E$ effects in reactions in which the electrical needs of the reaction centre are of the right sign, but only weak $-E$ effects in reactions in which the electrical requirements are of the opposite sign. Similarly, $-M$ groups will give strong $-E$ effects in reactions in which the forces are in the right direction, and only weak $+E$ effects where the forces are in the opposite direction.

In these cases, electromeric polarisability will be limited by electrostatic forces much in the same way as mesomeric polarisation. Thus the $+E$ effect of a substituent will be reduced by a positive ionic charge, and reduced by electronegativity for identically charged atoms in the same Mendeléjeff period. But it is increased, like inductomeric polarisability, with high period number in the same Mendeléjeff group.[88] The $-E$ effect of a substituent will be increased by a positive ionic charge, increased by a high group number along a Mendeléjeff period, and increased by a high period number in a Mendeléjeff group. These conclusions are summarised in the first two sections of Table 7-5.

As we have noted, these rules hold when the substituents are singly associated with an unsaturated hydrocarbon residue, to form systems having a somewhat small mesomeric energy. Other rules will apply to systems with a large mesomeric energy, that is, systems in which the normal mesomeric state does not closely approximate to one valency structure. In order to understand this, it is necessary to recall again that polarisability is a quantised property, and that since only certain positions and motions are allowed to the electrons in the quantum theory, the electrons in a molecule will not yield before an applied electric force as they would yield if the molecule were a structure of

[88] The reason is again quantal, *viz.*, that upper states, which control ground-state polarisability, and are approximately represented by the dipolar structures written above, are more accessible when, for instance, X = I than when X = F, because in molecules, as in atoms, electronic states are less widely separated in energy when electrons of higher principal quantum numbers are involved.

TABLE 7-5.—ELECTROMERIC POLARISABILITIES OF GROUPS.

+E Effects of ·X in Vinyl-X, etc.

$-\overset{-}{O}$ > $-OR$ > $-\overset{+}{O}R_2$; etc.

$-NR_2$ > $-OR$ > $-F$; etc.

$-I$ > $-Br$ > $-Cl$ > $-F$; etc.

−E Effects of :Y in Vinyl-C:Y, etc.

$=\overset{+}{N}R_2$ > $=NR$; etc.

$=O$ > $=NR$ > $=CR_2$; etc.

$=S$ > $=O$; etc.

+E Effects of ·X in Carbonyl-X, etc.

$-OR$ > $-\overset{-}{O}$; etc.

$-F$ > $-OR$ > $-NR_2$; etc.

$-I$ > $-Br$ > $-Cl$ > $-F$; etc.

−E Effects of :Y in R_2N-C:Y or $RO-C$:Y

$=NR$ > $=\overset{+}{N}R_2$; etc.

$=NR$ > $=O$; etc.

$=S$ > $=O$; etc.

±E Effects of C=C in $(C=C)_n$; etc.

$C=C-C=C-C=C$ > $C=C-C=C$ > $C=C$; etc.

$Ph-C=C$ > $C=C$; etc.

---

charges obeying classical electrostatic and electrodynamic laws. All that an imposed electric field can do in order to deform a normal molecular state is to mix in with the positions and motions of the electrons, as they are in the undeformed normal state, certain proportions, the proportions increasing with the strength of the field, of the positions and motions that characterise one or more of the quantally al-

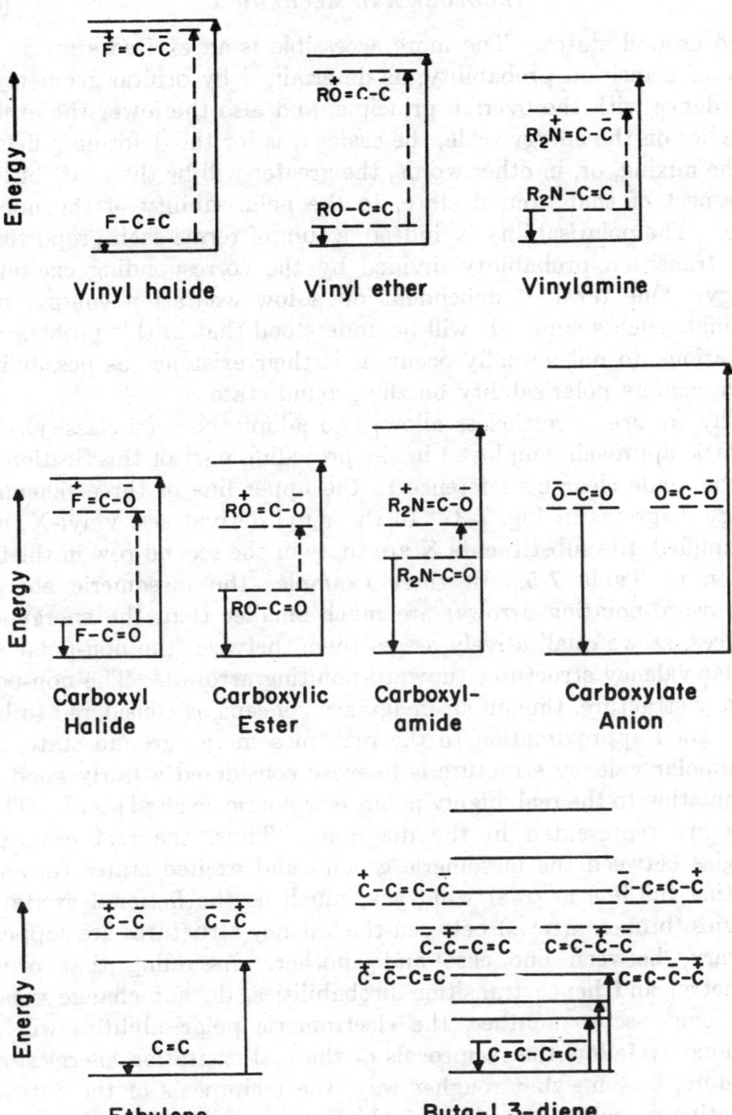

FIG. 7-3.—Schematic energy levels of mesomeric systems, drawn to illustrate main factors of electromeric polarisability of the ground states.

Note. As Professor A. Halevi pointed out to the writer, it would be unsatisfactory with higher principal quantum numbers and hence more crowded energy levels to rely on the dominance for polarisability of a single upper state.

lowed excited states. The more accessible is an excited state in the sense of transition probability, as determined by orbital geometry in accordance with the overlap principle, and also the lower the excited state lies on the energy scale, the easier it is for the deforming field to do the mixing, or, in other words, the greater will be the contribution, in respect of that excited state, to the polarisability of the normal state. The polarisability is, indeed, a sum of terms each proportional to a transition probability divided by the corresponding excitation energy. One term, if dependent on a low excitation energy, may dominate such a sum. It will be understood that in this problem the excitations do not actually occur: it is their existence as possibilities which confers polarisability on the ground state.

Why we are nevertheless allowed to adopt the semi-classical electrostatic approach, employed in the preceding part of this Section **7g**, will be made clear by reference to the upper line of three schematic energy diagrams in Fig. 7-3. In the vinyl derivatives, vinyl-X, here exemplified, the substituents X are those of the second row in the first section of Table 7-5. In these examples the mesomeric energies (downward-pointing arrows) are much smaller than the energy differences, as we qualitatively assess them, between the non-polar and dipolar valency structures (upward-pointing arrows). The non-polar valency structure, though an imaginary concept, is considered to be a fairly good approximation to the real, mesomeric, ground state, and the dipolar valency structure is likewise considered a fairly good approximation to the real, highly polar, mesomeric, excited state. These ideas are represented in the diagrams. Thus, the real excitation energies between the mesomeric ground and excited states (upward-pointing full-line arrows) will vary, much as the fictional excitation energies (broken arrows) between the valency structures are supposed to vary, between one case and another. Assuming that orbital geometry, and hence transition probabilities, do not change greatly from one case to another, the electromeric polarisabilities will approximately follow the reciprocals of the real excitation energies, and therefore, in somewhat rougher way, the reciprocals of the fictitious excitation energies—our ideas of which result from our having ranked them on the basis of qualitative electrostatic considerations. That is why we reach the qualitatively correct result (that the $+E$ electromeric polarisabilities of groups X in structures vinyl-X follow the order $F < RO < R_2N$) by employing the simple electrostatic argument already set out. The remaining results, summarised in the first section of Table 7-5 can be given a similar quantal confirmation.

But as soon as mesomeric energy becomes comparable to, or larger than, the energy separation of the valency structures, our electrostatic short-cut breaks down, as will be made clear by the second row of illustrations in Fig. 7-3. These are of carboxylic types, carbonyl-X, in which corresponding pairs of valency structures are energetically less separated than in the series just considered; and so, as X takes the successive forms F, OMe, NMe_2, they converge closely, and finally coincide when X becomes O^-. However, mesomerism is strong, and, during the successive changes in X, becomes stronger, with the result that the mesomeric states move apart in energy, as the diagrams illustrate. Electromeric polarisabilities will approximately follow the reciprocals of these real energy intervals, and thus, in contradistinction to the vinyl-X series, the $+E$ electromeric polarisabilities of X in the carbonyl-X series will follow the order $F > OR > NR_2 > O^-$. It is necessary to adopt such a quantal approach in order to deduce consistently the results set out in the third section of Table 7-5.

The results of the second section of Table 7-5, written for systems such as vinyl-C:Y and aryl-C:Y, were deduced above in the semi-classical electrostatic way, as they could be, because the mesomeric energy in such systems is sufficiently small. We could illustratively confirm them by setting up three diagrams just like those in the first row of Fig. 7-3, but now labelled as applying, in order, to C═C—C═NR, C═C—C═O, and C═C—C═NR_2^+. Again, the energies of the mesomeric states, following the energies of the valency structures, will converge along the series, and therefore the $-E$ electromeric polarisabilities of the illustrated groups Y will rise in the order $:NR < :O < :NR_2^+$, consistently with the entries in the second section of Table 7-5.

However, the conclusions in the fourth section of Table 7-5 have to be derived by the more correct quantal approach, because, in the derivative carboxyl types there represented, the mesomeric energies are large. We could illustrate the process of deduction by setting up schematic energy diagrams just like the last three in the second row of diagrams in Fig. 7-3, but now labelling them for application, in order, to R_2N—C═NR, R_2N—C═O, and R_2N—C═NR_2^+, that is, to an amidine, an amide, and an amidinium ion, respectively. As would be seen in such diagrams, the energies of the pairs of valency structures will converge along the series, but, because of the large and growing mesomeric energy, the energies of the pairs of mesomeric states will diverge. Thus we shall find that the $-E$ electromeric polarisabilities of the groups Y, in these carboxyl types R_2N—C═Y, will decrease in the order $:NR > :O > :NR_2^+$, consistently with the entries in the fourth section of Table 7-5.

A different type of problem arises in conjugated polyenes, the subject exemplified in the fifth section of Table 7-5. Here, strong interaction among the often numerous excited dipolar structures depresses the energies of some of the resulting excited states to near the energy of the non-polar, maximally double-bonded, structure. This enhances the mesomeric energy separation between that structure and the ground state of the system. The excited states have reduced double-bonding, with concentrations of non-bonding electrons towards the ends of the conjugated systems; and the electromeric polarisability of the ground state depends on the ease with which a polarising field can mix some proportion of these excited states, or of some of them, with the ground state. Of course, the lower of the excited states are the more available, and hence the more effective, for this purpose. As the third row of diagrams in Fig. 7-3 shows, an extension of conjugation greatly increases the number of low-lying excited states, and hence must increase the electromeric polarisability of the ground state, by increasing the number and reducing the energy of those excited states most able to provide paths of polarisation of the ground state by a deforming field.

One sees why electromeric polarisability is so much more important than inductomeric. Electromeric polarisability involves conjugated π electrons whose ground orbitals are usually the highest occupied orbitals in the molecule, and whose first excited orbitals are the lowest of the unoccupied orbitals. These electrons are therefore highly polarisable. Inductomeric polarisability involves σ electrons whose ground orbitals lie lower, and first excited orbitals higher, than any of the π orbitals mentioned. The σ electrons are therefore much less polarisable.

It seems occasionally to have been overlooked that a discussion of the extra polarisation needed to pass from an initial to a transition state is inadequate without a discussion of polarisability, *i.e.*, of the mobility of the electrons involved, which controls the ease or difficulty of introducing the required extra polarisation.

(7h) Stereochemistry of Electromeric Polarisability.[89]—Since the wave-functions of molecular excited states prescribe the paths of polarisability in molecular ground states, the polar reagents that call out the electromeric effect will attack preferentially those positions at which the excess or defect of electrons that they require presents itself in some low-lying excited state. As we saw in Section **7g**, these posi-

[89] C. K. Ingold, *J. Chim. Phys.*, 1956, **53**, 473; L. Burnell, *Tetrahedron*, 1964, **20**, 2403; 1965, **21**, 49.

tions are terminal, or mainly terminal, in conjugated unsaturated systems. As we shall see in Chapter XIII, addition commences almost entirely terminally in conjugated unsaturated systems.

There is an important difference between polarisability before a photon, as measured by optical refraction, and polarisability before a polar reagent, as is material to chemical reactivity. Because of the high frequencies of optical photons, they polarise only the electronic system of the substrate molecule; but the slow-moving chemical reagent will polarise the much more inertial nuclear system, as well as the electrons. Thus, electromeric polarisability has a stereochemical aspect. Because the lower excited states of the substrate molecule prescribe the important paths of polarisation in its ground state, it is important to learn what one can of the stereochemistry of excited states.

Not many type-cases, that is, cases typifying parent forms of unsaturation, have yet been quantitatively worked out, but acetylene is one that has.[90] Its ground state is linear, with its six-electron CC-bond, and dimensions as shown on the left in Fig. 7-4. The first excited state, to which transition from the ground state is spin-allowed, is like the ground state of ethylene from which two *trans*-hydrogen atoms have been removed, their places being taken by non-bonding orbitals, containing (interchangeably within the Pauli restriction) approximately three electrons derived from the original triple bond, which becomes correspondingly reduced in electron content, and so lengthened. This electron distribution and the experimentally measured dimensions are shown to the right in Fig. 7-4. On the left in Fig. 7-4, it is shown by means of arrows how an electron-seeking

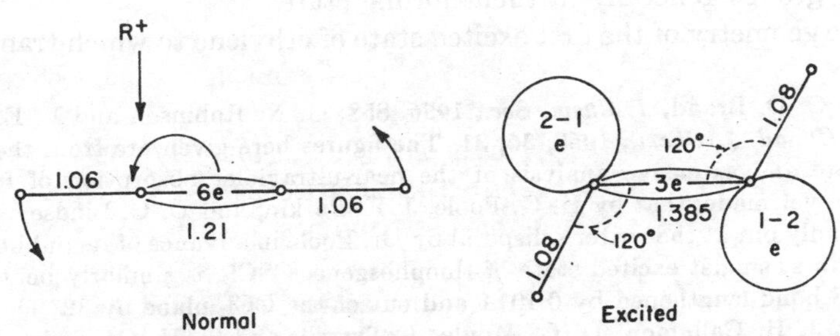

FIG. 7-4.—Electron and nuclear distribution in the normal and first excited states of acetylene. Deduced form of electron and atom polarisability in the normal state. Distances in *A*.

[90] C. K. Ingold and G. W. King, *Nature*, 1952, **169**, 1101; *J. Chem. Soc.*, 1953, 2702; K. K. Innes, *J. Chem. Phys.*, 1954, **22**, 863.

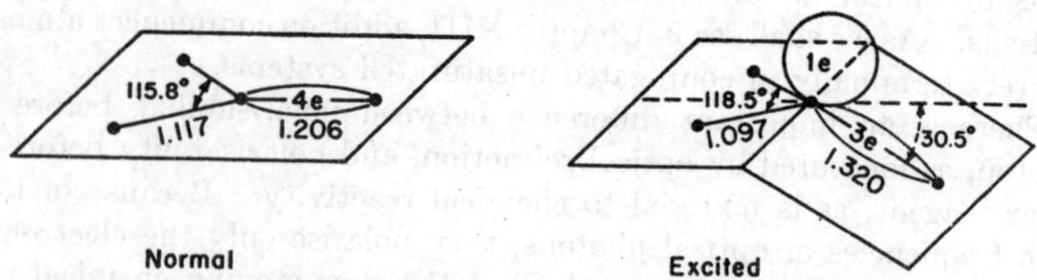

FIG. 7-5.—Electron and nuclear distributions in the normal state, and in the first excited state (the upper inversion level), of formaldehyde. Distances in *A*.

reagent, written R^+, on approaching one end of the acetylenic bond, will displace, not only π-shell electrons, not only the adjacent proton, but also the remote proton, and this last in a direction that, classically, would not have been expected. This means that any follow-up reaction, as by X^- in an addition, if it occurred soon enough after the initial attack by R^+, would lead to a *trans*-adduct.[89]

The first excited state of formaldehyde to which transition from the ground state is spin-allowed has also been quantitatively elucidated. It is pyramidal, with the line of the considerably lengthened CO bond some 30° out of the plane of the CH_2 group,[91] as illustrated in Fig. 7-5. Here, the electron configuration has moved about half-way towards that of a methanol molecule from which two hydrogen atoms have been removed, the unshared-electron orbital now on the carbon atom containing approximately one electron, derived at the expense mainly of the original double bond.[92] This extra-pyramidal orbital in the excited state will mark the direction of attack by reagents on carbonyl groups generally in their normal states.

The geometry of the first excited state of ethylene to which transition

[91] J. C. D. Brand, *J. Chem. Soc.*, **1956**, 858; G. N. Robinson and V. E. Digiorgio, *Canad. J. Chem.*, 1958, **36**, 31. The figures here given are from the most accurate and extensive analysis of the near-ultraviolet absorption of formaldehyde yet made, that by H. G. Poole, J. E. Parkin, and D. C. Lindsey, which was kindly put at the writer's disposal by Dr. Poole in advance of its publication.

The first singlet excited state of thiophosgene, $CSCl_2$, is similarly bent, with the CS bond lengthened by 0.10 *A* and out of the CCl_2 plane by 32° (J. C. D. Brand, J. H. Callomon, D. C. Moule, J. Tyrrell, and T. H. Goodwin, *Trans. Faraday Soc.*, 1965, **61**, 2365.)

[92] This description is not inconsistent with the spectroscopic conclusion that, in the excitation of formaldehyde, a non-bonding oxygen electron is partly transferred to carbon. The partial uncoupling of the π bonding shell, as the molecule goes out of plane, will recoup from the unshared-electron shell of the oxygen atom and will contribute to the occupancy of the new unshared-electron orbital on carbon.

from ground state is allowed is not yet completely elucidated. Neither is that of the first excited state of benzene to which transition from the ground state is electronically allowed; though it is generally believed that this state has two equilibrium configurations, one having the ring elongated along a line through para-positions, and the other having it elongated in the perpendicular direction. In either case, there will be a concentration of electrons towards the more acute angles.

(7i) Hyperconjugation.[93]—This is a second-approximation subject. It has been mentioned that the classification of molecular electrons as σ and π is an approximation, and that σ electrons should possess in vestigial form some of the delocalising properties of π electrons. These include the ability to conjugate, when symmetry allows, in second approximation with π electrons, or their generating p electrons or orbitals, and in third approximation with other σ electrons. The second-order interaction, with which alone we shall be here concerned, is called *hyperconjugation.* To what extent σ electrons will possess this capacity must depend on the lateral spread of the σ-bond orbital, and hence the extent is expected to be different for every type of σ bond. Bonds to hydrogen atoms probably have a large lateral spread, if we may judge from the fact that CH bonds are nearly isotropic, whereas CC bonds, in common with most bonds in which hydrogen does not participate, are much more polarisable along their length than transversely. Whether in any bond hyperconjugation is large enough to be detectable in physical and chemical properties is a matter for experiment.

Hyperconjugation involving σ electrons of CH bonds, the first recognised, best established, and certainly one of the most important forms of hyperconjugation, was discovered by Baker and Nathan[94] in 1935. They had been studying the combination of substituted benzyl bromides with pyridine to give benzyl-pyridinium bromides, a reaction which was shown to be facilitated by electron accession to the reaction zone. They found that p-alkyl substituents accelerated the reaction, as electron-releasing groups should, but not in the order required by the inductive mode of electron displacement, viz., $(CH_3)_3C\text{—}>(CH_3)_2CH->CH_3\cdot CH_2->CH_3$. The actual order was the opposite; and it was therefore concluded that in the p-alkylbenzyl system there exists an additional mechanism of electron release by alkyl groups, a mechanism which is most strongly developed in methyl, but becomes impeded when the methyl hydrogen atoms are replaced by carbon. Baker and Nathan knew that this type of anomaly would disappear, if the para-linked benzene ring were omitted from their

[93] J. W. Baker, "Hyperconjugation," Oxford University Press, Oxford, 1962.
[94] J. W. Baker and W. S. Nathan, *J. Chem. Soc.*, **1935**, 1844.

systems; and therefore they associated the anomaly with the presence, adjacently to the alkyl groups, of the conjugated system in the benzene nucleus. They suggested that the electron pairs of the CH bonds of methyl are appreciably less localised than are the electrons of CC bonds, and are able, somewhat like unshared electron pairs, to conjugate with an unsaturated system:

$$H—CH_2—C═C—C═C—$$

This new mode of electron release acts in the same direction as the inductive effect; but since its effectiveness depends on the number of suitably situated CH bonds, its magnitude decreases in the order,

$$CH_3— > CH_3{\cdot}CH_2— > (CH_3)_2CH— > (CH_3)_3C—$$

When these differences are more important than the differences in the inductive effect, then the alkyl groups will show an overall electron release in the order stated.

So the theory of conjugation, proposed by Thiele in 1898, underwent, not only its first major extension by Flurscheim for phenomenological reasons in 1902, to include partial-bond donation by latent valencies, but also a second extension, again for evidential reasons, by Baker and Nathan in 1935 to embrace partial-bond donation by hydrogen-binding valencies. In the latter extension, a *hyperconjugative mode* of electron displacement was assumed, which, originating in CH bonds, was electropositive, $+K$.

Baker and his associates at once set themselves to determine whether hyperconjugation was a factor of permanent polarisation, a *hypermesomeric effect*, $+M$, in principle significant for chemical equilibria as well as for physical properties and chemical reaction rates, or whether it was only a factor of polarisability, that is, a *hyperelectromeric effect*, $+E$, needing the stimulus of either a photon or a reagent molecule, and hence significant only for optical properties and chemical reaction rates, but not for other physical properties or for chemical equilibria. With Nathan and Shoppee, evidence was obtained, still in 1935, that hyperconjugation does include a hypermesomeric effect, $+M$, because it will retard a reaction which requires electrons to be withdrawn from the reaction centre.[95] The base-catalysed prototropic interconversion of diarylazomethines was known to be such a reaction, and it was shown that this conversion is retarded most by a *p*-methyl group and least by a *p*-*t*-butyl group:

[95] J. W. Baker, W. S. Nathan, and C. W. Shoppee, *J. Chem. Soc.*, 1935, 1847.

$$p\text{-}RC_6H_4\cdot CH{:}N\cdot CH_2\cdot C_6H_5 \rightleftarrows p\text{-}RC_6H_4\cdot CH_2\cdot N{:}CH\cdot C_6H_5$$

The same conclusion was later confirmed by a study of the equilibrium between substituted benzaldehydes and their cyanohydrins:

$$p\text{-}RC_6H_4\cdot CHO + HCN \rightleftarrows p\text{-}RC_6H_4\cdot CH(OH)\cdot CN$$

It was found[96] that the thermodynamic stability of the aldehyde, relatively to its cyanohydrin, is increased by *p*-alkyl groups, but most by the methyl group and least by the *t*-butyl group. This is to be expected if a mesomeric effect of the alkyl groups predominates over the inductive effect: for in the aldehyde the conjugation extends into the carbonyl side-chain, and therefore stabilises the aldehyde relatively to the cyanohydrin. Further details will be found in Chapter XIII.

The existence of a hyperconjugative electromeric effect $+E$ of alkyl groups has also been established. It follows from the observation[97] that, in a very strongly electron-demanding reaction, such as the aqueous hydrolysis of benzhydryl halides, which is known to depend on a preliminary separation of the molecule into its ions, the kinetic effects to be expected from the hyperconjugation of *p*-alkyl substituents are greatly increased:

$$p\text{-}RC_6H_4\cdot CHPh\cdot Cl \rightarrow p\text{-}RC_6H_4\cdot \overset{+}{C}HPh + Cl^-$$

These reactions are strongly accelerated by the alkyl substituents, and considerably more by methyl than by *t*-butyl. The reaction is further discussed in Chapter VII. We need not continue the history. It is one of extensive further experimental exemplification,[98] of numerous arguments about interpretation, and of various proposals for approximate quantal treatment. References to hyperconjugation involving CH electron-donor bonds will be found in Chapters VI, VII, IX, XI, and XIII. A strong case for an analogous $+K$ type of hyperconjugation involving NH and OH as electron-donor bonds, in place of CH bonds, has been presented by de la Mare,[98] as is mentioned in some of the same places.

The participation of the electron-pairs of CHal bonds in electronegative hyperconjugative electron-displacements, $-K$, has been postulated,[99] as a hypermesomeric polarisation, $-M$, in explanation of certain chemical equilibria:

[96] J. W. Baker and M. L. Hemming, *J. Chem. Soc.*, **1942**, 191.

[97] E. D Hughes, C. K. Ingold, and N. A. Taher, *J. Chem. Soc.*, **1940**, 949.

[98] P. B. D. de la Mare, *Tetrahedron*, 1959, **5**, 107; E. Berliner, *ibid.*, p. 202.

[99] M. Lora-Tamayo, *Cons. Sup. Inv. Cien.*, *Inst. Alonso Barba*, Madrid, 194[illegible], 3; P. B. D. de la Mare, E. D. Hughes, and C. K. Ingold, *J. Chem. Soc.*, 194[illegible], 17[illegible]

$$C{=}C{-}C{=}C{-}C{-}Hal$$

One simple chemical argument relates to the relative thermodynamic stabilities of the interconvertible dihalogeno-olefins, which are produced by 1,2- and 1,4-addition of halogens to conjugated di-olefins. It is always found (Chapter XIII), unless ordinary conjugation is present in the dihalogeno-olefins to make a difference, that the 1,4-dihalide is thermodynamically more stable than its 1,2-isomer, even when hydrogen-hyperconjugation should make the 1,2-dihalide the more stable, as in the example,

$$CH_3{-}CHBr{-}CH{=}CH{-}CHBr{-}CH_3 \rightleftarrows CH_3{-}CHBr{-}CHBr{-}CH{=}CH{-}CH_3$$

Therefore it seems necessary to assume that mesomerism dependent on halogen hyperconjugation is present, and is energetically more important than the hydrogen-hyperconjugation.

Physical data on dipole moments and on bond lengths, which can consistently be associated with the $+M$ hypermesomerism involving CH bonds, or with the $-M$ hypermesomerism involving CHal bonds, are mentioned in Chapter III.

CHAPTER III

Physical Properties of Molecules

As THE simplest field of application of the theories of binding discussed in the two preceding chapters, we shall consider in this chapter and the next some of the physical properties of molecules in their normal electronic states. The properties will be electrical polarity, electrical polarisability, diamagnetic polarisability, internal energy, geometry, and elasticity. We cannot get far with this programme without requiring a discussion of aromatic character; and the next chapter opens with one. That chapter also includes a discussion of ring-strain, another factor of significance for internal energy. All these discussions apply to electronic ground states, although excited states have to be mentioned in connexion with the electrical polarisability of ground states. But the study of the physical properties of excited states, and therewith the study of electronic transitions and the phenomena of colour—absorption, fluorescence, and phosphorescence —would lead so far that it has had to be put out of bounds.

(8) ELECTRIC DIPOLE MOMENTS

(8a) Significance of Experimental Dipole Moments.—Measurement of the electric dipole moment of molecules constitutes one of the most important methods of obtaining information about molecular electronic distribution. The principles of the measurement were established by Debye.[1] His absolute method depends on the determination of the temperature coefficient of the dielectric constant of the gaseous substance. He also invented an approximate method, which involves the use of the dielectric constant, measured at one temperature, in conjunction with the refractive index. The second of these methods is often applied, not to the gaseous substance, but to its dilute solution in some non-polar solvent, such as benzene. However, the results of measurements made in solution are inevitably approximate, because what is measured is, at best, the moment of the molecule, plus the moment it induces in the surrounding solvent: correction for this induced contribution, which may increase or decrease the apparent moment, is difficult, and is not usually attempted. On the other hand, the moments of many of the compounds cannot, for experimental reasons, be measured, or cannot be accurately measured, in the gaseous

[1] P. Debye, *Physik. Z.*, 1912, **13**, 97; "Polare Molekeln," Hirzel, Leipzig, 1929.

state; and therefore, we often have to be content with approximate moments measured in solution.

In order to secure adequate comparisons, two values, if they are available, will usually be cited for the dipole moment of a molecule, namely, that measured in the gaseous substance by the temperature-coefficient method (labelled G), and that measured in solution in benzene by the refractive-index method (labelled B). In the former method, the errors are entirely experimental. In the latter, the main errors are in the method itself; but we try to standardise the solvent error to some extent by maintaining the same solvent.

Dipole moments can be measured by another method which, when applicable, is very accurate, *viz.*, by the Stark displacement of rotational lines in the microwave spectrum. The main limitation on the method is that the spectrum must have been analysed, and the relevant rotational transitions identified. Dipole moments thus obtained apply to the gas phase.

Dipole moments are expressed in Debye units (*D*), one of which equals 10^{-18} electrostatic c.g.s. units.

(8b) Moments of Compounds with Dipolar Bonds.—In general, the dipole moments of compounds with dipolar bonds are considerably larger than those of compounds without; and thus the dipolar bond, when present, must be considered the main source of the observed moment. A number of moments for dipolar-bonded compounds are given in Table 8-1, where they are arranged in three series.[2]

All the moments of Series 1 lie in the range 5–7 *D*. The first one to consider is that of trimethylamine-oxide: nearly all of it must be due to the NO group. The length of the NO bond[3] is 1.36 *A*, and if an electron, of charge -4.80×10^{-10} e.s.u., were transferred through this distance, the moment would be 6.53 *D*. The difference between this figure and the observed one, 5.02 *D*, arises from the back-polarisation, in the N—O group, induced by its own dipole; but it under-estimates this polarisation, because small induced moments in the methyl groups will be included in the observed moment. Such defects in the moments of dipolar bonds, below those computed for the transference of an electron between non-polarisable atoms, are general. The higher values of the other moments of Series 1 must be attributed, in part, to moments produced by the electronegative halogen atoms, and in

[2] The moments of Series 1 and 3 are all recorded or quoted by G. M. Phillips, J. S. Hunter, and L. E. Sutton in their paper, *J. Chem. Soc.*, **1945**, 146. The moments of Series 2 are taken from the compilation by L. G. Wesson, "Tables of Electric Dipole Moments," Technology Press, Cambridge, Mass., 1948.

[3] G. M. Phillips, J. S. Hunter, and L. E. Sutton, *loc. cit.*

TABLE 8-1.—DIPOLE MOMENTS OF MOLECULES WITH DIPOLAR BONDS.

Series 1				Method
$Me_3\overset{+}{N}\overset{-}{O}$	$Me_3\overset{+}{N}\overset{-}{B}F_3$	$Me_3\overset{+}{N}\overset{-}{B}Cl_3$	$EtH_2\overset{+}{N}\overset{-}{Al}Cl_3$	
5.02	5.76	6.23	6.94	B
$(Et_2\overset{+}{O})_2\overset{-}{Be}Cl_2$	$Et_2\overset{+}{O}\overset{-}{B}F_3$	$Et_2\overset{+}{O}\overset{-}{B}Cl_3$	$Et_2\overset{+}{O}\overset{-}{Al}Cl_3$	
6.71	5.29	5.98	6.68	B
$Me_3\overset{+}{P}\overset{-}{B}Cl_3$	$Ph_3\overset{+}{P}\overset{-}{B}Cl_3$	$Et_2\overset{+}{S}\overset{-}{B}Cl_3$		
7.03	7.01	6.00	—	B
Series 2				
$Et\overset{+}{N}{\equiv}\overset{-}{C}$	$Ph\overset{+}{N}{\equiv}\overset{-}{C}$	$Me\overset{+}{N}\overset{-}{O}_2$	$Ph\overset{+}{N}\overset{-}{O}_2$	
—	—	3.54	4.19	G
3.47	3.53	3.15	4.03	B
Series 3				
$Ph_3\overset{+}{P}\overset{-}{O}$	$Ph_3\overset{+}{P}\overset{-}{S}$	$Ph_3\overset{+}{P}\overset{-}{Se}$	$Me_2\overset{+}{S}-\overset{-}{C}$	
4.28	4.73	4.83	6.2	B
$i\text{-}Bu_2\overset{+}{S}\overset{-}{O}$	$Ph_2\overset{+}{S}\overset{-}{O}$	$Me_2\overset{++}{S}\overset{=}{O}_2$	$Ph_2\overset{++}{S}\overset{=}{O}_2$	
—	—	4.44	—	G
3.90	4.00	—	5.14	B
$Ph_3\overset{+}{As}\overset{-}{O}$	$Ph_2\overset{+}{Se}\overset{-}{O}$	$Ph_3\overset{+}{Sb}\overset{-}{S}$	$(p\text{-}MeC_6H_4)_2\overset{+}{Te}\overset{-}{O}$	
5.50	4.44	5.40	3.93	B

part to the greater length of the bonds in the phosphorus, sulphur, and aluminium compounds. The moment of the beryllium compound can, if the minor contributions are neglected, be regarded as the vector sum of two dipolar-bond moments, each of which, assuming tetrahedrally oriented bonds, would be 5.81 *D*, this figure including the disturbances due to one chlorine atom and one ethyl group.

The moments of Series 2 are considerably smaller. The length of the triple bond[4] in *iso*cyanides being 1.17 *A*, their calculated electron-transfer moment is 5.62 *D*. The unusually large defect in the measured moments can plausibly be ascribed to a great back-polarisation in the highly polarisable triple bond in these structures.

The nitro-compounds are in a different case: a low electron-transfer moment is here to be expected from the mesomeric splitting of the negative charge between two oxygen atoms separated by a wide valency angle: the NO bond length[5] being 1.21 *A*, and the $\widehat{ONO}$ angle 127°, the calculated moment is only 2.59 *D*, so that the observed moments are abnormally *large*. This can be attributed to a combination of two causes. The first, and the less important, is the expected low polarisability in the nitro-group, owing to the stiffening effect of the high mesomeric energy arising from the symmetry, as discussed in Sections **7g** and **10c**. The second, and chief, cause is that, in addition to the usual inductive polarisation of the hydrocarbon residues, the nitro-groups involve these residues in a hyperconjugative or conjugative mesomeric system, which increases the dipole moments (Sections **7e** and **7f**):

$$H_3C{-}\overset{+}{N}({=}O){-}O^- \qquad C_6H_5{-}\overset{+}{N}({=}O){-}O^-$$

Naturally, the conjugative system in nitrobenzene does so more than the hyperconjugative system in nitromethane. None of the other molecules so far discussed can exhibit this effect—not even the *iso*cyanides, in which it would be stopped by the negative charge already on the carbon atom. Consistently, we find that the dipole moments of trimethylphosphine-borontrichloride and triphenylphosphine-borontrichloride are the same, and likewise, that the moments of ethyl *iso*cyanide and phenyl *iso*cyanide are the same, quite unlike the moments of nitromethane and nitrobenzene.

The compounds of Series 3 are a different case again. For all the compounds already considered, it is true, either that the positive atom of the dipolar bond could not increase its covalency, having no *d* orbitals in its valency shell (nitrogen, oxygen), or that it could (phosphorus, sulphur), but the negative atom (boron) has no electrons to put into the orbitals. In Series 3, the positive atoms (phosphorus, arsenic, antimony, sulphur, selenium, tellurium) have the orbitals, and

[4] L. O. Brockway, *J. Am. Chem. Soc.*, 1936, **58**, 2516.

[5] L. O. Brockway, J. Y Beach, and L. Pauling, *J. Am. Chem. Soc.*, 1935, **57**, 2693; A. J. Stosick, *ibid.*, 1939, **61**, 1127.

the negative atoms (oxygen, sulphur, selenium, carbon) have the electrons; and therefore the represented dipoles can, in greater or less degree, become neutralised by an additional electron-sharing or partial sharing involving the *d* orbitals of the positive atoms, and the electrons of the negative ones. This would produce, or partly produce, a double bond having as its second component a bond of π type between a *p* orbital on the negative atom and a *d* orbital on the positive one. Such a *p*—*d* π bond is naturally different in its physical and chemical properties from the *p*—*p* π bond familiar as a component of the double bonds of organic chemistry. Pauling and Brockway first suggested[6] that double bonds involving *d* orbitals are present in oxy-acids of the heavier elements: their main evidence was that the XO bonds in these acids are considerably shorter than dipolar single bonds should be. Phillips, Hunter, and Sutton have powerfully supported[7] the case for a partial formation of such bonds on the basis of the data of Series 3.

The calculated electron-transfer moment for a phosphine-oxide is 7.44 *D*. For a sulphoxide it is 6.86 *D*. For a sulphone, assuming two independent transfers along tetrahedrally inclined directions, it is 7.90 *D*. The observed moments are not much more than half those calculated: similar or greater defects are found in most of the other cases. This can be understood as arising from the partial formation of *pd* double bonds. Dimethylsulphonium-fluorenylide is the "exception which proves the rule." Here the sulphur atom has the orbitals and the carbon atom the electrons, so that, constitutionally, this compound belongs to Series 3. But its dipole moment, 6.2 *D*, places it with the compounds of Series 1. The evident reason, as Phillips, Hunter, and Sutton observe, is that the carbon electrons are rendered unavailable to the sulphur atom by their mesomeric involvement in the aromatic system—in a manner to be discussed in Chapter IV.[8]

(8c) Dipole Moment and Electronegativity.—The changes which occur in the dipole moments of methyl compounds, when their single substituent atom is allowed to vary along a period and down a group of the Mendeléjeff table, are illustrated[9] in Table 8-2.

The effect of variation along a period is illustrated by the figures of

[6] L. Pauling and L. O. Brockway, *J. Am. Chem. Soc.*, 1937, 59, 13.

[7] G. M. Phillips, J. S. Hunter, and L. E. Sutton, *J. Chem. Soc.*, 1945, 146.

[8] Dr. D. P. Craig suggests that, even here, there is appreciable double bond formation with sulphur *d* orbitals, his reason being that, in the absence of any such tendency, the negative charge would be so distributed by mesomerism over the aromatic nucleus as to produce a much larger moment than 6.2 *D* (personal communication).

[9] The values in this table, and in the following tables of Section 8, are taken from L. G. Wesson's "Tables of Electric Dipole Moments," except where specially noted.

TABLE 8-2.—DIPOLE MOMENTS OF METHYL COMPOUNDS.

Series 1

				Method
$CH_3 \cdot CH_3$	$CH_3 \cdot NH_2$	$CH_3 \cdot OH$	$CH_3 \cdot F$	
0.0	1.32	1.69	1.81	G
—	1.46	1.66	—	B
	$(CH_3)_2NH$	$(CH_3)_2O$		
	1.02	1.29		G
	1.17	—		B
	$(CH_3)_3N$			
	0.65			G
	0.86			

Series 2

$CH_3 \cdot F$	$CH_3 \cdot Cl$	$CH_3 \cdot Br$	$CH_3 I$	
1.81	1.83	1.79	1.64	G
—	1.86	1.82	1.48	B

Series 1. As the nuclear charge is progressively centralised in the isoelectronic groups $—CH_3$, $—NH_2$, $—OH$, $—F$, the dipole moment increases, as it should; but the first interval is much larger than the following ones. This is obviously to do with the angular structure of methylamine and methyl alcohol. It is only the component of the moment along the bond of the substituent that we should expect to increase in a fairly regular manner with increase in the periodic group number. Methylamine and methyl alcohol, alone of the four compounds in the top line of the table, have a transverse moment component, which heightens the observed, resultant moment.

It is improbable that the reductions in moment from methylamine to trimethylamine, and from methyl alcohol to methyl ether, are due mainly to changes in bond angle. Though the angles are not known accurately, they are unlikely to differ by more than a few degrees: in trimethylamine and methyl ether they are given as 108° and 111°, respectively, with an uncertainty of about 3°, while the angle in ammonia is 107° and in water 105°. The probable main cause of the changes in moment is that NH and OH bonds are associated with larger moments than NC and OC bonds. If we hypothetically associate with the NC and OC bonds the longitudinal moments 0.6 *D* and 1.2 *D*, respectively (taken as one-third and two-thirds of the methyl fluoride moment, disregarding the small differences of bond length), and with the NH and OH bonds the moments 1.3 *D* and 1.5 *D*, respectively (chosen to give the correct moments for ammonia and water), and if we take all bond angles in the methyl compounds as tetrahedral, then the computed resultant moments come out fairly correctly: $CH_3 \cdot NH_2$ 1.25, $CH_3 \cdot OH$ 1.58, $(CH_3)_2NH$ 1.05, $(CH_3)_2O$ 1.38, and $(CH_3)_3N$ 0.60 *D*. (In this analysis, as elsewhere in Section **8**, any moments which might have been assigned to the unshared electrons are treated as being shared among the bonds.)

The figures of Series 2 exhibit a less regular pattern: the moments of methyl fluoride, chloride, and bromide are about the same, while that of methyl iodide is appreciably smaller. One may plausibly interpret this as the result of two opposing influences in combination, namely, an inductive effect diminishing from fluorine to iodine (Section **7c**), and a concurrent lengthening of the CHal bond.

(8d) Dipole Moments of Alkanes.—In Section **7c** it was said that, because σ bond electrons are slightly delocalised, methyl groups in an alkane should in principle be electronegative relatively to methylene and methine groups.

Lide has determined the dipole moments of propane[10] and *iso*butane by the microwave method. His values are for propane 0.083 *D*, and for *iso*butane 0.132 *D*, the error of measurement being ± 0.001 *D*. We are interested in the direction of the dipole moments, but let us first note their consistency. The moment of propane, for which the $\widehat{CCC}$ bond angle is known to be 112.4°, could be compounded from two CH_3—CH_2 bond moments of 0.073 *D*. We should expect the CH_3—CH bond moment to be twice as great, 0.146 *D*. Three such bond moments, mutually inclined at 111.15°, the known $\widehat{CCC}$ bond angle of *iso*butane, build up a molecule of moment of 0.133 *D*, in good agreement with the value observed.

Another result of Lide's determines the directions of these moments, if we set it beside the evidence from effects of deuteration on acidity constants, that deuterium is electropositive relatively to ordinary hydrogen. Lide found that the dipole moment of 2-deutero*iso*butane was numerically larger than that of ordinary *iso*butane. Application of the vector-addition principle requires that the methyl groups in *iso*butane must be acting electronegatively towards the methine carbon atom, as was theoretically anticipated:

```
CH3                      CH3
   ↖                        ↖
CH3←C—H                  CH3←C←D
   ↙                        ↙
CH3         0.132 D      CH3         0.141 D
```

[10] D. R. Lide and D. E. Mann, *J. Chem. Phys.*, 1959, **29**, 914; D. R. Lide, *ibid.*, 1960, **33**, 1514, 1519.

TABLE 8-3.—DIPOLE MOMENTS OF HOMOLOGUES.

In each example, the upper figure is for the gas, and the lower for solution in benzene.

		Series 1			
CH_3Cl 1.83 1.86	C_2H_5Cl 2.00 —	n-C_3H_7Cl 2.04 1.94	n-C_4H_9Cl 2.04 1.93	i-C_3H_7Cl 2.15 2.04	t-C_4H_9Cl 2.13 —
CH_3Br 1.79 1.82	C_2H_5Br 2.01 1.88	n-C_3H_7Br 2.15 1.93	n-C_4H_9Br 2.15 1.93	i-C_3H_7Br 2.19 2.04	t-C_4H_9Br — 2.21
CH_3I 1.64 1.48	C_2H_5I 1.87 1.78	n-C_3H_7I 1.97 1.84	n-C_4H_9I 2.08 1.88	i-C_3H_7I — 1.84	t-C_4H_9I — 2.13
		Series 2			
CH_3NO_2 3.54 3.15	$C_2H_5NO_2$ 3.70 3.19	n-$C_3H_7NO_2$ 3.72 —	n-$C_4H_9NO_2$ (3.35) 3.29	i-$C_3H_7NO_2$ 3.37 —	t-$C_4H_9NO_2$ 3.71 —
$CH_3\cdot CN$ 3.94 3.51	$C_2H_5\cdot CN$ 4.03 3.57	n-$C_3H_7\cdot CN$ 4.05 3.57	n-$C_4H_9\cdot CN$ 4.09 3.57	i-$C_3H_7\cdot CN$ — 3.61	t-$C_4H_9\cdot CN$ — 3.65
		Series 3			
CH_3OH 1.69 1.66	C_2H_5OH 1.69 1.66	n-C_3H_7OH 1.64 1.71	n-C_4H_9OH 1.63 1.66	i-C_3H_7OH 1.68 1.70	t-C_4H_9OH — 1.66
CH_3NH_2 1.33 1.46	$C_2H_5NH_2$ — 1.38	n-$C_3H_7NH_2$ — —	n-$C_4H_9NH_2$ — 1.40	i-$C_3H_7NH_2$ — —	t-$C_4H_9NH_2$ — 1.29
		Series 4			
CH_3CHO 2.69 2.49	C_2H_5CHO 2.73 2.54	n-C_3H_7CHO 2.72 2.57	n-C_4H_9CHO — 2.57	i-C_3H_7CHO — 2.56	t-C_4H_9CHO — —

Laurie and Muenter have confirmed this conclusion in further microwave measurements of dipole moments.[11] First, they have confirmed the electropositivity of deuterium by noting the differences of moment

[11] V. W. Laurie and J. S. Muenter, *J. Am. Chem. Soc.*, 1966, **88**, 2883; *idem*, *J. Chem. Phys.*, 1966, **45**, 825.

which arise when it is substituted into a molecule of known polar sense, such as methyl fluoride:

$$CH_3F,\ 1.847\ D \qquad CD_3F,\ 1.858\ D$$

They then examined three propanes, with the following results:

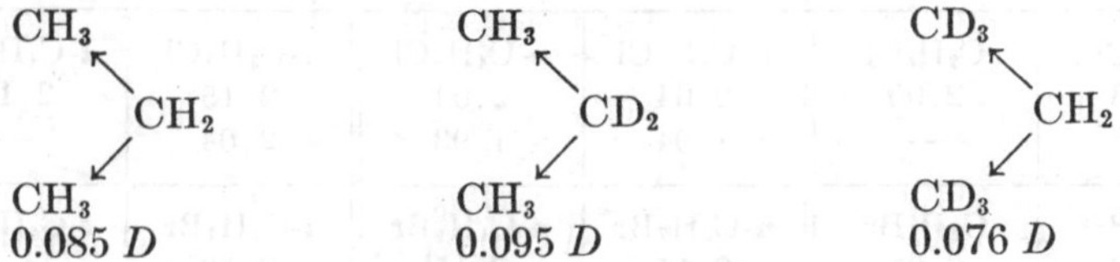

From these figures it follows that the CH_3—CH_2 bond moment is 0.075 *D* and has the direction shown by the arrows in the formulae. The value is close to that obtained from Lide's earlier work, 0.073 *D*.

Lide's work gave an estimate of the magnitude of the electropositivity of deuterium: measured as a difference of CH and CD bond moments, it is 0.009 *D*. Laurie and Muenter's work allows two estimates to be made, if we assume that all DCD bond angles are tetrahedral (as is unlikely to be exactly true). These estimates are 0.008 *D* and 0.009 *D*.

(8e) Dipole Moments of Homologues.—The dipole moments of some singly substituted paraffin compounds are arranged in homologous series in Table 8-3. The table is divided vertically into three parts: the left-hand and middle parts, taken together, illustrate effects of normal homology from methyl to normal butyl; and the left-hand and right-hand parts, read together, show the influence of branching homology from methyl to tertiary butyl. Four series of substituents are distinguished as follows:

Series 1: single-bonded substituents with no transverse moment.

Series 2: multiple-bonded substituents with no transverse moment.

Series 3: single-bonded substituents having a transverse moment.

Series 4: multiple-bonded substituents having a transverse moment.

In Series 1 there is a general increase of moment with homology; and the increases encountered in the branching homologues are more marked than those found in the normal-chain homologues. This is in accord with the theory of the inductive effect (Section 7a).

In Series 2, the increases are much smaller: this seems specially remarkable when we reflect that, as the moments of the methyl compounds are about twice those of Series 1, we might have expected the increases to be twice as great. But in Series 2, there is a small rise from methyl to ethyl, and after that no notable change up to *t*-butyl. This can be explained as a disturbance due to hyperconjugation. Nitromethane, as we have seen already, has its dipole moment increased by hyperconjugation, and the same must be true for methyl cyanide:

$$\begin{array}{c} H \\ H—C—C{\equiv}N \\ H \end{array}$$

This effect will diminish with homology, while the inductive effect increases, the overall result being that there is little change in the resultant moments.

We may note in passing that the unexpected direction of the Group IV moments,

$$\underset{0.735\ D}{(\delta+)CH_3—SiH_3(\delta-)} \quad \text{and} \quad \underset{0.642\ D}{(\delta+)CH_3—GeH_3(\delta-)}$$

which Laurie and Muenter determined[11] by the deuterium substitution method as applied in the microwave technique, may arise from hyperconjugative absorption of the CH_3 electrons into the valence-shell *d* orbitals of the Si and Ge atoms.

In Series 3 compensating effects of another kind can be discerned. These substituents have both longitudinal and transverse components in their electric moments; and, while a longitudinal component must be reinforced by the moments it induces in the hydrocarbon residue, a transverse component will be opposed by the moments which it induces: this is obvious, when one thinks of the pattern of electric force around a dipole. Thus one can understand that the overall result of induction is to produce no perceptible change in the moments of the alcohols, and an actual diminution with homology in the apparent moments of the amines, in which, as we have seen, the longitudinal component of the moment is relatively much weaker than in the alcohols.

In Series 4 we must expect both the forms of compensation recognised separately in Series 2 and 3. The data are consistent with this view.

(8f) Dipole Moments and Conjugation.—It was predicted[12] for mesomeric systems, before any relevant measurements were available, that they would possess an electric moment, which could oppose, and might in some cases outweigh, the electrostatic moment, producing

[12] C. K. Ingold, *Ann. Repts. on Progress Chem.* (Chem. Soc. London), 1926, **23**, 144

in the latter case an inversion in the direction of the overall electron displacement, as the following formulae illustrate:

$$(\delta+)\text{Alkyl}\rightarrow\text{NR}_2(\delta-) \qquad (\delta-)\text{Aryl}\rightarrow\text{NR}_2(\delta+)$$

Höjendahl[13] was one of the first to determine the directions of moments associated with the introduction of substituents into the benzene ring, by studying both mono- and poly-substituted benzenes, and employing Thomson's approximate vector-addition principle (Section **6b**). He thus found that the group NH_2 is the positive end of the aniline dipole.

A more general test for mesomeric moments in aromatic compounds was devised by Sutton.[14] He showed that, even when, as often, the mesomeric moment does not actually outweigh the inductive, there are highly significant differences between the dipole moments of two molecules Alkyl-R and Aryl-R with like substituents R: independently of the directions of the individual moments, the direction of the difference in their moments, the aromatic moment minus the aliphatic moment, always corresponds to the direction of the expected mesomeric effect in the aromatic compound. To illustrate this, we attach plus and minus signs to the moments, according to whether the substituent is acting electropositively or electronegatively. Then alkyl fluorides and phenyl fluoride both have negative moments; but that of phenyl fluoride is numerically the smaller; and so its extra moment is positive, in agreement with the structurally permitted $+M$ effect of the fluorine substituent (Section **7e**). Alkyl cyanides and phenyl cyanide also both have negative moments, but that of phenyl cyanide is numerically the larger; and hence its extra moment is negative, in agreement with the expected $-M$ effect of the substituent (Section **7e**):

$$(-I_s + M)\ \text{Ar}\rightarrow\text{F} \qquad \text{Ar}\rightarrow\text{CN}\ (-I_s - M)$$

The dipole moments in Table 8-4 further exemplify the matter. Here methyl and *t*-butyl compounds are taken as alternative aliphatic series with which the phenyl series may be compared. We try to secure straightforward comparisons by choosing substituents whose bonding directions are axes of symmetry: then, the mesomeric and inductive moments both lie along the symmetry axis, so that one is allowed to add or subtract their magnitudes. Such simplification is obviously provided by the monatomic and trigonal substituents. It is given for both the aliphatic and aromatic nitro-groups, and also, at

[13] K. Höjendahl, "Studies of Dipole Moments," Bianco Lunos Bagtrikkeri, Copenhagen, 1928.

[14] L. E. Sutton, *Proc. Roy. Soc.* (London), 1931, A, 133, 668.

TABLE 8-4.—COMPARISONS OF THE MOMENTS OF ALIPHATIC COMPOUNDS WITH THOSE OF AROMATIC COMPOUNDS.

R	Dipole moments			Method	Differences	
	MeR	Bu^{t}R	PhR		PhR−MeR	PhR−Bu^{t}R
NMe_2	−0.65 −0.86	—	+1.61 +1.58	G B	+2.26 +2.44	— —
CH_3	0.0 (0.0)	(0.0) (0.0)	+0.37 +0.34	G B	+0.37 +0.34	+0.37 +0.34
F	−1.81	—	−1.57	G	+0.24	—
Cl	−1.83 −1.86	−2.13 —	−1.70 −1.57	G B	+0.13 +0.29	+0.43 —
Br	−1.78 −1.82	 −2.21	−1.71 −1.55	G B	+0.08 +0.27	— +0.66
I	−1.48	−2.13	−1.38	B	+0.10	+0.75
CCl_3	−1.57	—	−2.07	B	−0.50	
CN	−4.03 −3.51	— −3.65	−4.39 −3.94	G B	−0.36 −0.43	— −0.29
NO_2	−3.54 −3.15	−3.71 —	−4.19 −4.03	G B	−0.65 −0.88	−0.48

least approximately, for the aromatic dimethylamino-group, by the stereochemical consequences of mesomerism (Section **7f**). The same simplification is not obtained for the aliphatic dimethylamino-group; but here the observational moments differ from our estimated longitudinal moment (0.6 *D*) by little enough to make it nearly immaterial which figure one takes for comparison with the widely different aromatic moment.

The group NMe_2 shows an outstandingly large moment difference,[15] or mesomeric moment, $+M$; the halogens show small mesomeric moments of the same sign, $+M$; and these, on the whole, diminish, as they should (Section **7e**), from F to I; while CN and NO_2 exhibit mesomeric

[15] The cases, $R = NMe_2$, NHMe, NH_2, have been re-examined by J. W. Smith, who used various comparison aliphatic amines, and concluded that the mesomeric moments of these groups R in phenyl-R are +2.06 *D*, +1.93 *D*, and +1.67 *D*, respectively (*J. Chem. Soc.*, **1961**, 81).

moments of the opposite sign, $-M$. All these moments are presumed to arise by conjugative electron displacement. A hyperconjugative mesomeric moment $+M$, probably contributes to the moment difference shown by CH_3, though this case needs further discussion; while a hyperconjugative moment, $-M$, is assumed to be the main cause of the moment difference given by CCl_3 (Section **7i**).[16]

It is an important general point that all these mesomeric moments are small in comparison with the moments (11-26 D) which would arise from complete conversions to dipolar structures, such as

$$\mathrm{Me_2\overset{+}{N}{=}C_6H_4^{-}} \quad \text{or} \quad \mathrm{\overset{-}{N}{=}C{=}C_6H_4^{+}}$$

This establishes the relatively early arrest of mesomeric electron displacement by the electrostatic forces (Section **7e**); and it is this early arrest of displacement which gives to the electromeric effect in these systems its strong dissymmetry, amounting almost to one-way character, for strong deforming forces (Section **7g**).[17]

The number of comparable aliphatic and olefinic systems with a symmetry axis is limited; but keten and acetone, for which the data are in Table 8-5, provide a straightforward example. If we recall that the stable form of acraldehyde is, like that of buta-1:3-diene (Section **6e**), the *trans*-form, then any mesomeric moment it might have, would make so small an angle with the resultant moment, tha

[16] The case R=CF_3 has been studied by J. D. Roberts, R. L. Webb, and E. A. McElhill, who found the following dipole moments in benzene: for *cyclo*hexyl-R, -2.40 D; for phenyl-R, -2.60 D; difference, -0.20 D (*J. Am. Chem. Soc.*, **1950, 72,** 408).

[17] Similar estimates can in some cases be obtained by other physical means—for instance, for circularly symmetrical substituents having a nuclear quadrupole moment, such as Cl, by the *nuclear quadrupole coupling coefficient,* as deduced from microwave spectra. Thus, if there were no mesomeric displacement of electrons from Cl to NO_2 in nitryl chloride Cl—NO_2, the electron density about the chlorine nucleus would be circularly symmetrical about the Cl—N bond as axis, and the nuclear quadrupole, regarded as an assembly of charges $\overset{-}{\underset{-}{+\quad+}}$, superposed on a spherical positive charge, would have no preferred orientation about the line of the bond. However, mesomeric displacement reduces the electron density around the Cl nucleus, above and below the NO_2 plane, and hence the nucleus will have a different energy according as the two positive charges or the two negative charges of the quadrupole lie in that plane. The energy difference, picked up as a splitting of lines in the microwave spectrum, shows that 5% of one π electron has been lost from the chlorine atom to the nitro group (D. J. Millen and K. M. Sinnott, *J. Chem. Soc.*. **1958,** 380).

TABLE 8-5.—COMPARISONS OF THE MOMENTS OF SATURATED AND UNSATURATED CARBONYL COMPOUNDS.

Substance	Moment	Substance	Moment	Method	Difference
$O{=}C(CH_3)_2$	−2.85	$O{=}C{=}CH_2$	−1.45	G	+1.40
	−2.74		−1.43	B	+1.31
$O{=}CH{-}CH_3$	−2.69	$O{=}CH{-}CH{=}CH_2$	−3.04	G	−0.35
	−2.49		−2.85	B	−0.38

we may, as an approximation, apply our simple treatment to a comparison of acraldehyde with acetaldehyde. As is shown in Table 8-5, the carbonyl oxygen atom of keten is exerting a $+M$ effect,[18] and that in acraldehyde a $-M$ effect, consistently with theoretical prediction:

$$O{=}C{=}CH_2 \qquad O{=}CH{-}CH{=}CH_2$$

(8g) Dipole Moments and the Secondary Steric Effect.—Hampson and his coworkers discovered a phenomenon[19] which illustrates very well the stereochemical necessity for planarity in a mesomeric system (Section **7f**). They found that when, in a benzene derivative, two ortho-methyl groups would prevent a polyatomic, and not too small, $+M$ or $-M$ substituent (such as a dimethylamino- or nitro-substituent) from attaining planarity with the aromatic ring, much of the mesomeric moment disappears, the dipole effect of the substituent going back a long way towards its aliphatic value. This does not happen to any marked extent with the simple amino-substituent, which is not large enough to be prevented by the ortho-methyl groups from attaining at least approximate planarity with the ring; and it does not happen with monatomic substituents, such as bromine.

This was the original discovery of the general phenomenon that steric repulsions break down conjugation by causing part of the conjugated system to twist, with the result that all the consequences of

[18] A. A. Hukins and R. J. W. LeFèvre have confirmed this by measurement of the moments of higher ketens, and comparison of the results with those for ketones (*Nature*, 1949, **164**, 1050; C. L. Angyal, G. A. Barclay, A. A. Hukins, and R. J. W. LeFèvre, *J. Chem. Soc.*, **1951**, 2583).

[19] R. H. Birtles and G. C. Hampson, *J. Chem. Soc.*, **1937**, 10; C. E. Ingham and G. C. Hampson, *ibid.*, **1939**, 981; see also A. V. Few and J. W. Smith, *ibid.*, 1949, 2663 H. Kopod, L. E. Sutton, W. A. de Jong, P. E. Verkade, and B. M. Wepster, *Rec. trav. chim.*, 1952, **71**, 521; H. Kopod, L. E. Sutton, P. E. Verkade, and B. M. Wepster, *ibid.*, 1959, **78**, 790.

conjugation, both the mesomeric and the electromeric effect, are weakened or lost. It will be convenient to call this type of interplay, however manifested, between steric pressure and conjugation, the *secondary steric* effect. Further reference will be made to it later in this Chapter, and in Chapters VI and XIV.

Some of Hampson's data are in the upper part of Table 8-6. In order to secure simple comparisons, derivatives of mesitylene or durene were compared with those of benzene, because one has not then to take account of the moments arising from direct interaction of the methyl groups with the benzene ring: they cancel for reasons of symmetry.

TABLE 8-6.—COMPARISON OF MOMENTS (IN BENZENE) OF DERIVATIVES OF MESITYLENE AND DURENE WITH THOSE OF BENZENE.

Substituents		Mesitylene derivatives	Durene derivatives	Benzene derivatives
		Mono-substituted derivatives		
NMe_2		1.03	—	1.58
NO_2		3.67	3.62	4.03
NH_2		1.40	1.39	1.54
Br		1.52	1.55	1.55
		p-*Di-substituted derivatives*		
NMe_2	NO_2	—	4.11	6.87
NH_2	NO_2	—	4.98	6.10
Br	NO_2	—	2.36	2.65

When strong $+M$ and $-M$ substituents occupy para-positions in benzene derivatives, as in *p*-nitroaniline, the resulting dipole moments are particularly large, because, not only are both the substituents conjugated with the ring, producing reinforcing moments from that cause, but also the two substituents are conjugated with each other through the ring, thereby making yet another contribution to the total moment:

$$R_2N—C_6H_4—\overset{+}{N}(=O)—\overset{-}{O}$$

In dimethyl-*p*-nitroduridine all these effects are largely annulled by the action of the four methyl groups in preventing either the dimethylamino-group or the nitro-group from orienting itself suitably for conjugation; and so a large fall in moment is observed when comparison is made with dimethyl-*p*-nitroaniline. In *p*-nitroduridine two of the three effects are wiped out, while the amino-group, because it is small, is still permitted to exert its mesomeric moment; and so a smaller fall in moment is found on making comparison with *p*-nitroaniline. The bromine substituent conjugates only very weakly, and therefore the drop in moment from *p*-bromonitrodurene to *p*-bromonitrobenzene is smaller still, and is, indeed, similar to the fall observed without the bromine substituent. These points are illustrated in the lower part of Table 8-6.

(8h) Moments of Unsaturated Hydrocarbons.—The dipole moments of a number of unsaturated hydrocarbons, including aromatic hydrocarbons are set out below (bz. means determined in benzene solution). In each case an indication of the determined or assumed direction of polarisation is given:

$CH_3{\rightarrow}CH{:}CH_2$	$CH_3{\rightarrow}CH{:}CH{\cdot}CH{:}CH_2$	$CH_3{\rightarrow}C{\vdots}CH$
$+0.35\ D$ (gas)	$+0.68\ D$ (gas)	$+0.75\ D$ (gas)
$CH_3{\rightarrow}C_6H_5$	$(CH_3)_3C{\rightarrow}C_6H_5$	$HC{\vdots}C{\leftarrow}C_6H_5$
$+0.34\ D$ (bz.)	$+0.56\ D$ (bz.)	$-0.78\ D$ (bz.)

The directions of polarisation are consistent with the idea that the polarisations are inductive, and arise from a primary inequality of hybridisation of the atomic orbitals from which that bond is formed, to which an arrow-head is attached in the formulae. This theory assumes that the electrons of a bond between two like atoms, *i.e.*, atoms of the same atomic number, will be concentrated towards the generating atomic orbital with the higher *s* content, that is, towards the more unsaturated of the two atoms (Section **4b**). The directions of the polarisations in toluene and phenylacetylene have been checked experimentally by introducing a substituent such as a halogen or a nitro-group, the direction of polarisation in which is known, into the para-position of the benzene ring, measuring the moments of the substituted hydrocarbons, and applying the approximate vector-addition principle.

As to the magnitudes of the moments, the acetylenic compounds provide the greatest dissymmetries of hybridisation, and hence their larger moments are not unexpected. It is more difficult to understand the larger moment of piperylene (penta-1,3-diene) than of propylene, and the larger moment of *t*-butylbenzene than of toluene: both of these differences should be in the observed direction, but they seem unexpectedly large.

This suggests that hyperconjugation contributes to the dipole moments of alkyl-unsaturated hydrocarbons, and contributes very substantially to those which have methyl bound to the unsaturated residue. The application of this idea to the effect of lengthening the unsaturated residue, as from propylene to piperylene, is obvious: in hyperconjugative electron displacement, the electrons do not stay in their bonds, but pass from bond to bond, and in the longer, unsaturated system these transfers can go further.

An application of the same idea to the effect of elaborating the alkyl group, as from toluene to *t*-butylbenzene, must accommodate the circumstance that in alkyl cyanides and nitro-alkanes, the better hyperconjugation of methyl than of *t*-butyl approximately balances the stronger inductive effect of *t*-butyl than of methyl (Section **8e**), whereas in the alkylbenzenes no such balancing is achieved. The explanation may be that, in alkyl cyanides and nitro-alkanes, the alkyl group owes its polarity to the polar group bound to it (Section **7c**), that is, to a source external to itself, a circumstance which will give to the inductive and hyperconjugative effects in these compounds a large degree of independence, so that it is correct to consider them as additive in first approximation. In alkyl-unsaturated hydrocarbons, on the other hand, the inductive and hyperconjugative effects are by no means independent, because the inductive polarisation depends on a hybridisation difference, which hyperconjugation will reduce. Thus, in toluene, for example, hyperconjugation will reduce the inductive component of the electric moment, as well as supplying a hyperconjugation contribution—with what net effect we cannot foresee. It could well be to make the moment of toluene substantially smaller than the more purely inductive moment of *t*-butylbenzene.

(9) HEATS OF FORMATION AND REACTION

(9a) Significance of Bond Energy Terms.—In accordance with Hess's law, the heat of combustion of a compound, the heats of formation of its combustion products from their elements, and the heats of atomisation of the elements, can be combined to give the heat of formation of the compound from its atoms. All molecules and atoms are taken to be in their normal states. Ideally the heats should be corrected to 0°K., but the data required for the correction are often unavailable, and for most purposes the correction is not important.

Fajans was the first to attempt[20] to represent the heats of formation of polyatomic molecules in terms of additive constants for the bonds. The fundamental point here is that the dissociation energy of a bond

[20] K. Fajans, *Ber.*, 1920, **53**, 643; 1922, **55**, 2836.

in a polyatomic molecule includes, and cannot be separated from, the energy of reorganisation of the dissociated fragments, which are, in general, atoms or free radicals. For example, the heats of the four stages of the atomisation of methane,

$$CH_4 \rightarrow CH_3 + H \rightarrow CH_2 + 2H \rightarrow CH + 3H \rightarrow C + 4H$$

will all be different for this reason. The average of the four heats, that is, one quarter of the heat of atomisation (or of formation from atoms) of methane, is frequently called the "bond energy" of the CH bond. However, following another modern practice, we shall call it the *energy term* of the bond, because it is not the dissociation energy of any particular bond, but, like a bond dipole moment, or an atomic refraction-constant, is a mean value, obtained by assuming, and adopted to illustrate, an additive principle. Like other additive principles, this one is, and must in principle be, inaccurate (Section **6b**); but like the others, it is nevertheless a convenient starting point for the study of those deviations which are so strong that no amount of averaging can obscure them.

The example given is representative of the most direct way of obtaining the energy terms of those bonds of polyatomic molecules to which it can be applied: the energy term of the single bond XY is taken as $(1/n)$th of the heat of formation of the compound XY_n. For carbon compounds, this method is restricted almost entirely to the bonds CH and CHal containing hydrogen or halogen atoms.

Other single bonds, CN, CO, and CS, for example, cannot be treated in this way. Their energy terms have to be obtained by difference, using the heat of formation of a molecule which contains one such bond, and deducting the energy terms, determined as described, of the other bonds. Thus, the energy term of the single bond CN, as derived from the heat of formation of methylamine, is taken to be what is left after the energy terms for three CH bonds and two NH bonds, obtained as described from the heats of formation of methane and ammonia, have been deducted. Naturally, the difference will not represent the dissociation energy of the CN bond of methylamine; but, having been obtained by the use of the additive principle, it should be suitable to illustrate that principle, which is the object of the analysis.

The energy terms of all the double and triple bonds of polyatomic organic molecules, C=C, C≡C, C=O, C=N, C≡N, etc., have to be determined by this difference method.

In order to bring the principle of the approximate additivity of bond energy terms into the most useful form possible, Pauling has employed a procedure[21] quite similar to that used in the treatment of refraction and other additive constants: first, molecules containing those features, namely, formal charges and conjugative unsaturation, which are associated with quite gross deviations from additivity are excluded from consideration; and then, the best average, additively computed, constants are found from the experimental data for other molecules. These molecules should then constitute the most favourable field for exhibiting the additive properties of the terms. Apparent conformity is further increased by allowing several values to the carbonyl and cyano-bonds, just as, in the classical treatment of molecular refraction on an additive basis, several atomic constants are allowed to the oxygen atom, and to the nitrogen atom, a tacit recognition of non-additivity. Some of Pauling's bond energy terms are reproduced in Table 9-1. They apply to the temperature 25°C.

TABLE 9-1.—PAULING'S BOND ENERGY TERMS (E IN KCAL./MOLE).

Bond	E	Bond	E	Bond	E
		Single bonds			
C—C	83.1	H—H	104.2	C—H	98.8
C—N	69.7	N—N	38.4	N—H	93.4
C—O	84.0	O—O	33.2	O—H	110.6
C—S	62.0	S—S	50.9	S—H	81.1
C—F	105.4	F—F	36.6	F—H	134.6
C—Cl	78.5	Cl—Cl	58.0	Cl—H	103.2
C—Br	65.9	Br—Br	46.1	Br—H	87.5
C—I	57.4	I—I	36.1	I—H	71.4
		Double bonds			
C=C	147	C=O (H_2CO)	164	C=O (R_2CO)	174
C=N	147	C=O(RCHO)	171	C=S	174
		Triple bonds			
C≡C	194	C≡N (HCN)	207	C≡N (RCN)	213

It is important for later application to have some estimate of the degree of accuracy with which such terms can be expected to reproduce heats of formation in the absence of major disturbances. The matter has been tested for hydrocarbons by the accurate measurements,

[21] L. Pauling, "Nature of the Chemical Bond," Cornell University Press, Ithaca, New York, 3rd Edn., 1960, pp. 73 and 188.

TABLE 9-2.—HEATS OF FORMATION OF PARAFFINS (ROSSINI).

	$-\Delta H$ (kcal./mole)	Diff. for CH_2
CH_4	17.86	—
$CH_3\cdot CH_3$	20.19	2.33
$CH_3\cdot CH_2\cdot CH_3$	24.75	4.56
$CH_3\cdot CH_2\cdot CH_2\cdot CH_3$	29.71	4.96
$CH_3\cdot CH_2\cdot CH_2\cdot CH_2\cdot CH_3$	34.74	5.03
$CH_3\cdot CH_2\cdot CH_3$	24.75	
$CH_3\cdot CH\cdot CH_3$ | CH_3	31.35	6.60
$CH_3\cdot CH_2\cdot CH_2\cdot CH_3$	29.71	
$CH_3\cdot CH\cdot CH_2\cdot CH_3$ | CH_3	36.67	6.9
CH_3 | $CH_3\cdot CH\cdot CH_3$	31.35	
CH_3 | $CH_3\cdot C\cdot CH_3$ | CH_3	39.41	8.06

which have been made by Rossini and his collaborators, of their heats of combustion.[22] The data for paraffins are in Table 9-2: they represent exothermicities of formation ($-\Delta H$) from graphite and molecular hydrogen at 25°C, not from atoms at 0°K; but the molecular state of the elements has no bearing on the constancy, or deviations from constancy, of the heat differences associated with a constant formula difference; and, although a correction for temperature would reduce all the heat differences, the corrections (0.4–0.6 kcal./mole) are only a little larger than (about twice) the experimental error. It is apparent that the heat of formation is not increased by a constant amount each time that one CC and two CH bonds are introduced during a formula increase by CH_2: the heat increase is about 2, 5, 7, or 8 kcal./mole, according as the new CH_3 group is replacing H in

[22] F. D. Rossini, *Chem. Revs.*, 1940, 27, 1.

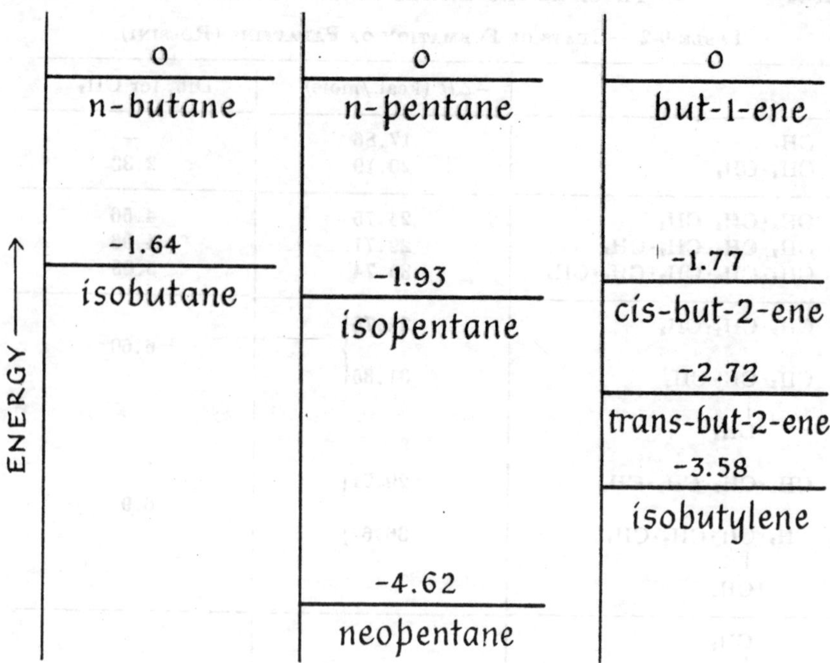

Fig. 9-1.—Stability sequences of the isomeric butanes, pentanes, and butenes. Energies are in kcal./mole. The zeros are arbitrary and non-identical.

CH_4, in a CH_3 group, a CH_2, or a CH group; that is, it is constant only to within ±3 kcal./mole, which for these compounds measures the degree of accuracy of the additive principle. Whether the deviations are to be associated mainly with variations in the properties of the replaced CH bonds, or of the replacing CC bonds, the data do not tell us. They do show that branching stabilises a paraffin (Fig. 9-1). Pitzer considers[23] that most of this effect arises from the greater electrokinetic attraction between the non-directly-bonded parts of the more branched hydrocarbon. This may be an important factor. We should also expect the tendency of alkane electrons slightly to concentrate in methyl groups (Sections **7c** and **8d**) to confer a stability increasing with the number of methyl groups. This factor would work in the same direction; but it is difficult to estimate its importance.[24]

Rossini and his coworkers have also studied olefins; and Kistiakow-

[23] K. S. Pitzer and E. Catalano, *J. Am. Chem. Soc.*, 1956, **78**, 4844. K. S. Pitzer, "Advances in Chemical Physics," Interscience Publishers, New York, 1959, Vol. 2, p. 59.

[24] This is the conclusion of Dr. L. D. Schaad from some quantal calculations he has done on the subject.

sky[25] and his collaborators have measured with precision the heats of hydrogenation of olefins, thus enabling their heats of formation to be evaluated with the aid of Rossini's data for the heats of formation of paraffins. The derived exothermicities, $-\Delta H$, are in Table 9-3. They show that the effect of homology at a distance from the double bond is much as for paraffins. They also show, however, that the substitution of CH_3, in place of H in unsaturated CH_2 or CH, increases the heat of formation by 7–8 kcal./mole, that is, by just about as much as if the CH_2 or CH were saturated, as in a paraffin.

TABLE 9-3.—HEATS OF FORMATION OF OLEFINS (ROSSINI, KISTIAKOWSKY).

	$-\Delta H$ (kcal./mole)			Diff. for CH_2		
	(*cis-*)	(—)	(*trans-*)	(*cis-*)	(—)	(*trans-*)
$CH_2{=}CH_2$		−12.56			—	
$CH_2{=}CH \cdot CH_3$		−4.96			7.60	
$CH_2{=}C(CH_3)_2$		+3.20			8.16	
$CH_3 \cdot CH{=}CH_2$		−4.96			—	
$CH_3 \cdot CH{=}CH \cdot CH_3$	+1.39		+2.34	6.35		7.30
$CH_3 \cdot CH{=}C(CH_3)_2$		+9.99		8.60		7.65
$CH_2{=}CH \cdot CH_3$		−4.96			—	
$CH_2{=}CH \cdot CH_2 \cdot CH_3$		−0.38			4.58	
$CH_2{=}CH \cdot CH_2 \cdot CH_2 \cdot CH_3$		+4.64			5.20	
$CH_3 \cdot CH{=}CH \cdot CH_3$	+1.39		+2.24	5.01		5.01
$CH_3 \cdot CH{=}CH \cdot CH_2 \cdot CH_3$	+6.40		+7.35			
$CH_2{=}C(CH_3)_2$		+3.20			5.22	
$CH_2{=}C(CH_2 \cdot CH_3)(CH_3)$		+8.42				
$CH_2{=}CH \cdot CH_2 \cdot CH_3$		−0.38			6.96	
$CH_2{=}CH \cdot CH(CH_3)_2$		+6.58				

[25] G. B. Kistiakowsky, H. Romeyn jr., J. R. Ruhoff, H. A. Smith, and W. E. Vaughan, *J. Am. Chem. Soc.*, 1935, 57, 65; G. B. Kistiakowsky, J. R. Ruhoff, H. A. Smith, and W. E. Vaughan, *ibid.*, p. 876.

The interpretative problem can be illustrated by reference to the butenes (Fig. 9-1). Besides the appreciable stability difference between the geometrically isomeric but-2-enes, there is general increase in stability along the series,

$$EtCH{=}CH_2 \qquad MeCH{=}CHMe \qquad Me_2C{=}CH_2$$

One would be tempted to interpret this as measuring the energy of hyperconjugation between the alkyl groups and the double bond, but for the circumstance that Rossini's results for the heats of formation of paraffins indicate that a similar increase in stability would be observed along the series,

$$\underset{\displaystyle CH_3\ \ CH_3}{EtCH{-}CH_2} \qquad \underset{\displaystyle CH_3\ \ CH_3}{MeCH{-}CHMe} \qquad \underset{\displaystyle CH_3\ \ CH_3}{Me_2C{-}CH_2}$$

The real conclusion is therefore that the energy of hyperconjugation between an alkyl group and an ethylenic double bond is at best of the same order of magnitude as the energy of the interactions between the atoms and bonds of a paraffin; that is, it is of an order at most of 1 kcal./mole.

More definite conclusions can be derived from the heats of formation of acetylenes: some values, again obtained from the heats of hydrogenation,[26] by combination with the heat of formation of paraffins, are in Table 9-4. The differences between the homologues, 9–10 kcal./mole, are here distinctly greater than any observed in the paraffin or olefin series; and, furthermore, the substituents are too far apart to interact directly to any important extent. Therefore, the data clearly indicate an energetically significant interaction between the methyl substituents and the triple bond. They do not, however, determine

TABLE 9-4.—HEATS OF FORMATION OF ACETYLENES (ROSSINI, KISTIAKOWSKY).

	$-\Delta H$ (kcal./mole)	Diff. for CH_2
$HC{\equiv}CH$	−54.87	—
$CH_3{\cdot}C{\equiv}CH$	−44.95	9.92
$CH_3{\cdot}C{\equiv}C{\cdot}CH_3$	−35.87	9.08

the absolute, or even the relative, importance, in the overall effect, of energy of hyperconjugation, that is, of delocalisation of the methyl CH electrons, and of energy of the inductive electron displacement (Section 8c) in the single CC bonds.

[26] J. B. Conn, G. B. Kistiakowsky, and E. A. Smith, *J. Am. Chem. Soc.*, 1939, **61**, 1868.

(9b) Energies of Conjugated Unsaturated Systems.—No such doubts attach to the broad meaning of the thermal data relating to all kinds of conjugated unsaturated systems. As Pauling and Sherman first pointed out,[27] the exothermicities of formation of molecules containing such systems are always greater than would be computed from bond energy terms, and the deviations are usually larger, often much larger, than the limits of approximation, say ± 3 kcal./mole, to within which the energy constants are additive. Thus the exothermicities of formation ($-\Delta H$) of carboxylic acids are about 28 kcal./mole greater than would be computed additively from the energy constants of the CO double bond and the various single bonds in the ordinary valency formula.

The extra stability thus demonstrated cannot be attributed to the inductive effect. All the polar bonds had their polarity and therefore the resonance energy of the inductive effect, in the simple molecules from whose formation-heats the energy terms were deduced. The large increases in stability associated with conjugated systems must therefore arise essentially from the electron delocalisation permitted in conjugated systems: they are the mesomeric energies resulting from the conjugation.

Because formal charges create large disturbances, the principle of approximate additivity can be applied only to formally non-polar valency structures; and these are expected always to be more stable than the alternative dipolar structures. In case more than one non-polar structure exists, that with the greatest number of double bonds will be the most stable. Mesomeric energies are reckoned as the excess exothermicity of formation over the value computed for the most stable valency structure. This is always the conventional structure, for example, $\cdot CO \cdot NH_2$ for the amide group, and the Kekulé structure for benzene. Table 9-5 gives a number of mesomeric resonance energies computed in this way. Such a table was first given by Pauling and Sherman,[27] but the figures quoted are Pauling's revised values.[21] The table does not include data for condensed and heterocyclic aromatic nuclei: these will be considered separately in Chapter IV. But the value for benzene is included here, mainly in order that the energy effects of conjugation between a phenyl group and other phenyl groups, or between a phenyl group and side-chains of the $+M$ or $-M$ type, can be assessed by difference.

The strikingly large values are those for carbon dioxide and its analogues, for the carboxyl group in all its forms, and for the aromatic nucleus; and this accords with general chemical experience, inasmuch

[27] L. Pauling and J. Sherman, *J. Chem. Phys.*, **1933**, **1**, 606.

TABLE 9-5.—MESOMERIC ENERGIES FROM BOND ENERGY TERMS.

	kcal./mole		kcal./mole
Carbon dioxide	36	Styrene	37+ 5
Carbon oxysulphide	20	*trans*-Stilbene	2×37+ 7
Carbon disulphide	11		
Alkyl isocyanates	7	*trans-trans*-1,4-Di-phenyl-buta-1,3-diene	2×37+11
Carboxylic acids	28	Phenylacetylene	37+10
Carboxylic esters	24		
Carboxyl amides	21	Aniline	37+ 6
Carbonic esters	42	Phenol	37+ 7
Urea	37		
Tropolone	36	Benzaldehyde	37+ 4
		Acetophenone	37+ 7
Benzene	37	Benzophenone	2×37+10
		Phenyl cyanide	37+10
Biphenyl	2×37+ 5	Benzoic acid	37+28+ 4
1,3,5-Triphenyl-benzene	4×37+20		

as the properties of carbon dioxide are very different indeed from those of a diketone, those of a carboxylic acid from those of ketone-alcohols, and those of benzene from those of a tri-olefin. Even the considerably smaller energy effects of conjugation between ring and side-chain in aniline and phenol correspond to some quite marked effects on the chemical properties of both the ring and the side-chain.

An alternative, and probably more accurate, way of estimating mesomeric energies in conjugated systems is to measure, not the excess exothermicity of formation of the compound, but the defect in the exothermicity of destruction of the system. This method has been applied by Kistiakowsky and his collaborators to the estimation of some comparatively small mesomeric energies, using hydrogenation as the means of breaking down the conjugated system. The hydrogenation heat of the system is compared with the hydrogenation heats of the individual units of unsaturation when isolated in separate molecules: for example, the hydrogenation heat of buta-1,3-diene is compared with that of two molecules of *n*-but-1-ene, that of benzene with that of three molecules of *cyclo*hexene, that of vinyl ethers with that of propylene, and so on. The values[28] in Table 9-6 refer to the gaseous

[28] G. B. Kistiakowsky, J. R. Ruhoff, H. A. Smith, and W. E. Vaughan, *J. Am. Chem. Soc.*, 1936, **58**, 146; M. A. Dolliver, T. L. Gresham, G. B. Kistiakowsky, and W. E. Vaughan, *ibid.*, 1937, **59**, 831; M. A. Dolliver, T. L. Gresham, G. B. Kistiakowsky, H. A. Smith, and W. E. Vaughan, *ibid.*, 1938, **60**, 440; R. B. Williams, *ibid.*, 1942, **64**, 1395.

TABLE 9-6.—MESOMERIC ENERGIES FROM HEATS OF HYDROGENATION (KCAL./MOLE) (KISTIAKOWSKY, *et al.*).

Conjugated molecule	Mols. H_2	$-\Delta H$	Diff.	Comparison molecule	Mols. H_2	$-\Delta H$
Buta-1,3-diene	2	57.07	3.6	*n*-But-1-ene	1	30.34
n-Penta-1,3-diene	2	54.11	4.1	*n*-But-1-ene	1	30.34
				n-Pent-2-ene	1	27.95[3]
*cyclo*Pentadiene	2	50.86	3.0	*cyclo*Pentene	1	26.91
*cyclo*Hexa-1,3-diene	2	53.37	3.8	*cyclo*Hexene	1	28.59
Crotonaldehyde	1	25.16	2.9	*n*-But-2-ene	1	28.10[4]
Ethyl vinyl ether	1	26.74	3.4	Propylene	1	30.11
2-Ethoxyprop-1-ene	1	25.10	3.3	*iso*Butylene	1	28.39
2-Methoxy-*n*-but-2-ene	1	24.80	2.1	2-Methyl-*n*-but-2-ene	1	26.92
Divinyl ether	2	57.24	3.5	*n*-Penta-1,4-diene	2	60.79
Vinyl acetate	1	30.12	0.0	Propylene	1	30.11
Benzene	3	49.80	36.0[1]	*cyclo*Hexene	1	28.59
Styrene	4	77.50	38.4[2]	Propylene	1	30.11
				*cyclo*Hexene	1	28.59
1,2-Dihydro-naphthalene[5]	1	24.6	4.0	*cyclo*Hexene	1	28.6
			3.0	1,4-Dihydronaptha-lene[5]	1	27.6
trans-Stilbene[5]	1	20.6	7.0	*trans*-But-2-ene	1	27.6
cis-Stilbene[5]	1	26.3	2.3	*cis*-But-2-ene	1	28.6
1,4-Diphenylbuta-1,3-diene[5,6]	2	44.5	10.7[7]	*trans*-But-2-ene	1	27.6

[1] Cf. the value 37 kcal./mole from bond energy terms.

[2] Cf. the value 42 kcal./mole from bond energy terms.

[3] Value for mixture of *cis*- and *trans*-forms.

[4] Weighted mean of values for *cis*- and *trans*-forms. (In the experiments with crotonaldehyde, the aldehydo-group was not hydrogenated.)

[5] Measured at 29° in solution in acetic acid, and approximately corrected to correspond to gaseous substances at 82°, the conditions to which the other measurements refer.

[6] The *trans*-*trans*-isomer.

[7] Cf. the value 11 kcal./mole from from bond energy terms.

substances at 82°C, and are otherwise uncorrected for heat-content differences; but the corrections cannot be important.

The mesomeric energies, shown in the "Difference" column of Table 9-6, are approximately represented by the following summary (energies are given in kcal./mole):

C=C—C=C	3.6	Alkyl·O—C=C	2.7
Aryl—C=C	3.1	Acyl·O—C=C	0.0
C=C—C=O	2.9		

In Acyl·O—C=C, the vinyl group must spoil the carboxyl conjugation, and supply new conjugation with the oxygen atom, to energetically equivalent extents. In *trans*-stilbene the observational mesomeric energy is more than 2×3.1 kcal./mole by 0.9 kcal./mole; and in 1,4-diphenylbuta-1,3-diene it is more than 2×3.1+3.6 kcal./mole, by 0.9 kcal./mole. These differences we can take to measure the through-conjugation, *i.e.*, the extent to which each phenyl group "feels" the other through the intervening chain in these linearly conjugated systems.

In the reduced mesomeric energy of *cis*-stilbene, we are undoubtedly seeing another physical manifestation of Hampson's *secondary steric effect* (Section **8g**). Here, the mutual pressure between the phenyl groups twists them out of the plane of the central ethylenic bond, impairing the functional conjugation, and cutting away two-thirds of its energetic effect. This molecule is isoelectronic with, and must be stereochemically closely similar to, *cis*-azobenzene, the stereochemistry of which is exactly known, and is as indicated diagramatically in Fig. 11-2 (p. 170).

(10) ELECTRICAL POLARISABILITY

(10a) Significance of Refraction Constants.—The electrical polarisability of a molecule, expressed as a spherical average α, is given, apart from a constant factor, by the molecular refraction:

$$R = \frac{4\pi N}{3} \cdot \alpha$$

where N is Avogadro's number. The molecular refraction is connected with the optical refractive index n by the formula of H. A. Lorentz,

$$R = \frac{n^2 - 1}{n^2 + 2} \cdot \frac{M}{d}$$

where M is the molecular weight, and d the density at the temperature and pressure for which n is measured. This formula assumes isotropic local distributions of molecules, so that it holds for gases, cubic crystals, and those amorphous liquids and solids which, if not structureless, are at least locally isotropic. It is thus an approximation for real amorphous liquids and solids; but for very many liquids it is a good approximation. Polarisability depends on frequency, because the electrons have an inertia; and therefore, in order to obtain the polarisability in static fields, one should correct to zero frequency by means of a dispersion formula. However, for colourless substances, the frequency of red or yellow light (such as H_α or D light) is low enough to render this correction so unimportant that it is usually neglected. Molecular refractions, having the dimensions of volume, are expressed in cubic centimetres per mole.

Two systems have been proposed for the additive representation of molecular refractions. Both proceed by first excluding those molecules which have features associated with large and somewhat complex deviations from additivity, notably formal charges and conjugative unsaturation, and then analysing the refractions of other molecules, to give, as well as may be, a set of additive constants.

The classical method of Landolt, Brühl, Eisenlohr, and others produced atomic constants. Even over the restricted field taken, it was found unsatisfactory to assign only one constant to each kind of atom, because simple unsaturation, and the kinds of atoms bound to a given atom, made differences to the apparent contribution of the atom. The effects associated with ethylenic and acetylenic bonds were represented by extra constants (in effect making two allowances for the polarisability of the same electrons), those of other multiple bonds by assigning special constants to one or both of the participating atoms, and those attributable to the kinds of atoms bound to a given atom by assigning other special constants to the latter (Brühl gives more than 30 constants for nitrogen). Thus the simple idea of additivity had in practice to be much patched up; but in this form it provides a sufficient basis for considering the large deviations, due to polarity and conjugation, to which we shall presently turn. Some of Eisenlohr's atomic refraction constants, together with his carbon double bond and triple bond constants,[29] are given in Table 10-1.

The second system, introduced by von Steiger, and developed by Smyth, Fajans and Knorr, and Denbigh, is based on the consideration that, since polarisability must come almost wholly from the valency shells of the atoms, and only to a small extent from the strongly bound core electrons, it would be more reasonable to try to analyse molecular refractions into contributions by the bonds and unshared pairs. Such a system is naturally more flexible than the atomic system, because

[29] F. Eisenlohr, "Spektrochemie organischer Verbindungen," Enke, Stuttgart, 1912.

TABLE 10-1.—ATOMIC AND MULTIPLE BOND REFRACTION CONSTANTS (IN C.C./MOLE).

	H_α	D		H_α	D
H	1.092	1.110	N (prim. amines)	2.309	2.322
C	2.413	2.418	N (sec. amines)	2.475	2.499
CC double bond	1.686	1.733	N (tert. amines)	2.807	2.840
CC triple bond	2.328	2.398	F[1]	1.088	1.090
O (alcohols)	1.639	1.643	Cl	5.933	5.967
O (ethers)	1.522	1.525	Br	8.803	8.863
O (carbonyl)	2.189	2.221	I	13.757	13.900

[1] Later value, included for comparison with other halogens.

the number of constants automatically required is greater: the number of kinds of single bond between n kinds of atom is $n(n+1)/2$, and every kind of double and triple bond has to be given its own constant.[30] The difficulty in carrying this analysis to its logical conclusion is that

TABLE 10-2.—OCTET REFRACTION CONSTANTS (IN C.C./MOLE) FOR D LIGHT.

Octet	Refr. const.	Octet	Refr. const.
C in $C(H_4)$	6.80	Si in $Si(C_4)$	9.20
C in $C(C_4)$	4.84	P in $P(H_3)$	11.8
N in $N(H_3)$	5.65	P in $P(C_3)$	11.04
N in $N(H_2C)$	5.13	S in $S(H_2)$	9.57
N in $N(HC_2)$	4.81	S in S(HC)	9.40
N in $N(C_3)$	4.65	S in $S(C_2)$	9.18
O in $O(H_2)$	3.76	Cl in Cl(H)	6.68
O in O(HC)	3.23	Cl in Cl(C)	6.57
O in $O(C_2)$	2.85	Cl in Cl(Si)	7.04
F in F(C)	1.65	Ar	4.20
Ne	1.00		

no way has been devised for separating the contributions of shared and unshared electrons of the same atom. Therefore Smyth quotes octet refraction constants, that is, totals for the shared and unshared pairs of an octet. Some of his values are in Table 10-2. Denbigh divides the unshared-pair contribution among the bonds, including a part with the constant of each bond. Either method of closing the logical gap provides a system, which is not less satisfactory than the atomic system, as a basis for considering effects of polarity and conjugation.

[30] A. L. von Steiger, *Ber.*, 1921, **54**, 1381; C. P. Smyth, *Phil. Mag.*, 1925, **50**, 361; "Dielectric Constant and Molecular Structure," Chemical Catalog Co., New York, 1931, Chap. 8; K. Fajans, and C. A. Knorr, *Ber.*, 1926, **59**, 249; K. G. Denbigh, *Trans. Faraday Soc.*, 1940, **36**, 936.

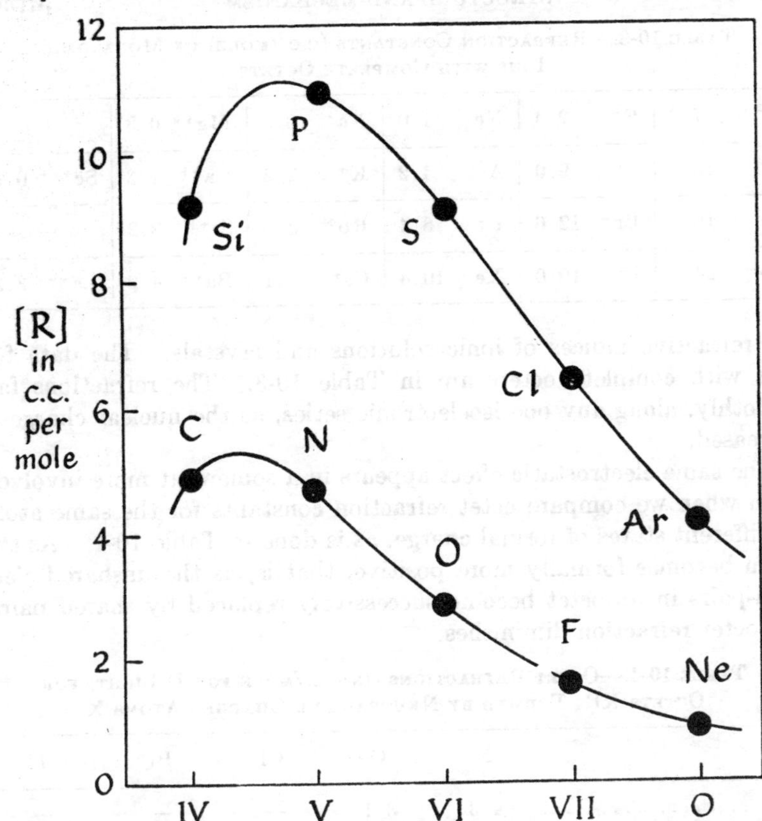

FIG. 10-1.—Octet refraction constants of neutral atoms forming bonds with carbon.

That unshared electrons in general contribute notably, like multiple bonds, to polarisability can be qualitatively shown in several ways, for instance, by comparing atomic or octet refractions along an isoelectronic series, such as CR_4, NR_3, OR_2, FR, Ne, or SiR_4, PR_3, SR_2, ClR, Ar (Fig. 10-1). Generally the refraction constants fall with increasing electronegativity along a series; but those of the nitrogen elements do not fall, while those of the oxygen elements, and even those of the halogens, except fluorine, do not fall by as much as would be expected on account of the increasing nuclear charge. These effects are obviously to be attributed to the unshared electrons.

(10b) Effects of Polarity on Refraction.—The effect of electronegativity on refraction is most simply illustrated by the refraction constants of monatomic ions, as deduced by Fajans and others[31] from

[31] J. A. Wasastjerna, *Z. physik. Chem.*, 1922, **101**, 193; *Soc. Sci. Fennica, Commentationes Phys. Math.*, 1933, **1**, 37; K. Fajans and G. Joos, *Z. Physik*,

Table 10-3.—Refraction Constants (c.c./mole) of Monatomic Ions with Complete Octets.

O^{--}	7.0	F^-	2.4	Ne	1.0	Na^+	0.5	Mg^{++}	0.3	—	
S^{--}	15	Cl^-	9.0	Ar	4.2	K^+	2.2	Ca^{++}	1.3	Sc^{+++}	0.9
Se^{--}	16	Br^-	12.6	Kr	6.4	Rb^+	3.6	Sr^{++}	2.2	—	
Te^{--}	24	I^-	19.0	Xe	10.4	Cs^+	6.1	Ba^{++}	4.2	La^{+++}	3.3

the refractive indices of ionic solutions and crystals. The data for ions with complete octets are in Table 10-3. The refractions fall smoothly, along any one isoelectronic series, as the nuclear charge is increased.

The same electrostatic effect appears in a somewhat more involved form when we compare octet refraction constants for the same atom in different states of formal charge, as is done in Table 10-4. As the atom becomes formally more positive, that is, as the unshared electron-pairs in its octet become successively replaced by shared pairs, the octet refraction diminishes.

Table 10-4.—Octet Refractions (in c.c./mole for D Light) for Octets XH_n Formed by Neutral and Charged Atoms X.

	N	O	Cl	Br	I
X^+	4.3	3.1	—	—	—
X (neutral)	5.6	3.8	6.7	9.1	13.7
X^-	—	5.1	9.0	12.6	19.0
X^{--}	—	7.0	—	—	—

In dipolar bonds the effect of the formal positive charge predominates, as would be expected, because it has the more central situation. The effect may be shown by comparing the refraction constant for a group containing a dipolar bond, with that of an isomeric group without the formal charges: the former refraction constant is found to be the smaller. It may also be shown by comparing the refraction of a whole molecule, or of a group, containing a dipolar bond, with that of another molecule, or group, in which the dipolar bond has been destroyed by taking an atom away: although the loss of an atom would normally cause a fall in refraction, it is found that the refraction does

1924, **23**, 1; M. Born and W. Heisenberg, *ibid.*, 1924, **23**, 388; K. Fajans, H. Kohner, and W. Geffcken, *Z. Elektrochem.*, 1928, **34**, 1; K. Fajans, *ibid.*, p. 502; C. P. Smyth, "Dielectric Constant and Molecular Structure," Chap. 8.

TABLE 10-5.—REFRACTION CONSTANTS (IN C.C./MOLE FOR H_α) OF GROUPS WITH DIPOLAR BONDS.

Group	Compounds	R_α	Group	Compounds	R_α
	Comparison with Isomeric Groups				
NO_2	Nitro-compounds	6.52	NO_2	Alkyl nitrites	7.21
SO_3	Alkyl sulphonates	9.78	SO_3	Dialkyl sulphites	11.08
	Comparisons with Groups Having One Oxygen Atom Less				
Cl_3PO	Phosphorus oxychloride	25.24	Cl_3P	Phosphorus trichloride	26.31
PO_4	Trialkyl phosphates	10.64	PO_3	Trialkyl phosphites	11.87
SO_2	Dialkyl sulphones	8.58	SO	Dialkyl sulphoxides	8.53
SO_4	Dialkyl sulphates	11.07	SO_3	Dialkyl sulphites	11.08

not fall, and may rise. Examples[32] of both forms of comparison are given in Table 10-5.

(10c) Refraction of Conjugated Unsaturated Systems.—It was recognized by Brühl, and emphasized in the work of Auwers and Eisenlohr, that systems, such as C=C—C=C, C=C—C=O, and N≡C—C≡N, having conjugated multiple bonds, and also systems, such as Ar—C=O, and Ar—C=C, in which an aryl group is conjugated with a multiple bond, exhibit *exaltations* of refraction; that is, they are associated with larger molecular refractions than those which are additively calculated with inclusion of all allowances for the unsaturation of the separate units composing the conjugated system.[29]

The production of an exaltation of refraction is a very common, though not a universal, property of conjugated unsaturated systems in the generalised sense, that is, of mesomeric systems. We may illustrate it for $+M$ systems,

X—C=C—

using the method by which Sutton established mesomeric dipole moments, namely, that of comparing aromatic with aliphatic compounds having the same single substituents X. Such a comparison is shown in Table 10-6. The refraction constants of the substituent atoms X in the aromatic compounds are computed from the molecular refractions of the latter by difference, using the empirical constant for the phenyl group (the molecular refraction of benzene, minus the constant for a hydrogen atom). This is in order that the exaltations, in the last column of the table, shall refer only to the conjugation of X

[32] W. Strecker and P. Spitaler, *Ber.*, 1926, 59, 1754.

TABLE 10-6.—ATOMIC REFRACTION CONSTANTS (IN C.C./MOLE FOR H_α) OF $+M$ SUBSTITUENTS IN AROMATIC COMPOUNDS AND OF THE SAME SUBSTITUENTS IN ALIPHATIC COMPOUNDS.

(Alk, R = alkyl groups)

X	Aromatic System	R_X	Aliphatic System	R_X	ΔR_X
—N	Ph—NR_2	4.22	Alk—NR_2	2.81	+1.41
—N	Ph—NHR	3.69	Alk—NHR	2.47	+1.22
—N	Ph—NH_2	3.24	Alk—NH_2	2.31	+0.93
—O	Ph—OR	2.18	Alk—OR	1.64	+0.54
—O	Ph—OH	1.76	Alk—OH	1.52	+0.24
—S	Ph—SH	8.13	Alk—SH	7.64	+0.49
—F	Ph—F	0.92	Alk—F	1.05	−0.13
—Cl	Ph—Cl	6.03	Alk—Cl	5.93	+0.10
—Br	Ph—Br	8.88	Alk—Br	8.80	+0.08
—I	Ph—I	13.94	Alk—I	13.76	+0.18
—N—	Ph—NR—Ph	5.23	Alk—NR—Alk	2.81	+2.42
—O—	Ph—O—Ph	2.84	Alk—O—Alk	1.64	+1.20
—S—	Ph—S—Ph	9.45	Alk—S—Alk	7.92	+1.53
>P—	$(Ph)_2$P—Ph	12.70	$(Alk)_2$P—Alk	9.23	+3.47

with phenyl, and shall not include contributions by the phenyl groups themselves.

For systems, such as these, in which the mesomeric electron displacement is somewhat small (Section **8f**), as also is the mesomeric energy due to conjugation of the substituent (Section **9b**), the non-polar valency structure is an approximation to the normal mesomeric state, while the dipolar valency structures are approximations to excited mesomeric states (Section **7e**). Since the effect of a perturbing electric field is to deform the normal state in the direction of an excited state (mixing in a part of the Ψ function of the latter), our expectation must be that the electromeric polarisability of these mesomeric systems will depend generally on the stability of the dipolar structures (Section **7g**): the lower lying they are on the energy scale, the greater should be the contribution of the electromeric polarisability of the system to the total polarisability of the molecule; the greater, in short, should be the exaltations, as estimated in Table 10-6. Since stability among dipolar structures, $^+X{=}C{-}C^-$, etc., is greatest for amino-compounds and least for the halogen derivatives, one can understand the general trend in the exaltations, as indicated by the found sequence N > O,S > Hals. A multiplicity of equivalent dipolar structures, corresponding to conjugation in alternative directions, should also increase electromeric polarisability (Section 7g),[33] and hence we have to expect the exaltations due to a common substituting atom to follow the sequence. triple > double > single, conjugation: this is partly confirmed by the data.

The small negative exaltations produced by aromatically bound fluorine can be understood as an electronegativity effect. Fluorine exerts a strong attraction for electrons, a $-I$ effect, and therefore, like a positive charge, must be expected to reduce the polarisability of attached groups; and it is very likely to reduce the polarisability of the intrinsically more polarisable aromatic group by a greater amount than that by which it affects the less polarisable alkyl group. No doubt, this inductive effect is present in all the examples in Table 10-6: it is producing negative exaltations, with magnitudes in the descending order, Hals > O,S > N; but only in the case of fluorine does this negative exaltation, due to the inductive effect, actually outweigh the positive exaltation produced by the electromeric effect.

Exaltations developed in conjugated systems terminated by substituents of the $-M$ class

$$\mathrm{C{=}C{-}C{=}Y}$$

have been extensively demonstrated by Brühl, Auwers, and Eisenlohr.[29] In Table 10-7 a comparison is given between aromatic molecules hav-

Table 10-7.—Atomic Refraction Constants (in c.c./mole for H_α) of $-M$ Substituents in Aromatic and in Olefinic Compounds, and of the Same Substituents in Aliphatic Compounds.
(Alk, R = Alkyl groups)

Y	Aromatic or Olefinic System	R_Y	Aliphatic System	R_Y	ΔR_Y
=O	Ph—CH=O	3.37	Alk—CH=O	2.19	+1.18
=O	Ph—CR=O	3.08	Alk—CR=O	2.19	+0.89
=O	Ph—C(OR)=O	2.90	Alk—C(OR)=O	2.19	+0.71
≡N	Ph—C≡N	3.92	Alk—C≡N	2.98	+0.94
=O	CHR=CH—CH=O	3.48	Alk—CH=O	2.19	+1.29
=O	CHR=CH—CR=O	3.10	Alk—CR=O	2.19	+0.91
=O	CHR=CH—C(OR)=O	2.75	Alk—C(OR)=O	2.19	+0.56

[33] This case is to be distinguished from that of multiplicity of equivalent most-stable valency structures: given strong interaction, this can produce the opposite result (Section 7g, and later in this Section).

ing $-M$ systems and aliphatic molecules containing the same substituents; and also an analogous comparison between olefinic and aliphatic molecules. As before, the refractive effect of the phenyl group is empirically allowed for, and so also is that of the carboxyl group (not that this makes any difference, as we shall note below), in order to isolate the effect of the particular form of conjugation now being considered.

These $-M$ systems, like the $+M$ systems, fulfil the condition that their mesomeric electron displacements are small, as also are their mesomeric energies (Sections **8f** and **9b**); and that therefore their non-polar valency structures should approximately represent their normal mesomeric states, as their dipolar valency structures should their excited mesomeric states (Section **7g**). Accordingly, electromeric polarisability should depend generally on the stabilities of the dipolar structures, $^+$X—C═C—Y$^-$, etc. Thus the sequence of exaltations, CH:O>CR:O >C(OR):O, found in both the aromatic and the olefinic series, seems reasonable; for the stabilities of the dipolar valency structures might be expected to decrease in this order, since, in order to produce such structures, a hyperconjugated system has to be broken down in the second case, and a conjugated system in the third.

In the $\pm M$ systems, which carboxyl derivatives exemplify, we find exaltations falling along the series

$$—CO·Cl > —CO·OR > —CO·NR_2 > —CO·O^-$$

the exaltations becoming negative for the last two members. This is illustrated for three series of carboxylic acid derivatives in Table 10-8.

The general result is just what we should have expected (Sections **7e** and **7g**). So long as the mesomeric displacement and energy are small, as they surely must be in the group —CO·Cl, we find a positive exaltation, as for the systems already considered. But as mesomerism becomes progressively stronger, as in $—CO_2R$, $—CO·NR_2$, and, finally, $—CO_2^-$, the valency structures become successively poorer approximations to the mesomeric states; and the lower and upper states are pressed successively further apart by the mesomeric resonance, so that it becomes increasingly difficult for an external electric field to mix the character of the upper state with that of the lower. In short, the electromeric system becomes progressively stiffened.

A related case, in which the stiffening effect of strong mesomerism appears to rather more than wipe out the positive exaltation normal for a conjugated system, is carbon dioxide:

Obsd. $R_\alpha = 6.71$; Additive $R_\alpha = 6.79$; $\Delta R_\alpha = -0.08$ c.c./mole.

Brühl, Auwers, and Eisenlohr showed by many examples that con-

TABLE 10-8.—POSITIVE AND NEGATIVE EXALTATIONS OF REFRACTION (c.c./MOLE FOR H_α) ASSOCIATED WITH FORMS OF THE CARBOXYL GROUP. (R = alkyl)

G in G—CX:O	Carboxyl form —CX:O				
	—CO·Cl	—CO·OR	—CO·OH	—CO·NR_2[1]	—CO·O^-[2]
H—	—	+0.17	+0.10	−0.16	−0.7
CH_3—	+0.38	±0.00	−0.14	−0.36	−0.9
RO—	—	+0.23	—	−0.39	—

[1] Amides having the groups —CO·NHR and —CO·NH_2 show somewhat varying exaltations 0.2–0.5 c.c./mole more positive than the values given for —CO·NR_2. This may be due to tautomerism, since the forms —C(OH):NR and —C(OH):NH should have molecular refractions about 1.0 c.c./mole higher than the isomeric forms —CO·NHR and —CO·NH_2.

[2] Empirical molecular refractions for the anions were calculated by mixture-law methods from recorded data for the indices of refraction (D light) of aqueous solutions of alkali metal formates and acetates. This can be done only approximately, because the correction for the effect of the ionic charges in modifying the refractivity of the surrounding water is a little uncertain. Additively computed refractions were reckoned using Fajans's constant for the negative oxygen atom, and Eisenlohr's constants for the carbonyl oxygen atom and the other atoms. Thus the differences, listed as negative exaltations, should isolate the effect of conjugation within the carboxylate ion. The conversion from D to H_α values is trivial.

jugation between ethylenic double bonds, and between double or triple bonds and phenyl groups in unsaturated hydrocarbons, always produces positive exaltations of refraction. The most striking general feature of these exaltations is that they increase greatly in magnitude as the conjugated system is extended. Some examples are given in Table 10-9: as before, an empirical allowance is made for the refraction of the phenyl group.

In the simplest unsaturated hydrocarbon, there can be not less than two dipolar valency structures; and, even though they would lie some-

TABLE 10-9.—EXALTATIONS OF REFRACTION OF CONJUGATED UNSATURATED HYDROCARBONS.

Hydrocarbon	ΔR_α in c.c./mole
CH_2=CMe—CMe=CH_2	+0.72
CH_2=CH—CH=CH—CH=CH_2	+2.07
Ph—CH=CH_2	+1.20
Ph—CH=CH—CH=CH_2	+3.66
Ph—C≡CH	+1.30
Ph—C≡C—C≡C—Ph	+10.7

what high in energy, they will have either identical or very nearly identical energy among themselves, with the result that one of the excited mesomeric states will become considerably depressed towards the normal mesomeric state. The more extended a conjugated system becomes, the greater will be the number of such dipolar structures, and the more will their mixing depress the lowest excited mesomeric state towards the normal state (Section **7g**). This leads to increased electromeric polarisability, and hence to an increased exaltation in the total polarisability.

Benzene exhibits a small negative exaltation:

$$\text{Obsd. } R_\alpha = 25.93; \quad \text{Additive } R_\alpha = 26.09; \quad \Delta R_\alpha = -0.16 \text{ c.c./mole.}$$

This again illustrates the stiffening effect of strong mesomerism, which here depresses greatly the energy of the normal state, but has no such large effect in depressing excited states derived from polar structures.[37]

Heterocyclic aromatic molecules also show negative exaltations, as illustrated by the following values (c.c./mole for the red H_α line):

Pyridine	Pyrrole	Furan	Thiophen
−0.97	−0.85	−0.80	−1.34

(10d) Polarisability as a Function of Direction.—Polarisability is a symmetric tensor. In every molecule, considered classically, even in an asymmetric molecule, there exist three mutually perpendicular directions, each having the property that an electric field along it will displace the electrons along it, and not at an angle. These directions are called the *principal axes of polarisability*, and the polarisabilities along them are called the *principal polarisabilities*, and are usually denoted by a, b, and c. A knowledge of the magnitudes and orientation of a, b, and c determines polarisability completely as a function of direction.

If a molecule has a rotational or alternating axis of symmetry, or, having several, has one unique one, then one of the three principal axes of polarisability will lie along it. If a molecule has a plane of symmetry, or the plane associated with an alternating axis, then two of the three principal axes of polarisability will lie in it.

If a molecule has four, or more, three-fold or more-than-three-fold rotational axes, as in tetrahedral molecules like CCl_4, P_4O_{10}, $(CH_2)_6N_4$, octahedral like $Fe(CN)_6^{----}$, or spherical like Hg, Br^-, etc., then the three principal polarisabilities will be equal: $a=b=c$; and their axes may be chosen arbitrarily, so long as they remain mutually perpendicular. If a molecule does not fulfil this condition, but has one three-fold or more-than-three-fold rotational or alternating axis, as in $CHCl_3$ (3-fold rotational), CO_3^{--} (3-fold), IF_5 (4-fold rotational),

$CH_2:C:CH_2$ (4-fold alternating), $Ni(CN)_4^{--}$ (4-fold), IF_7 (5-fold), C_2H_6 (6-fold alternating), C_6H_6 (6-fold), Cl_2 (∞-fold), then two of the three principal polarisabilities will be equal: $a \neq b = c$; and the axis of the unique one, a, will lie along the three- or more-than-three-fold axis, while the axes of the equal ones, b and c, may be arbitrarily chosen, so long as the three axes remain mutually perpendicular. If the molecule does not fulfil these conditions, but still has three two-fold rotational axes, as in p-$C_6H_4X_2$, then all three principal polarisabilities will be unequal: $a \neq b \neq c$; but their axes will lie along the symmetry axes. For all lower symmetries, including asymmetry, $a \neq b \neq c$; but the general rule, that a unique axis of symmetry will coincide with one principal axis, and a plane of symmetry will contain two principal axes, of polarisability, will determine the directions of the latter completely if there is one two-fold axis in a plane of symmetry, as in phenanthrene; and it will do so partially if there is either one two-fold axis perpendicular to a plane of symmetry, as in chrysene, or a plane only, as in quinoline, or a two-fold rotational axis only, as in a substituted allene XHC:C:CHX. The remaining form of symmetry is that of a centre of symmetry only: here, and in asymmetry, we cannot orient the principal axes of polarisability with reference to the structure.

A molecule can have a non-vanishing dipole moment if its total symmetry consists of either (1) no symmetry, as in cholesterol, or (2) one rotational axis, as in 2,2′-diaminobiphenyl, or (3) one plane of symmetry, as in NOCl, HCO_2H, PhOH, coumarin, or (4) one n-fold rotational axis contained in n planes of symmetry, as in H_2O, CH_2O, $PhNO_2$ ($n=2$), or in NH_3, CH_3I, quinuclidine ($n=3$). In cases (2) and (4), the dipole moment will lie along the symmetry axis, and therefore also along one of the principal axes of polarisability.

The number of independent functions of a, b, and c, which must be determined experimentally in order completely to describe the polarisability as a function of direction, is obviously one, two, or three according as three, two, or none of the principal polarisabilities are equal.

The *average* polarisability α is defined by the equation

$$3\alpha = a + b + c$$

It is measured by the molecular refraction.

A quantity, called the *anisotropy* of polarisability, denoted by γ^2, and defined by the equation

$$4\gamma^2 = (a - b)^2 + (b - c)^2 + (c - a)^2$$

depends symmetrically on the differences between a, b, and c. It can be measured by a method, the principle of which is as follows.

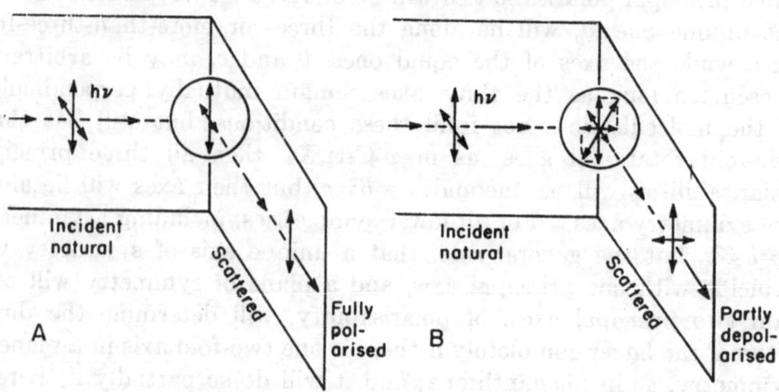

FIG. 10-2.—Perpendicular scattering of natural light. (A) Scattering by an isotropic molecule. (B) Scattering by an anisotropic molecule in an arbitrary orientation.

Natural light, perpendicularly scattered in the Tyndall effect, is completely plane-polarised, if the molecules are isotropic ($\gamma^2 = 0$); because then the forced vibrations of the electrons, which produce the scattered radiation considered, must be strictly perpendicular to the plane of scattering, that is, to the direction of propagation of both the light beams [Fig. 10-2(A)]. However, the radiation scattered by non-isotropic molecules will contain a second plane-polarised component, that is, one polarised in the plane of scattering: for the random orientations of non-isotropic molecules will lead to forced vibrations at various angles to the incident, alternating, electric field, which nearly always will not agree in direction with any principal axis of polarisability: these vibrations will have a component parallel to the direction of irradiation [Fig. 10-2(B)]. Therefore the degree of depolarisation of the scattered light, which can be measured, will depend on the anisotropy of polarisability of the molecules, and may be used to determine this quantity.

A third relation between a, b, and c can be evaluated only if the molecule possesses a non-vanishing dipole moment, μ, which agrees in direction with a principal axis of polarisability, say the axis of a. The significant quantity, χ, is then the excess of polarisability in the dipole direction over the mean polarisability in the plane at right-angles. It may be called the *polar anisotropy;* and it can be either positive or negative. It is defined by the equation,

$$2\chi = 2a - b - c$$

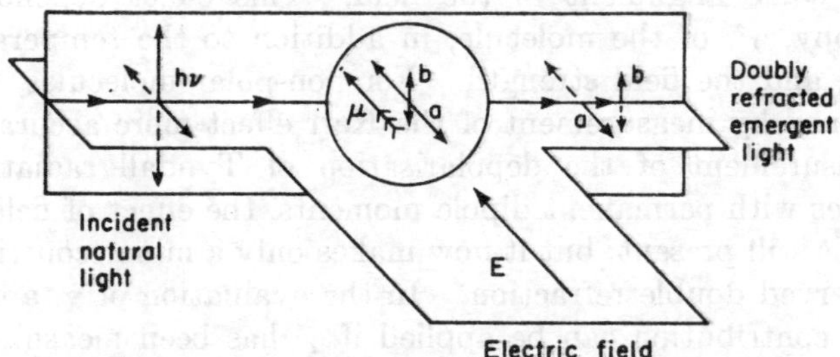

FIG. 10-3.—Electrical double refraction by an anisotropic molecule (shown as fully oriented in an electric field E), which is more polarisable (component a) in the dipole direction (μ) than it is transversely (component b). The emergent a-polarised light, having done more polarising in transit, is retarded (*i.e.*, refracted) more than is the emergent b-polarised light.

It can be determined by measurement of the Kerr effect. When a substance having a dipole moment is subjected to a strong electrostatic field, the molecules acquire a limited degree of alignment, and are therefore polarisable to different average extents by transversely travelling light plane-polarised in, and perpendicularly to, the field direction (Fig. 10-3). The resulting double refraction, that is, the amount of splitting of the refractive index, will evidently depend on both μ and χ, as well as on the temperature, the density, and the field strength. Thus, the dipole moment being known, the separation of refractive indices, that is, the Kerr effect, may be used to determine the polar anisotropy.

Even non-polar molecules, if not isotropic, will produce some double refraction in a strong electrostatic field, because the induced dipoles will have preferred directions in the molecules, and these directions will

TABLE 10-10.—DIRECTED POLARISABILITIES (IN A^3/MOLECULE) FOR D LIGHT IN LINEAR AND COMPARABLE MOLECULES.

The axis of a is the line containing the atoms (excepting the hydrogen atoms of methyl groups).

	a	$b=c$		a	$b=c$
H_2	0.68	0.89	CS_2	15.14	5.54
N_2	2.43	1.43	HCN	3.92	1.92
O_2	2.43	1.19	N_2O	5.32	1.83
Cl_2	6.60	3.62	C_2H_2	5.12	2.43
HCl	3.13	2.39	C_2N_2	7.76	3.64
HBr	4.23	3.32			
HI	6.58	4.89	$CH_3 \cdot CH_3$	5.50	4.05
CO	2.60	1.62	$CH_3 \cdot Cl$	5.42	4.14
CO_2	4.49	2.14	$CH_3 \cdot Br$	6.85	4.90

acquire some alignment in the field. This effect depends on the anisotropy, γ^2, of the molecule, in addition to the temperature, the density, and the field strength. For non-polar molecules, γ^2 can be determined by measurement of the Kerr effect more accurately than by measurement of the depolarisation of Tyndall radiation. For molecules with permanent dipole moments, the effect of field-induced dipoles is still present; but it now makes only a minor contribution to the observed double refraction. In the evaluation of χ, a correction for this contribution can be applied if γ^2 has been measured by the depolarisation method.

(10e) Directed Polarisabilities of Bonds.—Our knowledge of molecular polarisability as a function of direction is due mainly to the experimental work of H. A. Stuart[34] and of R. J. W. and C. G. LeFèvre.[35] In Table 10-10 some data are given for linear molecules, and for certain molecules which are linear except for the hydrogen atoms of methyl groups; and Table 10-11 contains some data for flat molecules, and for molecules which are flat except for the spread of their methyl groups.[34,36] The polarisabilities of individual molecules are conveniently expressed in cubic Angstrom units per molecule.

TABLE 10-11.—DIRECTED POLARISABILITIES (IN A^3/MOLECULE) FOR D LIGHT IN FLAT AND NEARLY FLAT MOLECULES.

The axis of *a* is the dipole axis. The axes of *a* and *b* lie in the plane containing the atoms[1] (excepting the hydrogen atoms of methyl groups).

	a	*b*	*c*		*a*	*b*	*c*
H_2S	4.01	4.04	3.44	Me_2O	4.88	6.30	4.31
				Me_2CO	7.08	7.10	4.82
C_6H_6	12.31	12.31	6.35				
C_6H_5Cl	15.93	13.24	7.58	C_6H_5Me	15.64	13.66	7.48
$C_6H_5\cdot NO_2$	17.76	13.25	7.75	*m*-$C_6H_4Me_2$	16.16	17.83	8.55
C_5H_5N	10.84	11.88	5.78				

[1] For benzene, the location of the axis of *b* rather than *c* in the plane of the atoms follows from symmetry, which requires two equal polarisabilities in the plane; and for the other molecules it follows from the polarisability values, read in the light of the approximate additivity principle.

From these figures it may be immediately concluded that, in general, bonds are more polarisable along their length than transversely: we see that, almost always, that line or plane which contains all or most of the bonds, or the most polarisable bonds, contains the larger prin-

[34] H. A. Stuart, "Molekulstruktur," Springer, Berlin, 1934.

[35] R. J. W. LeFèvre, C. G. LeFèvre and others, many papers, mainly in *J. Chem. Soc.*, since 1950. A summary of the position to 1965 is given by R. J. W. LeFèvre in "Advances in Physical Organic Chesmistry," ed. V. Gold, Vol. 3, p. 1.

[36] H. A. Stuart, *loc. cit.;* K. G. Denbigh, *Trans. Faraday Soc.*, 1940, **36**, 936.

cipal polarisabilities. The hydrogen molecule is the one exception; but the polarisability of hydrogen is so small that hydrogen atoms, whether in or off the line or plane of the other atoms, do not change the general distribution-in-direction of molecular polarisability.

As we noticed in Section **10a**, a satisfactory additive analysis of molecular polarisabilities in terms of bond contributions cannot be made when bonds and unshared electrons are together in the same valency shell: but this difficulty does not apply to CC and CH bonds, additive constants[35,37] for the directed polarisability of which are given in the upper part of Table 10-12.

TABLE 10-12.—LONGITUDINAL AND TRANSVERSE POLARISABILITIES OF BONDS (IN A^3/MOLECULE) FOR D LIGHT.

Bond	Longitudinal	Transverse
C—H	0.65	0.65
C—C	0.97	0.26
C=C	2.80	0.77, 0.73
C≡C	3.79	1.26
C—F (MeHal)	1.25	0.4
C—Cl (MeHal)	3.2	2.2
C—Br (MeHal)	4.6	3.1
C—I (MeHal)	6.8	4.7
C—O (Trioxan)	0.89	0.46
C=O (Me_2CO)	2.30	1.40, 0.46
N—H (NH_3)	0.50	0.83
N—C (NMe_3)	0.57	0.69

Although most bonds are less polarisable transversely than along their lengths, the CH bond is not measurably different from isotropic. The unusually large relative transverse polarisability is surely connected with the ability of CH bonds to hyperconjugate with π electrons, since conjugative interaction involves bond-orbital overlap laterally to the lines of the bonds (Sections **6e** and **7i**).

All forms of CC bond are some three or four times more polarisable along their lengths than transversely. Double bonds have two transverse polarisabilities, but those of the CC double bond are not far from equal.

The lower section of Table 10-12 contains some highly nominal polarisabilities of bonds between atoms one of which bears unshared electrons; but the figures are derived from molecules of such high symmetry that there is no doubt about the extent to which the polarisabilities of unshared electron-pairs are being included in the polaris-

[37] R. J. W. LeFèvre, *J. Proc. Roy. Soc. N. S. W.*, 1961, **95**, 1; R. J. W. LeFèvre, B. J. Orr, and G. L. D. Ritchie, *J. Chem. Soc.*, **1966**, *B*, 273, 281.

ability assigned to the bond under consideration. The polarisabilities assigned to the C—Hal bonds include those of all the unshared halogen electrons. The polarisabilities assigned to the carbonyl double bond include those of all the unshared electrons of the oxygen atom. And if these, in analogy with most bond electrons, are much more polarisable along the orbital axes than transversely, that would account for the large difference between the two transverse polarisabilities assigned to the carbonyl double bond. The NH and NC bond polarisability values each include a one-third share of the polarisabilities of the unshared nitrogen electrons. And if these electrons are anisotropic, as suggested for oxygen unshared electron pairs, this would explain why the transverse polarisabilities, assigned to the NH and NC bond, are so large, relatively to the longitudinal polarisabilities.

(10f) Directed Polarisabilities of Conjugated and Hyperconjugated Systems.—As we have seen already (Section **7g**), the excited electronic states which are important as prescribing the pathways of electromeric polarisability in the ground states of conjugated systems of double bonds can in first approximation be regarded as resonance hybrids of pairs of polar structures with reversed charges, the charges being concentrated towards the ends of the system. This picture requires that the observed exaltations of polarisability should be directed essentially in one way, namely, along the path of conjugation.

R. J. W. LeFèvre and C. G. LeFèvre have carried through a series of studies of the electrical double refraction and light-scattering depolarisation of comparable aromatic and aliphatic compounds, containing substituents which can conjugate with the benzene ring. Thus they compared PhX and MeX, with an identical substituent X of $+E$ type having unshared electrons; and PhY and MeY with the same substituent Y of $-E$ type, having an electronegative unsaturated group capable of conjugation. This has enabled them to determine, as a function of direction, the exaltations of polarisability, due to conjugation of the substituents with the aromatic ring, by a subtractive method, analogous to that used for developing Table 10-6 for such exaltations of spherical-average polarisabilities, as given by molecular refraction. Their data[38] are in Table 10-13.

The LeFèvres found generally, as should be expected, positive exaltations Δa of polarisability along the dipole axis, which is the axis of conjugation in all cases. The substituent fluorine exceptionally gave a small negative exaltation Δa; but as explained in connexion with spherical average polarisabilities, (Section **10c**), the effect of the electronegativity of fluorine on the polarisability of the groups attached

[38] C. G. LeFèvre and R. J. W. LeFèvre, *J. Chem. Soc.*, **1954**, 1577; R. J. W. LeFèvre and B. P. Rao, *ibid.*, **1958**, 1465.

TABLE 10-13.—DIRECTED POLARISABILITIES (IN A^3 PER MOLECULE FOR D LIGHT) OF THE SAME SUBSTITUENTS IN ALIPHATIC AND AROMATIC COMPOUNDS.

The axis *a* is the dipole axis. The axis *b* lies in the plane of the ring in aromatic compounds, and in the plane of the nitro-group in nitromethane.

	a	*b*	*c*	*a*	*b*	*c*	Δa	Δb	Δc
+E Substituents X									
X	MeX			PhX			Exaltations in PhX		
F	1.2	0.4	0.4	0.8	0.8	0.3	−0.4	+0.4	−0.1
Cl	3.2	2.2	2.2	4.3	2.0	1.5	+1.1	−0.2	−0.7
Br	4.6	3.1	3.1	6.3	2.5	2.2	+1.7	−0.6	−0.9
I	6.8	4.7	4.7	9.2	5.4	3.3	+2.4	−0.7	−1.4
−E Substituents Y									
Y	MeY			PhY			Exaltations in PhY		
CN	3.5	1.8	1.8	5.7	1.1	1.4	+2.2	−0.7	−0.4
NO_2	3.4	2.8	2.3	5.7	1.5	1.9	+2.3	−1.3	−0.4

to it is probably neither negligible, nor self-cancelling in the subtraction method.

We have seen that the inductomeric polarisability of the halogens stands in the order I>Br>Cl>F (Section **7d**, Table 7-3). The results of the LeFèvres show that the positive exaltations of polarisability, conferred by the conjugated halogens on their conjugated systems, along the axis of conjugation, stand in the same order. The reason is that, as explained already, polarisability is largely governed by the excitation energies of the relevant excited states; and these excitation energies are reduced, when electrons of higher principal quantum number are involved in the excitation (Section **7f**). In molecules, as in atoms, electronic energy levels lie closer together at higher quantum numbers.

A further most striking result in Table 10-13 is that the positive longitudinal exaltations Δa are accompanied by negative transverse exaltations Δb and Δc. These follow different rules in the two directions. Let us first consider the transverse exaltations Δb in the plane of the ring.

In the ground state of benzene the aromatic π shell has full hexagonal symmetry (Chapter IV): the electrons can move circumferentially with equal ease in all planar directions. In the ground states of the substituted benzenes here considered, mesomeric electron displacements are small, and hence the situation in the benzene π shell will not be very unlike that described for benzene itself. However, in those polar excited states which prescribe the paths of polarisability in the ground state, the π electrons in the ring are considerably localised on opposite sides of the ring. This follows, because the dipolar valency structures, to which the polar states approximate, have quinonoid bond distributions:

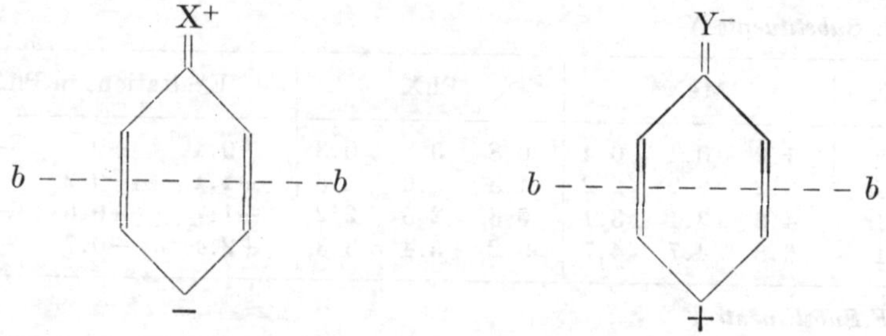

X^+ Y^-

b - - - - - - - - - b b - - - - - - - - - b

$-$ $+$

Such unevennesses of bond multiplicity round the ring must reduce the mobility of the electrons before a polarising field which seeks to move them from side to side of the ring in direction b.

The negative exaltations perpendicular to the plane of the ring, that is, in the c direction, are all small, unless electrons with principal quantum numbers greater than 2 are involved, as in chloro-, bromo-, and iodo-benzene, when the negative exaltations rise in magnitude with the principal quantum number of the halogen valency shell. This can be ascribed to the contractions, which the $3p$, $4p$, and $5p$ orbitals of chloro-, bromo-, and iodo-benzene, respectively, must undergo when they become $np\pi$ electrons in conjugation with the $2p\pi$ shell of benzene. The contractions will increase along the series $Cl < Br < I$, and, as they are in the c direction, they will produce negative exaltations in the c direction, increasing in magnitude along the series $Cl < Br < I$.

The LeFèvres' results for t-butyl chloride, bromide, and iodide are in Table 10-14. As compared with methyl halides, these t-butyl halides exhibit exaltations of polarisability along the a axis, that is, along the line of carbon-halogen bond. In the chloride, the exaltation is somewhat small, but for the bromide and iodide the exaltations are quite large. The a axis is the axis of resultant hyperconjugation. The exaltations increase with the atomic weight of the halogen, as in the benzene series. Again we would assume that polar excited states involving larger halogéns lie lower.

As in the benzene series, the positive longitudinal exaltations are accompanied by negative exaltations in the transverse directions: But in these aliphatic systems, the negative exaltations are small throughout. In particular, they do not increase with the atomic

TABLE 10-14.—DIRECTED POLARISABILITIES (IN A³ PER MOLECULE FOR D LIGHT) OF HALOGENS IN METHYL AND *t*-BUTYL HALIDES.

The axis *a* is the dipole axis. The axes *b* and *c* perpendicular to it are equivalent.

X	MeX		*t*-BuX		Exaltation in *t*-BuX	
	a	*b* = *c*	*a*	*b* = *c*	Δa	$\Delta b = \Delta c$
Cl	3.2	2.2	3.9	1.6	+0.7	−0.6
Br	4.6	3.1	6.0	2.6	+1.4	−0.5
I	6.8	4.7	8.8	4.2	+2.0	−0.5

weight of the halogen, as they should not on account of hyperconjugation, inasmuch as only $np\sigma$ halogen electrons, and not $np\pi$ as in the aromatic system, would be involved in conjugative interaction.

(11) SYMMETRY AND DIMENSIONS

(11a) Symmetry of Conjugated Unsaturated Molecules.—The most important methods by which information may be won concerning the geometry of molecules are through infra-red, micro-wave, and Raman spectroscopy, and by electron and X-ray diffraction. Spectroscopy, besides providing some very sensitive tests for molecular symmetry, can give highly accurate values for the dimensions of very simple molecules. Diffraction yields dimensional values of lower accuracy, but it can give them for a much larger variety of molecules.

The basis of all spectroscopic tests for symmetry is simply that symmetry leads to internal compensation between the interactions of the electromagnetic radiation with the "parts" of a symmetrical molecule, and so produces a null effect, exactly as when mesotartaric acid refuses to turn the plane of polarisation of light, although its separate "halves" would do so.

A molecule which can vibrate in some particular way will absorb light of the frequency of the vibration, if this motion produces an alternating electric moment (possibly superposed on a permanent dipole moment—but that is immaterial), as in the stretching vibrations of polar bonds. If we have two such bonds stretching and contracting in phase, if they are completely identical in length, elasticity, mass, polarity, and variation of polarity with length, and if they are oriented at precisely 180° to each other, then, and only then, will the alternating moments cancel, and there will be no absorption where we might have expected a band to appear. The same will happen if there are three exactly identical bonds arranged at exactly 120° to one another.

The carbonate and nitrate ions were originally thought to be non-trigonal molecules, each having one double bond and two single bonds.

Later, the theory of mesomerism represented them as trigonally symmetrical, each bond having a content of 8/3 electrons. Schaefer established, by the method explained, that they have, indeed, exact trigonal symmetry: their all-in-phase bond-stretching frequency, the so-called "breathing frequency," known from the Raman spectrum, is completely absent from the infra-red absorption spectrum.[39]

The Raman spectra of these ions show, in a similar way, that the ions are flat, though this is less interesting, because nobody ever thought otherwise. The transaction between radiation and molecule that produces a Raman spectrum is different from that which leads to absorption: a vibration will scatter Raman radiation if the vibration confers on the molecule an oscillating polarisability (of course, superposed on the permanent polarisability). If we suppose, at first, that the carbonate ion, in its equilibrium configuration, might be a pyramid of any height, then the polarisability will depend on the height, passing through a stationary value as the height passes through zero, that is, as the carbon atom is taken through the plane of the oxygen atoms. Therefore, when the carbon atom is executing small vibrations about its equilibrium position, up and down the trigonal axis, there will be a change of polarisability if the equilibrium configuration is pyramidal, but no change if it is planar: a Raman band should be produced in the former case, but not in the latter. In fact, the out-of-plane vibration frequency, known from the infra-red spectrum (because it produces an alternating electric moment), is absent from the Raman spectrum. The same is true for the nitrate ion.

Benzene has similarly been shown to have exact planar hexagonal symmetry (Chapter IV), and not any lower symmetry, such as that of a Kekulé structure, or that of the puckered hexagonal model which was at one time suggested. The forms of internal compensation which distinguish these symmetries are slightly more complicated than the forms illustrated above, but the general principles are the same.

(11b) Dimensions of Non-conjugated Molecules.—The most accurately known molecular dimensions are those obtained spectroscopically by the analysis of rotational frequencies. The more useful spectra are the infra-red and micro-wave spectra. The analysis directly yields the principal moments of inertia of the molecule, of which there are three, although in linear molecules one is almost zero, in planar molecules the sum of two almost equals the third, and in symmetrical molecules two, or all three, may have identical values: the symmetry laws governing identity of value, and location of axes, are exactly as

[39] C. Schaefer, *Trans. Faraday Soc.*, 1929, **24**, 841; C. Schaefer and C. Bormuth, *Z. physik*, 1930, **62**, 508.

for electrical polarisability (Section **10d**). From the measured, independent values of principal moments of inertia of a molecule, one can calculate the same number of interatomic distances. If the number of independent, non-symmetry-related, distances needed to determine the geometry of the molecule is greater than the number of independent principal moments of inertia, we can suitably multiply the number of measured moments of inertia by repeating the spectroscopic investigation with isotopic modifications of the molecule: isotopic substitution changes masses, and therefore moments of inertia, but it does not change the geometry of a molecule. Thus HCN, a linear molecule, has two equal, non-vanishing, principal moments of inertia, leading to only one finite value, while there are two independent interatomic distances to be found: one can find both if one investigates both HCN and DCN.

TABLE 11-1.—SOME SPECTRALLY-MEASURED BOND LENGTHS AND BOND ANGLES.

	X or XY length (A)	XH length (A)	$\widehat{HXH}$ angle
OH_2	—	0.957	105.0°
NH_3	—	1.014	106.8°
CH_4[1]	—	1.092	109.5°
$CH_3—CH_3$[1]	1.536	1.091	108.0°
$CH_3—OH$[2]	1.434	1.093	109.5°
$CH_2{=}CH_2$	1.338	1.085	117.4°
$CH_2{=}O$[3]	1.206	1.117	115.8°
$CH{\equiv}CH$	1.205	1.059	—
$CH{\equiv}N$	1.157	1.063	—

[1] D. W. Lepard, D. M. C. Sweeney, and L. H. Welsh, *J. Chem. Phys.*, 1962' **40**, 1567.

[2] E. V. Ivash and D. M. Dennison, *J. Chem. Phys.*, 1953, **21**, 1804. Their further results were that the OH length was 0.937 A and the COH angle 105.9°. They found that the symmetry axis of the CH_3 group passes between the hydroxyl O and H atoms 0.079 A from the O atom, *i.e.*, that the C—O bond is bent back from the tetrahedral direction by 3.0°.

[3] T. Oka, *J. Phys. Soc. Japan*, 1960, **15**, 2274.

This is how the quantitative geometrical knowledge has been obtained,[40] to which some reference has already been made, for example, that bond angles $\widehat{HXH}$ in H_2O, H_2S, and H_2Se are 105°, 92°, and 91°, respectively, in NH_3, PH_3, AsH_3, and SbH_3 are 107°, 94°, 92°, and 91°, respectively, and in ethylene and formaldehyde are 117° and 116°, respectively; that CH bond lengths diminish along the series, ethane, ethylene, acetylene (the values are 1.102, 1.085, and 1.059 A, respec-

[40] G. Herzberg, "Infra-red and Raman Spectra," Van Nostrand, New York, 1945, Chap. 4.

tively); and that CC bond lengths diminish strongly along the same series (1.543, 1.338, and 1.205 *A*, respectively). Some important spectrally measured bond lengths and bond angles are given in Table 11-1.[40,41]

Many more individual bond lengths than these have been measured by diffraction methods: values obtained by X-ray diffraction in solids are good to about ±0.01 *A* at best, or, more usually, ±0.02 *A*, while those derived by the method of electron diffraction in gases involve uncertainties which are often between ±0.02 *A* and ±0.04 *A*. It is suspected that, in measurements on crystals, bond lengths are sometimes rendered slightly anomalous by lattice forces.

The most general result which has emerged from a large body of diffraction measurements is that, excepting in the presence of conjugated unsaturated systems, and of some hyperconjugated systems, the length of a bond is, often to within the estimated error of measurement, though sometimes less exactly, characteristic of its *type* (that is, of the pair of atoms involved) and of its *multiplicity* (whether it is single, double, or triple).

As to the effect of the nature of the two atoms on the length of a bond of given multiplicity, it has been noticed that, provided that conjugated systems are excluded, the length of a bond AB often approximates to the arithmetic mean of the lengths of the bonds AA and BB: this means that bond lengths can be analysed into a set of radii, which are characteristic of the atoms and of the multiplicities of the bonds, and when added together reproduce the bond lengths. The best documented set of *covalent bond radii* is that given by Pauling,[42] some of whose figures are reproduced in Table 11-2. It is to be understood that the additive relation does not pretend to be more than approximate; but it is a very useful, and often a close, approximation.

As to the effect of bond multiplicity on the length of a bond between the same pair of atoms, the strong trend, illustrated in Table 11-1 by the CC bond lengths of ethane, ethylene, and acetylene, is quite general. It is accommodated in the scheme of bond radii by assigning to each atom that forms multiple bonds different radii according to the multiplicities of the bonds. This is made clear in Table 11-2.

(11c) Dimensions of Conjugated Molecules.—Along the series ethane, ethylene, and acetylene, the CC bond shortens with a contraction proportional to the logarithm of the multiplicity of the bond, and from methanol to formaldehyde the CO bond suffers a parallel con-

[41] C. C. Costain and B. P. Stoicheff, *J. Chem. Phys.*, 1959, **30**, 777. This is a compilation of precision data for CC and CH bond lengths. Full references are given to the original literature. But for certain molecules, use is here made of more recent data contained in the references under the table.

[42] L. Pauling, "Nature of the Chemical Bond," 3rd Edn., p. 221.

TABLE 11-2.—PAULING'S COVALENT RADII OF ATOMS (IN A).

	C	N	O	F
Single bond	0.772	0.70	0.66	0.64
Double bond	0.667	0.60	0.55	
Triple bond	0.603	0.55		
	Si	P	S	Cl
Single bond	1.17	1.10	1.04	0.99
Double bond			0.94	
Triple bond		0.93		
	Ge	As	Se	Br
Single bond	1.22	1.21	1.17	1.14
	Sn	Sb	Te	I
Single bond	1.40	1.41	1.37	1.33

traction (Fig. 11-1). The term "bond order" is not used here, because different definitions of it derive from different approximate quantal treatments. The term "bond multiplicity" derives only from the common expression "multiple bond," and means one-half of the electron content of the bond.

When mesomerism introduces symmetry into a molecule, we can assign to the bonds a proper-fractional multiplicity, such as $\frac{3}{2}$ and $\frac{4}{3}$ for the CC bonds of benzene and graphite, respectively, or for the CO

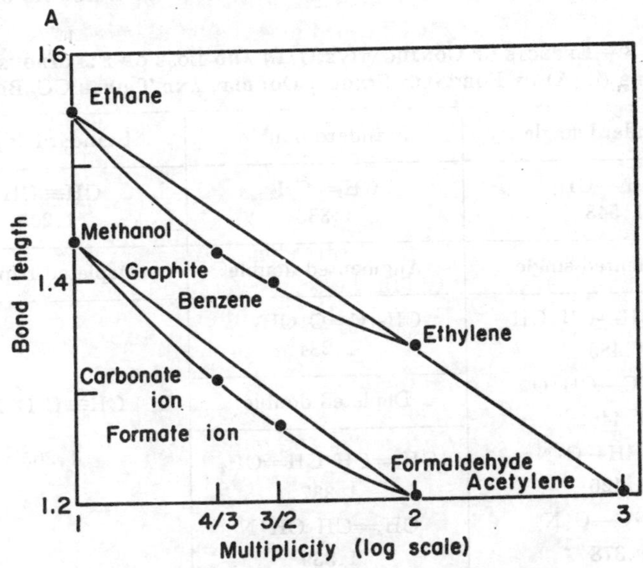

FIG. 11-1.—Bond length versus bond multiplicity.

bonds of the formate and carbonate ions, respectively. From ethane or methanol to these compounds, the CC or CO bonds show a greater contraction than the semi-logarithmically linear ones with increasing bond multiplicity. This is because we have not only added more electrons to the bonds, but also delocalised the added electrons, so making the binding stronger on two counts.

When mesomerism, without introducing new symmetry, makes a somewhat small, and not exactly known, addition of delocalised electrons to a formally single bond, we may expect a relatively large shortening of the bond for the same two mutually reinforcing reasons. When mesomerism makes a correspondingly small reduction in the electron content of a formally double bond or formally triple bond, and at the same time delocalises the electrons that are left behind, we do not expect much, if any, increase in the length of the bond, because the depletion and the delocalisation work in opposite ways. When hyperconjugative mesomerism reduces the electron content of a single bond, there is more likelihood of a substantial increase in length, because the deviation from the single bond is towards a "no-bond" structure of indefinite extension. Some of these qualitative deductions are illustrated by the curved lines in Fig. 11-1. Some experimental results for CC bonds are shown in Table 11-3.[41] When conjugation supplies extra electrons which are delocalised to a single or a double CC bond, the bond is shortened by 0.05–0.16 *A*. When conjugation depletes but delocalises the electrons of a double or triple

TABLE 11-3.—EFFECTS OF CONJUGATIVE GAIN AND LOSS OF ELECTRONS IN THE LENGTHS (IN A) OF FORMALLY SINGLE, DOUBLE, AND TRIPLE CC BONDS.

Standard single	Standard double	Standard triple
CH_3—CH_3 1.543	CH_2=CH_2 1.338	CH≡CH 1.205
Augmented single	Augmented double	Depleted triple
CH_2:CH—CH:CH_2 1.483	CH_2:C=C:CH_2 1.284	
CH⋮C—CH:O 1.446	Depleted double	CH≡C·C⋮N 1.205
CH_2:CH—C⋮N 1.426	CH_2=CH·CH=CH_2 1.337	
CH⋮C—C⋮N 1.378	CH_2=CH·CH⋮N 1.339	

CC bond, the bond is not detectably changed in length, that is, not by more than 0.005 *A*.

Suggestions have been made that the observed bond shortenings owe nothing to electron redistribution and delocalisation, but are due entirely to changes in the hybrid constitution, as from sp^3 to sp^2 or *sp*, of the carbon orbitals used to form the bond. Of course, such hybridisation changes of atomic orbitals are involved; but if they were given total responsibility for the molecular phenomena, then, on passing along the series —C—A, ═C—A, ≡C—A, the C—A shortenings, if we may use bond radii, should be independent of A. They are not. And if we may not use bond radii, the first simple explanation of the molecular property of bond lengths to suffer would be one which relies wholly on the purely atomic property of orbital hybridisation. For A-H, we know with some precision[41] the CH bond lengths given in Table 11-4, which also shows the differences. From them it follows by the orbital interpretation that a single bond, between two double bonds, between a double and a triple bond, and between two triple bonds, should be shortened by 0.014, 0.04, and 0.06 *A* in the respective cases. The observed shortenings, as will be seen from Table 11-3, are three or four times larger than these values, *viz.*, 0.06, 0.12, and 0.17 *A*, respectively.[43]

The compilation of bond lengths in Table 11-5 further illustrates points already made. Single bonds which fractionally gain multi-

TABLE 11-4.—EFFECTS OF CARBON UNSATURATION ON THE LENGTHS (IN A) OF CH BONDS.

$H—CH_2 \cdot CH_3$	$H—CH{:}CH_2$	$H—C⋮CH$
1.0914	1.085	1.059
	$H—C_6H_5$	$H—C⋮N$
	1.084	1.063
	0.007	0.023
	0.030	

[43] C. A. Coulson, "Volume Commémoratif Victor Henri," Maison Desoir, Liège, 1948, p. 15. The single CC-bond length of gaseous butadiene is a difficult measurement. If we go by the consistent X-ray values for the corresponding bond of crystalline all-*trans* sorbamide, methyl muconate, and mucononitrile, *viz.*, 1.452 ± 0.002 *A* (S. E. Filippakis, L. Leiserowitz, and G. M. J. Schmidt, *J. Chem. Soc.*, **1967**, B, 290, 297, 305), the shortening of the single bond becomes 0.09 rather than 0.06 *A*.

TABLE 11-5.—BOND LENGTHS IN CONJUGATED COMPOUNDS.

Compound	Bond	Calc. from radii (*A*)[1]	Found (*A*)		Method[2]	Ref.
			Unsaturated Halogen Compounds			
$C_6H_5 \cdot Cl$	C·Cl	1.76	1.69	±0.02	E	3
o-, *m*-, *p*-$C_6H_4Cl_2$	C·Cl	1.76	1.69–1.71	±0.02	E	3
C_6Cl_6	C·Cl	1.76	1.70	±0.02	E	3
$CH_2:CH \cdot Cl$	C·Cl	1.76	1.69	±0.02	E	4
1:1-, 1:2-$C_2H_4Cl_2$	C·Cl	1.76	1.67–1.71	±0.02	E	4
C_2Cl_4	C·Cl	1.76	1.73	±0.02	E	4
$CH\vdots C \cdot Cl$	C·Cl	1.76	1.68	±0.04	E	5
$CH\vdots C \cdot Br$	C·Br	1.91	1.80	±0.03	E	5
$N\vdots C \cdot Cl$	C·Cl	1.76	1.629	—	S	6
$N\vdots C \cdot Br$	C·Br	1.91	1.790	—	S	6
			Nitro-compounds			
$CH_3 \cdot NO_2$	N·O	1.36	1.22	±0.02	E	7
	N:O	1.15	1.22	±0.02	E	7
$C(NO_2)_4$	N·O	1.36	1.22	±0.02	E	8
	N:O	1.15	1.22	±0.02	E	8
			Carboxylate Ion			
$H \cdot CO_2Na$	C·O	1.43	1.27	±0.01	X	9
	C:O	1.22	1.27	±0.01	X	9
$\overset{+}{N}H_3 \cdot CH_2 \cdot CO_2^-$	C·O	1.43	1.26	±0.02	X	10
	C:O	1.22	1.26	±0.02	X	10
			Carbonate and Nitrate Ions			
$CaCO_3$	C·O	1.43	1.31	±0.01	X	11
	C:O	1.22	1.31	±0.01	X	11
$NaNO_3$	N·O	1.36	1.21	±0.01	X	11
	N:O	1.15	1.21	±0.01	X	11
$N_2O_5(NO_3^-$ ion)	N·O	1.36	1.243	±0.01	X	18
	N:O	1.15	1.243	±0.01	X	18
			Carboxylamide			
$CH_3 \cdot CO \cdot NH_2$	C·N	1.47	1.38	±0.05	X	12
	C:O	1.22	1.28	±0.05	X	12
			Carbonamide			
$CO(NH_2)_2$	C·N	1.47	1.37	±0.01	X	13
	C:O	1.22	1.25	±0.01	X	13

[1] Radii from Table 11-2.
[2] E = electron diffraction. X = X-ray diffraction. S = spectroscopy.
[3] L. O. Brockway and K. J. Palmer, *J. Am. Chem. Soc.*, 1937, 59, 2181.
[4] L. O. Brockway, J. Y. Beach, and L. Pauling, *ibid.*, 1935, 57, 2690.

TABLE 11-5.—(Continued)

Compound	Bond	Calc. from radii (A)[1]	Found (A)		Method[2]	Ref.
Azo-Compounds						
trans-Ph·N:N·Ph	C·N	1.47	1.41	±0.03	X	14
	N:N	1.20	1.23	±0.03	X	14
cis-Ph·N:N·Ph	C·N	1.47	1.46	±0.03	X	15
	N:N	1.20	1.23	±0.03	X	15
Carbon Dioxide and the Azide and Nitronium Ions						
O:C:O	C:O	1.22	1.1632	±0.0003	S	16
NaN_3, KN_3, NH_4N_3	N:N	1.20	1.15–1.16	±0.02	X	17
NO_2ClO_4	N:O	1.15	1.10	±0.01	X	18

[5] L. O. Brockway and I. E. Coop, *Trans. Faraday Soc.*, 1938, **34**, 1429.
[6] C. H. Towers, A. N. Holden, and F. R. Merritt, *Phys Rev.*, 1948, **74**, 113.
[7] F. Rogowski, *Ber.*, 1942, **75**, 244.
[8] A. J. Stosick, *J. Am. Chem. Soc.*, 1939, **61**, 1127.
[9] L. Pauling and L. O. Brockway, *Proc. Nat. Acad. Sci.* (U. S.), 1934, **20**, 336.
[10] W. H. Zachariasen, *Phys. Rev.*, 1938, **53**, 917.
[11] N. Elliot, *J. Am. Chem. Soc.*, 1937, **59**, 1380.
[12] F. Senti and D. Harker, *ibid.*, 1940, **62**, 2008.
[13] R. W. J. Wykoff and R. B. Cory, *Z. Krist.*, 1934, **89**, 462.
[14] J. J. de Lange, J. M. Robertson, and I. Woodward, *ibid.*, 1939, **A**, **171**, 398; J. M. Robertson, *J. Chem. Soc.*, **1939**, 232.
[15] G. C. Hampson and J. M. Robertson, *J. Chem. Soc.*, **1941**, 409.
[16] E. F. Barker and A. Adel, *Phys. Rev.*, 1933, **44**, 185; G. Herzberg, "Infra-red and Raman Spectra," pp. 394, 398.
[17] L. K. Frevel, *Z. Krist.*, 1936, **94**, 197; *J. Am. Chem. Soc.*, **1936**, **58**, 779.
[18] P. E. Grison, K. Ericks, and de Vries, *Acta Cryst.*, 1950, **3**, 290; M. R. Truter, D. J. Cruickshank, and G. A. Jeffery, *Acta Cryst.*, 1960, **13**, 855.

plicity by conjugation are always substantially shortened, whilst double bonds which fractionally thus lose multiplicity are either not lengthened or not much lengthened.

We have defined the term *secondary steric effect* (Section **6f**), and have referred to its discovery by Hampson, through its manifestation in dipole moments (Section **8g**). We also noted a second physical manifestation of it in heats of reaction (Section **9b**). We now find a physical manifestation of it in the field of bond lengths, as illustrated in Table 11-5 by the CN bond lengths in *cis*- and *trans*-azobenzene. The theory is just the same as for the heats of hydrogenation of *cis*- and *trans*-stilbene (Section **9b**). *trans*-Azobenzene is a planar molecule: mesomerism, involving the addition of delocalised electrons to the formally single CN bonds, is not stereochemically restricted; and hence these bonds should be shortened, as, indeed, they are—by 0.06 *A*. However, *cis*-azobenzene cannot attain planarity, because the ortho-CH-groups of the benzene rings would overlap. The crystal analysis shows that the planes of the benzene rings are twisted (Fig. 11-2) at angles of 56° out of the plane defined by the four atoms C·N:N·C, so providing a clearance of 3.3 *A* between ortho-carbon atoms, a clearance almost equal to the graphite layer-plane separation (3.4 *A*). This inhibits mesomeric electron redistribution between the azo-group and the benzene rings, and, consistently, Hampson and Robertson found that the CN bonds are not significantly shortened.

Further reference will be made to the dimensions of aromatic molecules in Chapter IV.

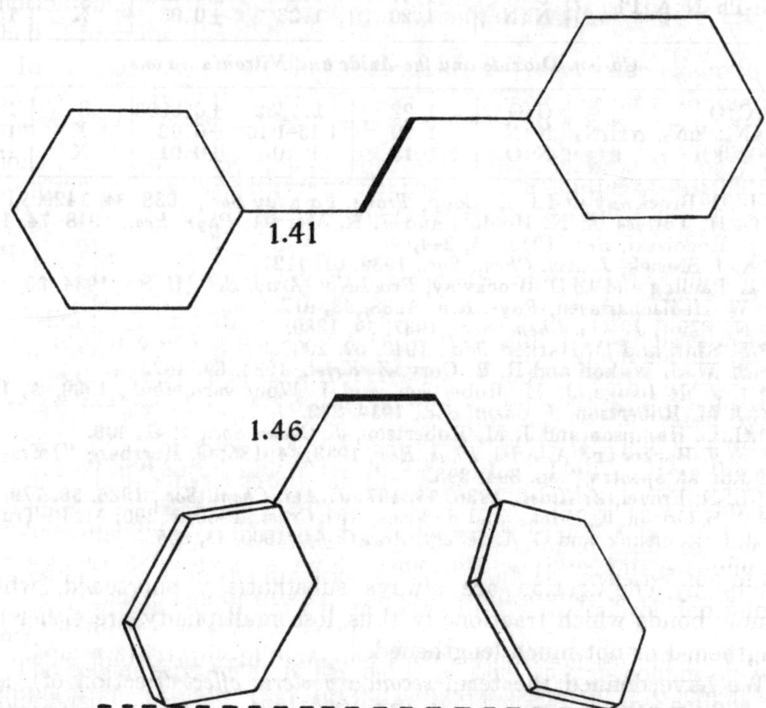

Fig. 11-2.—Geometrical forms of *trans*- and *cis*-azobenzene. The *trans*-compound is planar, but the planes of the benzene rings in the *cis*-compound are twisted (like a three-blade fan, with one blade removed) to give a clearance between ortho-positions about equal to the graphite layer-plane separation. The twisting stops conjugation between the rings and the nitrogen atoms, and thus the CN bonds are not shortened, as they are in the *trans*-isomeride.

(11d) Dimensions of Hyperconjugated Molecules.—As Table 11-6 will illustrate, the single CC bond between a methyl group and doubly or triply bonded carbon is shortened relatively to the bond between a methyl group and an alkyl residue. For doubly bonded carbon, this has been adequately established by the microwave method, in the example, no. 1 in the table, of acetaldehyde. The CC bond is here shortened by 0.042 *A*. For triply bonded carbon, the greater shorten-

TABLE 11-6.—SINGLE CC BOND LENGTHS (IN A) IN MOLECULES ALLOWING CH-BOND HYPERCONJUGATION (+M).

No.	Example	Length	Shortening	Method[1]
	Single Bond between Methyl and Alkyl			
—	$CH_3—CH_3$	1.543	—	S
	Single Bond between Methyl and Double-bonded Carbon			
1	$CH_3—CH{:}O$	1.501	0.042	S
	Single Bond between Methyl and Triple-bonded Carbon			
2	$CH_3—C\vdots CH$	1.46 ±0.02		E
		1.459	0.084	S
3	$CH_3—C\vdots N$	1.49 ±0.03		E
		1.458	0.085	S
4	$CH_3—C\vdots C\cdot C\vdots N$	1.454	0.089	S
5	$CH_3—C\vdots C—CH_3$	1.47 ±0.02	~0.07	E
6	$CH_3—C\vdots C\cdot C\vdots C—CH_3$	1.47 ±0.02	~0.07	E

[1] S = Spectroscopic data from ref. 41. E = electron-diffraction results by L. Pauling, H. D. Springall, and K. J. Palmer. *J. Am. Chem. Soc.*, 1939, **61**, 927.

ing of the single bond was originally demonstrated by Pauling, Springall, and Palmer by an electron-diffraction study of examples 2, 3, 5, and 6 in Table 11-6. Microwave studies by Trambarulo, Gordy, and others have since provided data of precision in examples 2, 3, and 4. The comparison of figures in examples 2 and 3 confirms that the electron diffraction results were reliable to within the accuracy claimed for them, and this increases our confidence in results 5 and 6. The accurately measured shortenings range from 0.084 *A* in methylacetylene to 0.089 *A* in methylcyanoacetylene.

We have encountered evidence of hyperconjugation in other physical properties, *e.g.*, in dipole moments (Sections **8b** and **8e**), and in heats of reaction (Section **9a**); and these bond-length changes seem best interpreted similarly, as in the example

$$H_3C—C\equiv CH$$

We assume that an addition of delocalised electrons to the single CC bond shortens the bond and is responsible for more than one-half of the observed shortening. The greater shortening with triply than with doubly bound carbon is easily understood. We could not confidently expect the electron depletion concurrent with delocalisation in the flanking bonds to have any observable effects on these lengths; and no such effect is observed.

Again a case has been pressed for interpreting these bond shortenings by changes in the hybrid constitution of the carbon atomic orbitals, without hyperconjugation, that is, without electron redistribution and delocalisation. But the previous answer applies, *viz.*, that, if this were true, the shortenings from —C—A to =C—A and to ≡C—A should be independent of A; whereas the observed shortenings are more than twice as great as those which would be deduced on these principles. Once again, the conclusion is, not that atomic orbital hybridisation makes no difference to the bond lengths, but that the shortenings owe much of their magnitude to hyperconjugation.[44]

TABLE 11-7.—SINGLE BOND LENGTHS (IN A) IN MOLECULES ALLOWING BOTH CH AND CHAL HYPERCONJUGATION (+M AND −M)[1].

Example	CC Length	Shortening[2]	CHal Length	Lengthening[2]
$ClCH_2 \cdot C \vdots CH$	1.47 ± 0.02	∼0.07	1.82 ± 0.02	∼0.06
$BrCH_2 \cdot C \vdots CH$	1.47 ± 0.02	∼0.07	1.95 ± 0.02	∼0.04
$ICH_2 \cdot C \vdots CH$	1.47 ± 0.02	∼0.07	2.13 ± 0.03	∼0.03

[1] Electron-diffraction data by L. Pauling, W. Gordy, and J. H. Saylor (*J. Am. Chem. Soc.*, 1942, **64**, 1733).

[2] The deviations of bond length are relative to the summed covalent radii from Table 11-2.

The results of Pauling, Gordy, and Saylor's electron-diffraction measurements on propargyl chloride, bromide, and iodide are summarised in Table 11-7. The CC single bonds in these compounds had the uniform length 1.47 ± 0.02 *A*. They are therefore significantly shortened. Having regard to the authors' estimate of error, the shortenings are not significantly different from what would be expected from CH hyperconjugation, $+M$, involving the two hydrogen atoms available for such in these examples. But neither are they distinguishably different from what might result from the combined effect of this CH hyperconjugation, $+M$, and a CHal hyperconjugation, $-M$. Both forms of hyperconjugation should contribute to the shortening:

[44] This was D. P. Craig's view in 1951, before the micro-wave precision data on bond lengths had become available (*cf.* the first edition of this book, p. 148, footnote).

$$H_2C(Hal)—C≡CH$$

The presence of the —*M* type hyperconjugation, involving the halogen atom, is suggested by the observed lengthenings of the CHal bonds, in two cases by more than the limits of experimental error, as Table 11-7 shows. It seems possible that electron depletion in the CHal bonds, where the bonding electrons become partly non-bonding, dominates the bond length.

(12) MECHANICAL ELASTICITY

(12a) Significance of Elastic Constants.—Spectroscopically observed vibration frequencies can be used to measure the stiffness of molecules. The main quantitative measure of stiffness is the Hooke's-law constant, or elastic modulus, or *force constant* (to give it its usual name), applying to a specified type of small deformation.

For diatomic molecules there is no uncertainty about what is meant by a force constant: it is the constant k which, for small deformations, in accordance with Hooke's law, connects the potential energy of deformation, V, with the displacement, Δx, of the one internal co-ordinate, x, namely, the length of the bond:

$$2V = k(\Delta x)^2$$

An equivalent statement is that the constant k is the restoring force per unit length-change. It is measured directly by the vibration frequency, ν, the formula being as follows,

$$4\pi^2\nu^2 = \frac{k}{m} = k\left(\frac{1}{m_1} + \frac{1}{m_2}\right)$$

where m is the "reduced mass" of the molecule, m_1 and m_2 being the masses of the atoms. If the vibrational amplitude is not small, we should make a correction for "anharmonicity," that is, for deviations from Hooke's law: such deviations take the form of admitting a partial dependence of V on higher powers of Δx than the second.

In the general case of an n-atomic molecule, the potential energy is a function of all the $3n-6$ internal co-ordinates;[45] and since, under Hooke's law, it is a quadratic function, it will be the sum of $(3n-6)(3n-5)/2$ terms, like $k(\Delta x)^2$ or $k'(\Delta x \cdot \Delta y)$, each with its own force constant k. The number of vibration frequencies, $3n-6$, even supposing

[45] There is one more internal co-ordinate in the special case of linear molecules.

they are all observed, is not enough[46] to determine all these k's. There are two ways out of this difficulty. The most satisfactory procedure is to measure the vibration frequencies of a sufficient number of isotopically different forms of the molecule, to make the total number of observed frequencies at least as great as the number of force constants (which are not changed by isotopic substitution). However, the usual plan, and often the only feasible plan, is to neglect those terms in the potential-energy function which are believed to be the least important, retaining not more terms than the number of the frequencies, indeed, fewer terms, if, by a judicious choice, they can be made to give a reasonably good account of the frequencies.

If such a choice includes, as it does in the much-used, approximate, potential-energy function known as the *valency force field*, one term, $k(\Delta x)^2$, for each bond, where Δx is the length-change for that bond, then k is said to be the *force constant for the bond*. In contrast to their status with respect to diatomic molecules, the bond force constants of polyatomic molecules are essentially approximation concepts: one must not try to express them too accurately. They depend on what parts of the potential energy function were chosen for discard, what other terms, besides the $k(\Delta x)^2$ terms, have been retained. The existence, in the full function, of terms like $k'(\Delta x \cdot \Delta y)$ implies that the energy of deformation cannot really be parcelled out additively among the bonds.

In the valency force field, another set of terms is included. They are of the form $\delta(\Delta\theta)^2$, and apply one to each valency angle, $\Delta\theta$ being the angular deformation: the constant δ, which is the restoring moment per unit angle-change, is called the *moment constant*, or, more often, the *bending force constant* for the valency angle. When resisted torsion is believed to be present, terms like $\gamma\phi^2$ are added, ϕ being the angle of twist: γ, the restoring moment per radian of twist, is called the *twisting force constant*. These angular force constants are, on the whole, cruder approximations, and less characteristic of the structural features to which they apply, than are the bond force constants.

The valency force field has been elaborated in many ways to suit special circumstances, for example, by the addition of terms in respect of the repulsive energy of near, but not directly bonded, atoms, such as the chlorine atoms in carbon tetrachloride.

(12b) Bond Force Constants and Bond Type.[47]—The force constants

[46] The numbers of different force constants, and different vibration frequencies, are both reduced in symmetrical molecules, but always the former number exceeds the latter.

[47] B. L. Crawford jr. and S. R. Brinkley, *J. Chem. Phys.*, 1941, **9**, 69; H. D. Noether, *ibid.*, 1942, **10**, 664; G. Herzberg, "Infra-red and Raman Spectra," 1945, p. 192; J. W. Linnett, *J. Chem. Phys.*, 1940, **8**, 91; *T. Faraday Soc.*,

of bonds are expressed in dynes/cm. The values obtained are of the order 10^4–10^6 dynes/cm., the majority being near the upper end of this range. Accordingly we shall quote, as is customary, values of $10^{-5}k$, in effect using 10^5 dynes/cm. as a "practical unit" of force constant.

Bond force constants are approximately characteristic of the type of bond, that is, the pair of atoms involved, and of bond multiplicity. They depend also, however, on the state and surroundings of the atoms, particularly their polarity and unsaturation, quite apart from any recognised effects which these factors may have on the multiplicity of the bond concerned.

The dependence of bond force constants on the chemical nature of the atoms may be illustrated by the constants for XH bonds in hydrides XH_n. There is a connexion with the position of the atom X in the Mendeléjeff table, as the following values show:

XH···	B	3.6[48]	C	5.0	N	6.5	O	7.6	F	9.7
			Si	2.7	P	3.1	S	4.0	Cl	5.2
							Se	3.1	Br	4.1
									I	3.1

The trend in the halogen series is repeated in the constants of XC bonds in the methyl halides, CH_3X:

XC..........F 5.6 Cl 3.4 Br 2.9 I 2.3

The simplest illustration of the effect of polarity on an XH bond constant is that given by the NH constants of ammonia, and of the ammonium ion:

NH....................NH_3 6.5 NH_4^+ 5.4

Induced polarity appears to have an appreciable influence on the force constants of CH bonds, as is shown by the following values for methyl compounds:

	$CH_3 \cdot CH_3$	$H \cdot CH_3$	$I \cdot CH_3$	$Br \cdot CH_3$	$Cl \cdot CH_3$	$F \cdot CH_3$
CH	5.1	5.0	5.0	4.95	4.9	4.7

For illustration of the effect of carbon unsaturation, or the combined influence of polarity and unsaturation, on the force constants of CH bonds, the following values are available:

	H—CH_3	H—CH:CH_2	H—C⋮CH	H—Ph	H—CH:O	H—C⋮N
CH	5.0	5.1	5.9	5.1	4.4	5.9

They are not easy to understand. The rise in the series, methane, ethylene, acetylene, might be attributed to the changing hybridisation

1941, **37**, 469; *Quart. Rev. Chem. Soc.*, 1947, **1**, 13. Linnett's values are quoted in Sections 12b and 12c.

[48] This is the value for the four exterior hydrogen atoms of B_2H_6.

(Section 4b). However, the gaps are curiously unequal; though it is consistent that the ethylene and benzene figures should agree. As the value for acetylene and hydrogen cyanide are identical, it is not obvious why those for ethylene and formaldehyde are not.

However, these are all small matters compared with that next to be noticed, namely, the effect of bond multiplicity. This is a major influence as the following figures show:

	$H_3C—CH_3$	$H_2C═CH_2$	$HC≡CH$
CC	4.5	9.8	15.6

	$H_2C═O$		$HC≡N$
CO	12.3	CN	18.1

The constants for the single, double, and triple CC bonds stand in the ratio 1:2·2:3·5. Good values are not available for the force constants of single CN and CO bonds; but if these constants may be taken as lying between those applying to CC and CF bonds, that is, in the neighbourhood of 5, then quite similar ratios would express the effect of multiplicity on the force constants of CN and CO bonds.

(12c) Force Constants, Conjugation, and Hyperconjugation.—The strong dependence of force constants on bond multiplicity leads to the expectation that the constants will reflect the altered bond multiplicities in mesomeric systems, possibly with some extra stiffening of the bonds, just as there is extra shortening, when the mesomeric energy is considerable.

The available data bear out these anticipations. The following is a list of CC bond constants, arranged, as far as possible, in order of increasing bond multiplicity:

CC	$H_3C—CH_3$	Me—C⋮CH	Me—C⋮N	N⋮C—C⋮N	C_6H_6	$H_2C═CH_2$
Mult...	1	1+	1+	1++	1.5 (m)	2
Const..	4.5	5.3	5.3	6.7	7.6	9.8

CC	$H_2C═CH_2$	$H_2C═C═CH_2$	O:C═C═C:O	MeC≡CH	HC≡CH
Mult...	2	2	2 (m)	3−	3
Const..	9.8	9.7	14.9	15.3	15.6

The upper row of entries contains two examples in which hyperconjugation (1+), and one in which ordinary conjugation (1++) should increase the multiplicity of a formal single bond: we see that the bonds are stiffened in these circumstances, which, however, do not separate the effect of the increased electron content from that of the changed orbital hybridisation. But this difficulty of interpretation does not arise in any of the examples considered below. The benzene molecule (symmetrically mesomeric, labelled m) shows somewhat more stiffening of its bonds than would be expected from a nominal multiplicity of 1.5. The lower set of entries contains allene, with no conjugation, and no stiffening of its double bonds, carbon suboxide, with conjugation (m), and much stiffening, even though there can be no increase in multiplicity in the CC bonds, because the central carbon atom has not the orbitals. In methylacetylene hyperconjugation should reduce the multiplicity of the formal triple bond (3—), and we do observe a decrease in the force constant. Here, no question of a hybridisation change can arise.

The carbonyl force constants listed below appear to be similarly related, except that one would have expected the constant for keten to bracket itself more evenly between the constants for formaldehyde and carbon suboxide:

CO	$H_2C{=}O$	$H_2C{:}C{=}O$	$O{=}C{:}C{:}C{=}O$	$O{=}C{=}O$
Mult.	2	2++	2++ (m)	2 (m)
Const.	12.3	12.3	14.2	15.5

The stiff bond of carbon dioxide is evidently to be associated with the very large mesomeric energy of that molecule (m): the multiplicity of the bonds cannot be increased, since the carbon atom has no suitable orbitals.

The force constants of the cyano-group show some interesting effects of hyperconjugation with methyl, and of conjugation with either a second cyano-group or with halogen atoms. All these forms of hyperconjugation (3 –), or of conjugation (3 – –), reduce the multiplicity of the formal triple bond, and are associated with decreases in its force constant. The decreases cannot be ascribed to hybridisation changes without electron transfer in any of these examples.

CN	$HC{\equiv}N$	$Me{\cdot}C{\equiv}N$	$N{\equiv}C{\cdot}C{\equiv}N$	$I{\cdot}C{\equiv}N$	$Br{\cdot}C{\equiv}N$	$Cl{\cdot}C{\equiv}N$
Mult.	3	3 –	3 – –	3 – –	3 – –	3 – –
Const.	18.1	17.5	17.5	16.8	16.8	16.7

The theory of hyperconjugation was introduced as the result of observations of reaction rates and equilibria (Section **7i**), but we have now noted four physical properties that the concept helps us to interpret (Sections **8b**, **8e**, **9a**, **11d** and this Section). In spite of some criticism, the idea does seem too useful to be discarded.

As a final illustration, we may compare the CHal force constants of cyanogen halides with those of methyl halides:

CHal					
Cl—CN	5.3	Br—CN	4.2	I—CN	2.9
$Cl{-}CH_3$	3.4	$Br{-}CH_3$	2.9	$I{-}CH_3$	2.3

The constants for the cyanogen halides are the larger; and although this might be in part an effect of polarity, the difference is so great for the chlorides, and falls so sharply towards the iodides, as to suggest strongly that conjugation, with increase in bond multiplicity, is an important cause of the difference, at least in the case of the chlorides: for such conjugation should be the more effective the smaller the halogen (Section **7e**).

CHAPTER IV

Aromaticity, and More on Physical Properties

(13) THEORY OF AROMATIC CHARACTER

(13a) Development of the Theory of Benzene Structure.[1]—In 1825 Faraday isolated benzene from coal gas. In 1834 Mitscherlich obtained it by distilling benzoic acid with lime. These investigators could not know that their substance was to become recognised as the parent of by far the largest series of organic chemical compounds. The rapid extension which this branch of chemistry underwent in later decades was dependent on the success in the first steps taken to develop a theory of the structure of benzene.

In the early 1860's organic chemistry was emerging from the type theory. Through the efforts of Frankland, Williamson, Kekulé, and others, the rules of valency, and of formulation of structures, had been made clear, largely by reference to compounds of the aliphatic series. However, there also existed a group of "aromatic" substances, not yet very numerous, which in composition and behaviour differed from aliphatic compounds, and seemed to form a notable exception to the rules of structure, and of valency. In 1865, Kekulé showed how this anomaly might be removed, pointing out that aromatic compounds could be brought within the established rules, if it were assumed that all contained a common "nucleus" of six carbon atoms.[2] He then proceeded to develop his hypothesis that the atoms formed a ring of alternate single and double bonds, leaving each atom with one unit of combining power. He believed, though he admitted that he could not prove, that the six combining positions were equivalent.

The next few decades were characterised by intense activity in the building of the main frame of aromatic chemistry. By 1874 Ladenburg had completed a proof of Kekulé's postulate of six-fold equivalence: the demonstration was improved and simplified in 1878 by Wroblewsky, and in 1879 by Hübner.[3]

[1] The earlier development is charmingly reviewed by A. Lachmann, "The Spirit of Organic Chemistry," Macmillan, New York, 1899, Chap. 3.

[2] F. A. Kekulé, *Bull. soc. chim.* (France), 1865, **3**, 98; *Ann.*, 1866, **137**, 169; "Lehrbuch der organische Chemie," Enke, Erlangen, 1866, **2**, 493.

[3] A. Ladenburg, *Ber.*, 1869, **2**, 140; *Ann.*, 1874, **172**, 344; E. Wroblewsky, *Ber.*, 1872, **5**, 30; *Ann.*, 1873, **168**, 153; 1878, **192**, 196; H. Hübner and A. Peterman, *ibid.*, 1869, **149**, 130; H. Hübner, *ibid.*, 1879, **195**, 1.

Wroblewky's demonstration still ranks as one of the best examples of the method and logic of organic-chemical structure-determination. He prepared the five then conceivable monobromobenzoic acids in order to see how many of them were different. The starting point for all preparations was *p*-toluidine, whose methyl group marked the position of the final carboxyl group. The principle of the method was to introduce bromine, either directly or by way of a nitro-group, and then to use the bromine, or the nitro-group, or a conversion product of the latter, such as an amino-group or iodine, in order to block the position or positions occupied, while bromine, or a substituent that could be converted to bromine, was introduced elsewhere in the molecule, all blocking groups being afterwards replaced by hydrogen. First one position, then this and a second, then these two and a third, and, finally, these three and a fourth, were thus blocked. The five final products contained two identical pairs. Ladenburg had already shown that such a demonstration of the presence of two pairs of positions equivalent for a second substituent, could be used to complete a proof of the equivalence of all six positions for a first substituent. For the three hydroxybenzoic acids gave the same phenol on decarboxylation and the same benzoic acid by reduction, and the phenol could be converted, by way of bromobenzene, into the benzoic acid. This showed that four positions were equivalent for a first substituent. And now it was known that two of the hydroxybenzoic acids had this property, namely, that each contained its hydroxyl group in one of a pair of equivalent positions. Since equivalence for a second substituent must be preserved when the first is specialised to hydrogen, so that what was the second substituent becomes the first, this result showed that the fifth and sixth positions in benzene were each equivalent to any of the first four.

In the same period, the problem of determining the relative positions of substituents was solved in principle. At first there was great confusion. Then Kekulé proposed that all compounds whose substituents were considered to be in the same relative positions as those of a standard "ortho-compound" should be called "ortho-," and similarly for other such designations. Originally the designations were used without any accepted implication as to the positional relations to which they corresponded. When later it was found that most compounds which had been classified as ortho- had their substituents in 1,2-positions, the prefix "ortho-" was reserved for 1,2-compounds, and similarly for the other prefixes.

The proposed principle of classification was simple. Fixed standards had first to be secured; and this could be done in a limited number of favourable cases. Thus, Graebe in 1869 deduced the formula of naphthalene, and therefrom that phthalic acid is a 1,2-derivative of benzene. It followed that those disubstituted benzenes whose substituents could be genetically connected with the carboxyl groups of phthalic acid were 1,2-compounds. But though the principle was simple, it worked badly. The reason was that some of the reactions which were used to establish genetic connexion, notably hydroxylations by treatment of sulphonic acids with alkali, and cyanisations by the reaction of halogeno-nitro-compounds with alkali cyanides, frequently involved rearrangements (for reasons which are even now not fully understood): such disturbances were at the outset difficult to recognise and locate. Then, in 1874, a secure basis for the orientation of substituents in benzene compounds was offered by Griess, Salkowsky, and Koerner, independently.[4] It involved demonstrating relations, not between one disubstituted benzene and another, but between di- and tri-substituted benzenes. Thus, of the six known diaminobenzoic acids, two on decarboxylation gave one diaminobenzene, while three gave another, and the remaining acid the third; and therefore, the first diaminobenzene had to be ortho-, the second meta-, and the third para-. In studying such relations one was not at the mercy of unrecognised rearrangements. Subsequent work on the orientation of substituents in benzene derivatives has been based on this method.

Thus the two problems, of symmetry, and of orientation, were solved in the first decade after the publication of Kekulé's fundamental paper. In the same period the attack was opened on the much greater problem, one which was to occupy chemists for many years afterwards, namely, that of the actual disposition and function of the six carbon valencies of benzene, which are not required to maintain the ring or to hold the hydrogen atoms.

Kekulé's assignment, in 1865, of the six valencies to three double bonds was provisional: for the symmetry question was then unsettled. In 1872, Kekulé issued a supplementary hypothesis to the effect that an oscillation occurred between the two possible arrangements of double bonds:[5]

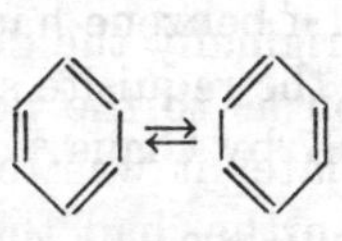

$$\rightleftarrows$$

His reason was that, as Ladenburg had already pointed out, the original formula admitted unrealised possibilities of isomerism in benzene de-

[4] P. Griess, *Ber.*, 1874, **7**, 1226; H. Salkowsky, *Ann.*, 1874, **173**, 66; W. Koerner, *Gazz. chim. ital.*, 1874, **4**, 305.

[5] F. A. Kekulé, *Ann.*, 1872, **162**, 77.

rivatives. It soon became clear that the additional symmetry introduced by the oscillation hypothesis was demanded by the observed extent of isomerism.

Subsequently to the original theory, but before its emendation, two other attempts were made to represent the symmetry that seemed to be indicated by the observed isomerism. One is expressed in the prism formula for benzene (below), first seriously advocated in 1869 by Ladenburg.[6] This formula requires the correct numbers of all the different kinds of substitution products. But the symmetry properties of the combining positions are such that these positions have to be correlated with those of a simple ring formula as indicated by the numbering:

Ortho-positions (6 pairs) are at the ends of face-diagonals, meta-positions (2 trios) at the corners of triangular faces, and para-positions (3 pairs) at the ends of longitudinal edges. Thus, in the prism structure, ortho-positions are not directly bound, while meta- and also para-positions are directly bound, in contrast to the bonding arrangements in the simple ring structure. One result of this was an exceedingly awkward formula for naphthalene.

In 1886 Baeyer commenced a series of experimental researches designed to determine the arrangement of the valencies of benzene, his method being to reduce benzene derivatives to *cyclo*hexadiene, *cyclo*hexene, or *cyclo*hexane compounds, and to determine the constitutions of the reduction products by the standard methods of aliphatic chemistry.[7] This work disproved the prism structure. For ortho-, meta-, and para-benzene compounds gave *cyclo*hexane-1,2-, -1,3-, and -1,4-derivatives, respectively; and one compound, ethyl 2,5-dihydroxyterephthalate, in which all three pairs of para-positions are labelled, gave a reduction product, ethyl succinosuccinate, having all substituents where they would be expected if benzene had the simple ring structure.

The other early formula of the requisite symmetry was the diagonal formula, first advanced in 1867 by Claus:[8]

[6] A. Ladenburg, *Ber.*, 1869, **2**, 141, 272.

[7] A. v. Baeyer, *et al.*, *Ann.*, 1887, **245**, 103; *Ber.*, 1888, **19**, 1797; *Ann.*, 1889, **251**, 257; *Ber.*, 1890, **23**, 1277; *Ann.*, 1890, **256**, 1; 1892, **266**, 169; 1893, **276**, 259.

[8] A. Claus, "Theoretische Betrachtungen und deren Anwendung zur Systematik der organischen Chemie," Freiburg, 1867, p. 207.

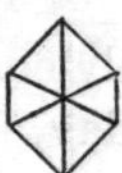

Originally Claus assumed the para- and ortho-bonds to have identical properties, so that each carbon atom was bound to three others in exactly the same way. (The difficulty of arranging for this in Euclidean space was not seriously felt at a time when formulae were considered essentially as symbols of chemical relationships, without much regard for any metrical properties the molecules might possess.) But in 1882 Claus suggested that the para-bonds should be regarded as radically different from all other known bonds, thus taking the first step in admitting, by the use of a special symbol, a difficulty insoluble in terms of already established concepts.[9]

Essentially the same view was represented more explicitly in the modified symbol known as the centric formula:

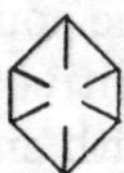

It was first used by Armstrong,[10] was at once adopted by Baeyer[11] as the best symbolic representation of his results, and was finally accepted by Claus as a suitable expression of his ideas.

Originally, the centric formula expressed the symmetry of benzene, but was agnostic with respect to all other properties. However, in 1891 Bamberger used it in a discussion of stability.[12] He attempted to correlate stability in different aromatic types by means of the assumption that the six-fold character of the centric valency group was the essential factor of stability. Since, he argued, pyridine could form a sextuple valency group without employing the salt-forming valencies of its nitrogen atom, while pyrrole could do so only by making use of all its nitrogen valencies, one could understand why pyridine had the basic properties of a tertiary amine, while pyrrole was practically non-basic:

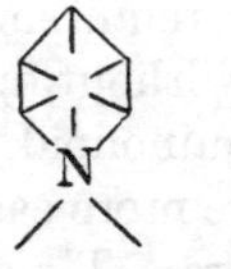

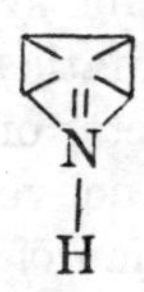

[9] A. Claus, *Ber.*, 1882, **15**, 1407; 1887, **20**, 1423.
[10] H. E. Armstrong, *J. Chem. Soc.*, 1887, **51**, 254.
[11] A. v. Baeyer, *Ann.*, 1887, **245**, 118.
[12] E. Bamberger, *Ber.*, 1891, **24**, 1758; 1893, **26**, 1946; *Ann.*, 1893, **273**, 373.

As far as it goes, this is completely correct: reading electrons for valencies, it is what we should say today.

Quite the most advanced of the early attempts to interpret aromatic stability, while still satisfying the symmetry condition, was that made in 1898 by Thiele.[13] Through a general study of unsaturation, he had been led to assume the reactive valencies of double bonds to be in principle continuously divisible, and to exist in most circumstances partly bound and partly in the free state; and he had shown how, in a chain of alternate single and double bonds, the possibilities of division could lead to what he called "conjugation" between the double bonds, that is, a more even spread of affinity over the double bonds and intervening single bonds, so that the main opportunities for reaction appeared at the ends of the chain, where un-neutralised free affinity was available. Thus he interpreted terminal addition to conjugated unsaturated systems in the aliphatic series. Then he pointed out that in Kekulé's benzene structure the conjugation is cyclic: there being no ends, there can be but little additive reactivity. The symmetry condition was fulfilled by starting with either of Kekulé's oscillating structures, and allowing the affinity redistribution to proceed equally to coincidence, so that all ring bonds became equivalent:

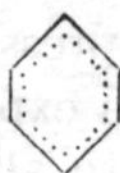

The outstanding merit of this theory was that it dealt with aromatic stability on the basis of concepts developed outside the aromatic series.

The main general characteristics of aromatic systems with which a structural theory should be concerned are its symmetry, its stability, and its transformations. The centric formula expresses the symmetry, and is not inconsistent with the stability. Thiele's formula expresses the symmetry, and interprets the stability. But any consideration of the modes in which benzenoid systems are disrupted, indicates appeal to Kekulé's formula, of course, in association with his dynamic hypothesis in order to satisfy the symmetry requirements. Transformations which destroy the aromatic system, without opening the ring, produce either addition products, or ortho-quinonoid, or para-quinonoid, derivatives; and all such conversions are more easily understood in terms of Kekulé's formula than of the others. Thus it came about that the last of the pre-electronic attempts to make a theory of benzene structure took the form of an expansion of Kekulé's dynamic hypothesis. At a very early date Dewar had proposed, as a possibility, the bridged

[13] J. Thiele, *Ann.*, 1898, **306**, 125.

formula for benzene:[14] as a static formula, it was quite unacceptable, lacking the necessary symmetry. In 1922 the writer revived it,[15] interpreting the para-bond as qualitatively comparable to the reactive component of a double bond; and he proposed to incorporate Dewar's formula with Kekulé's, each with the orientations (two or three) needed to fulfil the symmetry condition, in a more complex dynamical system:

(2) 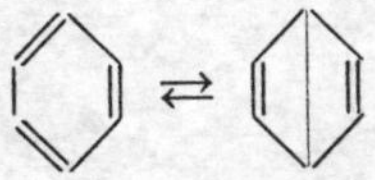 ⇄ (3)

The argument focussed attention on the transformations of the aromatic system, the main object of including the two types of structure being to permit parallel interpretations of ortho- and para-quinonoid conversions. However, the stability problem was not dealt with, except through the undeveloped idea that the interconversion of forms might be rapid enough to restrict reaction in any one form.

This was the apparent *cul de sac* to which classical chemical considerations led: the symmetry condition could be fulfilled in various ways; but no one way satisfactorily interpreted both the stability and the transformations. According to which of these characteristics was taken as guide, either of two roads would be followed; and, historically, they ended in different places, the one in Thiele's theory, the other in the expanded dynamic hypothesis. A decade after the promulgation of the latter, the electronic theory of chemical binding brought about the reconcilation that had seemed invisibly distant, showing that the two theories could be considered to represent complementary aspects or appearances of the same interior physical situation.

(13b) Mesomerism in the Benzenoid Nucleus.—Only for the sake of continuity of narrative do we refer again, but now as mere headings, to the discovery of the electronic theory of valency (1916), of the physical nature of covalency (1927), of mesomerism as a general phenomenon (1926), and of its interpretation by an extension of that of covalency (1929): all this is described in Chapters I and II.

The mesomerism of benzene was first discussed explicitly and in detail by E. Hückel[16] in 1931–32. He applied to the problem two approximate formalisms. One of them, known as the molecular orbital method, had been invented by Lennard-Jones somewhat earlier; and it has been much developed by Mulliken and others since. This treatment characteristically under-emphasizes the covalent nature of binding in molecules, and for that reason is not very simply correlated with

[14] J. Dewar, *Proc. Roy. Soc.* (Edinburgh), **1866**, 84.

[15] C. K. Ingold, *J. Chem. Soc.*, 1922, **121**, 1133.

[16] E. Hückel. *Z. Physik*, 1931, **70**, 204; **72**, 310; 1932, **76**, 626.

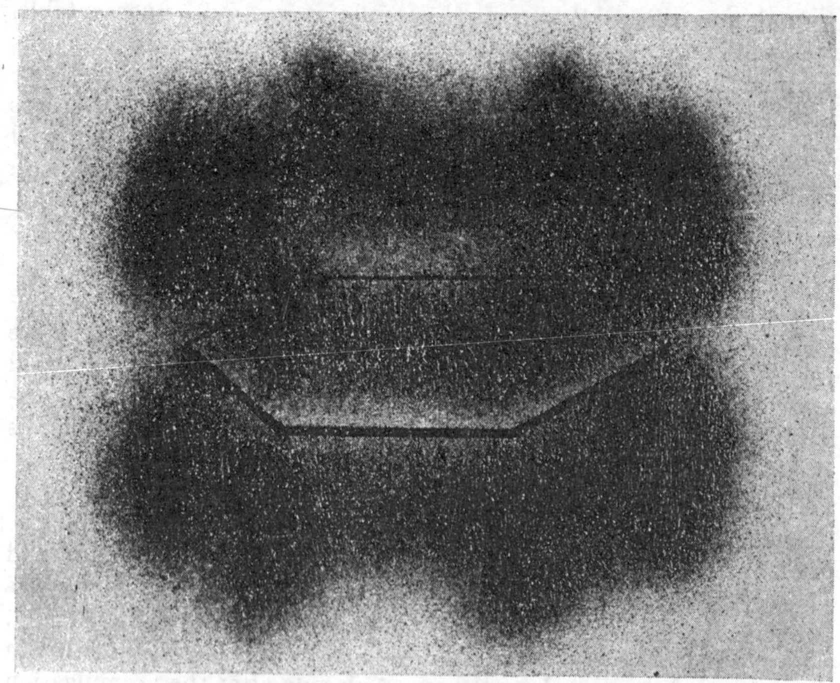

Fig. 13-1.—Illustrating the charge distribution of the π electron shell in benzene.

valency concepts. The second method, which Hückel himself invented, is known as the valency-bond treatment. It goes to the other extreme, over-emphasizing the covalent character of the binding; and, for that very reason, it appears particularly easily in the role of an interpretation of valency concepts. The technique of this method was simplified by Pauling and Wheland, who applied it to benzene and other aromatic hydrocarbons.[17]

In setting up the problem, Hückel, and likewise Pauling and Wheland, assumed that each carbon atom of benzene supplies one electron in an atomic p orbital, having its symmetry axis at right angles to the molecular plane, to form a molecular group of six π electrons. The remaining electrons are left to hold, with single σ bonds, the regular hexagonal frame of six CH carbonium-ionic centres. Each π electron is then considered as moving in the combined potential field of the framework and the smoothed-out field of the remaining π electrons. It is easily shown that the plane of the atomic nuclei is a nodal plane for all the π electrons, which together must produce a charge-density

[17] L. Pauling and G. W. Wheland, *J. Chem. Phys.*, 1933, **1**, 362; J. Sherman, *ibid.*, 1934, **2**, 488; G. W. Wheland, *ibid.*, 1935, **3**, 356.

distribution having total hexagonal symmetry, as illustrated in Fig. 13-1.

The common object of these techniques is to compute the mesomeric energy, or aromatic resonance energy, that is, the extra stability that arises from not confining the electrons to three static double bonds, as in a Kekulé formula. The answer depends on the assumptions made about the extra motion permitted to these electrons. In the molecular orbital treatment, interaction between the π electrons is neglected during the computation of the orbitals available to any one such electron as it moves among the atoms in the total molecular field: only afterwards is Pauli's principle introduced, the electrons being assigned in pairs to the more stable of the orbitals thus computed: and at no stage in the simplest treatment is π electron interaction allowed for. One might feel surprised that such a calculation gives a sensible result. But the calculated energies are derived in terms of an unevaluated energy-quantity, called β: in principle, β represents the energy effect of allowing one atomic p electron to spread its motion into one adjacent p orbital: in practice, β is a disposable constant, into which much of the error of method can be absorbed by choosing it to give the best possible fit with empirical data. The calculated energies for benzene, naphthalene, anthracene, and phenanthrene, are 2.00β, 3.68β, 5.32β, and 5.45β, respectively. These coefficients are approximately in the right ratios. If β is given the value 20 kcal./mole, the comparison with thermochemically determined mesomeric energies works out as shown in Table 13-1. In considering this comparison, it must be remembered that what are called "observed" mesomeric energies themselves involve interpretative factors of an arbitrary nature, as explained in Section **9b**.

In the valency-bond method, Pauli's principle, and electron interaction, are introduced from the outset. The electrons are assumed to remain as three spin-coupled pairs, never belonging, in Hückel's, or in Pauling and Wheland's treatment, to fewer than two atoms. They are, indeed, bonds having the internal energies and mutually repulsive interactions of two-electron bonds. But they are mobile bonds, always changing among the positions between which they were assumed to move in the earlier dynamical representations of benzene. It was found necessary to include not only the Kekulé but also the Dewar structures, in defining the limits of mobility of the mobile bonds: no other structures are involved, because bonds cannot cross.[18] The wave-function M of the normal mesomeric state is therefore constituted from those of Kekulé and Dewar structures, K and D, taken with two and three orientations, respectively, as is required by symmetry.

[18] More exactly: spin-pairing arrangements, which are included among the non-crossed structures, would result from crossing.

Pauling and Wheland's coefficients for them are as indicated in the following equation:

$$M = 0.625(K_1 + K_2) + 0.271(D_1 + D_2 + D_3)$$

They show that the Kekulé structures are more important than the Dewar structures, but that the latter are not negligible, in the composition of the mesomeric state. The Dewar structures contribute about 20% of the calculated mesomeric energy. The mesomeric energy is expressed in terms of an energy quantity called α: in principle, α represents the energy effect of allowing two adjacent atomic p electrons to undergo exchange, as in the formation of the π component of a static double bond; in practice α is a disposable constant, chosen to give the best fit with experimental data. The calculated energies for benzene, naphthalene, anthracene, and phenanthrene, are 1.11α, 2.04α, 3.09α, and 3.15α. respectively, the last two values involving a minor algebraic approximation. The coefficients have again approximately the right ratios. If α is chosen as 35 kcal./mole, the agreement with experiment is as shown in Table 13-1. Again however, we have the position that, not only do the "calculated" values depend heavily on empirical data, but also the "observed" values depend in part on interpretative assumption.

TABLE 13-1.—CALCULATED MESOMERIC ENERGIES (IN KCAL./MOLE) OF AROMATIC HYDROCARBONS: COMPARISON WITH THERMOCHEMICAL VALUES.

	Observed		Calculated	
	Energy constants	Hydrogenation	M.O. method (with $\beta=20$)	V.B. method (with $\alpha=35$)
Benzene	37	36	40	39
Naphthalene	75	—	74	71
Anthracene	105	—	106	108
Phenanthrene	110	—	109	110

The valency-bond method has since been considerably refined within its own framework, though it has not yet proved possible to eliminate its dependence on a disposable constant. (To calculate α non-empirically would be a heavy task.) What was inadequate in the earlier applications of the method was the specification of mesomerism exclusively in terms of fully covalent structures: and what is needed is the inclusion of dipolar structures: in general, the more that are included, the better the results should be. There are two types of singly dipolar structures with adjacent charges, A with 12 orientations, and

B with 12, and three types with non-adjacent charges, *P* with 6, *Q* with 24, and *R* with 6 orientations, as well as doubly and trebly dipolar types, to cite them in the probable order of diminishing importance:

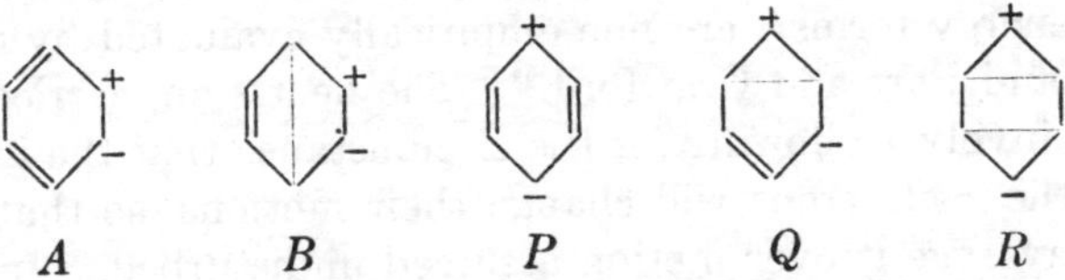

Work on the inclusion of such polar structures in the valency bond treatment was initiated by Sklar,[19] and has been developed by Craig,[20] who has solved the problem, with inclusion, besides the five non-polar structures *K* and *D*, of the twenty-four adjacent-charge structures *A* and *B*. His wave-function for the normal mesomeric state is as follows:

$$M = 0.39(K_1 + K_2) + 0.17(D_1 + D_2 + D_3) + 0.07(A_1 + A_2 + \cdots A_{12}) + 0.03(B_1 + B_2 + \cdots B_{12})$$

The energy is calculated to lie 17 kcal./mole below Pauling and Wheland's normal mesomeric state. This shows that quite large uncertainties are involved in the treatment based on non-polar structures only; but it suggests that higher approximations would shift the energy by only a few kcal./mole further. However, for the present any really close agreement with experiment must remain dependent on making the final result of calculation partly dependent on experiment.

The molecular orbital method has been developed, not entirely within its original framework, in ways which are theoretically interesting, inasmuch as they constitute, in principle, a technique for the non-empirical evaluation of the energies of π electron states. At the moment, the numerical accuracy of the calculations is insufficient to give quantitative agreement with experimental values; but the treatment of benzene does give a qualitatively satisfactory account of its energy levels, and has been of value in classifying some of its spectroscopically known, excited electronic states. The original steps were taken by Goeppert-Mayer and Sklar.[21] First, they formed the product wave-functions, as calculated by simple molecular orbital theory, into "antisymmetric" additive combinations, thereby placing the motion of the π electrons under the restriction that not more than two could be together in the same atom, so satisfying Pauli's principle in the atoms. Then, having assigned the electrons in pairs to the three

[19] A. L. Sklar, *J. Chem. Phys.*, 1937, 5, 669.
[20] D. P. Craig, *Proc. Roy. Soc.* (London), 1950, A, **200**, 272, 390, 401.
[21] M. Goeppert-Mayer and A. L. Sklar, *J. Chem. Phys.*, 1938, **6**, 645.

lowest orbitals, and made the wave-functions totally antisymmetric, to satisfy Pauli's principle fully, they allowed for the energy of mutual repulsion of the π electrons by averaging it over the orbitals. The necessary energy terms were non-empirically evaluated by Sklar and Lyddane[22] and Parr and Crawford.[23] The next step, carried through by Craig,[24] involves allowing for the circumstance that the interaction energy of the π electrons will change their motions, so that it is not correct to average it over motion assumed undisturbed. Indeed, the π electron pairs have not to be firmly assigned to three antisymmetrical orbitals, but must be allowed to move among all the orbitals, changing the total electronic wave-function, as in every resonance problem, until the energy is minimised. In principle this method, which is described as allowing for "configuration interaction," and was first developed in its molecular applications by Craig, gives molecular wave-functions as good as any that could be formed by the initial use of only p atomic wave-functions.

It will easily be understood why, despite the mesomerism of the aromatic nucleus, valency-bond formulae, particularly those of the relatively stable Kekulé structures, retain their usefulness for the interpretation of the transformations of the aromatic nucleus, why, for instance, we attach the curved-arrow signs to Kekulé formulae, even though such formulae could not by themselves account for the stability of the nucleus. If, in a chemical transformation affecting an aromatic nucleus, or in the transition state of such a transformation, the electron pairs are regarded as largely localised, then it is convenient, for the purpose of following the reaction mechanism, to think of those electron pairs as having immediately come from localised positions. Such a concept is possible if it is agreed to dissect the total transformation into two superposed processes, namely, (*a*) an excitation of the normal mesomeric state into a valency structure, and (*b*) a chemical reaction on ordinary lines involving the valency structure. The component processes have to be considered as simultaneous and not successive—like the bond-breaking and bond-forming processes in the bimolecular substitutions of saturated compounds (Section **6d**)—so that the whole of the energy of mesomerism has not to be supplied, in order to complete process (*a*), before process (*b*) can commence. But the activation energy of any process which permanently, or temporarily, breaks up the mesomeric system will be increased by the mesomerism, even if not by the full amount of the mesomeric energy. Thus does the theory

[22] A. L. Sklar and R. H. Lyddane, *ibid.*, 1939, **7**, 374.

[23] R. G. Parr and B. L. Crawford jr., *ibid.*, 1948, **16**, 1049.

[24] D. P. Craig, *Proc. Roy. Soc.* (London), 1950, **A, 200,** 474; R. G. Parr, D. P. Craig, and I. G. Ross, *J. Chem. Phys.*, 1950, **18**, 1561.

of mesomerism fulfil the three main requirements in the problem of aromatic nuclei, namely, to interpret their symmetry, their stability, and their transformations.

The theory of benzene provides a basis for modification to give a qualitative pattern for that of pyridine. But the possibilities of a satisfactory quantitative calculation of the energy states of pyridine are very much reduced by the need, created by the hetero-atom, for new but unknown energy integrals.

Observation shows that the introduction of the hetero-atom does not much change the size and shape of the molecule (Section **14b**), or those properties, chiefly the mesomeric energy (Section **15b**), and exaltation of diamagnetic susceptibility (Section **16e**), which arise primarily from π electron delocalisation. The hetero-atom does, however, create a dipole moment, $-2.26\ D$ in pyridine, the negative sign meaning that, as one should expect, the electrons have concentrated towards the electronegative nitrogen atom.[25] On the basis of our analysis of the dipole moments of simple alkylamines, and of the effects of carbon chain extension (Sections **8c** and **8d**), a moment of only about $-1.0\ D$ would be expected to arise from the effect of the electronegativity of the nitrogen atom on the σ bond electrons in pyridine. We are thus led to assume that a moment of $-1.2\ D$ arises from a displacement of the electrons of the π shell, an average displacement of 0.04 *A*, several times more than the average from the σ electrons. Quinoline has a moment of $-2.29\ D$, and *iso*quinoline $-2.73\ D$.[25] These moments are also due to the electronegativity of the nitrogen atom, which in *iso*quinoline acts appreciably on the electrons of the more remote ring.

(13c) Condensed Polycyclic Benzenoid Systems.—On passing from benzene to naphthalene, the π electron problem loses much of its symmetry, and becomes very much more complicated. Corresponding to the two Kekulé formulae for benzene, there are three Kekulé-like formulae for naphthalene, one with a centre of symmetry (*A*), and two without, these last (B_1, B_2) being identical but for orientation:

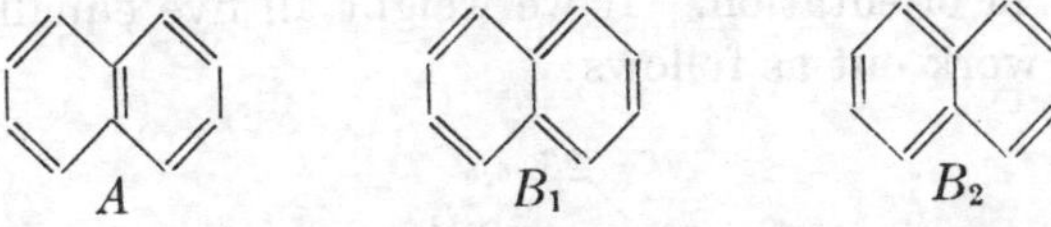

There are also 39 non-polar structures with trans-annular bonds, and many more polar structures. The whole system is so complicated that one is tempted to see whether any useful considerations can be set down after simplification on very drastic lines. The most drastic ap-

[25] A. D. Buckingham, J. Y. H. Chau, H. C. Freeman, R. J. W. LeFèvre, D. A. A. S. N. Rao, and J. Tardif, *J. Chem. Soc.*, **1956**, 1405.

proximation that one can make is to neglect the bridged and polar structures completely, in spite of their large numbers. If we do this, there still remains the problem of weighting the A- and B-type Kekulé structures in the mixed wave-function; but, after what has been done, it is an insignificant further step to take these weights as equal. The interesting conclusion then follows that the multiplicity of the 1,2-bonds of naphthalene is 5/3, and is greater than that of the other bonds, all of which have the multiplicity 4/3:

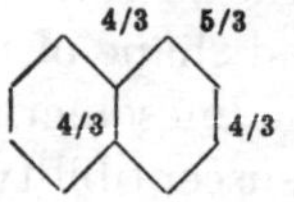

4/3 5/3
4/3 4/3

From this it appears that the 1,2-bonds of naphthalene should be more like double bonds than any of the bonds of benzene; and also that the whole 1,2,3,4-system in naphthalene should be somewhat similar to buta-1,3-diene, and probably still more similar to 1,4-diphenylbuta-1,3-diene.

These conclusions bring to mind much general chemical experience. 2-Naphthol halogenates and diazo-couples in the 1-position, as if its phenolic system preferred to resemble an enolic system with a double bond in the 1,2-position, rather than one having its double bond located in the 2,3-position. Naphthalene adds chlorine, not as easily as an olefin would, but much more readily than benzene.[26] Naphthalene is reduced by sodium dissolving in alcohol, just as 1,4-diphenylbutadiene is, and the two added hydrogen atoms appear in the 1,4-positions, in naphthalene, leaving an unattacked double bond in the 2,3-position exactly as in the case of 1,4-diphenylbutadiene. Metrical evidence supporting the above distribution of bond multiplicities will be mentioned later.

Phenanthrene is another example in which these simple considerations lead to chemically reasonable results. Phenanthrene has five Kekulé-like structures, which are of four different types, two structures differing only in orientation. If we weight all five equally, the bond multiplicities work out as follows:

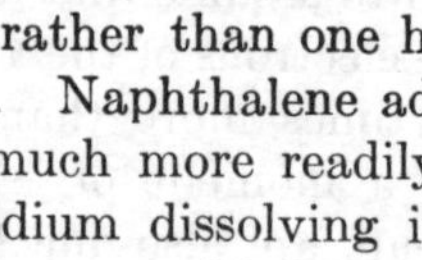

9/5 6/5
7/5
6/5 7/5 8/5
7/5 7/5
8/5

[26] In the older literature, naphthalene is reported to give a dichloride, but recent attempts to repeat this preparation have not met with success. Naphthalene does give several stereo-isomeric tetrachlorides (cf. Chapter XIII).

The 9,10-bond has the multiplicity 9/5, and therefore should be closely similar to a double bond. The non-angular bonds of the lateral rings show alternating multiplicities, as in naphthalene, though the alternations are less pronounced than those of naphthalene.

The conclusion concerning the 9,10-bond certainly agrees with its chemistry. Phenanthrene adds bromine in the 9,10-positions; it is readily reduced to give a 9,10-dihydro-derivative; and it is easily oxidised in the 9,10-positions (to give phenanthraquinone and diphenic acid). In all these properties the 9,10-bond resembles fairly closely the double bond of stilbene.

Anthracene lies on the reverse side of the picture. If we work out the bond multiplicities from the four Kekulé-like structures, which are of two types, each type having two orientations, we obtain, allowing all the structures equal weight, the following values:

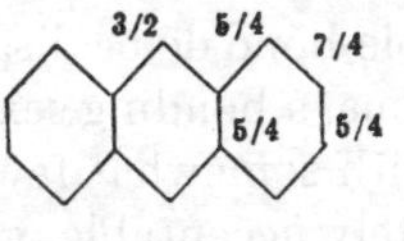

3/2 5/4 7/4
5/4 5/4

They suggest that the additive reactivity of the lateral rings, in which the bond multiplicities alternate, as in naphthalene but more strongly, should completely overshadow that of the central ring, in which the bonds of the CH-groups are as in benzene.

The reverse is the case. Anthracene is reduced by sodium amalgam to 9,10-dihydroanthracene. Chlorine, bromine, and nitrating agents substitute anthracene, first in the 9- and then in the 10-position; but by nitration in acetic acid an intermediate addition compound, 9-nitro-9,10-dihydroanthryl-10-acetate, can be isolated, which readily undergoes further conversion to 9-nitroanthracene. 9-Anthranol and 9-anthrone are separately isolable, but easily interconvertible, tautomers; and so also are 9,10-anthrahydroquinone and 9-hydroxy-10-anthrone.

It is desirable thus to *test* the qualitative reliability of so simple an approach as that of mixing all and only Kekulé structures equally. But having tested it, we should accept the answer, *viz.*, that it is not only unsound in theory, as we knew, but also untrustworthy in practice. This approach should not be used, as it has on occasion been, as a foundation on which to build an argument. Attempts have been made to calculate electron distributions in polycyclic aromatic systems quantitatively. Such calculations are sometimes qualitatively suggestive, but none commands confidence in its quantitative validity, inasmuch as the uncertainties introduced by the approximations made are nearly always of the order of magnitude of the quantities being calculated.

The general relationships between benzene and pyridine, described at the end of Section **13b,** are expected to apply as between naphthalene and quinoline or *iso*quinoline, or as between anthracene and acridine, and so on.

(13d) Non-benzenoid Closed-Conjugated Systems.[27]—In his original application of molecular orbital theory to benzene[16] Hückel observed that, for π electrons arranged on a circle, the successively occupied molecular π orbitals started with a single one and then went on to higher energies in successive degenerate pairs. Thus he developed the idea of molecular electron shells, analogous to the electron shells of an atom. Filled shells would occur with two π electrons (ethylene), with six (benzene), and, in general, with $4n+2$ electrons, but not with four π electrons (*cyclo*butadiene), with eight (*cyclo*-octatetraene), or, in general, with $4n$ electrons. Thus, the benzene group of six electrons, the aromatic sextet, should be the first π electron group to show closed-shell stability through double-bond delocalisation. The idea of a stable bonding group of six electrons, a bonding sextet, implying the tendency of a system which starts with somewhat fewer than six to build up six such electrons, is immediately acceptable, going back, as it does in its empirical aspect, to Bamberger (Section **13a**), with all the weight of his incorporation, on essentially that basis, of the five-membered heterocyclics in the aromatic family. Hückel rationalised the idea.

Hückel's $4n+2$ rule applies only to monocyclic π electron systems, though some authors have applied it to polycyclic systems, to which, in view of its derivation, it can have no direct relevance. It is not, for example, an objection to the rule that it does not predict the stability of acenaphylene, which has twelve π electrons. In the monocyclic series, the rule is valid up to the eight-membered ring; and, in view of the simple nature of the theory from which it was derived, we should probably not expect much more from it. *Cyclo*butadiene is too unstable to be kept. *Cyclo*-octatetraene can be kept, but it is a highly reactive, non-planar polyolefin. Monocyclic closed-conjugated rings from ten-membered upwards are incompletely known, but for these rings it would seem that the Hückel principle is not the dominating factor in their stability, or lack of it.

Hückel's classification of π electron systems was based on elementary molecular orbital theory, which in the next stage of refinement should be made to take account of interelectronic repulsion. In attempting this, Coulson and Rushbrooke were led to another useful classification, in which π electron systems are classed as "alternant" ("Alt.," under

[27] For an authoritative and more complete account, see D. P. Craig, in Chapter I of "Non-benzenoid Aromatic Compounds," Editor D. Ginsberg, Interscience Publishers, New York, 1959, p. 1.

the formulae, below), if spin-labels (α and β) could be attached to the π electron centres in an unbrokenly alternating way, and "non-alternant" (a "Non.," below) otherwise. The significance of the classification is that, in non-alternant hydrocarbons, the π electrons are distributed unevenly among the π centres, with an increase of charge at one end of a bond at the expense of the other. Thus, in azulene, the π electrons not only concentrate, as dipole moments show, towards the five-membered ring from the seven-membered (as if each ring were striving after a sextet), but also, according to calculation, they concentrate at alternate atoms in the separate rings. Such concentrations of charge on certain π centres may be expected to limit delocalisation; but the effect is not large. Many non-alternant molecules are known, and their mesomeric energies are not abnormally low. Alternant character, in short, is not closely associated with aromaticity.

The annexed illustrations show these two classifications, together with a third, described below.

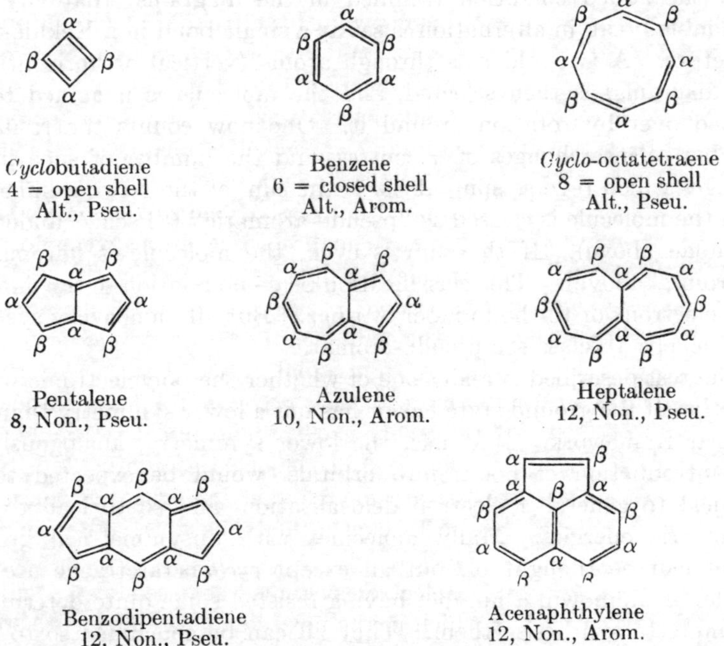

*Cyclo*butadiene
4 = open shell
Alt., Pseu.

Benzene
6 = closed shell
Alt., Arom.

Cyclo-octatetraene
8 = open shell
Alt., Pseu.

Pentalene
8, Non., Pseu.

Azulene
10, Non., Arom.

Heptalene
12, Non., Pseu.

Benzodipentadiene
12, Non., Pseu.

Acenaphthylene
12, Non., Arom.

The elementary molecular orbital and valency bond calculations made by Hückel on benzene lead to consistent results in that case, but markedly discrepant results when applied to his open-shell $4n$ systems. Thus the valency bond calculation predicts large mesomeric energies for *cyclo*butadiene and *cyclo*-octatetraene. Such discrepancies must diminish as the methods are refined, as they have been in the treatment of benzene (Section **13b**). Craig has investigated the factors underlying the discrepancies, and has shown that, in calculations made by molecular orbital and valency bond methods which have been freed from certain approximations inherent in the simple treatments, very low mesomeric energies are predicted for *cyclo*butadiene and for *cyclo*-octatetraene. Although such calculations are feasible only in the simplest cases, Craig was led by this study to suggest a more general criterion, based on symmetry, for recognising the circumstances in which only small mesomeric energies arise, and thus to propose a classification of π electron systems, which is aimed specifically at the conditions for aromaticity.

This criterion is limited to molecules with at least one two-fold rotational axis of symmetry passing through at least two π electron centres. The rule can be followed with the aid of any of the above diagrams. The molecule is first spin-labelled, as described already, with the added condition (fulfilled in the diagrams) that any unavoidable break in alternation is set at a single bond in a Kekulé-type structure. A two-fold axis through atoms (vertical or horizontal in the diagrams) is then selected, and the molecule is imagined to be turned over by rotation around it. One now counts the resulting number of interchanges of π centres, and the number of such interchanges which reverse spin-labels. If the sum of these two numbers is odd, the molecule is classed as "pseudo-aromatic" ("Pseu.," under the formulae above). If the sum is even, the molecule is "aromatic" ("Arom.," above). This classification bears no relation to the number of π electrons or to the number of rings. But all monocyclic systems of Hückel's $4n$ class are pseudo-aromatic.

The test described is really one of whether the polyelectronic wavefunction of the ground state has or has not a lower symmetry than the nuclear framework. If it has, the lower symmetry, analogously to the introduction of nodes into orbitals, would be expected to be inimical to general π electron delocalisation, and so to lead to low mesomeric energies. Many molecules with unsymmetrical ground states can be thought of, but all except *cyclo*-octatetraene are unstable, or unknown, a number having resisted some quite determined attempts to synthesise them. They all can be concluded so to lack aromatic stability that they can fairly be called "pseudo-aromatic." The elementary molecular orbital and valency bond approaches would then assign to their ground states different lower symmetries, and hence no argreement in calculated energies could be expected. According to Craig, the main need is to make the calculations less empirical, that is, less dependent on numerical data obtained empirically from other molecules, which, in calculations on pseudo-aromatic molecules, are always of a different symmetry class, *viz.*, the truly aromatic molecules.

The symmetry test is applicable only if the necessary symmetry is present in the molecular model. It cannot, for example, be applied to phenanthrene, generally regarded as typically aromatic, nor to the stable non-olefinic diphenylene, nor to the typically diolefinic dibenzopentalene; for none of these molecules has a two-fold axis through atoms. The last two of these compounds are formulated below.[28]

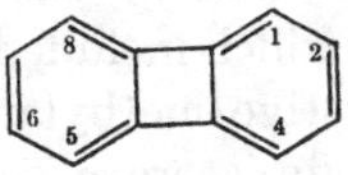

Diphenylene
(12, Alt.)

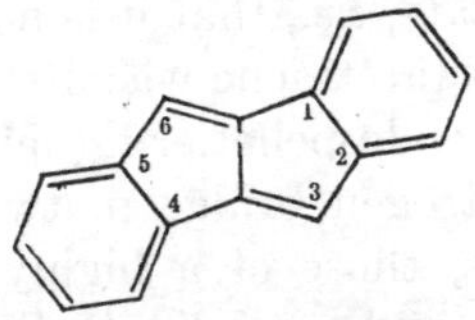

Dibenzopentalene
(16, Non.)

In such cases we can only try to judge which simpler and more symmetrical "parent" will control the stability of the derivative. In the two molecules formulated, we assume control by the benzene rings: that is, we assume that the benzene rings are not strongly conjugated with each other through the intervening rings.

Diphenylene must involve to an important degree the destabilising factor of ring, "strain," a factor which we consider more generally in Section **15a.** Ring strain can in principle affect all types of rings, including π electron rings. Its most prevalent component is the stress in bent bonds; and, in closed-conjugated systems, this is at its maximum in four-membered rings. An occasionally important component is trans-annular non-bonding pressure between ring atoms; and this component too must be at its maximum in four-membered rings. A third factor, one which can arise only in much larger rings, involves trans-annular non-bonding pressures between atoms which are at-

[28] The single Kekulé structures shown are probably the most important, because they best suit the internal angles of the non-benzenoid rings. (The single-single-bond angle, outside a double bond, is smaller than the single-double-bond angle.) W. H. Mills and I. G. Nixon demonstrated this type of factor, by showing that the indanol and tetralol formulated below diazo-couple where the represented enol groups would require, as shown by the arrows (*J. Chem. Soc.*, **1930,** 2510):

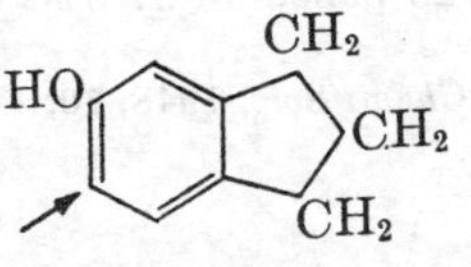

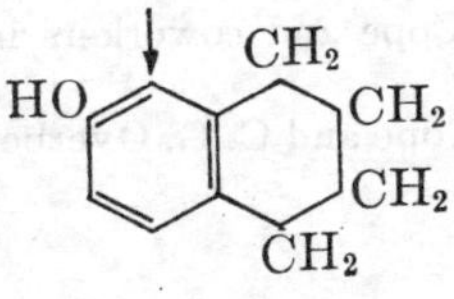

HO, CH_2, CH_2, CH_2

HO, CH_2, CH_2, CH_2, CH_2

tached to the rings and find themselves turned inwards in rings of a certain size.

A brief indication will now be given of the observational chemistry of some of the compounds which have been discussed above in theoretical terms.

*Cyclo*butadiene has not been isolated in a free state, but it has, as some derivatives have, been obtained in the form of metal complexes, such as $(C_4H_4)Fe(CO)_3$. On attempting to liberate the hydrocarbon, one obtains only products of its polymerisation or addition reactions.[29] These are stereospecific enough to show that *cyclo*butadiene has a singlet ground state, *i.e.*, that it is not a di-radical.

Cyclo-octatetraene was first prepared by Willstätter,[30] who obtained it from pseudo-pelletierin (below) by reactions which included removal of the nitrogen bridge in two steps of exhaustive methylation. Its properties, those of a highly reactive polyolefin, were a surprise to everyone; and accordingly Willstätter's work was repeatedly, though never justifiably, called in question.[31] Then Rappe obtained the substance by polymerisation of acetylene in the presence of nickel cyanide in tetrahydrofuran, a method allowing the production of large quantities.[32] Reppe confirmed Wilstätter's findings; and he, and later Cope and his coworkers, have greatly extended our knowledge of the physical properties and chemical transformations of *cyclo*-octatetraene.[33] And Cope, in order to get the record straight, prepared the substance again by Wilstätter's route.[34]

CH_2—CH——CH_2
| | |
CH_2 NMe CO
| | |
CH_2—CH——CH_2

Pseudopelletierin

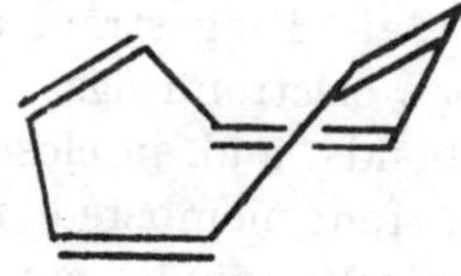

Cyclo-octatetraene

Cyclo-octatetraene is a saddle-shaped molecule (above), composed of four flat and essentially strainless ethylene units, so rotated about

[29] G. F. Emerson, L. Watts, and R. Petitt, *J. Am. Chem. Soc.*, 1965, **87**,153; *idem* and J. D. Fitzpatrick, *ibid.*, 3253; 3254; L. Watts, J. D. Fitzpatrick, and R. Petitt, *ibid.*, 1966, **88**, 623.

[30] R. Willstätter and E. Weser, *Ber.*, 1911, **44**, 3442; R. Willstätter and M. Heidelburger, *Ber.*, 1913, **46**, 517.

[31] For a summary, see W. Baker, *J. Chem. Soc.*, **1945**, 258.

[32] J. W. Reppe, reported in B.I.O.S. Reports, 1935, **137**, No. 22.

[33] A. C. Cope and coworkers in more than 20 papers in *J. Am. Chem. Soc.*, since 1950.

[34] A. C. Cope and C. G. Overberger, *J. Am. Chem. Soc.*, 1948, **70**, 1433.

the single bonds between them that there is only slight π orbital overlap between the units.[35] The molecule thus achieves strainlessness; and it has nothing to gain in compensation for the loss of strainlessness which it would suffer, if it should go into a single plane, like benzene; for the unsymmetrical π electron ground state of the flat molecule cannot supply a compensating amount of mesomeric energy. The CC bond lengths alternate, and, by an X-ray study[36] of the monocarboxylic acid, are 1.322 and 1.470 *A*, each ± 0.005 *A*. The ring angle is $126.4° \pm 0.4°$. The C:C stretching frequency, 1639 $cm.^{-1}$, is normal for an isolated, *i.e.*, non-conjugated, double bond.[37] The molecule shows scarcely any exaltation of refraction.[32] It also shows no exaltation of diamagnetic susceptibility[38] such as would be diagnostic of cyclic electron delocalisation (Section **16e**). Heats of formation and reaction allow it only a little mesomeric energy,[39] less than would be expected for an open-chain, normally conjugated, tetra-ene. It is a yellow liquid, but its visible colour arises only because the long vibrational tail of an absorption band, centred well up in the ultraviolet, encroaches on the visible region of the spectrum.

Cyclo-octatetraene is isomerised by heat to styrene, and is converted by numerous reagents to benzene derivatives, for instance, by chromic oxide to terephthalic acid.[40] It is reduced catalytically in the expected stages to *cyclo*-octane. It is reduced by alkali metals, and adds hydrogen halides, and halogens. Willstätter had noticed ring-bridging during additions, and Reppe and Cope have carefully elucidated some of these processes.[41] The underlying phenomenon of intra-annular valency tautomerism is discussed in Chapter XI (Section **49d**). It has been shown by Anet and by Roberts and their coworkers by the method of nuclear magnetic resonance that in *cyclo*-octatetraene itself, and in various of its simple substitution products,

[35] I. Tanaka and S. Shuda, *Bull. Chem. Soc. Japan*, 1950, **23**, 54; W. B. Pearson, G. C. Pimental, and K. S. Pitzer, *J. Am. Chem. Soc.*, 1952, **74**, 3437.

[36] D. P. Shoemaker, H. Kindler, W. G. Sly, and R. C. Srivastava, *J. Am. Chem. Soc.*, 1965, **87**, 482.

[37] E. R. Lippincott, R. C. Lord, and R. S. McDonald, *J. Am. Chem. Soc.*, 1951, **73**, 3370.

[38] R. C. Pink and A. R. Ubbelohde, *Trans. Faraday Soc.*, 1948, **44**, 708.

[39] R. B. Turner, W. R. Meador, W. von E. Doering, L. H. Knox, J. R. Mayer, and D. W. Wiley, *J. Am. Chem. Soc.*, 1957, **79**, 4127; and references cited therein.

[40] For a summary of the chemical properties of *cyclo*-octatetraene, see R. A. Raphael, in "Non-benzenoid Aromatic Compounds," Editor D. Ginsberg, Interscience Publishers, New York, 1959, Chap. 8, p. 465.

[41] J. W. Reppe, O. Schlichting, K. Klager, and T. Toepel, *Ann.*, 1948, **560**, 1; cf. also Section **49d**.

such as the fluoro- and deutero-carbethoxy-derivatives, the double bonds move round the ring; but that, because nuclear deformations are involved, an activation barrier resists the movement:[42]

For *cyclo*-octatetraene itself, the energy of activation of the cyclic bond shift is 13.7 kcal./mole, the lives of the successive stable conformations being of the order of a centisecond at 0°. In some substitution products the barriers are somewhat higher, and the individual conformers may live for several seconds at that temperature.

Several closed-conjugated large rings have been prepared, by Sondheimer and his coworkers, by the general method of oxidatively cyclising, or cyclicly polycondensing, alkane or alkene $\alpha\omega$-di-ynes, and subjecting the formed cyclic poly-ynes to graduated prototropic rearrangements and reductions.[43] $C_{14}H_{14}$ and $C_{18}H_{18}$, [14]-annulene and [18]-annulene, as they are called, are the best known. They are $4n+2$ hydrocarbons. Their nuclear magnetic resonance spectra show that they attain, and retain, the flat conformations represented below, at sufficiently reduced temperatures, $-60°$ for [14]-annulene and room temperature for [18]-annulene. At higher temperatures, for instance, room temperature for [14]-annulene and $+60°$ for [18]-annulene, these conformations become unstable. We can understand this, and also the greater stability of the flat conformation of [18]-annulene, inasmuch as the interior hydrogen atoms must be under a mutual compression which is strong in flat [14]-annulene, and appre-

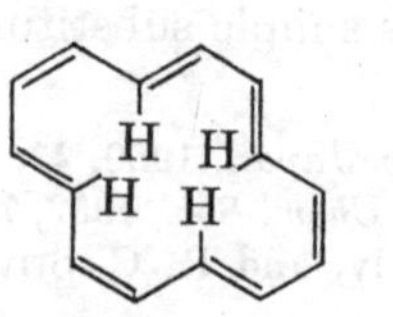

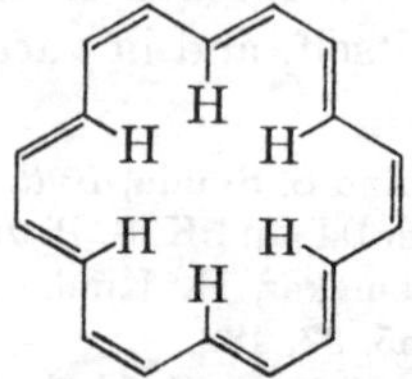

42 F. A. L. Anet, *J. Am. Chem. Soc.*, 1962, **84**, 671; *idem*, A. S. R. Bourn, and Y. S. Lin, *ibid.*, 1964, **86**, 3576; D. E. Gwynn, G. M. Whitesides, and J. D. Roberts, *ibid.*, 1965, **87**, 2862.

43 F. Sondheimer, Y. Amiel, and R. Wolovsky, *J. Am. Chem. Soc.*, 1957, **79**, 4247; F. Sondheimer and R. Wolovsky, *ibid.*, 1959, **81**, 1771, 4755; *idem* and Y. Guomi, *ibid.*, 1960, **82**, 755; F. Sondheimer and Y. Guomi, *ibid.*, p. 5765; F. Sondheimer, R. Wolovsky, and Y. Amiel, *ibid.*, 1962, **84**, 274; *idem*, L. M. Jackman, D. A. Ben-Effraim, Y. Guomi, and A. A. Bothner-By, *ibid.*, p. 4307; Y. Guomi and F. Sondheimer, *Proc. Chem. Soc.*, 1964, 299; *idem*, A. Malera, and R. Wolovsky, *ibid.*, p. 397; A. E. Beezer, C. T. Mortimer, H. D. Springall, F. Sondheimer, and R. Wolowsky, *J. Chem. Soc.*, **1965**, 216.

ciable in flat [18]-annulene. The mesomeric energy by heat of combustion of the latter is 100 kcal./mole. [24]-Annulene is of the $4n$ series, but [30]-annulene is a $4n+2$ hydrocarbon, and both are described as unstable. Probably Hückel's rule loses some of its force in such attenuated π electron systems as these very large rings present.

Pentalene and benzodipentadiene are so far unknown, despite many attempts to synthesize them, though heptalene (formulae, p. 195) has been obtained as a coloured, unstable, readily polymerising polyolefin.[44]

Azulene is well known and is, indeed, the parent of a great series of compounds, having a wide natural distribution in essential oils. Azulene is a blue solid, and an X-ray analysis of the crystal has shown[45] that the molecule is flat, and has the bond lengths given below (A):

1.39 1.39 1.39 1.48 1.40 1.41

7 8 9 1 6 10 2 5 4 3

The average bond length is as in benzene, 1.40 A, but the bridge-bond, which is single in both Kekulé structures (above), though it becomes double in some polar structures, is considerably longer, 1.48 A. Azulene has a dipole moment equal to 1.0 D; and measurements on 2-chloro-, 2-bromo-, and 2-cyano-azulene show that the electron displacement in the parent hydrocarbon is from the seven-membered to the five-membered ring. Azulene has an exaltation of diamagnetic susceptibility almost equal to that of its isomer naphthalene (Section 16c).[46] This means that cyclic electron delocalisation is approximately as good in azulene as it is in naphthalene. Azulene has a large, though not yet closely agreed, mesomeric energy. It has been estimated as being 30 kcal./mole less than that of naphthalene, and this, along with Pauling's figure for the latter molecule, would give 45 kcal./mole to azulene;[47] but an independent measurement by hydrogenation has given the value 31 kcal./mole.[39] It can probably be said that the uncorrected mesomeric energy of azulene must be approximately one-half that of naphthalene: and to the uncorrected value, a term of the order of 10 kcal./mole for the strain in the azulene ring would have to be added, in order to reach an estimate of the mesomeric energy in azulene.

Azulenes undergo most of the typical electrophilic aromatic substitutions, Friedel-Crafts acylations, nitrations, sulphonations, and

[44] H. Dauben and D. J. Bertelli, *J. Am. Chem. Soc.*, 1961, **83**, 4659.

[45] J. M. Robertson, H. M. M. Shearer, G. A. Sim, and D. G. Watson, *Acta Cryst.*, 1962, **15**, 1.

[46] W. Klemm, *Ber.*, 1957, **90**, 1051.

[47] E. Heilbronner and K. Wieland, *Helv. Chim. Acta*, 1947, **30**, 947.

diazo-couplings, though sometimes the conditions have to be carefully regulated, for the molecule is somewhat sensitive to drastic reagents.[48] The substitutions occur successively in the 1- and 3-positions; that is, they occur, as they should, in the five-membered ring, which we know to carry the negative dipole charge of the hydrocarbon; indeed, they occur where maxima of π electron densities have been placed by calculation.

The physical properties of acenaphthylene (formula, p. 195) seem not yet to have been studied. But it is a very stable hydrocarbon, formed in numerous high-temperature reactions, including the pyrolytic loss of hydrogen, above 700°, from its dihydro-derivative, acenaphthene (with a $\cdot CH_2 \cdot CH_2 \cdot$ bridge); and it is also formed from the latter by mild oxidising agents. It is produced, with an abnormal loss of hydrogen, when various acenaphthene-sulphonic and disulphonic acids are desulphonated with alkali. The $\cdot CH{:}CH \cdot$ bridge in acenaphthylene, rather like the $\cdot CH{:}CH \cdot$ bridge in phenanthrene, is mainly a centre of additions, as of halogens; and substituted derivatives are formed only after a subsequent elimination. Strong oxidation leads to naphthalic acid.

Diphenylene (formula, p. 197) was first prepared by Lothrop[49] from 2,2′-di-iodobiphenyl and cuprous oxide at 350°. It has a considerable mesomeric energy, about 22 kcal./mole, as deduced from its heat of combustion;[50] and when the strain energy, which cannot be much less than 30 kcal./mole, is added, the term properly attributable to π electron delocalisation (more than 50 kcal./mole) becomes a large fraction of that in biphenyl (about 79 kcal./mole). On the other hand, the electronic spectrum shows that there must be considerable interaction between the benzene rings.[51]

As to its chemical properties, Wilson Baker writes[52] that "it is not possible to handle diphenylene without becoming convinced that in nearly all respects it is a typical polynuclear aromatic compound." Nearly all its known reactions are normal electrophilic aromatic substitutions.[53] It can be halogenated, nitrated, and with mixed acid dinitrated, acetylated, and with excess of reagents diacetylated, and disulphonated. The first substituent enters the 2-position only, and the second the 6-position only, as far as is known.

[48] A. G. Anderson jr. and J. A. Nelson, *J. Am. Chem. Soc.*, 1950, **72**, 3824; A. G. Anderson jr., J. A. Nelson, and J. J. Tazuma, *ibid.*, 1953, **75**, 4980.

[49] W. C. Lothrop, *J. Am. Chem. Soc.*, 1941, **63**, 1187.

[50] R. C. Cass, H. D. Springall, and P. G. Quincey, *J. Chem. Soc.*, **1955**, 1188.

[51] E. P. Carr, L. W. Pickett, and D. Voris, *J. Am. Chem. Soc.*, 1941, **63**, 3031.

[52] W. Baker and J. F. W. McOmie in "Non-benzenoid Aromatic Compounds," Editor D. Ginsberg, Interscience Publishers, New York, 1959, p. 73.

[53] W. Baker, M. P. V. Boarland, and J. F. W. McOmie, *J. Chem. Soc.*, **1954**, 1476.

1,2:4,5-Dibenzopentalene (formula, p. 197), described by Blood and Linstead,[54] is a compound of a very different type. Its known reactions are all of the central butadiene residue. This residue is terminally dihydrogenated with sodium amalgam, tetrahydrogenated with hydrogen and palladised charcoal, and broken up completely on ozonolysis to form benzil-2,2′-dicarboxylic acid. All these reactions leave the benzene rings untouched.

(13e) Odd-Membered Aromatic Nuclei.—The valency bond structures in odd-membered rings cannot be closed-conjugated. Thus the mesomerism of the five-membered heterocyclic nuclei, as in pyrrole, differs qualitatively from that of the six-membered nuclei of the type of benzene and pyridine. Dipolar structures, which have to be included only in second approximation in the treatment of benzene, are quite fundamental to the mesomerism of a nucleus such as that of pyrrole. The principal structures which are required in order to express the mesomerism of a pyrrole are as follows:

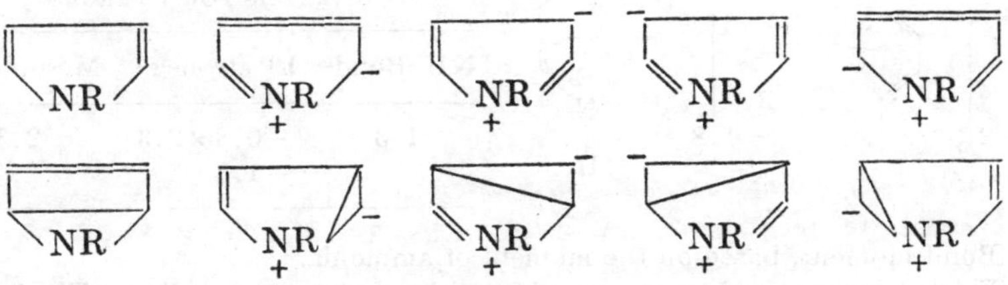

These structures allow the π electrons to circulate completely round the ring, but one pair of electrons remains continuously unshared. Thus the clockwise electron movement,

NR → NR

shifts the unshared pair one step anticlockwise; and the process can be continued as indicated by the arrows in the second formula. This means that, in the mesomeric state, the unshared electrons are spread all round the ring, so that the carbon atoms are partly anionic, and the nitrogen atom is, to a considerable extent, cationic. The same theory applies to other five-membered aromatic nuclei, such as those of thiophen, furan, glyoxaline, oxazole, etc., and to the five-membered components of condensed systems, such as those of indole, carbazole, thionaphthen, purine, etc.

Pyrrole has a large mesomeric energy, but it is smaller than that of

[54] C. T. Blood and R. P. Linstead, *J. Chem. Soc.*, **1952**, 2663.

benzene or pyridine; and the same difference runs through a comparison of analogous polynuclear compounds, as of indole with naphthalene or quinoline; and the distinction shows in heterocyclic molecules with other hetero atoms, molecules such as furan and thiophen (Section **15b**). The exaltation of diamagnetic susceptibility of pyrrole seems not to have been measured; but for furan the exaltation is large, though smaller than for benzene or pyridine. For thiophen the exaltation is as large as for benzene and pyridine (Section **16e**).

Pyrrole has the dipole moment +1.80 *D*, in the opposite direction to the dipole moment of pyridine.[55] The pyrrole moment can be approximately analysed as below. The analysis shows that a moment of +2.3 *D* arises from a mesomeric transfer of nitrogen electrons to the ring, spreading negative charges round the carbon atoms of the ring, and leaving the nitrogen atom with a positive charge, as the above polar valency structures would indicate:

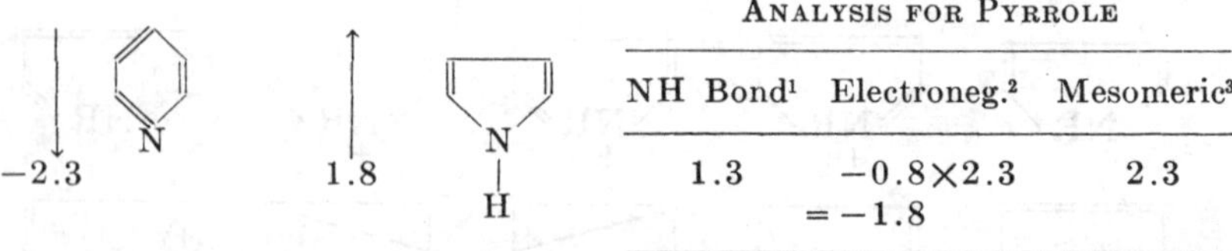

Analysis for Pyrrole

NH Bond[1]	Electroneg.[2]	Mesomeric[3]
1.3	−0.8×2.3 = −1.8	2.3

[1] Bond moment, based on the moment of ammonia.

[2] Electronegativity effect computed from the moment of pyridine. The factor 0.8 is a round allowance for the different numbers of σ and π electrons, and for the different geometry of the pyrrole molecule.

[3] By vector addition.

Although pyridine, quinoline, and acridine are bases, of the same order of basic strength as aniline, their odd-ring analogues, pyrrole, indole, and carbazole, are practically nonbasic. The theory of their mesomerism explains this, somewhat in the same way as Bamberger's theory did: the unshared nitrogen electrons are fundamentally involved in the aromatic system. The imino-hydrogen atoms of pyrrole, indole, and carbazole are distinctly acidic, like the imido-hydrogen atoms of succinimide and phthalimide. The theory accounts for this also: in each case, mesomerism confers a positive charge on the nitrogen atom.

The carbon positions in the pyrrole nucleus are enormously more reactive than those of the pyridine nucleus, or of benzene. As one standard text-book of organic chemistry remarks (twice on the same page): "The great reactivity of the methine hydrogens in pyrrole is

[55] H. Kofod, L. E. Sutton, and J. Jackson, *J. Chem. Soc.*, **1952**, 1467.

quite remarkable. They can be replaced by the most diverse atoms and groups with the same facility as the imine hydrogen, or even more." This is just what should be concluded from the theory that the unshared nitrogen electrons are spread all round the ring. To give one example, the action of halogens on pyrrole is extremely energetic, and, in order to secure sufficient control for preparative purposes, it is usual to work in very dilute solution: even then, in general, four or five hydrogen atoms are replaced. This behaviour is, of course, completely different from that of benzene and much more different from that of pyridine.

It has been shown[56] that 2,5-dimethylpyrrole and 1,2,5-trimethylpyrrole, on ozonolysis, give both glyoxal and methylglyoxal. This shows clearly that carbon unsaturation is not localised in the 2,3- and 4,5-bonds, but is distributed all round the ring as the preceding formulae illustrate.

The capacity of *cyclo*pentadiene to yield stable sodium and other alkali metal salts (the property used to separate it from the light fraction from coal tar) is evidently associated with the same type of mesomerism. The free hydrocarbon is not aromatic—its mesomeric energy is about the same as that of buta-1,3-diene. But the anion is aromatic, in the same way as is pyrrole. And thus the anion is much less unstable than hydrocarbon anions usually are. The valency structures are shown below, the anionic charge being equally divided between the five carbon atoms in the mesomeric state:

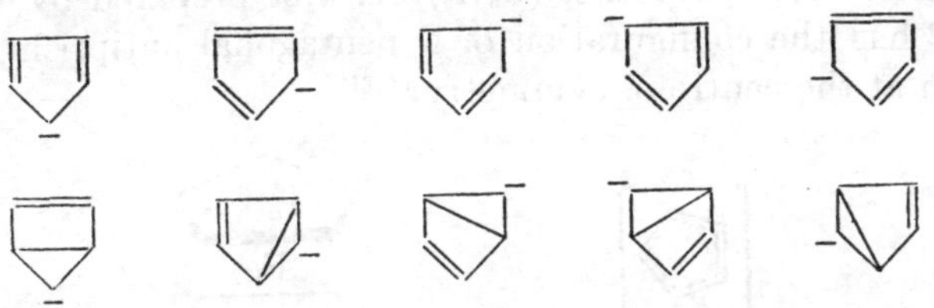

Indene and fluorene also form alkali metal salts. When an aqueous solution of a quaternary 9-fluorenylammonium salt, or of a 9-fluorenylsulphonium salt, is made alkaline, highly coloured, somewhat unstable compounds are produced. The coloured substance from dimethyl-9-fluorenylsulphonium salts has been investigated in some detail, and shown to be dimethylsulphonium-9-fluorenylide:[57]

[56] J. P. Wibaut and A. R. Gulje, *Proc. Koninkl. Akad. Nederland. Wetenschap.*, 1951, **B**, **54**, 330; J. P. Wibaut, *ibid.*, 1965, **B**, **68**, 117. Incidentally, J. P. Wibaut and S. Herzberg have shown that 2, 6-dimethylpyrone on ozonolysis gives glyoxylic acid, as well as methylglyoxal (*ibid.*, 1953, **56**, 333), thus vindicating Arndt's idea (Section **7b**) that the pyrone molecule is partly converted to pyrylium form.

[57] C. K. Ingold and J. A. Jessop, *J. Chem. Soc.*, **1929**, 2357; *ibid.*, **1930**, 713.

$$\text{(fluorenyl)}CH-\overset{+}{S}Me_2 \xrightarrow{\overset{-}{O}H} \text{(fluorenyl)}\overset{-}{C}-\overset{+}{S}Me_2$$

The reason for its formation is evidently that the anionic centre is stabilised by mesomerism of the *cyclo*pentadienide-ion type. As we noticed in Section **8b**, the large dipole moment of the compound shows that the unshared carbon electrons are not absorbed into the sulphur atom to a predominating extent, even though the latter has unoccupied orbitals. Krollpfeiffer and Schneider prepared the corresponding pyridinium-'ylide, and Wittig and his coworkers have made the trimethylammonium-, trimethylphosphonium-, and trimethylarsonium-'ylides:[58]

$$(C_6H_4)_2\overset{-}{C}H-\overset{+}{N}C_5H_5 \qquad (C_6H_4)_2\overset{-}{C}H-\overset{+}{X}Me_3 \quad (X = N, P, As)$$

In the nitrogen compounds no question of absorption of the 'ylide electrons into the cationic centre can arise.

The free *cyclo*pentadienylide ion should have full pentagonal symmetry. What has been proved convincingly by X-ray analysis is that its iron derivative, ferrocene, $(C_5H_5)_2Fe$, first prepared by Kealy and Pauson,[59] has the configuration of a pentagonal antiprism, with the iron atom at the centre of symmetry.[60,61]

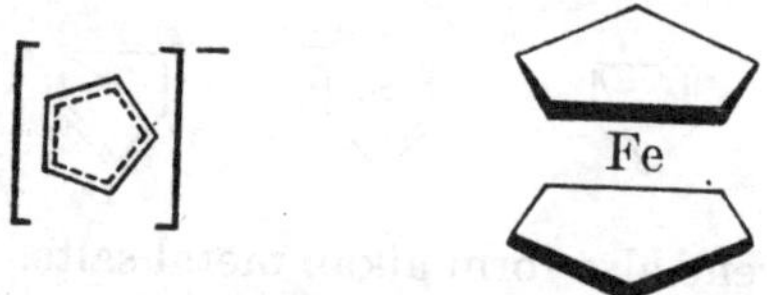

The extent of observed isomerism among derivatives of ferrocene has created the impression that no large barrier exists to rotation of the separate rings around the pentagonal axis. The substance is volatile, and stable to heat, sensitive to oxidising agents, but stable towards reducing agents. It is not prone to additions, but can undergo some electrophilic substitutions, for instance, sulphonations and Friedel-

[58] F. Krollpfeiffer and K. Schneider, *Ann.*, 1937, **530**, 34; G. Wittig and F. Felletschin, *Ann.*, 1944, **555**, 133; G. Wittig and H. Laib, *Ann.*, 1953, **580**, 57.

[59] T. J. Kealy and P. L. Pauson, *Nature*, 1951, **168**, 1039.

[60] J. D. Dunitz and L. E. Orgel, *Nature*, 1953, **171**, 121.

[61] P. L. Pauson, *Quart. Revs.*, 1955, **9**, 391.

Crafts acylations.[61] In these reactions, the first two substituents enter one in each ring. But an alkyl substituent, already in one ring, in part attracts an entering acyl group to the 2- and 3-positions of the same ring. All this suggests a considerable degree of aromaticity. But just how the iron atom absorbs the anionic charges without seriously impairing their delocalisation is not completely clear, though it is obvious that the 3*d* orbitals of the iron atom must be involved.

*Cyclo*heptatriene (tropilidene) is a polyolefin of no very special stability. But, as Doering and Knox showed,[62] it adds Br_2, and the adduct loses HBr, to give the ionic bromide of the *cyclo*heptatrienylium (tropylium) ion, an outstandingly stable carbonium ion.[63]

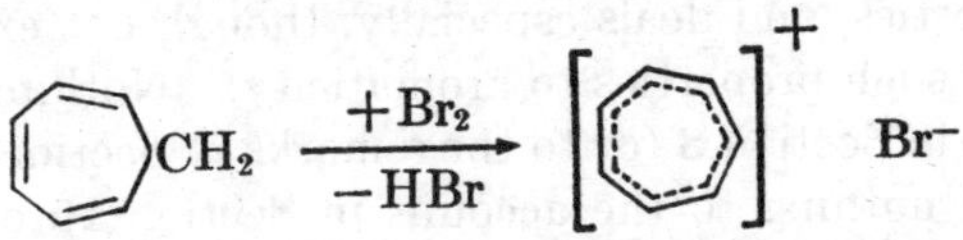

$$C_7H_6 \cdot CH_2 \xrightarrow[-HBr]{+Br_2} [C_7H_7]^+ \; Br^-$$

The tropylium ion should have full heptagonal symmetry, with a delocalised π sextet, to which several sets of seven equivalent valency structures can be assigned, the unbridged set being as shown below:

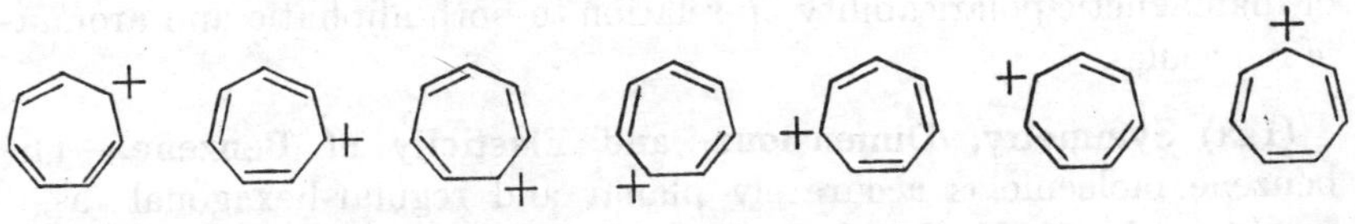

Most carbonium ions (see Chapter VII) are destroyed instantly and irreversibly by water, and indeed by any basic substance, neutral or anionic. But the tropylium ion has considerable stability in water, reacting with it reversibly, and qualitatively in the manner of the cation of a pseudo-base (Chapter XI), but here only to a small equilibrium extent, to form pseudo-basic *cyclo*heptatrienol (tropenol):

$$C_7H_7^+ + H_2O \rightleftharpoons C_7H_7 \cdot OH + H^+$$

Even in dilute solution, the tropylium ion is the more stable species; and, in view of the strong contrast with the properties of carbonium ions in general, this is a striking illustration of the stabilising effect of a delocalised six-electron π shell.

[62] W. von E. Doering and L. H. Knox, *J. Am. Chem. Soc.*, 1954, **76**, 3203.

[63] The text illustrates the naming of carbon cations and anions. The names are formed by adding "ium" or "ide" to the name of the radical:

$CH_3\cdot$	CH_3^+	CH_3^-
methyl	methylium	methylide

It is obvious that a whole series of seven-membered hetero-aromatic systems, typified by boratropylene and beryllatropylene, the electron-deficient counterparts of pyrrole and furan, remain undiscovered at the present time:

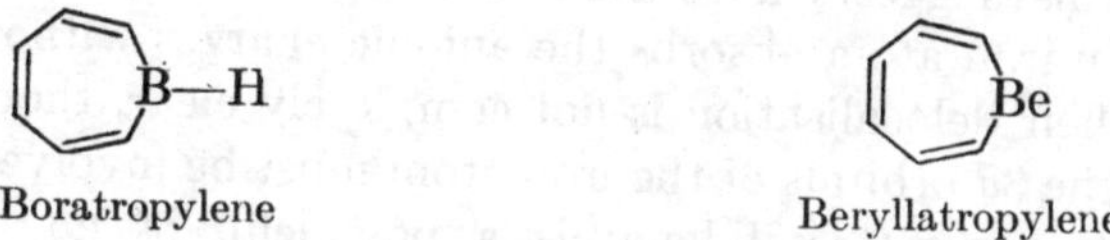

Boratropylene Beryllatropylene

(14) SYMMETRY, DIMENSIONS, AND ELASTICITY OF AROMATIC MOLECULES

The rest of this Chapter continues the treatment in Chapter III of physical properties, and deals especially, though not exclusively, with the relation of such properties to aromaticity. Nothing will be added to the account in Section **8** (or to the remarks in Section **13e**) on dipole moments, and nothing to the account in Section **10** of electrical polarisability. In this Section we shall deal with the symmetry, dimensions, and elasticity of aromatic molecules, and in the next Section with energy in rings, both aliphatic and aromatic. Then there will follow a separate Section on the property, not treated at all in Chapter III, of diamagnetic polarisability, in relation to both aliphatic and aromatic molecules.

(14a) Symmetry, Dimensions, and Elasticity of Benzene.—The benzene molecule is accurately planar and regular-hexagonal (as it would not be, if it had a single Kekulé formula). This result was first given by electron diffraction measurements to the not very narrow limits of accuracy of that method.[64] This conclusion was at one time seriously questioned, on what in principle was more precise spectroscopic evidence. It has, however, been confirmed with all the precision of the spectroscopic method: no frequencies that this strict symmetry would forbid are present in the vibration-rotation spectra of the gaseous substance.[65] Benzene has 20 fundamental frequencies, and the molecular symmetry forbids all but four in the infra-red, and all but seven others in the Raman spectrum, so that nine are totally

[64] R. Wierl, *Ann. Physik*, 1931, **8**, 521; P. L. F. Jones, *Trans. Faraday Soc.*, 1935, **31**, 1036; V. Schomaker and L. Pauling, *J. Am. Chem. Soc.*, 1939, **61**, 1769.

[65] W. R. Angus, C. R. Bailey, J. B. Hale, C. K. Ingold, A. H. Leckie, C. G. Raisin, J. W. Thompson, and C. L. Wilson, *J. Chem. Soc.*, **1936**, 912, *et seq.*; C. R. Bailey, A. P. Best, S. C. Carson, R. R. Gordon, J. B. Hale, N. Herzfeld, J. W. Holden, C. K. Ingold, A. H. Leckie, H. G. Poole, L. H. P. Weldon, and C. I Wilson, *ibid.*, **1946**, 222, *et seq.*

forbidden. It was once thought that a deviation from strictly regular-hexagonal symmetry was established by the appearance of some of these forbidden frequencies. But the appearances which seemed so to indicate were traced to the very small (and fluctuating) deformations which are produced by van der Waals forces in the liquid substance.[66] The frequencies in question had been determined by calculation from observed frequencies of dissymmetrically deuterated benzenes;[65] and so, when they were made visible by intermolecular forces in a condensed phase, their identity was known. Intermolecular forces act similarly, but less indiscriminately, in the solid substance. The molecule in the crystal will still be very nearly planar and regular-hexagonal; but the arrangement of neighbours around a given molecule is such as to reduce the strict symmetry to that of a centre of symmetry only. In the spectra, the molecule registers accordingly; and thus in the infra-red spectrum, six of the nine totally forbidden frequencies can be seen.[67] A powerful way of bringing out the forbidden frequencies is to put the benzene into a solvent, such as carbon disulphide, which exerts strong electrokinetic forces.[68] All the 20 frequencies of benzene can then be seen in the infra-red spectrum. All but the four allowed ones disappear completely from the spectrum of the gas.

The dimensions of benzene are given most accurately by the rotational Raman spectrum.[69] The bond lengths are CC = 1.397 *A* and CH = 1.084 *A*.

The elastic properties of benzene have been computed from the determined vibration frequencies, on the assumption that the energy of deformation can be represented in terms of six Hooke's-law constants.[70] These comprise a CC stretching force constant F, a CH stretching force constant f; also two moment constants for bending in the molecular plane, one of these, Δ, for bending of the ring angle, and the other, δ, for planar CH bending from the bisector of the ring angle; also included are two moment constants for bending out of the molecular plane; one of these, Γ, is for CC bond twisting by unequal out-of-plane bending of attached carbon atoms, and unequal out-of-plane bending of attached hydrogen atoms; and the other, γ, is for CH bend-

[66] W. R. Angus, C. R. Bailey, J. B. Hale, C. K. Ingold, A. H. Leckie, C. G. Raisin, and C. L. Wilson, *J. Chem. Soc.*, **1936**, 966.

[67] R. D. Mair and D. F. Hornig, *J. Chem. Phys.*, 1949, **17**, 1236.

[68] J. K. Thomson and A. D. E. Pullin, *J. Chem. Soc.*, **1957**, 1658; E. E. Ferguson, *J. Chem. Phys.*, 1957, **26**, 1265.

[69] A. Langseth and B. P. Stoicheff, *Canadian J. Phys.*, 1956, **34**, 350.

[70] E. B. Wilson, *Physical Rev.*, 1934, **45**, 706; R. P. Bell, *Trans. Faraday Soc.*, 1945, **41**, 293; F. M. Garforth, C. K. Ingold, and H. G. Poole, *J. Chem. Soc.*, **1948**, 492; 508.

ing out of the plane of the nearest three carbon atoms. The calculated force and moment constants are as follows:

$F = 7.61 \times 10^5$ dyne/cm. $f = 5.06 \times 10^5$ dyne/cm.
$\Delta = 13.7 \times 10^{-12}$ dyne-cm./radian $\delta = 8.0 \times 10^{-12}$ dyne-cm./radian
$\Gamma = 1.02 \times 10^{-12}$ dyne-cm./radian $\gamma = 2.62 \times 10^{-12}$ dyne-cm./radian

These force and moment constants reproduce the fundamental frequencies of benzene, and of its various deutero-derivatives, fairly well on the whole; but there is one strongly discrepant vibration. For benzene, the root-mean-square deviation of the calculated frequencies is under 8%, provided that we omit one frequency, for which the error is 40%. There is nothing complicated about the calculation of this particular frequency, which, like the "breathing frequency," 992 cm.$^{-1}$, shown below, depends on only one force constant, the CC stretching constant F, in the six-constant force system above. The value of this constant quoted above is taken from the frequency of the "breathing" vibration, in which six CC bonds stretch in phase. When the value is applied in order to calculate the frequency of the trigonal vibration shown below, in which three CC bonds stretch while three contract, all ring angles remaining 120°, and the molecule remaining flat, as before, the calculated frequency works out to 1837 cm.$^{-1}$. The observed frequency[67] is 1310 cm.$^{-1}$.

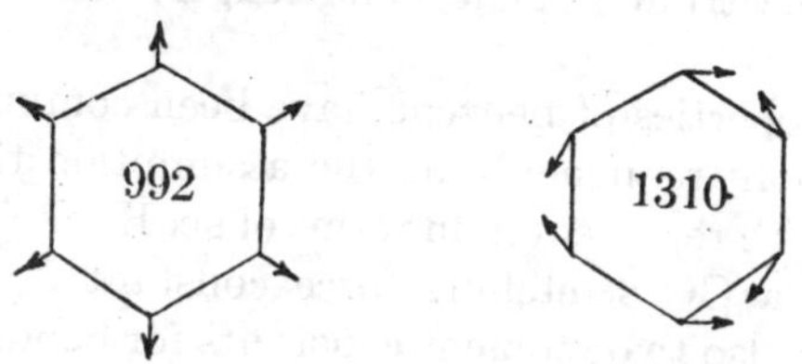

This large discrepancy is clearly connected with the circumstance that the trigonal vibration, in both directions of its amplitude, changes the nuclear framework towards those of canonical structures—structures that would exist, were it not that the delocalisation energy of π electrons makes another structure still more stable. These are the Kekulé structures, which would have alternate long and short bonds, but unchanged ring angles, and unchanged planarity. We may suppose that, as the nuclear framework changes towards that of such a structure, the electronic wave-function will follow it, to give bonds of alternating multiplicities, and therefore alternating bond-stretching force constants, such as will reduce the restoring forces, and thus lower the frequency. The restoring forces are reduced by the factor $(1310/1837)^2$, that is, by about one-half.

According to figures given in Section **13b,** the stretching force constants of CC bonds are roughly proportional to bond multiplicity.

The force constant F, given above for benzene, can be included in this statement, if a multiplicity of 1.5 is assigned to the benzene bond:

Multiplicity of CC bond	1	1.5	2	3
F in 10^5 dyne/cm.	4.5	7.6	9.8	15.6

The most notable feature of the bending moment constants is the smallness of the out-of-plane constants. The CC twisting moment constant of benzene, $10^{12}\Gamma = 1.0$ dyne-cm./radian, is only about one-fifth of the twisting constant for ethylene (5.3 in the same units),[71] whilst the out-of-plane CH bending constant of benzene, $10^{12}\gamma = 2.7$ dyne-cm.-radian, is only one-third of the corresponding in-plane bending constant of benzene. So much emphasis is laid on the planarity of benzene, that one tends to forget how easily that molecule can suffer out-of-plane deformations. For example, there was general surprise when paradixylylene (formula below) was found to be a stable substance. For since the van der Waals distance between two parallel benzene rings must approximate to the graphite layer-plane separation, 3.4 *A*, much out-of-plane bending is required to close the cyclophane ring in paradixylylene. An X-ray examination of this substance by C. J. Brown has given the results shown below.[72] The benzene rings are found to be squeezed to within the graphite separation by 0.3 *A*. However, they have each developed the two dihedral angles of 10.7°, marked below, and the bonds to the methylene groups have each become bent further in the same direction by 13.9°. The ring deformation is exactly that which produces the lowest of all the fundamental frequencies of benzene, 400 cm.$^{-1}$, the classical amplitude of which, in its zero-point vibration, is more than one-quarter of the deformation found in para-dixylylene.

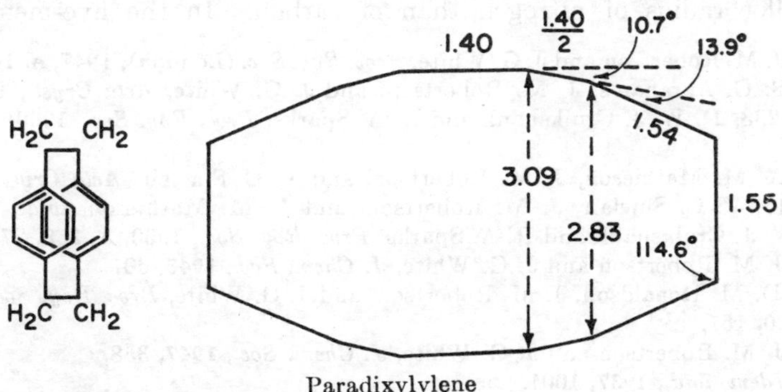

Paradixylylene

[71] R. L. Arnett and B. L. Crawford jr., *J. Chem. Phys.*, 1950, **18**, 118.
[72] C. J. Brown, *J. Chem. Soc.*, 1953, 3265.

(14b) Dimensions of Aromatic Molecules.—A series of measurements by the X-ray method of the CC bond lengths of polynuclear aromatic hydrocarbons has been made by Robertson and others. The general accuracy, carefully estimated by Robertson and White, is ±0.02 *A*.[73] For naphthalene,[74] anthracene,[75] coronene,[76] and ovalene,[77] all the carbon atomic positions have been determined; for pyrene,[78] 1,2:5,6-dibenzanthracene,[79] and perylene,[80] a proportion of them have been determined and others deduced from the assumed molecular symmetry. It is established that all the CC distances are not identical in any of these hydrocarbons, and it is of interest to compare the observed variations with the bond multiplicities as computed, with neglect of trans-annular binding, in the simple way illustrated in Section **13c**. This is done in Table 14-1 (lengths in *A*).

In naphthalene, perylene, coronene, and ovalene there is qualitative agreement between the variations of bond length and the simply computed multiplicities. In naphthalene there is an alternation of length in the external bonds of each ring. In coronene the interior bonds have the graphite length, while the exterior ones have lengths varying, according to type, about the benzene length. In anthracene there is a significant lack of agreement, inasmuch as the 2,3-bond is shorter than would be expected. In 1,2:5,6-dibenzanthracene and in pyrene there are notable qualitative divergences, particularly with respect to the bond which corresponds to the 9,10-bond of phenanthrene: this should be almost a double bond, but its length is practically the same as that of a benzene bond.

Some recorded dimensions of heterocyclic aromatic nuclei are set out in Table 14-2. Except that the CC bonds of pyrazine are unexpectedly short, the figures contain no great surprises. In the six-membered rings, the lengths are as for benzene, allowing for the smaller radius of nitrogen than of carbon. In the five-membered

[73] J. M. Robertson and J. G. White, *Proc. Roy. Soc.* (London), 1947, **A, 190,** 329.

[74] S. C. Abrahams, J. M. Robertson, and J. G. White, *Acta Cryst.*, 1949, **2,** 233, 238, D. W. J. Cruikshank and R. A. Sparks, *Proc. Roy. Soc.*, 1960, **A, 258,** 270.

[75] A. M. Mathieson, J. M. Robertson, and V. C. Sinclair, *Acta Cryst.*, 1950, **3,** 245; V. C. Sinclair, J. M. Robertson, and A. M. Mathieson, *ibid.*, p. 251; D. W. J. Cruikshank and R. A. Sparks, *Proc. Roy. Soc.*, 1960, **A, 258,** 270.

[76] J. M. Robertson and J. G. White, *J. Chem. Soc.*, **1945,** 607.

[77] D. M. Donaldson, J. M. Robertson, and J. G. White, *Proc. Roy. Soc.*, 1953 **A, 220,** 157.

[78] J. M. Robertson and J. G. White, *J. Chem. Soc.*, **1947,** 358.

[79] *Idem. ibid.*, **1937,** 1001.

[80] D. M. Donaldson, J. M. Robertson, and J. G. White, *Proc. Roy. Soc.*, 1953, **A. 220,** 311.

TABLE 14-1.—CARBON BOND LENGTHS IN AROMATIC HYDROCARBONS.

Hydrocarbon	Carbon bond length (A)	Bond multiplicity
Benzene	1.397	3/2
Naphthalene	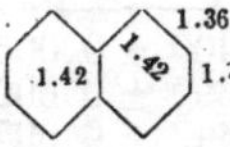 1.36, 1.42, 1.42, 1.41	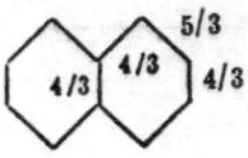 5/3, 4/3, 4/3, 4/3
Anthracene	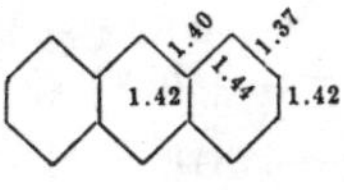 1.40, 1.37, 1.42, 1.44, 1.42	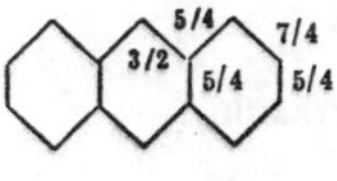 5/4, 7/4, 3/2, 5/4, 5/4
1,2:5,6-Dibenzanthracene	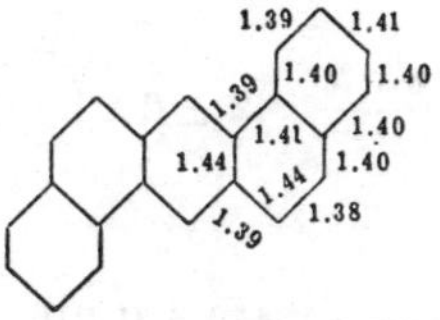 1.39, 1.41, 1.40, 1.40, 1.39, 1.41, 1.40, 1.44, 1.40, 1.44, 1.39, 1.38	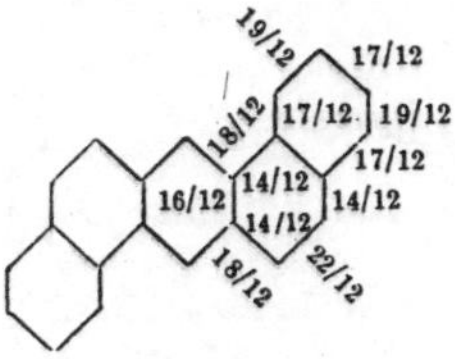 19/12, 17/12, 17/12, 19/12, 18/12, 17/12, 16/12, 14/12, 14/12, 14/12, 18/12, 22/12
Pyrene	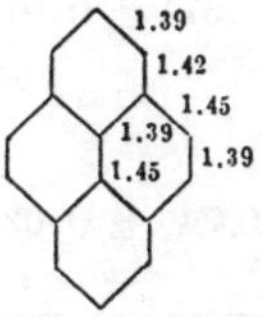 1.39, 1.42, 1.45, 1.39, 1.45, 1.39	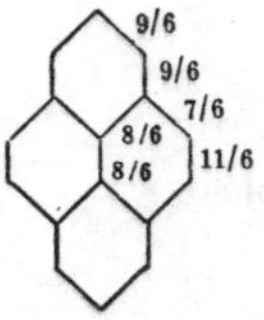 9/6, 9/6, 7/6, 8/6, 8/6, 11/6
Perylene	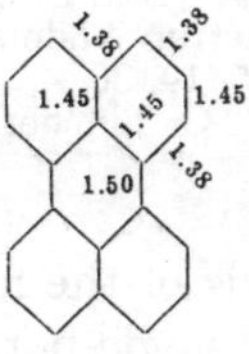 1.38, 1.38, 1.45, 1.45, 1.45, 1.38, 1.50	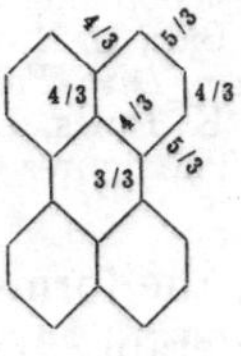 4/3, 5/3, 4/3, 4/3, 4/3, 5/3, 3/3
Coronene	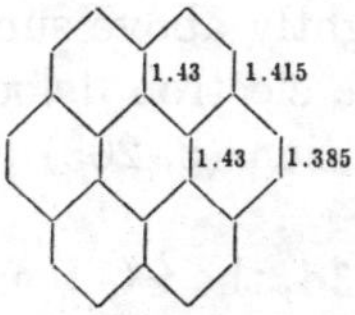 1.43, 1.415, 1.43, 1.385	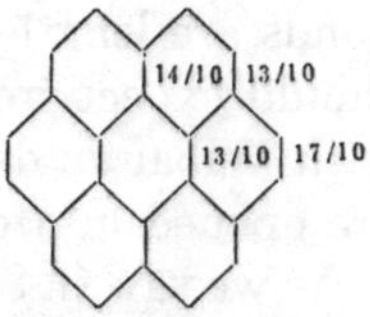 14/10, 13/10, 13/10, 17/10
Ovalene	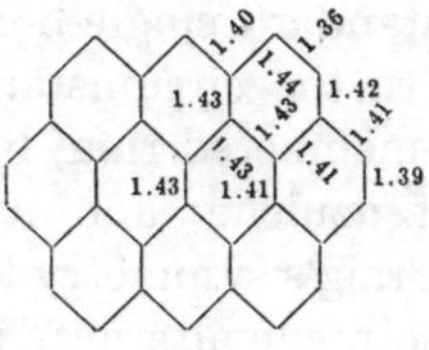 1.40, 1.36, 1.44, 1.43, 1.42, 1.43, 1.41, 1.43, 1.41, 1.43, 1.41, 1.39	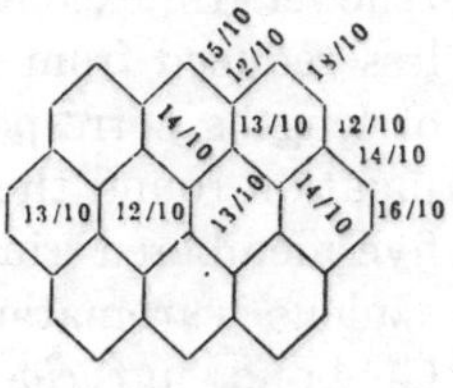 15/10, 12/10, 18/10, 14/10, 13/10, 12/10, 14/10, 13/10, 14/10, 13/10, 12/10, 16/10
Graphite	1.42	4/3

TABLE 14.2—DIMENSIONS OF HETERO-AROMATIC RINGS.

Compound	Bond lengths (A)	Hetero-angle	Ref.
Pyridine	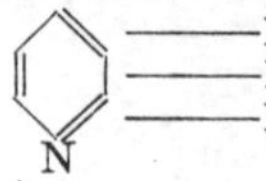 1.400 ± 0.005 1.390 ± 0.005 1.340 ± 0.005	116.7°	2
Pyrazine	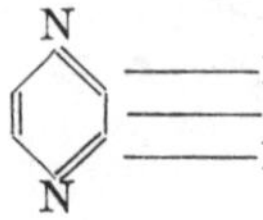 1.341 1.335 1.341	116°	4
Pyrrole	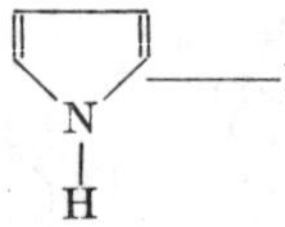 1.42 ± 0.02	105° ± 4°	1
Furan	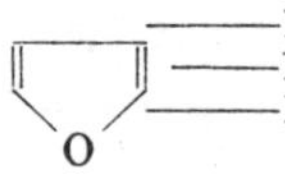 1.440 ± 0.016 1.354 ± 0.016 1.371 ± 0.016	106.1° ± 0.6°	3
Thiophen	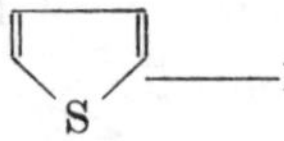 1.74 ± 0.03	91° ± 4°	1

[1] V. Schomaker and L. Pauling, *J. Am. Chem. Soc.*, 1939, **61,** 1769.
[2] B. Bak, L. Hansen, and J. Rastrup-Andersen, *J. Chem. Phys.*, 1954, **22,** 2013.
[3] *Idem, Disc. Faraday Soc.*, 1955, **19,** 30.
[4] K. K. Innes, J. A. Merritt, W. C. Tincher, and S. G. Tilford, *Nature*, 1960, **187,** 500. The figures are provisional.

rings, the formal single bonds of the non-polar structures are reduced considerably below sums of single-bond radii, and the formal double bonds are lengthened slightly above sums of double-bond radii, as we should expect from cyclic electron delocalisation, and as is consistent with Wibaut's demonstration (p. 205) that all CC bonds in a pyrrole are opened in ozonolysis.

As we saw in Section **13d,** the CC bonds in azulene all have the benzene length, except the bridge bond, which has a length, 1.48 *A*, much less reduced from the standard single-bond value. This distribution of lengths corresponds to the circumstance that there is closed-conjugation round the ten-membered ring, but not round the seven- and five-membered rings of azulene; and it agrees with the fact that azulene is aromatic by Craig's symmetry test. Again, we saw that the CC bonds in *cyclo*-octatetraene alternate in length between the mildly reduced single-bond length, 1.47 *A*, and the standard double-bond length, 1.32 *A*. This suggests that only a little functional conjugation is present, as follows from the multiplanar character of the molecule, and, as we shall see, its trivial mesomeric energy. It is consistent with the classification of *cyclo*-octatetraene, on grounds of electronic symmetry, as pseudo-aromatic.

(15) ENERGY IN ALIPHATIC AND AROMATIC RINGS

(15a) Steric Energy in Aliphatic Rings.—As was illustrated in Section **6e**, the heats of combustion of the *cyclo*alkanes do not increase with homology by equal increments, as do those of normal open-chain alkanes once these molecules are long enough to eliminate end-effects on the differences. The variations in the heats for the *cyclo*alkanes show that the rings must contain an energy term dependent on ring size. As Spitzer and Huffman originally found over the range *cyclo*pentane to *cyclo*octane, this energy is minimal in *cyclo*hexane. If we assume that the energy term is zero in *cyclo*hexane, we can assign values to the ring-dependent term in the other cases.

Measurements of the heats of combustion of *cyclo*alkanes have since been considerably extended, largely by Coops, whose values agree well with Spitzer and Huffman's, where there is overlap. Relatively to *cyclo*hexane as zero, the ring energy terms, E_r, of the *cyclo*alkanes, C_nH_{2n}, from *cyclo*propane to *cyclo*heptadecane, are as given below (kcal./mole).[81] They are graphically represented in Fig. 15-1.

n	3	4	5	6	7	8	9	10
E_r	27.9	26.6	6.0	0.0	5.9	9.7	12.1	12.8

n	11	12	13	14	15	16	17
E_r	12.3	5.1	7.1	3.6	5.0	4.3	4.5

Three sources of energy, due to ring formation in aliphatic rings, have been recognised: each shows itself prominently in various parts of the trace in Fig. 15-1. In 1885, Baeyer recognised stress in bonds, due to the deviations of ring angles from the tetrahedral angle.[82] Apart from double and triple bonds, which he considered as rings, Baeyer was concerned mainly with the apparently smaller stability of three- and four-membered rings than of five- and six-membered rings. Baeyer carried his comparisons only up to six-membered rings; and even they became

[81] Data for C_3H_6 by J. W. Knowlton and F. D. Rossini, *J. Res. Nat. Bur. Standards*, 1949, **43**, 113; for C_4H_8 by S. Kaarsenmaker and J. Coops, *Rec. trav. chim.*, 1950, **69**, 1364; for C_5H_{10} to C_8H_{16} by R. Spitzer and H. M. Huffman, *J. Am. Chem. Soc.*, 1947, **60**, 211; for C_4H_8 to C_9H_{18} by J. Coops and S. Kaarsenmaker, *Rec. trav. chim.*, 1952, **71**, 261; and for $C_{10}H_{20}$ to $C_{17}H_{34}$ by J. Coops, H. van Kamp, W. A. Lambregts, B. J. Visser, and H. Dekker, *ibid.*, 1960, **79**, 1226. Collation after D. P. Craig in "Non-benzenoid Aromatic Hydrocarbons," Editoı D. Ginsberg, Interscience Publishers, New York, 1959, p. 20; and J. Sicher in "Progress in Stereochemistry," Editors P. B. D. de la Mare and W. Klyne, Butterworths, London, 1962, Vol. 3, p. 202.

[82] A. von Baeyer, *Ber.*, 1885, **18**, 2277.

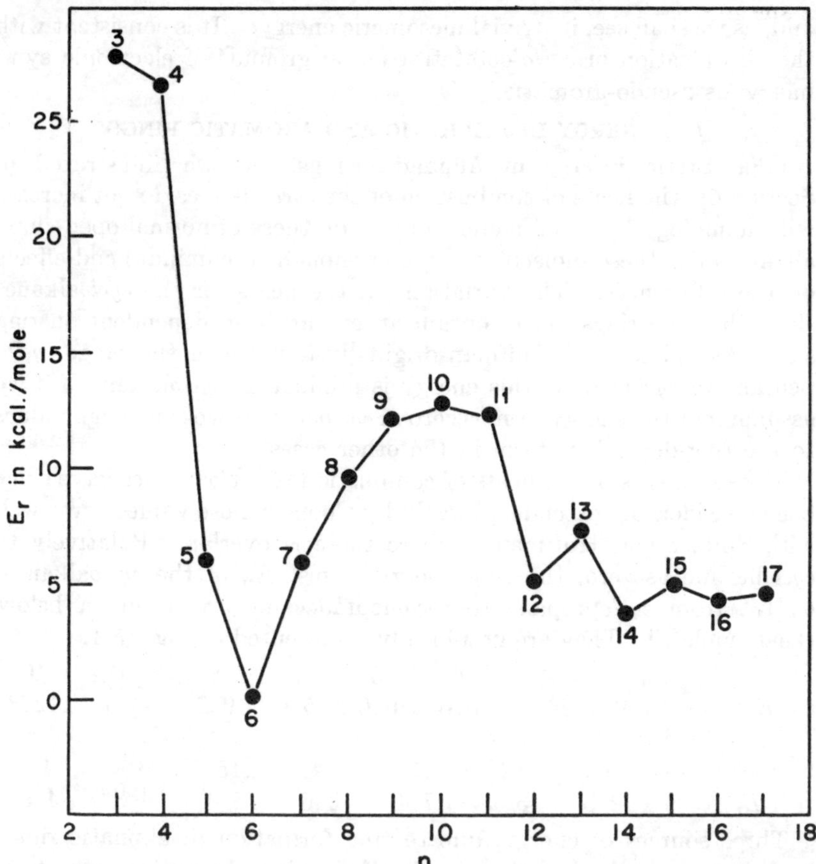

FIG. 15-1.—Ring energy terms of *cyclo*alkanes. (The errors range from 0.5 kcal./mole at $n = 17$, downwards approximately proportionally to n.)

disqualified for inclusion in the theory, when, in 1890, Sachse pointed out that they could assume strainless conformations.[83] But for three-, four-, and five-membered rings, the Baeyer thesis held, except that, as experience accumulated, four-membered rings seemed not to have the expected markedly greater stability than three-membered.[84] Thus the idea became current that other influences would have to be admitted. Baeyer called his source of energy "*Spannung*," which means stress, but was translated as "strain," the term which then became commonly used in English;[85] but now that other stereochemical energy

[83] H. Sachse, *Ber.*, 1890, **23**, 1362.

[84] W. H. Perkin and J. Simonsen, *J. Chem. Soc.*, 1907, **91**, 816.

[85] The same common confusion of stress with strain caused abandonment of the term "electronic strain" (meaning a displaced electron distribution) (1926).

terms have to be distinguished, it is conveniently called "Baeyer strain."

The next influence to be recognised was the application to rings of the difference of stability of staggered and eclipsed conformations around the ring bonds. As explained in Section **6e,** the existence of such conformational energy differences was established in the basic case of ethane by Kemp and Pitzer in 1936, and its direction was first determined from the pattern of variation of energy in *cyclo*alkane homologues by Spitzer and Huffman in 1947. They concluded that the staggered conformation was the more stable, because they found that an energy minimum in the homologous series occurred at *cyclo*hexane, the only homologue that had a totally staggered conformation free from Baeyer strain. *Cyclo*pentane and *cyclo*heptane contained ring energy, presumably minimised by partition between Baeyer strain and the energy of non-staggered conformations. The latter energy term has been given the matching designation "Pitzer strain." This form of strain will also be a source of instability, on the one hand, in *cyclo*butane and *cyclo*propane, and, on the other, in *cyclo*-octane and other homologues above *cyclo*heptane, though it must finally fade out in large enough rings.

But before this happens, a third influence shows itself, in the relative instability of nine- to eleven-membered rings. The first indication of this appeared in Ruzicka's work of the 1920's on the preparation of large-ring ketones by pyrolysis of thorium and other heavy-metal salts of alkane-$\alpha\omega$-dicarboxylic acids: the yields fell sharply, from the six-membered ring ketone, to a very low minimum at the nine- to eleven-membered rings, and then rose slowly towards the still larger rings.[86] In the 1930's, Ziegler achieved considerably higher yields of the large-ring ketones by using Thorpe's reaction[87] in conditions of high dilution. These conditions were set up in order to counteract the competition of intermolecular coupling, a competition which grows with increasing length of the chain to be intramolecularly cyclised;[88] but

[86] L. Ruzicka, M. Stoll, and H. Schinz, *Helv. Chim. Acta*, 1926, **9,** 249.

[87] This is a base-promoted cyclisation of dinitriles to imino-nitriles, hydrolysable to cyclic ketones:

$$(CH_2)_{n-2}\begin{cases} CH_2CN \\ CN \end{cases} \rightarrow (CH_2)_{n-2}\begin{cases} CH\cdot CN \\ | \\ C{:}NH \end{cases} \rightarrow (CH_2)_{n-2}\begin{cases} CH_2 \\ | \\ CO \end{cases}$$

[88] K. Ziegler, H. Emde, and H. Ohlinger, *Annalen*, 1933, **504,** 94.

Ziegler did not overcome the low yields of "medium-sized" rings, as the eight- to twelve-membered rings are called.

After a survey of such matters, and some study of the properties of medium-sized rings, which had in the meantime been obtained in good yields by the acyloin reaction,[89] Prelog suggested in 1950 that medium-sized rings have a special source of instability, due to trans-annular pressures of ring-bound atoms, which, in order to relieve excessive strain in other forms, become turned inward on ring-formation: in small rings the atoms are not turned inward, and in large rings they do not have to be, or, if they are, find space enough not mutually to interfere.[90] Since then, this special factor of instability has been thermochemically demonstrated,[81] and its identification as trans-annular non-bonding energy—"Prelog strain" as it has been called—has been supported by a large weight of chemical and physical evidence.

The chemical evidence consists in trans-annular reactions between atoms or groups which would not interact, if, with their immediate environments, they were presented to each other in separate molecules. In the *cyclo*decane series, reactions of the types known to proceed through carbonium ions (Chapters VII and IX), for instance, nucleophilic substitutions and eliminations by acetolysis of toluene-*p*-sulphonates ($X = \cdot O \cdot SO_2 \cdot C_6H_4Me$, in the formula below) in acetic acid, and by deamination of amines ($X = NH_2$) by nitrous acid, involve trans-annular hydride-ion shifts. The result is that, to a major extent, as was proved by isotopic labelling, the new substituent ($Y = OAc$, OH), or the introduced double bond, appears remotely from where the old substituent (X) departed.[91] Details concerning the mechanism remain to be filled in, but a first approximate formulation, given below, expresses the essential discovery:

[89] By the use of sodium, this reaction couples two carboxylic ester groups, either of different molecules or of the same molecule, to give either an open-chain or cyclic acyloin. Large-ring acyloins are thus obtained easily and without working at high dilutions. A possible route is as follows:

$$C_n\begin{cases}CO_2Et\\ CO_2Et\end{cases} \xrightarrow{2Na} C_n\begin{cases}C(ONa)(OR)\\ |\\ C(ONa)(OR)\end{cases} \longrightarrow C_n\begin{cases}CO\\ |\\ CO\end{cases} \xrightarrow{2Na} C_n\begin{cases}C\cdot ONa\\ \|\\ C\cdot ONa\end{cases} \xrightarrow{H_2O} C_n\begin{cases}CH\cdot OH\\ |\\ CO\end{cases}$$

[90] V. Prelog, *J. Chem. Soc.*, **1950**, 420.

[91] V. Prelog, H. J. Urech, A. A. Bothner-By, and J. Wünsch, *Helv. chim. Acta*, 1955, **38**, 1095; H. J. Urech and V. Prelog, *ibid.*, 1957, **40**, 477.

$$\begin{array}{c} \overset{1}{\mathrm{C}}\mathrm{H_2\cdot CHX\cdot CH_2\cdot CH_2} \\ \mathrm{CH_2} \qquad\qquad\qquad \mathrm{CH_2} \\ \mathrm{CH_2\cdot \underset{5}{C}H_2\cdot \underset{6}{C}H_2\cdot CH_2} \end{array} \longrightarrow \begin{array}{c} \mathrm{CH_2\cdot \overset{+}{C}H\cdot CH_2\cdot CH_2} \\ \mathrm{CH_2} \qquad\qquad\qquad \mathrm{CH_2} \\ \mathrm{CH_2\cdot CH_2-CH_2\cdot CH_2} \end{array}$$

$$\begin{array}{c} \mathrm{CH_2\cdot CH_2\cdot CH_2\cdot CH_2} \\ \mathrm{CH_2} \qquad\qquad\qquad \mathrm{CH_2} \\ \mathrm{CH_2\cdot \underset{+}{C}H-CH_2\cdot CH_2} \end{array} \longrightarrow \left\{ \begin{array}{c} \mathrm{CH_2\cdot CH_2\cdot CH_2\cdot CH_2} \\ \mathrm{CH_2} \qquad\qquad\qquad \mathrm{CH_2} \\ \mathrm{CH_2\cdot \underset{5}{C}HY\cdot CH_2\cdot CH_2} \\ \\ \mathrm{CH_2\cdot CH_2-CH_2\cdot CH_2} \\ \mathrm{CH_2} \qquad\qquad\qquad \mathrm{CH_2} \\ \mathrm{CH_2\cdot \underset{5}{C}H=\underset{6}{C}H\cdot CH_2} \end{array} \right.$$

Such trans-annular reactions are probably characteristic of the rings around the central hump in Fig. 15-1; for with *cyclo*dodecane compounds (at which point in the homologous series Prelog strain should have disappeared) only "local," that is completely normal, substitutions and eliminations were found.[92]

The most important physical evidence consists in the X-ray determinations by Dunitz and his collaborators of the structures of *cyclo*nonylamine hydrochloride, *trans*-1,6-diamino*cyclo*decane dihydrochloride, and *cyclo*dodecane.[93] In the nine- and ten-membered rings, six hydrogen atoms are so turned inward that in the nine-membered ring three 1,4- or 1,5-pairs, and in the ten-membered ring two 1,5-pairs, are only 1.8 *A* apart, that is, 0.4 *A* within the "touching" separation, 2.2 *A*. In the twelve-membered ring, eight hydrogen atoms are turned somewhat inward, but no two of them come closer together than 2.2 *A*. Slightly conventionalised representations of the ten- and twelve-membered rings are given below:

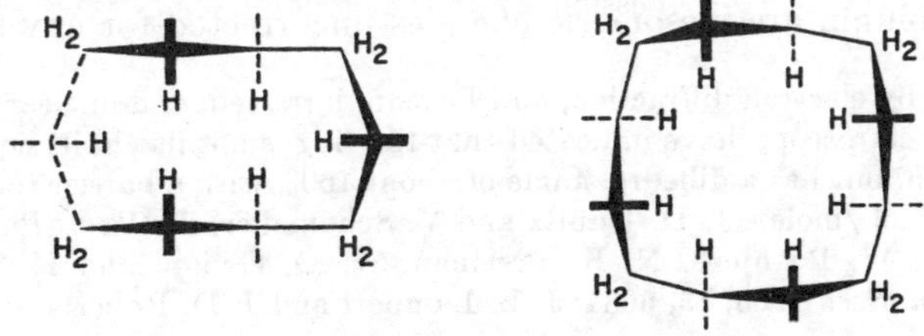

[92] W. Küng and V. Prelog, *Croat. Chim. Acta*, 1957, **29**, 357.

[93] R. F. Bryan and J. D. Dunitz, *Helv. Chim. Acta*, 1960, **43**, 3; E. Huber-Buser and J. D. Dunitz, *ibid.*, p. 760; J. D. Dunitz and H. M. Shearer, *ibid.*, p. 18.

It is simple now to go back to the dilemma of the beginning of the century, that the *cyclo*butane ring seemed more unstable than Baeyer strain alone should make it, a conclusion well supported by the subsequent thermochemical data already cited. Trans-annular pressures between the ring atoms themselves should occur in *cyclo*butane, which may, indeed, be the only *cyclo*alkane in which such pressures are large. A single trans-annular compression between carbon atoms at the separation of a *cyclo*butane diagonal would amount only to about 0.2 *A*. But in *cyclo*butane two such compressions are centred on the same point (or near it, if the ring is not flat[94]), and this must make the total compression energy much more than twice that of a single compression of the magnitude stated.

The only multiple bonds possible in small rings are *cis*-double bonds; but medium-sized and large rings can contain triple bonds, and even *trans*-double bonds. When a medium-sized ring is large enough to contain a *trans*-double bond, but is not large enough to allow it to rotate around the flanking single bonds as trunnions, chiral enantiomers can be formed, with such optical stability that they can be prepared and kept. Such optical stability arises in *trans-cyclo*-octene, as Cope has shown;[95] but it fades out very quickly with further increases in ring size: *trans-cyclo*-nonene can be optically resolved at low temperatures, but racemises at room temperature.

(15b) Mesomeric Energy in Aromatic Rings.—The main interest of thermochemical measurements on aromatic systems is that such determinations lead to estimates of the mesomeric energies of the systems. As mentioned in Section **9b**, such estimates have been made starting from heats of hydrogenation, and starting from heats of combustion. In the former method, the heats are compared with the heats of hydrogenation of fiducial molecules containing each double bond in a non-conjugated situation. Some mesomeric energies deduced in this way are given in Table 15-1. The figures in the "Difference" column are mesomeric energies uncorrected for any strain in

[94] Studies by electron diffraction, and Raman, infra-red, and nuclear magnetic resonance spectroscopy have indicated that the ring is not flat in its equilibrium configuration, but has a dihedral angle of about 160°, with a barrier to inversion of about 1 kcal./mole. (J. D. Dunitz and V. Schomaker, *J. Chem. Phys.*, 1952, **20**, 1703; G. W. Rathjens, N. K. Freeman, W. D. Gwinn, and K. S. Pitzer, *J. Am. Chem. Soc.*, 1953, **75**, 5634; J. B. Lambert and J. D. Roberts, *ibid.*, 1965, **87**, 3884).

[95] A. C. Cope, C. R. Ganellin, and H. W. Johnson, jr. *J. Am. Chem. Soc.*, 1962, **84**, 3191; *idem*, T. W. Van Auken and H. J. S. Winkler, *ibid.*, 1963, **85**, 3276; A. C. Cope, K. Banholzer, H. Keller, B. A. Pawson, J. H. Whang, and J. S. Winkler, *ibid.*, 1965, **87**, 3644; A. C. Cope and B. A. Pawson, *ibid.*, p. 3649.

TABLE 15-1.—MESOMERIC ENERGIES FROM HEATS OF HYDROGENATION.

Aromatic molecules				Comparison molecules		
	Mols. of H_2	$-\Delta H$, kcal./mol.	Diff., kcal./mol.		Mols. of H_2	$-\Delta H$, kcal./mol.
Benzene[1]	3	49.8	36.9	*Cyclo*pentene	1	26.9
Furan[2]	2	36.6	17.2	*Cyclo*hexene	1	28.9
Azulene[3]	5	99.0	32.5	*Cyclo*heptene	1	25.9

[1] G. B. Kistiakowsky, J. R. Ruhoff, H. A. Smith, and W. E. Vaughan, *J. Am. Chem. Soc.*, 1936, **58,** 146.

[2] M. A. Dolliver, T. E. Gresham, G. B. Kistiakowsky, H. A. Smith, and W. E. Vaughan, *J. Am. Chem. Soc.*, 1938, **60,** 440.

[3] R. B. Turner, W. R. Meador, W. von E. Doering, L. H. Knox, J. R. Mayer and D. W. Wiley, *J. Am. Chem. Soc.*, 1957, **79,** 4127.

the rings; but the only molecule for which an appreciable addition to the figure given ought to be made on this account is azulene, for which, however, it is unlikely to be more than 10 kcal./mole.

The second method of deriving mesomeric energies is by comparing heats of formation, deduced from measured heats of combustion, with sums of bond energy terms. A number of mesomeric energies, nearly all of them Pauling's values, deduced in this way, are in Table 15-2. The only one of these molecules for which a large addition to the apparent mesomeric energy ought to be made on account of ring strain is diphenylene: the necessary correction here might be about 30 kcal./mole.

The more obvious features of these figures are that the introduction of a nitrogen atom into the six-membered aromatic ring makes but little difference to its mesomeric energy, that the mesomeric energy of condensed six-membered rings increases fairly smoothly with the num-

TABLE 15-2.—MESOMERIC ENERGIES FROM BOND ENERGY TERMS (KCAL./MOLE).

Benzene	37	Pyridine	43
Naphthalene	77	Quinoline	69
Anthracene	105	Pyrrole	31
Phenanthrene	110	Indole	54
Cyclo-octatetraene	5	Carbazole	91
Azulene	45	Furan	23
Diphenylene[2]	22	Thiophen	31

[1] The figures, except that for diphenylene, are from L. Pauling, "Nature of the Chemical Bond," Cornell University Press, Ithaca, N.Y., 3rd Edn., 1960, p. 195.

[2] R. C. Cass, H. D. Springall, and P. G. Quincey, *J. Chem. Soc.*, 1955, 1188.

ber of rings (or the number of π electrons), and that the mesomeric energies of five-membered heterocyclic rings, though smaller than those of six-membered rings, are still quite large. The non-benzenoid hydrocarbons, *cyclo*-octatetraene, azulene, and diphenylene, have been discussed individually in Section **13d**.

(16) DIAMAGNETIC SUSCEPTIBILITY IN ALIPHATIC AND AROMATIC MOLECULES

(16a) Significance of Diamagnetic Susceptibility.—An atom or molecule may possess a permanent magnetic moment through two main causes: first, it may have one or more electrons with unpaired spins; secondly, the electrons may be moving in their orbitals with a resultant angular momentum. Molecular oxygen has a magnetic moment which arises from the first cause only (two unpaired spins). Nitric oxide has one, arising from both effects in combination (one unpaired spin, and one quantum of orbital angular momentum).[96]

When a magnetic field acts on matter whose molecules have permanent magnetic moments, the molecular moments become oriented in the direction of the field, and we observe the phenomenon of *paramagnetism*; that is, the magnetic susceptibility is positive; it is also large compared with the susceptibilities which arise from the magnetic effect next to be considered.

Almost all stable organic molecules (free radicals, with their unpaired electron spins, are the chief exception) have no permanent magnetic moments: thus they do not exhibit paramagnetism. They do, however, exhibit a residual, much weaker effect of opposite sign, which in principle is present in all matter, though it stands isolated only in the absence of permanent molecular magnetic moments. This is the phenomenon of *diamagnetism*, which is measured by a negative magnetic susceptibility. It arises, as was shown by Larmor, and in more detail by Langevin, because a magnetic field tends to induce circuit currents, whose magnetic fields oppose the inducing field. This happens even in an isolated atom, in which the electrons are given a circular motion in planes perpendicular to the field. It happens with more effect when larger conducting circuits can be established in polyatomic systems. Each electron, acting as a little circuit current, makes its own contribution to the induced magnetic polarisation of the

[96] Nitric oxide has no magnetic moment at low temperatures, because there the two effects cancel. Temperature enters into the matter, because the normal state of nitric oxide really consists of two states, separated by 0.344 kcal./mole. There are two states, because the spin moment can be oriented either with, or against, the orbital moment. In the latter case, the magnetic moments cancel. The state having the moments in opposition is the lower lying of the two, and at low temperatures is the only occupied state.

substance. And the contribution of any one electron is easily shown to be proportional to the mean area of the *orbit* it describes. (The induced electronic motion is, of course, superposed on the unperturbed motion; but we can dissect out from the total motion that part which is due to the magnetic field, and speak of it as motion in an "orbit.")

Magnetic *susceptibility*, as ordinarily measured and expressed, is really the susceptibility per c.c. If we divide this quantity, κ, by the density, and multiply by the molecular weight, we obtain the susceptibility per mole, called the *molecular susceptibility*, χ:

$$\chi = \kappa \cdot \frac{M}{d}$$

For a monatomic substance with spherical atoms, the Larmor-Langevin theory leads to the formula,

$$\chi = -\frac{Ne^2}{6mc^2} \sum_n \overline{r_i^2}$$

where N is Avogadro's number, m is the mass and e the charge of an electron, c is the velocity of light, and $\overline{r_i^2}$ is the mean value of the square of the radius of the magnetic orbit of the i'th electron, the sum being taken over all the n electrons in the atom. To mention now another geometrical model which will be needed later, if the atoms are imagined to be, not spheres, but circular cylinders or plates of the same radius, and if the plates are assumed to be fixed perpendicularly to the field, then the average areas of the circuits will evidently be larger, in the ratio of the volumes of a cylinder and inscribed sphere, and the above formula will have to be modified to

$$\chi = -\frac{Ne^2}{4mc^2} \sum_n \overline{r_i^2}$$

The magnetic susceptibility of an individual molecule is a tensor quantity. Diamagnetic spherical atoms, tetrahedral molecules XY_4, and a few other classes of molecules, are magnetically isotropic: their magnetic susceptibilities, now reckoned per individual molecule,

$$\xi = \chi/N$$

are the same for all directions. Most diamagnetic molecules are not isotropic: their magnetic susceptibilities, ξ, as measured in the gaseous, liquid, or powdered solid substances, are *average magnetic susceptibilities*, and are related in the usual way to three *principal magnetic susceptibilities*, x, y, and z, directed along three, mutually perpendicular *principal axes of magnetic susceptibility*:

$$3\xi = x + y + z$$

The symmetry rules for locating the principal axes are exactly as for electrical polarisability (Section **10d**). We shall restrict attention, at first, to average magnetic susceptibilities.

(16b) Pascal's Additivity Principle: Diamagnetic Constants.—In polyatomic molecules which are saturated, or contain only isolated centres of unsaturation, the electrons are largely localised: a magnetic field will cause them to circulate mainly locally, that is, within the atoms or bonds to which they belong. If they were to circulate strictly within non-interacting, magnetically isotropic atoms or other local units, the magnetic susceptibility would be accurately calculable by the addition of values appropriate to the units. About 1910, it was experimentally established by Pascal that the average molecular magnetic susceptibilities of diamagnetic molecules can, like molecular refractions, be approximately expressed in terms of additive constants for the atoms, together with certain constitutive corrections.[97]

Since the molecular magnetic susceptibility, χ, is negative in diamagnetic compounds, it is more convenient to discuss the positive quantity, $-\chi$, which may be called the *molecular diamagnetic susceptibility*. Diamagnetic susceptibilities are of the order of $10^{-6} - 10^{-4}$ c.g.s. electromagnetic units per mole, and hence it is simpler to quote values of $-10^6\chi$, that is, to take 10^{-6} e.m.u./mole as a "practical unit" of diamagnetic susceptibility, as is done below.

Pascal's atomic and multiple bond constants are set out in Table 16-1, though not entirely in the form in which he gave them. The atomic constants are those which were, or can be, deduced from his measurements on saturated aliphatic substances; and only one constant is given for each atom. The multiple bond constants are such that they have to be added into the total for the molecule only after all the atoms, including the multiply bonded atoms, have been taken into account.[98] In general, the constants are given to two figures only,

[97] P. Pascal's three most comprehensive papers are the following: *Ann. chim. phys.*, 1910, **19**, 5; 1912, **25**, 289; 1913, **29**, 218. There are also a number of contemporaneous papers by him in *Bull. soc. chim.* (France), some earlier ones in *Ann. chim.*, and many short papers from 1908 to 1914 and from 1921 to 1925 in *Compt. rend.* The whole work has been reviewed by S. S. Bhatnagar and K. M. Mathur in their book, "Physical Principles and Applications of Magnetochemistry," Macmillan, London, 1935, Chap. 4.

[98] To aid comparison with Pascal's papers, some further notes may be added concerning the derivation of the present list of constants.

First, the automatic correction of -4% has to be applied to Pascal's early experimental values, which were based on a figure, in error to that extent, of the magnetic susceptibility of water, taken as standard.

TABLE 16-1.—DIAMAGNETIC CONSTANTS OF ATOMS AND MULTIPLE BONDS.

Atom	$-10^6\chi$	Multiple bond (excluding atoms)	$-10^6\chi$
H	2.9		
C	6.0	(C)=(C)	−5.5
N	5.6	(C)=(N)	−8.2
O	4.6	(C)=(O)	−6.3
S	15.0	(N)=(N)	−4.0
F	6.3	(N)=(O)	−8.0
Cl	17.2		
Br	26.5	(C)≡(C)	−0.8
I	40.5	(C)≡(N)	−0.8

since the accuracy of the additive principle, and probably the accuracy of the experimental data, would not justify greater precision. In the presence of ionic charges, formal dipolar charges, or other sources of strong polarity, such as accumulated halogen atoms, and in the presence of some forms of conjugation, particularly the conjugation in aromatic systems, deviations arise which are well outside the otherwise allowable limits, as we shall note later.

The diamagnetic susceptibility of a free hydrogen atom can be exactly calculated:[99] it is 2.37 in our units. We should not expect it

Secondly, Pascal obtained most of his atomic constants (not those for N, O, or F) from measurements on the free elements. The values thus obtained for C (cane-sugar carbon) and S check well with those derived from measurements on organic compounds. Other values, notably those for Cl, Br, and I, do not agree well with the values which can be derived from his measurements on alkyl compounds. The halogen elemental values happen to agree with halogen values derived from aromatic halides, and therefore Pascal regarded the latter compounds as magnetically normal, and the alkyl halides as abnormal; while the opposite is done here, on account of the conjugative interaction between halogens and aromatic nuclei and the expected conjugative interaction in Cl_2, Br_2, and I_2, by employment of *d* orbitals.

Thirdly, Pascal dealt with unsaturation much as Brühl had done in relation to molecular refraction. He introduced constants for the CC double and triple bonds, but dealt with a number of other multiple bonds by assigning a special constant to one of the participating atoms (O in C:O for example). In the text the constants are so expressed that each atom has only one constant, while each multiple bond has a constant, which is to be added after all the atoms have been counted. Again, Pascal assigned a certain number of special constants to atoms involved in systems that we should regard as mesomeric (O_2 in carboxyl, N combined to aryl, etc.). It seems preferable, first, to allow for all the atoms and multiple bonds as if there were no mesomeric system, and then to treat the remaining deviation as belonging to the mesomeric system. In particular, this applies to aromatic systems, which Pascal treated as having centric formulae, without, however, allowing the centric valencies a magnetic effect.

[99] J. H. van Vleck, "The Theory of Electric and Magnetic Susceptibilities," Clarendon Press, Oxford, 1932, p. 206

to be the same as the diamagnetic constant for a hydrogen atom in combination. As to the other atomic constants, there is an obvious connexion with atomic size, particularly with period number in the Mendeléjeff table. In several cases, as we shall later observe, the constants can be related to the atomic radius, that is, to the permitted size of the magnetic orbits, in an approximately quantitative manner. Comment on the multiple bond values is offered in Section **16d.**

(16c) Diamagnetic Constants of Ions: Effects of Polarity.—The simplest illustration that can be given of the effect of polarity on diamagnetic susceptibility is that obtained by comparing the diamagnetic constants of monatomic, isoelectronic atoms and ions. This is done[100] in Table 16-2. Each increase in nuclear charge reduces the size of the electron shell, and hence reduces the area of the magnetic orbits, and the diamagnetic susceptibility.

TABLE 16-2.—DIAMAGNETIC CONSTANTS ($-10^6\chi$) OF MONATOMIC IONS, AND INERT GAS ATOMS.

	He, 1.9	Li^+, 1.0	
F^-, 9.0	Ne, 7.6	Na^+, 6.5	Mg^{++}, 5.0
Cl^-, 23.5	Ar, 19.2	K^+, 15.0	Ca^{++}, 11
Br^-, 34.5	Kr, 28.5	Rb^+, 22.5	Sr^{++}, 19
I^-, 50.5	Xe, 43.2	Cs^+, 35.0	Ba^{++}, 30

(16d) Effects of Unsaturation on Diamagnetism.—It will have been noticed in Table 16-1 that the diamagnetic constants of all multiple bonds are negative: apart from possible effects of conjugation, which we have not yet considered, unsaturation reduces diamagnetism. Furthermore, the constants belong to two distinct orders of magnitude: double bond constants are large and negative, of the same order of magnitude, sign apart, as atomic constants; while triple bond constants are small and negative, approximately an order of magnitude smaller than atomic constants.

One may associate these relations qualitatively with the geometrical forms of the electron distributions in double and triple bonds (Section **4b**, Fig. 4-4). The K shells of the atoms are, of course, too small to accommodate magnetic orbits of an effective size: nearly all the diamagnetic effect of any atom comes from its valency shell. In the double bond, the σ component may be expected to exhibit somewhat

[100] The experimental values for the inert gases are collected by P. W. Selwood, "Magnetochemistry," Interscience, New York, 1943, p. 33. A summary of data on ions is given by W. R. Angus, *Ann. Repts. on Progress Chemistry* (Chem. Soc. London), 1941, **36**, 33.

smaller magnetic effects than would be normal for single bonds, because of the compression exerted on it by the π component. The important point, however, is that the π component is unfavourable to the development of magnetic orbits of atomic size, because it is cut into two by a plane of zero electron density, across which the electrons cannot freely pass. Thus the diamagnetic susceptibility drops sharply when two valencies "collapse" on to an intervening single bond to form a double bond. In the triple bond, the compression of the σ orbital about the internuclear line is doubtless greater than in a double bond. But now the π shell contains, not a plane, but only a line of zero electron density; and that is very much less restricting. Therefore, a considerable restoration of diamagnetic susceptibility occurs when two valencies "collapse" on to a double bond to form a triple bond. Admittedly this is a rough picture; but in the absence of data concerning the directional magnetic properties of non-conjugated double and triple bonds, it is hardly profitable to try to go into the matter more quantitatively.

(16e) Effects of Conjugation and of Aromaticity on Diamagnetism.—These effects are conveniently described by the *exaltations*, observed in $-10^6\chi$, above the values additively computed from the constants for the atoms and multiple bonds in the reference valency structure, for example the Kekulé structure for benzene, the two-double-bond structure for furan, $R_2N—\overset{|}{C}=O$ for the carboxylamide group, $O^-—\overset{|}{N^+}=O$ for the nitrogroup, and so on. Exaltations computed in this way are listed in the left-hand part of Table 16-3. When one of the systems here entered is involved in a more extended form of conjugation, or when two of them are conjugated with each other, one may take the sum of the atomic and multiple bond constants as before, and add to that the exaltations listed on the left of Table 16-3, leaving out of account only such effects as may arise from the new or extended conjugation. The observed excess of $-10^6\chi$ over the value thus computed is the *extra exaltation* due to the additional conjugation. Extra exaltations obtained in this manner are given in the right-hand half of Table 16-3. The exaltations are all rounded to half a unit, since finer distinctions would not be reliable.

The first point to be noted is that the effect of multiple-bond conjugation in open chains is insignificant. One may conclude that the decreases and increases in bond multiplicity produce approximately compensating effects, and that the electrons circulate under a magnetic field essentially in one bond at a time.

A very different situation arises when there is complete cyclic con-

TABLE 16-3.—CONJUGATIVE EXALTATIONS OF DIAMAGNETIC SUSCEPTIBILITY.

	Exaltations in $-10^6\chi$		Extra exaltations[1] in $-10^6\chi$
C═C—C═C	+0.5	Aryl—Aryl	+0.5
C≡C—C≡C	0	Aryl—C═C	+1
N≡C—C≡N	0	Aryl—C≡C	+1.5
Benzene	+18	Aryl—NH_2, Aryl—NHR, Aryl—NR_2	−1
Pyridine	+18.5	Aryl—OH, Aryl—OR	+1
Naphthalene	+36	Aryl—Cl	+2.5
Anthracene	+55	Aryl—Br	+3.5
Phenanthrene	+53.5	Aryl—I	+3.5
Chrysene	+67.5	Aryl—CHO, Aryl—CO·R, Aryl—CO_2R, Aryl—$CONH_2$	+1.5[2]
Furan	+14	Aryl—NO_2	+0.5[3]
Thiophen	+18		
Cyclo-octatetraene	+2.5		
Azulene	+35.5		
HO—Ċ═O, RO—Ċ═O	+5		
H_2N—Ċ═O	+3.5[2]		
Ō—Ṅ═O	+2[3]		

[1] The aryl groups are all mononuclear phenyl or substituted phenyl groups.
[2] The values for amides may be partly the result of tautomerism.
[3] These values will include effects due to the formal charges in the NO_2-group.

jugation as in aromatic molecules, in which large positive exaltations of diamagnetism are observed. These effects are understood to arise from the circumstance that the electrons of the π shell are able to circulate round the whole molecule, thereby executing orbits of much more than atomic dimensions. Pascal noticed that condensed aromatic systems, such as naphthalene and pyrene, showed markedly heightened exaltations. This can be understood on the grounds that some of the electrons in such systems are able to execute orbits encompassing several rings. We note that, in the six-membered ring hydrocarbons, the exaltation increases smoothly with the number of rings. In the five-membered hetero-aromatic rings, the exaltation is as high, or nearly as high, as in benzene. In *cyclo*-octatetraene it is trivial. In azulene the exaltation is as high as in its isomer naphthalene. Some of these effects have since been more thoroughly studied, taking into account the directional variation of diamagnetic susceptibility, as will be described in Section **16f**.

The only other significant exaltations, noted on the left-hand side of Table 16-3, are the much smaller ones applying to the different forms of the carboxyl group, and to the nitro-group. Here it is relevant to observe that both atomic p orbitals, and double-bond π orbitals, are bisected by a nodal plane; but we may assume that the merging of p

and π orbitals in the conjugated systems allows the development of somewhat enlarged magnetic orbits.

Among the extra exaltations listed on the right of Table 16-3, there is one negative one: all the others are positive, and can be qualitatively understood as arising from the increased accommodation for magnetic orbits which is provided by the merging of the aromatic π orbitals with the p or π orbitals of the side chains. It seems reasonable to assume that a positive exaltation, due to this cause, is also present in the one case, that of aniline derivatives, in which the observed exaltations are negative; but that, superposed on the positive exaltation, there is a negative exaltation of larger magnitude, due to another cause. A possible cause is the changed hybridisation of the orbital of the unshared electrons of nitrogen. The atomic constant of nitrogen was derived from the diamagnetic susceptibilities of aliphatic amines, in which the unshared electrons are in tetrahedral orbitals: such orbitals are very unequally divided by their conical nodal surfaces (Section **4a**, Fig. 4-2); and they have one region, which can accommodate magnetic orbits of approximately atomic dimensions. In the aromatic amines, however, there is a change of hybridisation which can be described as consisting of two steps: first, the tetrahedral orbital goes into a p orbital, which is bisected by its planar nodal surface; then, the p orbital conjugates with the aromatic π orbitals. The first step would produce a negative exaltation, as on going from a single to a double bond (Section **16d**), and the second would produce a positive one: we observe the overall result of both steps. These considerations will apply also to phenol derivatives, but with quantitative differences, which might produce the observed small positive exaltations. They would not apply to the halogenobenzenes (or to thiophenol derivatives), because the halogen (and sulphur) unshared electrons are believed to be in nearly unhybridised p orbitals. The rather larger positive exaltations shown by aryl halides is consistent with this interpretation; and it has to be remembered that the larger size of the halogen valency shells will make the magnetic susceptibility somewhat sensitive to any spatial extension they undergo by conjugation with the aromatic system.

(16f) Directed Diamagnetism in Aromatic Systems.—Pascal adopted the value 6.0 for the diamagnetic constant of carbon in saturated aliphatic compounds. He obtained this value from the magnetic susceptibility of elemental carbon prepared from cane sugar. Subsequently measured values for diamond carbon yield practically the same figure. If, to this figure, we apply the Larmor-Langevin formula, taking the carbon atom as spherical, and as having four magnetically effective electrons, the root-mean-square radius of the magnetic orbits works out to 0.73 *A*. Corrections for the neglected core electrons would reduce the computed radius only to about 0.72 *A*. Thus it approximates fairly closely to the single-bond radius of carbon, 0.77 *A*: we conclude that here, the magnetic orbits are certainly of atomic dimensions.

Graphite has a much higher diamagnetic susceptibility than amorphous carbon, or diamond: the diamagnetic constant of a carbon atom, as deduced from the susceptibility of graphite, is 42 in our units. If we should calculate a mean radius for the magnetic orbits, on the basis of this figure, the value would be $\sqrt{7}$ times larger than before, that is, much larger than the radius of a carbon atom. This is clearly a special case of Pascal's general result that aromatic molecules exhibit an abnormally large diamagnetism. However, the qualitative interpretation of these effects, namely, that the π electrons are not confined to magnetic orbits within the atoms, but are able to describe larger orbits round the rings, cannot be raised to a quantitative status without taking into account the directional properties of the molecular diamagnetism. For the theory describes the excess of diamagnetism as being very unequally distributed in direction: it is, indeed, limited to one only of the three principal diamagnetic susceptibilities of the molecule, all three of which are averaged in the diamagnetic measurements discussed in the preceding Sections.

The magnetic susceptibility of a molecule can be studied as a function of direction by means of measurements made on a single crystal, provided that the crystal structure is known, and is suitable, that is, provided the molecules are not so oriented that their individual anisotropies cancel in the crystal as a whole. A number of measurements of this kind have been made by Raman, Krishnan, and Lonsdale; and their significance had been discussed by Pauling and by Lonsdale.[101]

From the magnetic data, Lonsdale has calculated the root-mean-square radii of the magnetic orbits described by each of the two main classes of valency electrons in a number of aromatic molecules. Some of her figures are reproduced in Table 16-4.

The simplifying assumptions made were (1) that the magnetic effect of the inner-core electrons may be neglected; (2) that the σ electrons can be taken as magnetically isotropic, the radii of their magnetic orbits being given by the Larmor-Langevin formula for the isotropic case; and (3) that the π electrons have negligible diamagnetism for

[101] C. V. Raman and K. S. Krishnan, *Proc. Roy. Soc.* (London), 1927, **A, 113,** 511; K. Lonsdale and K. S. Krishnan, *Proc. Roy. Soc.* (London), 1936, **A, 156,** 597; L. Pauling, *J. Chem. Phys.*, 1936, **4,** 673; K. Lonsdale, *Proc. Roy. Soc.* (London), 1937, **A, 159,** 149.

TABLE 16-4.—RADII OF MAGNETIC ORBITS OF AROMATIC ELECTRONS (AFTER LONSDALE).

σ Framework	σ Electrons		π Electrons	
	Number	Radius (A)	Number	Radius (A)
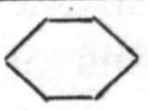	24	~0.71	6	~1.51
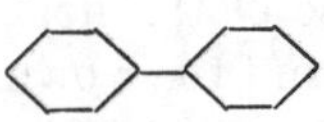	46	0.70	12	1.53
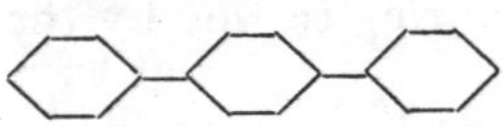	68	0.70	18	1.52
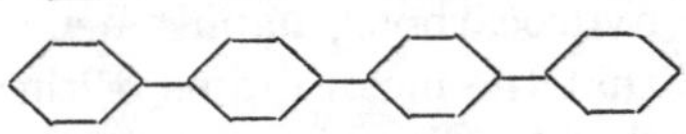	90	0.68	24	1.57
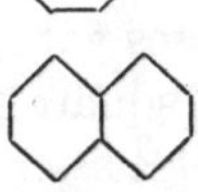	38	0.71	10	1.64
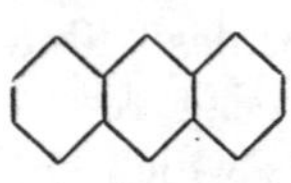	52	0.69	14	1.75
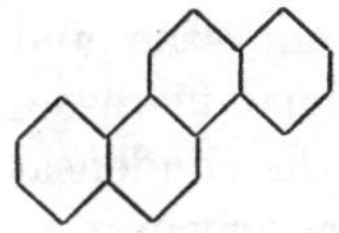	66	0.68	18	1.72
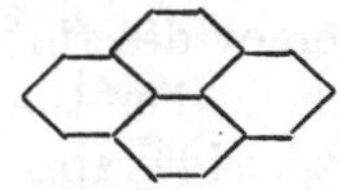	58	0.70	16	1.86
Graphite	∞	~0.79	∞	7.80

fields in the molecular plane, so that their magnetic orbits, developed only in the plane of the molecule, under the influence of fields normal to that plane, have to be calculated by the Larmor-Langevin formula as modified for plate-like molecules (Section 16a). The first assumption is certainly well justified. The second and third probably involve compensating errors; for we should expect the σ electrons of the CC bonds, owing to compression by the π shell, to have a reduced diamagnetic susceptibility towards fields in the molecular plane; and the π electrons should have a finite, if small, susceptibility for fields in the molecular plane. However, the overall result of the calculations is very satisfying.

For all types of aromatic nuclei, the mean radius of the magnetic orbits of the σ electrons is close to 0.70 A. This figure is identical with the average covalent radius of an aromatic carbon atom.

For benzene, and the non-condensed polynuclear hydrocarbons, biphenyl, *p*-diphenylbenzene, and di-*p*-biphenylyl, the mean radius of the magnetic orbits of the π electrons in the molecular plane is nearly constant and equal to about 1.53 *A*. This is a little longer, as might be expected, than the radius of a benzene ring measured only to the nuclei of the carbon atoms (1.40 *A*). Evidently the π electrons of benzene circulate completely round the ring; while those of the non-condensed polynuclear hydrocarbons circulate mainly round their own rings, and are not to any great extent driven from ring to ring by the magnetic field.

Turning to the condensed polynuclear hydrocarbons, naphthalene, anthracene, chrysene, and pyrene, we see that the mean radius of the magnetic orbits of the π electrons in the molecular plane increases with the number of rings. It does not increase as rapidly as the square-root of their number, which is what would happen if all the π electrons travelled exclusively round the peripheries of their molecules. One must conclude that some of the π electrons are circulating round their own rings, while some of them are describing orbits which encompass several rings. As the comparison between chrysene and pyrene shows, the mean radius, for a fixed number of rings, increases with the degree of condensation of the rings: the more the condensation, the greater is the fraction of the π electrons which are driven from ring to ring under the influence of the magnetic field, thereby describing orbits which enclose several rings. The limit is reached when the condensed aromatic network is of indefinitely large extent, as in graphite, for which the magnetic data indicate the average area of the magnetic orbits of the electrons to be that of about 30 benzene rings.

CHAPTER

Classification of Reagents and Reactions

(17) SIFICATION OF REAGENTS

CHEMICAL reactions are electrical transactions. Accordingly, when a reagent acts on an organic molecule, it may be assumed to do so by virtue of some predominating constitutional affinity either for atomic nuclei or for electrons; or, perhaps, for both in equivalence, that is, for atoms. Most reagents which have an even number of electrons belong to one of the first two categories; while odd-electron reagents belong to the third, more specialised, class.

(17a) Generalisation of the Concepts of Reduction and Oxidation.—A convenient, and historically valid, approach to the classification of even-electron reagents, as attackers of nuclei or of electrons, is through a progressive generalisation of the concepts of reduction and oxidation. The ideas can be traced to the pre-electronic theories of Michael and Lapworth; while, after the promulgation of the electronic theory of the atom and of valency, Fry and Stieglitz were among the first to interpret and develop this group of concepts.[1]

Long before the introduction of the electronic theory of valency, the terms reduction and oxidation had ceased to be restricted to reactions which removed or introduced oxygen. Hydrogen or a metal became oxidised when it was converted into a cation corresponding to an oxide, that is, into an acid or salt; and the cation was reduced when it was reconverted to hydrogen or the metal. Similarly, a halogen or other non-metal was reduced when it was converted into a halide ion or other anion of an acid or of a metal salt; and the anion was oxidised when reconverted to the halogen or other non-metal. An electronic formulation of any such reduction-oxidation, in this stage of generalisation of the term, shows that the reducing agent donates electrons to the oxidising agent. In some reactions there is an actual transfer of electrons, as in the example,

$$\text{Fe(metal)} + \text{Cu}^{++} \rightarrow \text{Fe}^{++} + \text{Cu(metal)}$$

Other reduction-oxidation processes involve only partial electron trans-

[1] H. S. Fry, "The Electronic Conception of Valence and the Constitution of Benzene," Longmans, Green, and Co., London and New York, 1921; J. Stieglitz, *J. Am. Chem. Soc.*, 1922, **44,** 1293.

fers: the reducing agent donates a share in its electrons without parting from them, while the oxidising agent receives a share without appropriating them, as in the example,

$$I^- + Cl{-}Cl \rightarrow I{-}Cl + Cl^-$$

This amount of generalisation of the reduction-oxidation concept has long been a commonplace. What its electronic interpretation showed was that, having once begun to generalise, there is no logical point at which one may stop short of including all cases of the donation and reception of electrons. Thus, the neutralisation process,

$$H\overset{-}{O} + H{-}\overset{+}{O}H_2 \rightarrow HO{-}H + OH_2$$

would not in pre-electronic times have been regarded as a reduction-oxidation. But it can be linked with the original, limited concept of reduction-oxidation by an argument only slightly more tortuous than that which has to be applied, say, in the above halide-halogen exchange. The hydroxide ion becomes converted into a bound hydroxyl radical, which, as a free hydroxyl radical, would be an admitted oxidising agent, even in the limited sense: therefore the hydroxide ion has undergone a change so nearly related to oxidation, and has itself behaved so like a reducing agent, that these terms might be allowed to cover the case. Again, the solvated hydrogen ion becomes a bound hydrogen atom, which, as a free hydrogen atom, would be an acknowledged reducing agent; and thus the hydrogen ion may be said to have been reduced, or to have behaved as an oxidising agent. The argument might be continued by reference to the addition process,

$$F^- + BF_3 \rightarrow BF_4^-$$

in which the connexion with reduction-oxidation in its original meaning is slightly more indirect still. A description of the connexion would commence by pointing out that the fluoride ion becomes converted into a bound fluorine atom, which, as a free fluorine atom, could, by the old generalisation, be regarded as an oxidation-equivalent for the free hydroxyl radical.

So one may proceed outwards, from the central concept of reduction-oxidation, in small, indeed, by the use of more examples, almost imperceptible, degrees; and there is no obvious point for stopping short of the boundary at which all cases of the donation and reception of electrons have been included. This is the approach to the polar classification of reagents which we shall use. As will be mentioned later, there are two other approaches, which lead essentially to the same classification.

(17b) Nucleophilic Reagents.—Reagents which act by donating their electrons to, or sharing them with, a foreign atomic nucleus will be called *nucleophilic reagents*, or sometimes *nucleophiles*. Table 17-1 contains a short list of examples, which are selected in order to illustrate some general features in the chemistry of such reagents.

TABLE 17-1.—SOME NUCLEOPHILIC REAGENTS.

No	Reagent	Notes	Number of active electrons	
1	$[Fe(CN)_6]^{---}$	R	1	completely donated
2	Na(metal)	R	1	completely donated
3	Sn^{++}	R	2	completely donated
4	SO_2	R	1 pair	share donated
5	S^{--}	R, B	1, 2, 3, 4 pairs	share donated
6	CN^-	(R), B	1 pair	share donated
7	OH^-	B	1, 2 pairs	share donated
8	NH_3	B	1 pair	share donated
9	$[Co(H_2O)_5(OH)]^{++}$	B	1 pair	share donated

R = Reducing agent, in the pre-electronic sense (see text).
B = Base, accordng to the Brönsted-Lowry definition (see text).

The main division in this table is between the first three and the last six reagents. Reagents nos. 1–3 act by donating one or more of their electrons completely: they are typical reducing agents in the restricted sense of the term. The examples given include three very different states of electric charge: they show that nucleophilic character is not simply related to the charge, but depends in a much more detailed way on the electronic constitution of the reagent.

The reducing property, in the ordinary pre-electronic sense of the term, cuts across the main division of the table and extends over part of the second series of reagents, those, nos. 4–9, which act by donating only a share in one or more of their unshared electron pairs. Reagents nos. 4 and 5 are reducing substances in the ordinary sense, and no. 6 is marginally so, but nos. 7–9 are not so.

This second series contains another sub-series, overlapping with the reducing agents, and represented by examples nos. 5–9. The identity of behaviour of reagents such as these with respect to combination with a proton was pointed out by Brönsted[2] and by Lowry,[3] who founded a broadened definition of the terms "acid" and "base" on the analogy between such equilibria as the following:

[2] J. N. Brönsted, *Rec. trav. chim.*, 1923, **42,** 718.
[3] T. M. Lowry, *J. Soc. Chem. Ind.* (London), 1923, **42,** 43.

$$S^{--} + H^+ \rightleftarrows SH^-$$

$$CN^- + H^+ \rightleftarrows HCN$$

$$OH^- + H^+ \rightleftarrows H_2O$$

$$NH_3 + H^+ \rightleftarrows NH_4^+$$

$$[Co(H_2O)_5(OH)]^{++} + H^+ \rightleftarrows [Co(H_2O)_6]^{+++}$$

The defining equation is

$$Base + H^+ \rightleftarrows Acid$$

and any base and acid thus related are said to be *conjugate* with respect to each other. Of the bases represented on the left of the above equation, only NH_3 would, in earlier times, have been accepted as a base. Among the acids formulated on the right, only HCN, and, marginally, H_2O, would previously have been admitted as acids. Brönsted and Lowry pointed out, however, that the differences of nett electric charge were trivial in comparison with the analogies of chemical behaviour on which they based their definition, which is now universally accepted. Basicity bears no simple relation to charge. Neither does acidity. Both properties depend in much more detailed ways on the electronic constitutions of the reagents.

The sub-series, illustrated by reagents nos. 5–9, comprises the typical bases. Of course, all bases are nucleophiles. Basicity, that is, affinity for a hydrogen nucleus, is a special manifestation of nucleophilic character, or *nucleophilic strength*, that is, affinity for atomic nuclei in general. And nucleophilic strength in every form, including basicity, is profoundly constitutional, cutting across all differences of electric charge.

(17c) Electrophilic Reagents.—Reagents which act by acquiring electrons, or a share in electrons, which previously belonged exclusively to a foreign molecule will be called *electrophilic reagents*, or sometimes *electrophiles*. Table 17-2 contains a list of selected examples.

The main division in this table is again between the first three reagents and the remainder. Reagents nos. 1–3 act by completely appropriating electrons from another molecule. They are all typical oxidising agents in the ordinary sense. The examples given include very different states of electric charge; and this is an illustration of the fact that electrophilic strength is not simply related to charge.

This first main series contains two sub-series. They arise from the circumstance that, since electrons are being acquired by the reagent, it makes a difference whether all the electron shells of the latter are complete, or whether some are incomplete. In the former case, repre-

TABLE 17-2.—SOME ELECTROPHILIC REAGENTS.

No.	Reagent	Fragments: Transferred	Fragments: Liberated	Notes	Active electrons	
1	$S_2O_8^{--}$	—	$2SO_4^{--}$	Ox	2	completely acquired
2	$[Fe(CN)_6]^{---}$	(No splitting)		Ox	1	completely acquired
3	$[Fe(H_2O)_6]^{+++}$	(No splitting)		Ox	1	completely acquired
4	O_3	O	O_2	Ox	1 pair	share acquired
5	SO_5^{--}	O	SO_4^{--}	Ox	1 pair	share acquired
6	Cl_2	Cl^+	Cl^-	Ox	1 pair	share acquired
7	HOCl	Cl^+, H^+	OH^-, OCl^-	Ox, A	1 pair	share acquired
8	HNO_3	O, NO_2^+, H^+	HNO_2, OH^-, NO_3^-	Ox, A	1 pair	share acquired
9	H_3O^+	H^+, $2H^+$	H_2O OH^-	A	1, 2 pairs	share acquired
10	HCl	H^+	Cl^-	A	1 pair	share acquired
11	HSO_4^-	H^+	SO_4^{--}	A	1 pair	share acquired
12	$HgCl_3^-$	(No splitting)		—	1 pair	share acquired
13	$AlCl_3$	(No splitting)		—	1 pair	share acquired
14	$SnCl_4$	(No splitting)		—	2 pairs	share acquired
15	NO_2^+	(No splitting)		—	1 pair	share acquired
16	Be^{++}	(No splitting)		—	4 pairs	share acquired
17	Co^{+++}	(No splitting)		—	6 pairs	share acquired

Ox = Oxidising agent, in the pre-electronic sense.
A = Acid, according to the Brönsted-Lowry definition.

sented by reagent no. 1, the acquired electrons can be accommodated only through the splitting of the reagent. In the latter situation, illustrated by reagents nos. 2 and 3, the additional electrons can be accommodated without splitting, and so splitting does not take place.

The second main division of the table contains reagents nos. 4–17, which act by acquiring only a share in some of the electrons of a foreign molecule. The oxidising property extends into this series, but does not run completely through it: reagents nos. 4–8 are oxidising in the usual sense, while reagents nos. 9–17, apart from a few marginal cases, are not normally regarded as oxidising agents.

This second main series also contains two sub-series, depending on whether all the electron shells are complete, or whether some are incomplete. The former situation is demonstrated by reagents nos. 4–11. In this sub-series, the acquired electrons can be accommodated only through the splitting of the reagent; and since only a share in the additional electrons is acquired by the reagent, it follows that, when the reagent splits, a part is transferred to, and bound in the reaction product, while a part is set free. The part transferred may be any molecular fragment capable of accepting a new electron pair into its valency shell: the examples given illustrate the transference of a neutral oxygen atom, a proton, a chlorinium ion, and a nitronium ion. When the fragment transferred is a proton, the reagent is behaving as an acid, according to the Brönsted-Lowry definition. Thus the electrophiles include the acids. Power to transfer a proton is evidently a special case of power to transfer an atomic nucleus carrying fewer electron pairs than it could take into its valency shell; and, therefore, acidity is a special case of electrophilic character, or *electrophilic strength*, affinity for external electrons in general. The electrophiles of this sub-series, whether they act by transferring a neutral atom such as oxygen, or a positive ion such as the proton, may be in various states of electric charge: what Brönsted and Lowry pointed out for acids is evidently true of the wider group of reagents, namely, that their chemical function bears no simple relation to their charge.

In the last sub-series, represented by reagents nos. 12–17, additional electron pairs can be accepted into the valency shells, and therefore these reagents combine with the molecule attacked, without splitting. Their normal action is to co-ordinate either with the unshared electron pairs of an atom, or with the π electron pairs of an unsaturated molecule. Again the state of charge is trivial in comparison with the analogy of behaviour of these reagents.

(17d) Alternative Approaches to the Classification of Reagents.— While we shall prefer to use the approach based on Fry's and Stieglitz's recognition of the electronic nature of oxidation and reduction, two other approaches have been made and supported, which lead, or could lead, to the same final result.

One is that of Lapworth.[4] He proceeded from the idea of ions: he was one of the very few who had realised since the beginning of the century that many organic reactions proceed through ions. He likened all reagents either to anions or to cations: an "anionoid" reagent was one which behaved analogously to an anion; and a "cationoid" reagent was one which behaved similarly to a cation. The difficulty with this approach is that it lays too much emphasis on charge, neglecting the teaching of Brönsted and of Lowry that similarities in reactivity cut across differences of charge. For example, one cannot say with

[4] A. Lapworth, *Mem. and Proc. Manchester Lit. & Phil. Soc.*, 1925, **69**, p. xviii; *Nature*, 1925, **115**, 625.

any firm conviction that the permanganate ion, as an oxidising agent, is behaving like a cation, or that a stannous ion, when reducing, is behaving like an anion. What may be done is so to amend the stated definitions that an anionoid or cationoid reagent becomes one which behaves as an anion or cation *would* behave *if* charge were the dominating determinant of reactivity. The classification is then equivalent to that given in the preceding sections: "anionoid" becomes synonymous with "nucleophilic," and "cationoid" with "electrophilic."

The other approach is that of Lewis.[5] He starts with the classical concept of bases and acids, and proceeds progressively to widen these terms. As we have seen, Brönsted and Lowry removed the original restriction to neutral substances, but retained, as essential, the connexion with proton transfers. Lewis proposed to abandon the restriction to proton reactions, and to apply the term "acid" to any bond-forming electrophiles, that is, any substance which will accept a share in the electrons of another molecule: "the basic substance furnishes a pair of electrons for the chemical bond, and the acidic substance accepts such a pair." Relevant examples are in the second main sections of Tables 17-1 and 17-2. Lewis was concerned primarily with the capacity of reagents for co-ordination, but it would not be an unnatural step to widen the terms "base" and "acid" a little further still, so as to include those reagents which donate or accept electrons completely. Lewis may have contemplated such an extension, which, although not specifically illustrated by him, could be read into at least one of the alternative definitions he gives. Relevant illustrations will be found in the first main sections of Tables 17-1 and 17-2. With this degree of extension the term "base" becomes synonymous with "nucleophile," and "acid" with "electrophile." No criticism can be offered of this chain of considerations; but as to the nomenclature, one feels that the Brönsted-Lowry definition of bases and acids is much too useful to be subsumed. We shall, without further explanation, employ the terms "basic" and "acidic" in the Brönsted-Lowry sense, leaving the terms "nucleophilic" and "electrophilic" to describe the broader classes of reagents.[6]

[5] G. N. Lewis, "Valence and the Structure of Atoms and Molecules," Chemical Catalog Co., New York, 1923, p. 141; *J. Franklin Inst.*, 1938, **226**, 293.

[6] It would have been possible to broaden the significance of the terms "reducing" and "oxidising" so that they became synonymous with "nucleophilic" and "electrophilic," respectively. But this has not been proposed, for a similar reason, namely, that the meanings which, since pre-electronic times, have been attached to the terms "reducing" and "oxidising" have given to these words a great practical utility, and that, therefore, it would be inconvenient to subsume their well-understood significance in wider connotations.

(18) CLASSIFICATION OF REACTIONS

(18a) Homolytic and Heterolytic Reactions.—Reactions form and break bonds; and by far the most important kind of bond that they can produce or destroy is the covalent bond. As was noted in Chapter I, the covalent bond may be formed, or broken, in two different ways.

First, it can be formed from electrons supplied one by each of the combining species, that is, by colligation, and broken by the reverse process homolysis:

$$A\cdot + B\cdot \underset{\text{homolysis}}{\overset{\text{colligation}}{\rightleftarrows}} A{:}B$$

In this type of reaction th[illegible] A· and B· are normally odd-electron molecules[illegible], either odd-electron atoms, such as H· or [illegible], such as HO· or $CH_3\cdot$, where the single dot represents the unpaired electron. Few odd-electron molecules are stable in ordinary conditions, though many can be transiently produced by one-electron redox processes, either homogeneously, or at an electrode, or by thermal, or photolytic, or other radiative dissociation of a covalent bond. Surface catalysis also may cause such dissociation, as of hydrogen on platinum, though the dissociation products, hydrogen atoms or ionised atoms, remain bound to the surface. Reactions which form and break covalent bonds by colligation and homolysis are called *homolytic reactions*. Many such reactions start with a one-electron reaction or a thermal, or radiative, or surface-catalysed homolysis. Some appear to be initiated by the mutual homolysis of two bonds to form a stronger bond or bonds. If either initiation process produces odd-electron species, the latter tend not only to colligate with each other, but also to attack even-electron molecules, liberating new odd-electron species, and thereby setting up reaction chains.

Secondly, the covalent bond can be formed by co-ordination, and broken by the opposite process, heterolysis:

$$A{:} + B \underset{\text{heterolysis}}{\overset{\text{co-ordination}}{\rightleftarrows}} A{:}B$$

In this type of process, the species A: and B are, normally, both even-electron molecules; and a high proportion of them are ordinary stable substances. Reactions which form and break bonds by co-ordination and heterolysis are known as *heterolytic reactions*. Most such low-temperature reactions, apart from those which start with a redox process or with a thermal, radiative, or surface-catalysed dissociation, are heterolytic reactions. The simplest affect only one bond; that is, they involve a single co-ordination or a single heterolysis. But many affect two or more bonds, and involve both co-ordination and heterolysis. The general pattern of organic chemistry, as we now see it after a century of development since the acceptance of structural theory, is based largely on heterolytic reactions, although homolytic reactions have become important in the latter part of that period. We shall next proceed to classify heterolytic reactions in more detail.

(18b) Nucleophilic and Electrophilic Reactions.—The distinction of function, and complementary character, of the species formulated A: and B, in the above-written equation for co-ordination and heterolysis, is evidently to be correlated with our classification of the even-electron reagents as nucleophilic and electrophilic: species A: belongs to the former category, and B to the latter.

It is, of course, a pure convention as to which of two interacting substances is regarded as "the reagent," and which "the substrate," that is, the substance on which the reagent acts. However, in many of the reactions of organic chemistry a definite convention concerning this is established. When bromine reacts with naphthalene, bromine is regarded as the reagent; and when phenylhydrazine reacts with acetone, phenylhydrazine is normally considered the reagent. Provided that there can be no ambiguity as to which substance is "the reagent," it is convenient to label reactions according to the class to which the reagent belongs. Since bromine is electrophilic, the bromination of naphthalene is termed an *electrophilic reaction*, naphthalene being considered the substrate; and since phenylhydrazine is a nucleophile, the conversion of acetone into its phenylhydrazone is classified as a *nucleophilic reaction*, acetone being regarded as the substrate.

(18c) Nucleophilic and Electrophilic Substitutions.—The above type of classification is particularly easy to make for *substitutions*, because, in this case, a knowledge of the reaction mechanism is not required. Consider the formation of methyl ethyl ether by the action of ethoxide ion on methyl iodide:

$$\mathrm{OEt^- + CH_3{-}I \rightarrow CH_3{-}OEt + I^-} \qquad (\mathrm{S_N})$$

The reaction is evidently a substitution: I is replaced by OEt. By convention, the ethoxide ion is regarded as the reagent: it is here the *substituting agent*. Independently of any question of mechanism, the substituting agent has supplied both the electrons of the bond by which it is bound in the product of this reaction: it has behaved as a nucleophile. Therefore the reaction would be correctly described as a substitution by a nucleophilic reagent: for brevity, we call it a *nucleophilic substitution*. Frequently, we contract this designation further to the symbol S_N, as is done above: the purpose here is to furnish a basis for compactly indicating mechanistic particulars by the addition of further symbols, as will be illustrated later.

Next, consider the formation of nitrobenzene by the reaction between nitronium ion and benzene:

$$NO_2^+ + Ph—H \rightarrow Ph—NO_2 + H^+ \qquad (S_E)$$

This reaction is a substitution, and nitronium ion is the substituting agent. Aside from mechanistic details, the new substituent, the nitro-group, is bound into the reaction product by a pair of electrons which originally belonged to the substrate, benzene: clearly, the substituting agent has behaved as an electrophile. Therefore we classify this reaction as an *electrophilic substitution*; and we may label it S_E, as is done above.

Let us consider how far considerations of this simple type can be generalised. In the example of nucleophilic substitution already given, the mechanism is actually one of the simpler known mechanisms by which the halogen of an alkyl halide can be replaced by a group of the form OR. We might, however, consider, as a second example, the conversion of *t*-butyl chloride in an aqueous solvent to *t*-butyl alcohol:

$$H_2O + t\text{-}C_4H_9—Cl \rightarrow t\text{-}C_4H_9—OH + H^+ + Cl^-$$

The mechanism is more complex than before; but it is not necessary to know this for the purposes of the present broad classification. However many steps this reaction may contain, and however many molecules may in some way be transiently involved in furthering the conversion of a particular molecule, it remains true that the electrons which bind the new substituent came from the substituting agent, and not from the substrate. Therefore this reaction is still a nucleophilic substitution. Even if we should assist the reaction by the addition of a silver or mercuric salt, the same statements hold, and the same conclusion follows; for the catalysing cation is not the substituting agent.

Quite generally, the replacements of halogen in alkyl halides, or in sufficiently reactive aryl halides, by the groups OH, OR, SH, SR, SR_2^+, SeR_2^+, etc., through the agency of water, alcohols, hydrogen sulphide, alkyl thiols, dialkyl sulphides, dialkyl selenides, etc., or the anions of these substances when available, are nucleophilic substitutions. Similarly, the reactions which replace bound halogen by the groups NH_2, NHR, NR_2, NR_3^+, PR_3^+, AsR_3^+, etc., through the agency of ammonia, amines, amides, imides, phosphines, arsines, etc., or the anions of such substances when available, are nucleophilic substitutions. Again, the replacement of halogen by halogen, either the same one, which might be isotopically marked, or a different one, through the agency of halide ions, is a form of nucleophilic substitution. So also is the replacement of halogen by CN, $CH(CO_2Et)_2$, etc., by the action of the appropriate anions.

The above-written hydrolysis of *t*-butyl chloride is a balanced reaction in acid solution. Everything that was said of the forward reaction applies without modification to the back reaction:

$$t\text{-}C_4H_9\text{—}OH + H^+ + Cl^- \rightarrow t\text{-}C_4H_9\text{—}Cl + H_2O$$

It also is a nucleophilic substitution. The reaction of ethers with halogen acids, as in Zeisel's analytical process,

$$CH_3\text{—}OR + H^+ + I^- \rightarrow CH_3\text{—}I + HOR$$

is equally a nucleophilic substitution. Generally, those reactions which replace hydroxyl groups in alcohols, or alkoxyl or aroxyl groups in ethers, by halogen are nucleophilic substitutions.

The reactions which produce sulphonium, selenonium, ammonium, phosphonium ions, etc., from alkyl halides are reversible processes. Again, the considerations which apply to the forward, hold for the reverse, reactions. Thus the replacement of an 'onium ionic group by halogen in a reaction such as the following,

$$Alk\text{—}SR_2^+ + Cl^- \rightarrow Alk\text{—}Cl + SR_2$$

is a nucleophilic substitution, in which the anion of the salt is the substituting agent, and the cation the substrate. The replacement of an 'onium ionic group by a hydroxyl, or alkoxyl, or aroxyl, or acyl group in the substitutive decomposition of an 'onium hydroxide, alkoxide, aryloxide, or carboxylate, as in the example,

$$Alk\text{—}SR_2^+ + OH^- \rightarrow Alk\text{—}OH + SR_2$$

is evidently analogous. Further, it is not necessary that the anion of the 'onium salt should be the substituting agent: for one may decompose a salt, having a weakly nucleophilic anion, by means of an added, more strongly nucleophilic, but neutral reagent, as in the following illustration:

$$Alk\text{—}SR_2^+ + NR_3 \rightarrow Alk\text{—}NR_3^+ + SR_2$$

All these reactions are nucleophilic substitutions. Generally, the reactions which replace 'onium ionic groups by Hal, OR, NR_2, NR_3^+, etc., are nucleophilic substitutions.

In earlier times the general reactions mentioned in the last four paragraphs, dealing as they do with different types of substances, were regarded as belonging to different departments of organic chemistry. The incorporation of all these general reactions into one great family, with the family bond of common mechanisms, became established,[7] and for the most part generally accepted (though there was at first no agreement about one of the mechanisms), in 1933–35.

Turning to electrophilic substitutions, the example already given, namely, the nitration of benzene by a nitronium ion, assumed to be supplied as such in an ionised nitronium salt, is mechanistically one of the simplest that could have been chosen; but this was not essential for the purposes of the present classification. When the nitrating agent is supplied as nitric acid, further steps are added to the nitration mechanism. But still the nitro-group is bound in the product with a pair of electrons which previously belonged, not to the nitric acid, but to the benzene, that is, to the substrate rather than the substituting agent:

$$\text{Ph—H} + \text{HNO}_3 \rightarrow \text{Ph—NO}_2 + \text{H}_2\text{O}$$

Thus the nitration is still an electrophilic substitution. In general, nitration, if it is a heterolytic substitution at all, as aromatic nitration certainly is under all ordinary conditions, is an electrophilic substitution.

By an argument which is the complete counterpart of that developed above concerning nucleophilic substitution, it can be shown that, not only aromatic nitration, but also aromatic nitrosation, halogenation, sulphonation, Friedel-Crafts alkylations and acylations, hydrogen exchange between aromatic compounds and strong acids, aromatic diazo-couplings, and aromatic mercurations, are all electrophilic substitutions, independently of mechanism, even though a number of these general reactions of substitution have several known mechanisms.

Table 18-1 summarises the results of these discussions of the classification of heterolytic substitutions as nucleophilic or electrophilic substitutions. Actually, we have illustrated nucleophilic substitution only in the aliphatic field; but as we shall see in Chapter VI, an important group of aromatic nucleophilic substitutions exists. Equally, we have illustrated electrophilic substitution only in the aromatic field; but, as is described in Chapter VII, aliphatic electrophilic substitutions have been established as an important family of reactions.

[7] E. D. Hughes, C. K. Ingold, and C. S. Patel, *J. Chem. Soc.*, **1933**, 526; E. D. Hughes and C. K. Ingold, *ibid.*, p. 1571; J. L. Gleave, E. D. Hughes, and C. K. Ingold, *ibid.*, **1935**, 235; E. D. Hughes and C. K. Ingold, *ibid.*, p. 244.

TABLE 18-1.—SOME NUCLEOPHILIC AND ELECTROPHILIC SUBSTITUTIONS.

Alk = almost any alkyl group, including an aralphyl group; and in a few cases it can additionally signify a suitably substituted, generally an *o*- or *p*-nitro-substituted, aryl group; Ar = almost any aryl group; R = either hydrogen, or alkyl including aralphyl, or, in some cases, acyl, and in others aryl.

Nucleophilic Substitutions

Reagent	Substrate	Substitution product
Hal^-	Alk·Hal′	Alk·Hal
OR^-, OHR	Alk·Hal	Alk·OR
SR_2	Alk·Hal	Alk·SR_2^+
NHR_2	Alk·Hal	Alk·NR_2
NR_3	Alk·Hal	Alk·NR_3^+
CN^-	Alk·Hal	Alk·CN
HHal	Alk·OR	Alk·Hal
Hal^-	Alk·SR_2^+, Alk·NR_3^+, etc.	Alk·Hal
OR^-, OHR	Alk·SR_2^+, Alk·NR_3^+, etc.	Alk·OR
NR_3	Alk·SR_2^+	Alk·NR_3^+
NOHal	Alk·NH_2	Alk·Hal
NO·OR	Alk·NH_2	Alk·OR

Electrophilic Substitutions

Reagent	Substrate	Substitution product
NO_2^+, HNO_3, etc.	ArH, R_2NH, ROH	$ArNO_2$, $R_2N·NO_2$, RO·NO_2
Hal^+, Hal_2, etc.	ArH, R_2NH, ROH	ArHal, R_2NHal, ROHal
SO_3, H_2SO_4, etc.	ArH, R_2NH, ROH	$ArSO_3H$, $R_2N·SO_3H$, RO·SO_3H
RCO^+, RCO·Cl, etc.	ArH, R_2NH, ROH	ArCOR, R_2N·COR, RO·COR
$Ar'N_2^+$	ArH, R_2NH, ROH	ArN_2Ar', $R_2N·N_2Ar'$, RO·N_2Ar'
NO^+, HNO_2, etc.	ArH, R_2NH, ROH	ArNO, R_2N·NO, RO·NO
Alk^+, Alk·Hal, etc.	ArH, R_2NH, ROH	ArAlk, R_2NAlk, ROAlk
Deutero-acids	ArH	ArD
HgX_2 salts	ArH	ArHgX

However, our purpose now is to illustrate the contrast between the two types of heterolytic substitution, and not to define completely their fields of application.

(18d) Nucleophilic and Electrophilic Additions.—Unlike substitutions, heterolytic *additions* cannot in general be classified without knowing, or making assumptions about, the mechanism of addition. However, this is not as great a difficulty as might appear. For, first, the mechanisms of some of the more important and typical additions have been established by specialised experimental investigations; secondly, many other additions are so clearly analogous to those whose mechanisms are proved as to leave no doubt about the broad classes to which these other processes belong; and, thirdly, considerable guidance can be obtained from the general chemical behaviour of the reagents involved. One would naturally approach any new case by developing these types of argument in the reverse order.

In further explanation of the method of approach, let us consider the addition of an addendum A·B, to an acceptor X:Y, to give the addition product A·X·Y·B. We wish to know whether A becomes bound to X by the electrons of AB, leaving B to become bound to Y by electrons of XY, or *vice versa*. We also wish to know whether AB adds because it is nucleophilic, so that reaction is incepted by the combination of electrons of AB with a nucleus of XY, or because it is electrophilic, so that a nucleus of AB attacks the electrons of XY, the rest of the process, in either case, being energetically downhill. The general chemical classification of AB will give a presumptive reply to the second of these questions, and this will usually carry with it an answer to the first. It will also indicate the classification of the addition process; and the indication should be followed up by appeal to analogy, and eventually, by specialised investigation.

Consider, as a first example, the addition of ammonia to acetaldehyde to give acetaldehyde-ammonia:

$$NH_3 + CH_3{\cdot}CH{=}O \rightarrow CH_3{\cdot}CH\begin{cases}OH\\NH_2\end{cases} \qquad (Ad_N)$$

The addendum, ammonia, has been classified as a nucleophilic reagent (Section **17b**, Table 17-1). Presumably it adds because it is nucleophilic, the unshared nitrogen electrons attacking the carbon kernel of the carbonyl group, leaving the reaction to be completed by the facile transference of a proton to the unshared oxygen electron. This description classifies the reaction as a *nucleophilic addition*, a conclusion which is supported by analogies with more closely studied examples. As a basis for the symbolic addition of mechanistic particulars, we may designate it Ad_N, as is done above.

As a second example, consider the addition of hydrogen chloride to propene to give *iso*propyl chloride:

$$HCl + CH_3{\cdot}CH{=}CH_2 \rightarrow CH_3{\cdot}CHCl{-}CH_3 \qquad (Ad_E)$$

The addendum, hydrogen chloride, has been classed as an electrophilic reagent (Section **17c**, Table 17-2). Let us assume that it adds because it is electrophilic, combining through its proton and the π electrons with one carbon atom, and leaving reaction to be completed by the facile addition of chloride ion to the other, now electron-depleted, carbon atom. Our assumption classifies the process as an *electrophilic addition*, and this is supported by analogy with more specifically studied cases. We may express the classification by the symbol Ad_E, as is done above.

It is implied in these conclusions that the carbonyl group, considered as a reagent, is predominantly electrophilic, and that the ethylenic system, as a reagent, is essentially nucleophilic. We have in mind here simply unsaturated, not conjugated, double bonds. The deductions certainly agree with general chemical experience to the effect that carbonyl compounds are especially vulnerable to many nucleophilic reagents (dissolving metals, dissolved reducing agents, cyanide ions, hydrogen sulphite ions, amines, hydrazines, hydroxylamine, etc.), while olefins are particularly sensitive to many electrophilic reagents (oxidising agents of all kinds, halogens, strong acids, etc.). The distinction can be linked with the constitutional difference that the electrons of the carbonyl group, including those of the π shell, are strongly displaced towards the oxygen atom, thereby exposing a thinly screened carbon nucleus; whereas both the carbon nuclei of the ethylenic group are well covered by their outer double-layer of π electrons.

(While reduction by dissolving metals, such as sodium, is a form of nucleophilic addition, and operates, as it should, upon the carbonyl and cyano-groups, but not upon simple olefins, the hydrogenation of olefins by elemental hydrogen on the surface of a transition metal, such as platinum, has different characteristics, and may well be a homolytic process. The oxidation of olefins by elemental oxygen, so-called autoxidation, is likewise a homolytic process, dependent on the di-radical nature of oxygen, which is a triplet molecule, having parallel electron spins.)

Without going here into more detailed arguments, which in some specific instances will be given later, we may refer to the list in Table 18-2 of some of the more important nucleophilic and electrophilic addition reactions. Again, the illustrations are representative, and not even approximately exhaustive.

The last entry in the first section of the table may require a word of further explanation. It includes the aldol addition reaction, which investigation has shown to depend on the acceptance, by one carbonyl molecule, of the anion of the other. As is well known, the addition products often undergo a subsequent elimination of water to form an $\alpha\beta$-ethylenic carbonyl compound. The last entry in the second section of the table represents Tilden's addition reaction: the formed nitroso-compound usually undergoes tautomeric change to give an oxime.

When ethylenic and carbonyl double bonds are conjugated with each other, C=C—C=O, the former acquires electrophilic properties, partly in addition to, and partly in replacement of, its normal nucleo-

TABLE 18-2.—SOME NUCLEOPHILIC AND ELECTROPHILIC ADDITIONS.

R = H, or alkyl, or aryl; X = R, or OR, or NR_2; Y = CO·R, or CN, or NO_2.

Nucleophilic Additions

Addendum	Acceptor	Addition product
Dissolving metals	$R_2C{=}O$, $RC{\equiv}N$	$R_2CH \cdot OH$, $RCH_2 \cdot NH_2$
Cr^{++}, H_2O	$RC{\equiv}N$	$RCH_2 \cdot NH_2$
Grignard reagents	$R_2C{=}O$	$R_2C(OMetal) \cdot Alkyl$
OH^-, H_2O	$R_2C{=}O$	$R_2C(OH)_2$ [$\rightleftarrows R_2CO$]
OH^-, H_2O	$RC{\equiv}N$	RCO_2^-
H_2S	$RC{\equiv}N$	$RCS \cdot NH_2$
NH_2X	$R_2C{=}O$	$R_2C(OH) \cdot NHX$ [$\rightarrow R_2C{:}NX$]
CN^-, ROH	$R_2C{=}O$	$R_2C(OH) \cdot CN$
$[CR_2 \cdot Y]^-$, ROH	$R_2C{=}O$	$R_2C(OH) \cdot CR_2 \cdot Y$

Electrophilic Additions

Addendum	Acceptor	Addition product
MnO_4^-, H_2O	$R_2C{=}CR_2$	$R_2C(OH) \cdot CR_2(OH)$
H_3O^+	$R_2C{=}CR_2$	$R_2CH \cdot CR_2(OH)$
H_2SO_4	$R_2C{=}CR_2$	$R_2CH \cdot CR_2(O \cdot SO_3H)$
Hal_2	$R_2C{=}CR_2$	$R_2CHal \cdot CR_2Hal$
Hal_2, ROH	$R_2C{=}CR_2$	$R_2CHal \cdot CR_2(OH)$
HOHal, H_3O^+	$R_2C{=}CR_2$	$R_2CHal \cdot CR_2(OH)$
HHal	$R_2C{=}CR_2$	$R_2CH \cdot CR_2Hal$
NOHal	$R_2C{=}CR_2$	$R_2C(NO) \cdot CR_2Hal$

philic character. This may be interpreted as indicating an appreciable displacement of the whole conjugated π shell towards the carbonyl oxygen atom, with partial exposure of the carbon nucleus at the other end of the system. Hence a number of nucleophilic additions of the simple carbonyl group occur also with the conjugated system, the terminal carbon atom of which acts like a carbonyl carbon atom. Thus, to the aldol additions of simple carbonyl compounds, there corresponds the Michael addition reactions of conjugated systems terminated by carbonyl groups:

$$R_2C{=}O + H{-}CR_2 \cdot CO \cdot R \rightarrow R_2C\begin{cases} OH \\ CR_2 \cdot CO \cdot R \end{cases}$$

(aldol)

$$R_2C{=}CR{-}CR{=}O + H{-}CR_2 \cdot CO \cdot R \rightarrow R_2C\begin{cases} CHR{-}CR{=}O \\ CR_2 \cdot CO \cdot R \end{cases}$$

(Michael)

(18e) Classification of Eliminations.—Eliminations could in principle be classified according to a similar plan, but at present this is hardly a practical necessity, for the reason that all the most important, and best investigated, eliminations would fall into one class: the *eliminant* is of the form HB throughout; of which the portion H is transferred, as a proton, to some basic molecule, either a specially introduced one, or the solvent; while the portion B is liberated, without forming a new covalent bond in the elimination process, though it may or may not form one subsequently. These statements apply without modification to the large group of *olefin-forming eliminations*, some examples of which are represented by the following equations:

$$OEt^- + (CH_3)_2CHBr \rightarrow HOEt + CH_3{\cdot}CH{:}CH_2 + Br^-$$

$$H_2O + (CH_3)_3CBr \rightarrow H_3O^+ + (CH_3)_2C{:}CH_2 + Br^-$$

$$OH^- + C_2H_5{\cdot}NMe_3^+ \rightarrow H_2O + CH_2{:}CH_2 + NMe_3$$

$$H_2O + (CH_3)_3C{\cdot}SMe_2^+ \rightarrow H_3O^+ + (CH_3)_2C{:}CH_2 + SMe_2$$

As these equations show, the only new covalent bond which, in this elimination process, is established between an external molecule and either fragment of the eliminant, is the bond between the proton and the nucleophilic molecule which accepts the proton. According to our system, these eliminations would all be classified as nucleophilic: this being appreciated, it is not necessary to emphasize it in the nomenclature. Thus, when symbolising the characteristic forms, we shall take E, rather than the more explicit E_N, as the basic symbol for elimination processes of the types illustrated.

There are differences of mechanism, but not of polar classification, when we go over to *carbonyl-forming eliminations*. These are the reactions which, as the following formulae illustrate, reverse the formation of the carbonyl addition compounds, such as cyanohydrins, aldols, and ketols:

$$OH^- + HO{\cdot}C(CH_3)_2{\cdot}CN \rightarrow H_2O + O{=}C(CH_3)_2 + CN^-$$

$$OH^- + HO{\cdot}C(CH_3)_2{\cdot}CH_2{\cdot}CO{\cdot}CH_3 \rightarrow H_2O + O{=}C(CH_3)_2 + [CH_2{\cdot}CO{\cdot}CH_3]^-$$

Using our knowledge of the mechanism of the corresponding addition processes, and the idea that the same reaction surface, and the same reaction co-ordinate on it, will apply to the forward and reverse reactions (the so-called principle of microscopic reversibility),[8] we believe

[8] The general form of this principle is that, if there are many reaction paths from given factors to given products, then, in equilibrium, as many molecular systems will pass forwards as backwards in each individual path. The only type of application with which we shall be concerned is simply that the *easiest* path forwards is the easiest backwards.

that, initially, these elimination processes, besides transferring a proton to an external base, liberate anions. These anions are either moderately strong, or very strong, bases (cyanide ion, the weakest of them, is roughly comparable to trimethylamine), and thus they will take an early opportunity to acquire protons: hence, with the possible exception of cyanide ion, they are normally isolated as their conjugate acids. However, the carbonyl-forming eliminations produce only one covalent bond with an external reagent, and that reagent is nucleophilic, just as with the olefin-forming eliminations.

Eliminations analogous to those of the carbonyl-forming series take place with the production of ethylenic double bonds conjugated with carbonyl groups. The reversal of Michael addition is a reaction of this type: it is a close relative of the reversal of aldol addition. The following formulation of an example will illustrate the correspondence:

$$OEt^- + H\cdot\underset{}{\overset{CO_2Et}{\overset{|}{C}}}H—C(CH_3)_2\cdot CH(CO_2Et)_2$$

$$\rightarrow HOEt + \overset{CO_2Et}{\overset{|}{C}}H{=}C(CH_3)_2 + [CH(CO_2Et)_2]^-$$

All these reactions are nucleophilic eliminations.

(18f) Production of Radicals for Homolytic Reactions.—The only immediately and plentifully available material of any great importance as a free-radical for producing homolytic reactions is molecular oxygen. Most of the radical reagents have to be produced *in situ*, or at least produced and used within their quite short life-times. There are several types of process by which they can be thus obtained.

One-electron *redox* processes are widely used for the controlled production of radicals. As an example, the mixture of hydrogen peroxide and a ferrous salt, long known as Fenton's reagent, owes its properties, as Haber and Weiss elucidated,[9] to the one-electron reduction of hydrogen peroxide to hydroxyl radicals:

$$e\text{ (from }Fe^{++}) + HO\cdot OH \rightarrow HO^- + OH^\cdot$$

Ferrous or cobaltous salts act analogously on the perdisulphate ions and on organic hydroperoxides.

Radicals can be formed by redox electron transfers on an electrode. The formed radicals usually react at the electrode surface. The classical reaction of Kolbe, in which dimerised alkyl chains are built by

[9] F. Haber and J. Weiss, *Proc. Roy. Soc.*, 1934, **A, 147**, 332; cf. N. Uri, *Chem. Rev.*, 1952, **50**, 375.

the anodic oxidation of carboxylate ions, almost certainly goes by way of radicals:

$$R\cdot CO\cdot O^- \rightarrow e \text{ (to anode)} + R\cdot CO\cdot O^\cdot \rightarrow CO_2 + R^\cdot \rightarrow R_2$$

The *thermal homolysis* of covalent bonds can be used to produce radicals of many types. The required temperatures depend on the strengths of the bonds to be broken. Roughly speaking, bonds having dissociation energies in the range 40–50 kcal./mole require temperatures in the neighbourhood of 200–400°, as in the examples,

$$Br_2 \rightarrow 2Br^\cdot$$

$$I_2 \rightarrow 2I^\cdot$$

$$HO{-}NO_2 \rightarrow HO^\cdot + NO_2$$

$$CH_3{-}N{:}N\cdot CH_3 \rightarrow CH_3^\cdot + N_2 + CH_3^\cdot$$

whilst bonds with energies in the range 30–40 kcal./mole will break at convenient rates in the neighbourhood of 50–200°, as in the examples,

$$F_2 \rightarrow 2F^\cdot$$

$$(CH_3)_3C\cdot O{-}O\cdot C(CH_3)_3 \rightarrow 2(CH_3)_3C\cdot O^\cdot \rightarrow 2CH_3^\cdot + 2(CH_3)_2CO$$

$$C_6H_5\cdot CO\cdot O{-}O\cdot CO\cdot C_6H_5 \rightarrow 2C_6H_5\cdot CO\cdot O^\cdot \rightarrow 2C_6H_5^\cdot + 2CO_2$$

$$(CH_3)_2C(CN){-}N{:}N\cdot C(CH_3)_2\cdot CN \rightarrow 2(CH_3)_2C(CN)^\cdot + N_2$$

$$(CH_3)(C_6H_5)_2C{-}C(C_6H_5)_2(CH_3) \rightarrow 2(CH_3)(C_6H_5)_2C^\cdot$$

A number of bond dissociation energies, relevant to the thermal formation of radicals, and also to their reactions of substitution and addition, are assembled in Table 18-3.[10]

[10] The values for the diatomic and some triatomic molecules are accurate, but the other values are approximate. Most of them are as given by T. L. Cottrell, "Strengths of Chemical Bonds," Butterworths Scientific Publications, London, 1958, Chap. 9, p. 173. The values for the halogens are from L. Pauling's "Nature of the Chemical Bond," Cornell University Press, Ithaca, New York, 3rd Edn., 1960, Chap. 3, pp. 79, 83. The value for the side-chain C—H bond of toluene and that for the C—I bond of iodobenzene are as given by A. H. Schon and M. Szwarc (*Ann. Rev. Phys. Chem.*, 1957, **8**, 439). The value for C–N in azobis*iso*butyronitrile and for N—O in nitric acid are approximate activation energies of homolysis determined by J. P. van Hook and A. V. Tobolsky (*J. Am. Chem. Soc.*, 1958, **80**, 779), and by H. S. Johnston, L. Foering, Y. S. Tao, and G. S. Moserly (*J. Am. Chem. Soc.*, 1951, **73**, 2319), respectively. The value for N—O in methyl nitrite is from P. Gray and A. Williams (*Chem. Rev.*, 1959, **59**, 239). The O—O values for hydrogen peroxide and *t*-butylhydroperoxide are from S. W. Benson (*J. Chem. Phys.*, 1964, **40**, 1007). All the values given for C—S and S—S are as determined by T. F. Palmer and F. P. Lossing (*J. Am. Chem. Soc.*, 1962, **84**, 4661).

TABLE 18-3.—SOME BOND DISSOCIATION ENERGIES (KCAL./MOLE).

Bond	kcal./mole	Bond	kcal./mole
H—H		**C—Hal**	
H—H	104	H_3C—F	108
H—C		F_3C—F	121
H—CH_3	101	H_3C—Cl	80
H—$CH_2 \cdot CH_3$	96	Cl_3C—Cl	68
H—$CH(CH_3)_2$	92	$CH_2{:}CH \cdot CH_2$—Cl	60
H—$C(CH_3)_3$	89	H_3C—Br	67
H—C_6H_5	102	Cl_3C—Br	50
H—$CH_2 \cdot C_6H_5$	83	C_6H_5—Br	71
H—CH:O	76	$C_6H_5 \cdot CH_2$—Br	51
H—N		$CH_2{:}CH \cdot CH_2$—Br	46
H—NH_2	102	H_3C—I	54
H—O		C_6H_5—I	61
H—OH	117	$C_6H_5 \cdot CH_2$—I	39
H—O·OH	90	$CH_2{:}CH \cdot CH_2$—I	36
H—S		**N—N**	
H—SH	90	H_2N—NH_2	60
H—Hal		**N—O**	
H—F	135	O_2N—OH	40
H—Cl	103	O_2N—O·CH_3	38
H—Br	87	**O—O**	
H—I	71	HO—OH	48
C—C		HO—O·$C(CH_3)_3$	42
H_3C—CH_3	83	$(CH_3)_3C \cdot O$—$O \cdot C(CH_3)_3$	37
H_3C—C_6H_5	87	$CH_3 \cdot CO \cdot O$—$O \cdot CO \cdot CH_3$	30
H_3C—$CH_2 \cdot C_6H_5$	63	**O—Hal**	
H_3C—$CH_2 \cdot CH{:}CH_2$	61	HO—Cl	60
H_2C═CH_2	~152	HO—Br	56
C—N		**S—S**	
H_3C—NO_2	57	$CH_3 \cdot S$—$S \cdot CH_3$	69
H_3C—$N{:}N \cdot CH_3$	46	**Hal—Hal**	
$(CH_3)_2(CN)C$—$N{:}N \cdot C(CN)(CH_3)_2$	31	F—F	37
C—O		F—Cl	61
H_3C—OH	90	Cl—Cl	58
HCO—OH	90	Cl—Br	52
$CH_3 \cdot CO$—OH	90	Cl—I	50
C—S		Br—Br	46
CH_3—SH	70	Br—I	42
$(CH_3)_3C$—SH	65	I—I	36

Catalytic hydrogenation with the group-VIII metals having filled *d* shells, namely, the metals nickel, palladium, and platinum, almost certainly depends on the *surface homolysis* of hydrogen molecules. The mechanism is obscure, but it obviously involves exposed metal atoms having deficient metal-metal binding, and the energetics presumably depend on getting two weak metal-hydrogen bonds for the price of the one strong bond in the hydrogen molecule, so that only weak bonds have to be broken by a substrate able to pick off the hydrogen atoms one at a time. It is known that some square complexes of group-VIII metals will at room temperature take up a hydrogen molecule, as two atoms which become bound to the remaining octahedral positions. This is a possible molecular model for what goes on at the metal surface.

The non-ionising *photolysis* of molecules constitutes another important means of producing radicals. The photolysing light must be in the spectral range of a continuous, visible or near ultra-violet band, absorption in which gives a dissociating upper electronic state. The four halogens have absorption bands of this nature, and so can be photolytically atomised. In each case, one of the $p\pi$-type unshared (non-bonding) electrons becomes promoted, without or with spin inversion, to a $p\sigma$-type, anti-bonding orbital, that is, one of the same symmetry as the upper orbital described for the excited hydrogen molecule in Section **3d**, an orbital circularly symmetrical about the bond, but with a nodal plane between the nuclei. Just as in the hydrogen molecule, the anti-bonding effect of an electron in this anti-bonding orbital is so strong that the excited halogen molecules spontaneously dissociate. Singlet and triplet dissociating states are possible. The spin inversions, which produce triplet states—states more stable than the singlet in accordance with Hund's rule (Section **3b**)—are difficult to accomplish in transitions of electrons of the lighter elements (wherein the magnetic fields, needed to invert a spin, are weak), and are accordingly infrequent accompaniments of the excitation of fluorine and chlorine; but such spin inversions are predominating in the excitations of the heavier halogens, bromine and iodine. However, all these upper states, whether singlet or triplet, are dissociating:

$$Cl_2 \text{ (normal)} \xrightarrow{h\nu} Cl_2 \text{ (excited, singlet)} \rightarrow 2Cl\cdot$$

$$Br_2 \text{ (normal)} \xrightarrow{h\nu} Br_2 \text{ (excited, triplet)} \rightarrow 2Br\cdot$$

Azomethane and bromotrichloromethane are examples of more complex molecules which can be photolytically dissociated to give radicals:

$$CH_3\cdot N:N\cdot CH_3 \xrightarrow{h\nu} 2CH_3\cdot + N_2$$

$$Cl_3C\cdot Br \xrightarrow{h\nu} Cl_3C\cdot + Br\cdot$$

The only dissociating upper state of the hydrogen molecule is the lowest triplet state (Section **3d**). But this is inaccessible from the ground state by light absorption, because of the strong inhibition in such a very light atom to spin inversion. However, excitation by *electron-impact* is not subject to that inhibition. Electron impact can raise the hydrogen molecule to a number of excited singlet and triplet states. All excited singlet states will radiatively return to the ground state, and all triplet states above the lowest one will radiatively degrade to the lowest triplet state. This has one of its electrons in an anti-bonding $2p\sigma$ orbital, and so it dissociates, as described in Section **3d**. This is the mechanism in outline of formation of hydrogen atoms in the hydrogen discharge tube, and in the Langmuir hydrogen-atom arc, or welding torch:

$$\begin{array}{ccl} & \nearrow & e\ H_2 \text{ (upper triplets)} \\ H_2 \text{ (normal)} & & \quad\downarrow -h\nu \\ & \searrow & e\ H_2 \text{ (lowest triplet)} \rightarrow 2H^{\cdot} \end{array}$$

By processes which are not well understood, *ionising radiolysis*, as by X-rays, can produce radicals and cations in great variety, even from simple alkanes. It is generally considered that the first step is always the discharge of an electron, to leave an odd-electron cation, which can break down to a cation and a radical, either in one way, as in the example of water,

$$H_2O \xrightarrow{-e} H_2O^+ \longrightarrow OH^{\cdot} + H^+$$

or in two ways, as in that of methane, in which the second way formulated,

$$CH_4 \xrightarrow{-e} CH_4^+ \begin{array}{l} \nearrow CH_3^{\cdot} + H^+ \\ \searrow CH_3^+ + H^{\cdot} \end{array}$$

is the more important. Higher alkanes undergo additional degradation to give various "cracked" products, including odd-electron cations, and even-electron neutral molecules, notably olefins.

(18g) Homolytic Substitutions.—The substitutions in which a supplied radical can engage are of two kinds, depending broadly on whether the substrate is saturated or unsaturated. If it is saturated, substitution can only commence with the extraction of an atom in order to create a radical centre with which colligation can subsequently occur. If the substrate is unsaturated, an opportunity is provided for the reagent radical to open up the π electron system, without the need to break a σ bond in order to secure a point for combination. If this reagent radical cannot attack the π electron system, as the oxygen molecule normally cannot, then it is thrown back on the first method of substitution, namely, to start by breaking a σ bond.

We shall call the first of these modes of substitution, that which starts with the extraction of an atom, *saturated homolytic substitution*. The atom extracted is usually an exterior, and hence a univalent, atom. The common case is that of the preliminary extraction of a hydrogen atom; but the preliminary extraction of a halogen atom has been observed. Whether a particular supplied "initiating" radical will or will not be able to extract a certain atom from a substrate, is first of all a thermodynamic question; and then, if thermodynamics permits, it becomes a kinetic question. Thermodynamically, the atom transfer must be exothermic or only slightly endothermic. An idea about this can be obtained from approximate bond dissociation energies, such as those in Table 18-3. One can see, for example, that thermodynamics would favour the extraction of a hydrogen atom from methane by a hydroxyl radical or a chlorine atom, but not by a thiol radical or a bromine atom. But even if thermodynamics would permit reaction, kinetics may present an obstacle. The bond-breaking and -making processes may be energetically self-balancing or better, but yet may need a certain energy investment in order to start them off; and thus, an exothermic reaction may still have a finite activation energy, and an endothermic process may require an activation energy exceeding its endothermicity.

Supposing that the external supply of substituting radicals is quite small, the second step of substitution requires that the radical, derived by loss of an atom from the substrate, shall be able to wrest a radical from some plentiful molecular source of radicals. The thermodynamic possibility, or impossibility, of a particular second step of this nature, may be checked by reference to data such as those in Table 18-3, in the manner already illustrated.

When the second step produces, as the residue set free from the molecular source of radicals, the same radical as that which took an atom from the substrate in the first step of substitution, then the first step can be repeated, and, by continuation, the steps can follow each other alternately, radical begetting radical in a prolonged kinetic chain, leading to high rates, and a conversion of material large out of all proportion to the original supply of radicals. This is the situation in that celebrated prototype of all homolytic chlorinations, the chlorination of hydrogen: for which, on the basis of experiments by Bodenstein and others, Nernst proposed[11] the first specific chain mechanism, which all subsequent investigations have confirmed.[12] It is expressed, if R = H, in the following formulae:

$$\left.\begin{aligned} RH + Cl^{\cdot} &\rightarrow R^{\cdot} + HCl \\ R^{\cdot} + Cl_2 &\rightarrow RCl + Cl^{\cdot} \end{aligned}\right\} \text{Chain}$$

This chain reaction with R = H is thermodynamically favoured, because the dissociation energy of HCl is greater than both that of H_2 and that of Cl_2. If R = alkyl, so that the equations represent the chlorination of an alkane, the chain reaction is still thermodynamically favoured, because, not only is the dissociation energy of HCl greater than the bond dissociation energy of R—H, but also the bond dissociation energy of R—Cl is greater than the dissociation energy of Cl_2. All this can be checked in Table 18-3.

The kinetic chains in the chlorine-hydrogen reaction and also in the chlorination of alkanes are very long. The length of a kinetic chain depends on the frequency of terminating processes, that is, of reactions which destroy either of the radicals that by regenerating each other maintain the chains. The gaseous nitration of alkanes by nitric acid has a homolytic mechanism of short kinetic chains. They are kept short by the side reactions which lead to concurrent oxidation.

In reactions of autoxidation, the oxygen molecule substitutes by a process which comprises two steps completely analogous to those of the substitutions just treated, and comprises also an additional step necessitated by the circumstance that the oxygen molecule is a diradical (a triplet molecule), so that its primary substitution product is itself a radical. As we have noted, the oxygen molecule, for some reason not clearly understood, has little capacity for attacking closed π electron shells. Characteristically, it starts reaction by extracting either in gas reactions one, or in liquid phases one or two, weakly bound hydrogen atoms. In particular, hydrogen atoms bound to carbon in a benzyl or allyl situation, or to carbon adjacent to oxygen, especially in carbonyl (see Chapter VII), as, for example, in *iso*-propylbenzene, drying oils, and aldehydes, are most readily extracted to yield a benzyl, allyl, or acyl radical. The radical thus created then takes up a second oxygen molecule. This completes the primary substitution of H by O_2. But the product is a peroxy-radical, and it

[11] W. Nernst, *Z. Elektrochem.*, 1918, 24, 335.

[12] C. N. Hinshelwood, "Kinetics of Chemical Change in Gaseous Systems," Clarendon Press, Oxford, 1933, p. 1001; N. N. Semenoff, "Chemical Kinetics and Chain Reactions," Clarendon Press, Oxford, 1935, p. 89.

generally engages in the further step of extracting a hydrogen atom from another substrate molecule to yield a hydroperoxide and a radical identical with the original radical. Thus the conditions for a chain reaction are established:

$$RH + O_2 \rightarrow R\cdot + HO\cdot O\cdot$$

$$2RH + O_2 \rightarrow 2R\cdot + HO\cdot OH$$

$$\left.\begin{array}{l} R\cdot + O_2 \rightarrow RO\cdot O\cdot \\ RO\cdot O\cdot + RH \rightarrow RO\cdot OH + R\cdot \end{array}\right\} \text{Chain}$$

The kinetic chains are often long. The product hydroperoxide is generally rather unstable under the conditions of its formation. It decomposes homolytically to produce more chain-initiating radicals, and in this way generally becomes the major source of radicals even at very low extents of oxidation. That is, hydroperoxides, even at very low concentrations, are more effective radical sources than is the direct reaction between molecular oxygen and the substrate. Since radicals, produced from the molecular product of the chain reaction, themselves start chains, the overall oxidation is autocatalytic, the rate increasing with time and with increasing extent of oxidation. Thus autoxidation is a branching chain reaction, a form of reaction kinetics which commonly leads to explosions, when restriction of reagent supply or access does not set a limit to the reaction rate.

Let us now turn to the second mode of homolytic substitution, which we shall call *unsaturated homolytic substitution*. Here, the substrate contains a shell of π electrons, for instance a double or triple bond, or a benzene ring, and the attacking radical colligates with the aid of one electron of the π shell. The resulting radical may then either lose an atom, or gain a second radical. In the former case we have overall a substitution, and in the latter case an addition.

Experience has shown that aromatic substrates can engage in either substitutions or additions: which they will do in a given situation depends on what reagents are available that can take an atom from, or supply a second radical to, the first-formed addition-radical. Substitution is in principle open also to olefinic substrates, but in observations made up to the present, they have been found always to engage in additions only. In this Section we are concerned with substitutions, and therefore, for the moment, with aromatic substrates.

When aromatic substrates are attacked by methyl, higher alkyl, phenyl, or substituted phenyl radicals—all radicals which can be generated in quantity, for instance, by the pyrolyses of peroxides or azo-compounds—substitution occurs in two steps, of which the first is slow:

$$C_6H_6 + R\cdot \xrightarrow[\text{slow}]{} C_6H_6R\cdot$$

$$C_6H_6R\cdot + R\cdot \longrightarrow C_6H_5R + HR$$

A contrasting reaction of addition is illustrated in the next Section.

We shall sometimes find it convenient to label homolytic substitutions S_H. It is possible then to add further symbols to indicate mechanism.

(18h) Homolytic Additions.—Three kinds of homolytic additions are recognised, two of them quite different, and the third a mixture of the other two. To the first kind we shall apply the name *homolytic mono-addition.* They arise when the unsaturated substrate, on taking up a supplied radical, produces an addition radical, which instead of losing an atom to an external radical, so leading to overall substitution, takes up a second radical from the supplied source of radicals, so completing an addition. If the liberated residue of the radical source is a radical identical with that originally taken up, a chain reaction will be established. Benzene photolytically adds chlorine by this mechanism.

$$\left.\begin{array}{l} C_6H_6 + Cl\cdot \rightarrow C_6H_6Cl\cdot \\ C_6H_6Cl\cdot + Cl_2 \rightarrow C_6H_6Cl_2 + Cl\cdot \end{array}\right\} \text{Chain}$$

The formed dichloride continues similarly to add chlorine until the hexachloride is finally formed.

Olefins generally undergo homolytic additions to the exclusion of substitution. Ethylene photolytically adds chlorine by the same homolytic chain mechanism as that which benzene employs. It adds hydrogen bromide also by the same mechanism in oxidising conditions, which will produce from the hydrogen bromide the necessary chain-initiating bromine atom:

$$\left.\begin{array}{l} CH_2{=}CH_2 + Br^{\cdot} \rightarrow Br{\cdot}CH_2{-}CH_2{}^{\cdot} \\ Br{\cdot}CH_2{-}CH_2{}^{\cdot} + HBr \rightarrow Br{\cdot}CH_2{-}CH_2{\cdot}H + Br^{\cdot} \end{array}\right\} \text{Chain}$$

It is easy to see from Table 18-3 that the addition radical must extract H and not Br from HBr.

Organic molecules may act as addenda in this mechanism, for instance, bromotrichloromethane, adding in the parts Cl_3C and Br, and aldehydes, adding in the parts RCO and H. Bromotrichloromethane can be added to olefins, either, like chlorine, with photolytic initiation, or, like hydrogen bromide, with the aid of a chemical radical-chain initiator, originally supplied, or at least originally acting, in quite small amount. The chemical initiator could, for example, be a small supply of methyl radicals, produced in any of the standard ways. As can be understood from Table 18-3, the methyl radical will extract bromine from bromotrichloromethane, and so will produce a chain-initiating trichloromethyl radical. Whether the initiation is photolytic or chemical, the homolytic monoaddition follows the standard pattern:

$$\left.\begin{array}{l} CH_2{=}CH_2 + Cl_3C^{\cdot} \rightarrow Cl_3C{\cdot}CH_2{-}CH_2{}^{\cdot} \\ Cl_3C{\cdot}CH_2{-}CH_2{}^{\cdot} + Cl_3CBr \rightarrow Cl_3C{\cdot}CH_2{-}CH_2{\cdot}Br + Cl_3C^{\cdot} \end{array}\right\} \text{Chain}$$

Aldehydes add to olefinic substrates, after chemical initiation, as by a methyl or phenyl radical. The products are ketones.

We shall call the second of the three types of homolytic additions undergone by olefinic substrates *homolytic polyaddition*[13]. Its product is a polymer.[14] Homolytic polyaddition is a form of self-addition. It arises when, after chemical initiation, the first-formed addition radical, instead of extracting a second radical from some radical source, which is often not available, or not sufficiently available, adds to another molecule of the olefinic substrate. The product is another addition radical, which, being in much the same position as its predecessor, adds to yet

[13] This allows the term "polymerisation" broadly to cover both polyadditions and polycondensations, as seems to have become the custom.

[14] The products of polycondensations are properly called "polycondensates," but they too are frequently called "polymers."

another olefinic molecule. So, by the successive addition of olefin molecules long structural chains may be built up, the process coming to an end only when the growing radical reacts with a radical. Many olefinic substances, especially those with a terminal methylene group, behave in this way, as is illustrated below for styrene:

$$\mathrm{R\cdot + CH_2{:}\underset{\substack{|\\ Ph}}{CH} \rightarrow RCH_2{\cdot}\underset{\substack{|\\ Ph}}{CH}{\cdot}}$$

$$\mathrm{RCH_2{\cdot}\underset{\substack{|\\ Ph}}{CH}{\cdot} + CH_2{:}\underset{\substack{|\\ Ph}}{CH} \rightarrow RCH_2{\cdot}\underset{\substack{|\\ Ph}}{CH}{\cdot}CH_2{\cdot}\underset{\substack{|\\ Ph}}{CH}{\cdot}}$$

$$\mathrm{RCH_2{\cdot}\underset{\substack{|\\ Ph}}{CH}{\cdot}CH_2{\cdot}\underset{\substack{|\\ Ph}}{CH}{\cdot} + CH_2{:}\underset{\substack{|\\ Ph}}{CH} \rightarrow RCH_2{\cdot}\underset{\substack{|\\ Ph}}{CH}{\cdot}CH_2{\cdot}\underset{\substack{|\\ Ph}}{CH}{\cdot}CH_2{\cdot}\underset{\substack{|\\ Ph}}{CH}{\cdot}}$$

$$\mathrm{------------ \rightarrow RCH_2{\cdot}\underset{\substack{|\\ Ph}}{CH}{\cdot}\left[CH_2{\cdot}\underset{\substack{|\\ Ph}}{CH}\right]_n{\cdot}CH_2{\cdot}\underset{\substack{|\\ Ph}}{CHR'}}$$

Kinetically, this is not a chain reaction in the original connotation of that term. But the successive steps are so similar to one another that, by a natural extension of terminology, it may be called a chain reaction; and, for the mathematical analysis of its kinetics, it can be treated as such. This terminology has, of course, nothing to do with the fact that the reaction produces structural carbon chains.

We shall call the third type of homolytic addition undergone by olefinic substances *homolytic teleaddition*. Its product is called a *telemer*. Homolytic teleaddition arises when, after radical chain initiation, the first-formed addition radical finds comparable opportunities of extracting a radical from a source of radicals, as in monoaddition, and of adding to another olefinic substrate molecule, as in polyaddition. In these circumstances, a few steps of polyaddition may become interposed between the first step of monoaddition and its second and final step. To put it otherwise, polyaddition chains are started, but they are cut so short by the ample opportunities for chain termination, that the groups which would be added in monoaddition, and which become the structural end-groups in polyaddition, are a very important part of the constitution of the low polymers, called telemers, which are formed.

As examples, we may refer to the addition of carbon tetrachloride, and of acetaldehyde, to ethylene, under initiation by phenyl radicals. The telemeric products are

$$\left.\begin{array}{l} Cl_3C\cdot CH_2\cdot CH_2\cdot [CH_2\cdot CH_2]_n\cdot CH_2\cdot CH_2\cdot Cl \\ CH_3\cdot CO\cdot CH_2\cdot CH_2\cdot [CH_2\cdot CH_2]_n\cdot CH_2\cdot CH_2\cdot H \end{array}\right\} n = 0, 1, 2, \cdots$$

It will be convenient in some discussions shortly to denote homolytic additions by the symbol Ad_H.

(18i) Other Reactions to be Treated.—The unit processes of heterolysis and homolysis have mechanisms as simple as any found in organic chemistry. These reactions also offer a field for the study of equilibrium relations, which, because of the simplicity of the relations between factors and products, give basic information on the relative stabilities, *i.e.*, the free-energy differences, of molecules, ions, and radicals.

The data obtained in this way allow us to go somewhat further than before in correlating structural effects on reactivity in the substitutions, additions, and eliminations already studied.

Molecular rearrangements arise largely as elaborations of the processes of substitution, addition, and elimination. We shall find it convenient to classify rearrangements, first, according as they occur in reactions of saturated, or unsaturated, or of specifically aromatic systems. Within each of these fields we shall divide the rearrangements into nucleophilic and electrophilic. These terms refer, as usual, to the nature of the reagent responsible for the reaction in which rearrangement occurs; and we use these terms for classification. But for the subdivisions of unsaturated rearrangements, we use equivalent historical names, which call attention to the nature of the group that shifts, rather than to the nature of the responsible reagent—the names prototropy and anionotropy in particular.

Some reactions of addition and elimination, and some of molecular rearrangement, cannot be classified as nucleophilic, electrophilic, or homolytic, not because we do not know enough about their mechanisms but for reasons of fundamental principle. These reactions are those which require no external reagent, and, somewhere along the reaction co-ordinate, though not necessarily at a maximum or minimum of energy, pass through a cyclic intermediate configuration. The reaction re-locates bonds in this configuration, as in the examples formulated below. We know that this relocation involves peripheral electronic movements in the cyclic intermediate configuration; but we cannot know whether the electrons remain paired during the readjustment or whether they unpair and re-pair; and we cannot know which way round they go, in moving from their old bond locations to their new ones:

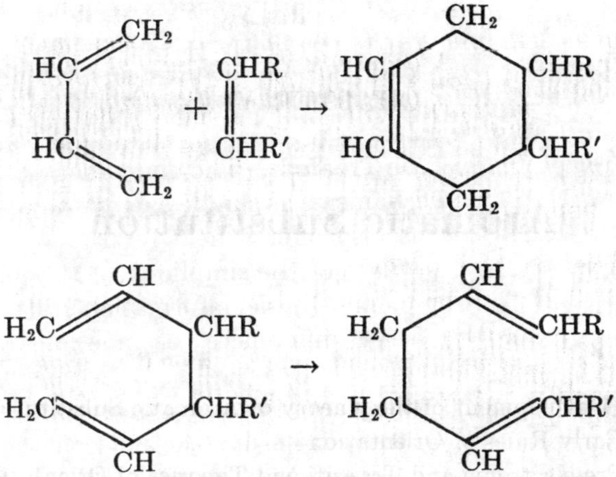

$$HC(=CH_2)\text{–}HC(=CH_2) + CHR{=}CHR' \rightarrow \text{cyclo-}[CH_2\text{–}HC{=}HC\text{–}CH_2\text{–}CHR'\text{–}CHR]$$

$$\text{cyclo-}[CH\text{–}H_2C{=}\ldots] \rightarrow \ldots$$

We shall be concerned only with homogeneous reactions, whether in the gas phase or in solution. These are the reactions for which the quantitative laws arise from energetics and the laws of chance, operating on large numbers of molecular systems. We shall not concern ourselves with reactions within crystalline solids, on solid surfaces, or on enzymes, reactions in which at least some of the interacting atoms are permanently in defined positions, so that the reactions are not dependent on the production by chance of favourable positions and velocities of all such atoms: the topochemical factor has become highly important. Topochemical reactions comprise a large field, indeed several large fields, of reactions, which, however, because of their extent, we shall have to regard as outside our scope.

CHAPTER VI

Aromatic Substitution

THE DISCUSSION of organic reactions now to be commenced will broadly follow the survey of types of reaction given in Chapter V. Thus we shall start with substitutions, and immediately with electrophilic aromatic substitutions, because, as a matter of history, it was directly through their study that the electronic theory of organic chemistry, especially of the co-operation of polarisation and polarisability effects, each involving inductive and conjugative electronic interactions, took the shape described in Chapter II. In electrophilic aromatic substitution the significant observations relate to the orientation and rate of substitution. Their study led to the generalisations of Chapter II many years before kinetic investigations had been carried far enough to disclose the actual mechanism of any particular substitution, even of nitration, the substitution most extensively employed.

(19) DEVELOPMENT OF THE THEORY OF AROMATIC SUBSTITUTION

(19a) Early Rules of Orientation.—One of the first results of the introduction in 1874 of sound methods for the determination of the positions of substituents in the benzene nucleus was the discovery of regularities concerning the orientation of substitution. It appeared that there were two broadly contrasting types of orientation, one towards ortho- and para-positions, and the other towards meta-positions. It also appeared that the nature of the substituent already present determined the position or positions which a new substituent must take up. Already in the middle 1870's attempts were being made to reduce the known facts to a rule.

The notion that atoms and groups have an electrochemical character had survived from the teachings of Berzelius. The first three of the proposed rules of orientation in aromatic substitution, those of Koerner,[1] Hübner,[2] and Noelting,[3] were essentially forms of the same rule; and it expressed the conclusion that the significant property of an orienting group was its electropolar nature. Negative groups, said this rule, that is, those which confer or enhance acidic properties, will,

[1] W. Koerner, *Gazz. chim. ital.*, 1874, 4, 305, 446.

[2] H. Hübner, *Ber.*, 1875, 8, 873.

[3] E. Noelting, *Ber.*, 1876, 9, 1797.

provided that their electronegativity is strong enough, direct a new substituent to the meta-position; and positive groups, that is, those that confer or enhance basic properties, as well as neutral, and even sufficiently weakly negative, groups, will direct new substituents into the ortho- and para-positions. It was appreciated, and regarded as causal, that the substituents that can readily be introduced in place of hydrogen, and are thus oriented, themselves have a pronounced electronegative character, as, for example, halogen, nitro-, and sulphonic acid substituents.

This group of rules made a positive contribution to the subsequently developed theory of the subject: for it foreshadowed the part played by the inductive effect in the modern theory of orientation in aromatic substitution. Electronegative groups are those whose nuclei are under-screened: they are the groups which, for this electrostatic reason, attract electrons, reducing the electron density in an attached residue, thus exerting what we now term the negative-inductive ($-I$) effect. Electropositive groups electrostatically raise electron density in an attached residue, that is, they exert a positive-inductive ($+I$) effect. The rules of Koerner, Hübner, and Noelting mean, then, that groups which attract electrons strongly ($-I$ effect) direct substituents to the meta-positions, while other groups direct them to the ortho- and para-positions; and this is broadly true.

In the succeeding decades, rules of a different nature were advanced: they directly or indirectly connect orientation with the state of saturation or unsaturation of the directing substituent. In 1887 Armstrong noted[4] that substituents attached to the benzene ring by an atom involved in a multiple bond were meta-directing, whereas other substituents were ortho- and para-directing. Essentially the same correlation was later stressed by Vorländer.[5] In 1892, Crum Brown and Gibson announced their famous rule[6] to the effect that a substituent X would be meta-directing if HX could be directly oxidised to HOX, and ortho- and para-directing otherwise. Neither rule is accurate, but the second is considerably more accurate than the first.

Now although the connexion was never made clear, these rules are closely related; and they foreshadow the part played by the mesomeric effect in the modern theory of aromatic orientation. A substance HX will be the more easily oxidisable to HOX, if the latter contains some special factor of stability denied to the former, for instance, a very stable mesomeric system in which the unshared electrons of oxygen

[4] H. E. Armstrong, *J. Chem. Soc.*, 1887, **51**, 258.
[5] D. Vorländer, *Ann.*, 1902, **320**, 122.
[6] A. Crum Brown and J. Gibson, *J. Chem. Soc.*, 1892, **61**, 367.

participate; and this condition is fulfilled when the group —X is of the form —Y═Z, having a multiple bond, provided that Z will readily accept electrons:

H—O—Y═Z

These are the groups which become meta-orienting, if the power of the system to withdraw aromatic electrons by an analogous mechanism is sufficient:

Ar—Y═Z

Armstrong and Vorländer's rule points to unsaturation as the condition for meta-orientation; but that condition alone is not sufficient. Crum Brown and Gibson's rule provides the second condition, that of electron attraction accompanying unsaturation; and this will produce meta-orientation: therefore their rule is the more accurate. But it is still not accurate, because, although the two conditions together are sufficient, they are not necessary: for strong electron attraction, even without unsaturation, will produce meta-orientation.

(19b) Pre-electronic and Transitional Theories of Orientation.—In 1902 the first serious theory (as distinct from a rule) of orientation was advanced by Flürscheim.[7] He used Werner's idea that chemical affinity, even apart from unsaturation, is continuously divisible, and is partly in the bonds, and partly free. He assumed that an atom, such as "bivalent" oxygen, which has the intrinsic ability to increase its valency, would, when bound to an aromatic carbon atom, make a large affinity-demand on the latter, leaving it with relatively little affinity for its other bonds, and little free affinity. This atom would accordingly make only a small affinity-demand on the next atoms; and thus the disturbance would be propagated, and an alternating distribution of bound, and of free, affinity would be set up, as indicated in the left-hand diagram below. This would lead to ortho- and para-orientation, the assumption being that a substituting agent would be attracted preferentially to the positions having the most free affinity. A substituent atom in its highest valency state, such as the "pentavalent" nitrogen atom of a nitro-group, was regarded as an atom whose resources of affinity were already over-strained: it would be unable to make more than a small affinity-demand on the nuclear atom to which it was bound, and this would produce a different affinity distribution. leading to meta-orientation, as indicated in the right-hand diagram:

[7] B. Flürscheim, *J. prakt. Chem.*, 1902, **66**, 321; 1905, **71**, 497; *Ber.*, 1906, **39**, 2015; *Chemistry & Industry*, 1925, **44**, 246; *J. Chem. Soc.*, **1926**, 1562.

OR

O O
N

ortho- and para-Orientation meta-Orientation

(Flürscheim's diagrams: bonds of high and low affinity-content are denoted by thick and thin bond-signs; while atoms with much and little free affinity are labelled by the long and short, dotted lines.)

Carbon was considered to have a fixed valency: therefore, a carbon atom, directly bound to the benzene ring, would behave as determined by the atoms of variable valency bound to it. Thus benzotrichloride, benzaldehyde, and phenyl cyanide, should be predominantly meta-orienting (as they are), and phenylnitromethane should be mainly ortho- and para-orienting (as it is not). If the carbon atom bound to the nucleus were bound to another carbon atom by a multiple bond, as in styrene, then, as an unsaturated atom, it would make a high affinity-demand on the benzene ring, and so produce ortho- and para-orientation (as it does—contrary to the Armstrong-Vorländer rule). If it were bound by single bonds only to hydrogen and carbon atoms only, as in toluene or ethylbenzene, then the main determinant of the behaviour would be the unsaturation, and resulting considerable affinity-demand, of the benzene ring itself, and again ortho- and para-orientation should result (as is the case).

Flürscheim's theory fulfilled a distinguished role in the development of the modern theory. For, first, it embodied a widened idea of unsaturation and of conjugation, recognising in the power of an atom to increase its valency (to share its unshared electrons, as we should now say) a condition which could, similarly to a double or triple bond, disturb the distribution of affinity in its neighbourhood. Secondly, it describes the affinity redistribution resulting from this kind of unsaturation quite correctly in its formula covering ortho- and para-orientation. This formula could be (and was) directly translated into electronic terms; and thus, as we shall see more clearly later, it foreran the part played by the electromeric effect in the modern theory of aromatic substitution.

However, difficulties arose in the interpretation of meta-directive effects. Already in 1902, one meta-orienting compound was known, namely, phenylnitromethane, for which the theory could not account;

and Flürscheim was forced into a highly unconvincing (and, as was later proved, incorrect)[8] explanation of the case. During the 1920's many such examples were demonstrated, which could not be explained away. The cause of the trouble was partly that Flürscheim's theory, as a pre-electronic theory, treats electrochemical character as a property separable from valency distribution; and partly that, based as the theory is on Werner's view of valency, it does not recognise the major difference of mobility that exists between unsaturated and saturated valencies (that is, between π and σ bonds).

Holleman gave an important criterion by which all theories of orientation must be judged. In 1910 his book appeared.[9] In it, he set forth the known facts of orientation, including numerous quantitative findings of his own. He also offered a theoretical treatment, in which he assumed that the first step in substitution is addition to a Kekulé double bond; and that substituents orient by modifying the additive reactivity of double bonds. But he did not attempt to complete a theory of orientation, by correlating the presumed effects on reactivity with the constitutions of the substituents. The valuable element in his discussion is his insistence on the connexion between orientation and the reactivity of the aromatic nucleus. He points out that ortho- and para-orienting substituents usually increase the rate at which substitution takes place, whereas meta-orientation is definitely associated with a diminished rate of substitution. Therefore no theory can be satisfactory if it modifies meta-carbon atoms in meta-orientation exactly as it modifies ortho- and para-carbon atoms in ortho- and para-orientation. Flürscheim's theory fails by this test; for the theory would suggest activated meta-carbon atoms in meta-orientation, whereas the rate relations show that all nuclear positions are deactivated.

Over the next fifteen years, a group of closely related theories, often known, individually or collectively, as the "theory of alternate polarities," secured a very notable amount of attention.[10] The first form of this theory, due to Fry, assumed that the atoms of benzene had alternating charges, in two equivalent, rapidly interconvertible forms, called "electromers":

[8] J. W. Baker and C. K. Ingold, *J. Chem. Soc.*, **1926**, 2462; *ibid.*, **1929**, 423

[9] A. F. Holleman, "Die direkte Einführung von Substituenten in den Benzolkern," Veit, Leipzig, 1910.

[10] H. S. Fry, *J. Am. Chem. Soc.*, 1912, **34**, 664; 1914, **36**, 248, 262, 1038; 1915, **37**, 855; "The Electronic Conception of Valence and the Constitution of Benzene," Longmans Green and Co., London and New York, 1921; D. Vorländer, *Ber.*, 1919, **52**, 263; 1925, **58**, 1893; A. Lapworth, *Mem. Proc. Manchester Lit. & Phil. Soc.*, 1920, **64**, iii, 2; *J. Chem. Soc.*, 1922, **121**, 416; W. O. Kermack and R. Robinson, *ibid.*, p. 427; T. M. Lowry, *ibid.*, 1923, **123**, 826

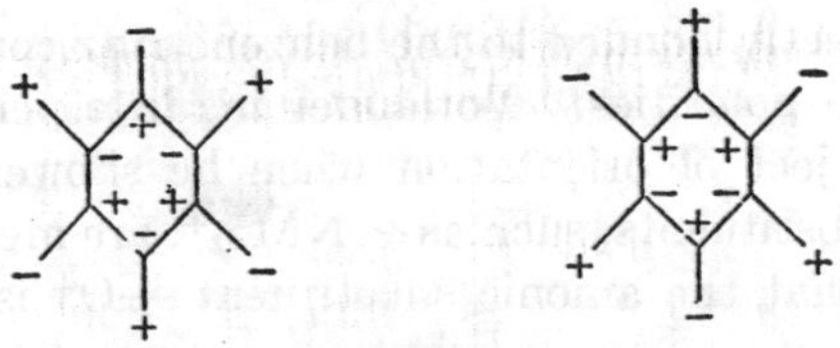

Fry's electromers of benzene

In most derivatives of benzene one electromer predominated; and since substitution preferentially replaced positive hydrogen, a favoured electromer required a favoured orientation, as the following expressions indicate:

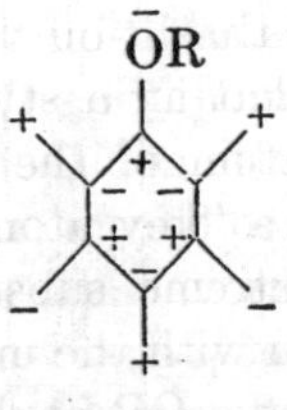

Favoured electromer requiring ortho-para-orientation

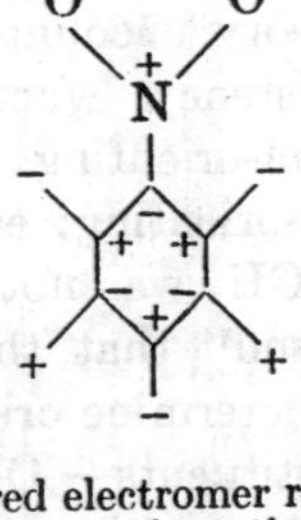

Favoured electromer requiring meta-orientation

Which arrangement of the alternating charges would be favoured by a given substituent was deduced from Crum Brown and Gibson's rule in the following way. Oxidation involves electron release: therefore a facile reaction HX→HOX signifies that X tends to charge an attached atom negatively. For instance, the facile oxidation $HNO_2 \rightarrow HNO_3$ shows that the nitro-group will *repel* electrons to an adjacent atom, in particular, an adjacent nuclear carbon atom, charging it negatively, as in the diagram. It is interesting that so plausible an argument should have yielded the wrong inference: one sees that it was due to a neglected effect of unsaturation and resulting mesomerism in making the oxidation of nitrous to nitric acid a facile process. But, given this false start, the equally false assumption of alternate polarities yields the right orientation.

Vorländer and Lapworth obtained the same preferred sign distributions round the ring by allowing the most electrochemically extreme atom in the substituent, called by Lapworth the "key atom," to determine the form of the alternations. Thus O in —OR and $—NO_2$ had to be negative, so that N in $—NO_2$ became positive; and H in $—CH_3$ had to be positive so that the C atom became negative. Vorländer added the proposition that the sign of an ionic charge carried by an atom directly bonded to the benzene ring could be accepted as determining the polarities. Vorländer made a permanent contribution to the subject of orientation when he showed experimentally[11] that cationic substituents, such as $—NMe_3^+$, are meta-orienting, while it was known that the anionic substituent $—O^-$ is ortho- and para-orienting.

As to mechanism, Lapworth and Lowry insisted that the assumed charges arise only during reaction; and Lowry that the carbon atoms, but not the hydrogen atoms, of the benzene molecule receive charges; while Kermack and Robinson offered an electronic (but quite unphysical) picture of the production of charges by the alternate contraction and expansion of octets.

This theory encountered many difficulties. Vorländer pointed to an inconsistency, when Malherbe showed[12] that *t*-butylbenzene is mainly para-orienting. It was discovered[13] that an α-styryl ether is ortho-para-orienting: evidently the oxygen atom of the substituent $—C(OR){:}CH_2$ was not behaving properly as a "key atom." Again, it was found[14] that the electrochemically extreme substituent —F could not determine orientation in competition with the much less extreme substituents —OR and $—NR_2$, and that —OR could not do so in competition with $—NR_2$. And always Holleman's criterion had to be applied, namely, that a theory could not be sound which treats meta-orientation as implying meta-activation, and accordingly modifies meta-positions in meta-orientation exactly as it modifies ortho- and para-positions in ortho-para-orientation: by this test, the theory of alternate polarities was doomed from before its birth. In retrospect, the theory may be regarded as an expression of the widespread conviction that *somehow* electrochemical factors were fundamental in orientation, and that their basic position ought to receive explicit recognition in theory.

(19c) Inception of the Electronic Theory of Orientation.—In 1926, the theory of orientation took the direction from which it has not since deviated. In a sense, the problem was handled by including it in the larger one of constitutional effects on organic reactions generally; but it is equally true that the study of aromatic orientation became for some years the spearhead of the attack on this larger problem.

Already there existed much of the material required for the construc-

[11] D. Vorländer and E. Siebert, *Ber.*, 1919, **52**, 282; D. Vorländer, *ibid.*, 1925, **58**, 1893.

[12] D. F. du T. Malherbe, *Ber.*, 1919, **52**, 319.

[13] C. K. Ingold and E. H. Ingold, *J. Chem. Soc.*, 1925, **127**, 870.

[14] C. K. Ingold and E. H. Ingold, *J. Chem. Soc.*, **1926**, 1310; E. L. Holmes, C. K. Ingold, and E. H. Ingold, *ibid.*, p. 1328.

tion of a general theory of constitutional effects on reactivity. Lewis had established his form of electron displacement, as a permanent molecular condition, now called the inductive effect; and Lowry had proposed and illustrated his form of electron displacement, as an activation phenomenon, now called the electromeric effect (Section **7a**). In a discussion of additions to olefins Lucas had combined the inductive and electromeric effects, showing how the former could assist and give direction to the latter (Section **7b**). Reagents had been classified as seekers of electrons or of nuclei, electrophilic or nucleophilic reagents, as they are usually called today; and it was appreciated that the reagents participating in the aromatic substitutions to which the orientation rules apply are electrophilic reagents (Sections **17** and **18c**). Around this time, Robinson and the writer and their associates began to combine this group of ideas into a theory of aromatic orientation.[15] Early in this development, the idea of permanent electron displacements by the conjugative mechanism, the mesomeric effect, was introduced (Section **7a**); while somewhat later the concept of activating displacements by the inductive mechanism, the inductomeric effect, was incorporated into the general theory (Section **7a**).

It remained to test the theory by critical observations. And this was done, as will be described below, by the production of data allowing penetration at two depths into the mechanism of orientation. The first appeal was to quantitatively determined ratios in which isomerides are formed by substitution, data of the kind in whose production Holleman was the pioneer. Then, a deeper insight was sought by an analysis of the orientation ratios into component effects on rate, leading to an elucidation of the relationship between orientation and reactivity, a correlation of which Holleman had emphasized the importance. The developed theory, and the observations of both these kinds, are so mutually illuminating, that it is convenient to describe them together.

(20) ORIENTATION IN ELECTROPHILIC AROMATIC SUBSTITUTION[16]

(20a) Orienting Effects of Poles.—Vorländer made the important discovery[17] that a free positive ionic centre in direct union with the benzene nucleus leads to strongly predominating meta-orientation, independently of whether the element, which carries the positive

[15] J. Allen, A. E. Oxford, R. Robinson, and J. C. Smith, *J. Chem. Soc.*, **1926**, 401; C. K. Ingold and E. H. Ingold, *ibid.*, p. 1310; H. R. Ing and R. Robinson, *ibid.*, p. 1365; F. R. Goss, C. K. Ingold, and I. S. Wilson, *ibid.*, p. **2440**; C. K. Ingold, *Ann. Rept. on Progress Chem.* (Chem. Soc. London), 1926, **23**, **129**; C. K. Ingold and F. R. Shaw, *J. Chem. Soc.*, **1927**, 2918.

[16] C. K. Ingold, *Rec. trav. chim.*, 1929, **48**, 797.

[17] D. Vorländer and E. Siebert *Ber.*, 1919, **52**, 283; D. Vorländer, *ibid.*, 1925, **58**, 1893.

charge, is light or heavy, non-metal or metal.[18] The examples included the nitration of phenyltrimethylammonium nitrate, diphenyliodinium nitrate, diphenyl-lead dinitrate, and triphenylbismuth dinitrate. The list of elements which, as positive ionic centres bonded directly to the aromatic ring, have been shown to exhibit powerful meta-orientation, has since been extended to include mercury, thallium, and tin, by Challenger and Rothstein.[19] It has been further extended, as will be specified below, by the inclusion of a number of additional elements of the Mendeléjeff groups V and VI, so that the list of cations of this form which have been studied includes the following:

$PhHg^+$ Ph_2Tl^+ Ph_2Sn^{++} Ph_2Pb^{++} Ph_3Bi^{++} Ph_2I^+

$PhNMe_3^+$ $PhPMe_3^+$ $PhAsMe_3^+$ $PhSbMe_3^+$ $PhSMe_2^+$ $PhSeMe_2^+$

Substituents of this positive ionic type are amongst the strongest meta-orienting groups known. However, the degree of meta-orientation decreases generally with increasing length of a carbon chain interposed between the positive pole and the benzene nucleus. This has been established by comparing the behaviour of phenyl-, benzyl-, 2-phenylethyl-, and 3-phenyl-*n*-propyl-trimethylammonium ions in nitration.[20] The proportions of meta-nitro-products are as shown in Table 20-1. There is no appreciable dinitration, and thus the differences from 100% represent ortho- and para-nitro-products. We shall be dealing later with the general correlation of orientation with rate of nitration, but may note now that, as Ridd and others[21] have shown, the rate of mononitration rises with chain length in the similarly monatomic way illustrated in the table.

In the last example, very little of the effect of the positive pole appears to be felt at the benzene ring, the proportion of meta-product being scarcely greater than that obtained from toluene (3%). The

[18] An 'onium element of Mendeléjeff's first period, if it has unshared electrons, may furnish an exception. Whereas Ph_2Cl^+, and $_+Ph_2I^+$, give almost wholly meta-products, Ph_3O^+, which has no empty *d* orbitals able to give a $-K$ conjugation (cf. p. 276), gives predominatingly the para-product on nitration (A. N. Nesmeyanov, T. P. Tolstaya, L. S. Isaeva, and A. V. Grib, *Doklady Akad. Nauk S.S.S.R.*, 1960, **133**, 602.)

[19] F. Challenger and E. Rothstein, *J. Chem. Soc.*, **1934**, 1258.

[20] F. R. Goss, C. K. Ingold, and I. S. Wilson, *J. Chem. Soc.*, **1926**, 2440; F. R. Goss, W. Hanhart, and C. K. Ingold, *ibid.*, **1927**, 250; C. K. Ingold and I. S. Wilson, *ibid.*, p. 810; J. H. Ridd, *J. Tennessee Acad. Sci.*, 1965, **40**, 92.

[21] C. K. Ingold, F. R. Shaw, and I. S. Wilson, *J. Chem. Soc.*, **1928**, 2030; J. W. Baker and W. G. Moffitt, *ibid.*, **1930**, 1722; M. Brickman, S. Johnson, and J. H. Ridd, *Proc. Chem. Soc.*, **1962**, 228; F. L. Riley and E. Rothstein, *J. Chem. Soc.*, **1964**, 3872; M. Brickman, J. H. P. Utley, and J. H. Ridd, *ibid.*, **1965**, 6851; A. Gastaninza, T. A. Modro, J. H. Ridd, and J. H. P. Utley, *ibid*, **1968**, B, 534.

TABLE 20-1.—EFFECTS OF SIDE-CHAIN LENGTHENING ON THE RELATIVE RATE OF MONONITRATION OF AROMATIC AMMONIUM IONS AND ON THE PROPORTION OF META-PRODUCTS FORMED.

	$PhNMe_3^+$	$PhCH_2NMe_3^+$	$Ph(CH_2)_2NMe_3^+$	$Ph(CH_2)_3NMe_3^+$	$PhCH_3$
Rate	1	3.6×10^3	4.63×10^6	5.10×10^7	4.69×10^8
Meta	89%	85%	19%	5%	3.5%

series of results shows clearly that no effect producing an alternation in substitution type is transmitted through the side-chain. Any of the "alternating" theories, such as Flürscheim's, or the alternate-polarity theory, would require, for example, that, since the phenyltrimethylammonium ion is meta-orienting, the benzyltrimethylammonium ion should be predominantly ortho- and para-orienting. The position is the same as in the already mentioned case of nitrobenzene and phenylnitromethane, in which Flürscheim himself recognised the difficulty.

The effect of the position of the positive ionic element in the Mendeléjeff table has been illustrated by comparisons among phenyl and benzyl polymethyl 'onium ions of the elements of groups V and VI. The experiments again refer to nitration. The proportions of meta-products are set out, along with the already-given data for the related ammonium ions, in Table 20-2.

All this supports the conclusion that meta-orientation results from a withdrawal of aromatic electrons by the orienting side-chain: meta-orientation is a manifestation of electronegativity, just as was felt by the makers of the earliest orientation rules. The electron displacement mechanism at work is that of the negative-inductive effect, $-I$ (Section **7a**), the intensity of which at the aromatic nucleus is diminished by relay through a chain of saturated carbon atoms, becoming barely appreciable after relay through three intervening carbon atoms:

$$C_6H_5 \rightarrow \overset{\delta\delta\delta+}{C}H_2 \rightarrow \overset{\delta\delta+}{C}H_2 \rightarrow \overset{\delta+}{C}H_2 \rightarrow \overset{+}{N}Me_3 \quad (-I \text{ mode})$$

In all cases the main constitutional cause of the electron attraction is the cationic charge on the 'onium element. But for a fixed charge of one unit, the intrinsic electronegativity of the element also has an appreciable effect. In the benzyl-'onium series, meta-orienting power increases towards the right of the Mendeléjeff table among isoelectronic atoms (Section **7b**), that is, with increasing centralisation of the total nuclear charge:

$$\overset{+}{S} > \overset{+}{P}; \quad \text{and} \quad \overset{+}{Se} > \overset{+}{As}$$

Moreover meta-orienting power decreases towards heavier elements in a given Mendeléjeff group (Section **7b**), that is, diminishes with improvement in the nuclear screening:

$$\overset{+}{N} > \overset{+}{P} > \overset{+}{As}; \quad \text{and} \quad \overset{+}{S} > \overset{+}{Se}$$

Anomalies arise in the phenyl-'onium series. The most striking of these is that the proportion of meta-nitration by the phenyltrimethyl-

TABLE 20-2.—PERCENTAGES OF META-DERIVATIVES IN MONONITRATION OF PHENYL AND BENZYL 'ONIUM IONS.

Phenyl (group V)	Phenyl (group VI)	Benzyl (group V)	Benzyl (group VI)
$C_6H_5\cdot\overset{+}{N}Me_3$ 89%	—	$C_6H_5\cdot CH_2\cdot\overset{+}{N}Me_3$ 85%	—
$C_6H_5\cdot\overset{+}{P}Me_3$ 97%	$C_6H_5\cdot\overset{+}{S}Me_2$ 90%	$C_6H_5\cdot CH_2\cdot\overset{+}{P}Me_3$ 19%	$C_6H_5\cdot CH_2\cdot\overset{+}{S}Me_2$ 52%
$C_6H_5\cdot\overset{+}{As}Me_3$ 96%	$C_6H_5\cdot\overset{+}{Se}Me_2$ high	$C_6H_5\cdot CH_2\cdot\overset{+}{As}Me_3$ 7%	$C_6H_5\cdot CH_2\cdot\overset{+}{Se}Me_2$ 16%
$C_6H_5\cdot\overset{+}{Sb}Me_3$ 86%	—	—	—

ammonium ion is lower than would be expected from the general trends. This did not emerge from the older determinations; but they have been revised since 1962 by Ridd, Rothstein, and others, using more exact methods of isomer-analysis than were available formerly; and these authors' values are quoted as far as possible in the tables above. By far the most important difference which the new figures make is to the proportion of meta-nitration in the phenyltrimethylammonium ion.

Two anomalies require to be interpreted. The first relates to the position of nitrogen relatively to the other group-V elements, in the phenyl-'onium series. Ridd's interpretation of this is that a special factor of conjugative electronegativity operates in all these elements, excepting nitrogen, which has no valency-shell d orbitals, namely, $-K$ conjugation of the aromatic π electrons with the empty d orbitals of the valency shells of the elements, the $3d$ orbitals of phosphorus, the $4d$ of arsenic, and the $5d$ of antimony. The conjugation will be strongest with phosphorus, because this d orbital has to be less contracted in order to conjugate effectively than have the larger d orbitals of arsenic and antimony. The positive charges will contract the d orbitals.

Craig was the first to emphasize and illustrate[22] that *d*-orbital contraction in a potential field can greatly facilitate $d\pi$-$p\pi$ bonding as is here assumed. Similar effects must apply to the phenyl-'onium ions of the elements sulphur and selenium, of group VI.

The other anomaly is the smallness of differentiation in meta-orientation between the phenyl- and benzyl-trimethylammonium ions; but we shall leave the discussion of this matter until we have taken up the general subject of the relation of orientation to rate of substitution.

The powerful ortho-para-orienting effect of a free negative ionic centre is familiarly illustrated in the exclusive ortho-para-substitution of phenols in alkaline solution, as in diazo-coupling, and in chlorination with alkaline hypochlorite. Comparisons of the orienting powers of different anionic elements, $\bar{O}$, $\bar{S}$, $\bar{Se}$, etc., or of the same one in different positions relatively to the aromatic ring, have not yet been undertaken.

The orientation in phenoxide ions is presumed to be due to repulsion of electrons from the anionic substituent into the aromatic ring: it is an effect of electropositivity. Doubtless it includes the positive-inductive effect,

$$C_6H_5 \leftarrow \bar{O} \quad (+I \text{ mode})$$

though the co-operating effect of the $+K$ conjugation of the unshared oxygen electrons with the aromatic π electrons is also of great importance. We shall consider such conjugative effects later.

(20b) Orienting Effects of Dipolar Bonds.—The octet theory places one dipolar bond in the nitro-group (Section **2d**); and, though the theory of mesomerism divides the dipole between two bonds (Section **7c**), the electrochemical equivalent of one dipolar bond is present. Physical evidence shows (Section **8b**) that, although within the nitro-group the electrons must be considerably displaced towards the positive atom, yet a great amount of dipolar character remains to influence an adjacent residue. There is also double-bond unsaturation in the nitro-group, again divided between two bonds. While we must not in general neglect effects of unsaturation in the treatment of orientation, the orienting effects of dipolar bonds are so strong that, in the first stage of approximation, we shall disregard unsaturation.

The octet theory places two dipolar bonds in the sulphone group; and it provides no double-bond unsaturation (Section **2d**). Physical evidence shows that, within the sulphone groups, the electrons are considerably displaced towards the sulphur atom (Section **8b**); and that

[22] D. P. Craig, *Rev. Pure Appl. Chem.*, 1954, **4**, 4; D. P. Craig and E. A. Magnusson, *J Chem. Soc.*, **1956,** 4895.

there is some increase in sulphur covalency owing to the partial development of double bonds involving sulphur *d* orbitals. Yet much dipolar character remains to affect reactivity in an adjacent group. And again, in first approximation, we may disregard the unsaturation.

Any dipolar group, such as —NO_2 or —SO_2R, is always bound to an adjacent residue by the positive end of its dipolar bond or bonds. Hence the influence of a dipolar group is expected to be qualitatively like that of a positive pole, quantitatively diminished by the smaller contrary effect of the more distant negative end of the dipole.

The nitro-group is one of the strongest meta-orienting groups among those which have no nett ionic charge. The proportion in which meta-products are formed in the nitration of nitrobenzene,[23] phenylnitromethane,[24] and 2-phenyl-1-nitroethane,[20] are shown in Table 20-3. (The figure for phenylnitromethane confirms an early qualitative finding by Holleman,[25] who showed that phenylnitromethane was predominantly meta-orienting in nitration by isolating about 50% of the meta-nitro-derivative. This was the result against which Flürscheim found it necessary to put up a special defence of his theory in 1902, as noted in Section **19b**.) Again the figures relate to mononitration, the differences from 100% representing ortho- and para-nitro-products.

TABLE 20-3.—PERCENTAGES OF META-DERIVATIVES FORMED IN THE MONONITRATION OF NITROBENZENE AND ITS NORMAL SIDE-CHAIN HOMOLOGUES.

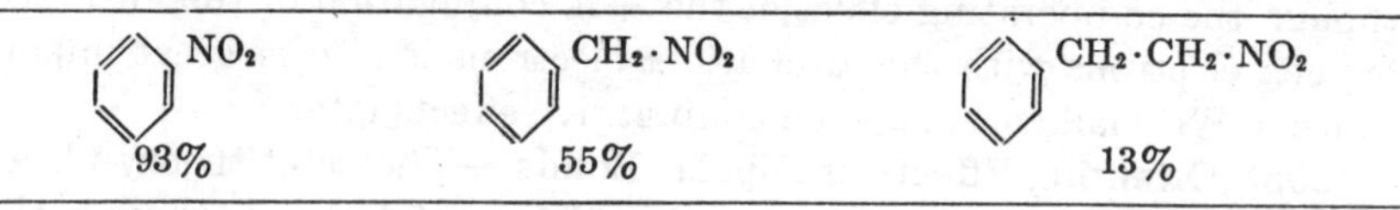

The gross effects are attributed to attraction of the aromatic electrons by the positive end of the dipolar bond, acting either directly, or through an intervening carbon chain, as with the above-mentioned trimethylammonium ions. The meta-orientation is evidently weaker in the nitro-compounds than in the trimethylammonium ions of identical carbon-chain length; and this is attributed to the influence of the negative end of the dipolar bond, including the effect which takes the form of an electron-displacement, or back-polarisation, within the nitro-group itself. However, as a whole, the nitro-group is electronegative, exerting a strong $-I$ effect in all cases. Its unsaturation co-operates producing a $-K$ conjugative effect.

The sulphone group is another strongly meta-orienting group: phenyl

[23] A. F. Holleman and B. R. de Bruyn, *Rec. trav. chim.*, 1900, **19**, 79; J. W. Baker, *J. Chem. Soc.*, **1929**, 2255; J. R. Knowles and R. O. C. Norman, *ibid.*, **1961**, 2938.

[24] J. W. Baker and I. S. Wilson, *J. Chem. Soc.*, **1927**, 842.

[25] A. F. Holleman, *Rec. trav. chim.*, 1895, **14**, 123.

TABLE 20-4.—PERCENTAGES OF META-DERIVATIVES FORMED IN THE MONONITRATION OF PHENYL AND BENZYL SULPHONYL COMPOUNDS.

$C_6H_5 \cdot SO_2 \cdot C_2H_5$	$C_6H_5 \cdot SO_2 \cdot OCH_3$	$C_6H_5 \cdot SO_2 \cdot \bar{O}$
89%	—	~60%
$C_6H_5 \cdot CH_2 \cdot SO_2 \cdot C_2H_5$	$C_6H_5 \cdot CH_2 \cdot SO_2 \cdot OCH_3$	$C_6H_5 \cdot CH_2 \cdot SO_2 \cdot \bar{O}$
22%	32%	14%

alkyl sulphones give a very high proportion of meta-nitro-compound,[26] but benzenesulphonic acid gives a considerably smaller proportion.[27] The same type of difference is seen in benzylsulphonyl compounds,[28] though the proportions of meta-isomer are now much smaller. The data are in Table 20-4.

The explanation assumes that the sulphonic acid nitrates through its anion. In the sulphone, and in the sulphonic ester, the partial compensation of the meta-orienting effect of the charged sulphur atom arises essentially from the two formally negative oxygen atoms of the sulphone group; but, in the sulphonic acid, ionic dissociation produces a third such oxygen atom, the effect of which is seen in the altered orienting power of the group.

(20c) Orienting Effects of Formally Neutral Groups without Unshared Electrons or Incomplete Electron Shells Adjacent to the Aromatic Nucleus.—Whereas it was possible, as an approximation, to discuss the powerful orienting effects of poles and dipolar bonds with only incidental reference to the unsaturation, which is present in some cases, either as unshared electron pairs or vacant valency orbitals, as in the dimethylsulphonium-ion group, or as double bonds as in the nitro-group, so much simplification cannot be attempted even in a preliminary discussion of the weaker orienting effects of neutral systems. Here we must from the outset take account at least of the conjugation of unshared electron pairs, or empty valency orbitals, with the aromatic nucleus, though it is still possible, as an approximation, to defer explicit consideration of the conjugation of multiple bonds. Accordingly, we shall first survey orienting effects by neutral systems which do not possess unshared electrons or valency orbitals conjugated with

[26] R. F. Twist and S. Smiles, *J. Chem. Soc.*, 1925, **127**, 1248: F. L. Riley and E. Rothstein, *J. Chem. Soc.*, 1964, 3860.

[27] J. Obermiller, *J. prakt. Chem.*, 1914, **69**, 70.

[28] C. K. Ingold, E. H. Ingold, and F. R. Shaw, *J. Chem. Soc.*, 1927, 813; F. L. Riley and E. Rothstein, *J. Chem. Soc.*, 1964, 3860.

the nucleus, and then study the altered situation which arises in the presence of such conjugation.

It is well established by observations on dipole moments, and by chemical arguments, that the replacement of aromatic hydrogen by an alkyl group causes a weak recession of electrons from the substituent: alkyl groups are weakly electropositive. It is similarly established that the replacement of hydrogen by typically electronegative elements, such as halogens, or by a carbonyl group, or by any non-ionised form of carboxyl group, or by a cyano-group, produces a considerable concentration of electrons towards the substituent: all these groups are strongly electronegative. It is in this form that we have classified the groups according to their expected inductive effects (Section **7c**):

$$\underset{+I}{\leftarrow\mathrm{Alk}} \qquad \underset{\text{(Standard)}}{-\mathrm{H}} \qquad \underbrace{\rightarrow\mathrm{Hal} \quad \rightarrow\mathrm{CO\cdot R} \quad \rightarrow\mathrm{CN}}_{-I}$$

It follows that alkyl groups should be essentially ortho-para-orienting, and carbonyl, carboxyl, and cyano-substituents predominantly meta-orienting; and this is indeed the case, as can be verified from the figures given in Table 20-5. (Halogen substituents directly bonded to the nucleus, which have unshared electrons conjugated with the aromatic ring, are considered later. It will also be noted later that the carbonyl, carboxyl, and cyano-substituents, and likewise the nitro-substituent, when directly bonded to the aromatic nucleus, owe part of their meta-directive power to the conjugation of their multiple bonds with the nucleus.)

A further consequence of the above electropolar classification is that the replacement of hydrogen in any position in a substituent by an alkyl group will make the substituent less meta-orienting; and that the replacement of the hydrogen by a halogen atom, or by a carbonyl, carboxyl, or cyano-group, will render the substituent more meta-orienting. Such effects should be the more important if the replacement is made close to the aromatic nucleus, since inductive effects suffer large losses by relay. For replacement in a given position, the magnitude of the effect should depend on the electronegativity of the replacing group. All these points are illustrated with reference to nitration in Table 20-5, the figures in which are again percentages of the meta-nitro-isomer in the mononitration product. Each row in the table represents a polar series, except the last row, which refers to two independent pairs of homologues.

The aromatic deuterium atom has no detectable orienting effect.[29]

[29] W. M. Lauer and W. E. Noland, *J. Am. Chem. Soc.*, 1953, **75**, 3689; T. G. Bonner, F. Bowyer, and Gwyn Williams, *J. Chem. Soc.*, 1953, 2650; P. B. D. de la Mare, T. M. Dunn, and J. T. Harvey, *ibid.*, **1957**, 923.

TABLE 20-5.—PERCENTAGES OF META-DERIVATIVES FORMED IN THE MONONITRATION OF LATERALLY SUBSTITUTED TOLUENES.

The numbers in parenthesis are references to the notes below.

$C_6H_5\cdot CO\cdot O—H$ 82% (1, 12)	$C_6H_5\cdot CO\cdot O \leftarrow CH_3$ 73% (1)	$C_6H_5\cdot CO\cdot O \leftarrow CH_2 \leftarrow CH_3$ 68% (1)	
$C_6H_5\cdot CH_2 \rightarrow F$ 18% (7)	$C_6H_5\cdot CH_2 \rightarrow Cl$ 14% (5, 6, 9)	$C_6H_5\cdot CH_2 \rightarrow Br$ 7% (5)	
$C_6H_5\cdot C(\leftarrow CH_3)_2 \rightarrow NO_2$ 29% (8)	$C_6H_5\cdot CH_2 \rightarrow NO_2$ 55% (9)	$C_6H_5\cdot C(\rightarrow Br)_2 \rightarrow NO_2$ 84% (8)	
$C_6H_5\cdot CH_2—H$ 3% (2, 3, 4)	$C_6H_5\cdot CH_2 \rightarrow Cl$ 14% (5, 6)	$C_6H_5\cdot HC(\rightarrow Cl)_2$ 34% (5)	$C_6H_5\cdot C(\rightarrow Cl)_3$ 64% (2, 5)
$C_6H_5\cdot CH_2—H$ 3% (2, 3, 4)	$C_6H_5\cdot CH_2 \rightarrow CO_2Et$ 13% (9)	$C_6H_5\cdot CH(\rightarrow CO_2Et)_2$ 23% (5, 10)	$C_6H_5\cdot C(\rightarrow CO_2Et)_3$ 57% (5)
$C_6H_5\cdot CO\cdot CH_3$ 68% (11)	$C_6H_5\cdot CO\cdot NH_2$ 70% (12)	$C_6H_5\cdot CO\cdot OH$ 82% (1, 12)	$C_6H_5\cdot CO\cdot Cl$ 90% (12)
$C_6H_5\cdot CN$ 81% (13)	$C_6H_5\cdot CH_2\cdot CN$ 20% (9)	$C_6H_5\cdot CH(CO_2Et)_2$ 23% (5, 10)	$C_6H_5\cdot CH_2\cdot CH(CO_2Me)_2$ 8% (14)

[1] A. F. Holleman, *Rec. trav. chim.*, 1899, **18**, 267.

[2] A. F. Holleman, J. Vermeulen, and W. J. de Mooy, *ibid.*, 1914, **33**, 1.

[3] C. K. Ingold, A. Lapworth, E. Rothstein, and D. Ward, *J. Chem. Soc.*. **1931,** 1959.

[4] H. Cohn, E. D. Hughes, and M. H. Jones, personal communication.

[5] B. Flürscheim and E. L. Holmes, *J. Chem. Soc.*, **1928,** 1067.

[6] C. K. Ingold and F. R. Shaw, *ibid.*, **1949,** 575.

[7] C. K. Ingold and E. H. Ingold, *ibid.*, **1928,** 2249.

[8] J. W. Baker and C. K. Ingold, *ibid.*, **1926,** 2462.

[9] J. R. Knowles and R. O. C. Norman, *ibid.*, **1961,** 2938.

[10] J. W. Baker and C. K. Ingold, *ibid.*, **1927,** 832.

[11] J. W. Baker and W. G. Moffitt, *ibid.*, **1931,** 314.

[12] K. E. Cooper and C. K. Ingold, *ibid.*, **1927,** 836.

[13] J. W. Baker, K. E. Cooper, and C. K. Ingold, *ibid.*, **1928,** 426; J. P. Wibaut and R. van Strick, *Rec. trav. chim.*, 1958, **77,** 316; G. S. Hammond and K. J. Douglas, *J. Am. Chem. Soc.*, 1959, **81,** 1184.

[14] J. W. Baker and A. Eccles, *ibid.*, **1927,** 2125.

Deuterium is slightly electropositive, but slightly less polarisable than protium: perhaps these two effects compensate: or they may each be too small to influence orientation appreciably. The trimethylsilyl group Me_3Si has very little orienting action. Phenyltrimethylsilane on nitration gives nitrobenzene and a mixture of the nitro-trimethylsilyl-isomers which contains 40% of the meta-isomer,[30] the statistical proportion.

(20d) Orienting Effects of Formally Neutral Groups Having Unshared Electrons Adjacent to the Nucleus.—A major effect of unsaturation is encountered when formally neutral substituents have unshared electrons capable of conjugation with the aromatic nucleus: such substituents are ortho-para-orienting, independently of the direction of the inductive effect. This influence of suitably placed unshared electrons is usually not enough to reverse the meta-orientation of substituents having a formal positive charge, such as the sulphonium-ion or the iodinium-ion substituents; but it does outweigh any meta-orientation which in neutral groups might otherwise have been expected, as in electron-attracting halogen and alkoxyl substituents. The effect is attributed to the development of negative charges on the ortho- and para-positions in consequence of conjugative electron displacements of the $+K$ type originating in the unshared electrons of the substituent (Section **7a**):

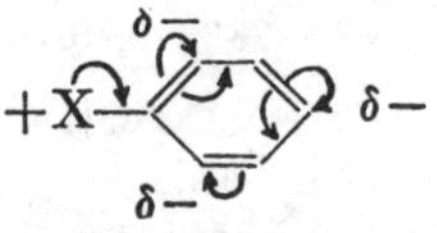

$\delta+$X (benzene ring) $\delta-$ (ortho), $\delta-$ (para), $\delta-$ (ortho) (+ *K*-mode)

This description[31] avoids a statement as to whether the conjugative displacement, which is effective in producing the result, is predominantly a permanent molecular condition ($+M$ effect), or is essentially an activation phenomenon ($+E$ effect). The point will be discussed in detail later; but the fact that even the halogenobenzenes are ortho- and para-orienting, although they are known to have large permanent displacements of electrons away from the ring and towards the halogen, shows already that the displacements, which are so effective in leading to the observed orientation, must actually be temporary.

Orientation of this type is exerted by the neutral forms of the elements of the Mendeléjeff groups V, VI, and VII. Along an isoelectronic series, the strength of the orientation follows the order of reactivity of the unshared electrons, and therefore decreases with increas-

[30] J. L. Speier, *J. Am. Chem. Soc.*, 1953, **75**, 2930.

[31] Concerning the use of Kekulé formulae in such representations, see Section **13b**.

TABLE 20-6.—COMPETITIVE ORIENTATION BY N, O, F IN THE NITRATION OF DISUBSTITUTED BENZENES.

Compound		Group	Yield
NHAc, OMe	Ortho- and para- to	NHAc:	76% isolated
		OMe:	13% isolated
NMeAc, OMe	Ortho- and para- to	NMeAc:	69% isolated
		OMe:	4% isolated
NHAc, OAc	Ortho- and para- to	NHAc:	71% isolated
		OAc:	0% isolated
OMe, F	Ortho- and para- to	OMe:	97% by analysis
		F:	3% by analysis

Example:— NHAc/OMe benzene with positions 2%, 13%, 74%, 0% — isolated mono-nitro-products (total 89%).

ing group number (Section **2e**). This was established[32] by placing the groups in competition with one another in pairs, with the results, for nitration, shown in Table 20-6.

In order to appreciate the comparisons between nitrogen and oxygen, it is necessary to realise that acylation of the nitrogen atom, the purpose of which was to prevent salt formation with the nitrating acid, diminishes the ortho-para-orienting power of the acylated group. This is empirically manifested in many known results. Thus acetylguaiacol nitrates exclusively para- to the methoxy-group:[33]

$$C_6H_4(OMe)(OAc) \rightarrow NO_2C_6H_3(OMe)(OAc)$$

Again, while a single acylation of nitrogen, as in aceto-*p*-toluidide, will not suffice to reduce the orienting power of the acylamino-group below that of the methyl group, double acylation, as in phthaloyl-*p*-toluidine will do so, with the result that the nitration of these compounds proceeds as indicated:[34]

[32] C. K. Ingold and E. H. Ingold, *J. Chem. Soc.*, **1926**, 1310; E. L. Holmes and C. K. Ingold, *ibid.*, p. 1328.

[33] F. Reverdin and P. Crépieux, *Ber.*, 1903, **36**, 2257; C. K. Ingold and E. H. Ingold, *J. Chem. Soc.*, **1926**, 1310.

[34] O. L. Brady, W. G. E. Quick, and W. F. Welling, *J. Chem. Soc.*, 1925, **127**, 2264.

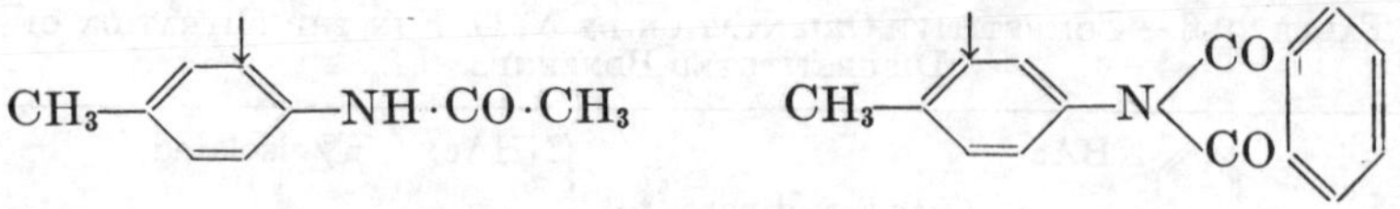

$CH_3-C_6H_4-NH\cdot CO\cdot CH_3$ $CH_3-C_6H_4-N(CO)_2C_6H_4$

The effect is also theoretically expected. For the acylation of an oxygen or nitrogen atom produces a form of carboxyl group, X—C=Y, the internal mesomerism of which must interfere with orientation due to conjugation of X with the aryl system (Section **7e**).

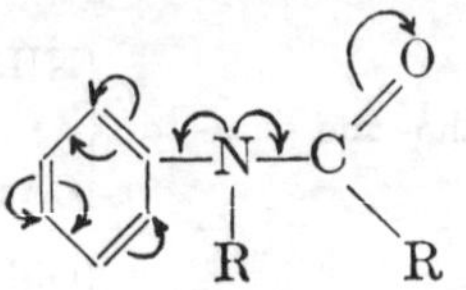

In spite of the handicap caused by acylation, the nitrogen atom evidently controls the orientation when in competition with oxygen, as the oxygen atom does when in competition with fluorine. Thus we find the order N > O > F expected for the $+M$ or $+E$ effect (Sections **7e** and **7f**).

The double-bond electrons of styrene conjugate with the aromatic nucleus, much as do unshared electrons. The resulting ortho-para-orientation is not destroyed by a terminal electron-attracting group, as in cinnamic acid,[35] styrene-ω-sulphonyl chloride,[35] or ω-nitrostyrene:[36] even this last-named gives only 2% of meta-derivative on nitration:

$Ph\cdot CH:CH\cdot CO_2H$	$Ph\cdot CH:CH\cdot SO_2Cl$	$Ph\cdot CH:CH\cdot NO_2$
0% meta-NO_2	<2% meta-NO_2	~2% meta-NO_2

The situation thus resembles that obtained in the halogenobenzenes, the ortho-para-orientation of which is not destroyed by the electronegativity of the halogen. As before, it follows that the electron displacements which lead to ortho-para-substitution in styrene derivatives, must be polarisability effects, and this again is confirmed by evidence to be mentioned later.

A more finely poised situation of the same nature, except that hyperconjugation takes the place of conjugation, occurs in benzyl compounds which are predominantly ortho-para-orienting in spite of the presence of a strongly electronegative side-chain substituent, for example, benzyl chloride or benzyl cyanide (cf. Table 20-5).[37] However, an analysis of the case requires reference to rate measurements, and therefore is given later.

[35] F. C. Bordwell and K. Rohde, *J. Am. Chem. Soc.*, 1948, **70**, 1191.

[36] J. W. Baker and I. S. Wilson, *J. Chem. Soc*., **1927**, 842.

[37] J. R. Knowles and R. O. C. Norman, *J. Chem. Soc.*, **1961**, 2938; F. L. Riley and E. Rothstein, *J. Chem. Soc.*, **1964**, 3860, 3872.

(20e) Orienting Effects of Groups Having Vacant Valency-Shell Orbitals Adjacent to the Aromatic Nucleus.—Harvey and Norman have added a whole class to the very few into which we formerly divided orienting substituents by providing the example of phenylboronic acid. Nitrated in a mixture of nitric and sulphuric acids, this gives 73% of the meta-nitro-derivative. The boronic acid side-chain is expected to be inductively slightly electropositive, and the cause of its strong meta-orientation is obviously the withdrawal of aromatic electrons from the ring by conjugation with the vacant $2p$ orbital of the boron atom.[38]

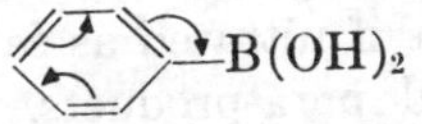

$$C_6H_5\text{—}B(OH)_2 \qquad (-K \text{ mode})$$

It has been noted (Section **20a**) that conjugation of aromatic π electrons with the vacant $3d$ orbitals in phenyltrimethylphosphonium and phenyldimethylsulphonium ions probably accounts for part of the strong meta-orientation shown by these ions; and also that similar but presumably weaker effects of the same nature, that is, effects of $-K$ conjugation, may contribute to the meta-orientation characteristic of the analogous cations of the higher elements of Mendeléjeff's groups V and VI.

(20f) Orienting Effects in Ionogenic Systems.—Apparent exceptions to the rule that neutral nitrogen and oxygen stand in the order $N > O$ with respect to their capacity for ortho-para-orientation are traceable to the development of ionic charges on one or other of these atoms under the conditions of substitution. The theoretical order of ortho-para-orienting power of nitrogen and oxygen in their neutral and charged forms is $\overset{-}{O} > NR_2 > OR > \overset{+}{N}R_3$; and this, as will appear later, is also the theoretical order for the rates of the substitutions. Hence phenols tend to substitute through their anions, and aniline derivatives through their neutral forms, even when very little of these more reactive forms is present. Thus "H-acid" is well known to diazo-couple ortho- to hydroxyl in alkaline solution, and ortho- to the amino-group in acid media, thereby giving two series of azo-dyes. The former mode of reaction illustrates the inequality $\overset{-}{O} > NR_2$, and the latter the inequality $NR_2 > OR$:

[38] D. R. Harvey and R. O. C. Norman, *J. Chem. Soc.*, **1962**, 3822. If bases are not kept away, they can fill up the electron-accepting boron orbital. The authors show that, on nitration in acetic anhydride, phenylboronic acid exhibits predominating ortho-para-orientation; they assume that in these conditions the reaction takes place in part through the adduct

$$Ph\overset{-}{B}(OH)_2\text{—}\overset{+}{O}Ac_2$$

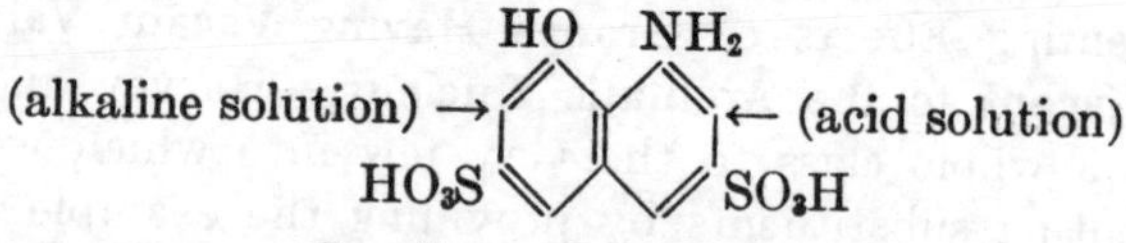

(alkaline solution) → [H-acid structure: HO, NH_2; HO_3S, SO_3H] ← (acid solution)

Coupling positions in H-acid

In pseudo-acidic systems, the negative charge produced by proton-loss becomes distributed, the anion being mesomeric; and, if part of the anionic charge reaches an atom adjoining the aromatic ring, increased ortho-para-orientation will result. Baker has illustrated this with respect to the nitration of phenylnitromethane and its derivatives:[39] these pseudo-acids, if nitrated as salts, give greatly increased proportions of ortho- and para-products. Evidently the anion of phenylnitromethane is an ortho-para-orienting ion; and when, say, the lithium salt of phenylnitromethane is added to nitric acid, nitration of the anion occurs sufficiently rapidly to be largely effective before proton-uptake has regenerated the predominantly meta-orienting, but more slowly substituting, pseudo-form of the neutral molecule:

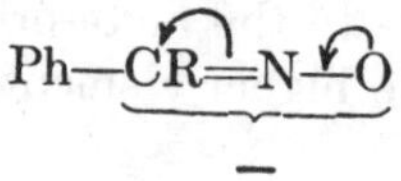

$$\text{Ph—}\underbrace{\text{CR=N—O}}_{-} \quad \text{(anion of a pseudo-acid)}$$

In a pseudo-basic system the positive charge formed by proton-uptake or anion-loss becomes distributed, the cation being mesomeric; and, if part of the cationic charge reaches the atom adjacent to the aromatic ring, increased meta-orientation will result. It has thus been explained[40] why benzaldehyde, acetophenone, and benzylidene-imines, on nitration in concentrated sulphuric acid, give notably high proportions of meta-products (about 90%):

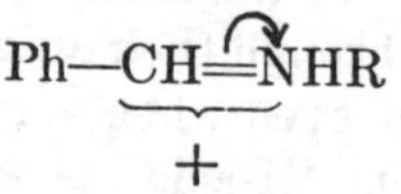

$$\text{Ph—}\underbrace{\text{CH=NHR}}_{+} \quad \text{(cation of a pseudo-base)}$$

Examples of another kind have been furnished by LeFèvre, who has shown[41] that 2-phenylbenzopyrylium and 2-phenyl-1-methylquinolinium nitrates are nitrated practically exclusively in the meta-position of the phenyl ring:

[39] J. W. Baker, *J. Chem. Soc.*, **1929,** 2257.

[40] J. W. Baker and C. K. Ingold, *J. Chem. Soc.*, **1930,** 431; J. W. Baker and W. G. Moffitt, *ibid.*, **1931,** 314.

[41] R. J. W. LeFèvre, *J. Chem. Soc.*, **1929,** 2771; R. J. W. LeFèvre and F. C. Mathur, *ibid.*, **1930,** 2236; R. J. W. LeFèvre and C. G. LeFèvre, *ibid.*, **1932,** 1988.

Me

O+ N+

(21) REACTIVITY IN ELECTROPHILIC AROMATIC SUBSTITUTION[42]

(21a) Object and Method of the Observations.—The reagents which effect the oriented aromatic substitutions under consideration are electrophilic (Section **18c**); and we must assume either that they are themselves, or that they produce, entities which preferentially attack those nuclear positions in which electrons are most available.

Three general deductions can therefore be drawn from the studies of orientation described in Section **20.** From the demonstrated influence of the electropolarity of substituents ($\pm I$ effects), it follows (i) that ortho-para-orientation is associated with the transfer of electrons from the substituent into the aromatic ring; and (ii) that meta-orientation involves the withdrawal of electrons from the ring. And from the illustrated orienting influence of unsaturation ($+K$ effects), it is deduced (iii) that activating negative charges are transferred selectively to the ortho- and para-positions in ortho-para-oriented substitutions. It seems natural to try to complete these statements by an assumption, which is (iv) that positive charges selectively deactivate the ortho- and para-positions when electrons are withdrawn from the ring in meta-oriented substitutions. This would imply that meta-oriented substitutions take place where they do, not because the meta-positions are rendered any more reactive by the orienting substituent, but because the ortho- and para-positions have been rendered less reactive. It would be consistent with Holleman's rule that a low reactivity is characteristic of meta-orientation. The three deductions and the completing assumption might be represented in symbolic fashion, as follows:

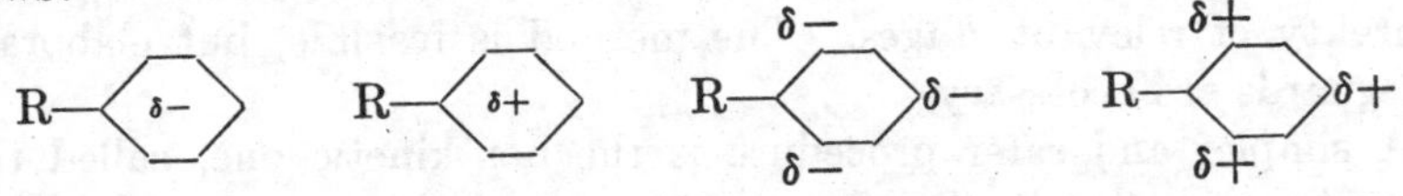

R—⟨ $\delta-$ ⟩	R—⟨ $\delta+$ ⟩	R—⟨ ⟩ with $\delta-$ at ortho, para, ortho	R—⟨ ⟩ with $\delta+$ at ortho, para, ortho
(i) ortho-para-	(ii) meta-	(iii) ortho-para-	(iv) meta-
(Deduced)			(Assumed)

It was realised at a comparatively early stage that, in order to obtain further insight into the electrical conditions in oriented substitutions,

[42] C. K. Ingold and F. R. Shaw, *J. Chem. Soc.*, **1927**, 2918; C. K. Ingold, *Rec. trav. chim.*, 1929, **48**, 797; *J. Chem. Soc.*, **1933**, 1120.

it would be necessary to consider this question of reactivity in more detail. It is not enough to know the proportions in which isomerides are formed: one must know how the orienting substituent influences those individual rates, of which the proportions of isomerides are ratios; and, in particular, one must know to what extent the rate of attack on each nuclear position is greater or less in the presence of the orienting substituent than it would have been in its absence, that is, in unsubstituted benzene. For example, toluene on nitration gives ortho-, para-, and meta-isomerides in the proportions 57%, 40%, and 3%, respectively. But this does not tell us whether the methyl group thus orients by activating the ortho- and para-positions and deactivating the meta-positions (alternation), or by activating the ortho- and para-positions and leaving the meta-positions unaffected, or by activating the ortho- and para-positions strongly and the meta-positions less strongly, or by acting in one of two other possible ways. In order to decide this question, one needs to know, in addition to the orientation data, the rate of nitration of toluene relatively to that of benzene.

This could conceivably be determined in either of two ways. The most obvious way is by the *kinetic method*: the kinetics of nitration of benzene and toluene could be separately studied, and rate constants compared. But this is an unsafe method unless the reaction mechanism is fully understood; for, in most aromatic substitutions, as in other reactions, the supplied reagents are converted into the analysed products in a series of reaction stages, only one of which, the attack of some active species on the aromatic ring, bears on the question of the intrinsic reactivity of the latter. For example, in nitration by nitric acid there are four steps, of which only the third is relevant to the present inquiry. One therefore has to make sure that neither of the compared reaction rates is being controlled by any of the irrelevant reaction stages, and that a ratio of experimental rate constants is identical with the ratio of the rates of the relevant stages. One also has to be sure that there are not several active species, leading to a plurality of relevant stages. The method is feasible, but elaborate safeguards are necessary.

A simpler and safer procedure is the non-kinetic one, called the *competition method*.[43] It is independent of control, even of highly unequal degrees of control, of reaction rate by irrelevant reaction stages. One allows the compounds under comparison, say, benzene and toluene, in known proportions, to compete, in the same homogeneous solution, for a small amount, in simplest principle, an indefinitely small amount, of the common reagent, say, nitric acid; and then,

[43] C. K. Ingold and F. R. Shaw, *J. Chem. Soc.*, **1927**, 2918.

without following what happens as a function of the time, one determines the proportions of the products, in our example, nitrobenzene and total nitrotoluenes, after the conclusion of the reaction. A readily evaluated correction can be applied for the circumstance that, in practice, the amount of supplied reagent, although small, is not indefinitely small, and that therefore the proportions of the competing substances undergo some change as one gets consumed faster than the other. The main assumption in this method is that the relevant reaction stage is of the same reaction order with respect to each of the two substances compared; and as it is scarcely conceivable that that number could ever be other than unity, the assumption of equality seems a very safe one. It is also assumed that there is not a multiplicity of parallel relevant stages dependent on different active entities; but this is a safe assumption for nitration under most conditions, since the reaction is entirely dominated by the ready formation and high electrophilic activity of the nitronium ion. The important condition, that the mixing of the reagents to homogenicity is complete before an appreciable amount of reaction has taken place, must, of course, be satisfied. (Attempts to use the method have been made with insufficient attention to this condition.)

(21b) Results and Their Interpretation apart from the Conjugative Effect.—Some relative rates of nitration, as measured by the competition method, are assembled in Table 21-1. They are totals for all nuclear positions, and are expressed on a scale such that the total rate of nitration of benzene is unity. The conditions of nitration are not quite the same in all cases, but experiment has shown that these relative rates are not very sensitive to the conditions.

If by multiplication we combined these rates with the proportions in which the isomerides are formed, we can arrive at comparable figures for the relative rates of attack on each individual nuclear position, that is, each ortho-, and each meta-, and the para-positions, of each of the compounds for which the necessary values are available. It is convenient to change the unit of rate, so that the total rate of nitration of benzene becomes six, instead of one, and the unit is the rate of attack on one individual position in benzene. Then, any figure applying to an individual nuclear position in a substituted benzene, if above unity, represents the activation of that position by the substituent, and, if below unity, measures the deactivation of the position. The figures thus reckoned are called *partial rate factors*. For a number of compounds, the results of this synthesis of relative rates and orientation ratios are given later in this Section and in the next Section.

For the purpose of discussing such data, substituents have been classified into four types, according to the polar effects through which

TABLE 21-1.—RELATIVE RATES OF MONONITRATION OF BENZENE DERIVATIVES.

Compound	Rate	Ref.	Compound	Rate	Ref.
Ph—H	1.00	—	Ph—$CH_2 \cdot CO_2Et$	3.75	5, 7
Ph—CH_3	24.5	1, 6, 7	Ph—$CH_2 \cdot Cl$	0.71	7
Ph—$C(CH_3)_3$	15.5	6, 7	Ph—$CH_2 \cdot CN$	0.345	7
Ph—CO_2Et	0.0037	2	Ph—$CH_2 \cdot NO_2$	0.122	7
Ph—$SO_2 \cdot C_6H_5$	0.0035	8	Ph—$CH_2 \cdot SO_2 \cdot C_2H_5$	0.24	8
Ph—F	0.15	3	Ph—$CH_2 \cdot NMe_3^+$	0.000026	10
Ph—Cl	0.033	3	Ph—$CH_2 \cdot PMe_3^+$	0.0066	8
Ph—Br	0.030	3	Ph—$CH_2 \cdot AsMe_3^+$	0.0127	8
Ph—I	0.18	3	Ph—NMe_3^+	1.2×10^{-8}	10
Ph—$CH{:}CH \cdot CO_2H$	0.11	4	Ph—PMe_3^+	5.8×10^{-8}	10
Ph—NO_2	6×10^{-8}	9	Ph—$AsMe_3^+$	4.6×10^{-7}	10
Ph—$CH_2 \cdot OMe$	6.5	7	Ph—$SbMe_3^+$	0.000018	10

[1] C. K. Ingold, A. Lapworth, E. Rothstein, and D. Ward, *J. Chem. Soc.*, **1931**, 1959.

[2] C. K. Ingold and M. S. Smith, *ibid.*, **1938**, 905.

[3] M. L. Bird and C. K. Ingold, *ibid.*, p. 918.

[4] F. G. Bordwell and K. Rohde, *J. Am. Chem. Soc.*, 1948, **70**, 1191.

[5] C. K. Ingold and F. R. Shaw, *J. Chem. Soc.*, **1949**, 575.

[6] H. Cohn, E. D. Hughes, M. H. Jones, and M. G. Peeling, *Nature*, 1952, **169**, 291.

[7] J. R. Knowles and R. O. C. Norman, *J. Chem. Soc.*, **1961**, 2938.

[8] F. L. Riley and E. Rothstein, *J. Chem. Soc.*, **1964**, 3860, 3872.

[9] J. G. Tillett, *J. Chem. Soc.*, **1962**, 5142.

[10] J. H. Ridd and J. H. P. Utley, *Proc. Chem. Soc.*, **1964**, 24; *idem* and M. Brickman, *J. Chem. Soc.*, **1965**, 6851; personal communication from Dr. J. H. Ridd.

NOTE: Some figures very different from those here given, all very much nearer to unity, have been published for hydrocarbons and halogenobenzenes by G. A. Olah and coworkers since 1961. These figures are for nitration with nitronium salts, usually in solvent tetramethylene sulphone (sulpholane). They are unacceptable, because they were obtained by a travesty of the competition method, inasmuch as the elementary condition of the method, that the rate of reaction is much smaller than the rate of mixing, was not shown (and cannot be shown) to be satisfied. Cf. also W. S. Tolgesi, *Canad. J. Chem.*, 1965, **43**, 343; S. Y. Caille and J. P. Corriu, *Chem. Comm.*, **1967**, 1251. The position thus set up has been discussed in detail by J. H. Ridd ("Studies in Chemical Structure and Mechanism," Methuen, London, 1966, Chap. 7; *cf.* P. J. Christy, J. H. Ridd, and N. Sears, forthcoming).

they are expected to influence orientation, as shown in Table 21-2. The classification is a simplified one, two obviously possible types, $+I-K$ and $-I-K$, having been omitted: what has been done is to include substituents of the omitted classes in the types $+I$ and $-I$, respectively, as though the $-K$ effect were of secondary importance This will be justified later as an approximation.

In the remainder of this Section, we shall consider interpretation

TABLE 21-2.—CLASSIFICATION OF ORIENTING SUBSTITUENTS.

Type	Electronic mechanism	Examples	Effect on: Orientation	Effect on: Reactivity
(1) $+I$	Ph←R	Ph—CH_3	ortho-para-	Activation
(2) $-I$	Ph→R	Ph—CO_2Et	meta-	Deactivation
(3) $-I+K$	Ph→R (curved arrow)	Ph—SMe_2^+	As in (2)	
		Ph—Cl	ortho-para-	Deactivation
		Ph—OMe	As in (4)	
(4) $+I+K$	Ph←R (curved arrow)	Ph—O^-	ortho-para-	Activation

within Types 1 and 2. First, we set down the partial rate factors for nitration in the examples of toluene and ethyl benzoate:

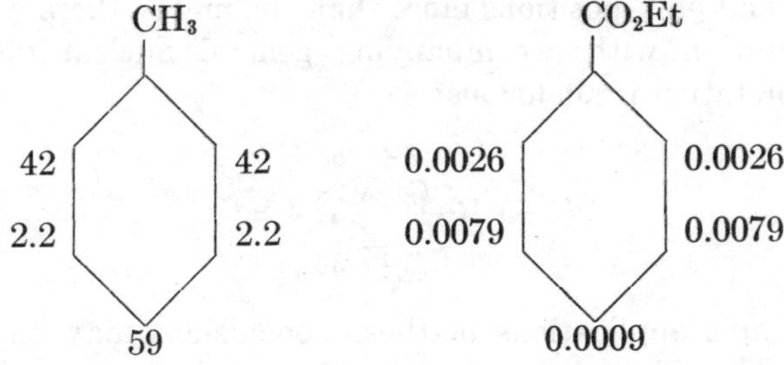

We do not essay more than two-figure accuracy, because the figures vary a little with the conditions, particularly the temperature. The figures we shall quote relate to temperatures not far from the ordinary temperature. Low isomer proportions tend to rise and high ones to fall as the temperature is raised, mainly because differences of activation energy become reduced in importance at higher absolute temperatures: the Arrhenius exponent depends on E_A/T. Experimentally, the matter has been carefully examined in several cases, *e.g.*, the nitration of toluene,[44] where the proportion of meta-isomer is raised from below 3% to more than 4% when the temperature is raised from $-30°$ to $+60°$.

Referring first to toluene as an example of Type 1, it will be apparent that the question, which was left open by the orientation ratios, is

[44] A. F. Hoheman and J. E. van der Arend, *Rec. trav. chim.*, 1909, **28**, 408; A. F. Hollemann, J. Vermeulen, and W. J. de Mooy, *ibid.*, 1914, **33**, 1; W. W. Jones and M. Russell, *J. Chem. Soc.*, **1947,** 921; R. M. Roberts, P. Heilberger, J. D. Watkins, H. P. Browder, and K. A. Kobe, *J. Am. Chem. Soc.*, 1958, **80,** 4285.

answered by the rate data: the methyl group activates *all* positions in the nucleus, the ortho- and para-positions somewhat strongly, and the meta-positions more weakly. This is believed to be a general effect of substituents of Type 1. The interpretation which is given is that the $+I$ effect first places a negative charge on the α-position, from which it is relayed conjugatively with great efficiency to ortho- and para-positions, and thence with inductive attenuation to meta-positions, so that ortho-para-orientation with general activation results. The polarisations are represented below:

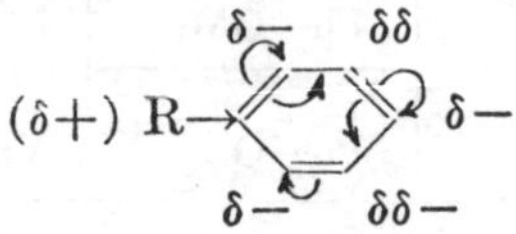

$$(\delta+)\ R\rightarrow C_6H_5 \quad \text{ortho: } \delta-,\ \text{meta: } \delta\delta,\ \text{para: } \delta-,\ \text{meta: } \delta\delta- \qquad (+I \text{ effect})$$

As is illustrated by the figures for ethyl benzoate, the effect of substituents of Type 2 is just the opposite: they deactivate all positions, the ortho- and para-positions more than the meta-, thereby producing meta-orientation with accompanying general nucleaı deactivation. The interpretation is analogous:

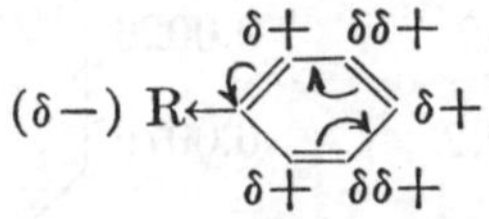

$$(\delta-)\ R\leftarrow C_6H_5 \quad \text{ortho: } \delta+,\ \text{meta: } \delta\delta+,\ \text{para: } \delta+,\ \text{ortho: } \delta+,\ \text{meta: } \delta\delta+ \qquad (-I \text{ effect})$$

Some simple applications of these conclusions may be mentioned here. (1) The chief reason why nitration has been so much employed in the quantitative study of aromatic substitution is that the nitro-group is a strongly deactivating substituent of Type 2, and that therefore it is particularly easy, in nitration, sharply to separate the stages of successive substitution, as is necessary in quantitative work on orientation ratios. Such sharp separation is more difficult to secure in most other substitutions. (2) In homocyclic polynuclear systems, such as biphenyl, naphthalene, or anthraquinone, activating substituents of Type 1 lead to further substitution in the ring already substituted, while deactivating substituents of Type 2 divert substitution into the other aromatic ring. Thus, 1-methylnaphthalene nitrates in the 4-position, while 1-nitronaphthalene further nitrates in the 5- and 8-positions. (3) The nitrogen atom of pyridine, if the latter is present as free base, as in halogenation under certain conditions, should act like a substituent of Type 2. Thus pyridine is halogenated preferentially in the 3-position (β-position). In the acid conditions usual in nitration and sulphonation, the cationic charge on the pyridinium ion must very strongly deactivate the whole nucleus, though such deactivation should be least strong in the 3-positions. In fact, pyridine has been nitrated and sulphonated but with great difficulty, and in the 3-position. (4) In the quinolinium ion, the deactivating effect of the cationic charge diverts substitution into the benzo-ring. Thus quinoline nitrates and sulphonates, without difficulty, in the 5- and 8-positions. In 2-phenylbenzopyrylium and 2-phenyl-1-methylquinolinium salts, the benzo-ring, to which the positive pole is adjacent, is more strongly deactivated than the phenyl ring. Hence substitution takes place in the meta-position of the latter, as was noted in Section **20f**.

The carbethoxyl and ethylsulphonyl groups, whose rates of nitration, relatively to that of benzene, are given in Table 21-1, are typical of deactivating and meta-orienting groups of Type 2. Approximate relative rate figures for a range of Type 2 groups have been estimated, largely indirectly, for chlorination and bromination by molecular halogens in organic solvents.[45] The order of reactivity among the Type 2 groups is

$$(H) > COPh > CO_2Et > CO_2H > CN > NO_2$$

and the range of rates in this series is something like a million. Logarithms of the partial rate factors for meta-substitution are given in Table 21-3. The spread of values probably increases in the order nitration, chlorination (by Cl_2), bromination (by Br_2).

TABLE 21-3.—LOGARITHMS OF PARTIAL RATE FACTORS FOR META-SUBSTITUTION IN MONO-SUBSTITUTED BENZENES WITH ORIENTING SUBSTITUENTS OF TYPE 2.

Reagent	Orienting substituents				
	COPh	CO_2Et	CO_2H	CN	NO_2
HNO_3 in Ac_2O		−2.10			
Cl_2 in HOAc	−2.64	−2.82	−3.11		−5.3
Br_2 in $MeNO_2$				−6.05	−7.0

(21c) The Conjugative Effect, the Holleman Anomaly, and the Distinctive Effects of Polarisation and Polarisability.—The special importance of substituents of Type 3, that is, of substituents of the

[45] K. J. L. Orton and A. E. Bradfield, *J. Chem. Soc.*, **1927,** 896; A. E. Bradfield and Brynmor Jones, *Trans. Faraday Soc.*, 1941, **37,** 726; P. W. Robertson, P. B. D. de la Mare and B. E. Swedlund, *J. Chem. Soc.*, **1953,** 782; "Aromatic Substitution," P. B. D. de la Mare and J. H. Ridd, Butterworths Scientific Pubs., London, 1959, pp. 140 and 146. Cf. P. B. D. de la Mare and C. A. Vernon, *J. Chem. Soc.*, **1943,** 246; and L. M. Stock and H. B. Brown, *J. Am. Chem. Soc.*, 1960, **82,** 1942.

$-I+K$ class, is that, because the inductive and conjugative effects are opposed, a study of situations in which they are more or less balanced brings out the differences in their modes of operation.

From these differences there arises what has been called the "Holleman anomaly." As noted in Section **19b**, Holleman enunciated in 1910 the widely true principle that ortho-para-orientation is associated with activation and meta-orientation with deactivation. The discovery[43] in 1927 that the halogenobenzenes combine ortho-para-orientation with deactivation provided a striking group of exceptions. It was realised then that, in the field of electrophilic substitution, such exceptions would have to belong to Type 3, and the opposite kind of anomaly, an association of meta-orientation with activation, would never be found. The observed anomaly pointed, as was noted at the time, to a dichotomy of polarisation and polarisability effects, and thus to that pattern of theory which is set out for organic chemistry generally in Section **7a**.

The kind of reactivity distribution created by a substituent of Type 3, when its inductive and conjugative effects are not too far off balance, may be illustrated by the partial rate factors set out below for the nitration of chloro- and bromo-benzene: all nuclear positions are deactivated, the meta-positions most:

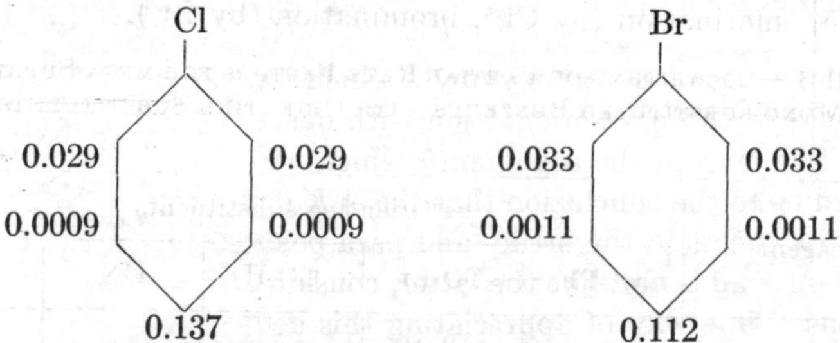

Suppose that substituents of Type 3 are arranged as a series, which starts with a group, such as $-SMe_2^+$, which has a strongly dominating $-I$ displacement, and a very weak $+K$ displacement. The series would continue through a number of intermediate cases, such as the halogens, and ω-carboxyvinyl, in which both forms of displacement are important. It could end with a substituent, such as $-OMe$, which has a weak $-I$ displacement together with a very strong $+K$ displacement. Then, at the beginning of such a series, we find meta-orientation associated with deactivation; and at the end we observe ortho-para-orientation associated with activation. But in between, the switch from dominating meta- to ortho-para-orientation occurs at an earlier point than does the switch from deactivation to activation; and, bracketed between these two points, is a band of groups, among them

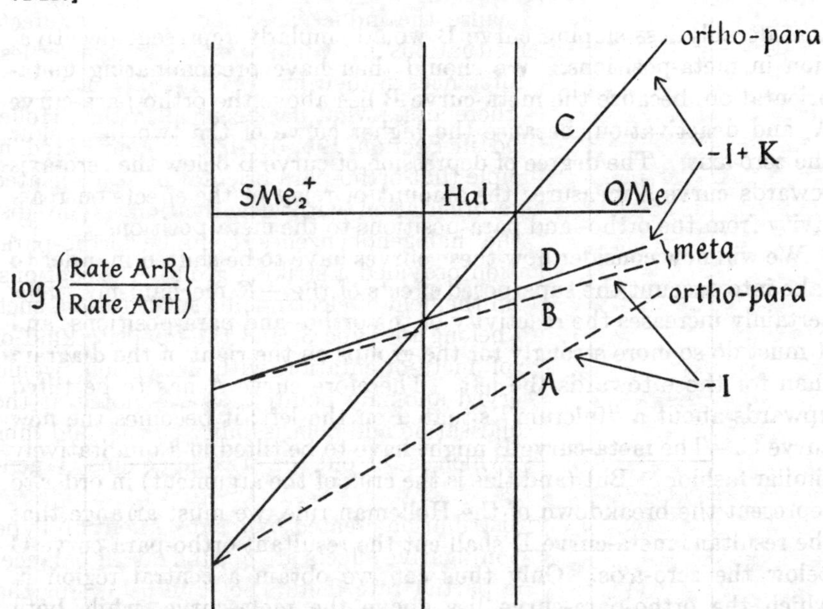

FIG. 21-1.—A schematic analysis of the effects of combined $-I+K$ mechanisms of electron displacement on orientation and reactivity in electrophilic aromatic substitution.

the halogens and ω-carboxyvinyl, which break Holleman's rule by associating ortho-para-orientation with deactivation (see Table 21-2).

The first step in the argument[43] which we shall base on these facts will lead us to the conclusion that the $+K$ displacement is more exclusive in its effects in the ortho- and para-positions, than is the $-I$ displacement, and is not, like the latter, considerably relayed to the meta-positions. One way of appreciating this deduction is with the aid of the schematic analysis set forth in Figure 21-1. The groups of Type 3 are supposed to be arranged horizontally in a series, as described above. Activation and deactivation of the nuclear positions are assumed to be measured upwards or downwards on a logarithmic scale from a zero axis, which represents the logarithm of the unit rate of substitution at one position in benzene.

Let us first consider how the effect of the $-I$ mechanism acting alone would have to be represented. We have seen that this form of displacement deactivates all nuclear positions, the ortho- and para- more than the meta-position. All this it must do more strongly for the groups on the left of the diagram than for those towards the right. We might then introduce curve A, as a locus of points representing deactivation in ortho-positions, or, alternatively, para-positions, since their condition is similar. Between this curve and the zero axis, a considerably less sloping curve B would similarly represent deactivation in meta-positions. We should then have predominating meta-orientation, because the meta-curve B lies above the ortho-para-curve A, and deactivation, because the higher curve of the two lies below the zero axis. The degree of depression of curve B below the zero-axis towards curve A measures the amount of relay of the effects on reactivity from the ortho- and para-positions to the meta-positions.

We will now consider how these curves have to be shifted in order to take into account the superposed effects of the $+K$ mechanism. This certainly increases the reactivity of the ortho- and para-positions; and it must do so more strongly for the groups on the right of the diagram than for those towards the left. Therefore curve A has to be tilted upwards about a "fulcrum" situated on the left: it becomes the new curve C. The meta-curve B might have to be tilted in a qualitatively similar fashion. But (and this is the crux of the argument) in order to represent the breakdown of the Holleman rule, we must arrange that the resultant meta-curve D shall cut the resultant ortho-para-curve C below the zero-axis. Only thus can we obtain a central region in which the ortho-para-curve lies above the meta-curve, while both curves lie below the axis, that is, a region of ortho-para-orientation associated with general nuclear deactivation. The diagram shows the two switch-points which divide the field into three sections. On the left, curve D lies above curve C, and the higher curve lies below the axis: here we have meta-orientation associated, as always, with deactivation. On the right, curve C lies above curve D, and the higher curve is above the axis: here ortho-para-orientation is associated, as is normal, with activation. In the centre we find the anomalous region.

All this shows that curve B must be shifted very little, if at all, to give the resultant meta-curve D. One way of stating the condition for representing the described anomalous correlation of orientation with reactivity is that the angular shift BD must bear a smaller ratio to the angular shift AC than the slope of B bears to the slope of A. In other words, the anomaly shows that the conjugative mechanism $+K$ acts with a distinguishing specificity on the ortho- and para-positions, and is not, like the inductive effect $-I$, considerably relayed to the meta-positions.

The second step of the argument involves consideration of the reason for this difference in ortho-para-selectivity between the conjugative and inductive mechanisms. We shall deduce that it indicates a difference in time-dependence of the displacements arising by the two mechanisms; and, in particular, that, while the inductive mechanism $-I$ represents, chiefly and typically, a permanent state of polarisation of the molecule, $-I_s$, the conjugative mechanism $+K$ has its main effect in a temporary process, $+E$, which arises when the attacking reagent is taking advantage of the polarisability of the system.

On the basis of a study of substituents of Types 1 and 2, we have already concluded that the free charges, which the $\pm I$ effects of these substituents place on ortho- and para-positions, are partly relayed to the meta-positions. Now if the $+K$ mechanism really placed *free* charges on the ortho- and para-positions, then these charges could not avoid being partly relayed to the meta-positions; and, in that case, the $+K$ mechanism would have no greater ortho-para-specificity than the $-I$ mechanism. We must conclude that the charges produced by the $+K$ mechanism *are not free*, but are locally neutralised as they are created. An equivalent statement is that the electron displacements by the $+K$ mechanism are essentially electromeric displacements, $+E$, stimulated by the electrophilic reagent, and that they therefore become important only at those moments at which the reagent is already at an ortho- or a para-position, and is there committed to ortho- or para-attack.

So we may expect this major difference of selectivity between polarisation and polarisability effects: the latter operate only *where* the reagent is and only while it is there. In electrophilic aromatic substitution, the conjugative displacements to reaction centres at ortho- or para-positions are essentially polarisability effects. One can discuss, as is sometimes done, the conjugative effect on the initial and transition states; but the system has to get from the initial to the transition state, and the ease of that process is dependent on the electromeric effect.

Substituents of Type 3 confer on the benzene ring an enormous range of reactivities. This has been made clear by the approximate scale of reaction rates, many established indirectly, for chlorination and bromination by molecular halogens in acetic acid and other solvents, over the ortho-para-orienting part of the Type 3 range of orienting groups, that is, from the right-hand edge of Fig. 21-1 as far as the second vertical rule leftward. The estimated partial rate factors for para-halogenation spread over a range of 10^{19}: their logarithms are in Table 21-4.[45] The fundamental activation sequence, N>O>F, stands out in strong relief, as does the important reduction of such activations by *N*- and *O*-acyl substituents (Sections **7e** and **7f**). The replacement of *N*- and *O*-hydrogen atoms by methyl groups effects smaller reductions of activation—effects which may be due, as Robertson, de la Mare, and Swedlund have suggested, to the loss of hyperconjugative electromeric effects originating in NH and OH bonds.

As will be seen in Table 21-1, rates of nitration in the halogenobenzene series go through a minimum: F>Cl≈Br<I. This may reflect

TABLE 21-4. LOGARITHMS OF PARTIAL RATE FACTORS FOR PARA-HALOGENATION IN MONOSUBSTITUTED BENZENES HAVING ORIENTING SUBSTITUENTS OF TYPE 3.

Substitution	Orienting substituents				
	NMe_2	NHAc	NMeAc	N:NPh	
Chlorination		+6.4	+3.3	+2.3	
Bromination	+19.5	+9.1	+6.15		
	OH	OMe	OPh	O·COPh	F
Chlorination	+7.7			+2.0	+0.8
Bromination	+11.7	+9.8	+7.9		

the conclusions that, among $+K$ effects of halogens, $+E$ is quite negligible for fluorine, and $+M$ maximal and so dominating in spite of its usually minor role, whereas $+E$ is maximal and, hence, dominating for iodine. The same pattern among the halogens has been found again in several series of monohalogeno-polymethyl-benzenes by Illuminati,[46] who used bromination by molecular bromine in nitromethane as the substitution process. He has in part extended the investigation back from orienting substituents of Mendeléjeff's group VII to group VI, by showing that the rate order for the halogen orienting groups, F > Cl, is paralleled by that for the group VI substituents, MeO > MeS, though these substituents, unlike the halogens, are strongly activating. The data refer to the bromination by molecular bromine in acetic acid of methoxy- and methylthio-durene. They are expressed below as rates of bromination in the one available position in these compounds, relatively to the rate of bromination at one position in durene:

MeO; Me, Me, Me, Me — 164,000

MeS; Me, Me, Me, Me — 970

[46] G. Illuminati and B. Marino, *J. Am. Chem. Soc.*, 1956, 78, 4975; G. Illuminati, *ibid.*, 1958, 80, 4941, 4945.

We have no comparable quantitative information about substituents of Type 4, but the qualitative data are impressively consistent with theoretical expectation. In these groups the two modes of electron displacement collaborate, as represented in the symbol $+I+K$: the groups are very strongly electropositive, so that we expect exceptionally high rates and exclusive ortho-para orientation. The rates of electrophilic substitutions of the phenoxide ion are so high that feasible methods of measurement, or competitive comparison with rates for other benzene derivatives, have not yet been found. Orientation is exclusively ortho and para. The following symbols represent the $+E$ effect as stimulated by an electrophilic reagent attacking an ortho- or a para-position (the reagent is indicated by ⊕):

(+*E* effects under ortho- and para-attack)

One can now explain the simplification which is involved in our fourfold classification of orienting substituents. As is known from physical evidence (Chapter III), the $+K$ mechanism of electron displacement involves a part, the $+M$ effect, which can be measured as a permanent polarisation of the molecule. We have just concluded that it is the other part, the $+E$ effect, that is, the temporary polarisability effect stimulated by the electrophilic reagent, which is of outstanding importance in electrophilic aromatic substitution. It is therefore clear why, in our approximate classification of orienting groups, the $-K$ mechanism was neglected. It also has, in principle, two parts, a $-M$ effect and a $-E$ effect. But electrophilic reagents are not the right kind to stimulate a $-E$ effect. And thus there remains only the $-M$ effect, which, as a simplification, was regarded as included, by subtraction or addition, in the greater permanent polarisations constituting the $+I$ and $-I$ effects of Types 1 and 2. In a more detailed classification, these two types would be split up as indicated in Table 21-5.

Expressions are given below for the electron displacements involved in $+M$ and $-M$ effect:

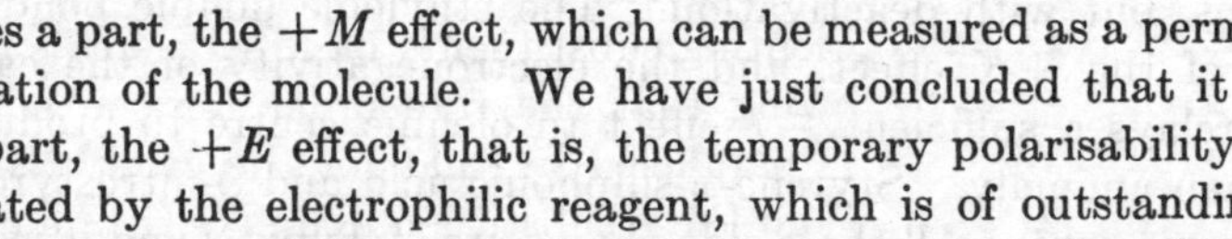

+*M* effect

−*M* effect

It is not essential that the inductive and conjugative modes of elec-

TABLE 21-5.—EXTENDED CLASSIFICATION OF ORIENTING SUBSTITUENTS.

Type	Electronic mechanism	Example	Effect on Orientation	Effect on Reactivity
(1) $+I$	Ph←R	$Ph{\leftarrow}CH_3$	ortho-para-	Activation
(1′) $+I-M$	Ph↶R	$Ph{\leftarrow}CO_2^-$	ortho-para- or meta-	Activation or Deactivation
(2) $-I$	Ph→R	$Ph{\rightarrow}NH_3^+$	meta-	Deactivation
(2′) $-I-M$	Ph↷R	$Ph{\rightarrow}CO_2Et$	meta-	Deactivation
Types 3 and 4, as in Table 21-2.				

tron displacement, which when critically balanced, produce the Holleman anomaly, should originate in the same atom, as they do in the halogen atom. The conjugative effect $+K$ must start from an atom adjacent to the aromatic ring, but the inductive effect $-I$ could originate further away and become relayed to the atom conjugated with the ring. This is what happens in the side-chain of cinnamic acid, a substance that nitrates almost entirely in the ortho- and para-positions, but with deactivation. The ethylenic double bond is the source of the $+K$ effect, and the electronegativity of the carboxyl group relays a sufficient $-I$ effect to olefinic centre to produce the Holleman anomaly. Styrene-ω-sulphonic acid and ω-nitrostyrene are in the same case. All three side-chains are of Type 3; and it would be easy to arrange that $+I$ effect, as of a carboxylate-ion group, co-operated with a $+K$ conjugative effect in a side-chain of Type 4.

(21d) Hyperconjugation and the Holleman Anomaly.—As Knowles and Norman and also Riley and Rothstein have shown,[37] the relay of inductive electronegativity can balance electropositive CH hyperconjugation in benzyl compounds sufficiently to produce another set of cases of the Holleman anomaly. A series, qualitatively like the series SMe_2^+, · · · Hal, · · · OMe, which illustrated the gradations of orientation and rate treated in Fig. 21-1, but one showing much smaller overall variations of these properties, can be made from groups of the form CH_2X, where X is any of a series of groups in order of diminishing electronegativity, as in the examples,

$Ph{-}CH_2{\cdot}NO_2$	$Ph{-}CH_2{\cdot}CN$ $Ph{-}CH_2{\cdot}Cl$	$Ph{-}CH_2{\cdot}OMe$
m-direction	*o,p*-direction	*o,p*-direction
deactivation	deactivation	activation

In this series, the two middle members show the Holleman anomaly. The partial rate factors are set out below. (In order to save space the ortho- and meta-factors are entered only once.)

	$CH_2 \cdot NO_2$	$CH_2 \cdot CN$	$CH_2 \cdot Cl$	CH_2OMe
ortho	0.082	0.25	0.72	10.0
meta	0.200	0.21	0.30	1.3
para	0.167	1.15	2.24	16.3

Evidently the whole argument of the preceding Section can be applied to this series of examples. The corresponding conclusion, already drawn by the authors mentioned, is equally inevitable. In its first stage it is that, within the overall $-I+K$ effect of these Type 3 groups, the $+K$ hyperconjugative portion is distinguishingly specific for ortho- and para-positions, whereas the $-I$ inductive portion suffers the normal relay from ortho- and para- to meta-positions. From this, it follows that, whereas the $-I$ inductive effect is predominantly a polarisation, the $+K$ hyperconjugative effect is essentially a polarisability effect, called into operation when, and only when, an electrophilic substituting agent is present either at an ortho- or at a para-position.

(21e) Interpretations Involving Field Effects.—The field effect of an electropolar substituent will agree in electropolar sign with its inductive effect, but will have a different spatial distribution, diminishing with the direct distance from its source to the point at which it re-enters the substrate molecule. It is to be expected that field effects will be highly sensitive to the dielectric medium, provided, of course, that at least one polar, re-orientable solvent molecule can get into the track of the field.

In electrophilic aromatic substitution, the field effect is difficult to distinguish from the inductive, first because the field effect is of the same sign as the inductive effect, and secondly because, once either effect reaches and enters the aromatic ring, further distribution is taken over with great efficiency by the conjugated system of the ring itself. As to where to look for evidence that could indicate the field effect in a distinctive way, it was said in the first edition of this book that the field effect, "if it were strong enough, could reverse, as between meta- and para-positions, an orientation determined by the inductive effect." "But" the conclusion then was (and still is) "it is not strong enough." Nevertheless in some more recent work by Ridd and his collaborators[47] one seems to see the field effect doing its best in the direction of the potentiality ascribed to it.

The inductive and field effects are at their simplest when they originate from an ionic charge. The distribution over the ring of such effects arising from a positive ionic charge in a side-chain, the case considered by Ridd, is as follows. The inductive effect enters at the α-carbon atom, and is distributed with little loss (for schematic simplicity, the diagram of Fig. 21-2 shows no loss) to ortho- and para-positions, and then from there, with heavy loss, to the meta-positions. The field effect enters mainly (and other points of entry can be neglected in comparison) at the ortho-carbon atoms, from which it is distributed with little loss (the diagram shows no loss) to the positions ortho- and para- to them (that is, α- and meta- to the substituent), and therefrom, with heavy loss to the one remaining nuclear position (that para- to the substituent). Thus the inductive and field effects contribute reversed orientations at the meta- and para-positions, though they combine to deactivate ortho-positions.

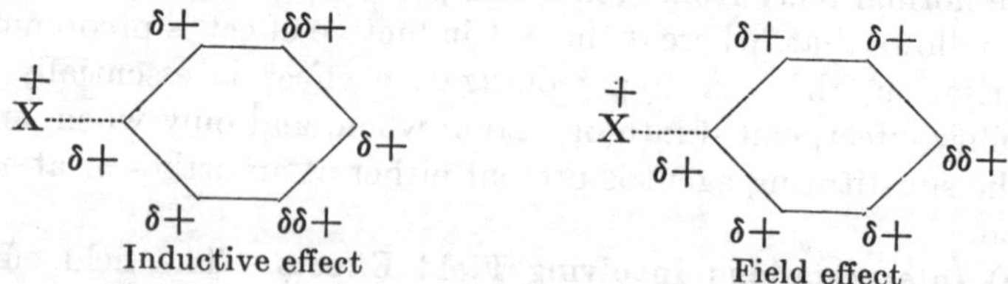

Inductive effect Field effect

One of the comparisons made by Ridd and his coworkers was of the nitration of the phenyl- and benzyl-trimethylammonium ions in mixed acid. Contrary to an early report that the phenyl cation gave nothing but the meta-nitro-derivative, the two cations give about the same proportions of meta- and para-products, namely, 89% and 85% of the meta-nitro-products and 11% and 13% of the para-derivatives. However, the similar product ratios come from reactions having very different rates. The data[47] are included, with others for later discussion, in Table 21-6.

In explanation, it is assumed that, in the phenyltrimethyl-ammonium ion, the field effect is strong, though it is still somewhat weaker than the inductive effect. The great strength of the field effect is

[47] J. R. Knowles and R. O. C. Norman, *J. Chem. Soc.*, **1961**, 2938; M. Brickman, S. Johnson, and J. H. Ridd, *Proc. Chem. Soc.*, 1962, **228,** M. Brickman and J. H. Ridd, *J. Chem. Soc.*, **1965,** 6845; *idem* and J. H. P. Utley, *ibid.*, p. 6851; F. L. Riley and E. Rothstein, *ibid.*, **1964,** 3860, 3872; J. H. Ridd, *Tetrahedron*, **1964,** 43; personal communication from Dr. J. H. Ridd.

TABLE 21-6.—RELATIVE RATES AND PRODUCT PROPORTIONS IN THE NITRATION OF PHENYL AND BENZYL 'ONIUM IONS AND PHENYLNITROMETHANE.

		$Ph \cdot NMe_3^+$	$Ph \cdot NH_3^+$	$Ph \cdot CH_2 \cdot NO_2$
Rates ($C_6H_6 = 1$)		1.2×10^{-8}	9.4×10^{-7}	12.2×10^{-2}
Proportions	*o*-	0.05%	1.5%	22%
	m-	89%	62%	55%
	p-	11%	37%	23%
		$Ph \cdot CH_2 \cdot NMe_3^+$	$Ph \cdot CH_2 \cdot PMe_3^+$	$Ph \cdot CH_2 \cdot AsMe_3^+$
Rates ($C_6H_6 = 1$)		4.3×10^{-5}	6.6×10^{-3}	12.7×10^{-3}
Proportions	*o*-	2%	13%	17%
	m-	85%	19%	7%
	p-	13%	68%	76%

ascribed to the difficulty of putting a reorientable solvent molecule into the space between the ammonium pole and the ortho-positions on which mainly it acts, and hence to the absence of the commonly experienced dielectric loss of field intensity. In the benzyltrimethylammonium ion, on the other hand, the field originating at the charged centre traverses part of the polar medium before reaching the ortho-positions, with a resulting loss of intensity. To keep within a first approximation, let us neglect this relatively weak effect, and also neglect the expected weak para-reactivation in the benzyl cation by the CH-hyperconjugation.[37] Taking account of the stronger effects only, we can draw a simplified, schematic, free-energy diagram, as in Fig. 21-2, which shows how a strong field effect in the phenyl cation could produce approximately identical meta-para product-ratios in substitutions of the phenyl and benzyl cations, despite a great difference of nuclear deactivation in the two cations, a difference which, indeed, the field effect enhances. When a growing chain of methylene groups is interposed between the ring and the ionic centre, both the internal inductive effect and the coulombic field effect fall rapidly, but the former exponentially and more rapidly, with the result that the weak effects now reaching the ring are mainly field effects.

The same workers studied the nitration of the anilinium ions in mixed acid, that is, of the protonated, rather than the methylated, phenylammonium ions. Some of their results are also summarised in Table 21-6. The protonated cations were shown to be nitrated as such, and not through their conjugate bases, which were present in such minute proportions, that even substitution at every encounter with the reagent could not account for more than a minute proportion of the observed rates of substitution. The protonated cation shows the weaker deactivation and the weaker meta-orienting action. Ridd ascribes this to removal of the low-dielectric envelope of methyl groups from around the cationic charge, and the consequently increased dispersal of effective charge and its field in the high-dielectric medium.

A comparison of the rate and orientation figures, due to Riley and Rothstein, for benzyl-trimethylphosphonium and benzyl-trimethylarsonium ions, on the one hand, with those, due to Knowles and Norman,

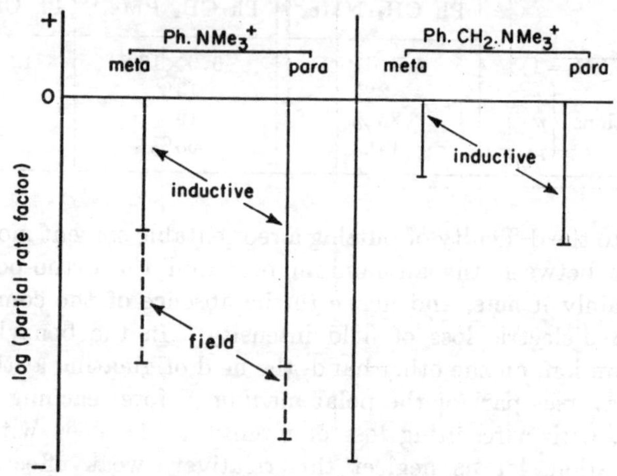

FIG. 21-2.—Schematic free-energy diagram for the nitration of phenyl- and benzyl-trimethylammonium ions, illustrating how a strong field effect in the phenyl ion can enhance deactivation, while reducing the proportion of meta-product, even to near identity with that given by the much less deactivated benzyl ion. For simplicity, the small field effect, and the small hyperconjugative effect, in the benzyl ion are not represented.

for phenylnitromethane, on the other, is also made by Ridd. Although the nitro-compound is less deactivated for nitration than either of these two 'onium ions, the nitro-compound gives more meta-product (Table 21-6). Ridd sees in this the faster fading out with increasing distance, in accordance with general electrostatic principles, of the field effect emanating from a dipole than of the field effect emanating from a pole. One can see theoretically that to leave out or much weaken the field effect represented in Fig. 21-2 would increase rate and yet increase the proportion of meta-product.

We have been discussing what may be termed the *substrate field effect*, because it is exerted by the substituents on another part of the substrate. These must exert also a field effect on the attacking reagent, a *reagent field effect* as we may call it. For the field, by attracting or repelling the polar reagent, will change its local concentration in the vicinity of the potential centres of reaction and hence affect reaction rates at these centres. This type of field effect was first described by Bjerrum in connexion with acid-base equilibria, as we shall note in Chapter XIV.

The reagent field effect is likely to be significant in nitration, in which the reagent is a cation, the nitronium ion, and not a neutral molecule. In the nitration of the phenyl- and benzyl-ammonium ions discussed above, the ammonium-ion field will repel nitronium ions, and hence rates will be reduced by this cause, reduced most in the ortho-positions, and relatively little in the meta- and para-positions, though more in the meta- than in the para-positions. Qualitatively, this distribution of kinetic effects over the ring is the same as that expected for the substrate field effect. At present we have no way to separate these components of the field effect in aromatic substitution, even though they conceptually operate in very different ways. We do, however, expect that in other systems, in which no benzene ring can conjugatively carry to the reaction-centres any effect which reaches the ring, the reagent field effect will often be more important than the substrate field effect. These matters will be discussed and illustrated in Chapters XIV and XVI.

(22) ORTHO-TO-PARA PRODUCT RATIOS IN ELECTROPHILIC AROMATIC SUBSTITUTION

(22a) Factors Affecting the ortho-para-Ratio.—The theory which considers ortho- and para-orientation collectively against the contrast of meta-orientation deals with constitutional factors of a gross kind. On turning from this question to that of ortho- versus para-substitution, alike in relation to ortho-para-orienting compounds as a class and to the ortho- and para-by-products formed in the substitutions of predominantly meta-orienting compounds, it is found that more subtle influences are at work. For instance, it is no longer possible to treat the nature of the entering group as a relatively unimportant detail.

A general analysis of the data concerning ortho- versus para-substitution was made in 1926 by the writer, who deduced the existence of a primary steric effect, as Holleman had previously,[48] and also of inductive and conjugative effects,[49] which work as follows:

[48] A. F. Holleman, *Chem. Revs.*, 1925, 1, 218.

[49] C. K. Ingold, *Ann. Repts. on Progress Chem.* (Chem. Soc. London), 1926, 23, 140.

Primary steric effect decreases *o*-reactivity.

$$\text{Inductive}\begin{cases}-I \text{ effect decreases}\\ +I \text{ effect increases}\end{cases} o\text{-} > p\text{-reactivity.}$$

$$\text{Conjugative}\begin{cases}-M \text{ effect decreases}\\ +E \text{ effect increases}\end{cases} p\text{-} > o\text{-reactivity.}$$

In 1928 the explanation was added[50] that the inductive effects are electrostatic, acting essentially through the associated field effects, and in 1949 the complementary explanation was given[51] that the conjugative effects arise from quantally caused differences of stability of ortho- and para-quinonoid bonding arrangements. We shall follow this classification, first analysing the data in terms of the factors indicated, and then going into the physical mechanisms of the polar factors.

(22b) Evidence for the Primary Steric Effect.—Unlike polar orientation, which depends much more on the orienting than on the entering substituent, steric orientation is a matter of space-sharing between the orienting substituent and the carrier of the entering group, and hence the effective volume of each of these competitors for space should be comparably important in the production of a steric effect. In advancing his proposition concerning the importance of the primary steric effect in aromatic substitution, Holleman gave some figures,[48] assembled in Table 22-1, which seem to confirm this assumption. The figures show that, independently of the substituent already present, the proportion of ortho-substitution falls and that of para-substitution rises, as the group introduced successively becomes Cl, NO_2, Br, SO_3H. This is a sequence in which no polar origin can be recognised. On the

TABLE 22-1.—EFFECT OF THE ENTERING SUBSTITUENT ON THE PERCENTAGES OF ORTHO- AND PARA-PRODUCTS FORMED FROM SEVERAL BENZENE DERIVATIVES.

Group introduced	Compound substituted and percentages of products							
	Toluene		Chlorobenzene		Bromobenzene		Phenol	
	ortho-	para-	ortho-	para-	ortho-	para-	ortho-	para-
Cl	—	—	39.0	55.0	45.1	52.5	49.8	50.2
NO_2	56.0	40.9	30.1	69.9	37.6	62.4	40.0	60.0
Br	39.7	60.3	11.2	87.2	13.1	85.1	9.8	90.2
SO_3H	31.9	62.0	0.0	100.0	0.0	100.0	—	—

[50] C. K. Ingold and C. C. N. Vass, *J. Chem. Soc.*, **1928**, 417; A. Lapworth and R. Robinson, *Mem. Proc. Manchester Lit. & Phil. Soc.*, 1928, **72**, 243.

[51] P. B. D. de la Mare, *J. Chem. Soc.*, **1949**, 2871.

other hand, it could, as Holleman suggested, be an order of increasing effective size for steric hindrance in these reactions.

A somewhat clearer separation of the primary steric effect from polar effects is possible when the orienting group is only weakly polar, and, without changing that character, can be varied largely in size. The alkylbenzenes have been widely studied in this connexion. LeFèvre explained, as an effect of the steric restriction of ortho-substitution, the higher proportions in which para-compounds are formed in the nitration of the more branched side-chain homologues of toluene.[52] The data, more complete now than were available to him, are in Table 22-2.

TABLE 22-2.—PROPORTIONS OF PRODUCTS FORMED IN THE MONONITRATION OF MONOALKYLBENZENES.

	$Ph\cdot CH_3$ (1)	$Ph\cdot CH_2\cdot CH_3$ (2)	$Ph\cdot CH(CH_3)_2$ (3)	$Ph\cdot C(CH_3)_3$ (4)
Ortho-....	57	45	30	12
Meta-....	3.2	6.5	7.5	8.5
Para-.....	40	48	62	79

[1] A. F. Holleman, J. Vermeulen, and W. J. de Mooy, *Rec. trav. chim.*, 1914, **33,** 1; C. K. Ingold, A. Lapworth, E. Rothstein, and D. Ward, *J. Chem. Soc.*, **1931,** 1959; H. Cohn, E. D. Hughes, M. H. Jones, and M. G. Peeling, *Nature*, 1952, **169,** 291.

[2] E. L. Cline and E. E. Reid, *J. Am. Chem. Soc.*, 1927, **49,** 3150; H. C. Brown and W. H. Bonner, *ibid.*, 1954, **76,** 605.

[3] G. Vavon and A. Collier, *Bull. soc. chim.* (France), 1927, **41,** 357; H. C. Brown and W. H. Bonner, *loc. cit.*

[4] H. Cohn, E. D. Hughes, M. H. Jones, and M. G. Peeling, *loc. cit.*

For toluene and *t*-butylbenzene the ratios of meta- to para-nitro-products are roughly the same. The great differences are in the ratios of ortho- to meta-, or of ortho- to para-products. This indicates that the distinction is especially associated with the ortho-position. The simplest interpretation is that the polar effects of the two alkyl groups are not very different, and that the changes in all the percentages are to be ascribed mainly to a selective repression, presumably a steric repression, of substitution in the position ortho- to the larger alkyl group.

LeFèvre has similarly explained the favoured substitution in the positions adjacent to the methyl groups of the *p*-alkyltoluenes. Such substitution has been established for the nitration of *p*-ethyltoluenes,[53] for the nitration, halogenation, and sulphonation of *p*-cymene,[52] and for the nitration of *p*-*t*-butyltoluene:[54]

[52] R. J. W. LeFèvre, *J. Chem. Soc.*, **1933,** 980; *ibid.*, **1934,** 1501.

[53] O. L. Brady and J. N. E. Day, *J. Chem. Soc.*, **1934,** 114.

[54] M. Battegay and P. Haeffely, *Bull. soc. chim.* (France), 1924, **35,** 981.

$CH_3C_6H_4CH_2{\cdot}CH_3$ $CH_3C_6H_4CH(CH_3)_2$ $CH_3C_6H_4C(CH_3)_3$

Until recently one was not compelled to accept these interpretations, particularly those relating to the *p*-alkyltoluenes. The alternative view was possible (and was advanced) that, owing to hyperconjugation, the methyl group has, among alkyl groups, the strongest ortho-para-orienting polar effect. But this is not the case: Cohn, Hughes, Jones and Peeling disproved it by showing that the rates of mononitration of toluene and of *t*-butylbenzene stand in the ratio 100:64. If we combine this figure with the relevant orientational proportions (Table 22-2), and with the already noted rate value for toluene (Table 21-1), then the rates of attack on the individual nuclear positions of toluene and *t*-butylbenzene (the rate for one position of benzene being taken as unity) present the following comparison:

	CH_3	$C(CH_3)_3$
ortho	42, 42	5.5, 5.5
meta	2.2, 2.2	4.0, 4.0
para	59	75

This shows that, hyperconjugation notwithstanding, the *t*-butyl group is slightly more activating than is the methyl group for substitution in all positions—except ortho-positions. But, relatively to the methyl group, the *t*-butyl group greatly represses ortho-substitution; and such a selective repression can scarcely be regarded otherwise than as a steric effect.

The products and the rates of halogenation of toluene and of *t*-butylbenzene by two chlorinating agents, Cl^+ and Cl_2, and two brominating agents, Br^+ and Br_2, have been studied by P. B. D. de la Mare, H. C. Brown, and others.[55] The work constitutes a combination of the Holleman approach of varying the substituting agent, and the LeFèvre-Hughes approach of studying orientation and rate of substitution of weakly polar alkylbenzenes, to the problem of distinguishing steric effects from polar. Unlike electrophilic nitration, in which the nitronium ion is almost always the attacking species, electrophilic chlorination may, according to the conditions, depend on

[55] P. B. D. de la Mare and J. T. Harvey, *J. Chem. Soc.*, **1956**, 63; **1957**, 131; *idem*, M. Hassan and S. Varma, *ibid.*, **1958**, 2756; H. C. Brown and L. M. Stock, *J. Am. Chem. Soc.*, 1957, **79**, 1421, 5175; "Aromatic Substitution," by P. B. D. de la Mare and J. H. Ridd, Butterworths Scientific Pubs., London, 1959, Chaps. 8–10; L. M. Stock and H. Himoe, *J. Am. Chem. Soc.*, 1961, **83**, 1937.

The most striking result here is that the change in the orienting group from methyl to *t*-butyl reduces the rate of ortho-bromination by Br^+ by a factor of 5, and reduces the rate of ortho-chlorination by Cl_2 by a factor of 9, and of ortho-bromination by Br_2 by a factor of more (probably much more) than 20.

(22c) Evidence for Participation by the Inductive Effect.—The conclusion that polar effects exist whereby $+I$ substituents increase ortho-reactivity more than they do para-, while $-I$ substituents decrease ortho-reactivity more than para-, has been generally accepted; but the evidence concerning $+I$ groups rests primarily on the example of toluene. The ratio of ortho- to para-nitro-products given by toluene, 1.5, is certainly larger than that given by most ortho-para-orienting substances; but it is still less than 2, the ratio of the numbers of positions of each kind. It is supposed that the ratio would be greater than 2 if the methyl group did not afford some degree of steric shielding of the ortho-positions.[57] Strong evidence in favour of this view has been forthcoming from de la Mare's studies of the chlorination of toluene by chlorinium ion and of its bromination by brominium ion, with the results recorded in Table 22-3, above. With these smaller substituting agents, as we believe them to be, the ortho/para ratios rise to 3.3 and 2.5 in the respective cases.

The evidence that $-I$ groups deactivate ortho- more than they do para-positions is substantial. In Table 22-5 will be found some figures for the proportions in which isomerides are formed in nitration for several series of compounds. Along the series PhF, PhCl, PhBr, PhI, we see a rising proportion of ortho-substitution. This is contrary to what would be expected on account of an effect of steric hindrance; but it is consistent with the idea that a selective polar deactivation of the ortho-positions by halogens, with an intensity which follows the order of electronegativity, $F > Cl > Br > I$, overrides the expected effect of steric hindrance. A rising ortho-proportion is likewise seen in the benzyl series BzF, BzCl, though the separation is much smaller, as might be expected. This confirms that it is indeed the $-I$ effect, and not the $+K$ effect, of the halogens with which the observed trends are more closely correlated. And one has only to turn to data for the nitration of other groups of benzyl compounds, for instance, BzCN, $BzCO_2Et$, having substituents suitably related as to electronegativity and size, in order to discover that the effect illustrated is not peculiar to halogen compounds. For evidential purposes, a suitable relation between electronegativity and size is essential. A comparison which lacks such a relation is that of the falling ortho-proportion along the

[57] P. B. D. de la Mare, *J. Chem. Soc.*, **1949**, 2871.

apparent in Table 22-3. This suggests that the extra participation is electromeric,[56] which in itself, as we shall see in Section **22d**, is expected to increase para-substitution at the expense of ortho-, and so might have inverted the orders as between Cl_2 and NO_2^+ in Table 22-3, for the less sterically formidable molecule toluene, for which the ortho- and para-figures are in fact very similar.

TABLE 22-4.—RELATIVE RATES OF SUBSTITUTION OF TOLUENE AND OF *t*-BUTYLBENZENE BY VARIOUS ELECTROPHILIC SUBSTITUTING AGENTS.

(The rate of substitution of benzene with each substituting agent is taken as unity for substitutions by that reagent.)

Substituting Agents	Cl^+	Br^+	NO_2^+	Cl_2	Br_2
Toluene	60	36	24.5	345	605
t-Butylbenzene	—	12	15.5	110	125

By combining the data of Tables 22-3 and 22-4, we can set down for halogenation, as we previously did for nitration, the partial rate-factors for toluene and *t*-butylbenzene, that is, the rate of attack of a reagent on each individual nuclear position in these molecules, relatively to the rate of its attack on one individual position in benzene. As shown above, the data allow us to do this completely for two of the four halogenating agents, and partly for one of the others:

Bromination by Br^+: CH_3 — ortho 76, 76; meta 2.5, 2.5; para 59. $C(CH_3)_3$ — ortho 14, 14; meta 2.6, 2.6; para 39.

Chlorination by Cl_2: CH_3 — ortho 620, 620; meta 5, 5; para 820. $C(CH_3)_3$ — ortho 72, 72; meta 7, 7; para 505.

Bromination by Br_2: CH_3 — ortho 600, 600; meta 5.5, 5.5; para 2400. $C(CH_3)_3$ — ortho 30, 30; meta ?, ?; para 750.

[56] P. B. D. de la Mare in "Progress in Stereochemistry," Editors W. Klyne and P. B. D. de la Mare, Butterworths Scientific Pubs., London, 1958, Vol. 2, p. 72, and references (since 1945) there cited.

TABLE 22-5.—PERCENTAGES OF ISOMERIDES FORMED ON MONONITRATION OF SOME ELECTRONEGATIVELY SUBSTITUTED AROMATIC COMPOUNDS.

	PhF (1)	PhCl (2, 11)	PhBr (3, 11)	PhI (4, 11)
Ortho	12	30	37	38
Meta		0.9	1.2	1.8
Para	87	69	62	60
	$PhCH_2F$ (5)	$PhCH_2Cl$ (6)	$PhCH_2 \cdot CN$ (7)	$PhCH_2 \cdot CO_2Et$ (8)
Ortho	28	32	17	32
Meta	18	14	14	10
Para	54	54	69	58
	$PhCH_3$ (9)	$PhCH_2Cl$ (6)	$PhCHCl_2$ (10)	$PhCCl_3$ (10)
Ortho	57	32	23	6.8
Meta	3.2	14	34	64
Para	40	54	43	29

[1] A. F. Holleman, *Rec. trav. chim.*, 1905, **24**, 140.
[2] A. F. Holleman and B. R. de Bruyn, *ibid.*, 1900, **19**, 189.
[3] A. F. Holleman and B. R. de Bruyn, *ibid.*, p. 364.
[4] A. F. Holleman, *ibid.*, 1913, **32**, 134.
[5] C. K. Ingold and E. H. Ingold, *J. Chem. Soc.*, 1928, 2249.
[6] A. F. Holleman, J. Vermeulen, and W. J. de Mooy, *Rec. trav. chim.*, 1914, **33**, 1; B. Flürscheim and E. L. Holmes, *J. Chem. Soc.*, 1928, 1607; C. K. Ingold and F. R. Shaw, *ibid.*, 1949, 575.
[7] J. W. Baker, K. E. Cooper, and C. K. Ingold, *ibid.*, 1928, 426.
[8] B. Flürscheim and E. L. Holmes, *loc. cit.*; J. W. Baker and C. K. Ingold, *ibid.*, 1927, 832.
[9] A. F. Holleman, J. Vermeulen, and W. J. de Mooy, *loc. cit.*; C. K. Ingold, A. Lapworth, E. Rothstein, and D. Ward, *J. Chem. Soc.*, 1931, 1959; H. Cohn, E. D. Hughes, and M. H. Jones, personal communication.
[10] A. F. Holleman, J. Vermeulen, and W. J. de Mooy, *loc. cit.*; B. Flürscheim and E. L. Holmes, *loc. cit.*
[11] Meta proportions by radioactive dilution: J. D. Roberts, J. K. Sanford, F. L. J. Sixma, H. Cerfontain, and R. Zeigt, *J. Am. Chem. Soc.*, 1954, **76**, 4525.

series $PhCH_3$, $PhCH_2Cl$, $PhCHCl_2$, $PhCCl_3$: this has been variously claimed as support for selective ortho-deactivation by steric hindrance and by electronegativity; but, just because it fits either interpretation, it is evidence for neither.

Just as the chief product is the para-compound in cases of predominating ortho-para-orientation by electronegative substituents, so for benzotrichloride, in which the electronegativity of the side-chain is great enough to make the main product of substitution the meta-derivative, the chief by-product is the para-compound. This result is not wholly dependent on the spatial form of the side-chain: for in the nitration of the phenyl- and benzyl-trimethylammonium ions, and the anilinium and benzylammonium ions, the chief by-product is the para-compound, as we saw in Section 21e. This appears to be the rule for

The most striking result here is that the change in the orienting group from methyl to *t*-butyl reduces the rate of ortho-bromination by Br^+ by a factor of 5, and reduces the rate of ortho-chlorination by Cl_2 by a factor of 9, and of ortho-bromination by Br_2 by a factor of more (probably much more) than 20.

(22c) Evidence for Participation by the Inductive Effect.—The conclusion that polar effects exist whereby $+I$ substituents increase ortho-reactivity more than they do para-, while $-I$ substituents decrease ortho-reactivity more than para-, has been generally accepted; but the evidence concerning $+I$ groups rests primarily on the example of toluene. The ratio of ortho- to para-nitro-products given by toluene, 1.5, is certainly larger than that given by most ortho-para-orienting substances, but it is still less than 2, the ratio of the numbers of positions of each kind. It is supposed that the ratio would be greater than 2 if the methyl group did not afford some degree of steric shielding of the ortho-positions. Strong evidence in favour of this view has been forthcoming from de la Mare's studies of the chlorination of toluene by chlorinium ion and of its bromination by brominium ion, with the results recorded in Table 22-3, above. With these smaller substituting agents, as we believe them to be, the ortho/para ratios rise to 3.3 and 2.5 in the respective cases.

The evidence that $-I$ groups deactivate ortho- more than they do para-positions is substantial. In Table 22-5 will be found some figures for the proportions in which isomerides are formed in nitration for several series of compounds. Along the series PhF, PhCl, PhBr, PhI, we see a rising proportion of ortho-substitution. This is contrary to what would be expected on account of an effect of steric hindrance; but it is consistent with the idea that a selective polar deactivation of the ortho-positions by halogens, with an intensity which follows the order of electronegativity, $F > Cl > Br > I$, overrides the expected effect of steric hindrance. A rising ortho-proportion is likewise seen in the benzyl series BzF, BzCl, though the separation is much smaller, as might be expected. This confirms that it is indeed the $-I$ effect, and not the $+K$ effect, of the halogens with which the observed trends are more closely correlated. And one has only to turn to data for the nitration of other groups of benzyl compounds, for instance, BzCN, $BzCO_2Et$, having substituents suitably related as to electronegativity and size, in order to discover that the effect illustrated is not peculiar to halogen compounds. For evidential purposes, a suitable relation between electronegativity and size is essential. A comparison which lacks such a relation is that of the falling ortho-proportion along the

[57] P. B. D. de la Mare, *J. Chem. Soc.*, **1949**, 2871.

apparent in Table 22-3. This suggests that the extra participation is electromeric,[56] which in itself, as we shall see in Section **22d,** is expected to increase para-substitution at the expense of ortho-, and so might have inverted the order as between Cl_2 and NO_2^+ in Table 22-3, for the less sterically formidable molecule toluene, for which the ortho- and para-figures are in fact very similar.

TABLE 22-4.—RELATIVE RATES OF SUBSTITUTION OF TOLUENE AND OF *t*-BUTYLBENZENE BY VARIOUS ELECTROPHILIC SUBSTITUTING AGENTS.
(The rate of substitution of benzene with each substituting agent is taken as unity for substitutions by that reagent.)

Substituting Agents..	Cl^+	Br^+	NO_2^+	Cl_2	Br_2
Toluene............	60	36	24.5	345	605
t-Butylbenzene.....	—	12	15.5	110	125

By combining the data of Tables 22-3 and 22-4, we can set down for halogenation, as we previously did for nitration, the partial rate-factors for toluene and *t*-butylbenzene, that is, the rate of attack of a reagent on each individual nuclear position in these molecules, relatively to the rate of its attack on one individual position in benzene. As shown above, the data allow us to do this completely for two of the four halogenating agents, and partly for one of the others:

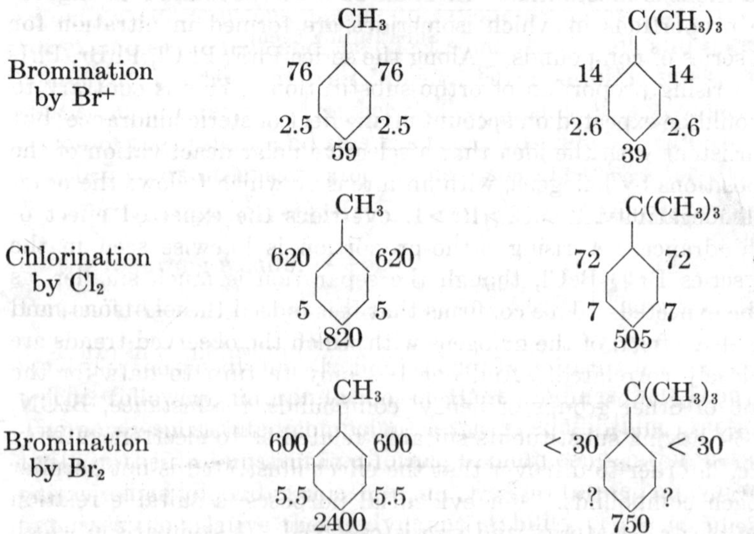

[56] P. B. D. de la Mare in "Progress in Stereochemistry," Editors W. Klyne and P. B. D. de la Mare, Butterworths Scientific Pubs.. London, 1958, Vol. 2, p. 72, and references (since 1949) there cited.

of the orienting substituent with the para-position of common concern to the two ratios. The required constitutional feature of conjugation between the ring and the orienting substituent shows that the interaction must be a selective conjugative effect.

Thus the arguments of 30 years take us full-circle, so increasing our confidence in the first conclusion that, in contrast to $-I$ orienting groups, the $-I-M$ groups exert on the ortho/para ratio a polar effect, due to the $-M$ character of the groups, and having the form of a selective para-deactivation.

(22e) Evidence for Participation by the Conjugative $+E$ Effect.—We touched the fringe of this subject in the last two lines of Table 22-7. In order to examine the situation in which polarisability in the form of an electromeric effect $+E$ is entirely dominating, we must enter the field of oxy- and amino-substituents. Orientation by these substituents is an almost pure polarisability effect, and we can therefore expect the nature of the substituting agent to have special importance.

The existence of a pattern of dependence of orientation on the substituting agent in substitutions of hydroxy- and amino-compounds was first pointed out by Lapworth and Robinson.[59] They cited Gattermann and Liebermann's finding[62] that 1-naphthol-3- and -5-sulphonic acids, and also 1-naphthylamine-3- and -5-sulphonic acids, couple with negatively substituted (for example, nitro-substituted) diazonium ions essentially in the 4-position, but with unsubstituted diazonium ions largely in the 2-position:

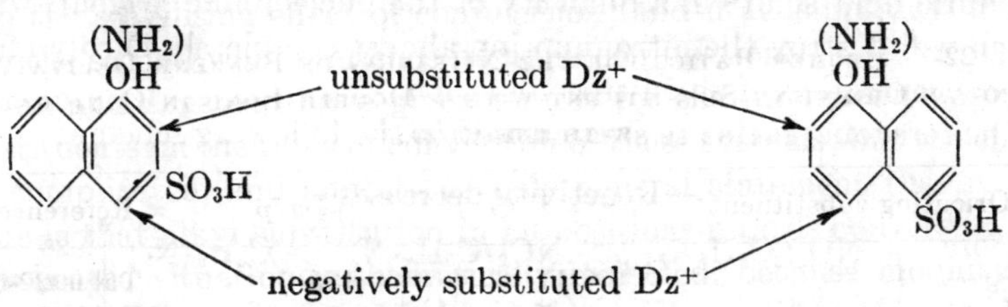

(NH$_2$) OH — SO_3H ← unsubstituted Dz$^+$ → (NH$_2$) OH — SO_3H

← negatively substituted Dz$^+$ →

This is not an effect for which steric hindrance can be held responsible. Lapworth and Robinson noted that the electrophilic reactivity of a diazonium ion is increased by negative substitution:[63] there is, for instance, a strong increase along the series

$$C_6H_5\cdot N_2^+ \qquad NO_2\cdot C_6H_4\cdot N_2^+ \qquad (NO_2)_2C_6H_3\cdot N_2^+$$

[62] L. Gattermann and H. Liebermann, *Ann.*, 1912, **393**, 198.

[63] This was qualitatively well known, and has since been quantitatively confirmed, as described in Section **24e**.

Therefore the conclusion was drawn that the shift from ortho- to para-coupling was to be correlated with the increasing activity of the reagent.

However, let us take as a second example one which tends in the opposite direction. Phenol is nitrosated mainly in the para-position: only about 8% of the ortho-nitroso isomeride is formed.[64] But when phenol is nitrated, under conditions which minimise intervention by nitrous acid, much more ortho-compound, never less than 40%, is produced.[65] Qualitatively similar statements could be made about dimethylaniline.

OH(NMe$_2$)

NO_2^+ and carriers

NO^+ and carriers

This effect likewise cannot be attributed to steric hindrance; and, as to reactivity, the opposite situation obtains. It is qualitatively evident, since so many aromatic compounds can easily be nitrated which cannot be nitrosated, that nitrating agents are in general more active than nitrosating agents: electrophilic activity increases in the order $NO^+ < NO_2^+$. Millen[66] has confirmed this, by showing spectroscopically that, when equivalent amounts of nitronium and nitrosonium ions are present in sulphuric acid solution, a quantity of the nucleophilic reagent, water, which will destroy the nitronium ion almost completely hardly affects the concentration of the nitrosonium ion.

The foregoing facts are summarised in the following scheme:

more para-seeking $\left\{ (NO_2)_2C_6H_3{\cdot}N_2^+ > NO_2{\cdot}C_6H_4{\cdot}N_2^+ > C_6H_5{\cdot}N_2^+ \right\}$ less para-seeking

—Reactivity decreases→

$NO^+ < NO_2^+$

—Reactivity increases→

Now there is one respect in which the more para-seeking reagents of both series agree. And that is that the $-M$ mesomeric systems formed by the groups they introduce into the aromatic nucleus involve stronger interactions with the $+E$ orienting substituents than do those pro-

[64] J. Veibel, *Ber.*, 1930, **63**, 1577.

[65] E. D. Hughes, C. K. Ingold, D. I. H. Jacobs, M. H. Jones, G. F. Minkoff, and R. I. Reed, *J. Chem. Soc.*, 1950, 2628.

[66] D. J. Millen, *J. Chem. Soc.*, 1950, 2600.

selves make specific para-deactivation seem much more probable than specific ortho-activation. The reason is that by no plausible addition to the speed of ortho-substitution can we reduce the proportions of para-substitution to as little as is observed, and yet allow the proportion of meta-substitution to remain as large as is observed. It is a simple arithmetical exercise to show that it is impossible to build up figures of the pattern of the isomer proportions in Table 22-6, from the isomer proportions given by saturated orienting substituents, by adding to the corresponding partial rates of substitution an extra rate of ortho-substitution. The conversion can be made only by subtracting a rate of para-substitution.

The third idea was advanced at a later time and supported by quantum mechanical calculations of an all-too-common grossly approximated type. It was that the high ortho/para ratios arising in the presence of a double bond conjugated with the ring require no special explanation, the lower ratios observed in other cases being the result of steric hindrance.[60] De la Mare and Ridd have dealt with this argument,[61] pointing out that the ratios $\frac{1}{2}$(ortho)/para and $\frac{1}{2}$(meta)/para decrease together along a series of orienting substituents having a double bond conjugated with the nucleus, and that the two ratios pass through unity at the same point if the series is extended to run through from conjugatively electronegative to conjugatively electropositive ($-M$ to $+E$) substituents. Their figures are in Table 22-7. As they remark, the result illustrated can hardly be a coincidence. Its common cause cannot be steric hindrance, and is evidently an interaction

TABLE 22-7.—ISOMER RATIOS FOR THE NITRATION OF BENZENE DERIVATIVES HAVING AN ORIENTING SUBSTITUENT WITH A DOUBLE BOND IN CONJUGATION WITH THE RING

Orienting substituent	$\frac{1}{2}o/p$	$\frac{1}{2}m/p$	Reference
NO_2	11	135	Table 22-6
CO_2H	7	31	Table 22-6
$CO{\cdot}NH_2$	4.5	12	Table 22-6
CO_2Et	4.3	10	Table 22-6
CHO	1.6	4	Table 22-6
$CH(NO_2){:}CH{\cdot}C_6H_4NO_2(p)$	0.32	0.22	1
$CH{:}CH{\cdot}NO_2$	0.23	0.015	1

[1] J. W. Baker and I. S. Wilson, *J. Chem. Soc.*, 1927, 842.

[60] J. D. Roberts and A. Streitwieser, *J. Am. Chem. Soc.*, 1952, **74**, 4723; R. D. Brown, *ibid.*, 1953, **75**, 4077.

[61] P. B. D. de la Mare and J. H. Ridd, "Aromatic Substitution," Butterworths Scientific Publications, London, 1959, p. 82.

all meta-orienting compounds which yield small amounts of by-products—with one striking group of exceptions, which we now proceed to consider.

(22d) Evidence for Participation by the Conjugative $-M$ Effect.—The exceptions arise whenever the meta-orienting substituent contains a multiple bond so situated that it could conjugate with the ring, the substituent being of the $-I-M$ type, that is, Type 3 in the expanded classification of Table 21-5. Groups having the form COR, CO_2R, CN, NO_2, etc., belong to this class. For these orienting groups the ortho-para ... illustrated in Table 22-6.

TABLE 22-6.—PERCENTAGES OF ISOMERS FORMED ON MONONITRATION OF SOME BENZENE DERIVATIVES WITH UNSATURATED ELECTRONEGATIVE SUBSTITUENTS.

	PhCHO (1)	PhCO·CH₃ (2)	PhCO₂H (3)	PhCO₂Et (3)
Ortho	~19	~30	18.5	28.3
Meta	72	68	80.2	68.4
Para	~9	—	1.3	3.3

	PhCO·NH₂ (4)	PhCO·Cl (4)	PhCN (5)	PhNO₂ (6)
Ortho	27	8	15	6.4
Meta	70	90	83	93.3
Para	~3	<2	2	0.3

[1] O. L. Brady and S. Harris, *J. Chem. Soc.*, 1923, **123**, 484; J. W. Baker and W. G. Moffitt, *ibid.*, 1931, 1722.
[2] R. Camps, *Arch. Pharm.*, 1901, **240**, 1; J. W. Baker and W. G. Moffitt, *loc. cit.*
[3] A. F. Holleman, *Rec. trav. chim.*, 1899, **18**, 267.
[4] J. W. Baker, K. E. Cooper, and C. K. Ingold, *J. Chem. Soc.*, 1927, 836.
[5] J. W. Baker and C. K. Ingold, *ibid.*, 1928, 436; J. P. Wibaut and R. van Strik, *Rec. trav. chim.*, 1958, **77**, 316.
[6] A. F. Holleman and B. R. de Bruyn, *Rec. trav. chim.*, 1900, **19**, 79.

Three interpretations have been placed on this phenomenon. From inspection of the figures, the writer assumed it to be the result of an interference with para-substitution (by the $-M$ effect of the substituent).[58] Lapworth and Robinson suggested the alternative of a special facilitation of ortho-substitution (their theoretical picture being that the multiple bond in the side-chain adds the reagent and passes it internally to an ortho-position).[59] However, the data them-

[58] C. K. Ingold, *Ann. Repts. on Progress Chem.* (Chem. Soc. London), 1926, **23**, 140.
[59] A. Lapworth and R. Robinson, *Mem. Proc. Manchester Lit. & Phil. Soc.*, 1928, **72**, 243.

of the orienting substituent with the para-position ... concern to the two ratios. The required constitutional feature of conjugation between the ring and the orienting substituent shows that the interaction must be a specific conjugative effect.

Thus the arguments of 30 years take us full-circle, but increasing our confidence in the first conclusion that, in contrast to $-M$ effect, the groups, the $-I-M$ groups exert on the ortho/para ratio a polar effect, due to the $-M$ character of the groups, and having the form of selective para-deactivation.

(22e) Evidence for Participation by the Conjugative $+E$ Effect.—We touched the fringe of this subject in the last two lines of Table 22-7. In order to examine the situation in which polarisability in the form of an electromeric effect $+E$ is entirely dominating, we must enter the field of oxy- and amino-substituents. Orientation by these substituents is an almost pure polarisability effect, and we can therefore expect the nature of the substituting agent to have special importance.

The existence of a pattern of dependence of orientation on the substituting agent in substitutions of hydroxy- and amino-compounds was first pointed out by Lapworth and Robinson.[59] They cited Gattermann and Liebermann's finding[62] that 1-naphthol-3- and -5-sulphonic acids, and also 1-naphthylamine-3- and -5-sulphonic acids, couple with negatively substituted (for example, nitro-substituted) diazonium ions essentially in the 4-position, but with unsubstituted diazonium ions largely in the 2-position:

(NH₂) OH — unsubstituted Dz⁺ — (NH₂) OH; SO₃H — negatively substituted Dz⁺ — SO₃H

This is not an effect for which steric hindrance can be held responsible. Lapworth and Robinson noted that the electrophilic reactivity of a diazonium ion is increased by negative substitution:[63] there is, for instance, a strong increase along the series

$$C_6H_5N_2^+ < NO_2C_6H_4N_2^+ < (NO_2)_2C_6H_3N_2^+$$

[62] L. Gattermann and H. Liebermann, *Ann.*, 1912, **393**, 198.
[63] This was qualitatively well known, and has since been quantitatively confirmed, as described in Section 24c.

selves make specific para-deactivation seem much more probable than specific ortho-activation. The reason is that by no plausible addition to the speed of ortho-substitution can we reduce the proportions of para-substitution to as little as is observed, and yet allow the proportion of meta-substitution to remain as large as is observed. It is a simple arithmetical exercise to show that it is impossible to build up figures of the pattern of the isomer proportions in Table 22-6, from the isomer proportions given by saturated orienting substituents, by adding to the corresponding partial rates of substitution an extra rate of ortho-substitution. The conversion can be made only by subtracting a rate of para-substitution.

The third idea was advanced at a later time and supported by quantum mechanical calculations of an all-too-common grossly approximated type. It was that the high ortho/para ratios arising in the presence of a double bond conjugated with the ring require no special explanation, the lower ratios observed in other cases being the result of steric hindrance.[60] De la Mare and Ridd have dealt with this argument,[61] pointing out that the ratios $\frac{1}{2}$(ortho)/para and $\frac{1}{2}$(meta)/para decrease together along a series of orienting substituents having a double bond conjugated with the nucleus, and that the two ratios pass through unity at the same point if the series is extended to run through from conjugatively electronegative to conjugatively electropositive ($-M$ to $+E$) substituents. Their figures are in Table 22-7. As they remark, the result illustrated can hardly be a coincidence. Its common cause cannot be steric hindrance, and is evidently an interaction

TABLE 22-7.—ISOMER RATIOS FOR THE NITRATION OF BENZENE DERIVATIVES HAVING AN ORIENTING SUBSTITUENT WITH A DOUBLE BOND IN CONJUGATION WITH THE RING.

Orienting substituent	$\frac{1}{2}o/p$	$\frac{1}{2}m/p$	Reference
NO_2	11	135	Table 22-6
CO_2H	7	31	Table 22-6
$CO\cdot NH_2$	4.5	12	Table 22-6
CO_2Et	4.3	10	Table 22-6
CHO	1.6	4	Table 22-6
$CH(NO_2):CH\cdot C_6H_4NO_2(p)$	0.32	0.22	1
$CH:CH\cdot NO_2$	0.23	0.015	1

[1] J. W. Baker and I. S. Wilson, *J. Chem. Soc.*, **1927**, 842.

[60] J. D. Roberts and A. Streitwieser, *J. Am. Chem. Soc.*, 1952, **74**, 4723; R. D. Brown, *ibid.*, 1953, **75**, 4077.

[61] P. B. D. de la Mare and J. H. Ridd, "Aromatic Substitution," Butterworths Scientific Pubs., London, 1959, p. 82.

localisation during a charge transfer, should involve a larger uncertainty of electron position than the resonance system (*a*)—(*c*), in which two π bonds could remain static during a transfer; and that, therefore, in accordance with the uncertainty principle, energy is minimised by including structure (*b*) with a larger coefficient than (*c*) in the mesomeric system. (The greater stability of para- than of ortho-benzoquinones can be similarly understood.[70])

The conclusion that this type of mechanism produces deactivation receives further support from orientational data. For example, it is well known that when an ortho-para-orienting substituent of the $+E$ type and a strongly meta-orienting substituent of the $-I-M$ type stand in a meta-relation to each other, then, despite the opposition of steric hindrance, a third substituent often enters in the position between them. Thus, *m*-nitroanisole nitrates mainly in the 2-position, though also partly in the 4- and 6-positions;[71] while *m*-hydroxybenzaldehyde chlorinates mainly in the 2-position,[72] nitrates in the 2-, 4-, and 6-positions,[73] and brominates in the 4- and 6-positions, mainly the latter[74] (the conventional numbering is as indicated):

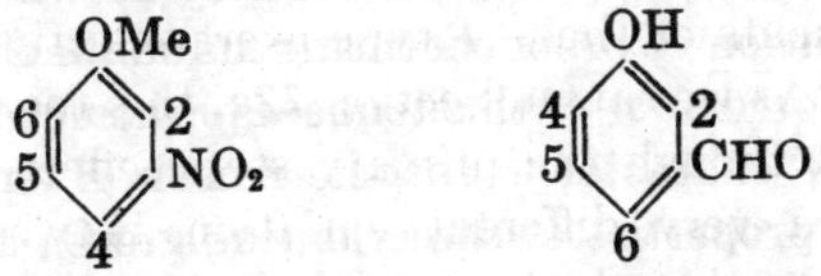

OMe (ring positions 2, 4, 5, 6; NO_2)   OH (ring positions 2, 4, 5, 6; CHO)

Substitution in the 2-position would be expected if dipolar structures such as (*b′*), of the general type of (*b*), were especially important in the mesomeric states of these molecules; for then the electromeric electron displacement, originating in the methoxyl or hydroxyl group, would have to emerge mainly in the 2-position:

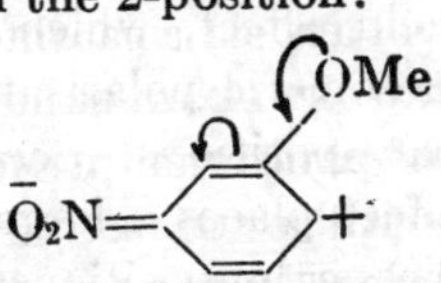

$$\bar{O}_2N{=}\langle\;\rangle{\overset{+}{}}\text{OMe} \qquad (b')$$

The fact that, although chlorination does take place almost entirely in the 2-position, nitration is diverted partly, and bromination almost wholly, to the 4- and 6-positions, can be ascribed to steric hindrance.

[70] The matter has been treated with quantal formalism in several variations, with results which are consistent with but, because of the assumptions and approximations made, add little to the conclusions derived from qualitative reasoning.

[71] A. F. Holleman, *Rec. trav. chim.*, 1903, **22**, 263.

[72] H. H. Hodgson and H. G. Beard, *J. Chem. Soc.*, **1926**, 147.

[73] P. Friedländer and O. Schenk, *Ber.*, 1914, **47**, 3040; H. H. Hodgson and H. G. Beard, *loc. cit.*

[74] H. H. Hodgson and H. G. Beard, *J. Chem. Soc.*, 1925, **127**, 876; **1926**, 147.

The series $Cl < NO_2 < Br$ is part of Holleman's series $Cl < NO_2 < Br < SO_3H$ for steric hindrance in its dependence on the entering group, and the reappearance here of dissimilar behaviour between two usually similar halogens is confirmation of Holleman's interpretation.

(22h) Physical Mechanism of the Electromeric Effect on the ortho-para-Ratio.—Orientation by the polarisability effect $+E$ obviously cannot be discussed except in relation to the reagent which stimulates the effect. As Waters has emphasized,[75] the transition state of substitution and the initial state of the aromatic system should be treated differentially in all discussions of orientation; and the need for this strictly correct approach will certainly be increased when an orienting group of $+E$ type produces a special factor of difference between the transition and initial states.

With this provision, and with suitable sign inversions, we may apply to the electromeric effect $+E$ on the ortho-para-ratio a physical theory which is just a simple extension of that outlined in the preceding Section in relation to the mesomeric effect $-M$.

We have to interpret the general tendency in $+E$ oriented substitutions to the formation of preponderating amounts of para-compounds; and also the reinforcement of this tendency when the introduced group has a strong $-M$ character. For the reason given in the preceding Section, the $+E$ properties of the orienting group, and the $-M$ character of the introduced group, are expected to co-operate more effectively to form a stable mesomeric state if these groups are para-situated, so that the shortest route through the conjugated system is as long as it can be, than if they are ortho, when the shortest route is shorter; and some part of such a difference of stability in the final ortho- and para-products will appear as a difference in the stabilities of the transition states of ortho- and para-substitution. This interprets the general predominance of para-orientation. If now the introduced group is changed to one with a stronger $-M$ character, say, from phenylazo- to *p*-nitrophenylazo-, or from nitro- to nitroso-, then we may expect that all energy effects due to conjugation between the orienting and entering groups will be scaled up, including the difference in the energies of the ortho- and para-transition states of substitution. This interprets the heightened tendency towards para-orientation of the stronger $-M$ substituents.

(23) MECHANISMS OF AROMATIC NITRATION

Having discussed the factors which determine the orientation in electrophilic aromatic substitution, we can be led on to consider the actual processes taking place at the localities thus determined. [illegible]

[75] W. A. Waters, *J. Chem. Soc.*, 1948, [illegible].

localisation during a charge transfer, should involve a larger uncertainty of electron position than the resonance system (c), in which two π-bonds could remain stationary during the transfer, and that, therefore, in accordance with the uncertainty principle, energy is minimised by including structure (b) with a larger coefficient than (c) in the mesomeric system. (The greater stability of para- than of ortho-benzoquinones can be similarly understood.[70])

The conclusion that this type of mechanism produces deactivation receives further support from orientational data. For example, it is well known that when an ortho-para-orienting substituent of the +E type and a strongly meta-orienting substituent of the −I−M type stand in a meta-relation to each other, then, despite the opposition of steric hindrance, a third substituent often enters in the position between them. Thus, m-nitroanisole nitrates mainly in the 2-position, though also partly in the 4- and 6-positions,[71] while m-hydroxybenzaldehyde chlorinates mainly in the 2-position,[72] nitrates in the 2-, 4-, and 6-positions,[73] and brominates in the 4- and 6-positions, mainly the latter[74] (the conventional numbering is as indicated):

OMe (6, 2, 5, 4; NO_2)   OH (4, 2, 5, 6; CHO)

Substitution in the 2-position would be expected if dipolar structures such as (b′), of the general type of (b), were especially important in the mesomeric states of these molecules, for then the electromeric electron displacement, originating in the methoxyl or hydroxyl group, would have to emerge mainly in the 2-position:

OMe, O_2N (b′)

The fact that, although chlorination does take place almost entirely in the 2-position, nitration is diverted partly, and bromination almost wholly, to the 4- and 6-positions, can be ascribed to steric hindrance.

The matter has been treated with quantal formalism in several variations, with results which are consistent with, but, because of the assumptions and approximations made, add little to the conclusions derived from qualitative reasoning.

[71] A. F. Holleman, Rec. trav. chim., 1903, 22, 263.

[72] H. H. Hodgson and H. G. Beard, J. Chem. Soc., 1926, 147.

[73] P. Friedländer and O. Schenk, Ber., 1914, 47, 3040; H. H. Hodgson and H. G. Beard, loc. cit.

[74] H. H. Hodgson and H. G. Beard, J. Chem. Soc., 1925, 127, 876; 1926, 147.

For the nitroso- and nitro-groups the theoretical argument is quite similar to that already given for the simple carbonyl group and the carboxyl group (Section 7e); the nitro-group (like the carboxyl group) contains an internal mesomeric system, which limits the extent to which the group as a whole can conjugate with the aromatic system, while the nitroso-group (like the carbonyl group) involves no such limitation:[67]

HO—⟨ ⟩—N=O   HO—⟨ ⟩—N—O (O)

Our conclusion up to this point is, then, that +E substituents, while they activate both ortho- and para-positions, selectively activate para-positions; and that they do this more strongly the more effectively the entering group can conjugate, through the aromatic ring, with the orienting substituent.

(22f) Physical Mechanism of Inductive Effects on the ortho-para-Ratio; and the Field Effect.—We must now take up the question of the physical mechanisms underlying polar effects on the ortho-para-ratio; and we begin with the inductive effects ±I.

The general view about this is that the influences on the ortho-para-ratio, which appear to be correlated with the inductive effect of the orienting substituent, are really due to its associated field effect,[68] that is, to the direct action of its electrostatic field (Sections 6f and 19e). As we saw in Section 21e, the inductive effect of an orienting substituent, operating on the reactive positions of the substrate molecule entirely through the intervening electronic system of the molecule, and the associated field effect, which makes use of partly external paths, [illegible] sign and magnitude, from one orienting group to another, in the same kind of

[67] An explicit demonstration of this difference between the nitroso- and nitro-group has been given by [illegible], 1931, 810.

[68] C. K. Ingold and C. C. N. Vass, J. Chem. Soc., 1928, 417; A. Lapworth and R. Robinson, Mem. Proc. Manchester Lit. & Phil. Soc., 1928, 72, 243.

way, wherefore they are often considered together under a generalised connotation of the term "inductive effect." However, in favourable circumstances, the inductive effect in its more specific sense, and the field effect, are phenomenologically distinguishable by reason of their differing distributions over the reactive positions. In electrophilic aromatic substitution, the field effect is outstandingly strong in ortho-positions, relatively to other positions: it is much weaker in meta- and para-positions, weakest in the latter. This makes its effect on the ortho/para ratio important in a way not affected by the circumstance that, theoretically, the field effect itself has two components, as discussed in Section **21e;** for these two components have qualitatively the same distribution over the reactive positions, and hence are not now phenomenologically separated.

The electropositive field effect on the ortho/para ratio is that orienting substituents of the $+I$ type will confer selective activation on ortho-positions. This, as we saw in Section **22c**, can be recognised in the observations, in spite of the opposing action of the primary steric effect. The electronegative field effect on the ortho/para ratio is that orienting substituents of the $-I$ type exert selective deactivation on ortho-positions. As we saw in Section **22c,** this too can be recognised in the data, even though the primary steric effect acts in the same sense (but with a very different variation between orienting substituents), and even though the special class of unsaturated orienting substituents, next to be considered, exert a selective deactivation on para-positions.

(22g) Physical Mechanism of the Mesomeric Effect on the ortho-para-Ratio.—This must be a selective *internal* polar effect: for, outweighing the associated field effect, which would selectively deactivate ortho-positions, a mesomeric polarisation $-M$ selectively and dominantly deactivates para-positions (Section **22d**). It must be concluded that the $-M$ effect places a larger positive charge on the para-position than on the ortho-positions. In other words, the mesomeric effect must produce a mesomeric state containing as component structures, besides non-polar structures (*a*), also dipolar structures (*b*) and (*c*); and it must contain structure (*b*) with a larger mixing coefficient than (*c*):

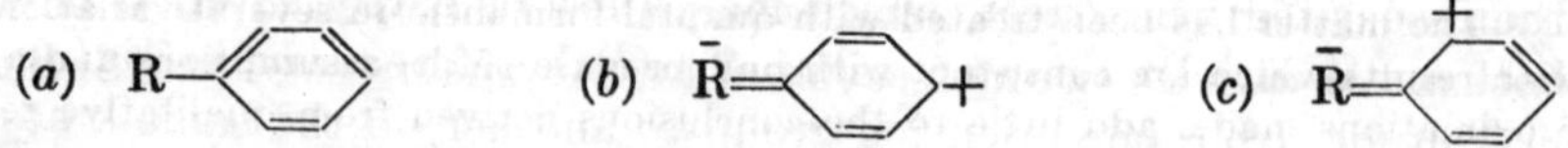

This conclusion has been emphasized by de la Mare especially.[69] A plausible theoretical argument can be indicated by noting that the resonance system (*a*)—(*b*), in which only one π bond can avoid de-

[69] P. B. D. de la Mare, *J. Chem. Soc.*, **1949, 2871.**

first of these equations is seen to represent the overall reaction which would result from an ionic dissociation of the oxide:

$$N_2O_5 = NO_2^+ + NO_3^-$$

(ii) The spectroscopic identification of the nitronium ion is concerned with two frequencies, 1400 and 1050 cm.$^{-1}$, which, in the Raman spectra of certain mixtures containing nitric acid, appear with such intensity that they could not belong to the nitric acid molecule. Médard first observed them[86] in the spectrum of mixtures of nitric and sulphuric acids. Susz and Briner obtained them[87] from solutions of dinitrogen pentoxide in nitric acid. Chédin investigated them extensively,[88] and most of our detailed knowledge of them is due to him. He discovered their weak appearance in the spectrum of nitric acid itself, thereby showing that they belong to a product of a self-reaction of nitric acid molecules. He proved that their source is a dehydration product of nitric acid, and is destroyed, with regeneration of molecular nitric acid, by water. All this indicated dinitrogen pentoxide as the source; but Chédin found that solutions of this substance in aprotic solvents gave quite a different spectrum. The conclusion was therefore drawn that the two frequencies arise from dinitrogen pentoxide in a special form. It was suggested that the special form might be an ionised form,[89] the frequency 1400 cm.$^{-1}$ belonging to the nitronium ion, and 1050 cm.$^{-1}$ to the nitrate ion, or, in the presence of sulphuric acid, to the hydrogen sulphate ion, consistently with the known spectra of these anions. Further spectroscopic study[90] confirmed these interpretations. The other Raman frequencies of the nitrate and hydrogen sulphate ions were found in the spectra of the relevant solutions. Strong appearances of the frequency 1400 cm.$^{-1}$ were obtained, without the simultaneous production of 1050 cm.$^{-1}$, by mixing nitric acid with perchloric or selenic acid: the spectra of the perchlorate or hydrogen selenate ions appeared, but they contain no frequency near 1050 cm.$^{-1}$ Finally, a close examination of spectra recorded under widely varying conditions showed that the source of the frequency 1400 cm.$^{-1}$ had only that frequency in its Raman spectrum. This limits the source to a diatomic molecule or a linear triatomic molecule with like end-

[86] L. Médard, *Compt. rend.*, 1934, **199**, 1615.

[87] B. Susz and E. Briner, *Helv. Chim. Acta,* 1935, **18**, 378.

[88] J. Chédin, *Compt. rend.*, 1935, **200**, 1397; 1935, **201**, 552, 714; 1936, **202**, 220, 1067; 1936, **203**, 772, 1509; *Ann. chim.*, 1937, **8**, 243.

[89] G. M. Bennett, J. C. D. Brand, and G. Williams, *J. Chem. Soc.*, **1946**, 869.

[90] C. K. Ingold, D. J. Millen, and H. G. Poole, *Nature*, 1946, **158**, 480; *J. Chem. Soc.*, **1950**, 2576.

Similar cryoscopic results have been recorded since.[79] Ultraviolet absorption spectra,[80] and electrical conductance values,[81] have been adduced in support of Hantzsch's conclusions. However, with the aid of improved cryoscopic technique, it has been found that the depression, by nitric acid, of the freezing-point of sulphuric acid is, not 3, but approximately 4 times that of an ideal solute;[82] and this points unmistakably to the conclusion that nitric acid is transformed into the nitronium ion, in accordance with the equation

$$HNO_3 + 2H_2SO_4 = NO_2^+ + H_3O^+ + 2HSO_4^-$$

There is no other way in which a 4-fold depression could be produced. As to the small deviation from an exactly 4-fold value, it was found that interionic attraction has a negligible effect on the freezing-points of the solutions;[83] but that water, although a strong base towards sulphuric acid, is not infinitely strong,[84] so that whenever those ions are formed, which appear on the right-hand side of the equation,

$$H_2O + H_2SO_4 = H_3O^+ + HSO_4^-$$

they partly recombine. From the independently evaluated equilibrium constant of this reaction, it was computed that the freezing-point depression given by nitric acid, when corrected for the small amount of reassociation of the water ions, becomes an exactly 4-fold depression. It follows that the conversion of nitric acid to nitronium ion is quantitative. In the same study it was found[85] that dinitrogen pentoxide, tetroxide, and trioxide give depressions close to 6 times that of an ideal solute; and that, when similarly corrected, these depressions become exactly 6-fold depressions. This shows that the three oxides are quantitatively converted into nitronium and nitrosonium ions, according to the following equations:

$$N_2O_5 + 3H_2SO_4 = 2NO_2^+ + H_3O^+ + 3HSO_4^-$$

$$N_2O_4 + 3H_2SO_4 = NO_2^+ + NO^+ + H_3O^+ + 3HSO_4^-$$

$$N_2O_3 + 3H_2SO_4 = 2NO^+ + H_3O^+ + 3HSO_4^-$$

Taking into account the reaction of nitric acid with sulphuric acid, the

[79] C. R. de Robles and E. Moles, *Anales fís. y quím.* (Madrid), 1935, 32, 474.

[80] A. Hantzsch, *Ber.*, 1925, 58, 941.

[81] M. Usanovich, *Acta Physicochim. U. R. S. S.*, 1935, 2, 239; 1935, 3, 703.

[82] R. J. Gillespie, J. Graham, E. D. Hughes, C. K. Ingold, and E. R. A. Peeling, *Nature*, 1946, 158, 480.

[83] R. J. Gillespie, E. D. Hughes, and C. K. Ingold, *J. Chem. Soc.*, 1950, 2473.

[84] R. J. Gillespie, *J. Chem. Soc.*, 1950, 2493.

[85] R. J. Gillespie, J. Graham, E. D. Hughes, C. K. Ingold, and E. R. A. Peeling, *J. Chem. Soc.*, 1950, 2504.

and nitrate ions.[92]

(iii) Hantzsch first showed that nitric and perchloric acids interact to form solid, salt-like compounds, which he believed to be the perchlorates of his protonated cations of nitric acid, $(H_2NO_3)^+(ClO_4)^-$ and $(H_3NO_3)^{++}(ClO_4)^-_2$. These experiments have been repeated with improved technique.[93] It has been found that the solids are really mixtures of nitronium perchlorate and hydroxonium perchlorate $(NO_2)^+(ClO_4)^-$ and $(H_3O)^+(ClO_4)^-$, formed by the reaction

$$HNO_3 + 2HClO_4 = NO_2^+ + H_3O^+ + 2ClO_4^-$$

Dinitrogen pentoxide and perchloric acid give the same two salts in other proportions.

$$N_2O_5 + 3HClO_4 = 2NO_2^+ + H_3O^+ + 3ClO_4^-$$

By crystallisation from nitromethane the pure nitronium salt $(NO_2)^+(ClO_4)^-$ was obtained. Other pure nitronium salts, including $(NO_2)^+(FSO_3)^-$, $(NO_2)^+(HS_2O_7)^-$, and $(NO_2)_2^+(S_2O_7)^{--}$ were prepared.[95] All these salts were shown to have ionic constitutions, the Raman spectra of the crystals consisting simply of the superposed known spectra of the ions indicated.[96] As Millen, Poole, and the writer recognised,[97] on the basis of Chédin and Pradier's spectral

[91] D. J. Millen, *J. Chem. Soc.*, 1950, 2606.

[92] C. K. Ingold and D. J. Millen, *J. Chem. Soc.*, 1950, 2612.

[93] A. Hantzsch, *Ber.*, 1925, 58, 953; A. Hantzsch and K. Berger, *Ber.*, 1928, 61, 1328.

[94] D. R. Goddard, E. D. Hughes, and C. K. Ingold, *Nature*, 1946, 158, 480; *J. Chem. Soc.*, 1950, 2559.

[95] It has been shown, both cryoscopically by R. J. Gillespie (*J. Chem. Soc.*, 1950, 2516), and spectroscopically by D. J. Millen (*ibid.*, p. 2589), that oleum contains at least two sulphuric acids higher than H_2SO_4 and $H_2S_2O_7$, namely, $H_2S_3O_{10}$ and $H_2S_4O_{13}$, together with the ions of all these acids. A nitronium salt of one of the higher acids has been prepared, namely, $(NO_2)_2^+(S_3O_{10})^{--}$.

[96] D. J. Millen, reported by D. R. Goddard, E. D. Hughes, and C. K. Ingold, *Nature*, 1946, 158, 480; D. J. Millen, *J. Chem. Soc.*, 1950, 2606.

[97] C. K. Ingold, D. J. Millen, and H. G. Poole, *Nature*, 1946, 158, 480.

separate problem for every kind of substitution, though we must expect a sufficient resemblance between the different reactions to justify their common classification as electrophilic substitutions. Nitration has played such an outstanding part in the development of the theory of orientation that it is natural to take it as a leading example in the study of mechanisms of substitution.

(23a) Existence of the Nitronium Ion.—Reference has been made several times already to nitration through the nitronium ion, NO_2^+. This is an old theory, having been proposed by Euler in 1903, and frequently supported on indirect grounds since that date,[76] but it was not established, and even the existence of the ion was not conclusively demonstrated, until 1946.[77] Since then many details have been filled in, as will be noted below.

The existence of the nitronium ion has been proved in four ways which do not depend on its behaviour in nitration. Its formation in large concentrations in certain solutions, notably in sulphuric acid solution, has been demonstrated (i) by cryoscopic measurements, and (ii) by spectroscopic studies on such solutions. Its identification as the cationic unit in ionic crystals has been established (iii) by the preparation, and spectroscopic study, of crystalline nitronium salts, and (iv) by X-ray analyses of certain nitronium salts. We will first review this evidence.

(i) Hantzsch made an extensive study of the effect of solutes on the freezing-point of sulphuric acid, and one of the solutes in which he was particularly interested was nitric acid, which he assumed to be converted into protonated forms:

$$HNO_3 + H_2SO_4 = H_2NO_3^+ + HSO_4^-$$

$$HNO_3 + 2H_2SO_4 = H_3NO_3^{++} + 2HSO_4^-$$

He obtained a range of depressions, by solute nitric acid, of the freezing-point of solvent sulphuric acid. They bracketed a value of 3 times that of an ideal solute.[78] Accordingly, he concluded that, in excess of sulphuric acid, nitric acid exists chiefly as the divalent cation $H_3NO_3^{++}$.

76 H. Euler, *Ann.*, 1903, **330**, 280; *Z. angew. Chem.*, 1922, **35**, 580; P. Walden, *ibid.*, 1924, **37**, 390; [illegible] and H. Eyring, *J. Chem. Phys.*, 1940, **8**, 433; C. C. Price, *Chem. Revs.*, 1941, **29**, 51; F. H. Westheimer and M. S. Kharasch, *J. Am. Chem. Soc.*, 1946, **68**, 1871; G. M. Bennett, J. C. D. Brand, and G. Williams, *J. Chem. Soc.*, 1946, 869.

77 E. D. Hughes, C. K. Ingold, and R. I. Reed, *Nature*, 1946, **158**, 448; R. J. Gillespie, J. Graham, E. D. Hughes, C. K. Ingold, and E. R. A. Peeling, *ibid.*, p. 480; C. K. Ingold, D. J. Millen, and H. G. Poole, *ibid.*; D. R. Goddard, E. D. Hughes, and C. K. Ingold, *ibid.* For a review see R. J. Gillespie and D. J. Millen, *Quart. Rev. Chem. Soc.*, 1948, **2**, 277.

78 A. Hantzsch, *Z. physik. Chem.*, 1908, **65**, 41.

first of these equations is seen to represent the overall reaction which would result from an ionic dissociation of the oxide:

$$N_2O_5 = NO_2^+ + NO_3^-$$

(ii) The spectroscopic identification of the nitronium ion is concerned with two frequencies, 1400 and 1050 cm.$^{-1}$, which, in the Raman spectra of certain mixtures containing nitric acid, appear with such intensity that they could not belong to the nitric acid molecule. Médard first observed them[86] in the spectrum of mixtures of nitric and sulphuric acids. Susz and Briner obtained them[87] from solutions of dinitrogen pentoxide in nitric acid. Chédin investigated them extensively,[88] and most of our detailed knowledge of them is due to him. He discovered their weak appearance in the spectrum of nitric acid itself, thereby showing that they belong to a product of a self-reaction of nitric acid molecules. He proved that their source is a dehydration product of nitric acid, and is destroyed, with regeneration of molecular nitric acid, by water. All this indicated dinitrogen pentoxide as the source; but Chédin found that solutions of this substance in aprotic solvents gave quite a different spectrum. The conclusion was therefore drawn that the two frequencies arise from dinitrogen pentoxide in a special form. It was suggested that the special form might be an ionised form,[89] the frequency 1400 cm.$^{-1}$ belonging to the nitronium ion, and 1050 cm.$^{-1}$ to the nitrate ion, or, in the presence of sulphuric acid, to the hydrogen sulphate ion, consistently with the known spectra of these anions. Further spectroscopic study[90] confirmed these interpretations. The other Raman frequencies of the nitrate and hydrogen sulphate ions were found in the spectra of the relevant solutions. Strong appearances of the frequency 1400 cm.$^{-1}$ were obtained, without the simultaneous production of 1050 cm.$^{-1}$, by mixing nitric acid with perchloric or selenic acid: the spectra of the perchlorate or hydrogen selenate ions appeared, but they contain no frequency near 1050 cm.$^{-1}$. Finally, a close examination of spectra recorded under widely varying conditions showed that the source of the frequency 1400 cm.$^{-1}$ had only that frequency in its Raman spectrum. This limits the source to a diatomic molecule or a linear triatomic molecule with like end-

86 L. Médard, *Compt. rend.*, 1934, **199**, 1615.

87 D. Susz and E. Briner, *Helv. Chim. Acta*, 1935, **18**, 378.

88 J. Chédin, *Compt. rend.*, 1935, **200**, 1397; 1935, **201**, 552, 714; 1936, **202**, 220, 1067; 1936, **203**, 772, 1509; *Ann. chim.*, 1937, **8**, 243.

89 G. M. Bennett, J. C. D. Brand, and G. Williams, *J. Chem. Soc.*, 1946, 869.

90 C. K. Ingold, D. J. Millen, and H. G. Poole, *Nature*, 1946, **158**, 480; *J. Chem. Soc.*, 1950, 2576.

Similar cryoscopic results have been recorded since.[79] Ultraviolet absorption spectra,[80] and electrical conductance values,[81] have been adduced in support of Hantzsch's conclusions. However, with the aid of improved cryoscopic technique, it has been found that the depression, by nitric acid, of the freezing-point of sulphuric acid is, not 3, but approximately 4 times that of an ideal solute;[82] and this points unmistakably to the conclusion that nitric acid is transformed into the nitronium ion, in accordance with the equation

$$HNO_3 + 2H_2SO_4 = NO_2^+ + H_3O^+ + 2HSO_4^-$$

There is no other way in which a 4-fold depression could be produced. As to the small deviation from an exactly 4-fold value, it was found that interionic attraction has a negligible effect on the freezing-points of the solutions;[83] but that water, although a strong base towards sulphuric acid, is not infinitely strong,[84] so that whenever those ions are formed, which appear on the right-hand side of the equation,

$$H_2O + H_2SO_4 = H_3O^+ + HSO_4^-$$

they partly recombine. From the independently evaluated equilibrium constant of this reaction, it was computed that the freezing-point depression given by nitric acid, when corrected for the small amount of reassociation of the water ions, becomes an exactly 4-fold depression. It follows that the conversion of nitric acid to nitronium ion is quantitative. In the same study it was found[85] that dinitrogen pentoxide, tetroxide, and trioxide give depressions close to 6 times that of an ideal solute; and that, when similarly corrected, these depressions become exactly 6-fold depressions. This shows that the three oxides are quantitatively converted into nitronium and nitrosonium ions, according to the following equations:

$$N_2O_5 + 3H_2SO_4 = 2NO_2^+ + H_3O^+ + 3HSO_4^-$$
$$N_2O_4 + 3H_2SO_4 = NO_2^+ + NO^+ + H_3O^+ + 3HSO_4^-$$
$$N_2O_3 + 3H_2SO_4 = 2NO^+ + H_3O^+ + 3HSO_4^-$$

Taking into account the reaction of nitric acid with sulphuric acid, the

[79] C. R. de Robles and E. Moles, *Anales fís. y quím.* (Madrid), 1935, **32**, 474.

[80] A. Hantzsch, *Ber.*, 1925, **58**, 941.

[81] M. Usanovich, *Acta Physicochim.*, *U. R. S. S.*, 1935, **2**, 239; 1935, **3**, 703.

[82] R. J. Gillespie, J. Graham, E. D. Hughes, C. K. Ingold, and E. R. A. Peeling, *Nature*, 1946, **158**, 480.

[83] R. J. Gillespie, E. D. Hughes, and C. K. Ingold, *J. Chem. Soc.*, **1950**, 2473.

[84] R. J. Gillespie, *J. Chem. Soc.*, **1950**, 2493.

[85] R. J. Gillespie, J. Graham, E. D. Hughes, C. K. Ingold, and E. R. A. Peeling, *J. Chem. Soc.*, 1950, 2504.

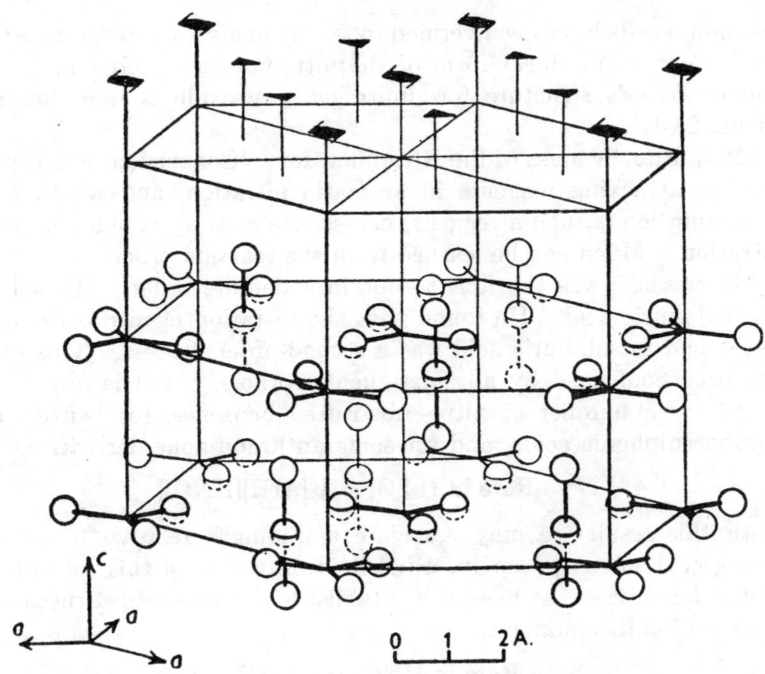

FIG. 23-1.—Schematic representation of the structure of N_2O_5. (Reproduced with permission from Grison, Ericks, and de Vries, *Acta Cryst.*, 1950, **3**, 293.)

data,[98] crystalline dinitrogen pentoxide is nitronium nitrate, $(NO_2)^+(NO_3)^-$. No covalency change occurs when it dissolves in nitric acid, the pre-formed ions simply falling apart, as when sodium chloride dissolves in water. However, it evaporates as covalent molecules, also like sodium chloride.[99] Other, conveniently stable, nitronium salts have since been prepared by Schmeisser and Elischer, and extensively by Olah and his collaborators.[100] Some of these salts are nowadays obtainable commercially, *e.g.*, $(NO_2)^+(BF_4)^-$, $(NO_2)^+(PF_6)^-$, $(NO_2)^+(AsF_6)^-$, and $(NO_2)^+(SbF_6)^-$.

(iv) In two examples, namely, nitronium perchlorate, and nitronium nitrate (dinitrogen pentoxide),[101,102] the ionic constitutions of

[98] J. Chédin and J. C. Pradier, *Compt. rend.*, 1936, **203**, 722.

[99] Concerning the energy relations involved in these comparisons, especially with reference to the volatility differences, see D. J. Millen, *loc. cit.*

[100] M. Schmeisser and S. Elischer, *Z. Naturforsch.*, 1952, **7b**, 583; S. J. Kuhn and G. A. Olah, *J. Am. Chem. Soc.*, 1961, **83**, 4570.

[101] F. G. Cox, G. A. Jeffery, and M. R. Truter, *Nature*, 1948, **162**, 259; M. R. Truter, D. J. Cruikshank, and G. A. Jeffery, *Acta Cryst.*, 1960, **13**, 855.

[102] P. E. Grison, K. Ericks, and J. L. de Vries, *Acta Cryst.*, 1950, **3**, 290.

nitronium salts have been verified by X-ray analyses. Both investigations confirm the linear form of the nitronium ion. Grison, Ericks, and de Vries's structure for dinitrogen pentoxide is reproduced in Figure 23-1.

(23b) Effectiveness of the Nitronium Ion.—Conclusions about what are the attacking reagents in aromatic nitration, and whether the nitronium iòn is such a reagent, necessitate a study of the kinetics of nitration. Much can be learned from the reaction order.

Martinsen[103] was the first to obtain a definite order. His solvent was sulphuric acid. He found that the nitration of nitrobenzene by nitric acid in sulphuric acid was a second-order process. This result has been confirmed by all subsequent workers,[104] and is now established for a number of nitro-substituted benzenes, for benzoic and benzenesulphonic acids, and for some anthraquinone derivatives:

$$\text{Rate in } H_2SO_4 = k_2[\text{ArH}][\text{HNO}_3] \qquad (1)$$

With this result we may associate a finding[105] relative to another strong-acid solvent, namely, nitric acid: nitration in this solvent is a first-order process, as has been established for nitro-substituted benzenes and anthraquinones:

$$\text{Rate in } HNO_3 = k_1[\text{ArH}] \qquad (2)$$

This equation is what the previous one would become if nitric acid were in constant excess, as it necessarily is, when it is the solvent.

These results show only that the attacking reagent, if not nitric acid, is formed so rapidly from it as to bear a constant ratio to it. One cannot deduce from the kinetic results alone whether the ratio is large or small.

More informative results have been secured by the study of nitration in organic solvents, especially nitromethane and acetic acid, usually with nitric acid in constant excess over the aromatic compound.[106] The reaction order now depends on the reactivity of the benzene derivative as found by the competition method (Section **21a**). For aro-

[103] H. Martinsen, *Z. physik. Chem.*, 1904, **50,** 385; *ibid.*, 1907, **59,** 605.

[104] A. Klemenc and K. Schöller, *Z. anorg. u. allgem. Chem.*, 1924, **141,** 231; K. Lauer and R. Oda, *J. prakt. Chem.*, 1936, **144,** 176; *Ber.*, 1936, **69,** 1061; R. Oda and U. Ueda, *Bull. Inst. Phys. Chem. Research* (Tokyo), 1941, **20,** 335; F. H. Westheimer and M. S. Kharasch, *J. Am. Chem. Soc.*, 1946, **68,** 1871; G. M. Bennett, J. C. D. Brand, D. M. James, T. J. Saunders, and G. Williams, *J. Chem. Soc.*, **1947,** 474.

[105] E. D Hughes, C. K. Ingold, and R. I. Reed, *J. Chem. Soc.*, **1950,** 2400.

[106] G. A. Benford and C. K. Ingold, *J. Chem. Soc.*, **1938,** 929; E. D. Hughes, C. K. Ingold, and R. I. Reed, *Nature*, 1946, **158,** 448; *J. Chem. Soc.*, **1950,** 2400.

matic compounds more reactive than benzene, and in some conditions for benzene itself, the reaction order is zeroth. This means that nitration proceeds at a constant rate, independently of the concentration of aromatic compound, coming to a sudden stop only when no more of the latter is left. All compounds which obey this law—benzene, toluene, ethylbenzene, *p*-xylene, mesitylene, and *p*-chloroanisole have been compared—nitrate at the same rate:

Rate for sufficiently reactive aromatic compounds in organic solvents
$$= k_0 \text{ (with } HNO_3 \text{ in constant excess)} \quad (3)$$

For benzene itself in some conditions, and always for fluoro- and iodobenzene, which by the competition test are somewhat less reactive than benzene (see Section **21a**, Table 21-1), there is a slight degree of dependence of rate on concentration; and for chloro- and bromo-benzene, which are somewhat less reactive still (Table 21-1), there is more dependence. So, the degree of dependence increases as the reactivity decreases; but there is a limit. The limit is attained with two deactivating halogen substituents, as in a dichlorobenzene; and it is a definite limit, not surpassed, for instance, in a trichlorobenzene. It can be reached by the use of a single, more strongly deactivating, substituent, such as the carbethoxyl group of ethyl benzoate (Table 21-1). This limiting dependence of rate on concentration is simple proportionality; that is, the reactions are of first order. And, naturally, the rate constants for those compounds which obey the law are different, standing in the relation to be expected from the deactivating effects of the substituents, as determined by the competition method:

Rate for sufficiently unreactive aromatic compounds in organic
$$\text{solvents} = k_1 [ArH] \text{ (with } HNO_3 \text{ in constant excess)} \quad (4)$$

Of the results summarised in equations (1)–(4) above, it is those of equation (3) which directly give the answer to the mechanistic problem. Zeroth-order nitration means that the reaction being measured, the slow process, is one in which the aromatic compound takes no part; and that something which that process produces is taken up, as fast as it becomes available, by the aromatic compound, which thereby becomes nitrated. The slow process is not specific to the solvent, because chemically different solvents give the same kinetic phenomena. It must therefore be a process of the nitric acid. Now it cannot be simply a proton transfer, if, as we believe, proton transfers are instantaneous in oxy-acids. It has an activation energy, and therefore must break a bond of nitric acid. Further, the process must be heterolytic, because it has to produce an electrophilic nitrating agent, that is, an even-electron fragment containing the group NO_2 with electron-deficient nitrogen. There is only one possibility: instantaneous proton transfers being disregarded, the fundamental heterolysis must be as shown; and its product, which the reactive benzene derivatives consume as it is formed, is the nitronium ion:[107]

$$H{-}O{-}\vdots N(=O){-}O \rightarrow HO^- + NO_2^+$$

The results summarised in equations (1), (2), and (4) are consistent with this conclusion, though they could not alone have produced it. In the strong acid solvents the nitronium ion is rapidly formed, and constitutes a constant fraction of the stoicheiometric nitric acid. We know from physical evidence that in sulphuric acid that fraction is close to unity, while in nitric acid it is fairly close to zero; but this distinction does not emerge from the kinetic evidence.[108] The kinetic orders depend simply on the rapidity of the conversion (equations 1 and 2).

In organic solvents, however, the nitronium ion is formed at a measurable rate, that is, just as fast as one would measure it in any zeroth-order reaction. But by using sufficiently unreactive aromatic compounds, one can allow it, even at this speed, to set up a stationary concentration, from which the aromatic compound takes what it needs, according to its concentration and reactivity (equation 4).

Water as a solvent acts much like the organic solvents considered above. The important common properties of these solvents are, first, that they are polar and so able to solvate ions, and second that, not being acids stronger than nitric acid, they are media in which the nitronium ions can be formed measurably slowly. In order to identify

[107] Proton transfers subsequent to a slow stage are kinetically insignificant. Therefore if we should consider heterolysing one of the other oxygen atoms to give O^{--} and HNO_2^{++}, an instantaneous proton transfer would regenerate NO_2^+: and so the conclusion is still that the formed, and effective, reagent is NO_2^+.

[108] W. H. Lee and D. J. Millen have shown by a study of its electrical conductance that analytically pure nitric acid contains dissociation products in the concentrations

$$[NO_2^+] = [NO_3^-] = [H_2O] = \begin{cases} 0.51\ M \text{ at } -10° \\ 0.61\ M \text{ at } -20° \end{cases}$$

This means that 4–5% by weight of analytically pure and dry nitric acid is dissociated according to the equation

$$2HNO_3 \rightarrow NO_2^+ + NO_3^- + H_2O$$

at these temperatures (*J. Chem. Soc.*, **1956**, 4463).

the nitrating agent in an aqueous medium, one must work with aromatic compounds which, besides being water-soluble, are reactive enough to allow them, if they are indeed nitrated by the nitronium ion, to seize this entity before the much more plentiful water turns it back again into nitric acid. This considerable feat was accomplished by Bunton and Halevi.[109] Their media were mixtures of about 40 moles of nitric acid with 60 moles of water, and their water-soluble substrates were sodium arylalkanesulphonates, such as the mesitylene-1*a*-sulphonate and the *iso*durene-2*a*-sulphonate, which contain several activating methyl substituents:

$$\text{3,5-}(CH_3)_2C_6H_3{-}CH_2\cdot SO_3^- \qquad \text{2,4,6-}(CH_3)_3C_6H_2{-}CH_2\cdot SO_3^-$$

These substrates were nitrated in two kinetic forms depending on substrate concentration. At concentrations in the millimolar range, the kinetic order was first in the substrate; but at concentrations of several tenths molar, the order in substrate became zeroth.

Rate at low substrate concentrations in aqueous nitric acid $= k_1$ [ArH] (with HNO_3 in constant excess) (5)

Rate at high substrate concentrations in aqueous nitric acid $= k_0$ (with HNO_3 in constant excess) (6)

The two results together establish nitration by the nitronium ion, even under these aqueous conditions, in which the stationary concentration of nitronium ion must be far below the limits of the known methods of spectroscopic detection. At low concentrations these substrates, as equation (5) represents, are not able to trap the nitronium ions, each as it is formed in the aqueous medium, and most of these ions fall victim to the surrounding water. But at high concentrations, as equation (6) shows, the substrates can and do seize nearly all the nitronium ions, despite the enveloping water. The measured rate of nitration is then the rate of the purely inorganic bond-breaking process, in which the nitronium ion is produced.

As we shall note in Chapter VIII, this zeroth-order rate is identical with the rate of ^{18}O-exchange between the nitric acid and the water—an independent proof that the bond broken is indeed an N—O bond

[109] C. A. Bunton, E. A. Halevi, and D. R. Llewellyn, *J. Chem. Soc.*, **1952**, 4913; C. A. Bunton and E. A. Halevi, *ibid.*, p. 4917; C. A. Bunton and G. Stedman, *ibid.*, **1958**, 2420.

of nitric acid, and that the nitrating agent is produced by that bond-breaking process.

(23c) Mechanism of Formation of the Nitronium Ion.—In the absence of definite evidence, it could have been supposed that the nitronium ion is formed from nitric acid by a single-stage bimolecular heterolysis:

$$HNO_3 + HNO_3 \rightarrow NO_2^+ + NO_3^- + H_2O$$

A transition state, capable of breaking in the required way, is easily conceivable.

It has been shown, however, that two stages are involved, as follows:

$$HNO_3 + HNO_3 \overset{\text{fast}}{\rightleftharpoons} H_2NO_3^+ + NO_3^-$$

$$H_2NO_3^+ \xrightarrow{\text{slow}} H_2O + NO_2^+$$

In its first stage, the scheme, as written, represents a special case of a more general mechanism. For the two molecules of nitric acid function differently: the first merely supplies a proton to the second, which is the real source of the nitronium ion. So the first molecule could be replaced by a molecule of any sufficiently strong acid, and the mechanism would, in essence, be the same. The second stage can be pictured in the form

$$O_2N\text{—}\overset{+}{O}H_2 \rightarrow O_2N^+ + OH_2$$

which is a unimolecular heterolysis, analogous to some in carbon chemistry that lead to carbonium ions, as we shall observe in Chapter VII.

The actual evidence on the matter comes from the study[105] of the effect of added strong acids, of added ionised nitrates, and of added water, on rates of zeroth-order nitrations, and on rates of first-order nitrations, in organic solvents. The main results are as follows: (1) Very small amounts of sulphuric acid strongly accelerate both reactions, the rates increasing linearly with the concentrations of added acid over certain ranges. (2) Very small amounts of nitrate ions strongly retard both reactions, the reciprocals of the rates now increasing linearly with added nitrate over certain ranges. (3) Alike in zeroth- and first-order nitrations, the large rate changes produced by added acid or nitrate do not entail any disturbance to the reaction order. (4) Relatively to these effects, water has a negligible effect on the rate of the zeroth-order reaction; but the addition of much more water reduces the rate; and, accompanying a strong reduction, the zeroth-order reaction goes over into a first-order reaction.

Results (1) and (2) would be consistent with either the one-step or the two-step mechanism of formation of nitronium ion. These results show that the mechanism contains a reversible step, in the forward direction of which one proton is taken up and one nitrate ion is produced. The key to the mechanistic problem lies among the four findings summarised as result (3). The crucial finding is that nitrate ions strongly retard zeroth-order nitrations without disturbing their zeroth-order character. This shows that the formation of nitronium ion, which is rate-controlling for zeroth-order nitration, must itself consist of two steps. For one step, *viz.*, that in which nitrate ion is produced, is easily and strongly reversed. But another step, *viz.*, that in which nitronium ion is produced, is not so reversed, because, in zeroth-order nitration, the nitronium ion is trapped, as it is produced, by the aromatic compound. So there must be two steps, the first nitrate-ion-producing, and the second and final step nitronium-ion-producing. This being the case, material balance and charge balance fully determine the stoicheiometry, as written above for the two-step mechanism. The remaining experimental results are consistent with this mechanism. Water is not produced in the easily reversed stage; and therefore water does not affect the rate, comparably to nitrate ion. But when much more water is added, then the second stage becomes reversed, and nitration is strongly retarded; and then nitration goes over, as it should, from a zeroth-order into a first-order reaction.

These observations prove that the nitric acidium ion, $H_2NO_3^+$, has a separate existence, although it is not in itself a nitrating agent in the conditions, and has, indeed, never been shown to be a nitrating agent in any conditions, not even of aqueous nitration. The nitric acidium ion has not been proved to be present in high concentration in any solution; nor has any of its salts been isolated.

(23d) Mechanism of Attack by the Nitronium Ion.—Two theories have been set up concerning the process by which the nitronium ion attaches itself to the aromatic ring with expulsion of the proton. One is that the introduction of the nitronium ion, and the transference of the proton to an external base, constitute a single-stage termolecular process, which we may label S_E3. In formulating it, the proton-accepting base is written A^-, in recognition of the circumstance that, in acid media, the strongest available base is usually the anion of the acid:

$$NO_2^+ + ArH + A^- \rightarrow NO_2\cdot Ar + HA \qquad (S_E3)$$

This apparently plausible theory is no longer entertained.[110]

[110] It has been pointed out that the secondary rate phenomena which were held to support the termolecular mechanism have other explanations (R. J.

The second, and the accepted, theory is that two stages are involved,[111] a slow uptake of nitronium ion being followed by rapid transfer of the proton. Since the rate-determining stage is bimolecular, we label this mechanism S_E2:

$$\left.\begin{array}{l} NO_2^+ + ArH \xrightarrow{\text{slow}} \overset{+}{Ar}\Big\langle{}^{H}_{NO_2} \\ \overset{+}{Ar}\Big\langle{}^{H}_{NO_2} + A^- \xrightarrow{\text{fast}} ArNO_2 + HA \end{array}\right\} \qquad (S_E2)$$

One reason why the termolecular mechanism was never really tenable is that, by a well-established theory, to be outlined and illustrated in Chapter VII, concerning solvent effects on reaction rate, a process, such as S_E3, in which ionic charges disappear, should be impeded by polar solvents; but aromatic nitrations go particularly well in polar solvents. It is true that this effect is due essentially to solvent action on the processes which produce the nitronium ion; but it could not control the solvent effect on the overall nitration, if the effect on the last stage, or on any essential forward stage, were strongly in the opposite direction. A more detailed analysis,[105] based on a study of solvent effects on the zeroth- and first-order reactions, and on reaction-order itself, has shown that, while an increase in polarity of the solvent does, indeed, accelerate strongly the formation of the nitronium ion, such solvent changes have a relatively negligible effect on the rate of attack by the nitronium ion on the aromatic molecule. This excludes mechanism S_E3, but is consistent with mechanism S_E2, the rate-controlling stage of which neither creates nor destroys ionic charges.

A succinct proof that the proton-transfer stage in nitronium-ion attack is a separate step, because it is not kinetically significant in the nitronium-ion nitrations investigated, has been provided by Melander.[111] He used the principle that bonds holding isotopic hydrogen atoms differ considerably in zero-point energy, while only part of such difference appears in the transition states of reactions which break the bonds, because the partly broken bonds have smaller vibrational quanta: this leads to differences of activation energy, and of rate. It is experimentally well established that protium and deuterium are displaced from similar states of combination, in a variety of reactions, at

---

Gillespie and D. J. Millen, *Quart. Rev. Chem. Soc.*, 1948, **2,** 277; R. J. Gillespie, E. D. Hughes, C. K. Ingold, D. J. Millen, and R. I. Reed, *Nature*, 1949, **163,** 599; R. J. Gillespie and D. G. Norton, *J. Chem. Soc.*, **1952,** 971).

[111] L. Melander, *Nature*, 1949, **163,** 599; *Acta Chem. Scand.*, 1949, **3,** 95; *Arkiv Kemi*, 1950, **2,** 213; cf. T. G. Bonner, F. Bowyer, and Gwyn Williams, *J. Chem. Soc.*, **1953,** 2650.

widely different rates; protium usually from 3 to 10 times faster then deuterium. The corresponding factors of difference for protium and tritium would range from about 5 to about 25. Melander used tritium, his method being to nitrate a benzene compound containing tritium in one of two or more otherwise equivalent positions, benzene with one tritium atom, toluene with one ortho-tritium atom, and so on. He found that, to within his experimental error, there was no selection of protium rather than tritium for displacement by the entering nitro-group. This proves conclusively that the expulsion of the aromatic proton is not involved in the rate-determining stage of nitronium ion attack. The same point is shown just as conclusively in Bonner, Bowyer, and Gwyn Williams's demonstration[111] that the rate of nitration of nitrobenzene and of pentadeuteronitrobenzene in mixed acids are identical.

As to the geometrical form of the intermediate cation, it seems very probable that the groups H and NO_2 are bound by tetrahedral bonds:

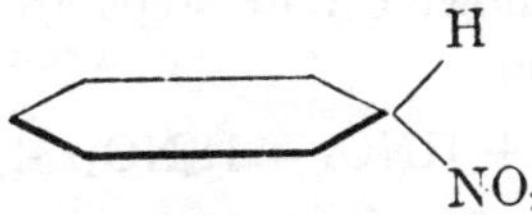

H

NO_2

The structure is that of a *cyclo*hexadienylium ion, and the ionic charge is distributed between the ortho- and para-positions. An equivalent statement is that the ion is mesomeric, with the following principal valency structures:

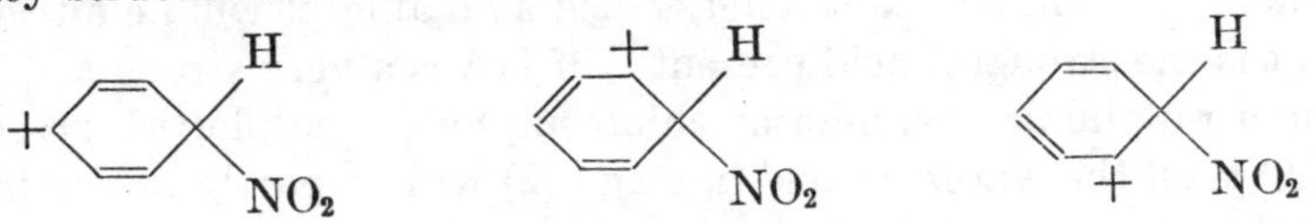

H + H H

\+

NO_2 NO_2 + NO_2

The assumption of intermediates of this type in aromatic substitution generally was first made by Pfeiffer and Wizinger.[112] It has been supported by Wheland on theoretical grounds.[113] Salts of such intermediate cations have been isolated, in some cases by the use of low temperatures, for several types of electrophilic aromatic substitution. Thus, on nitrating benzotrifluoride with nitryl fluoride and boron trifluoride (which make nitronium tetrafluoroborate), Olah and Kuhn obtained the intermediate formulated below as a yellow crystalline salt, which was stable below $-50°$, but above that temperature decomposed by proton transfer to give *m*-nitrobenzotrifluoride.[114]

[112] P. Pfeiffer and R. Wizinger, *Ann.*, 1928, **461**, 132.
[113] G. W. Wheland, *J. Am. Chem. Soc.*, 1942, **64**, 1900.
[114] G. A. Olah and S. J. Kuhn, *J. Am. Chem. Soc.*, 1958, **80**, 6541.

$$C_6H_5CF_3 + NO_2F + BF_3 \rightarrow \left[C_6H_5(CF_3)(NO_2)(H)^+ \right] BF_4^- \rightarrow CF_3C_6H_4NO_2 + HF + BF_3$$

The occurrence of additive intermediates does not affect our designation of the mechanism as S_E2, which implies no more than it expresses, *viz.*, an electrophilic substitution in which two reactants are covalently involved in the transition state. The symbol is silent about the number of steps in the mechanism, and, if several, about which is rate controlling. It is designedly silent about much else, and, like other such symbols, is a class designation, unelaborate because it does not seek to distinguish varieties within its class.

To summarise, the following four steps are recognised as essential to nitration by nitric acid:

$$HA + HNO_3 = H_2NO_3^+ + A^- \quad (1)$$

$$H_2NO_3^+ = NO_2^+ + H_2O \quad (2)$$

$$NO_2^+ + ArH = ArHNO_2^+ \quad (3)$$

$$ArHNO_2^+ + A^- = ArNO_2 + HA \quad (4)$$

The acid HA will be the strongest acid available: it will be nitric acid, if that is the strongest acid present. If HA is a very strong acid, such as fluorosulphonic, perchloric, chlorosulphonic, sulphuric, or selenic acid,[114] then the water formed in stage (2) will be partly or completely ionised:

$$HA + H_2O = H_3O^+ + A^- \quad (5)$$

Nitric acid is not a strong enough acid thus to ionise water as a base to an appreciable degree under nitration conditions; but the nitric acidium ion is, and the equilibrium

$$H_2NO_3^+ + H_2O = H_3O^+ + HNO_3 \quad (6)$$

has been shown to have a minor, but appreciable, effect on nitration kinetics.[105]

(23e) Carriers of the Nitronium Ion.—Structures more complex than NO_2^+ can attack, and leave a nitro-group in an aromatic molecule: it is convenient to call such structures "carriers" of the nitronium ion. A carrier NO_2X is expected to be a better nitrating agent the more strongly X attracts electrons, and thus the series,

$$NO_2^+, \quad NO_2 \cdot OH_2^+, \quad NO_2 \cdot ONO_2, \quad NO_2 \cdot OBz, \quad NO_2 \cdot OH$$

should illustrate progressively decreasing nitrating power. It is interesting to try to observe how far along the series a practical degree of nitrating power survives: the difficulty in doing so is to distinguish direct nitration by NO_2X from nitration by NO_2^+ formed from NO_2X.

As we have seen, the nitric acidium ion seems not to be a nitrating agent in any known conditions. It acts only by generating nitronium ion.

Covalent dinitrogen pentoxide in carbon tetrachloride solution appears to be a nitrating agent, though complications arise from the ease with which this molecule gives the nitronium ion, when any species is present that can solvate an ion.[115] Simple second-order kinetics can be realised:

$$\text{Rate by } N_2O_5 \text{ in } CCl_4 = k_2[N_2O_5][ArH]$$

But, normally, this reaction is overlaid by an autocatalytic process, or rather, a family of autocatalytic processes, of high order, depending on the nitric acid formed during nitration. The kinetic equation is

$$\text{Rate by } N_2O_5\text{—}HNO_3 \text{ in } CCl_4 = k[N_2O_5][ArH][HNO_3]^n$$

where n is typically 3, and probably has the range 2–4. The second-order reaction can be isolated from the catalysed reaction by using low concentrations (for obvious reasons), and not too low temperatures (since high-order reactions have low temperature-coefficients). It is held to represent direct nitration by molecular dinitrogen pentoxide. The catalysed processes can be given practically exclusive importance by adding extra nitric acid. They are ascribed to nitration by the nitronium ion, which is produced when either formed or added nitric acid ionises some of the dinitrogen pentoxide. The minimal number of nitric acid molecules that we can imagine as effective in ionising a dinitrogen pentoxide molecule is two, that is, one molecule to "solvate" each ion. The total number which solvate the pair of ions in solvent nitric acid is four.[116] Thus the estimated values of the exponent n seem not unreasonable.

The series of directly acting nitrating agents appears to stop here. An investigation[117] of benzoyl nitrate, to which acetyl nitrate seems closely similar, has shown that it acts, not as such, but as a regulating

[115] V. Gold, E. D. Hughes, C. K. Ingold, and G. H. Williams, *J. Chem. Soc.*, **1950**, 2452.

[116] R. J. Gillespie, E. D. Hughes, and C. K. Ingold, *J. Chem. Soc.*, **1950**, 2552.

[117] V. Gold, E. D. Hughes, and C. K. Ingold, *J. Chem. Soc.*, **1950**, 2467.

medium for the supply of low-concentration dinitrogen pentoxide, through the acid-catalysed disproportionation,

$$2NO_2 \cdot OBz = N_2O_5 + Bz_2O$$

In its turn, the dinitrogen pentoxide acts, as shown above, almost entirely by ionising to give nitronium ion. Paul's observation that very small amounts of added sodium nitrate strongly reduce the rate of nitration by nitric acid in solvent acetic anhydride, that is, by acetyl nitrate, is consistent with this finding.[118]

No evidence has been forthcoming that molecular nitric acid, as such, nitrates any substance in any circumstances.

The short summary is that compounds NO_2X which nitrate at all do so predominantly or exclusively by the ionizing mechanism:

$$NO_2X \rightarrow NO_2^+ + X^-$$

$$NO_2^+ + ArH \rightarrow ArNO_2 + H^+$$

The channelling of the reactions of all substituting agents through their common cationic intermediate is characteristic of aromatic nitration and is not a common property of electrophilic aromatic substitutions generally.

(23f) Effect of Nitrous Acid on Nitronium-Ion Nitration.—By "nitrous acid" is meant material in a nitration solution which, after dilution with water, may be estimated as nitrous acid. The effect of added, or of adventitious, nitrous acid on rate of nitration by the nitronium-ion mechanism constitutes a complication in the elucidation of the mechanism, which is easily avoided by the use of media free from nitrous acid. This is why it has not been mentioned hitherto. But it is a necessary part of the background of the investigation of the group of nitration processes next to be described.

Nitrous acid retards nitration by the nitronium-ion mechanism. Before the explanation was known, it was empirically discovered[106] that the law of the retardation, for low concentrations of nitrous acid, is expressed by including in the kinetic equations for the zeroth- and first-order processes, a further common factor, so that they read,

$$\text{Rate} = k_0(1 + a[\text{HNO}_2]^{\frac{1}{2}})^{-1}$$

$$\text{Rate} = k_1[\text{ArH}](1 + a[\text{HNO}_2]^{\frac{1}{2}})^{-1}$$

nitric acid being in constant excess (HNO_2=*analytical* HNO_2).

The cause of this anticatalysis is now understood.[105] It depends on the following inorganic-chemical relations, which have been inde-

[118] M. A. Paul, *J. Am. Chem. Soc.*, 1958, **80**, 5329; cf. J. H. Ridd, "Studies in Chemical Structure and Mechanism," Methuen, London, 1966, Chap. 7.

pendently established,[119] partly by spectroscopic means and partly by electrical conductance and transport measurements. Nitrous acid exists in excess of nitric acid essentially in the form of dinitrogen tetroxide. To a small extent this is homolysed to nitrogen dioxide, but that is not important in the present connexion. It is also heterolysed, that is, ionised, nearly completely in a pure nitric acid solvent, but only as a weak electrolyte in organic solvents containing nitric acid; and the ions are the nitrosonium ion and the nitrate ion:

$$2NO_2 \rightleftarrows N_2O_4 \rightleftarrows NO^+ + NO_3^-$$

In a nitration, the nitrate ions thus formed deprotonate nitric acidium ion, the precursor of the nitronium ion, as already described for added ionising nitrates; and thus nitrous acid retards nitration. It is easy to verify that this mechanism leads to the kinetic equations given.

With higher concentrations of nitrous acid, and in the presence of some water, a stronger form of anticatalysis by nitrous acid sets in. The explanation is that, in the circumstances indicated, a small, but kinetically effective, fraction of the nitrous acid exists as dinitrogen trioxide, formed in the balanced reaction

$$2N_2O_4 + H_2O \rightleftarrows N_2O_3 + 2HNO_3$$

This oxide is also slightly homolyzed, and appreciably heterolysed, the ions being the nitrosonium ion and the nitrite ion:

$$NO + NO_2 \rightleftarrows N_2O_3 \rightleftarrows NO^+ + NO_2^-$$

The nitrite ion, as the stronger base, is specifically much more effective, than is the nitrate ion, in deprotonating the nitric acidium ion, and thus depressing the rate of nitration. A short calculation shows that this new effect should be expressed by adding to the anticatalytic factor another term, so that the generalised factor reads

$$(1 + a[H\dot{N}O_2]^{\frac{1}{2}} + b[HNO_2]^{\frac{3}{2}})^{-1}$$

By suitably adjusting concentrations, it is readily possible to arrange that the last term in this polynomial is so large that the others may be neglected; and in this simplified form the expanded kinetic expression has been experimentally verified.

(23g) Nitration through Nitrosation.—It has long been known that there are two groups of aromatic compounds in whose nitrations nitrous acid is often a positive catalyst, in sharp contrast to what has just been stated about the nitration of aromatic compounds in general. These two groups are the derivatives, including the alkylation products,

[119] J. D. S. Goulden and D. J. Millen, *J. Chem. Soc.*, **1950**, 2620.

of phenol and aniline. Two questions are hereby raised: How does this happen? And why is it special to phenol and aniline derivatives?

Before the first of these questions can be answered on experimental grounds, a troublesome complication has to be eliminated. It is that some of those aromatic compounds, whose nitrations are positively catalysed by nitrous acid, are also appreciably oxidised under nitration conditions. This is a side-reaction, in which we have no immediate interest; but it produces nitrous acid, and so the positive catalysis becomes an autocatalysis. Phenol behaves like this, and so also, to a smaller degree, does anisole. But through a judicious amount of deactivation of the nucleus by substitution, oxidation can be stopped, while the positive catalysis by nitrous acid remains. This happens, for example, in *p*-nitrophenol and *p*-chloroanisole.

An investigation[120] of the kinetics of nitration of these and similar compounds by nitric acid in constant excess in solvent acetic acid has shown that the total reaction, although at first sight complicated, actually consists of two concurrent reactions, which, separately, are simple. They can be separated nearly completely by suitable adjustments of conditions. One of them is found to have the familiar form,

$$\text{Rate} = k_0(1 + a[\text{HNO}_2]^{\frac{1}{2}})^{-1}$$

which is diagnostic of nitronium-ion nitration: that it is the zeroth-order variety of this process is to be expected from the high reactivities of the aromatic compounds. The other is a new reaction, which has the following form (again HNO_2 means *analytical* HNO_2):

$$\text{Rate} = k_2[\text{ArH}][\text{HNO}_2]$$

Evidently this is the reaction to which the positive catalysis is due. It can be made almost negligible by cutting out the nitrous acid as completely as possible, and raising the nitric acid concentration sufficiently to make nitronium ion freely available; or it can be made dominating by working with much nitrous acid, and reducing the nitric acid concentration.

The kinetics of the catalysed process give strong support to the theory that they depend on an initial nitrosation, followed by a rapid oxidation of the formed nitroso-compound by the nitric acid, with restoration of the nitrous acid consumed in the initial slow stage:

$$\text{ArH} + \text{HNO}_2 \xrightarrow{\text{slow}} \text{ArNO} + \text{H}_2\text{O}$$

$$\text{ArNO} + \text{HNO}_3 \xrightarrow{\text{fast}} \text{ArNO}_2 + \text{HNO}_2$$

[120] C. A. Bunton, E. D. Hughes, C. K. Ingold, D. I. H. Jacobs, M. H. Jones, G. J. Minkoff, and R. I. Reed, *J. Chem. Soc.*, **1950**, 2628.

This raises the question of the mechanism of nitrosation, and, in particular, the question of which of the family of nitrosonium-ion carriers is at work in the conditions of the kinetic investigation. A priori, NO^+, $H_2NO_2^+$, N_2O_4, N_2O_3, and HNO_2 all qualify for consideration; for although the free nitrosonium ion should be the most reactive of these, so much more of one of the others may be present as to give it a dominating kinetic importance.

We noticed in Section **23f** that, in organic solvents containing excess of nitric acid, analytical nitrous acid is stored mainly as N_2O_4. The equilibria which connect this mixed anhydride with other species, present in small amount, are

$$N_2O_4 = NO^+ + NO_3^-$$

$$N_2O_4 + H_2O = HNO_2 + HNO_3$$

$$N_2O_4 + H_2O = H_2NO_3^+ + NO_3^-$$

$$2N_2O_4 + H_2O = N_2O_3 + 2HNO_3$$

Obviously, we can identify the nitrosating agent by studying the effect of added nitrate ions and added water on the second-order rate constant k_2. Small amounts of added water have no effect, but comparably small amounts of added nitrate ion markedly reduce the rate constant. This shows that only the first of the four equilibria written above is important for regulating the concentrations of nitrosating agents. The mathematical form of the dependence of the rate constant on the nitrate ion concentration is

$$k_2 = k_2' + k_2''[NO_3^-]^{-1}$$

This shows that part of the catalysed rate, that measured by k_2', is due to attack by N_2O_4 molecules on the aromatic compounds, whilst the rest of it, measured by k_2'', is due to attack by NO^+ ions, which, although in much lower concentration, have a much higher specific reactivity than the dominating species N_2O_4.[121]

There remains the question of why positive catalysis by nitrous acid is a familiar feature of the nitrations only of aromatic compounds containing substituents of the form OR or NR_2. A reasonable view as to this is that it is due, not to any direct participation by these side-chains, but to the circumstance that the aromatic nuclei in these systems are highly reactive towards electrophilic reagents: so much so that, in order to isolate mononitration from polynitration, it is necessary to choose conditions which render nitronium ion only difficultly available, with the result that the field is opened to the much less reactive (Section **22e**), but much more plentiful, carriers of the nitrosonium ion.

[121] E. Blackall, E. D. Hughes, and C. K. Ingold, *J. Chem. Soc.*, **1952,** 28.

Two demonstrations support this theory. The first consists in showing that compounds of the forms ArOR and $ArNR_2$ do not refuse to behave like other aromatic compounds towards nitronium ion, when competition by nitrosonium-ion carriers is not excessive: this has been established as described above. Secondly, it has been shown that aromatic compounds other than those of the forms ArOR and $ArNR_2$, aromatic hydrocarbons, for instance, provided only that a sufficient nuclear reactivity has been built up by substitution, will exhibit the special nitration characteristics of phenols and amines. This has been demonstrated in the example of mesitylene: its nitration by nitric acid in organic solvents shows strong positive catalysis by nitrous acid. And kinetic investigation has proved that, as with *p*-chloroanisole and similar compounds, so with mesitylene, the two nitration processes run concurrently, either of which can be made dominating by adjusting concentrations; and that these processes obey just the same kinetic equations.[122]

(24) MECHANISMS OF OTHER ELECTROPHILIC AROMATIC SUBSTITUTIONS

(24a) Chlorination, Bromination, and Iodination.—Any halogenating agent can be regarded as a "carrier" of the halogenium ion Hal^+; and one of the more interesting questions concerning the mechanism of aromatic halogenation is that of whether substitution ever takes place through the pre-formed free halogenium ion, or whether it is always conveyed to the aromatic nucleus by a carrier such as the hypohalous acidium ion $Hal \cdot OH_2^+$, elemental halogen Hal_2, or molecular hypohalous acid $Hal \cdot OH$, or even perhaps polyhalide anions, such as Hal_3^-.

The question of the existence of free halogenium ions Hal^+ was first

[122] The prevalent notion, that the nuclear nitration of phenol and aniline derivatives depends on direct interaction between the side-chains and the nitrating agent, probably arises from the circumstance that one alkyl group is frequently eliminated during nitrations of phenolic ethers and dialkylanilines. However, an examination of these processes has led to the conclusion that they occur concurrently with, or subsequently to, the rate-determining step of nuclear nitration. There are two mechanisms of elimination. One is a non-oxidative mechanism favoured by phenolic ethers, in which the alkyl group is presumably eliminated as carbonium ion, R^+, since, when acetic acid is the solvent it can be recovered as an alkyl acetate, ROAc. The other is an oxidative mechanism, favoured by dialkylanilines, from which an alkyl group is apparently eliminated as a radical-cation, such as CH_2^+, since it can be recovered as an aldehyde. For further details, reference may be made to the original papers: C. A. Bunton, E. D. Hughes, C. K. Ingold, D. I. H. Jacobs, M. H. Jones, G. J. Minkoff, and R. I. Reed, *loc. cit.*; J. Glazer, E. D. Hughes, C. K. Ingold, A. T. James, G. T. Jones, and E. Roberts, *J. Chem. Soc.*, **1950**, 2657; E. D. Hughes and G. T. Jones, *ibid.*, p. 2678.

discussed by Noyes and by Stieglitz.[123] Support for the existence of the iodinium ion I^+ was adduced when Lewis showed[124] that liquid iodine possesses a considerable electrical conductance. It was believed for a time[125] that the blue paramagnetic substance formed in a solution of iodine in sulphuric oleum by the addition of oxidising agents, such as iodate or persulphate, was I^+. Gillespie and Milne have shown, however, by several mutually confirmatory physical methods,[126] that it is the odd-electron ion I_2^+. They detected I_3^+ as a minor component, but not I^+. Such direct evidence, however, has not been forthcoming for the other halogens.

In an investigation of the kinetics of electrophilic halogenation, Soper and Smith identified two carriers of the chlorine substituent in 1926, *viz.*, the hypochlorous acid molecule and the chlorine molecule.[127] They studied the rate of aqueous chlorination of phenol by hypochlorite over a range of pH values, and obtained kinetics consistent with equation (1):

$$\text{Rate} = k[\text{ClOH}][\text{OPh}^-] \qquad (1)$$

An alternative equation, in which the reactants are represented as ClO^- and PhOH, though equally consistent with the kinetics, is so out of keeping with the recognised electrophilic nature of the substitution that it need not be considered. The same workers found that, among acids, hydrochloric acid, which quantitatively produces elemental chlorine, was specific in causing a great increase in the rate of chlorination. The new reaction followed equation (2):

$$\text{Rate} = k[\text{Cl}_2][\text{OPh}^-] \qquad (2)$$

The work shows that molecular chlorine is specifically a much more powerful carrier for chlorination than is molecular hypochlorous acid.

The kinetics of aqueous aromatic chlorination were taken up again in 1950 by de la Mare, Hughes, and Vernon.[128] They studied aromatic chlorination in aqueous hypochlorous acid, which was acidified with perchloric acid or sulphuric acid, and was kept free from chloride ion, and hence from molecular chlorine, by added silver ion. This system contained a strong chlorinating agent; and a situation could be set up, as was subsequently described both by Derbyshire and Waters[129] and

[123] W. A. Noyes, *J. Am. Chem. Soc.*, 1901, **23**, 460; J. Stieglitz, *ibid.*, p. 797.

[124] G. N. Lewis, *J. Am. Chem. Soc.*, 1916, **38**, 762.

[125] J. Arotsky, H. C. Mishra, and A. C. R. Symons, *J. Chem. Soc.*, **1961**, 15.

[126] R. J. Gillespie and J. M. Milne, *Chem. Comm.*, **1966**, 158.

[127] F. G. Soper and G. F. Smith, *J. Chem. Soc.*, **1926**, 1582.

[128] P. B. D. de la Mare, E. D. Hughes, and C. A. Vernon, *Research*, 1950, **3**, 192, 242.

[129] D. H. Derbyshire and W. A. Waters, *J. Chem. Soc.*, **1951**, 73.

by de la Mare *et al.*,[130] in which aromatic compounds of not too reactive a kind, for example toluene-ω-sulphonic acid, benzene, and toluene, were chlorinated according to equation (3):

$$\text{Rate} = k[\text{ArH}][\text{ClOH}][\text{H}^+] \tag{3}$$

If we knew no more, this would point to chlorination by either the hypochlorous acidium ion $ClOH_2^+$ or the chlorinium ion Cl^+; but the investigation as a whole showed that only the latter interpretation could be entertained. For de la Mare, Hughes, and Vernon had progressively increased the reactivity of their aromatic substrate, until the factor [ArH] faded out from the rate equation,[128,130] which then contained, or consisted wholly of, the term in equation (4):

$$\text{Rate} = k[\text{ClOH}][\text{H}^+] \tag{4}$$

Anisole, quinol dimethyl ether, and phenol, for example, were thus chlorinated at a rate which was independent of their concentration, and, within the class of compounds which behave thus, independent of their identity. It was found in the same work[128] that these solutions of hypochlorous acid and perchloric acid could be used to add the elements of hypochlorous acid to olefins; and that adequately reactive olefins, allyl fluoride and allyl ethyl ether, for example, underwent the additions at a rate which was independent of the concentration and nature of the olefinic substrate. Moreover this common rate of addition to olefins was identical with the common rate of substitution in the aromatic compounds.

The kinetic phenomena summarised in equations (3) and (4) are entirely parallel to those which disclosed the formation, and effectiveness in nitration, of the nitronium ion. They indicate that, following the pre-equilibrium protonation of the hypochlorous acid molecule, a slow, and therefore activated, purely inorganic process, the breaking of some inorganic bond, takes place, to produce the real chlorinating agent. De la Mare, Hughes, and Vernon's representation of these processes[128] was thus as follows:

$$\left.\begin{aligned} \text{ClOH} + \text{H}_3\text{O}^+ &\underset{\text{fast}}{\rightleftharpoons} \text{Cl}\cdot\text{OH}_2^+ + \text{H}_2\text{O} \\ \text{Cl}\frown\text{OH}_2^+ &\xrightarrow[\text{slow}]{} \text{Cl}^+ + \text{H}_2\text{O} \end{aligned}\right\} \tag{5}$$

As Millen pointed out,[131] it need not be thought strange that the

[130] P. B. D. de la Mare, A. D. Ketley, and C. A. Vernon, *J. Chem. Soc.*, **1954**, 1290; de la Mare, J. T. Harvey, M. Hassan, and S. Varma, *ibid.*, **1958**, 2756.

[131] Communicated to the writer by Professor D. J. Millen, and noted in the first edition of this book.

chlorinium ion and the hypochlorous acidium ion can co-exist as slowly interconvertible entities in aqueous solution, although in composition one is a hydrate of the other. The free chlorinium ion should by Hund's rule (Section **3b**) be in its triplet state, with two of its electrons in separate orbitals and with parallel spins (like the oxygen atom in Table 3-2). It would thus be unable to co-ordinate directly with a water molecule. In order to permit co-ordination, the chlorinium ion must be lifted to the more energised state, having all electron spins paired, and one $3p$ orbital left unoccupied. This energy of excitation is the essential source of the activation energy of hydration, though the latter then becomes quantitatively reduced by the London adiabatic principle (Section **6d**).

These interpretations have not been universally accepted, largely because of some calculations,[132] which are taken to show that the free-energy required for the formation of the chlorinium ion would be prohibitively large. History repeats itself: it was on an argument of the calculated unavailability of sufficient engergy that the concept of the carbonium ion was resisted throughout the 1930's, as the Arrhenius dissociation theory itself was through the 1890's and later. Perhaps an eventual reconciliation will involve, as twice before, a reappraisal of solvation energies.

Certainly no one has been able to suggest a plausible alternative explanation of the kinetic phenomena. The first attempt in this direction,[133] a proposed slow proton transfer to give $HO\cdot ClH^+$, the presumed chlorinating agent, fails (a) because $HO\cdot ClH^+$ would not be a chlorinating agent, and (b) because it requires that the slow formation of the chlorinating agent be slower in deuterium water. Swain and Ketley showed[134] that it is faster by a factor of two, a normal factor of acceleration for reactions which, as equations (5) require, depend on pre-equilibrium proton transfer. A second suggestion,[135] that of a slow transfer of positive chlorine from $ClOH_2^+$ to the AgCl molecule to give the $AgCl_2^+$ ion, the presumed chlorinating agent, also fails,[136] (a) because there are no AgCl molecules, silver chloride, whether in solution or as solid, consisting only of silver ions and chloride ions, and (b) because the rates of those chlorinations which are of zeroth-

[132] R. P. Bell and E. Gelles, *J. Chem. Soc.*, **1951**, 2734.

[133] By R. S. Mulliken, quoted and discussed by P. B. D. de la Mare and J. H. Ridd, "Aromatic Substitution," Butterworths Scientific Pubs., London, 1959, p. 118.

[134] C. G. Swain and A. D. Ketley, *J. Am. Chem. Soc.*, 1955, **77**, 3410.

[135] E. A. Shilov, F. M. Vainshtein, and A. A. Yasnikov, *Kinetika i Kataliz*, 1961, **2**, 214; J. Arotsky and M. C. R. Symons, *Quart. Rev. Chem. Soc.*, 1962, **16**, 194.

[136] J. H. Ridd, *Ann. Repts. Chem. Soc.*, 1961, **58**, 163.

order in substrate are substantially independent of the small concentration of silver ions.

De la Mare, Hughes, and Vernon found[128,130] that, on going to their most reactive substrates, the substrate concentration re-entered the rate expression, the kinetics returning, partly or wholly, from those of equation (4) to those of equation (3). Their interpretation of this was that these highly active substrates take their chlorine from the immediately formed hypochlorous acidium ion, refusing to wait for the slow formation of the chlorinium ion. Some phenol ethers show this effect, as do some reactive olefins, such as *iso*butylene.

There are two other lines of approach which aid recognition of the ionic chlorine carriers. One depends on the circumstance that the power of an aqueous strong acid to transfer, in equilibrium, a proton to a weakly basic solute molecule varies with a function of acidity, called by L. P. Hammett h_0, which equals $[H^+]$ at low acidities, but above a certain threshold of acidity rises more steeply than $[H^+]$. The rate of a reaction which depends on pre-equilibrium proton-uptake should therefore vary as h_0, rather than $[H^+]$, when these quantities differ. Wherever it has been tested, it has been found that the factor $[H^+]$ in the foregoing kinetic equations should be replaced by h_0, when the difference between these measures of acidity is significant.[130,137] This supports the first step in equations (5).

The other approach is that developed in Sections **20b** and **20c** with reference to ortho/para ratios in the substitutions of aromatic hydrocarbons, particularly toluene and *t*-butylbenzene, by various electrophilic substituting agents, including cationic and molecular chlorine and bromine. The interpretation of the observations there proposed would not work at all, if the cationic chlorinating agent, taken to be Cl^+, were in reality some polyatomic species, such as $HO \cdot ClH^+$ or $AgCl_2^+$. This consideration supports the second step of equations (5).

Four electrophilic carriers of chlorine have thus been recognized as effective in aqueous chlorination. In expected order of diminishing specific activity they are:

$$Cl^+ \qquad Cl \cdot OH_2^+ \qquad Cl \cdot Cl \qquad Cl \cdot OH$$

In non-aqueous media molecular chlorine is the most important chlorinating agent, but other carriers of chlorine may become important. The best known is chlorine acetate, $Cl \cdot O \cdot CO \cdot CH_3$, which is formed from either chlorine monoxide, or chlorine and mercuric acetate, in acetic acid.[138]

[137] P. B. D. de la Mare and J. H. Ridd, "Aromatic Substitution," Butterworths Scientific Pubs., London, 1959, p. 116.

[138] P. B. D. de la Mare, A. D. Ketley, and C. A. Vernon, *Research*, 1953, **6**, **12S**; P. B. D. de la Mare, I. C. Hilton, and C. A. Vernon, *J. Chem. Soc.*, **1960**, 4039; P. B. D. de la Mare, I. C. Hilton, and S. Varma, *ibid.*, p. 4044.

Francis found[139] that bromine water brominates *m*-nitrophenol about 1000 times more rapidly than does an equimolar solution of hypobromous acid at pH3; and he suggested (wrongly) that the free ion Br^+ might be the effective reagent in bromine water. Shilov and Kanjaev made the important discovery[140] that aqueous hypobromous acid in the presence of a strong acid, such as perchloric acid, becomes a much more active brominating agent than bromine water: for the bromination of anisole-*m*-sulphonic acid by acidified aqueous hypobromous acid, they established the rate equation,

$$\text{Rate} = k[\text{ArH}][\text{HOBr}][\text{H}^+] \tag{6}$$

The product $[HOBr][H^+]$ is evidently proportional to the concentration of hypobromous acidium ion, $BrOH_2^+$; and, since water is in excess, it could also, as the authors pointed out, be measuring the stationary concentration of brominium ion, Br^+. Wilson and Soper noted[141] that bromination by Br_2 requires a different dependence of the reaction rate on bromide ion from that of bromination through either $BrOH_2^+$ or Br^+; and by investigating this dependence in the example of the bromination of *m*-nitroanisole by bromine water, they showed that the active agent in bromine water is Br_2. But they confirmed the Shilov-Kanjaev equation for the bromination of *m*-nitroanisole by acidified aqueous hypobromous acid, as also did Derbyshire and Waters[142] for the bromination of benzylsulphonic acid and benzoic acid by the same reagent. All the authors recognise that this equation points to bromination by either $BrOH_2^+$ or Br^+, but does not distinguish between these possibilities. The bromination of aromatic compounds by bromine has been investigated in acetic acid as solvent,[143] and also in 70% aqueous acetic acid.[144] In these media it seems certain that molecular bromine is one of the effective bromine carriers; but there are complications which have not yet been fully elucidated; and it is not clear what part, if any, the expected carrier bromine acetate plays in these brominations.

We have two indications that in the investigated conditions the cationic brominating agent is Br^+ rather than $BrOH_2^+$, that is, that

139 A. W. Francis, *J. Am. Chem. Soc.*, 1925, **47,** 2340.

140 E. A. Shilov and N. P. Kanjaev, *Compt. rend. acad. sci., U.R.S.S.*, 1939, **24,** 890.

141 W. J. Wilson and F. G. Soper, *J. Chem. Soc.*, **1949,** 3376.

142 A. E. Derbyshire and W. A. Waters, *Nature*, 1949, **164,** 446; *J. Chem. Soc.*, **1950,** 564, 574.

143 P. W. Robertson, P. B. D. de la Mare, and W. T. G. Johnston, *J. Chem. Soc.*, **1943,** 276; P. B. D. de la Mare and P. W. Robertson, *ibid.*, **1948,** 100.

144 A. E. Bradfield, G. I. Davies, and E. Long, *J. Chem. Soc.*, **1949,** 1389; S. J. Branch and Brynmor Jones, *ibid.*, **1954,** 2317.

the dehydration of the latter enters into the overali pre-equilibrium:

$$\begin{aligned} BrOH^+ + H_3O^+ &\rightleftharpoons Br\cdot OH_2^+ + H_2O \\ Br_2OH_2^+ &\rightleftharpoons Br^+ + H_2O \end{aligned} \qquad (7)$$

A much smaller energy barrier between $BrOH_2^+$ and Br^+ than between $ClOH_2^+$ and Cl^+ would be expected, because the triplet-to-singlet promotion energy is certain to be considerably smaller in the $4p$ electron shell of bromine than in the $3p$ shell of chlorine.

In explanation of the first indication, we must refer again to the circumstance that the rate of a reaction depending on a simple pre-equilibrium proton-transfer, such as the pre-equilibrium step in equations (5), or the first step in equations (7), if it were the only pre-equilibrium step, should rise with acidity according to Hammett's h_0, above that threshold of acidity above which h_0 rises faster than $[H^+]$. There is yet another measure of acidity, called by V. Gold j_0, which, from low acidities upward, follows first $[H^+]$, then, after the threshold, h_0, and then, after a higher threshold, rises more steeply even than h_0; and this is the measure of acidity which should be followed by the rate of a reaction which depends on a proton uptake combined with a dehydration, all in pre-equilibrium, as illustrated by the combined pair of steps in equations (7). Now Derbyshire and Waters carried their kinetic study of the bromination of benzoic acid by acidified hypobromous acid to acidities high enough to show[142] that the rate followed h_0, except at the highest examined acidities, when it deviated from h_0 in the direction of j_0, though an investigation of still higher acidities would have been needed fully to confirm dependence on j_0.

The second argument is the same as one used in connexion with chlorination, namely, that the interpretations given in Sections **20b** and **20c** of ortho/para ratios in the electrophilic substitutions of toluene and *t*-butylbenzene would fail completely if the brominating agent, there taken as Br^+, were really $Br\cdot OH_2^+$.

The short summary is that, for aqueous bromination, the brominating entities in diminishing order of specific activity are a cationic form of bromine, which is probably the brominium ion, Br^+, and the molecular form of the halogen, Br_2. In bromine water, and in non-aqueous solutions of bromine, the most important brominating entity is the bromine molecule.

As to iodination, Soper and Smith studied[145] the aqueous iodination of phenol at various pH values in 1927. Their rates could be sum-

[145] F. G. Soper and G. F. Smith, *J. Chem. Soc.*, **1927**, **2757**.

marised in equation (8):

$$\text{Rate} = k[\text{IOH}][\text{PhOH}] \tag{8}$$

The interpretation offered at the time, namely, that molecular hypoiodous acid was attacking the phenol molecule, involved the surprising conclusion that hypoiodous acid is a stronger iodinating agent than molecular iodine. But, as Painter and Soper subsequently pointed out,[146] the above equation can be rewritten as at (9):

$$\text{Rate} = k'[\text{IOH}_2^+][\text{PhO}^-] \tag{9}$$

and interpreted as indicating that the hypoiodous acidium ion attacks the phenoxide ion. Moreover, since water is in constant active mass, the iodinium ion, in pre-equilibrium, will bear a constant ratio to the hypoiodous acidium ion, and therefore, the same equation can be written as at (10):

$$\text{Rate} = k''[\text{I}^+][\text{PhO}^-] \tag{10}$$

and interpreted as meaning that the iodinium ion attacks the phenoxide ion. However, one of these three possibilities is cut away in Berliner's study of the rate of aqueous iodination of aniline.[147] The kinetics are entirely similar, if the anilinium ion be taken as the analogue of the phenol molecule; and, if we had no other information, they could be interpreted similarly as resulting from the interaction of any of the three pairs of reagents indicated by the concentration-products in the following equivalent rate expressions:

$$\text{Rate} = k[\text{IOH}][\text{PhNH}_3^+] \tag{11}$$

$$\text{Rate} = k'[\text{IOH}_2^+][\text{PhNH}_2] \tag{12}$$

$$\text{Rate} = k''[\text{I}^+][\text{PhNH}_2] \tag{13}$$

But we know that iodination through the anilinium ion would be a meta-oriented process, whereas, actually, the iodination is a facile ortho-para-substitution, hence only the interpretations (12) and (13) are permissible. With the corresponding interpretations (9) and (10) for the iodination of phenol, it emerges that the rate of attack of the iodinating entity, either I^+ or IOH_2^+, on phenoxide ion, is much greater, as it should be, than the rate of attack of the entity on the aniline molecule.

Berliner also studied the kinetics of iodination of anisole and of some aniline derivatives by means of iodine monochloride in aqueous hy-

[146] B. S. Painter and F. G. Soper, *J. Chem. Soc.*, **1947**, 342.
[147] E. Berliner, *J. Am. Chem. Soc.*, 1950, **72**, 4003; 1951, **73**, 4307.

drochloric acid.[148] The conclusion again was that the iodinating entity was a cationic form of iodine, either I^+ or IOH_2^+.

Thus the only well-authenticated electrophilic iodinating agent is a cationic form of iodine. Whether this is the iodinium ion or the hypoiodous acidium ion is not established, though our arguments concerning the active bromine cation lead us to assume that the iodinium ion I^+ would be freely formed in pre-equilibrium, and therefore could be the effective iodinating agent.

We come now to the mode of attack of halogenating agents on the aromatic ring. As to the halogenium cations, what evidence we have points to the conclusion that their attack resembles that of the nitronium cation (Section **23d**). That is to say, the halogenium ion is taken up in a first step to give a *cyclo*hexadienylium ion (Pfeiffer-Wizinger adduct), which in a second step loses a proton much more rapidly than it can reverse its own formation:

$$\mathrm{Hal^+ + ArH} \underset{\text{slow}}{\rightleftharpoons} \overset{+}{\mathrm{Ar}}\begin{matrix}\diagup\mathrm{Hal}\\ \diagdown\mathrm{H}\end{matrix} \qquad (14)$$

$$\overset{+}{\mathrm{Ar}}\begin{matrix}\diagup\mathrm{Hal}\\ \diagdown\mathrm{H}\end{matrix} \xrightarrow[\text{fast}]{} \mathrm{ArHal + H^+}$$

In these circumstances, the last step does not affect the rate of halogenation, which will be either that of the formation of the *cyclo*hexadienylium ion, or that of formation of the halogenium ion, whichever is the slower; and so, when the proton to be lost is made a deuteron, or a triton, the measured rate will be the same. A demonstration of this nature has been given for bromination by cationic bromine by de la Mare, Dunn, and Harvey.[149] They showed that, when benzene and hexadeuterobenzene were brominated by acidified aqueous hypobromous acid in accordance with the kinetic equation (6), the rates were identical, as required by scheme (14).

Chlorinating by the chlorinium ion is expected to follow the same pattern, but iodination by the iodinium ion may not do so, because the considerable reversibility of aromatic iodination suggests that the cationic adduct of equation (14) may lose iodinium ion, that is, re-

[148] E. Berliner, *J. Am. Chem. Soc.*, 1956, **78**, 3632; 1958, **80**, 856.

[149] P. B. D. de la Mare, T. M. Dunn, and J. T. Harvey, *J. Chem. Soc.*, **1957**, 923.

verse its own formation, somewhat rapidly, and possibly more rapidly than it loses a proton.[150]

Aromatic chlorination by molecular chlorine in water,[127] and in acetic acid,[151] can be represented by the kinetic equation (15) below. So also can aromatic bromination by molecular bromine in water,[152] and, in sufficiently dilute solution, in acetic acid ($<M/1000$).[153]

$$\text{Rate} = k[\text{ArH}][\text{X}_2] \tag{15}$$

This equation implies that processes subsequent to the uptake of molecular halogen to form a neutral *cyclo*hexadienyl dihalide must be fast. Their sequence may plausibly be supposed to be as written at (16):

$$\overset{+}{\text{Ar}}\begin{smallmatrix}\diagup \bar{\text{X}}\text{—X} \\ \diagdown \text{H}\end{smallmatrix} \rightarrow \overset{+}{\text{Ar}}\begin{smallmatrix}\diagup \text{X} \\ \diagdown \text{H}\end{smallmatrix} + \text{X}^-$$

$$\overset{+}{\text{Ar}}\begin{smallmatrix}\diagup \text{X} \\ \diagdown \text{H}\end{smallmatrix} \rightarrow \text{ArX} + \text{H}^+ \tag{16}$$

Robertson has shown[154] that bromination by bromine at higher concentrations (to $M/40$) in acetic acid follows the third-order equation (17):

$$\text{Rate} = k[\text{ArH}][\text{Br}_2]^2 \tag{17}$$

No parallel kinetic form of chlorination is known: and this suggests that the function of the extra bromine molecule in equation (17) is not concerned with the extraction of the aromatic proton, but is a consequence of the power of the higher halogens to self-combine, with expansion of a valency electron-shell, especially in the presence of a nett negative charge, as in the perhalide ions. On these grounds, Gwyn

[150] For a discussion of the somewhat equivocal evidence, see P. B. D. de la Mare and J. H. Ridd, "Aromatic Substitution," Butterworths Scientific Pubs., London, 1959, p. 121.

[151] K. J. P. Orton and A. E. Bradfield, *J. Chem. Soc.*, 1927, **129**, 966. This was the first demonstration: it has been confirmed on many occasions since.

[152] A. Bertoud and M. Mosset, *J. Chim. phys.*, 1934, **36**, 272.

[153] I. K. Walker and P. W. Robertson, *J. Chem. Soc.*, **1939**, 1515.

[154] P. W. Robertson, N. T. Clare, K. J. McNaught, and G. W. Paul, *J. Chem. Soc.*, **1937**, 335; P. W. Robertson, P. B. D. de la Mare, and W. T. G. Johnston, *J. Chem. Soc.*, **1943**, 276.

Williams proposed[155] to interpret equation (17) by means of scheme (18):

$$\mathrm{Ar}^{+}\!\begin{smallmatrix}\diagup \overset{-}{\mathrm{Br}}\text{—}\mathrm{Br}\\ \diagdown \mathrm{H}\end{smallmatrix} + \mathrm{Br_2} \xrightarrow[\text{slow}]{} \mathrm{Ar}^{+}\!\begin{smallmatrix}\diagup \mathrm{Br}\\ \diagdown \mathrm{H}\end{smallmatrix} + \mathrm{Br_3^-} \qquad (18)$$

$$\mathrm{Ar}^{+}\!\begin{smallmatrix}\diagup \mathrm{Br}\\ \diagdown \mathrm{H}\end{smallmatrix} \longrightarrow \mathrm{ArBr} + \mathrm{H^+}$$

With more concentrated solutions of bromine in acetic acid (to $M/5$), Robertson and his coworkers[156] found a fourth-order reaction (19):

$$\text{Rate} = k[\mathrm{ArH}][\mathrm{Br_2}]^3 \qquad (19)$$

Quite generally, an effective order at a given bromine concentration in acetic acid was raised when a less polar co-solvent, such as chloroform, was added, and was lowered when water was added. Whether equation (19) should be interpreted by an extension of Gwyn Williams's polyhalide-ion scheme or, as has been suggested, by assuming attack by a pre-formed dimer of bromine, Br_4, has not yet been made clear.

Partial rate factors for the halogenation of mono-substituted benzenes are illustrated in Sections **22b** and **24j**.

The mechanism of halogenation of phenols, whether by cationic or molecular halogens, has analogies with the mechanism of reactions dependent on prototropy (Chapter XI), and, in particular, in the halogenation of keto-enolic systems (a phenol is a form of enol). As has been shown, the aqueous halogenation of phenols proceeds through the aryloxide anion, which is formed quickly, is reprotonated quickly, and may be halogenated quickly. If it is indeed halogenated quickly, then the final loss of a proton from the *cyclo*hexadienyl adduct may be the slowest step in the sequence of steps constituting halogenation. This has been illustrated by Zollinger and his coworkers for the aqueous bromination of G-acid.[157] The rate with acidified hypobromous acid was independent of pH (as a reaction of Br^+ with ArO^- would be), and was equal to the rate of bromination with elemental bromine as re-

[155] Gwyn Williams, *Trans. Faraday Soc.*, 1941, **39**, 729.

[156] P. W. Robertson, P. B. D. de la Mare, and W. T. G. Johnston, *J. Chem. Soc.*, **1943**, 276.

[157] M. Christen and H. Zollinger, *Helv. Chim. Acta*, 1962, **45**, 2057, 2066; M. Christen, W. Koch, W. Simon, and H. Zollinger, *ibid.*, p. 2077.

agent; and this rate was independent of the concentration of whichever reactant was in excess. Evidently the intermediate adduct was being formed rapidly, reversibly, and nearly as completely as the supply of materials allowed. It was, in fact, obtained in high enough concentration, and for long enough, to allow its constitution, as the expected bromo-enone of equation (20), to be determined from its ultraviolet absorption and nuclear magnetic resonance spectra. The measured process was the loss of its proton:

HO₃S, HO₃S —OH ⇌ (fast) —O⁻ ⇌ (Br⁺ or Br₂, fast) H Br =O

G-acid (20)

→ (slow) Br —O⁻ ⇌ (fast) Br —OH

(24b) Sulphonation.—The kinetics of aromatic sulphonation have been studied under three kinds of conditions. The first involves the use of slightly aqueous sulphuric acid. Systems of this kind were first studied by Stubbs, Williams, and Hinshelwood,[158] who used nitrobenzene as solvent; but the results were complicated by effects of reversibility. This difficulty was avoided by Cowdrey and Davies,[159] who examined the sulphonation of *p*-nitrotoluene using, as media, and therefore in large and constant excess, aqueous sulphuric acids 92–99% by weight in H_2SO_4. Davenport and Hughes[160] reverted to nitrobenzene as the solvent, but studied the sulphonation of toluene and ortho-xylene with a constant excess of various aqueous acids, 95–99% by weight in H_2SO_4, avoiding in this way trouble from reversibility. The results of the last two investigations are consistent; and they point to the conclusion that monomeric sulphur trioxide, or, possibly, a sulphuric acid solvate of it, is the active species contained in sulphonating media of this type.

The possible active species that have been considered in this or in other connexions are (1) the sulphuric acidium ion $H_3SO_4^+$, (2) monomeric SO_3 or a solvate, (3) the ion HSO_3^+, presumably with inclusion of possible solvates, and (4) dimeric sulphur trioxide S_2O_6. Reagents

[158] F. J. Stubbs, C. D. Williams, and C. N. Hinshelwood, *J. Chem. Soc.*, **1948**, 1065.

[159] W. A. Cowdrey and D. S. Davies, *J. Chem. Soc.*, **1949**, 1471.

[160] E. D. Hughes and D. A. Davenport, personal communication; cited in the first edition of this book.

(1) and (2) are known to be present in pure sulphuric acid, which, according to Gillespie,[161] is 0.013 molal in sulphuric acidium ion, and 0.0083 molal in the solvate, disulphuric acid, of monomeric sulphur trioxide. Reagent (3) is of importance in oleum, as we shall see. Reagent (4) occurs as its solvate, trisulphuric acid, in oleum.

All these possible reagents require the retardation of sulphonation by added water; but they require the retardation to obey different laws. Water is largely, and may for the present purpose be considered as completely, ionised in sulphuric acid, according to the equation,

$$H_2O + H_2SO_4 = H_3O^+ + HSO_4^-$$

The number of ions of water that have to be produced along with one molecule or ion of any of the possible reagents can be seen, from the following equations, to be 1, 2, 3, and 4, in that order:

$$(1) \qquad 2H_2SO_4 = H_3SO_4^+ + HSO_4^-$$

$$(2) \qquad 2H_2SO_4 = SO_3 + H_3O^+ + HSO_4^-$$

$$(3) \qquad 3H_2SO_4 = HSO_3^+ + H_3O^+ + 2HSO_4^-$$

$$(4) \qquad 4H_2SO_4 = S_2O_6 + 2H_3O^+ + 2HSO_4^-$$

It follows that attack by $H_3SO_4^+$ requires a rate proportional to the inverse first-power of the concentration of the water, by SO_3 a rate varying as the inverse square, by HSO_3^+ as the inverse cube, and by S_2O_6 as the inverse fourth-power. The experimental answer is unequivocal: the rate varies as the first power of the concentration of the aromatic compound, and as the inverse square of the concentration of the water. As can be seen from the equations, the effect of an added ionising hydrogen sulphate can be used to distinguish the first two possibilities from the last two: all the results are consistent with the conclusion that the active species is monomeric sulphur trioxide. In these conditions the transition state of sulphonation has the composition $ArH + SO_3$.

A different situation applies to sulphonation in oleum. Using nitrobenzene, the phenyltrimethylammonium ion, and their *p*-methyl or *p*-halogen derivatives, as substrates, Brand and Horning have conducted sulphonations in oleums containing 4–10% of "free" sulphur trioxide.[162] They found that the logarithms of the first-order rate-constants were linear functions, with slopes close to unity, of the sum of two logarithms, *viz.*, the logarithm, $-H_0$, of Hammett's measure of acidity h_0, and the logarithm of the partial pressure (*i.e.*, of the thermodynamic activity) of the sulphur trioxide. This was taken to mean

[161] R. J. Gillespie, *J. Chem. Soc.*, **1950, 2516.**

[162] J. C. D. Brand and W. C. Horning, *J. Chem. Soc.*, **1952,** 3622.

that the medium is supplying a proton as well as a sulphur trioxide molecule to the transition sate of sulphonation, which thus has the composition $ArH + SO_3 + H^+$.

We have here a picture of two mechanisms of sulphonation, dominant in different ranges of acidity, the mechanism of higher acidities carrying in its transition state an additional proton:

$$\text{ArH} \underset{-SO_3}{\overset{+SO_3}{\rightleftharpoons}} \text{Ar}^{+}(H)(SO_3^-) \rightleftharpoons \text{ArSO}_3\text{H}$$

(Cowdrey-Davies)

$$\text{ArH} \underset{-SO_3 - H^+}{\overset{+SO_3 + H^+}{\rightleftharpoons}} \text{Ar}^{+}(H)(SO_3H) \underset{+H^+}{\overset{-H^+}{\rightleftharpoons}} \text{ArSO}_3\text{H}$$

(Brand-Horning)

Sulphonation is reversible, the equilibrium favouring the forward process at high acidities, and the reverse process, that is, desulphonation, at low ones. A knowledge of the mechanism of a reversible reaction in one direction gives the mechanism in the other, to the extent prescribed by our knowledge that the transition state must be common to both (principle of microscopic reversibility). Long and Paul noted[163] that the mechanism of Cowdrey and Davies implies that desulphonation in 92–99% sulphuric acid would not be acid catalysed. The one-sided equilibrium at such acidities precludes a direct investigation of the point; but in more dilute sulphuric acid, say, 10–50%, desulphonation certainly is acid catalysed. Using results by Crafts,[164] applying to 15–45% sulphuric acid, Gold and Satchell,[165] and also Long and Paul, showed that the rate followed Hammett's h_0, an indication that a pre-equilibrium uptake of a proton is involved; and Gold and Satchell noted that this should be so according to the Cowdrey-Davies mechanism, as long as the sulphonic acid is stored in the medium mainly as sulphonate ion. But at concentrations above 50% of sulphuric acid ($\log h_0 > 3$) the form in which the sulphonic acid is stored is expected to shift over from sulphonate ion to sulphonic acid molecule, and then the dependence of the rate of desulphonation on h_0 should disappear. Using results by Pinnow[166] and by Lantz,[167]

[163] F. A. Long and M. A. Paul, *Chem. Rev.*, 1957, **57**, 935.

[164] J. M. Crafts, *Ber.*, 1901, **34**, 1350; *Bull. Soc. chim.* (France), 1907, **1**, 917.

[165] V. Gold and D. P. N. Satchell, *J. Chem. Soc.*, **1956**, 1635.

[166] J. Pinnow, *Z. Elektrochem.*, 1915, **21**, 380; 1917, **23**, 243.

[167] R. Lantz, *Bull. Soc. chim.* (France), 1945, **12**, 253, 1004.

Gold and Satchell showed that, at concentrations of sulphuric acid somewhat above 50%, the dependence of desulphonation rates on h_0 does fall off markedly. Subsequently, Fuller and the writer found that the dependence of the rate of desulphonation of 2,4-dimethoxy-benzene-sulphonic acid in aqueous perchloric acid upon h_0 begins to fail at $\log h_0 = 3$, and that the failure is almost complete at $\log h_0 = 4.3$.[168] That is, the acid catalysis of desulphonation has almost disappeared.

Hydrogen isotope effects have not been reported for sulphonation in aqueous sulphuric acid, but small ones have been observed in sulphonations in oleum. The rate of para-sulphonation of bromobenzene by oleum in nitrobenzene solution is reduced to something above half its value when the para-hydrogen atom is a tritium atom.[169] This suggests that the transition state of the second of the represented steps in the Brand-Horning mechanism is only a little less energised than that of the first step. The rate of sulphonation of the p-tolyltrimethylammonium ion in solution in oleum containing 7% of "free" sulphur trioxide is reduced to about three-quarters of its value when dideutero-sulphuric acid, instead of sulphuric acid, is used to make up the oleum.[170] This might mean any of several things, for instance, that the components of the addendum in the Brand-Horning mechanism are not pre-combined, the proton transfering itself to the sulphur trioxide molecule while the latter is being added to the substrate molecule.

The kinetics of sulphonation of benzene derivatives by sulphur trioxide in nitrobenzene as solvent have been studied by Hinshelwood and his collaborators.[171] The observed rates were proportional to the concentration of aromatic compound, and to the square of the concentration of sulphur trioxide. The conclusion was drawn that, while undoubtedly two molecules of sulphur trioxide were involved in the reaction, that might be so because a pre-formed dimer, S_2O_6, was the active reagent. However, if the sulphonation process, like other aromatic substitutions, involves two stages, then their rate relations *in an aprotic solvent* could be such that the overall kinetic effect of the incursion of one monomeric SO_3 molecule in each stage would lead to the observed rate law.

[168] M. W. Fuller and C. K. Ingold, not yet published.

[169] L. Melander, *Acta Chim. Scand.*, 1949, **3**, 95; *Arkiv. Kemi*, 1950, **2**, 213; U. Berglund-Larsson and L. Melander, *Arkiv. Kemi*, 1953, **6**, 219.

[170] J. C. D. Brand, J. W. P. Jarvie, and W. C. Horning, *J. Chem. Soc.*, 1959, 3844.

[171] D. R. Vicary and C. N. Hinshelwood, *J. Chem. Soc.*, **1939**, 1372; K. D. Wadsworth and C. N. Hinshelwood, *ibid.*, **1944**, 469; E. Dresel and C. N. Hinshelwood, *ibid.*, p. 649.

(24c) Hydrogen Exchange.—A qualitative study of the deuteration of the aromatic nucleus by deutero-acids has led to the conclusion[172] that the hydrogen exchange thus effected is a typical electrophilic substitution. Of course, it is a reversible substitution, completely balanced except for isotopic differences.

The evidence is as follows. First, deuterating acids were found to arrange themselves in the efficiency series,

$$D_2SO_4 > D_2SeO_4 > D_3O^+ > PhOD > D_2O$$

which is obviously an acidity series: in general, any member of the corresponding series of protium acids will transfer a proton extensively to the conjugate base of a member standing to its right, but only slightly to the conjugate base of one standing to its left.

Secondly, aromatic substituents so modified the reactivity of the aromatic nucleus towards such reagents as to give a rate sequence identical with that of such well-studied reactions as nitration, chlorination, and diazo-coupling:

$$—\bar{O} > —NR_2 > —OR > (H) > —SO_3H$$

The differences were large, so much so that all the reagents could not be used preparatively to deuterate all the benzene derivatives. Benzene sulphonic acid was not deuterated by sulphuric acid under conditions in which benzene itself could readily be deuterated by sulphuric or selenic acid. Anisole, aniline, and dimethylaniline were conveniently deuterated by aqueous acid, that is, by the deuteroxonium ion. Phenol was deuterated in alkaline aqueous solution; and a study of the dependence of the rate on pH showed that the phenoxide ion was simultaneously undergoing rapid deuteration through the attack of phenyldeuteroxide molecules, and slow deuteration by attack of deuterium oxide molecules—deuteroxide ions, as such, having no action.

Thirdly, some evidence was obtained that hydrogen exchange follows the usual orientation laws for electrophilic aromatic substitution. It was found that phenol, aniline, and anisole underwent facile deuteration with respect to three nuclear positions only, this number being determined by the deuterium uptake, with control of and allowance for, any side-chain deuteration. Best and Wilson proved formally,[173] in the examples of phenol and aniline, that the three exchanging positions were the ortho- and para-positions, by displacing the deuterium by

[172] C. K. Ingold, C. G. Raisin, and C. L. Wilson, *Nature*, 1934, **134**, 734; *J. Chem. Soc.*, **1936**, 915.

[173] A. P. Best and C. L. Wilson, *J. Chem. Soc.*, **1938**, 28.

bromine. Further proof was given[174] for aniline by eliminating the amino-group after deuteration and showing spectroscopically that the benzene recovered was pure 1,3,5-trideutrobenzene.

During the 1950's a question of difficulty arose over the mechanism of the transfer of the proton from the attacking acid to the aromatic substrate. The cause of the difficulty was that rates of aromatic hydrogen exchange were found approximately to follow h_0, Hammett's measure of the power of a medium to transfer protons in equilibrium to weak, electrically neutral bases. This correlation suggested that the transfer of the proton was a pre-equilibrium process, and was therefore complete, the proton having discarded the residue of its original carrier, so getting right into the exchanging system, before the latter had arrived at its transition state. The transition state would then have the composition of the substrate plus the proton, but would not contain the residue of the acid from which the proton had come. This made it difficult to imagine what could be the slow step in hydrogen exchange, *i.e.*, what could be going on in the transition state itself. Implausibly, two slowly interconvertible isomers of the protonated aromatic compound were "invented," and the slow process was taken to be an intramolecular shift of the newly added proton. Now this theory was never really tenable. For a transition state of the assumed composition requires a rate expression depending, apart from the substrate, only on hydrogen ions (as in specific hydrogen-ion catalysis), and therefore not containing any term in the complete, *i.e.*, the undissociated acid, which supplied the proton. But even the early demonstrations of aromatic hydrogen exchange with acids had shown that, not only the hydrogen ion, but each acid in a mixture of acids makes its own contribution to the rate (as in general acid catalysis). For example, the rate of exchange with phenoxide ion contains an important term in the undissociated phenol molecule acting as an acid. Such direct involvements of undissociated acids in aromatic hydrogen exchanges were documented afresh, and much more fully, in 1959 by Kresge and Chiang[175] in the example of 1,3,5-trimethoxybenzene and in 1960 by Colapietro and Long[176] with azulene as substrate. These investigations showed that in buffers the undissociated acid molecules

[174] C. R. Bailey, A P. Best, R. R. Gordon, J. B. Hale, C. K. Ingold, A. H. Leckie, L. H. P. Weldon, and C. L. Wilson, *Nature*, 1937, **139**, 880; C. R. Bailey, J. B. Hale, N. Herzfeld, C. K. Ingold, A. H. Leckie, and H. G. Poole, *J. Chem. Soc.*, **1946**, 255.

[175] A. J. Kresge and Y. Chiang, *J. Am. Chem. Soc.*, 1959, **81**, 5509; 1961, **83**, 2877; *Proc. Chem. Soc.*, **1961**, 81.

[176] J. Colapietro and F. A. Long, *Chem. and Ind.*, **1960**, 1056.

made substantial contributions to the exchange rates. It followed that the whole of the acid molecule contributed to the composition of the transition state of exchange, in which, therefore, the proton is only in process of being transferred. In other words, it followed that the proton transfer is itself the slow step of hydrogen exchange, which may be formulated (for deuterium introduction) thus:

$$\mathrm{ArH} + \mathrm{DX} \rightleftharpoons \overset{+}{\mathrm{Ar}}\!\begin{matrix}\diagup \mathrm{H}\\ \diagdown \mathrm{D}\end{matrix} + \mathrm{X}^- \rightleftharpoons \mathrm{ArD} + \mathrm{HX}$$

The nature of the original false scent was disclosed in Bunnett's study of the factors controlling acidity measures. Hammett's h_0, which is defined by measurements of the equilibrium proportions of proton transferences to representative nitrogen bases, applies moderately well to most nitrogen and oxygen bases, but not to carbon bases. It must be regarded as coincidental that it applies approximately to the partial proton transference in the transition states of proton transfers to aromatic carbon.[177]

The *cyclo*hexadienylium salts $ArH_2^+X^-$, such as the above-written mechanism assumes to be formed, are shown to be formed by the electrical conductivities of aromatic hydrocarbons in solution in liquid hydrogen fluoride,[178] by their depression of the vapour pressure of boron trifluoride in solvent hydrogen fluoride, and by their extraction from solutions in *n*-heptane by mixtures of hydrogen fluoride and boron trifluoride.[179] The extraction experiments provide estimates of the relative basicities of the aromatic hydrocarbons. Data for the relative conductances, and for the relative basicities (uncorrected for solubility differences of the non-ionised hydrocarbons), are in Table 24-1.[180] It will be obvious that methyl substituents promote proton uptake to form salts $ArH_2^+BF_4^-$, especially at ortho- and para-positions, so that meta-related methyl substituents reinforce one another strongly. It will be clear from the figures for hexamethylbenzene that the proton may be added not only at a hydrogen-carrying, but also at a methyl-carrying carbon atom. From toluene to the higher homologues, the

[177] J. F. Bunnett, *J. Am. Chem. Soc.*, 1961, **83**, 4056 (four papers). The same difficulty arose contemporaneously in connexion with acid-catalysed olefin hydration. Bunnett's solution covered both cases, and its general nature is explained in Section **52a** (Chapter XIII).

[178] M. Kilpatrick and J. E. Luborsky, *J. Am. Chem. Soc.*, 1953, **75**, 577.

[179] D. A. McCaulay and A. P. Lien, *J. Am. Chem. Soc.*, 1951, **73**, 2013.

[180] D. A. McCaulay and A. P. Lien, *Tetrahedron*, 1959, **5**, 186.

basicities are sufficient to allow the *cyclo*hexadienylium salts to be isolated as yellow or orange solids at −80°.[181] At higher temperatures from −70° to −10° they give electrically conducting melts, which slowly decompose. The salt formed from mesitylene, deuterium fluoride, and boron trifluoride gave off 60% of hydrogen fluoride and 40% of deuterium fluoride when decomposed. This primary deuterium isotope effect shows that the added deuteron achieves a condition of binding comparable to that of an originally aromatic proton, as required by the formula assigned to the cation (below). In the example of the salt from pentamethylbenzene, hydrogen fluoride, and boron trifluoride, the presence of a methylene group, as required by the formula (below), has been proved by the nuclear magnetic resonance spectrum of the salt.[182]

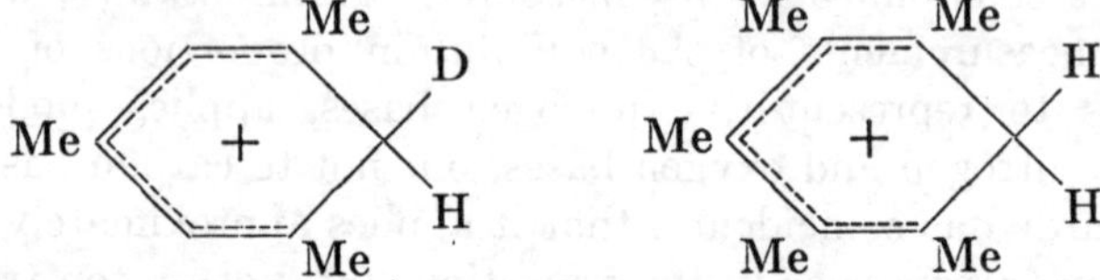

Klit and Langseth were the first to use a Friedel-Crafts system for

TABLE 24-1.—RELATIVE CONDUCTANCE IN HF, RELATIVE BASICITIES IN $HF—BF_3$, AND RELATIVE RATES OF HYDROGEN EXCHANGE IN $CF_3 \cdot CO_2H$, OF SOME AROMATIC HYDROCARBONS.

Hydrocarbon	Condy. in HF	Basicity in $HF—BF_3$	Rate H-exchange in $CF_3 \cdot CO_2H$
Benzene	—	—	0.0012
Toluene	—	—	0.20
p-Xylene	1	1	1
o-Xylene	1.1	2	1.2
m-Xylene	26	20	37
Pseudocumene (1,2,4)	63	40	100
Hemimellitene (1,2,3)	69	40	127
Durene (1,2,4,5)	140	120	330
Prehnitene (1,2,3,4)	400	170	—
Mesitylene (1,3,5)	13,000	2,800	11,300
Isodurene (1,2,3,5)	16,000	6,500	30,000
Pentamethylbenzene	29,000	8,700	32,000
Hexamethylbenzene	97,000	89,000	—

[181] G. A. Olah and S. J. Kuhn, *J. Am. Chem. Soc.*, 1958, **80**, 6535; G. A. Olah, A. E. Parleth, and J. A. Olah, *ibid.*, p. 6540.

[182] C. MacLean, J. H. van der Waals, and E. L. Mackor, *Mod. Phys.*, 1958, **1**, 247.

the purpose of effecting aromatic hydrogen exchange.[183] They preparatively deuterated benzene by the use of deuterium chloride and aluminium chloride, and by repetition produced hexadeuterobenzene.

Table 24-1 contains Lauer and Stedman's figures for the relative rates of deuteration of aromatic hydrocarbons in trifluoroacetic acid containing deuterium oxide.[184] It is noteworthy that the hydrocarbons stand in the same order for rate of deuteration as they do for equilibrium degree of protonation.

The patterns of activation or deactivation produced by orienting substituents in the aromatic ring for various isotopic forms of hydrogen exchange are illustrated by the partial rate factors set out below.

Me: 83, 1.9, 83 MeO: 23000, 0.25, 55000

H-for-D by aq.-H_2SO_4 or aq.-$HClO_4$[185]

Me: 250, 4, 420 *t*-Bu: 200, 7, 490

D-for-H by $CF_3 \cdot CO_2D$[186]

Me: 250, 5, 250 *t*-Bu: 170, 9, 180 Cl: 0.035, 0.002, 0.160 I: 0.043, 0.003, 0.112

H-for-T by aq.-H_2SO_4 or aq.-HOAc-H_2SO_4[187]

The patterns generally resemble those obtained for nitration and halogenation (Sections **21b**, **21c**, and **22b**). There seems to be only a mild steric retardation of ortho-hydrogen-exchange, even in exchanges in trifluoroacetic acid, where the substituting agent may be the molecu-

[183] A. Klit and A. Langseth, *Nature*, 1935, **135**, 956; *Z. Physik. Chem.*, 1936, A, **176**, 65.

[184] W. Lauer and G. Stedman, *J. Am. Chem. Soc.*, 1958, **80**, 6439.

[185] V. Gold and D. P. N. Satchell, *J. Chem. Soc.*, **1956**, 2743; D. P. N. Satchell, *ibid.*, p. 3911.

[186] E. L. Meakor, P. G. Smith, and J. H. van der Waals, *Trans. Faraday Soc.*, 1957, **83**, 1309; W. Lauer, G. Matson, and G. Stedman, *J. Am. Chem. Soc.*, 1958, **80**, 6433, 6437; R. Baker, C. Eaborn, and R. Taylor, *J. Chem. Soc.*, **1961**, 4927.

[187] C. Eaborn and R. Taylor, *J. Chem. Soc.*, **1961**, 247, 2388.

lar form of the acid; and there is still less selective ortho-retardation in the aqueous-acid reactions, in which the proton carrier is probably H_3O^+. The meta-deactivation in anisole is noteworthy: it is consistent with the classification of methoxyl as a $-I + K$ substituent (Section **21c**, and Fig. 21-1, which was drawn for the first edition of this book, when no such direct experimental check was available).

(24d) Alkylation.—This substitution is commonly effected by means of an alkyl halide and a Friedel-Crafts catalyst. The latter is an electron-deficient halide, such as aluminium chloride—in general, a halide of an element, boron, aluminium, titanium, iron, zinc, gallium, or the like, which has a strong tendency to form complex halides. Alternatively, alkylation may be effected by means of an olefin, a Friedel-Crafts catalyst, and a so-called co-catalyst, which is a proton-acid, usually either a hydrogen halide, or enough water to produce such. As the following equations illustrate, either of these systems could in principle produce an alkylium ion:

$$CH_3 \cdot CH_2 \cdot Cl + AlCl_3 \rightarrow CH_3 \cdot CH_2^+ + AlCl_4^-$$

$$CH_2{:}CH_2 + HCl + AlCl_3 \rightarrow CH_3 \cdot CH_2^+ + AlCl_4^-$$

It is generally believed that the alkylium ion, either free, or in an ion-pair, or in some other lightly associated form, is the entity which attacks and alkylates the aromatic ring. This idea was advocated by Meerwein in 1927.[188] Today the evidence for it is weighty in its extent and variety, though we still lack the confirmation of an ability to isolate carbonium-ion formation as the rate-controlling step of alkylation.

Aluminium chloride is insoluble in non-basic solvents, such as alkanes, and carbon disulphide; it has a limited solubility in benzene and the lower arenes; and it is freely soluble in basic solvents, such as ethers, ketones, nitriles, and nitro-compounds. Aluminium bromide is soluble in all solvents. Insofar as they dissolve, the two halides appear to exist in similar forms, as Al_2X_6 in alkanes and carbon disulphide, as coloured π- or charge-transfer complexes, arene . . . Al_2Cl_6, having a loose binding similar to that in benzene-picrate, in the lower arenes, and as highly dipolar co-ordinated adducts, such as $Et_2O^+ \cdot Al^-Cl_3$ (cf. Section **8a**), in basic solvents. The corresponding gallium halides behave quite similarly. These different forms, in which the aluminium and gallium halides exist in solution, may be regarded as different ways of holding the active entity, *i.e.*, monomeric un-co-ordinated AlX_3 or GaX_3, in an easily available state. When an alkyl halide is added, a dipolar co-ordination adduct, $RX^+—Al^-X_3$ or $RX^+—Ga^-X_3$,

[188] H. Meerwein, *Ann.*, 1927, **455**, 327.

is formed in an instantaneously established equilibrium. When the metal halide MX_3 was originally only lightly complexed, as in M_2X_6 or arene . . . M_2X_6, the new equilibrium may lie on the side of the new complex $RX^+—M^-X_3$, as we can tell from the change of vapour pressure of RX. When, however, the original complex was strong, as in a basic solvent, the new equilibrium may lie mainly on the side of the old complex. All this happens immediately. And then, somewhat slowly in systems formed from methyl and primary alkyl halides, but much more rapidly in systems from secondary and tertiary alkyl halides, a further change takes place, which is manifested by a mixing-up, as can be told by isotopic labelling, of the halogens in the alkyl halide and the metal halide.[189] Different halogens, chlorine and bromine, for instance, can thus be mixed up, and halogens can be exchanged between two alkyl halides, having different halogens and different alkyl groups, through the mediation of an aluminium halide. These halogen-mixing changes are most simply understood as ionisations of the co-ordination adduct, often according to the pattern,

$$\text{basic-solvent}\overset{+}{}—\overset{-}{\text{Al}}\text{X}_3 + \text{RX} \rightleftharpoons \text{R}\overset{+}{\text{X}}—\overset{-}{\text{Al}}\text{X}_3 \rightleftharpoons \text{R}^+ + \text{AlX}_4^-$$

Aluminium and gallium halides tend to add to residues of themselves, much as do sulphur trioxide and metaphosphoric acid; and so, in some conditions, the above equations should carry an extra AlX_3 molecule, as in the example,

$$\text{arene} \ldots \text{Al}_2\text{X}_6 + \text{RX} \rightleftharpoons \text{R}\overset{+}{\text{X}}—\overset{-}{\text{Al}_2}\text{X}_6 \rightleftharpoons \overset{+}{\text{R}} + \overset{-}{\text{Al}_2\text{X}_7}$$

We have already considered the circumstances in which the first of the represented equilibria should lie towards the left or towards the right. Little is known about the second equilibrium. One expects it to shift towards the right as carbonium-ion stability increases along the series, methylium, primary, secondary, tertiary alkylium (cf. Chapter VII). It should shift to the right towards higher perhalopolyaluminates or polygallates. The equilibrium materials have a small electrical conductance; but since, in the media used, the ions will exist almost wholly in ion-pair form, only a small conductance would in any case be expected.

When an aromatic hydrocarbon is added to this system, the reactions typical of Friedel-Crafts alkylations ensue. The alkylation is reversible. In the forward reactions hydrogen halides are formed, and through their agency dealkylations, as well as hydrogen exchanges, set

[189] F. Fairbrother, *J. Chem. Soc.*, **1937,** 313; **1941,** 293; **1945,** 503; *Trans. Faraday Soc.*, 1941, **37,** 763; F. L. J. Sixma, H. Hendricks, and D. Holzapffel, *Rec. trav. chim.*, 1956, **75,** 127.

in. Dealkylation is a simple extension of hydrogen exchange; for as we have noticed (Section **24c**), an acidic Friedel-Crafts system can add a proton, not only to a hydrogen-bearing, but also to an alkyl-bearing, aromatic carbon atom. This consideration prescribes the mechanism of alkylation. For the principle of microscopic reversibility teaches that a *cyclo*hexadienylium ion of the form established as an intermediate in hydrogen exchange, in particular, the alkyl derivative appropriate to dealkylation, must be a common intermediate for both dealkylation and alkylation:

$$\left.\begin{matrix} \overset{+}{R}X\text{—}\overset{-}{Al}X_3 \\ \upharpoonleft\downharpoonright \\ R^+AlX_4^- \end{matrix}\right\} + C_6H_5\text{—H} \rightleftharpoons \overset{+}{C_6H_5}\!\!<^{R}_{H} + AlX_4^- \rightleftharpoons C_6H_5\text{—R} + \left\{\begin{matrix} H^+AlX_4^- \\ \upharpoonleft\downharpoonright \\ HX + AlX_3 \end{matrix}\right.$$

With many Friedel-Crafts systems, those formed with aluminium bromide or gallium bromide, for example, aromatic alkylations can be run in homogeneous solutions, either in a non-basic solvent or in a basic one. But systems from boron fluoride and hydrogen fluoride, and from aluminium chloride and hydrogen chloride, with a hydrocarbon or other non-basic material as solvent, form two liquid layers. These are an acid-salt layer containing all the boron or aluminium, in which the reactions go on, and an organic layer in which organic factors and products of reaction are stored, insofar as they are not too strongly basic. The extent to which an arene will go into the acid-salt layer will depend on the basicity of the arene, and also on the temperature, inasmuch as a rise of temperature tends to break up salt-like solvation of the arene, thereby returning the latter to the hydrocarbon layer.[190]

Returning to the matter of mechanism, there is preparative evidence for the assumed *cyclo*hexadienylium intermediates in aromatic alkylation.[191] Using toluene, *m*-xylene, and mesitylene as the compounds to be alkylated, methyl, ethyl, *iso*propyl, and *t*-butyl fluorides as the alkyl halides, and boron fluoride as catalyst, the Olahs and Kuhn, employing low temperatures, prepared a number of the tetrafluoroborate addition salts, as yellow, orange, or red solids. At temperatures between −110° and −50° these salts became electrically conducting melts, which at somewhat higher temperatures decomposed to give the aromatic alkyl derivative. Doering and his collaborators

[190] Personal communication from Dr. D. E. Pearson.

[191] G. Olah, S. Kuhn, and J. Olah, *J. Chem. Soc.*, **1957**, **2174**; G. A. Olah and S. J. Kuhn, *J. Am. Chem. Soc.*, 1958, **80**, 6541; W. von E. Doering, M. Saunders, H. G. Boyton, H. W. Earhart, E. F. Wadley, and W. R. Edwards, *Tetrahedron*, **1958**, **4**, **1178**.

have shown that the final product of the polymethylation of benzene with methyl chloride and aluminium chloride is the remarkably stable heptamethyl*cyclo*hexadienylium tetrachloroaluminate. In water, at not too high acidities, the cation loses a proton to give methylene-hexamethyl*cyclo*hexadiene. But the deprotonation is reversible and the olefin is, in fact, so basic that it can be extracted by 4*N* aqueous hydrochloric acid to regenerate the original cation:

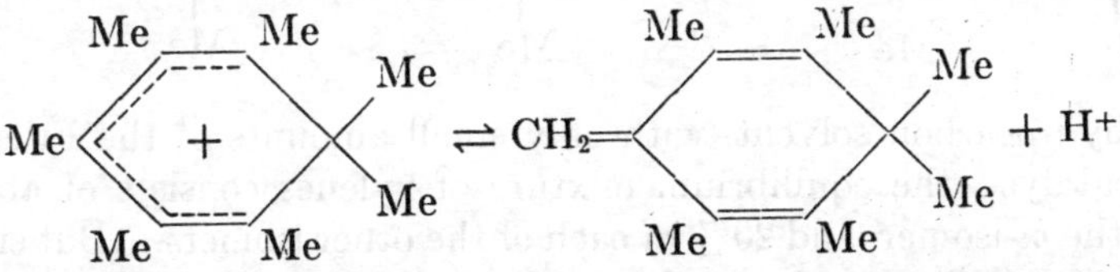

$$\text{(heptamethylcyclohexadienylium cation: Me groups on ring, } + \text{)} \rightleftharpoons CH_2{=}\text{(hexamethylcyclohexadiene: Me groups on ring)} + H^+$$

A notable feature of Friedel-Crafts alkylations consists in the accompanying isomerisations. Of course, isomerisations will occur which are dependent on the reversibility of the reaction, and consist in alternate de-alkylations and re-alkylations. These sequences lead in parallel to disproportionation, that is, the movement of alkyl groups from one alkylated aromatic molecule to another, as in the conversion of toluene to a mixture of benzene and the xylenes. Of more interest are the intramolecular isomerisations, which often take place at lower temperatures,[190] and, having the character of Wagner-Meerwein rearrangements, are not accompanied by disproportionations. These rearrangements are diagnostic of mechanisms dependent on carbonium-ion intermediates, inasmuch as they require the prior formation of carbonium ions. They consist in the shift, with its bond electrons, to the carbonium ionic centre, from an immediately adjoining carbon atom, of a hydrogen atom or of some substituent, commonly a methyl group, the former site of which becomes the new carbonium ionic centre (Chapter X). The xylenes, for example, can be interconverted in this intramolecular way by the acid constituted from a Friedel-Crafts catalyst and co-catalyst. Alternatively, a particular preformed xylene can be thus converted into its isomer. A study of the kinetics of this reaction has shown[192] that it consists only of 1,2-alkyl-shifts, as is characteristic of Wagner-Meerwein rearrangements: the four finite rate constants are those of the reactions ortho⇄meta and para⇄meta; and an attempt to evaluate the two rate constants of the interconversion ortho⇄para gave to both the value zero. The required carbonium ions are, of course, the *cyclo*hexadienylium ionic intermediates

[192] R. H. Allen, A. Turner, and L. D. Yates, *J. Am. Chem. Soc.*, 1959, **81**, 42; R. H. Allen and L. D. Yates, *ibid.*, p. 5289; *idem* and D. S. Early, *ibid.*, 1960, **82**, 4853; R. H. Allen, *ibid.*, p. 4856.

on which all Friedel-Craft alkylations depend. The para⇄meta conversion is here illustrated:

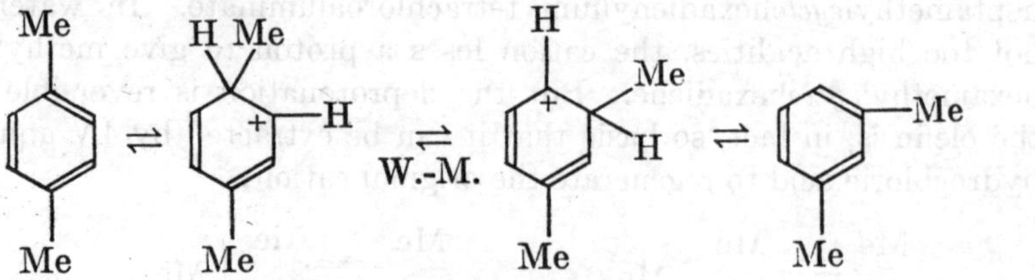

$$\text{p-xylene} \rightleftharpoons \text{[H, Me]}^+ \overset{}{\underset{\text{W.-M.}}{\rightleftharpoons}} \text{[H, Me]}^+ \rightleftharpoons \text{m-xylene}$$

In a hydrocarbon solvent, with only small amounts of the Friedel-Crafts catalyst, the equilibrium mixture of xylenes consists of about 60% of the *m*-isomer, and 20% of each of the other isomers. But since *m*-xylene is much more basic than either of its isomers (Table 24-1), one can "cheat" this equilibrium by the use of an excess of a strongly acidic Friedel-Crafts reagent, which will selectively sequester the most basic isomer, and so lead preparatively to nearly 100% of *m*-xylene.

The kinetics of alkylation have been studied by H. C. Brown and his collaborators.[193] Alkylation of benzene, toluene, and *m*-xylene by 3,4-dichlorobenzyl chloride and *p*-nitrobenzyl chloride, with aluminium chloride, in solvent nitrobenzene, followed the rate equation,

$$\text{Rate} \propto [\text{ArH}][\text{RCl}][\text{AlCl}_3]$$

Alkylation of benzene and toluene by ethyl bromide, with aluminium bromide, or by methyl and ethyl bromides, with gallium bromide, in 1,2,4-trichlorobenzene as solvent, followed a similar third-order equation. The kinetic form means that the transition state of alkylation in these solvents involves the whole material content of $RX + MX_3$, which in the initial state is stored as two kinetic particles—presumably because one of them is strongly complexed with the solvent: they are the entities represented on the left of the left-sided equilibrium,

$$\text{basic-solvent}\overset{+}{}\text{—}\overset{-}{\text{M}}\text{X}_3 + \text{RX} \rightleftharpoons \text{solvent} + \overset{+}{\text{R}\text{X}}\text{—}\overset{-}{\text{M}}\text{X}_3$$

In hydrocarbon solvents, however, other kinetics obtain, the significance of which is not clear.

That the active alkylating agent is a carbonium ion in some form—and, if this is so, the kinetic evidence points to an ion-pair form—in Friedel-Crafts alkylations generally is shown by the prevalence of

[193] H. C. Brown and M. Grayson, *J. Am. Chem. Soc.*, 1953, **75**, 6285; H. Jungk, C. R. Smoot, and H. C. Brown, *ibid.*, 1956, **78**, 2185; C. M. Smoot and H. C. Brown, *ibid.*, pp. 6245, 6249; S. U. Choi and H. C. Brown, *ibid.*, 1959, **81**, 3315; 1963, **85**, 2596.

Wagner-Meerwein rearrangements within the alkyl groups being introduced, when the structures of the latter are suitable. According to the theory of Wagner-Meerwein rearrangements, the rearranging alkyl groups must at some stage have been in a carbonium-ion condition. By this criterion, we can show that carbonium ions are formed from an alkyl halide and a Friedel-Crafts catalyst, without any aromatic substrate. It does not follow that the Wagner-Meerwein rearrangement observed in these circumstances will have time to occur before the first-formed carbonium ion reacts with an initially introduced aromatic substrate; whether it has time or not largely depends on the alkyl structure. Thus *n*-propyl chloride, on treatment with aluminium chloride, gives *iso*propyl chloride; and added deuterium chloride does not introduce deuterium into the product.[194] This is therefore not an elimination-addition sequence going by way of propylene, but is a Wagner-Meerwein rearrangement involving a shift of hydrogen from position-2 to position-1 in the *n*-propylium ion, to give the *iso*propylium ion:

$$CH_3 \cdot CH_2 \cdot CH_2 \cdot Cl \rightleftharpoons CH_3 \cdot CH_2 \cdot CH_2^+ \rightleftharpoons CH_3 \cdot \overset{+}{C}H \cdot CH_3$$
$$\rightleftharpoons CH_3 \cdot CHCl \cdot CH_3$$

But when *n*-propyl chloride and aluminium chloride are used to alkylate benzene, the product is *n*-propylbenzene. We assume that the primary alkylium ion is so reactive that it attacks the benzene before the 2-hydrogen atom has had time to shift over. For, if we now weaken the binding of the 2-hydrogen atom, which was secondary, by making it tertiary, as in *iso*butyl chloride, not only will treatment with aluminium chloride produce *t*-butyl chloride, but also treatment with aluminium chloride and benzene will give *t*-butylbenzene. The Wagner-Meerwein transformation has the same form as before:

$$(CH_3)_2CH \cdot CH_2Cl \rightleftharpoons (CH_3)_2CH \cdot CH_2^+ \rightleftharpoons (CH_3)_2\overset{+}{C} \cdot CH_3 \rightleftharpoons (CH_3)_3CCl$$

But now the 2-hydrogen atom shifts over faster than even the primary alkylium ion can attack the benzene ring, so that all the alkylating of the latter is done by the more stable, though more slowly reacting, tertiary alkylium ion. These examples illustrate the extremes of a conflict, which we can follow higher in the alkyl series,[195] between

[194] A. V. Topchev, B. A. Kreutsel and L. N. Andreef, *Dokl. Akad. Nauk, U.S.S.R.*, 1953, **92**, 781.

[195] Reviews by N. O. Calloway, *Chem. Rev.*, 1935, **17**, 237; H. Gilman and R. N. Meals, *J. Org. Chem.*, 1943, **8**, 126; cf. also L. Schmierling and J. P. West, *J. Am. Chem. Soc.*, 1954, **76**, 1917.

length of life and reactivity in interconvertible ions: they become more readily formed, but less reactive, along the series, primary, secondary, tertiary alkylium. Shifts of methyl, as well as of hydrogen, may contribute to the interconversions, the slowest steps of which are usually the shifts of either hydrogen or methyl from a secondary carbon atom. Secondary butyl halides give mixtures of *s*- and *t*-butylbenzenes, whereas *iso*butyl and *t*-butyl halides given only *t*-butylbenzene:

$$CH_3\cdot CH_2\cdot \overset{+}{C}H\cdot CH_3 \rightarrow \overset{+}{C}H_2\cdot CH(CH_3)_2 \rightarrow CH_3\cdot \overset{+}{C}(CH_3)_2$$

$$\overset{+}{C}H\ (\text{sec-butyl}) \xrightarrow{ArH} \text{Product} \qquad CH_3\cdot\overset{+}{C}(CH_3)_2 \xrightarrow{ArH} \text{Product}$$

Neopentyl, *s-iso*amyl, and *t*-amyl halides give identical mixtures of *s-iso*amyl- and *t*-amyl-benzenes:

$$(CH_3)_3C\cdot\overset{+}{C}H_2 \rightarrow (CH_3)_2\overset{+}{C}\cdot CH_2\cdot CH_3 \rightleftharpoons (CH_3)_2CH\cdot\overset{+}{C}H\cdot CH_3$$

$$(CH_3)_2\overset{+}{C}\cdot CH_2\cdot CH_3 \xrightarrow{ArH} \text{Product} \qquad (CH_3)_2CH\cdot\overset{+}{C}H\cdot CH_3 \xrightarrow{ArH} \text{Product}$$

And so on. There seems often to be easy reversibility, and a good balance of the combined effects of life and reactivity, between secondary and tertiary isomers of carbonium ions.

The patterns of reactivity distribution over the benzene ring in Friedel-Crafts alkylations are qualitatively similar to those already illustrated for nitration and halogenation but show generally smaller contrasts. For alkylations, toluene is relatively mildly activated, and chlorobenzene mildly deactivated; and in both substrates the positional discrimination is milder, more of the meta-isomers being produced. These findings are due to H. C. Brown and his coworkers,[196] who connect them theoretically on the basis that the more active reagent is less discriminating, whether between substrates or between positions in a substrate. Along a series of reactions, methylation, ethylation, and *iso*propylation, by means of the alkyl bromide and gallium bromide, of the same substrate, toluene, the rates increase, according to Allen and Yates,[196] in the ratios 1:14:20,000. Presumably the carbonium ion gets formed either more rapidly, or in greater

[196] L. M. Stock and H. C. Brown in "Advances in Physical Organic Chemistry," Editor V. Gold, Academic Press, London and New York, 1963, Vol. 1, p. 35; R. H. Allen and L. D. Yates, *J. Am. Chem. Soc.*, 1961, **83**, 2799.

equilibrium proportion, or both, along the series, and the rate of alkylation is controlled more by carbonium-ion availability than by the rate of carbonium-ion attack on the substrate.

Some figures by Brown and his collaborators for rates of substitution in benzene derivatives, relatively to the rates of substitution in benzene, and figures by Brown, and by Allen and Yates, for the proportions of isomers formed in the substitutions of benzene derivatives, are assembled in Table 24-2.[196] The data by Brown and coworkers are for the conditions stated in the table headings, and those (in italics) by Allen and Yates are for various Friedel-Crafts systems, which acted very similarly, and were carefully controlled to eliminate effects of isomerisation subsequent to substitution.

TABLE 24-2.—RELATIVE RATES AND ISOMER PERCENTAGES IN ALKYLATIONS, MAINLY WITH ALKYL BROMIDES AND GALLIUM BROMIDE (BROWN; ALLEN).

Substrate	Substitution	Solvent (25°)	Rel. rate ($C_6H_6 = 1$)	Percentages: Ortho	Meta	Para
PhMe	Methylation	PhMe	5.7	56, *60*	10, *14*	34, *26*
	Ethylation		2.5	38, *48*	21, *18*	41, *34*
	*Iso*propylation		1.8	26, *42*	27, *22*	47, *36*
PhF	Ethylation	$C_2H_4Cl_2$	0.28	43	14	43
PhCl			0.215	42	16	42
PhBr			0.133	24	22	54

Brown's partial rate factors for ethylation are shown below. The pattern given by toluene is qualitatively normal for an orienting substituent of Type (1) $(+I)$, as are those given by the halogenobenzenes for those substituents of Type (3) $(-I+K)$ which expose the Holleman anomaly. But all the contrasts are less sharp than those illustrated for nitration in Sections **21b** and **21c**:

	CH_3	F	Cl	Br
ortho	2.8	0.36	0.27	0.10
meta	1.6	0.12	0.16	0.087
para	6.0	0.74	0.39	0.43

Other ways of producing carbonium ions can be employed in aromatic alkylations. One is through the dehydrating protonation of an alcohol, such as benzhydrol:

$$Ph_2CH \cdot OH + H^+ \rightleftharpoons Ph_2CH^+ + H_2O$$

Bethel and Gold[197] have shown that benzhydrylation of mesitylene, anisole, and other aromatic compounds, by benzhydrol in acetic acid containing sulphuric acid, occurs with a rate which follows Gold's acidity measure j_0, the measure of the degree to which a medium will supply in equlibrium a proton to extract a hydroxide ion from a hydroxy-compound, as formulated above. Another method, examined by Pearson and his coworkers,[198] is through the deamination of primary aliphatic amines, such as *iso*propylamine, by means of nitrous acid:

$$Me_2CH \cdot NH_2 + HNO_2 + H^+ \rightarrow Me_2CH^+ + N_2 + 2H_2O$$

In the *iso*propylation of benzene or alkylbenzenes by this method, the yields are low, because other things happen to the carbonium ions in the media employed. However, the ratios in which the cymenes are formed from toluene are almost identical with those obtained by Allen and Yates under more ordinary conditions of alkylation.

(24e) Acylation.—Acylium ions RCO^+ are on the whole more stable, less reactive, and therefore are more easily produced than alkylium ions. In 1937 Treffers and Hammett[199] showed cryoscopically that mesitoic acid in solvent sulphuric acid is quantitatively heterolysed according to the equation:

$$C_6H_2Me_3 \cdot CO_2H + 2H_2SO_4 \rightarrow C_6H_2Me_3 \cdot CO^+ + H_3O^+ + 2HSO_4^-$$

Benzoic acid does not behave in this way: it simply becomes protonated: so also does acetic acid. But Gillespie showed,[200] again cryoscopically, that benzoic anhydride and acetic anhydride are quantitatively heterolysed in sulphuric acid, as illustrated by the equation

$$C_6H_5 \cdot CO \cdot O \cdot CO \cdot C_6H_5 + 2H_2SO_4 \rightleftharpoons C_6H_5 \cdot CO^+ + C_6H_5 \cdot COOH_2^+ + 2HSO_4^-$$

Burton and Praill showed that solutions of such anhydrides, along with sulphuric acid or perchloric acid, could be used for aromatic acylation.[201] They showed also that the solution obtained by mixing

[197] R. D. Bethel and V. Gold, *Chem. and Ind.*, **1956**, 741; *J. Chem. Soc.*, **1958**, 1905; *idem* and T. Riley, *ibid.*, **1959**, 313.

[198] D. E. Pearson, C. V. Breder, and J. C. Craig, *J. Am. Chem. Soc.*, **1964**, **86**, 5054.

[199] H. P. Treffers and L. P. Hammett, *J. Am. Chem. Soc.*, **1937**, **59**, 1708.

[200] R. J. Gillespie, *J. Chem. Soc.*, **1950**, 2997.

[201] H. Burton and P. F. G. Praill, *J. Chem. Soc.*, **1950**, 1203, 2034; **1951**, 522, 529, 726.

acetyl chloride and silver perchlorate in solution in nitromethane, and filtering off the silver chloride, contained an alkylating agent capable, for instance, of converting anisole into *p*-methoxyacetophenone readily and in high yield. The acylating agent here could only have been the acetylium ion, $CH_3 \cdot CO^+$, co-ordinated, of course, with the nitromethane.

Acylium salts of the complex perhalo-acids of importance in the Friedel-Crafts method of acylation have been isolated as crystalline solids, and characterised spectroscopically. Seel prepared and characterised one of them,[202] acetylium tetrafluoroborate, $CH_3 \cdot CO^+BF_4^-$, in 1943. Olah and his collaborators have prepared many acylium salts containing the anions BF_4^-, PF_6^-, AsF_6^-, SbF_6^-, and $SbCl_6^-$.[202] They have used a number of these for various *O*-, *N*-, and *S*-acylations; and they have used acetylium hexafluoroantimonate and acetylium hexachloroantimonate, $CH_3 \cdot CO^+SbF_6^-$ and $CH_3CO^+SbCl_6^-$, for aromatic acetylations.

The kinetics of Friedel-Crafts acylations have been studied by H. C. Brown and his collaborators.[203] The benzoylation of benzene and alkylbenzenes by means of benzoyl chloride and aluminium chloride, either in excess of benzoyl chloride, or in ethylene dichloride as solvent, and also the acetylation of these hydrocarbons by acetyl chloride and aluminium chloride in solvent ethylene dichloride, all follow the rate equation,

$$\text{Rate} \propto [\text{ArH}][\text{AlCl}_3]$$

In all cases the aluminium chloride is initially complexed almost stoicheiometrically with the acyl chloride, which is in excess, and is the most basic substance present. Presumably they form the ionising adduct,

$$\text{RCCl}:\overset{+}{\text{O}}\text{—}\overset{-}{\text{Al}}\text{Cl}_3 \rightleftharpoons \text{RCO}^+ + \text{AlCl}_4^-$$

The kinetics show that this adduct,[204] either in dipolar or ion-pair form, but not the acylium ion dissociated from it, enters into the composition of the transition state of aromatic acylation.

[202] F. Seel, *Z. anorg. Chem.*, 1943, **250**, 331; G. A. Olah, S. J. Kuhn, W. S. Tolgyesi, and E. B. Baker, *J. Am. Chem. Soc.*, 1962, **84**, 2733; *idem* and M. E. Moffatt, *ibid.*, 1963, **85**, 1328.

[203] H. C. Brown and F. R. Jenson, *J. Am. Chem. Soc.*, 1958, **80**, 2291, 2296; H. C. Brown and G. Marino, *ibid.*, 1959, **81**, 3308; *idem* and L. M. Stock, *ibid.*, p. 3210.

[204] That of benzyol chloride is certainly in dipolar form in the solid, as has been shown by an X-ray study (S. E Rasmussen and N. S. Broch, *Chem. Comm.*, **1965**, 289).

One of the main reasons for thinking that the active agent is the ion-pair is that it seems to make very little difference, as we shall see below, either to the relative reactivity for acylation of different aromatic compounds, or to the distribution of reactivity over a particular aromatic ring, whether we operate with one of the Friedel-Crafts acylating systems for which the kinetics of acylation have been studied, or with a pre-prepared acylium salt, such as a hexafluoroantimonate, in an inert but polar solvent. It is generally assumed that, however the acylium ion is carried and presented, it is first added to the aromatic molecule, to form an acyl*cyclo*hexadienylium ion, which subsequently becomes deprotonated:

$$\mathrm{RCO^+} + \text{—H} \rightleftharpoons \overset{\text{COR}}{\text{H}} \rightleftharpoons \text{—COR} + \mathrm{H^+}$$

So far, no well-characterised salts of an acyl*cyclo*hexadienylium ion have been isolated.

The relative reactivities of different aromatic molecules, and the distribution of reactivity over their aromatic rings, in acylations, has been investigated by H. C. Brown and by G. A. Olah, with their respective collaborators. Brown has studied benzyolation and acetylation, with acyl chlorides and aluminium chloride in various solvents, that is, with typical Friedel-Crafts reagents.[196] Olah has studied acetylation, using the same reagents, and also the pre-prepared salts, acetylium hexafluoroantimonate and acetylium hexachloroantimonate, in nitromethane as solvent.[205] The method, and within a method the solvent, or the anion of the salt, make little difference to the results. Samples of these authors' figures for rates of substitution relative to the rate for benzene, and for the proportions of isomers formed, are in Table 24-3. It is a point of interest that the differences from nitration are qualitative opposites of those shown by alkylation. That is to say, activations and deactivations are more pronounced, and isomer proportions are more uneven, in acylations than in nitration, and *a fortiori* than in alkylation. Brown links these effects with the mild reactivity of acylium ions, relatively to nitronium and alkylium ions.

The same characteristics may be brought out by the use of the partial rate factors, some examples of which, referring to acetylation with acetyl chloride and aluminium chloride in ethylene dichloride as

[205] G. A. Olah, M. E. Moffatt, S. J. Kuhn, and B. A. Hardie, *J. Am. Chem. Soc.*, 1964, **86**, 2198; G. A. Olah, S. J. Kuhn, S. H. Flood, and B. A. Hardie, *ibid.*, p. 2203.

TABLE 24-3.—RELATIVE RATES AND ISOMER PERCENTAGES IN BENZOYLATION WITH BENZOYL CHLORIDE AND ALUMINIUM CHLORIDE, AND IN ACETYLATION SIMILARLY, AND WITH ACETYLIUM HEXAHALOANTIMONATES (BROWN, OLAH).

Substrate	Reagent	Solvent (25°)	Rel. rate ($C_6H_6=1$)	Percentages		
				Ortho	Meta	Para
			Benzoylation			
Ph—Me	$PhCOCl+AlCl_3$	PhCOCl	110	9.3	1.4	89
Ph—Me	$PhCOCl+AlCl_3$	$C_2H_4Cl_2$	117	—	—	—
Ph—Bu-*t*	$PhCOCl+AlCl_3$	$C_2H_4Cl_2$	76	0.0	5.4	95
Ph—F	$PhCOCl+AlCl_3$	$C_2H_4Cl_2$	0.25	0.0	0.0	100
Ph—Cl	$PhCOCl+AlCl_3$	PhCOCl	0.0115	0.0	0.0	100
			Acetylation			
Ph—Me	$MeCOCl+AlCl_3$	$C_2H_4Cl_2$	128	1.2	1.2	98
Ph—Me	$MeCO^+SbF_6^-$	$MeNO_2$	125	1.4	0.9	98
Ph—Me	$MeCO^+SbCl_6^-$	$MeNO_2$	121	0.8	0.9	98
Ph—Bu-*t*	$MeCOCl+AlCl_3$	$MeNO_2$	114	0.0	3.8	96
Ph—Bu-*t*	$MeCO^+SbF_6^-$	$MeNO_2$	74	0.0	5.7	94
Ph—F	$MeCO^+SbF_6^-$	$MeNO_2$	0.51	—	—	—
Ph—Cl	$MeCOCl+AlCl_3$	$C_2H_4Cl_2$	0.021	0.0	0.5	99
Ph—Cl	$MeCO^+SbF_6^-$	$MeNO_2$	0.016	—	—	—
Ph—Cl	$MeCO^+SbF_6^-$	$MeNO_2$	0.02	—	—	—
Ph—Br	$MeCOCl+AlCl_3$	$C_2H_4Cl_2$	0.014	0.0	0.0	100
Ph—Br	$MeCO^+SbF_6^-$	$MeNO_2$	0.01	—	—	—

solvent, are set out below:

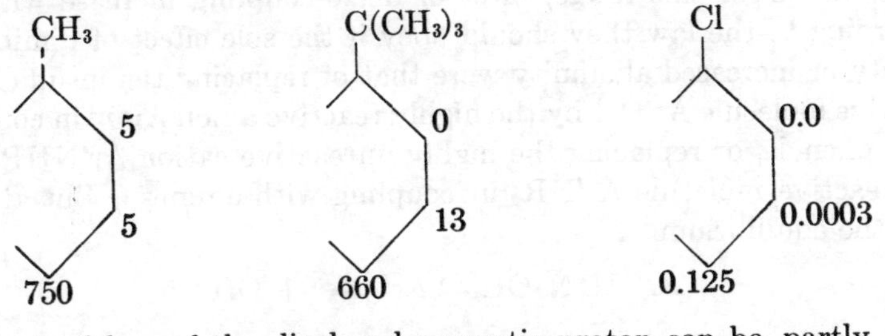

CH_3: 5, 5, 750

$C(CH_3)_3$: 0, 13, 660

Cl: 0.0, 0.0003, 0.125

The final loss of the displaced aromatic proton can be partly rate-controlling. This is shown by the observation[205] of reduced rates of acylation by pre-prepared acetylium hexafluoro- and hexa-chloro-antimonates in nitromethane solution, when aromatic deuterium has to be displaced. As compared with benzene, the rates of acetylation of hexadeuterobenzene were reduced by factors close to 2.2. Somewhat similar factors were obtained for the acylation of toluene and mesitylene. As primary deuterium isotope effects go, these are small effects. They probably signify that the energy barriers protecting the presumed intermediate acetyl*cyclo*hexadienylium ion from acetylium-ion loss and from proton loss are comparable.

(24f) Diazo-coupling.—It has been tolerably clear from orientation theory since 1926, that the active species in diazo-coupling is an electrophilic substituting agent, which could hardly be anything else than the diazonium ion ArN_2^+. However, this was not formally established until 1941.

The first comprehensive study of the kinetics of diazo-coupling with phenols was that of Conant and Peterson.[206] They represented the rate as proportional to $[ArN_2OH][Ar'OH]$, and thought of the process as a bimolecular reaction between the molecules indicated. However, since the active mass of the solvent water is constant, the kinetic laws are still satisfied if one molecule of water is removed from the transition state, the rate being set proportional to $[ArN_2^+][Ar'O^-]$, as an expression of the view that the bimolecular reaction is between the diazonium ion and the aryloxide ion. The kinetic study was extended, with the inclusion of coupling with aromatic amines, by Wistar and Bartlett[207] and by Hauser and Breslow.[208] They showed that the only generally consistent picture of the coupling process is that indicated by assuming $[ArN_2^+][Ar'O^-]$ to be the appropriate concentration product for coupling with phenols, and $[ArN_2^+][Ar'NR_2]$ for coupling with amines.

Most diazonium ions are thermodynamically stable, relatively to the non-ionised diazohydroxides, in acidic and weakly alkaline aqueous solution. Over this range, rates of diazo-coupling increase with pH according to the law they should obey if the sole effect of diminished acidity or increased alkalinity were that of replacing the insufficiently reactive molecule Ar′OH by the highly reactive anion ArO^- in coupling with phenols, or replacing the highly unreactive cation $Ar'NHR_2^+$ by the reactive molecule $Ar'NR_2$ in coupling with amines. But at high pH, the equilibrium

$$Ar'\cdot N{:}N\cdot OH \rightleftarrows Ar'\cdot N_2^+ + OH^-$$

moves appreciably to the left, reducing the active mass of the diazonium ion, and therefore reducing the accelerating effect of alkalinity on diazo-coupling.

That the phenyldiazonium ion is only a weak electrophile is shown by the fact that it will substitute the phenoxide ion and the aniline molecule, but not the less reactive anisole molecule, or the molecules of

[206] J. B. Conant and W. D. Peterson, *J. Am. Chem. Soc.*, 1930, **52**, 1220.
[207] R. Wistar and P. D. Bartlett, *J. Am. Chem. Soc.*, 1941, **63**, 413.
[208] C. R. Hauser and D. S. Breslow, *J. Am. Chem. Soc.*, 1941, **63**, 418.

still less reactive benzene compounds. However, the reactivity of a diazonium ion is enhanced by electronegative substitution. This is shown by Conant and Peterson's rate values, as reduced and summarised by Hammett.[209] The following relative rates for para-substituted phenyldiazonium ions hold to within 25% for coupling with five different phenols:

$—NO_2$	$—SO_3^-$	—Br	H	$—CH_3$	$—O{\cdot}CH_3$
1300	13	13	(1)	0.4	0.1

This kind of relationship is to be expected, because the nitro-group will increase, and the methoxyl group will decrease, the positive charge carried by the diazo-group, as indicated in the following expressions:

$$\left[O_2N—C_6H_4—N{\equiv}N\right]^+ \qquad \left[MeO—C_6H_4—N{\equiv}N\right]^+$$

Some time ago, Kurt Meyer and his associates discovered empirically that nitro-substituents could be used to extend the range of the coupling reaction.[210] The phenyldiazonium ion will couple freely with phloroglucinol ethers, but not with less reactive phenolic ethers. The *p*-nitrophenyldiazonium ion will couple with resorcinol ethers, though still not with simple phenolic ethers. However, the 2:4-dinitrophenyldiazonium ion will couple with anisole and phenetole. And the 2:4:6-trinitrophenyldiazonium ion will couple with mesitylene (which is comparable in reactivity to a negatively monosubstituted anisole, such as *p*-chloroanisole). These results make it clear that in principle the diazonium ion is a general reagent for electrophilic aromatic substitution.

It has been known since the last century[211] that the easy coupling of diazonium ions with *NN*-dialkylanilines fails with ortho-substituted derivatives of the latter. The cause of this became apparent only

[209] L. P. Hammett, "Physical Organic Chemistry," McGraw-Hill, New York, 1940, p. 314.

[210] K. H. Meyer and S. Leinhardt, *Ann.*, 1913, **398**, 66; K. H. Meyer, A. Irschick, and H. Schlösser, *Ber.*, 1914, **47**, 1741; K. H. Meyer and V. Schöller, *Ber.*, 1919, **52**, 1468; K. H. Meyer and H. Tochtermann, *Ber.*, 1921, **54**, 2283; They also showed that nitro-substituents would extend the range of diazo-coupling so that it included electrophilic olefinic substitution. Thus, although the phenyldiazonium ion would not couple with any of the simpler derivatives of buta-1:3-diene, the *p*-nitrophenyldiazonium ion coupled satisfactorily with 2:3-dimethylbuta-1:3-diene, but not with less reactive butadienes, while the 2:4-dinitrophenyldiazonium ion coupled with 2-methylbuta-1:3-diene, and even with buta-1:3-diene itself. In all cases, coupling occurred in the 1-position.

[211] P. Friedländer, *Monatsh.*, 1898, **19**, 627; cf. T. C. van Hoek, P. E. Verkade, and B. M. Wepster, *Rec. trav. chim.*, 1958, **77**, 559.

after the discovery of the secondary steric effect in 1937 (Section **8g**): pressure from the ortho-substituents twists the dialkylamino-group and so destroys its activating conjugation with the ring (cf. Section **24i**).

Zollinger has shown that diazo-coupling uses the bimolecular mechanism S_E2, involving a *cyclo*hexadienylium intermediate:[212]

$$Ar'N_2^+ + ArH \underset{(-1)}{\overset{(1)}{\rightleftharpoons}} \overset{+}{Ar}\begin{matrix} N_2Ar' \\ H \end{matrix}$$

$$\overset{+}{Ar}\begin{matrix} N_2Ar' \\ H \end{matrix} + B \xrightarrow[(2)]{} ArN_2Ar' + HB^+ \qquad (S_E2)$$

and does not employ the one-step termolecular mechanism S_E3:

$$Ar'N_2^+ + ArH + B \rightarrow ArN_2Ar' + HB^+ \qquad (S_E3)$$

His evidence relates to the kinetic effect of providing deuterium as the hydrogen atom to be replaced, and to the incidence of general base catalysis. In general, there is no kinetic isotope effect, and (once the reactive form of the substrate is fully supplied, *e.g.*, as the phenoxide ion, rather than the phenol molecule) there is no detectable basic catalysis. Both these observations indicate against mechanism S_E3, but can be reconciled with mechanism S_E2 on the assumption that its step (2) is so much faster than step (−1) that the proton loss does not affect the rate, which is simply that of the addition process (1).

But in special structural circumstances, in particular, when a sulphonate-ion substituent neighbours the coupling position, a reduction in rate is found when deuterium has to be displaced, and, concurrently, a base catalysis of coupling sets in. This is general base catalysis, each base in a mixture, *e.g.*, not only water, but also acetate ions, in an acetate buffer, contributing its own rate term. These effects mean that the proton loss, that is, its transference to a base, has become at least partly rate-controlling. The kinetic isotope effects in a series of three examples, along which rate-control by the proton loss is increasing from insignificance to dominance, are set out below. They refer to

[212] H. Zollinger, *Helv. Chim. Acta*, 1955, **38**, 1597, 1617, 1632; O. A. Stamm and H. Zollinger, *ibid.*, 1957, **40**, 1955; H. F. Hodson, O. A. Stamm, and H. Zollinger, *ibid.*, 1958, 41, 1816; R. Ernst, O. A. Stamm, and H. Zollinger, *ibid.*, p. 2274; H. Zollinger, *Angew. Chem.*, 1958, **70**, 2021.

coupling with diazotised *p*-chloroaniline in the positions marked by a deuterium atom in the formulae:

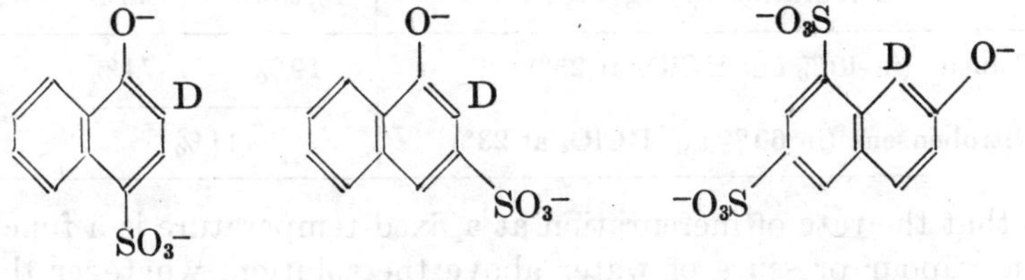

k/k_D · · · 1.04 3.10 6.55

Now we cannot assume that these effects are due to the incursion of mechanism S_E3, because, if that were so, the catalytic rate term due to a base would rise linearly with the concentration of the base, whereas in general it rises less than linearly, *i.e.*, on a diminishing gradient, according to a law noted below. The alternative interpretation is that the sulphonate ion groups are so reducing the rate of proton loss from the adduct-ion of mechanism S_E2, that this rate falls near to, or even below, the rate of reversal of the original addition. As this happens, there will be a rising isotope effect as illustrated, and, at the same time, a base catalysis will appear. The catalysed rate will now depend on base concentration through the factor $[B]/(c+[B])$, where c is a constant, equal to the ratio, k_1/k_2, of the rate-constants of the reactions between which the adduct is partitioned. This is the less-than-linear law mentioned. So all aspects of these phenomena support mechanism S_E2.

(24g) Mercuration.—There has been some doubt about the electropolar classification of this substitution in non-polar solvents, but in polar solvents it is certainly electrophilic. Klaproth and Westheimer showed that mercuration by mercuric perchlorate in water containing perchloric acid produces isomer ratios, as Table 24-4 illustrates, comparable to those given by other electrophilic substitutions.[213] The free acid present prevents hydrolysis, *i.e.*, deprotonation of the aqueous co-ordination shell of the mercuric ion; and it strongly increases the rate of substitution. The latter effect is not acid catalysis, because added sodium perchlorate does the same. Perren and Westheimer have shown[214] that this effect is due to activation of the mercuric ion, analogously to the activation of hydrogen ion, by the loss of water from its solvation shell, as the thermodynamic activity of solvent water becomes diminished by the added electrolytes. Their evidence

[213] W. J. Klaproth and F. H. Westheimer, *J. Am. Chem. Soc.*, 1950, **72**, 4461.
[214] C. Perren and F. H. Westheimer, *J. Am. Chem. Soc.*, 1963, **85**, 273.

TABLE 24-4.—ORIENTATION OF MERCURATION.

Mercuration by $Hg(ClO_4)_2$	ortho-	para-	meta-
Toluene (in 40% aq. $HClO_4$ at 25°)	19%	74%	7%
Nitrobenzene (in 60% aq. $HClO_4$ at 23°)	11%		89%

is that the rate of mercuration at a fixed temperature is a function of the vapour pressure of water above the solution, whatever the electrolyte may be that is controlling the vapour pressure.

Aqueous mercuration follows the kinetic law,

$$\text{Rate} \propto [\text{ArH}][\text{Hg}^{++}]$$

Perren and Westheimer found that the rate of mercuration of hexadeuterobenzene was 4.7–6.7 times smaller than the rate for benzene. The mechanism is not established, but the isotope effect shows that, if the mechanism is S_E2, with prior formation of a *cyclo*hexadienylium adduct, then proton loss from the adduct must be rate-controlling.

The distribution of reactivity conferred on the benzene ring by orienting substituents for mercuration by mercuric acetate in solvent acetic acid has been illustrated by Brown and his collaborators,[196] who have measured partial rate factors in these conditions for several mono-substituted benzenes. Some of their results are recorded here:

	CH_3	$C(CH_3)_3$	OMe	Cl
ortho	5.7	~0	186	0.075
meta	2.2	3.4	~1	0.060
para	23	17	2300	0.36

Qualitatively, these patterns of reactivity are much like those of other electrophilic substitutions, but the contrasts both between substrates, and between positions in a substrate, are somewhat mild—milder, for instance, than for nitration or hydrogen exchange.

(24h) Desilylation, Degermylation, Destannylation, and Deplumbylation.—Eaborn and his coworkers have shown that group-IV aromatic substituents of the form XR_3, where X = Si, Ge, Sn, Pb, and R = alkyl, can be replaced by hydrogen, bromine, mercury, and so on by use of the appropriate electrophilic substituting agents, *i.e.*, the same reagents as would be used to secure replacements of aromatic hydrogen. The replacement of the group-IV substituents by hydrogen through the agency of strong acids has been extensively investigated by these workers, and the results permit a new type of comparison.[215] Most previously studied electrophilic aromatic substitutions allow comparisons in which the substituting agent and the orienting group are varied, the group being replaced, namely, hydrogen, remaining the same. The acidolysis of group-IV substituents afforded an opportunity to maintain a common substituting agent, but to use a variety of expelled groups, and so to examine how aromatic reactivity, intrinsic, and as modified and redistributed by orienting substituents, vary with the expelled group.

The acidolysis of any of the compounds mentioned is usually effected with perchloric or sulphuric acid in an aqueous organic solvent. The stoicheiometry can be expressed by the equation

$$ArXR_3 + H_3O^+ \rightarrow ArH + XR_3^+ + H_2O$$

with the added note that the expelled XR_3^+ is converted to a hydroxide, alkoxide, or salt in the conditions.

The nature of the substituting agent, the stoicheiometry, and the patterns of reactivity produced by orienting substituents all make clear that the reactions are electrophilic substitutions. The detailed mechanisms are not unambiguously settled, but Eaborn and his coworkers have shown, for all four group-IV elements, that rates of acidolysis are reduced by factors from 1.6 to 3.1 when solvent water is replaced by deuterium oxide. This shows that the proton addition is at least partly rate-controlling, so that, if the mechanism is S_E2, the slow step is the formation of the substituted *cyclo*hexadienylium ion:

$$H_3O^+ + \text{(Ar–}XR_3) \xrightarrow[\text{slow}]{} \text{(cyclohexadienylium ion bearing } XR_3 \text{ and H)} \longrightarrow \text{(Ar–H)} + R_3X^+$$

Although the reactions run in the opposite direction, this conclusion corresponds to Westheimer's on similar evidence that in aromatic mercuration the final proton loss is rate-controlling.

The rate of replacement by acidolysis of XR_3 groups is dependent on

[215] C. Eaborn, *J. Chem. Soc.*, **1956,** 4856; F. B. Deans and C. Eaborn, *ibid.*, **1959,** 2299; *idem* and D. E. Webster, *ibid.*, p. 3031; C. Eaborn, Z. Lasocki, and D. E. Webster, *ibid.*, p. 3034; C. Eaborn and R. C. Moore, *ibid.*, p. 3640; C. Eaborn and K. C. Pande, *ibid.*, **1960,** 1566; **1961,** 297, 3715, 5082; C. Eaborn and J. A. Waters, *ibid.*, p. 542; R. W. Bott, C. Eaborn, and P. M. Greaseley, *ibid.*, **1964,** 4804; R. W. Bott, C. Eaborn, and D. R. M. Walton, *J. Organmetal. Chem.*, **1964, 2,** 154.

the Mendeléjeff period, especially towards higher periods, of the group-IV elements. Eaborn and Pande have estimated, partly indirectly because of the great range of the figures, the following relative rates:

H	SiR_3	GeR_3	SnR_3	PbR_3
	1	35	350,000	200,000,000
1	10^4	$10^{5.5}$	$10^{9.5}$	10^{12}

The rates, relative to the rate of replacement of hydrogen in hydrogen exchange, are in the lower line of figures. The nature of the alkyl groups R_3 is relatively unimportant: the three alkyl systems employed by Eaborn, trimethyl, triethyl, and tri*cyclo*hexyl, provide rates diminishing in that order, but all comprised within a range of the order of ten-fold.

A general idea of the activating or deactivating effects of substituents previously present in the aromatic compound can be obtained from the survey in Table 24-5 of the kinetic effects of para-substituents. They do produce a great range of rates, greatest when a silicontrialkyl group is to be expelled, and then diminishing along the series of germanium-, tin-, and lead-trialkyl groups. But even in the desilylations, the kinetic effects are smaller than in hydrogen exchanges, as far as we can judge from the comparisons available (Section **24c**).

TABLE 24-5.—EFFECT OF *p*-SUBSTITUENTS ON THE RELATIVE RATES OF ACIDOLYTIC REPLACEMENT OF XR_3 SUBSTITUENTS (EABORN).

Reagent	$HClO_4$, H_2O, MeOH, 51°		$HClO_4$, H_2O, 25°	
Expelled	$SiMe_3$	$GeEt_3$	$Sn(C_6H_{11})_3$	$Pb(C_6H_{13})_3$
p-Group				
NMe_2	30,000,000	20,000,000	20,000	—
OH	10,000	2,700	—	—
OMe	1,500	540	63	21
Me	21	14	6	3.4
t-Bu	16	11	7	
H	1	1	1	1
F	0.75	0.92	0.62	—
Cl	0.13	0.17	0.19	0.32
Br	0.10	0.17	0.15	—
I	0.10	0.13	0.14	—
CO_2H[a]	0.0015	0.0052	0.030	—
NMe_3^+[a]	0.00038	0.0011	0.0064	—
NO_2[a]	0.00012	0.00037	—	—

[a] Reagent for Si and Ge compounds: H_2SO_4, H_2O, $MeCO_2H$, 50°.

Thus a *p*-methoxyl group raises the rate of acidolytic dedeuteration by 55,000 times, but of desilylation by only 1500 times.

We see in Table 24-5 examples, additional to those mentioned in Section **21c,** of the stronger activating effect accompanying orientation by OH than by OMe, a very general phenomenon of electrophilic aromatic substitution, most consistently interpreted as an effect of HO-hyperconjugation, a matter to be further discussed in Section **24j.**

Relative rates of acidolytic displacements of XR_3 groups from various aromatic positions under the influence of methyl, methoxyl, phenyl, and chloro-groups, are set out below. It will be noted that, in accordance with H. C. Brown's generalisation, as the activations or deactivations become milder with increasing ease of expulsion of the XR_3 group, that is, with increasing power of the substituting agent relative to the task before it, so the distributions of reactivity over the ring become less uneven.

For all the reactions, methyl is a normal Type 1 $(+I)$ substituent; it activates all positions in the benzene ring, but with only weak *m*-activation. Methoxyl is a substituent of Type 3, $(-I+K)$, but is a near-extreme example in its strongly dominating conjugative effect; and it provides in these reactions, as it does in hydrogen exchange (Section **24c**), strong *o*- and *p*-activation, accompanied by weak *m*-de-activation. This would be so, if its conjugative action were a practically pure polarisability effect, therefore exerting a selectivity for *o*- and *p*-positions which is practically exclusive (Section **21c**), and so leaving unobscured at the *m*-positions the weak deactivating effect of inductive electronegativity. The phenyl substituent is also of Type 3, but has less unbalance between its electronegative inductive and electropositive conjugative components, though it has still too little electronegativity (or too much conjugation) to display the Holleman anomaly. Thus the distribution of reactivity is qualitatively like that produced by methoxyl, but is less extreme. Here again we have a substituent, which, unlike methyl, activates the *o*- and *p*-positions, and de-activates the *m*-positions. Chlorine is a substituent of Type 3, which commonly does display the Holleman anomaly; that is, it de-activates the whole benzene ring, but in such a way as to leave a dominating *o*-*p*-reactivity. Though the data are incomplete, there can be no doubt that chlorine is acting in that way in these reactions. In the representations below, the arrows bear a note of the nature of the expelled group; and they bear a letter-label indicative of the acidolysing agent, as follows: *a* means $HClO_4$, H_2O, MeOH, 51°; *b* means $HClO_4$, H_2O, EtOH, 25°; and *c* means H_2SO_4, H_2O, $MeCO_2H$, 50°

CH_3 — 17.8, 2.3, 21.3 — $SiMe_3$ ← *a*

CH_3 — 12.4, 2.1, 14.0 — $GeEt_3$ ← *a*

CH_3 — ?, 1.8, 5.6 — $Sn(C_6H_{11})_3$ ← *b*

OMe — 335, 0.23, 1510 — $SiMe_3$ ← *a*

OMe — 207, 0.51, 540 — $GeEt_3$ ← *a*

OMe — ?, 0.85, 63 — $Sn(C_6H_{11})_3$ ← *b*

Ph — 5.85, 0.33, 2.83 — $SiMe_3$ ← *c*

Cl — ?, 0.012, 0.19 — $SiMe_3$ ← *c*

Cl — ?, 0.019, 0.17 — $GeEt_3$ ← *c*

Cl — ?, 0.039, 0.19 — $Sn(C_6H_{11})_3$ ← *b*

Cl — ?, 0.125, 0.32 — $Pb(C_6H_{11})_3$ ← *b*

(24i) Nitrosation.—We observed in Section **23g** that highly reactive aromatic compounds, notably phenols, anilines, and their O- or N-alkyl derivatives, are *o*- and *p*-nitrosated by nitrous acid in excess of nitric acid, to give nitroso-compounds, which are at once oxidised by nitric acid to nitro-compounds. We noted also that the analytical nitrous acid exists in these acid mixtures mainly as dinitrogen tetroxide, though a very little of it is present as nitrosonium ion; and that both these entities act as carriers of the nitroso-group.

The kinetics of aromatic nitrosation, in such conditions that the formed nitroso-compound survives, has been investigated by Ridd and Qureshi in the example of dimethylaniline.[216] In aqueous solution, at acidities established by means of perchloric acid as the only strong acid, the kinetic pattern is exactly like that described more fully in Chapter VIII for diazotisation and some other reactions of nitrous acid: at low acidities, *e.g.*, $[H^+]=0.002M$, the rate is independent of the concentration of the substrate, and follows the second-order form of equation (1); whilst at higher acidities, *e.g.*, $[H^+]=0.075M$, the substrate concentration becomes kinetically significant, and the kinetic equation (2) is of third order overall:

[216] J. H. Ridd and E. Qureshi, *J. Chem. Soc.*, forthcoming.

$$\text{Rate} \propto [HNO_2]^2 \qquad (1)$$

$$\text{Rate} \propto [PhNMe_2][HNO_2]^2 \qquad (2)$$

The interpretation is that equation (1) represents the rate of formation of dinitrogen trioxide, and that this becomes the measured rate when, at low acidities, enough of the amine is present in free-basic form to trap the trioxide as fast as this is formed. In the following scheme reaction (1) is slow and reaction (2) is fast, in particular much faster than reaction (−1):

$$2HNO_2 \underset{(-1)}{\overset{(1)}{\rightleftharpoons}} N_2O_3 + H_2O$$

$$N_2O_3 + PhNMe_2 \xrightarrow[(2)]{} \text{Products}$$

At considerably higher acidities, so little of the amine is present in free-basic form that the rate of reaction (2) falls to well below that of reaction (−1). In these circumstances, reactions (1) and (−1) maintain an equilibrium reservoir of dinitrogen trioxide, from which the aromatic compound slowly draws off its requirements. Thus the substrate concentration appears in equation (2), whilst the quadratic factor now represents the stationary concentration of dinitrogen trioxide. It will be appreciated that the concentration factors in equations (1) and (2) mean exactly what they look like: $PhNMe_2$ means free basic amine, and HNO_2 means non-ionised nitrous acid: neither is a straight analytical concentration.

Dinitrogen trioxide, which is, of course, nitrosyl nitrite, is here the carrier of the nitroso-group. But if the required acidity is maintained, not by perchloric acid, whose anion cannot form a covalent nitrosyl compound, but by some other acid whose anion can do so, then the formed nitrosyl compound may also act as a carrier of the nitroso-group. Thus, added bromide ions catalyse the nitrosation, and a kinetic study by Ridd and Qureshi has shown that this is due to the formation and action of nitrosyl bromide:

$$HNO_2 + H^+ + Br^- \rightleftharpoons NOBr + H_2O$$

$$NOBr + PhNMe_2 \longrightarrow \text{Products}$$

The main nitrosation product, whatever the carrier, is *p*-nitroso dimethylaniline. But there is an accompanying oxidation, which can be very considerable in reactions run at high dilution. This does not affect the rate of disappearance of dimethylaniline at low acidities: the overall rate, that is of nitrosation plus oxidation, is simply the rate of production of the nitroso-carrier. Therefore the oxidation is due to a branching of the reaction path after the rate-controlling process is over, and the nitroso-carrier is both nitrosating and oxidising. It is assumed that the first product of attack of the carrier may split off either a proton to give the nitroso-product, or a nitric oxide molecule to give the one-electron-oxidation product, a radical whose dimer is tetramethylbenzidine (which was isolated). Each nitrosation followed by loss of nitric oxide extracts one electron, and by repetition until four electrons have been extracted from two original dimethylaniline molecules, the final oxidation product, the tetramethyldibenzoquiniminium ion, is obtained:

$$\left.\begin{matrix}\mathrm{Me_2N{-}C_6H_5} \\ +\,\mathrm{X{\cdot}NO}\end{matrix}\right\} \rightarrow \left[\mathrm{Me_2N{=}C_6H_4}\begin{matrix}\mathrm{H}\\ \mathrm{NO}\end{matrix}\right]^{+}\mathrm{X^-} \begin{matrix}\nearrow \mathrm{Me_2N{-}C_6H_4{-}NO} + \mathrm{H^+} + \mathrm{X^-} \\ \searrow \mathrm{Me_2N{=}C_6H_5^{+}}\cdot + \mathrm{NO} + \mathrm{X^-}\end{matrix}$$

$$\xrightarrow{-\mathrm{H^+}} \mathrm{Me_2N{-}C_6H_5}\cdot \xrightarrow[\text{steps}]{\text{several}} \mathrm{Me_2\overset{+}{N}{=}C_6H_4{=}C_6H_4{=}\overset{+}{N}Me_2}$$

As Friedländer discovered, dimethylanilines having ortho-substituents cannot be nitrosated.[211] As Hickinbottom found, the same is true of N-methyl-N-*t*-butylaniline.[217] These effects, which apply also to diazo-coupling (Section **24f**), have been shown by Verkade and Wepster,[218] by correlation with physical and thermodynamic properties of the bases, to arise from steric pressure between N- and *o*-substituents (even *o*-H if the N-groups are large enough), which so twists the basic groups as to destroy their activating conjugation with the ring (secondary steric effect).

(24j) Further Discussion of Hyperconjugative Effects.—We here continue the discussion in Sections **21c** and **21d** of the orienting effects, first of electropositive conjugation, and then of hyperconjugation, by commenting on those results, scattered through the previous subdivisions of Section **24,** which appear to depend on hyperconjugation involving N—H, O—H, and C—H bonds. The previous discussions

[217] W. J. Hickinbottom, *J. Chem. Soc.*, **1933,** 496.

[218] J. Burgers, M. A. Hoefnagel, P. E. Verkade, H. Visser, and B. M. Wepster, *Rec. trav. chim.*, 1958, **77,** 481; R. C. van Hoek, P. E. Verkade, and B. M. Wepster, *ibid.*, p. 559; J. A. C. Th. Brouwers, S. C. Bijlma, P. E. Verkade, and B. M. Wepster, *ibid.*, p. 1080; A. van Loon, P. E. Verkade, and B. M. Wepster, *ibid.*, 1960, **79,** 977.

showed that, in electrophilic aromatic substitution, not only the conjugative, but also hyperconjugative effects, are essentially electromeric polarisability effects ($+E$).

The extension of the concept of hyperconjugation, as advanced by Baker and Nathan in reference to C—H bonds, to embrace N—H and O—H bonds was initiated in 1953 by Robertson, de la Mare, and Swedlund.[219] Their evidence has been extended since, largely by de la Mare and by Eaborn, and the upholding of the concept against alternative proposals is due essentially to de la Mare.

Some examples are collected in Table 24-6. They show that the acceleration of *p*-substitution by orienting substituents is in the order NHAc>NMeAc, and OH>OMe, the inequality signs representing three or two orders of magnitude in rates of halogenation, and one order for acidic desilylation and degermylation.

The kinetic forms of the reactions show that the abnormally high rates of substitution of the NHAc and OH compounds are not due to substrate ionisation with reaction through the anion: the original substituents do not lose their protons but remain intact in the transition states of the substitutions.

TABLE 24-6.—LOGARITHMS OF THE PARTIAL RATE FACTORS FOR *PARA*-SUBSTITUTION IN RPH: COMPARISON OF NHAC WITH NMEAC AND OF OH WITH OME.

R	Bromination, Br_2, HOAc (Table 21-4)	Chlorination, Cl_2, HOAc (Table 21-4)	Desilylation, H_3O^+, aq. MeOH (Table 24-5)	Degermylation H_3O^+, aq. EtOH (Table 24-5)
NHAc	9.1	6.4		
NMeAc	6.1	3.3		
OH	11.7		4.0	3.4
OMe	9.8		3.2	2.7

It is not possible to assume that the methyl group, though electropositive when bound to aromatic carbon, is electronegative when bound to nitrogen or oxygen. In systems in which conjugation between the substituent and a distant reaction site is broken, the methylated substituent releases electrons more strongly than does its hydrogen-substituted parent. Thus *m*-methoxybenzoic acid is a weaker acid than *m*-hydroxybenzoic acid. The methyl group in Me—N and Me—O is inductively electropositive.

[219] P. W. Robertson, P. B. D. de la Mare, and B. E. Swedlund, *J. Chem. Soc.*, **1953**, 782.

As to another suggestion, de la Mare has shown,[220] in the examples of halogenation, that we have not to think of rates for the hydrogen-substituted parent compounds as normal, and those of their methylated derivatives as being rendered abnormally low—low by two or three orders of magnitude—by secondary steric effects, pressure between N- or O-methyl and ortho-hydrogen having so twisted the methylated groups as to impair their conjugation with the ring. The test is to interchange the positions of the supposedly pressed-together methyl groups and hydrogen atoms. When this was done the rates were changed only by small factors, such as 5, as might be expected to result from such nuclear substitution by methyl (meta to halogen).

De la Mare's views have not been universally accepted, largely because of an obscurely based prejudice to the effect that the different electron-pairs contributing to the overall conjugation of, say, phenolic OH, *viz.*, the two lone pairs and the OH-bond pair, have independent steric requirements. If the pairs did not act as a whole, but acted independently and additively through components in a common direction, then by twisting the group one could introduce OH-bond hyperconjugation only at the undue expense of lone-pair conjugation. But that assumed independence is not in the theory of hyperconjugation. It is not our incompetence, but nature's organisation, that prevents our separating the polarisability effects of shared and unshared electrons in the same atom (Section **10a**); and therefore, under Einstein's teaching, we should not imply such a separation in our theories. Provided that the atom has a stereochemically suitable path of conjugation, all its redistributable electrons will co-operate to produce the charge transfer.

De la Mare has pointed this out,[221] and has added to his case for the participation of OH-bond electrons in the activation involved in brominating phenol, by showing that, when the bond is an OD-bond, the rate of bromination is reduced by a factor of $k_{OH}/k_{OD} = 1.85$. This means that, although, as the kinetics show, the OH group remains undissociated in the transition state, its internal binding is substantially weakened, as it would be by partial loss of its bond-electrons.

Hyperconjugative effects involving CH bonds are small by comparison with those of NH and OH bonds. For alkyl groups they are of the same order of magnitude as inductive effects, from which they

[220] G. Chuchani, *J. Chem. Soc.*, **1959**, 1763; **1960**, 325; P. B. D. de la Mare, *Tetrahedron*, 1959, **5**, 107.

[221] P. B. D. de la Mare, O. M. H. el Dusouque, J. G. Tillett, and M. Zellner, *J. Chem. Soc.*, **1964**, 5306; P. B. D. de la Mare and O. M. H. el Dusouque, *ibid.*, **1967, B**, 251.

are distinguishable only through the inverted order of differences between branching homologues, and in a simple manner only when the hyperconjugative differences exceed the inductive differences. Distinction is made the harder inasmuch as the inductive and hyperconjugative effects of alkyl groups are not independent; for the former effect depends on differences of unsaturation, and hence of orbital hybridisation (Section **7c**), differences which the latter effect tends to smooth out, with the result that hyperconjugative effects are always underestimated (Section **8h**). In this situation, it is not surprising that interpretations intended as alternatives to hyperconjugation have been advanced. Berliner has carefully considered these,[222] with reference, not only to aromatic substitution, but to the whole range of heterolytic organic reactions, and has convincingly concluded that none can cover, as consistently as the concept of hyperconjugation can, the great complex of facts with which we are faced.

Two other expected characteristics of hyperconjugation should be mentioned, before we review the relevant data in the field of electrophilic aromatic substitution. One is that hyperconjugation requires a structurally conjugated system extending through to the reaction centre: when we break such a system, the hyperconjugation should disappear. The other is that, in the reactions under consideration, hyperconjugation should be essentially a polarisability effect, and hence would be expected to vary quite largely in intensity, relatively to the inductive effect, from one reaction to another, and from one substituting agent to another.

We can, without sacrifice of principle, restrict the orienting alkyl groups, which we shall compare, to methyl and *t*-butyl. Their inductive order for activation in all ring positions is *t*-Bu > Me. Their hyperconjugative order for activation in *o*- and *p*-positions is Me > *t*-Bu; and there should be no hyperconjugative activation at *m*-positions. In Table 24-7 we collect from preceding Sections the partial rate factors for various aromatic substitutions oriented by Me and *t*-Bu in *p*- and in *m*-positions. We do not tabulate the figures for *o*-positions, because steric effects would enter into them, so creating more superposed influences than we could hope to sort out.

It is at once apparent that the inductive order of activation, *t*-Bu > Me, applies to all meta-substitutions. There is no such qualitative uniformity in para-substitutions, into which therefore some additional factor must have entered with a relative importance which varies with

[222] E. Berliner, *Tetrahedron*, 1959, 5, 202.

TABLE 24-7.—PARTIAL RATE FACTORS FOR PARA- AND META-SUBSTITUTION IN RPH: COMPARISON OF ME WITH *t*-BU.

		para		meta	
	R.	Me	*t*-Bu	Me	*t*-Bu
1	Nitration, NO_2^+	59	75	2.2	4.0
2	Bromination, Br^+	59	39	2.5	2.6
3	Chlorination, Cl_2	820	500	5.0	6.9
4	Bromination, Br_2	2420	750	5.5	—
5	H-exchange, CF_3CO_2H	420	490	3.8	7.0
6	H-exchange, H_3O^+	250	180	5.0	9.3
7	Acetylation, $AcAlCl_4$	750	660	4.8	13.1
8	Benzoylation, $BzAlCl_4$	580	430	4.6	12.3
9	Mercuration, Hg^{++}	23.0	17.2	2.2	3.4
10	Desilylation, H_3O^+	21.3	11.9	2.3	3.0
11	Degermylation, H_3O^+	14.0	11.5	2.1	3.3
12	Destannylation, H_3O^+	5.6	7.0	1.85	—

the reaction. For nine of the reactions, para-substitution exhibits the hyperconjugative order of activation, Me$>$*t*-Bu. In three reactions (nos. 1, 5, 12) the overall para-activations are in the inductive order, but by a much smaller rate-ratio than applies (nos. 1, 5) to the corresponding meta-activations. We conclude that even those para-activations which display the inductive order involve a hyperconjugative components of a magnitude comparable with the inductive component, though its differences do not dominate over those of the inductive effect.

(25) NUCLEOPHILIC AROMATIC SUBSTITUTION[223]

The name in the title is given to those substitutions in which a nucleophilic reagent, such as Br^-, SR^-, or NR_3, combines with aromatic carbon, and a previously present substituent, such as $\cdot Cl$, $\cdot NO_2$, or $\cdot N_2^+$, becomes expelled along with its bonding electrons. With considerable difficulty, even $\cdot H$ may be expelled with its bonding electrons, that is, as H^-. In bimolecular nucleophilic substitution, an electron-attracting substituent, especially one conjugated with the aromatic system, such as a nitro-, carbonyl, cyano-, or sulphonyl group, aids the attack of the reagent; and a 2- or 4-situated hetero-atom, as in pyridine, acts in a similar way. The general nature of nucleophilic aromatic substitution will be clear from the following examples:

[223] The present section owes much to the broad perspective first given to this subject by J. F. Bunnett and R. E. Zahler's analysis of its literature (*Chem. Revs.*, 1951, 49, 273).

$$NO_2C_6H_3(NO_2)Br + \bar{O}Me \rightarrow NO_2C_6H_3(NO_2)OMe + Br^-$$

$$C_5H_4N\text{-}Cl + NH_3 \rightarrow C_5H_4N\text{-}NH_2 + HCl$$

$$C_6H_5N_2^+ + I^- \rightarrow C_6H_5I + N_2$$

Nucleophilic aromatic substitution can proceed by several mechanisms. The unimolecular and bimolecular mechanisms can definitely be recognised; and other mechanisms, some of which are understood, can be seen to exist. The unimolecular mechanism is limited to the replacement of those substituents which are sufficiently loosely bound to undergo spontaneous heterolysis in solution. The bimolecular mechanism is much more general, doubtless because it makes much less severe demands on the quality of the expelled group. There are a number of substitutions in which the introduced group does not take the place of the expelled group, so that a hydrogen shift is involved. We shall consider these divisions of the subject in turn.

(25a) Unimolecular Substitution.—The best established example of nucleophilic aromatic substitution by the unimolecular mechanism, S_N1, is the uncatalysed decomposition of diazonium ions, in hydroxylic solvents, to give phenols or phenolic ethers, accompanied often by aryl halides or other such substitution products, if the necessary nucleophilic anions are present in the solution:

$$\left.\begin{array}{l} ArN_2^+ \xrightarrow{\text{slow}} Ar^+ + N_2 \\ \left\{\begin{array}{l} Ar^+ + H_2O \xrightarrow{\text{fast}} Ar\cdot OH + H^+ \\ Ar^+ + ROH \xrightarrow{\text{fast}} Ar\cdot OR + H^+ \\ Ar^+ + Cl^- \xrightarrow{\text{fast}} Ar\cdot Cl \end{array}\right. \end{array}\right\} (S_N1)$$

It was suggested by Moelwyn-Hughes and Johnson,[224] and again by Waters,[225] that these reactions have the S_N1 mechanism. The clearest published statement of the argument for this view is that given by

[224] E. A. Moelwyn-Hughes and M. Johnson, *Trans. Faraday Soc.*, 1940, **36**, 948.
[225] W. A. Waters, *J. Chem. Soc.*, **1942**, 266.

Bunnett and Zahler,[223] who put the case as follows. The decomposition of benzenediazonium chloride in water has been shown to follow first-order kinetics.[224,226] Its rate is unaffected by the identity or concentration of the anion accompanying the diazonium cation, even when this anion enters largely into the formation of the product.[226,227] The rate of phenol production is almost the same[226] in D_2O as in H_2O. The kinetic effect of aromatic substituents[226] is characteristic, and completely different from that observed in any form of bimolecular nucleophilic substitution (Section **25b**); and this characteristic effect can readily be understood on the basis of the unimolecular mechanism.

Our theoretical preconceptions concerning the kinetic effects of substituents in unimolecular nucleophilic substitutions are as follows. First, as to polar effects, substituents which supply electrons should accelerate, and those which withdraw electrons should retard the rate-controlling heterolysis, and therefore the measured reaction. These effects should be generally stronger when the substituent is acting from an ortho- or para-position, than when it is acting from a meta-position. This statement neglects a special circumstance applying to diazonium ions, which is discussed below. Then, as to steric effects, a primary steric effect of an ortho-substituent should accelerate the heterolysis, and therefore the measured reaction. In the case of a conjugated ortho-substituent, the secondary steric effect could weaken whatever polar effect arises from the conjugation.

The data, obtained[226] by Crossley, Kienle, and Benbrook, are given in Table 25-1. Considering first the meta-substituents, it is evident that the $+I$ and $+K$ groups, including some (Ph, OR) which are of $-I+K$ type with a strong $+K$ component, increase the reaction rate, while the $-I$ and $-K$ groups, including one (Cl) which is of $-I+K$ type with a strong $-I$ component, retard the reaction. This is as expected. When we examine whether the same substituents act similarly, but more strongly, from ortho- and para-positions, we find that the electron-withdrawing ortho- and para-substituents do indeed retard the reaction very markedly, but that the electron-furnishing substituents, instead of accelerating more strongly when acting from ortho- and para-positions, usually retard the reaction, and, on the whole, retard it more strongly, the more strongly they might have been expected to accelerate it.

Although the retarding effect of ortho- and para-substituents of $+K$

[226] M. L. Crossley, R. H. Kienle, and C. H. Benbrook, *J. Am. Chem. Soc.*, 1940, **62**, 1400.

[227] J. C. Cain, *Ber.*, 1905, **38**, 2511; E. S. Lewis and J. E. Cooper, *J. Am. Chem. Soc.*, 1962, **84**, 3847.

TABLE 25-1.—EFFECT OF SUBSTITUENTS ON FIRST-ORDER RATE OF DECOMPOSITION OF BENZENEDIAZONIUM SALTS IN WATER AT 28.8°.

	$10^7 k_1$, with k_1 in sec.$^{-1}$		
Substituent	ortho-	meta-	para-
$\cdot$OH	6.8	9100	0.93
$\cdot OCH_3$	—	3400	0.11
$\cdot C_6H_5$	1100	1700	37
$\cdot CH_3$	3700	3400	91
$\cdot$H	740	740	740
$\cdot CO_2H$	140	410	91
$\cdot SO_3^-$	91	150	42
$\cdot$Cl	0.14	31	1.4
$\cdot NO_2$	0.37	0.69	3.1

type was not theoretically foreseen, Hughes has pointed out[228] that it ought to have been expected on account of the peculiar combination of charge and unsaturation in the diazonium group. Ortho- and para-substituents of $+K$ type, when exerting a $+M$ effect in the initial state of the diazonium ion, will work towards the attainment of neutrality in the N_2-group as a whole, but will do so by increasing the covalent multiplicity of the aryl-nitrogen bond, which is thereby rendered more difficult to heterolyse. For example, the $+M$ effect of a para-methoxyl group must cause some inclusion of the wave-function of the structure,

$$R\overset{+}{O}{=}\langle\;\rangle{=}\overset{+}{N}{=}\overset{-}{N}$$

in the mesomeric wave-function of the normal diazonium ion. Any corresponding modification of the wave-function of the transition state of heterolysis must be smaller. Therefore reaction will be retarded. Methyl groups could act in a qualitatively similar way, on account of hydrogen-hyperconjugation. The fact that ortho-methyl and ortho-phenyl groups do not retard the reaction, as the corresponding para-groups do, is probably due to a primary steric acceleration, that is, a steric squeezing-out of the N_2-group. In the case of ortho-phenyl, the secondary steric effect, producing a twist of the phenyl group, would act in the same direction.

(25b) Bimolecular Substitution.—Most nucleophilic substitutions, which involve the expulsion of an originally neutral substituent, notably of halogen, from the aromatic ring, at temperatures which are not

[228] E. D. Hughes, cited by J. F. Bunnett and R. E. Zahler, ref. 223.

particularly high, use the bimolecular mechanism, S_N2. This is established by their second-order kinetics, which are documented by many records. Reference may be made in illustration to an early kinetic study[229] by Lulofs of the reaction between 2,4-dinitrochlorobenzene and sodium methoxide and ethoxide in methyl or ethyl alcohol, and to a more recent investigation[230] by Sugden and Lu of the rate of the reaction of 2, 4-dinitrobromobenzene with lithium radiobromide in ethylene diacetate:

$$(NO_2)_2C_6H_3 \cdot Cl + OEt^- \rightarrow (NO_2)_2C_6H_3 \cdot OEt + Cl^-$$

$$(NO_2)_2C_6H_3 \cdot Br + \overset{*}{Br}{}^- \rightarrow (NO_2)_2C_6H_3 \cdot \overset{*}{Br} + Br^-$$

In substitutions of this type, the rate of attack by different reagents on the same aromatic molecule follows the general order of nucleophilic strength towards carbon. This is the conclusion to which Bunnett and Zahler come,[223] after having assembled data from many sources. Supplementary data have been provided by Bunnett and Davies.[231] For chlorine replacement in 2,4-dinitrochlorobenzene, the following rate-orders of nucleophilic reagents seem established:

$$SPh^- > OMe^- > OPh^- > OH^-$$

$$\text{Piperidine} > \text{Aniline} > I^- > Br^-$$

The kinetic effect of substituents in the aromatic molecule on bimolecular nucleophilic substitution was theoretically discussed[232] by the writer, who contrasted the expected polar effects with those applying to bimolecular electrophilic substitution in aromatic compounds. The outstanding accelerating effects should come from ortho- and para-situated groups of the $-I-K$ class, especially when they have a real or formal positive charge, as well as co-operating unsaturation, as in $\cdot N_2^+$ and $\cdot NO_2$. Weaker accelerating effects should be exerted by the same groups when meta-situated. Generally weaker accelerating effects, with a qualitatively similar positional dependence, should be shown by groups of the $-I$ class, such as $\cdot NR_3^+$. Weak accelerating effects are expected from meta-situated groups of the $-I+K$ type with sufficiently weak $+K$ properties, as in $\cdot Cl$. Retarding effects are expected from $+I$ or $+I+M$ groups, such as $\cdot Me$, or from ortho- or para-situated groups of $-I+M$ type with weak $-I$ properties, as in $\cdot NR_2$.

[229] P. K. Lulofs, *Rec. trav. chim.*, 1901, **20**, 292.

[230] J. J. Le Roux, C. S. Lu, S. Sugden, and R. W. K. Thomson, *J. Chem. Soc.*, **1945**, 586.

[231] J. F. Bunnett and G. T. Davies, *J. Am. Chem. Soc.*, 1958, **76**, 3011.

[232] C. K. Ingold, *Rec. trav. chim.*, 1929, **48**, 797.

A retarding primary steric effect is allowed in these substitutions, since they are bimolecular; but it is not expected to be very strong, because the reagent attacks laterally to the aromatic plane. Also, a secondary steric effect, that is, steric interference with conjugation, is expected to appear.

Most of these expectations can be illustrated from recorded observations. The outstanding effect of a diazonium-ion substituent in accelerating the nucleophilic replacement of an ortho or para-situated halogen, or nitro- or alkoxyl group, is well known for what Bunnett and Zahler call its "nuisance importance." During the diazotisation of anilines, such groups may become replaced by hydroxyl through reaction with water, or by chlorine if hydrochloric acid is used in the diazotisation. Thus 4,5-dinitro-*o*-anisidine, on diazotisation in acetic acid, gives a 1,4-diazo-oxide:[233]

$$\text{NH}_2\text{-C}_6\text{H}_2(\text{NO}_2)(\text{MeO})\text{-NO}_2 \rightarrow \overset{+}{\text{N}}_2\text{-C}_6\text{H}_2(\text{NO}_2)(\text{MeO})\text{-NO}_2 \rightarrow \overset{+}{\text{N}}_2\text{-C}_6\text{H}_2(\text{NO}_2)(\text{MeO})\text{-O}^-$$

The strong accelerating effects of ortho- and para-situated nitro-groups on the substitutions under consideration are well known. 2,4,6-Trinitrohalogenobenzenes react very easily[234] with water, alcohols, ammonia, and primary and secondary amines, to give picric acid or its esters or amides. Probably none of these reactions is unimolecular, for the reaction of 2,4,6-trinitrochlorobenzene with ethyl alcohol, although very fast, is greatly accelerated by added sodium ethoxide.[235] The 2,4-dinitrohalogenobenzenes interact with similar reagents more slowly, and the reactions with alkoxide ions in alcoholic solvents, for example, have been shown to follow second-order kinetics.[229,236] Ortho- and para-mononitrohalogenobenzenes undergo analogous reactions more slowly still, again, wherever tested, with second-order kinetics; while meta-nitrohalogenobenzenes react even more slowly.[237] With methyl alcoholic sodium methoxide, *m*-nitrochlorobenzene suffers no appreciable loss of halogen below temperatures at which the nitro-

[233] H. S. Forest and J. Walker, *J. Chem. Soc.*, **1948**, 1939.

[234] F. Pisani, *Compt. rend.*, 1854, **39**, 852; P. T. Austin, *Ber.*, 1875, **8**, 666; P. G. van de Vliet, *Rec. trav. chim.*, 1924, **43**, 606.

[235] J. Graham, E. D. Hughes, and C. K. Ingold, unpublished observations.

[236] A. F. Holleman and J. ter Weel, *Rec. trav. chim.*, 1915, **35**, 41.

[237] A. F. Holleman and J. W. Beekman, *Proc. Koninkl. Nederland. Akad. Wetenschap.*, 1903, **6**, 327; A. F. Holleman, *ibid.*, 1904, **6**, 659; A. F. Holleman and J. W. Beekman, *Rec. trav. chim.*, 1904, **23**, 225; A. F. Holleman and W. J. de Mooy, *ibid.*, 1915, **35**, 5; J. F. Bunnett and A. Levitt, *J. Am. Chem. Soc.*, 1948, **70**, 2778; C. W. L. Bevan and G. C. Bye, *J. Chem. Soc.*, 1954, 3091.

TABLE 25-2.—RELATIVE RATES OF NUCLEOPHILIC SUBSTITUTION OF HALOGEN.

Group R	R-C_6H_4-Br + piperidine in benzene at 99°	R-$C_6H_3(NO_2)$-Cl + NaOMe in MeOH at 25°	
	Scale: $k_{NO_2}=1,000$	Scale: $k_{NO_2}=1,000$	Scale: $k_H=1$
NO_2	1,000	1,000	170,000
SO_2Me	53	106	18,000
NMe_3^+	—	33	5,500
CN	31	—	—
COMe	13	12	2,100
Cl	—	0.07	11
H	—	0.006	1

group undergoes reduction to give *mm'*-dichloroazoxybenzene. With the same reagent, *m*-nitrofluorobenzene suffers a normal displacement of its halogen to give *m*-nitroanisole; but this reaction occurs much more slowly than do the corresponding reactions of the *o*- and *p*-nitrofluoro-compounds.

It has been known since 1890 that the ortho- or para-situated substituents, ·CHO, ·COPh, ·CO_2R, ·CO_2^-, ·CN, ·SO_2·NH_2, ·SO_3^-, are mildly activating for the bimolecular nucleophilic displacement of aromatic halogen. When any of these groups is introduced into an ortho- or para-position with respect to halogen in a nitrohalogenobenzene, the rate of displacement of halogen by interaction with ammonia or aniline is increased.[238] Quantitative data for a range of para-situated groups, including some strongly activating groups, some weakly activating or deactivating halogens, and some deactivating alkyl, hydroxyl, alkoxyl, amino- and dialkylamino-groups, have been provided by Bunnett and his coworkers,[239] as reproduced on a relative basis in Table 25-2, and by Berliner and Mottek,[240] as similarly given in Table 25-3.

In these tables the groups are arranged in order of their kinetic effect. The circumstance that NMe_3^+ stands below NO_2 testifies to the importance in these reactions of the $-E$ effect, which the former group

[238] M. Schöpff, *Ber.*, 1889, **22**, 3281; 1890, **23**, 3440: 1891, **24**, 3771; A. Grohmann, *Ber.*, 1890, **23**, 3445; 1891, **24**, 3808; P. Fischer, *Ber.*, 1891, **24**, 3785.

[239] J. F. Bunnett and A. Levitt, *J. Am. Chem. Soc.*, 1948, **70**, 2778; J. F. Bunnett, H. Moe, and D. Knutson, *ibid.*, 1954, **76**, 3936.

[240] E. Berliner and L. C. Mottek, *J. Am. Chem. Soc.*, 1952, **74**, 1574; cf. R. L. Heppolette and J. Miller, *ibid.*, 1953, **75**, 4205.

TABLE 25-3.—RELATIVE RATES OF NUCLEOPHILIC SUBSTITUTION OF BROMINE.

R-C₆H₃(NO₂)-Br in excess of piperidine at 25°

R	Scale $k_H = 1$	R	Scale $k_H = 1$
Br	7.82	*t*-Bu	0.170
Cl	5.59	Me	0.146
I	5.42	OMe	0.0180
CO_2H	2.52	OEt	0.0151
		NMe_2	0.00121
H	1	OH	0.00059
		NH_2	0.00013
F	0.260		

cannot exert. The position of SO_2Me indicates a $-E$ effect here, consistently with much other evidence (Chaper III) that sulphur is more than quadricovalent in the sulphonyl group. That Cl is less activating relatively to the heavier halogens than its electronegativity would warrant is probably due to its appreciable $+M$ effect. That F is deactivating is almost certainly due to its strong $+M$ effect. The order of the two deactivating alkyl groups may be ascribed to mesomeric hyperconjugation in methyl. The strongly deactivating groups are the strong $+M$ groups, OR and NR_2; and here, OH appears out of place, probably because, in the basic conditions, it is acting partly as O^-.

Weak primary steric effects can be discerned. Semi-quantitative work has shown[241] that when, into a *p*-nitrohalogenobenzene, first one, and then a second similar, halogen are introduced at ortho-positions with respect to the displaceable halogen, the following kinetic effects are produced. The first ortho-chlorine, or bromine, or iodine atom accelerates; the second ortho-chlorine or bromine atom produces no substantial further acceleration; while the second iodine atom actually reduces the rate of reaction.

The secondary steric effect can also be discerned. Thus it has been found,[242] for the reactions of substituted *o*-nitro-, *p*-nitro-, and 2,4-dinitro-chlorobenzenes with methyl alcoholic sodium methoxide, that, although a chlorine substituent normally accelerates reaction, it shows a distinctly weaker accelerating effect than corresponds to its position relatively to the displaced group, when it is ortho-situated with respect to an activating nitro-group; and it may show an actual retarding influence, when so situated, if there is already an ortho-

241 R. B. Sandin and M. Liskear, *J. Am. Chem. Soc.*, 1935, 57, 1304.
242 E. A. Kriuger and M. S. Bednova *J. Gen. Chem.* (U.S.S.R.), 1933, 3, 67.

TABLE 25-4.—RELATIVE RATES OF NUCLEOPHILIC SUBSTITUTION OF FLUORINE.

NO_2-C₆H₃(X)-F + Y^- in methanol at 0°.

Y^-	X: H	X: Me	X: Br
OH^-	1	1	1
OMe^-	36	23	47
SMe^-	48	208	298

substituent on the other side of the nitro-group. It has also been found[243] that an alkyl substituent meta- to the chlorine atom in 2,4-dinitrochlorobenzene reduces the rate of reaction with piperidine or with methoxide ion, fairly strongly if the alkyl group is in position-5, and very strongly if it is in position-3 (between the nitro-groups); and that both effects are markedly greater when the alkyl group is *t*-butyl than when it is methyl.

It has been plausibly suggested by Bunnett[244] that an effect of electrokinetic attraction can be seen in data, such as those of Table 25-4, which indicate that attack by a more highly polarisable reagent is relatively favoured by the introduction of a more highly polarisable substituent near the site of reaction.

The hetero-atom of pyridine has an activating effect for nucleophilic substitution in the 2- and 4-positions. This appears to be somewhat weaker than is the activating effect of a nitro-substituent in benzene for substitution in the ortho- and para-positions. Thus Mangini and Frenguelli showed[245] that the reactions of 2-chloro-5-nitropyridine with several amines and alkoxide ions went rather more slowly than the corresponding reactions of 2,4-dinitrochlorobenzene. Though the comparison is not at all simple theoretically, one may perhaps associate the difference with the smaller electronegativity that is available to assist the $-E$ effect in the pyridine system:

NO_2 ... N ... $\bar{X}$ Cl NO_2 ... $\overset{+}{N}$(O)O^- ... $\bar{X}$ Cl

[243] B. Capon and N. B. Chapman, *J. Chem. Soc.*, **1957**, 600.

[244] J. F. Bunnett, *J. Am. Chem. Soc.*, 1957, **79**, 5969; J. F. Bunnett and J. D. Richardson, *ibid.*, 1959, **81**, 315.

[245] A. Mangini and B. Frenguelli, *Gazz. chim. ital.*, 1939, **69**, 86.

The *Smiles rearrangement*,[246] in which, under basic conditions, an electronegative bridge ·X· separates from aromatic carbon, to be replaced by the conjugate-basic atom Y of some acidic centre YH situated beyond the bridge in the original molecule, can be regarded as an intramolecular nucleophilic aromatic substitution:

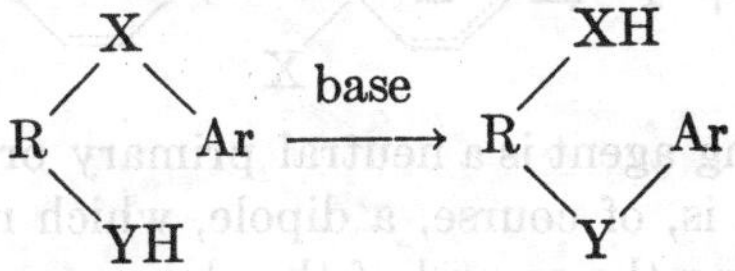

$$\text{R}\begin{matrix}\diagup \text{X} \diagdown \\ \diagdown \text{YH} \diagup\end{matrix}\text{Ar} \xrightarrow{\text{base}} \text{R}\begin{matrix}\diagup \text{XH} \\ \diagdown \text{Y} \diagup\end{matrix}\text{Ar}$$

The bridge —X— may be $—SO_2—$, —SO—, —S—, or —O—, and the acidic centre ·YH may be ·OH, ·SH, ·NHR, ·CO·NHR, or, $·SO_2·NHR$. Activation by a suitably situated nitro- or other such group is usually required.

The following example[247] is typical:

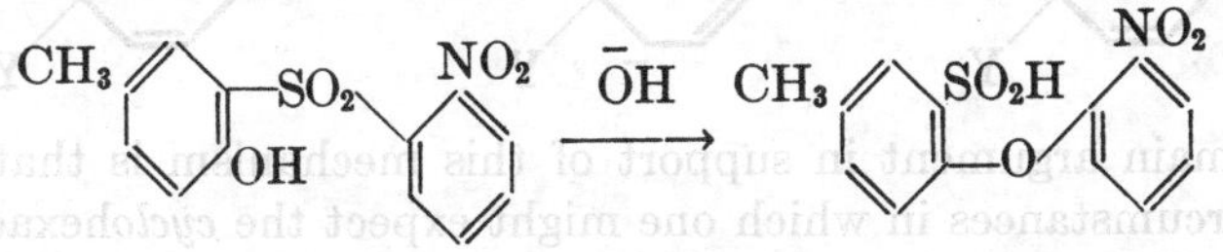

$$CH_3C_6H_3(OH)\text{-}SO_2\text{-}C_6H_4NO_2 \xrightarrow{\bar{O}H} CH_3C_6H_3(SO_2H)\text{-}O\text{-}C_6H_4NO_2$$

Observations on the relative value of different substituents, and of different positions of substitution, for facilitation of the rearrangement are in harmony with its classification as a nucleophilic substitution.

Rate of bimolecular nucleophilic substitution depends, of course, not only on the nucleophilic power of the attacking reagent, and on the polar and steric effects of substituents, but also on the nature of the expelled group. This is a complicated matter. Bunnett and Zahler,[223] on the basis of their very thorough study of the literature, suggest the following order of ease of expulsion; but they emphasize that it is an approximate order, liable to alteration in detail with changes in the substituting agent and in the influencing groups:

$$F > NO_2 > Cl, Br, I > N_3 > SO_3R > NR_3^+ > OAr > OAlk$$
$$> SR > SO_2R > NR_2$$

They conclude with evident justice that anionic stability is a facilitating factor, but that the various types of conjugation in which the group is involved before, and in some cases after, expulsion, have an important influence.

Bunnett and Zahler[223] were the first seriously to propose that bimolecular nucleophilic substitution normally went through an addition-

[246] S. Smiles and others; about a dozen papers in *J. Chem. Soc.*, from 1931 to 1938; first paper, *J. Chem. Soc.*, 1931, 914.

[247] A. A. Levy, H. C. Rains, and S. Smiles, *J. Chem. Soc.*, 1931, 3264.

elimination sequence, involving a *cyclo*hexadienylide adduct, corresponding to the *cyclo*hexadienylium adduct established for many electrophilic aromatic substitutions:

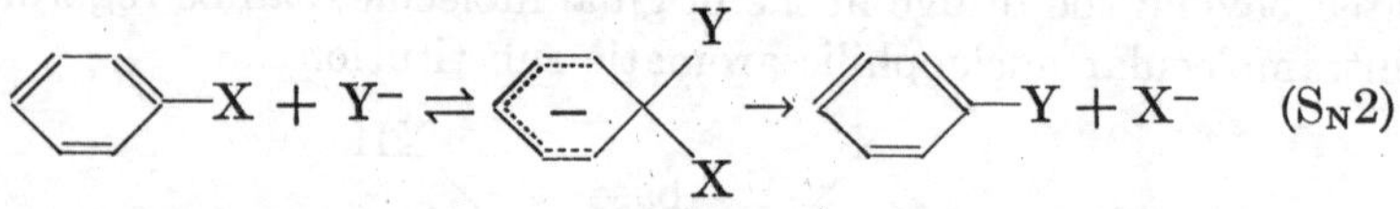

$$C_6H_5{-}X + Y^- \rightleftharpoons [C_6H_5(X)(Y)]^- \rightarrow C_6H_5{-}Y + X^- \qquad (S_N2)$$

When the substituting agent is a neutral primary or secondary amine, the assumed adduct is, of course, a dipole, which must lose a proton either before or during the second of the steps represented above; but this is only a minor variant of the mechanism. The *cyclo*hexadienylide intermediate is in either case mesomeric with its anionic charge divided in accordance with the three valency structures below:

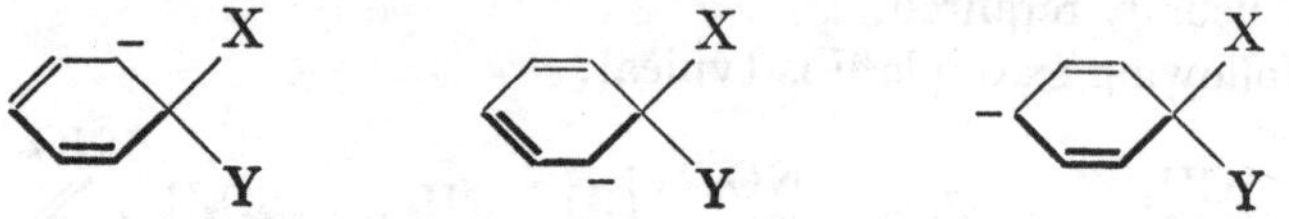

[Three valency structures of the cyclohexadienylide with X and Y on the same carbon, negative charge at the ortho, ortho and para positions respectively]

The main argument in support of this mechanism is that, in just those circumstances in which one might expect the *cyclo*hexadienylide intermediate to be most stable (or least unstable) relatively to the aromatic factor and product of the substitution, it can be isolated. The circumstances are, first, that the ability of the system to support a negative charge is strongly enhanced by the presence of a nitro-substitutent; and secondly, that neither of the groups X and Y has enough stability as an anion to be lost rapidly in that form from the adduct. This shows that the addition-elimination sequence does occur, but does not establish its degree of generality.

For this evidence, we go back to the beginning of the century, when Meisenheimer[248] established the nature of the coloured addition products of aromatic polynitro-compounds with metal alkoxides and cyanides, by showing, for example, that the same adduct was obtained from 2,4,6-trinitroanisole and potassium ethoxide as from 2,4,6-trinitrophenetole and potassium methoxide; and, furthermore, that the adduct, however produced, gave, on treatment with acid, the same mixture of the trinitroanisole and trinitrophenetole. In the following formulation, the position of the potassium atom is assigned arbitrarily:

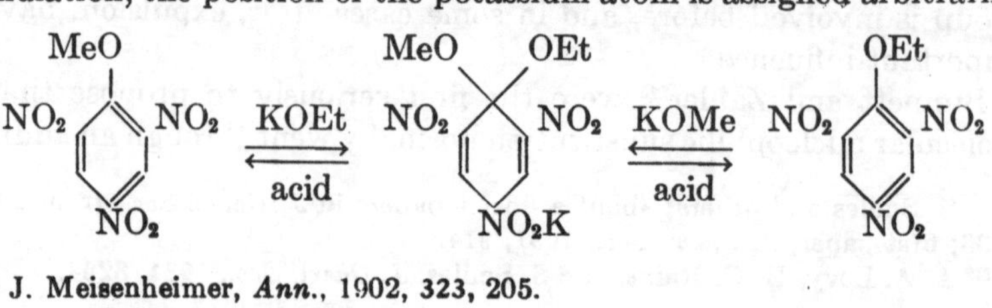

$$\text{MeO}C_6H_2(NO_2)_3 \underset{\text{acid}}{\overset{\text{KOEt}}{\rightleftharpoons}} (\text{MeO})(\text{OEt})C_6H_2(NO_2)_2(NO_2K) \underset{\text{KOMe}}{\overset{\text{acid}}{\rightleftharpoons}} \text{EtO}C_6H_2(NO_2)_3$$

[248] J. Meisenheimer, *Ann.*, 1902, 323, 205.

Crampton and Gold have established,[249] through proton magnetic resonance spectra, the mesomeric nature of the *cyclo*hexadienylide anions of the salts formed by addition of potassium methoxide to methyl picrate and to 1,3,5-trinitrobenzene:

MeO OMe; NO_2 NO_2; NO_2 MeO H; NO_2 NO_2; NO_2

In the heterocyclic series, the addition of Grignard reagents, or of lithium alkyls, to pyridines or quinolines, or of the carbanion of the metal compound to a quaternary 'onium ion derived from the aromatic base, leads to particularly stable adducts. This is not unnatural, since both the groups which could conceivably become eliminated as anions, hydrogen and alkyl, have very low anionic stabilities. They also have quite unequal anionic stabilities; and thus the nucleophilic substitution goes substantially in one direction, that of alkylation with loss of hydride ion. For example, lithium *n*-butyl and pyridine form a crystalline adduct, which at a higher temperature eliminates lithium hydride:[250]

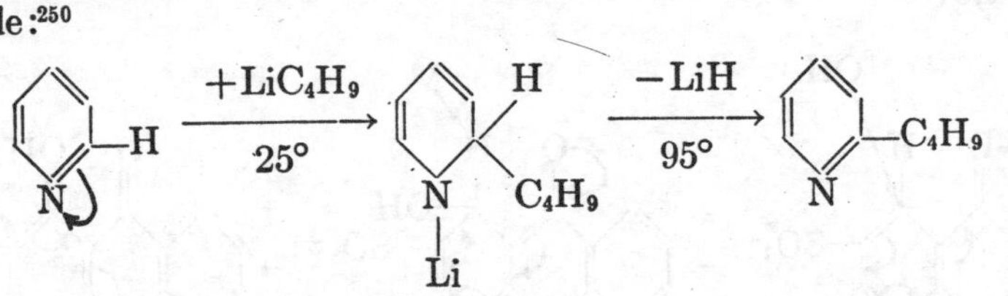

$$C_5H_5N \xrightarrow[25^\circ]{+LiC_4H_9} \text{(N-Li, 2-H, 2-}C_4H_9\text{ adduct)} \xrightarrow[95^\circ]{-LiH} 2\text{-}C_4H_9C_5H_4N$$

The reaction of pyridine with sodium amide at temperatures near 200°, as in the normal method of manufacture of 2-aminopyridine may pursue a similar course, except that, since the additive intermediate should lose amide ion more easily than hydride ion, an equilibrium would be expected to lie on the side of the factors. However, such an equilibrium would be disturbed by cation transfer between aminopyridine and sodium hydride. This gives hydrogen, the evolution of which carries the reaction to completion:

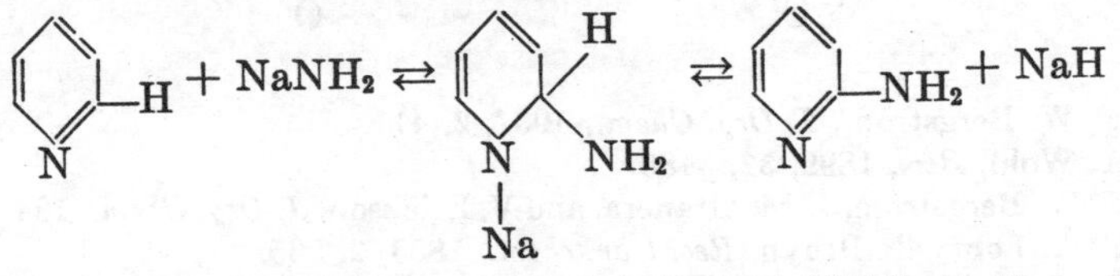

$$C_5H_5N + NaNH_2 \rightleftarrows \text{(N-Na, 2-H, 2-}NH_2\text{ adduct)} \rightleftarrows 2\text{-}NH_2C_5H_4N + NaH$$

$$C_5H_4N\cdot NH_2 + NaH \rightarrow C_5H_4N\cdot NHNa + H_2$$

249 M. R. Crampton and V. Gold, *J. Chem. Soc.*, 1964, 4293.

250 K. Ziegler and H. Zeiser, *Ber.*, 1930, **63**, 1874.

The most general procedure for overcoming a tardy elimination of a hydride ion from the additive intermediate in nucleophilic substitution is to add an oxidising agent. Thus the reaction between quinoline and potassium amide does not go forward to any substantial extent in liquid ammonia; but it gives a good yield of 2- and 4-aminoquinoline on the addition of potassium nitrate.[251]

In the reactions of aromatic nitro-compounds with strongly nucleophilic reagents, such as OR^-, NR_2^-, or CN^-, some of the nitro-compound itself will usually act as the oxidising agent. This is the case, for example, in the formation of *o*-nitrophenol from nitrobenzene and solid potassium hydroxide,[252] of *p*-nitrotriphenylamine from nitrobenzene and sodium diphenylamide,[253] or of 3-nitro-2-cyanoanisole from *m*-dinitrobenzene and methyl alcoholic potassium cyanide.[254] Loss of nitro-compound can often be avoided, and better yields obtained, if an independent oxidising agent is supplied, as in the conversion of *sym*-trinitrobenzene into picric acid by the action of alkaline aqueous ferricyanide.[255] When the aromatic compound cannot easily act as its own oxidising agent, it is all the more desirable to supply one, as in the manufacture of alizarin by heating anthraquinone-2-sulphonic acid with alkali hydroxide in the presence of a nitrate or chlorate:[256]

OH⁻ O +OH⁻
O H Ō H O OH
—SO₃⁻ → —OH —SO₃⁻ → —SO₃⁻
O O O

O OH OH O OH
—SO₃⁻ → —OH + SO₃⁻⁻
O⁻ O

[251] F. W. Bergstrom, *J. Org. Chem.*, 1937, 2, 411.

[252] A. Wohl, *Ber.*, 1899, 32, 3486.

[253] F. W. Bergstrom, I. M. Granera, and V. Erickson, *J. Org. Chem.*, 1942, 7, 98.

[254] C. A. Lobry de Bruyn, *Rec. trav. chim.*, 1883, 2, 205.

[255] P. Hepp, *Ann.*, 1882, 215, 344.

[256] Badische Anilin- und Soda-fabrik, German Patent, 186526.

The existence of additive intermediates does not disqualify the name "bimolecular nucleophilic substitution," or its symbol S_N2, in application to these reactions. These designations mean no more than they say, *viz.*, a nucleophilic substitution in which two reactants are covalently involved in the transition state. The name is silent as to the number of steps in the reaction, and, if several, as to which is rate-controlling. Like other such names, this is an unelaborate class title, and does not seek to particularise varieties within its class.

(25c) Cyanisations of Nitro-compounds (von Richter Reaction).—This is one of several types of nucleophilic aromatic substitutions with the common characteristic that the group introduced goes, or may go, into the aromatic molecule elsewhere than the position vacated by the expelled group: obviously a transfer of hydrogen from one aromatic position to another accompanies such substitutions.

It was mentioned in Section **13a**, that one of the reactions, which was considerably used in the attempts of the early 1870's to classify benzene derivatives with respect to the relative positions of their substituents, was the *replacement of a nitro- by a cyano-group*, and thence by a carboxyl group. These substitutions were discovered by von Richter,[257] who effected them by treating nitro-compounds with ethyl alcoholic potassium cyanide at temperatures between 120° and 270°. The reactions were at first thought to correlate the nitro-compound and the carboxylic acid with respect to the positions of their substituents. But in 1875 Richter reached the surprising conclusion that the carboxyl group does not appear in the position previously occupied by the nitro-group.[258] His observations have since been confirmed and extended by M. Holleman,[259] and again, more recently, by Bunnett, and his coworkers.[260]

The general pattern of the *von Richter reaction*, as it has been named by Bunnett, may be illustrated by the following examples:

$$\text{NO}_2\text{-C}_6\text{H}_4\text{-Br} + \text{KCN in EtOH at } 150° \rightarrow \text{CO}_2\text{H-C}_6\text{H}_4\text{-Br}$$

[257] V. v. Richter, *Ber.*, 1871, **4,** 21, 459, 553; 1874, **7,** 1145; 1875, **8,** 1418.

[258] V. v. Richter, *Ber.*, 1875, **8,** 1418.

[259] M. Holleman, *Rec. trav. chim.*, 1905, **24,** 194.

[260] J. F. Bunnett, J. F. Cormack, and F. C. McKay, *J. Org. Chem.*, 1950, **15,** 481; J. F. Bunnett, M. H. Rauhut, D. Knutson, and G. E. Russell, *J. Am. Chem. Soc.*, 1954, **76,** 5755; J. F. Bunnett and M. H. Rauhut, *J. Org. Chem.*, 1956, **21,** 934, 939, 944.

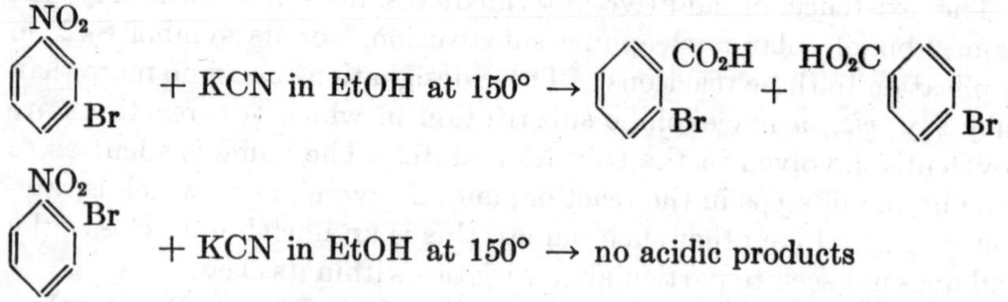

NO_2-C$_6$H$_4$-Br (meta) + KCN in EtOH at 150° → CO_2H, Br (ortho) + HO_2C, Br (para)

NO_2-C$_6$H$_4$-Br (ortho) + KCN in EtOH at 150° → no acidic products

Similar results have been recorded with Cl, I, and MeO, in place of the Br in the above illustrations. In none of these cases is the halogen atom displaced. The cyanide ion appears to have only a small tendency to attack halogen-bearing carbon, though it has a considerable affinity for hydrogen-bearing carbon, if this is ortho-situated, and perhaps if para-situated, with respect to a nitro-group.

Bunnett and Zahler discussed this reaction;[223] and they suggested a mechanism in which the first step is the addition of cyanide ion at the β-end of a carbon-carbon double bond conjugated with the nitro-group, the aliphatic analogy being the β-addition of cyanide ion to an $\alpha\beta$-unsaturated ester. After proton uptake from the alcoholic medium, the substitution is assumed to be completed by the loss of nitrous acid and hydrolysis of the cyano-group. The first step of this mechanism, the addition of cyanide ion, is accepted today, but the assumed modes of loss of the combined nitrogen have had to be modified.[261] Rosenblum showed that the combined nitrogen is lost essentially as N_2, rather than as HNO_2 plus NH_3. He confirmed that the N_2 is not formed by way of ammonium nitrite by running the von Richter reaction in the presence of ammonia isotopically labelled with $^{15}NH_3$: no ^{15}N appeared in the evolved N_2. Samuel labelled the solvent oxygen with ^{18}O, leaving the only other oxygen in the system, the oxygen of the nitro-group, unlabelled. He thus showed that the eventually obtained carboxyl group was not formed by hydrolysis, be cause only one of its two oxygen atoms comes from the solvent, the other coming from the nitro-group. The mechanism which accounts for these facts, and which Rosenblum attributes to R. B. Woodward, is shown below. Ullman and Bartkus have supported the assumed steps from the benzpyrazolone onward by observing the correct behaviour of a synthetic benzpyrazolone in the conditions of the von Richter reaction:

[261] M. Rosenblum, *J. Am. Chem. Soc.*, 1960, **82,** 3797; D. Samuel, *J. Chem. Soc.*, **1960,** 1318; E. F. Ullman and E. A. Bartkus, *Chem. and Ind.*, **1962,** 93.

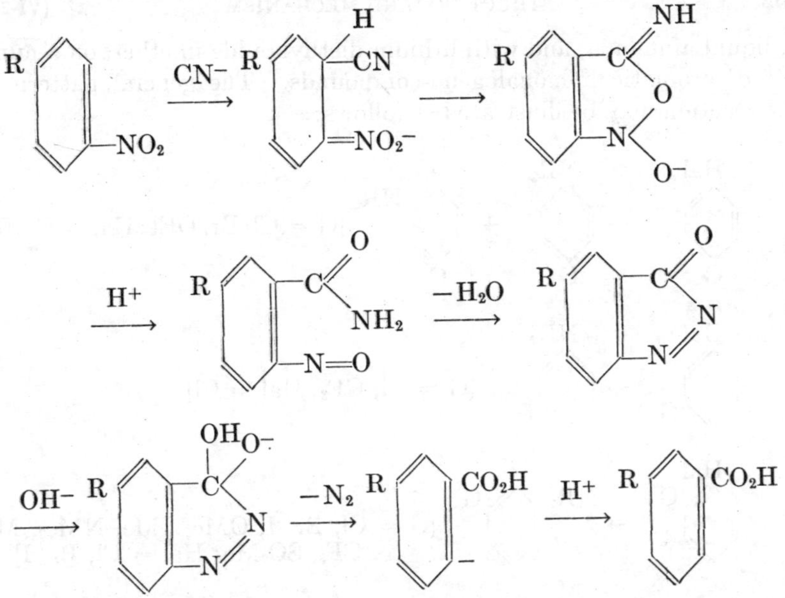

(25d) Substitution by Elimination (Benzyne Mechanism).—The *replacement of halogen by an amino-group* by the action of metal amides on aromatic halides leads frequently, though not invariably, to a rearranged product. It seems that the amide ion can attack either halogen-bearing aromatic carbon, or hydrogen-bearing carbon ortho-situated with respect to halogen. The basic discoveries were made by Kym and by Haeussermann.[262] Kym found that *p*-dibromobenzene, when heated with *p*-toluidine and soda-lime, gave NN′-di-*p*-tolyl-*m*-phenylenediamine. Haeussermann observed that *o*-, *m*- and *p*-di-chlorobenzenes, on reaction with potassium diphenylamide, all gave NNN′N′-tetraphenyl-*m*-phenylenediamine, though the *p*-dihalide gave also some of the *p*-diamine. The reaction has been extensively studied by Gilman and his coworkers,[263] who have operated with sodium amide

[262] O. Kym, *J. prakt. Chem.*, 1895, **51**, 325; O. Haeussermann, *Ber*, 1900, **33**, 939; 1901, **34**, 38.

[263] H. Gilman and S. Avakian, *J. Am. Chem. Soc.*, 1945, **67**, 349; H. Gilman, N. N. Grounse, S. P. Massie, R. A. Benkeser, and S. M. Spatz, *ibid.*, p. 2106; H. Gilman, R. H. Kyle, and R. A. Benkeser, *ibid.*, 1946, **68**, 143; H. Gilman and R. H. Kyle, *ibid.*, 1948, **70**, 3945; R. A. Benkeser and R. G. Severson, *ibid.*, 1949, **71**, 3838; G. A. Martin, *Iowa State Coll. J. Sci.*, 1946, **21**, 38; *Chem. Abs.*, 1947, **41**, 952.

in liquid ammonia, and with lithium diethylamide in ether, on a number of aromatic monohalogeno-compounds. The general pattern of the reaction may be illustrated as follows:

Hal / G → NR_2 / G + NR_2 / G [G = Cl, Br, OEt; Hal = Cl, Br]

Hal / G → NR_2 / G [G = Cl, CF_3; Hal = Cl]

Hal / G → NR_2 / G [G = Cl, Br, I, OMe, SMe, NMe_2, Me, CF_3, SO_2Me; Hal = Cl, Br, I]

Hal → NR_2 + NR_2 [Hal = F (may give either); Hal = Cl, Br, I (gives only 2-)]

Hal → NR_2 [Hal = F, Cl, Br, I]

The mechanism of these reactions was established by J. D. Roberts and his collaborators.[264,266] Their evidence shows that the reactions depend on a preliminary, base-promoted elimination to form a dehydrobenzene, or *benzyne*, as it is called, an intermediate of short but finite life, which subsequently adds on the elements of the amine, whose anion extracted a proton ortho to the halogen atom, so initiating the original elimination.

Roberts's first item of evidence consisted in showing that chloro- and iodo-benzene labelled with ^{14}C in the halogen-bearing position, on treatment with potassamide in liquid ammonia, give aniline with the ^{14}C label divided equally (to within the experimental error and the expected small isotope effect) between the amino-bearing position and a position ortho to it:

[264] J. D. Roberts, H. E. Simmons, L. A. Carlsmith, and C. W. Vaughan, *J. Am. Chem. Soc.*, 1953, **75**, 3290; J. D. Roberts, D. N. Semenow, H. E. Simmons, and L. A. Carlsmith, *ibid.*, 1956, **78**, 601.

$$\text{C}_6\text{H}_5^*\text{—Hal} \xrightarrow[\text{NH}_2^-]{} \text{Benzyne} \xrightarrow{\text{NH}_3} \text{C}_6\text{H}_5^*\text{—NH}_2 \ \text{and} \ o\text{-}^*\text{C}_6\text{H}_4\text{—NH}_2$$

Benzyne

(The asterisk denotes label of radioactive ^{14}C.)

The case for this interpretation was completed by a study of effects of ortho-deuteration. When ortho-deuterated chlorobenzene was aminated in the conditions mentioned above, the chlorobenzene, recovered before conversion to aniline was complete, was found to have exchanged its deuterium for protium from the solvent. When a similar experiment was done with bromobenzene, no such hydrogen exchange was found in residual bromobenzene. The mechanisms of elimination are therefore different. The bound chlorine can survive for a time the development of an anionic centre ortho to it, and the amide ion is a strong enough base to develop such a centre in these circumstances; thus the elimination occurs by a two-step mechanism, which we shall later describe as unimolecular elimination in the conjugate base of the substrate, and symbolise E1cB:

$$\text{C}_6\text{H}_4(\text{Cl})(\text{H}) \underset{\text{NH}_3}{\overset{\text{NH}_2^-}{\rightleftharpoons}} \text{C}_6\text{H}_4(\text{Cl})^- \xrightarrow{-\text{Cl}^-} \text{C}_6\text{H}_4 \ (\text{benzyne}) \qquad \text{(E1cB)}$$

The bound bromine, on the other hand, cannot withstand the development of an ortho negative charge, and so it separates, carrying away the negative charge as the latter develops, in a one-step process, which we shall later describe as bimolecular elimination, and symbolise E2:

$$\text{C}_6\text{H}_4(\text{Br})(\text{H}) \xrightarrow{\text{NH}_2^-} \text{C}_6\text{H}_4 \ (\text{benzyne}) + \text{Br}^- + \text{NH}_3 \qquad \text{(E2)}$$

In each mechanism the formed benzyne rapidly adds the elements of ammonia, probably as amide ion, followed by a proton. The experiment with chlorobenzene shows that the amination involves prior extraction of an ortho-proton. In the experiment with bromobenzene, this proton extraction becomes a part of the rate-controlling step of amination; and consistently, the substitution of ortho-deuterium for ortho-protium retards the amination by a factor $k_H/k_D = 5.7$; moreover, the substitutions without and with rearrangement are equally thus retarded.

Confirmation of the benzyne intermediate follows from experiments in which it is trapped by added nucleophiles. Bergstrom originally discovered,[265] and Roberts has extended and interpreted the observations,[266] that nucleophiles, which will do nothing by themselves to halogenobenzenes in liquid ammonia, replace the halogen if some sodamide is introduced. Thus, with phenoxide or phenylthiolate ion, as well as amide ion, in the liquid ammonia, much of the normal amination product, aniline, is replaced by diphenyl ether or diphenyl sulphide. The amide ion is the only one of these anions which can extract the aromatic proton. But, in the subsequent addition to unsaturated carbon, the phenoxide and phenylthiolate ions are competitive with, and, indeed, the phenylthiolate ion is more successful than, the amide ion.

The alkaline aqueous hydrolysis of aryl halides at high temperatures appears to proceed in part through a benzyne mechanism. Thus *m*-chlorotoluene gives a mixture of *o*-, *m*-, and *p*-cresol, and *p*-chlorotoluene gives a mixture of *m*- and *p*-cresol. However, in general, some mechanism of direct substitution, presumably S_N1 or S_N2, which does not involve rearrangement, appears to accompany the elimination mechanism, which, in simple phenyl halides, should involve 50% of rearrangement. Roberts found[267] that chlorobenzene labelled with ^{14}C at the halogen-bearing carbon atom, on hydrolysis with 4*N* sodium hydroxide in water at 340°, gave 58% of phenol with the label in the position substituted, plus 42% having the label in an ortho-position. From the way in which the proportion of rearrangement accompanying hydrolysis of the halogenotoluenes decreases as the basicity of the medium is weakened, it would seem likely that the main mechanism used, additionally to that of elimination, is mechanism S_N1.

Benzyne has been produced in other ways than by base-promoted eliminations, namely, by pyrolysis or photolysis of *o*-iodophenyl-

[265] F. W. Bergstrom, H. E. Wright, C. Chandler, and W. H. Gilkey, *J. Org. Chem.*, 1936, **1**, 170; H. E. Wright and F. W. Bergstrom, *ibid.*, p. 179; F. W. Bergstrom and R. Agostinho, *J. Am. Chem. Soc.*, 1945, **67**, 2152; P. H. Dirstine and F. W. Bergstrom, *J. Org. Chem.*, 1946, **11**, 55.

[266] E. F. Jenny, M. C. Caserio, and J. D. Roberts, *Experientia*, 1958, **14**, 349; J. D. Roberts, *Spec. Pubs. Chem. Soc.*, 1958, **12**, 115.

[267] A. T. Bottini and J. D. Roberts, *J. Am. Chem. Soc.*, 1957, **79**, 1458.

mercuric iodide, o-$IC_6H_4 \cdot HgI$,[268,272] or of diazotised anthranilic acid, *i.e.*, the inner salt, *o*-diazoniumbenzoate, *o*-$N_2^+ \cdot C_6H_4 \cdot CO_2^-$.[269,272] When thermally produced in the presence of furane, benzyne adds across the 2,5-positions of that substance, and with anthracene, across its 9,10-positions, to give the products formulated:[269,270]

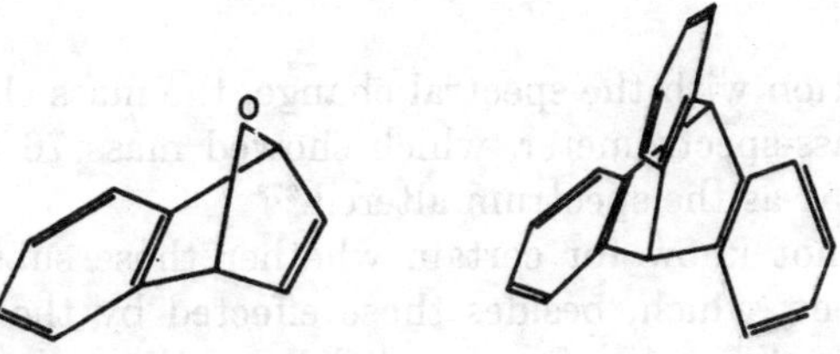

1,4-Dihydronaphthalene 1,4-oxide Triptycene

Produced in benzene it gives three isomeric hydrocarbons, the H-Ph adduct, biphenyl, and the 1,4-adduct, and valency isomer of the 1,2-adduct, formulated below:[271]

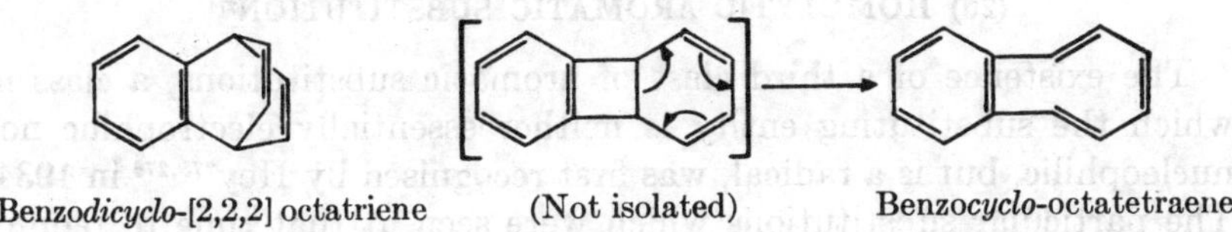

Benzo*dicyclo*-[2,2,2] octatriene (Not isolated) Benzo*cyclo*-octatetraene

Produced in a previously evacuated tube by flash photolysis of solid *o*-iodophenylmercuric iodide or *o*-diazoniumbenzoate, benzyne appeared after 10 μsec. as the main light-absorbing species, with a strong though structureless band in the region 230–270 mμ; and then, in the course of 1 msec., this spectrum became replaced by that of dipheny-

[268] G. Wittig and H. F. Ebel, *Angew. Chem.*, 1960, **72**, 554.
[269] M. Stiles and R. G. Miller, *J. Am. Chem. Soc.*, 1960, **82**, 3802.
[270] M. Stiles, R. G. Miller, and U. Burkhardt, *J. Am. Chem. Soc.*, 1963, **85**, 1792.
[271] R. G. Miller and M. Stiles, *J. Am. Chem. Soc.*, 1963, **85**, 1798.

lene, which hydrocarbon was subsequently collected in solid form and independently identified:[272]

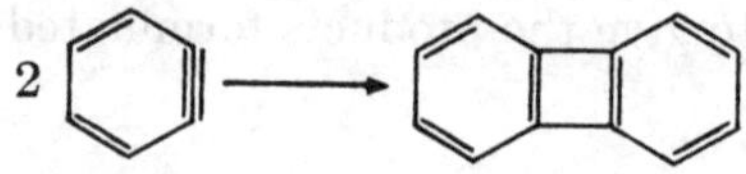

2 [benzyne] ⟶ [biphenylene]

In correlation with the spectral change, the mass change was followed with a mass-spectrometer, which showed mass 76 becoming replaced by mass 152 as the spectrum altered.[273]

We do not know for certain whether those substitutions with rearrangement, which, besides those effected by the von Richter reactions, made difficulties for the workers of the early 1870's, when they were attempting to orient disubstituted benzenes by genetic correlation (Section **13a**)—for example, the conversions of benzene-*p*-disulphonic acid and of *p*-bromophenol, by fusion with alkali, into resorcinol, and the conversion by similar means of *m*-bromophenol, and of *o*-bromophenol, into mixtures of catechol and resorcinol—owe their unexpected behaviour to the benzyne mechanism. But it is possible that they do; for the conditions are highly basic in all cases.

(26) HOMOLYTIC AROMATIC SUBSTITUTION[274]

The existence of a third class of aromatic substitutions, a class in which the substituting entity is neither essentially electrophilic nor nucleophilic, but is a radical, was first recognised by Hey[275,276] in 1934. The particular substitutions which were seen at that time to require such a classification were arylations.

(26a) Arylation.—Hey was concerned with Gomberg's method of preparing biaryls by thermal decomposition of aqueous diazonium

[272] R. S. Berry, G. N. Spokes, and M. Stiles, *J. Am. Chem. Soc.*, 1960, **82,** 5240; 1962, **84,** 3570.

[273] R. S. Berry, J. Clarty, and M. E. Schafer, *J. Am. Chem. Soc.*, 1964, **86,** 2738.

[274] Extensive use has been made in writing this Section of the review article by D. H. Hey, "Vistas in Free Radical Chemistry," Pergamon Press, London, 1959, p. 209, and of the monograph by G. H. Williams, "Homolytic Aromatic Substitution," *ibid.*, 1960, in the series "Organic Chemistry," edited by D. H. R. Barton and W. Doering.

[275] W. S. M. Grieve and D. H. Hey, *J. Chem. Soc.*, **1934,** 1797.

[276] D. H. Hey, *J. Chem. Soc.*, **1934,** 1966.

salts in the presence of a water-insoluble benzene derivative. For reasons which are mentioned below, Hey interpreted these reactions as homolyses of the covalent pseudo-salts, which were in equilibrium with the ionised salts in the aqueous phase, and were extracted therefrom by the non-aqueous aromatic phase, where they decomposed to provide aryl radicals, which attacked and replaced hydrogen in the aromatic solvent molecules:

$$ArN_2^+ + X^- \rightleftharpoons Ar\cdot N{:}N\cdot X \rightarrow \dot{Ar} + N_2 + \dot{X}$$

$$\xrightarrow{R\cdot C_6H_5} \begin{cases} R\cdot C_6H_4\cdot Ar \text{ and} \\ \text{other products} \end{cases} \qquad (X = Cl, OAc, OH, \text{etc.})$$

Grieve and Hey[275] improved the method, eliminating the aqueous phase by using the rearrangement of an acylarylnitrosoamine to produce the covalent diazo-acetate (X=OAc) directly in the benzenoid solvent, the molecules of which thus became arylated in a homogeneous system:

$$\underset{\displaystyle Ac}{Ar\cdot \overset{|}{N}}{-}N{=}O \;\rightarrow\; Ar\cdot N{=}N{-}\underset{\displaystyle Ac}{\overset{|}{O}}$$

Even in this modification, the products were somewhat complicated mixtures, and the analytical methods of the day were quite inadequate to cope with them: one simply had to isolate what one could. But in spite of his very imperfect knowledge of product compositions, Hey could see that substituents as different from one another in all polar characteristics as methyl, bromine, and nitroxyl, oriented similarly. Also the reactivities of the benzene derivatives with these substituents seemed much alike. (Actually, this was so because the slow step was the above isomerisation; but fortunately the conclusion was correct.) Hey examined[276] two other conceivable phenyl-producing reactions with respect to their ability to phenylate a benzenoid solvent, *viz.*, the pyrolysis of phenylazotriphenylmethane, and that of dibenzoyl peroxide:

$$Ph\cdot N{:}N\cdot CPh_3 \rightarrow \dot{Ph} + N_2 + \dot{C}Ph_3 \xrightarrow{R\cdot C_6H_5} R\cdot C_6H_4\cdot Ph, \text{ etc.}$$

$$(Ph\cdot CO\cdot O{-})_2 \rightarrow 2Ph\cdot CO\cdot \dot{O} \rightarrow 2\dot{Ph} + 2CO_2 \xrightarrow{R\cdot C_6H_5} R\cdot C_6H_4\cdot Ph, \text{ etc.}$$

These reactions arylated the benzenoid solvent much in the way that the acylarylnitrosoamines had done: and they appeared to show the same indifference to the polar qualities of the already-present substituent. These substitutions could not be electrophilic or nucleophilic: they had to be non-polar, that is, homolytic.

Several other phenyl-producing reactions have been subsequently studied, and shown to effect arylations in just the same pattern. They include the pyrolysis of phenyldimethyltriazen,[277] $Ph \cdot N{:}N \cdot NMe_2$, of phenyliodosodibenzoate, $PhI(O \cdot CO \cdot Ph)_2$,[278] and of lead tetrabenzoate, $Pb(O \cdot CO \cdot Ph)_4$,[279] and the photolysis of triphenylbismuth, $BiPh_3$.[280]

The most important subsequent work, however, has been the development, mainly by Hey and Gareth Williams since 1952, of the quantitative study of arylation, by the production, in correlation, of the relative rates of arylation of different monosubstituted benzenes, and of the proportions in which the three mono-aryl isomers of each are formed. These data, in combination, yield the partial rate factors for arylation in the different aromatic positions of the compounds, that is, the factors which measure the activating or deactivating effect of each orienting substituent on each of the remaining aromatic positions. Such figures disclose sharply the characteristics of homolytic aromatic substitution, and its very strong differences from electrophilic and from nucleophilic substitution.

The first necessity in quantitative work is to secure a sufficiently clean stoicheiometry. As to the choice of a radical-forming reaction, most of those mentioned above have been used with some success, but the decompositions of dibenzoyl peroxide and of acetylphenylnitrosoamine have been employed extensively. Successive substitutions, and other succeeding reactions leading to products of relatively high molecular weight, are minimised by working in solutions made as dilute as possible; and then the main problem is to avoid unwanted initial or early reactions. The pyrolysis of dibenzoyl peroxide has an advantage in that the two radicals which are final products of its self-decomposition are both phenyl-radicals. On the other hand, the intermediately formed benzoyloxy radicals, although they are probably incapable (cf. Section **18f**, Table 18-3) of extracting hydrogen from benzene, or the aromatic hydrogen from most simple benzene derivatives, can extract it from naphthalene, and from phenols and anilines; and it can extract benzylic hydrogen, α-alkoxyl hydrogen, aldehydic hydrogen, and probably tertiary hydrogen, from side-chains. Nevertheless, for many aromatic substrates, the stoicheiometry of the reaction with diaroyl peroxides approximates to that of the equation,

277 J. Elks and D. H. Hey, *J. Chem. Soc.*, **1943,** 441.

278 D. H. Hey, C. J. M. Stirling, and G. H. Williams, *J. Chem. Soc.*, **1956,** 1475.

279 D. H. Hey, C. J. M. Stirling, and G. H. Williams, *J. Chem. Soc.*, **1954,** 2747.

280 D. H. Hey, D. A. Shingleton, and G. H. Williams, *J. Chem. Soc.*, **1963,** 5612.

$$(Ar'\cdot CO_2)_2 + ArH = Ar\cdot Ar' + Ar'\cdot CO_2H + CO_2$$

and this means that a peroxide molecule is supplying just one aryl radical to enter the substrate, and one aroyloxy radical to take away the hydrogen atom displaced. In these reactions the formed Ar·Ar′ is not accompanied by any Ar_2, so confirming that the aryloxy radical is not taking away aromatic hydrogen independently of the aryl substitution. In naphthalene, for contrast, the recovery of acid is far in excess of the requirements of the equation, and the arylnaphthalenes are accompanied by the three isomeric binaphthyls, and by naphthyl benzoates. In the arylation of toluene, the amount of side-chain attack is tolerably small, and a correction for it can be reliably applied. But in the arylations of ethylbenzene, *iso*propylbenzene, and anisole, by the peroxide method, the side-chains are extensively attacked. In such cases one should find some other source of aryl radicals. The phenylation of naphthalene has been successfully studied by the use of acetylphenylnitrosoamine.

The use of contemporary methods of analysis, based on spectroscopy and chromatography, has confirmed early impressions that substitutions by the same radical derived from different sources at the same temperature are identically oriented. Thus the phenylation of nitrobenzene at 125° gives nitrobiphenyls in the proportions, ortho 56%, meta 15%, para 29%, to within ±1%, no matter whether the source of the phenyl radicals is dibenzoyl peroxide, phenylazotriphenylmethane, or phenyliodosodibenzoate.

The method used for the determination of relative rates of arylation is prescribed by the circumstance that the slow step of the reaction lies always among the steps that lead to the aryl radical, and is never the attack of the latter on the aromatic compound. Relative rates were therefore determined by the competition method (Section **21a**): a mixture of the substrates to be compared constitutes the solvent, within which the aryl radical is produced; and then the proportion in which each substrate is arylated is determined.

A number of results for the orientation and relative rate of phenylation, and the derived partial rate factors for that substitution, are assembled in Table 26-1.

The isomer percentages confirm early impressions that they are all comparable, and are not divided into strongly differing sets according to the polar characteristics of the orienting groups. The rates confirm the (imperfectly based) early impression that they are all of the same order of magnitude, and that great activations and deactivations do not arise. The similar behaviour of benzene and pyridine, which differ constitutionally by the displacement of a protonic charge along

TABLE 26-1.—ISOMER PERCENTAGES, RELATIVE RATES, AND PARTIAL RATE FACTORS FOR HOMOLYTIC AROMATIC PHENYLATION.

Substrate	Percentages[a]			Relative rates ($C_6H_5 = 1$)			Partial rate factors[e]		
	o or α	*m* or β	*p* or γ	A[b]	B[c]	C[d]	*o* or α	*m* or β	*p* or γ
Pyridine	58	28	14	1.04	—	1.0	1.8	0.87	0.87
Ph·F	54	31	15	1.03	—	—	1.7	0.95	0.86
Ph·Cl	50	32	18	1.06	1.4	1.5	1.6	1.0	1.2
Ph·Br	50	33	17	1.29	1.4	1.6	1.9	1.3	1.3
Ph·I	52	31	17	1.32	1.7	—	2.0	1.3	1.3
$Ph\cdot CH_3$	67	19	14	1.23[f]	—	1.9	2.5	0.71	1.0
$Ph\cdot CF_3$	29	41	30	—	1.0	—	0.87	1.2	1.8
$Ph\cdot CMe_3$	24	49	27	0.64	—	—	0.46	0.94	1.0
$Ph\cdot SiMe_3$	31	45	24	—	1.1	—	1.0	1.4	1.5
$Ph\cdot SO_3Me$	53	33	14	—	1.5	—	2.4	1.5	1.3
Ph·CN	60	10	30	—	3.7	—	6.5	1.1	6.5
$Ph\cdot NO_2$	62	10	28	2.94	—	3.0	5.5	0.86	4.0
$Ph\cdot CO_2Me$	58	17	25	1.78	—	—	3.1	0.93	2.7
$Ph\cdot C_6H_5$	49	23	28	2.94	—	3.0	2.1	1.0	2.5
Naphthalene	79	21	—	—	—	9.9	11.7	3.1	—

[a] The isomer percentages are from Hey's review article and Williams's monograph,[274] but the work on benzotrifluoride was subsequently published.[281] In all these determinations the phenyl radicals were produced from dibenzoyl peroxide at 80°, except that in the case of benzonitrile the temperature was 70°. The determinations were by Hey and Williams and their collaborators (1952–64), except those for pyridine, bromo- and iodo-benzene, and methyl benzenesulphonate, which were by Dannley and Gregg and their coworkers (1952), and that for phenyltrimethylsilane, which was by Rondesvedt and Blanchard (1956).

[b] The rates in column A were determined by Hey and Williams and their collaborators (1952–64), and are as restandardised by Hey, Orman, and Williams;[282] and they include the revised value by Hey, Saunders, and Williams for methyl benzoate.[283] The phenyl radicals were produced from dibenzoyl peroxide, initially in $0.01M$ concentration, at 80°.

[c] The rates in column B are by Dannley and Gregg (1954), as quoted in the monograph.[274] The radicals were from dibenzoyl peroxide, initially in 0.03–$0.06M$ concentration, at 70°.

[d] The rates in column C, except that for naphthalene, are by Huisgen and Grashey (1950, 1957), as quoted in the monograph.[274] The radicals were generated from acetylphenylnitrosoamine at 20°. The rate for naphthalene is by Davies, Hey, and Williams,[284] who employed the same radical source at 25°.

[e] The rates used in the calculation of the partial rate factors are from column A if available, otherwise from column B, and in the example of naphthalene from column C. They all apply to temperatures 70–80° except for naphthalene, for which figures for 25° and for 80° have, somewhat inappropriately, been combined. It has been shown[283] that the varying compositions of the mixed solvents used in determining relative rates make no difference either to the rates, or to the isomer proportions, and therefore none to the partial rate factors.

[f] This relative rate for toluene is corrected for 13% side-chain attack.

the length of a CH bond, is eloquent of the essentially non-polar nature of the substitution. The partial rate factors reflect the general monotony: except for the last five substrates in the table, they are all of the order of unity, the *m*-factors ranging from 0.7 to 1.5, the *p*-factors from 0.9 to 1.8, and the *o*-factors, more subject to local effects, from 0.5 to 2.5. For the last four benzenoid examples the *m*-factors are as before, but nearly all the *p*- and *o*-factors exhibit raised values, as also do the α- and β-factors for naphthalene.

The common structural feature of these *o*- and *p*-, or α- and β-activated substances is the existence of αβ-unsaturation in $2p\pi$ conjugation with the ring being substituted. (The inclusion of biphenyl in this statement may be rendered marginal by twisting.) This suggests that the activated step of arylation is an addition of the aryl radical. For the produced adduct-radical can then achieve some stability by conjugative distribution of its radical-centre over three aromatic positions, to which the distribution is limited in *o*-, *m*-, and *p*-adducts formed from substrates without the αβ-$2p\pi$ conjugation, as illustrated below for fluorobenzene. But in substrates having this conjugation, the limitation to three positions in the ring being substituted applies only to *m*-adducts, whilst *o*- or *p*-benzene adducts, or α- or β-naphthalene adducts can gain extra stability from a further conjugative spreading of the radical-centre, outside the ring being substituted, as illustrated below for benzonitrile. In these diagrams, the dots mark the possible positions of the radical-centre, and the variously distributable bonds of the $2p\pi$ system are omitted. Of course, rates are conditioned by the stabilisation of transition states, rather than of

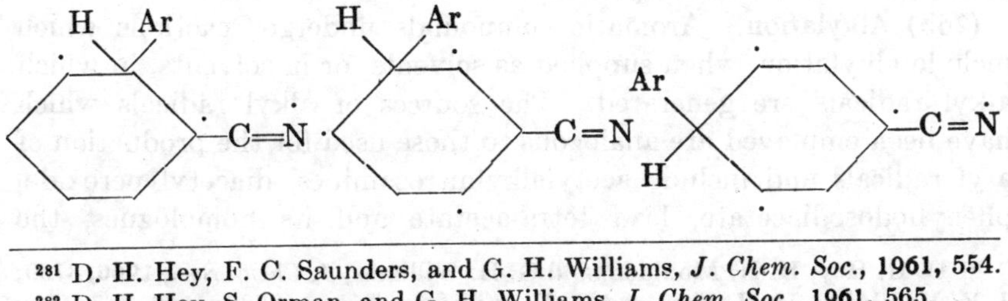

[281] D. H. Hey, F. C. Saunders, and G. H. Williams, *J. Chem. Soc.*, **1961**, 554.
[282] D. H. Hey, S. Orman, and G. H. Williams, *J. Chem. Soc.*, **1961**, 565.
[283] D. H. Hey, F. C. Saunders, and G. H. Williams, *J. Chem. Soc.*, **1964**, 3409.
[284] D. I. Davies, D. H. Hey, and G. H. Williams, *J. Chem. Soc.*, **1961**, 3112.

products; but the former effects are likely to follow the latter qualitatively in their variation from case to case.

Hey and Williams consider that substituted aryl radicals show signs of their polar nature in their arylations of substituted benzenes. The data[274,285] suggest that this may be one of several minor influences on product proportions and relative rates.

We have noticed that, under the conditions established as suitable for the quantitative studies described, loss of the displaced proton does not precede uptake of the aryl radical: it must either accompany or succeed it. We inferred from conjugative effects on the reaction that a slow step of radical uptake is succeeded by hydrogen loss. These conclusions are confirmed by the absence of the isotope effect in substrate hydrogen: arylation displaces protium and tritium without discrimination.[286] It follows that hydrogen loss is not part of the rate-controlling step, and therefore must constitute a final fast step.

Aromatic arylation is a typical *unsaturated* homolytic substitution in the classification of Section **18g.** If in describing it we refer, as usual, to the molecularity of the rate-controlling step, we shall call it a bimolecular, homolytic, aromatic substitution, and label it S_H2:

$$C_6H_6 + \dot{A}r \xrightarrow{\text{slow}} \dot{C}_6H_6\text{(Ar)(H)}$$

$$\dot{C}_6H_6\text{(Ar)(H)} + \dot{X} \xrightarrow{\text{fast}} C_6H_5\text{—Ar} + HX \qquad (S_H2)$$

The mechanism S_H2 obviously parallels the bimolecular electrophilic and nucleophilic mechanisms of aromatic substitution, S_E2 and S_N2. Its mesomeric *cyclo*hexadienyl-radical intermediate corresponds to the mesomeric *cyclo*hexadienylium-ion and *cyclo*hexadienylide-ion intermediates of the heterolytic mechanisms.

(26b) Alkylation.—Aromatic compounds undergo reactions which include alkylation, when supplied as solvents, or in solvents, in which alkyl radicals are generated. The sources of alkyl radicals which have been employed are analogous to those used for the production of aryl radicals and include acetylalkylnitrosamines, diacetyl peroxide, phenyliodosodiacetate, lead tetra-acetate and its homologues, the

[285] D. H. Hey, H. N. Moulden, and G. H. Williams, *J. Chem. Soc.*, **1960,** 3769; J. K. Hambling, D. H. Hey, and G. H. Williams, *ibid.*, p. 3782; **1962,** 487; *idem* and S. Orman, *ibid.*, **1961,** 3108; **1965,** 101.

[286] Chang Shih, D. H. Hey, and G. H. Williams, *J. Chem. Soc.*, **1959,** 1871.

anodic generation of radicals by electrolysis of carboxylic acids, and the photolysis of heavy metal alkyls. Some special methods are available for particular radicals, for instance, the decomposition of di-*t*-butyl peroxide, which gives methyl radicals along with acetone.

Most of the recorded yields of mono-alkyl substitution products of aromatic substrates are low: many other products are concurrently formed. With radical sources that first produce acyloxy radicals, these radicals may enter as ester groups. Naphthalene, treated with lead tetra-acetate, is reported to give no methylnaphthalenes but only naphthyl acetates. A circumstance which makes the occurrence of unwanted reactions generally more extensive in alkylation than in arylation is that, when we introduce an alkyl group, we introduce benzylic hydrogen, so that supplied alkyl radicals get consumed in dehydrogenating and further alkylating the first-formed side-chains.

Some isomer percentages for monomethylation are set down in Table 26-2. In the earlier determinations, in which the methyl radicals were obtained by pyrolysis of diacetyl or di-*t*-butyl peroxide, the yields of mixed isomers were small or unstated, wherefore one cannot feel confident that the reported compositions were not disturbed by succeeding reactions. But in the work of Corbett and Williams, in which methyl radicals were produced by photolysis of methylmercuric iodide, the yields of mixed isomers approached the yield of methane, as is required by the equations,

$$\dot{C}H_3 + ArH \rightarrow CH_4 + \dot{A}r$$

$$\dot{C}H_3 + \dot{A}r \rightarrow CH_3 \cdot Ar$$

TABLE 26-2.—ISOMER PERCENTAGES IN HOMOLYTIC AROMATIC METHYLATION.

Substrate	*o*	*m*	*p*	Note	Substrate	*o*	*m*	*p*	Note
PhF	57	37	6	*c*	$PhCH_3$	45	18	37	*c*
						57	26	17	*a*
PhCl	62	28	10	*c*					
	64	25	11	*b*	PhOMe	74	15	11	*b*
					PhCN	48	9	43	*b*
PhBr	62	28	10	*c*					
	67	23	10	*b*	$PhNO_2$	66	6	28	*b*

[a] E. L. Eliel, K. Rabindran, and S. H. Wilen, *J. Org. Chem.*, 1957, 22, 829 Radical source, $(CH_3 \cdot CO \cdot O)_2$ at 110°.

[b] B. R. Cowley, R. O. C. Norman, and W. A. Waters, *J. Chem. Soc.*, 1959, 1799. Radical source, di-*t*-butyl peroxide at 130–145°.

[c] G. E. Corbett and G. H. Williams, *J. Chem. Soc.*, **1964**, 3437. Radical source, $CH_3HgI + h\nu$ at b.p. of aromatic substrate.

wherefore the proportions of isomers found should fairly closely correspond to the proportions formed.

In the reaction with anisole, some demethylation of the side-chain occurs. In the reaction with toluene, some methylation in the side-chain takes place: according to Eliel and his coworkers, the proportion of ethylbenzene formed is about equal to that of *m*-xylene. The results in general can be summarised in the statement that they show the same monotony as those for phenylation, and also similar variations from case to case.

Thanks to Szwarc and his coworkers,[287] we have a body of data for the relative rates at which methyl radicals are taken up by different aromatic compounds, though those rates are not associated with determined product compositions. Szwarc's method is to bring each aromatic compound separately into competition with a common aliphatic solvent (*iso*-octane) for the radicals formed by decomposing diacetyl peroxide. From the pure solvent, the radicals extract hydrogen, giving carbon dioxide, and methane (together with a little ethane formed by radical dimerisation) as the gaseous products. When the solvent contains an aromatic substrate, the amount of methane evolved along with a given amount of carbon dioxide is reduced; and the shortfall is ascribed to retention of methyl radicals in the aromatic compound. It is attempted to minimise successive reactions by the use of dilute solutions. Typical data are in Table 26-3. The main difficulty in the way of a close interpretation of them is that

TABLE 26-3.—RELATIVE RATES OF AROMATIC METHYLATION BY DIACETYL PEROXIDE IN ISO-OCTANE AT 65° OR 85° (SZWARC).

C_6H_6	1	$C_6H_5\cdot CH_3$	1.7	$C_6H_5\cdot CO_2Et$	5.2
$C_6H_5\cdot F$	2.2	$C_6H_5\cdot OMe$	0.65	$C_6H_5\cdot NO_2$	10
$C_6H_5\cdot Cl$	4.2	$C_6H_5\cdot CN$	12	$C_6H_5\cdot COPh$	11
$C_6H_5\cdot Br$	3.6	$C_6H_5\cdot CO\cdot Me$	2.4	$C_6H_5\cdot C_6H_5$	5
naphthalene	22	anthracene	820	tetracene	9230
		phenanthrene	27	chrysene	57
pyridine	3	quinoline	29	carbazole	420
		*iso*quinoline	36		

[287] M. Levy and M. Szwarc, *J. Chem. Phys.*, 1954, **22**, 1621; *J. Am. Chem. Soc.*, 1955, **77**, 1949; M. Szwarc, *J. Polymer Sci.*, 1955, **16**, 367; R. P. Buckley, F. Leavitt, and M. Szwarc, *J. Am. Chem. Soc.*, 1956, **78**, 5557; W. J. Hellman, A. Rembaum, and M. Szwarc, *J. Chem. Soc.*, **1957**, 1127; M. Szwarc, *J. Phys. Chem.*, 1957, **61**, 40.

there were no analyses even of the total products (apart from isomer mixtures), and one therefore does not know to what stoicheiometries the determined relative rates apply.

The rates of methylation of phenyl derivatives recall the relative rates of phenylation, and it is possible that a similar discussion would apply (Section **26a**). The striking special feature of the present results is the great increase in affinity for a methyl radical shown by the condensed, and especially by the linearly polycondensed, aromatic ring-systems. Similar results have been reported by Smid and Szwarc for ethylation, *n*-propylation, and *iso*propylation.[288] It should be said that generally similar results were previously recorded by Kooyman and Farenhorst[289] for the relative rates of attack of the trichloromethyl radical on such aromatic compounds. Theoretical considerations offered by Coulson[290] make it highly probable that the broad pattern of the data is determined essentially by the extent to which the first-formed adduct-radicals of the S_H2 mechanism described in Section **26a,** can gain stability by delocalisation of their radical-centres over the $2p\pi$ conjugated systems. This is probably the weightiest evidence we now have that alkylation does indeed use the S_H2 mechanism, as established for arylation.

(26c) Hydroxylation.—The main sources of hydroxyl radicals with which aromatic hydroxylation has been effected are Fenton's reagent and the radiolysis of water (Section **18f**). Stein and Weiss were the first to show[291] that these reagents give generally similar products in aromatic hydroxylation. Subsequently, the photolysis of hydrogen peroxide[292] and the photo-induced interionic electron-transfer in ferric hydroxide[293] were added to the list of hydroxyl-producing reactions shown to behave thus.

The difficulty of securing a clean and simple stoicheiometry is on the whole greater with hydroxylation than with arylation or alkylation; for besides the usual profusion of succeeding reactions, we encounter in hydroxylation some additional early reactions.[294] This, as Stein and Weiss first made clear, is due to the changed situation concerning

[288] J. Smid and M. Szwarc, *J. Am. Chem. Soc.*, 1956, **78,** 3322; 1957, **79,** 1534; *J. Chem. Phys.*, 1958, **29,** 432.

[289] E. C. Kooyman and E. Farenhorst, *Trans. Faraday Soc.*, 1953, **49,** 58.

[290] C. A. Coulson, *J. Chem. Soc.*, **1955,** 1435; cf. J. A. Binks, J. Gresser, and M. Szwarc, *ibid.*, **1960,** 3944.

[291] (*a*) H. Loebl, G. Stein, and J. Weiss, *J. Chem. Soc.*, **1949,** 2074; (*b*) **1950,** 2704; (*c*) G. R. A. Johnson, G. Stein, and J. Weiss, *ibid.*, **1951,** 3275.

[292] E. Boyland and P. Sims, *J. Chem. Soc.*, **1953,** 2966.

[293] H. G. C. Betts, M. G. Evans, and N. Uri, *Nature*, 1950, **166,** 869; H. G. C. Betts and N. Uri, *J. Am. Chem. Soc.*, 1953, **75,** 2750.

[294] J. H. Merz and W. A. Waters, *J. Chem. Soc.*, **1949,** 2427.

bond strengths. The Ph—OH bond is probably a strong bond, rendered strong by conjugation. The H—OH bond is very strong, about 15 kcal./mole stronger than the H—Ph bonds (Section **18f**, Table 18-3). One of these early reactions is the hydroxylating displacement of the orienting group, so that, for example, nitrobenzene gives phenol, as well as the three nitrophenols, whilst the lost nitro-group appears as nitric acid.[294] Another early reaction is the formation of symmetrical biaryls, the dimers of aryl radicals formed by hydrogen loss from the substrate.[294] This means that a mechanism (it may not be the only one) is in operation in which the substrate loses its displaced hydrogen

TABLE 26-4.—ISOMER PERCENTAGES IN HOMOLYTIC AROMATIC HYDROXYLATION.

Substrate	Source of OH	o or α	m or β	p	Footnote
Ph·Cl	Fenton's reag.	45	25	30	291(*c*)
	H_2O, X-rays	30	30	40	291(*c*)
Ph·CO_2H	H_2O, X-rays	50	30	20	296
	H_2O_2, $h\nu$	50	25	25	292
	$Fe_3{}^+OH^-$, $h\nu$	40	40	20	293
Ph·NO_2	Fenton's reag.	25	50	25	291(*a*)
	H_2O, X-rays	30	30	40	291(*b*)
Naphthalene	Fenton's reag.	80	20	—	292
	H_2O_2, $h\nu$	75	25	—	292

to form an aryl radical, which in part dimerises before substitution can be completed by the uptake of a hydroxyl radical. Mechanisms of this type are, of course, quite distinct from S_H2 mechanisms, established or made probable for arylation and alkylation, in which the first step is addition, and the loss of the displaced hydrogen atom is the last step. A further practical complication referable to the great heat of formation of water is that the extraction of side-chain hydrogen is particularly prominent in hydroxylation. Toluene gives not only various side-chain oxidation products, notably benzaldehyde, but also dibenzyl.[294] Phenol appears first to lose its side-chain hydrogen; but then the formed radical-centre spreads to the *o*- and *p*-positions, where, exclusively, hydroxylation and further oxidation to quinonoid products takes place.[295]

[295] G. Stein and J. Weiss, *J. Chem. Soc.*, **1951**, 3264.

The other examined monosubstituted benzenes give all three hydroxy-isomers, but, because of the complex stoicheiometry, the determined proportions have only semi-quantitative significance. Values selected as being probably as good as any available are quoted in Table 26-4 to the nearest 5%. The results by Downes[296] for benzoic acid and irradiated water were obtained by precise analytical methods.

These figures show no strong differentiation according to the polar type of the orienting group, and they are, indeed, at least as monotonous as the figures for phenylation and methylation in Tables 26-1 and 26-2. This confirms the accepted conclusion that we are dealing with homolytic reactions. As to their details, all that we can say at present is that a mechanism is present in which loss of the displaced hydrogen is not the final step.

[296] A. M. Downes, *Austral. J. Chem.*, 1958, 11, 154.

CHAPTER VII

Aliphatic Substitution*

* This Chapter is an extension of three summaries of the subject by E. D. Hughes; *Trans. Faraday Soc.*, 1938, **34,** 185, 202; 1941, **37**, 603.

(27) MECHANISMS OF NUCLEOPHILIC ALIPHATIC SUBSTITUTION

(27a) Incorporation of Nucleophilic Aliphatic Substitution.—The reactions to be considered are covered by the general equation,

$$Y + Alk \,\vdots\!-X \rightarrow Alk-Y + X \qquad (S_N)$$

where the new bond is formed by co-ordination, and the old one broken by heterolysis, as indicated by the position of the dotted line. There is an electron transfer from the substituting agent Y to the centre of substitution in Alk, and from this centre to the expelled group X; so that, in consequence of the substitution, Y becomes formally one electronic unit more positive, and X one unit more negative. Subject to this, there need be no restriction on the states of electrification of the species involved.

The class of nucleophilic substitutions includes a number of well-known general reactions (Table 18-1, p. 246). Among them are the Finkelstein reaction, for example,

$$I^- + RCl \rightarrow RI + Cl^-$$

the Menschutkin reaction, for instance,

$$NR_3' + RCl \rightarrow R\cdot NR_3'^+ + Cl^-$$

and various forms of Hofmann degradation, such as the following,

$$OH^- + R\cdot NR_3'^+ \rightarrow R\cdot OH + NR_3'$$

$$I^- + R\cdot NR_3'^+ \rightarrow R\cdot I + NR_3'$$

Another series of examples is provided by the acid or alkaline hydrolysis or alcoholysis of alkyl halides,

$$H_2O + RCl \rightarrow R\cdot OH + HCl$$

$$OEt^- + RCl \rightarrow R\cdot OEt + Cl^-$$

and similar hydrolyses of oxy-esters, such as alkyl nitrates, sulphates, and sulphonates. The cyanisation of alkyl halides, the alkylation of phenols and thiols, and the alkylation of malonic and acetoacetic esters and similar compounds belong to the same class of substitutions. It includes, indeed, nearly all types of alkylation process in which the alkylating agent is either an alkyl halide, or an alkyl ester of an oxyacid, such as alkyl sulphate or sulphonate, or a fully alkylated ammonium or other 'onium ion, or a transiently formed alkyl diazonium ion. An 'onium-ion exchange-reaction which involves a different distribution of charges from any illustrated in the preceding equations is the following,

$$NR_3' + R{\cdot}SR_2^+ \rightarrow R{\cdot}NR_3'^+ + SR_2$$

Aqueous deamination by nitrous acid may be considered to proceed through the following substitution process:

$$H_2O + R{\cdot}N_2^+ \rightarrow R{\cdot}OH + N_2 + H^+$$

Finally, what has been called an alkyl group can be nearly any kind of substituted alkyl group; and it can be unsaturated.

Before 1927 the general reactions exemplified above were not regarded as having any relation one with another: they were treated as belonging to different departments of organic chemistry. But from this time they became incorporated in the super-family of reactions, now known as nucleophilic aliphatic substitutions. The family bond was a common pattern of mechanisms. Incorporation in this field was thus a consequence of the study of mechanism.

(27b) Development of the Theory of Nucleophilic Substitution.—Speculations concerning the mechanism of substitution at a saturated carbon atom were offered before the electronic character of the covalent bond was understood. One picture, which was advanced in several different forms,[1] was that substitution was initiated by an addition process between the substituting agent and the compound substituted, to form a molecular compound, from which the displaced group was subsequently eliminated. Another idea was that proposed by Le Bel,[2] namely, that the introduction of the replacing group and expulsion of the replaced group are interdependent features of a single synchronous process: this theory was later restated in electronic form by Lewis,[3] and was given a physical interpretation by London[4] (Section 6d). The third possible type of theory, namely, that of prior dissociation of the compound substituted, was first suggested in electronic terms by Lowry,[5] who assumed that such dissociation might produce a carbonium ion, which would later combine with the substituting agent.

[1] E. Fischer, *Ann.*, 1911, **381**, 123; A. Werner, *Ber.*, 1911, **44**, 873; *Ann.*, 1912, **386**, 1; P. Pfeiffer, *ibid.*, 1911, **383**, 92; J. Gadamer, *J. prakt. Chem.*, 1913, **87**, 312; J. Meisenheimer, *Ann.*, 1912, **456**, 126.

[2] J.-A. Le Bel, *J. chim. phys.*, 1911, **9**, 323.

[3] G. N. Lewis, "Valence and the Structure of Atoms and Molecules," Chemical Catalog Co., New York, 1923, p. 113.

[4] F. London, *Z. Elektrochem.*, 1929, **35**, 552.

[5] T. M. Lowry, *Inst inter. chim. Solvay, Conseil chim.* (Brussels), 1925, 130.

During the period 1927–30, Hanhart, Burton, Rothstein, Patel, and the writer employed forms of the last two theories, that of synchronous substitution and that of prior dissociation, sometimes with emphasis on one or the other, but sometimes in essential conjunction, for the purpose of interpreting observed characteristics of a number of nucleophilic substitutions, for instance, Hofmann degradations,[6] replacements in anionotropic systems,[7] and substitutions in the saturated side-chains of aromatic compounds.[8] Soon afterwards, Meer and Polanyi,[9] and also Olson, Long, and Voge,[10] discussed substitution at a saturated carbon atom, though only from the standpoint of the synchronous mechanism.[11] However, a convenient starting-point for the more detailed exploration of these reactions was established in 1933–35, when Hughes and the writer emphasized the common mechanistic pattern of all nucleophilic substitutions, and recognised as general the involvement and interplay of the synchronous and prior-dissociation mechanisms.[12]

(27c) The Bimolecular and Unimolecular Mechanisms.—The fundamental postulate is that a nucleophilic substitution, S_N, as a heterolytic reaction in solution, normally has available two reaction mechanisms. One of them contains only one stage, in which two molecules simultaneously undergo covalency change: we call this mechanism bimolecular, and label it S_N2. It resembles London's mechanism of homolytic substitution, inasmuch as bonds are formed and broken synchronously; and, as in that mechanism, the concurrence of the covalency changes is a major factor leading to a restriction of the activation energy to accessible values. However, unlike the London mechanism, in which covalency changes are effected by colligation and homolysis,

[6] W. Hanhart and C. K. Ingold, *J. Chem. Soc.*, **1927**, 997.

[7] H. Burton and C. K. Ingold, *J. Chem. Soc.*, **1928**, 904.

[8] C. K. Ingold and E. Rothstein, *J. Chem. Soc.*, **1928**, 1217; C. K. Ingold and C. S. Patel, *J. Indian Chem. Soc.*, 1930, **7**, 95.

[9] N. Meer and M. Polanyi, *Z. physik. Chem.*, 1932, **B**, **19**, 164.

[10] A. R. Olson, *J. Chem. Phys.*, 1933, **1**, 418; A. R. Olson and F. A. Long, *J. Am. Chem. Soc.*, 1934, **56**, 1294; A. R. Olson and H. H. Voge, *ibid.*, p. 1690.

[11] There was an attempt at this time to set up the position that the formation and fission of covalent bonds had, for energetic reasons, always to be synchronous that is, that the prior-dissociation mechanism was inapplicable. It was not appreciated that the electrostatic solvation and desolvation of ions in polar solvents can have an energetic importance comparable to that of the formation and fission of covalent bonds (E. D. Hughes and C. K. Ingold, *J. Chem. Soc.*, **1935**, 244).

[12] E. D. Hughes, C. K. Ingold, and C. S. Patel, *J. Chem. Soc.*, **1933**, 526; E. D. Hughes and C. K. Ingold, *ibid.*, p. 1571; J. L. Gleave, E. D. Hughes, and C. K. Ingold, *ibid.*, **1935**, 235; E. D. Hughes and C. K. Ingold, *ibid.*, p. 244; E. D. Hughes, *ibid.*, p. 255.

the bimolecular nucleophilic mechanism alters the bonding by co-ordination and heterolysis: it involves an electron transfer from the substituting agent to the seat of substitution, and from the latter to the displaced group. This can be expressed by the equation,

$$\text{Y} \curvearrowright \text{Alk—X} \rightarrow \text{Y—Alk} + \text{X} \qquad (\text{S}_\text{N}2)$$

in which ionic-charge labels have been omitted since there are several possibilities.

Alternatively, the difference may be described in terms of the transition state of substitution. In London's mechanism of homolytic substitution, the transition state involves two partial bonds, which are longer than fully formed covalent bonds. In the bimolecular mechanism of nucleophilic substitution, the transition state contains two partial and partially ionic bonds, which differ in length and polarity from fully formed bonds. In the transition state of a "symmetrical substitution," such as that effected by a bromide ion (which could be isotopically labelled) in an alkyl bromide molecule, the bonds undergoing change could be described as half-ionic half-bonds: each bromine atom-ion is held with a bond of multiplicity one-half, and carries half a unit of negative charge, supposing that we neglect the charge which induction will force upon the intervening carbon atom:

$$(-\tfrac{1}{2}e)\text{Br}\cdots\cdots\text{Alk}\cdots\cdots\text{Br}(-\tfrac{1}{2}e)$$

Another important difference between the London mechanism of gaseous homolytic substitution and the bimolecular mechanism of nucleophilic substitution in solution relates to the significance of solvation in the latter process: wherever there are charges, in the initial, the transition, or in the final state of substitution, there are strong electrostatic forces of solvation in any polar solvent. We do not show these forces in our formulae, though we do show bonds, essentially because the solvation forces, being electrostatic, are not usually directed; but energetically, such forces are, in general, of the same order of importance as the bonds, and, along with bond changes, must be regarded as primary determinants of activation energy.

The second mechanism of nucleophilic substitution involves two stages: a slow heterolysis of the compound substituted is followed by a rapid co-ordination between the formed carbonium ion and the substituting agent. The rate-determining stage is the first; and since in that stage only one molecule is undergoing covalency change, we call the mechanism *unimolecular*, and label it $\text{S}_\text{N}1$:

$$\left.\begin{array}{l} \text{Alk—X} \xrightarrow[\text{slow}]{} \text{Alk}^+ + \text{X} \\ \text{Y Alk}^+ \xrightarrow[\text{fast}]{} \text{Y—Alk} \end{array}\right\} \quad (\text{S}_\text{N}1)$$

Here again the charge signs of X and Y are omitted, since there are various possibilities.

The energy of the initial heterolysis has to be set off against the energy of solvation of the ions (both ions, not one of them only, as has been mistakenly asserted). The energy difference approximates to the heat of ionisation in solution (Fig. 27-1). Thus, in order that mechanism S_N1 shall operate with a practical degree of facility, a solvent of suitable polarity is essential (as has not always been fully appreciated).

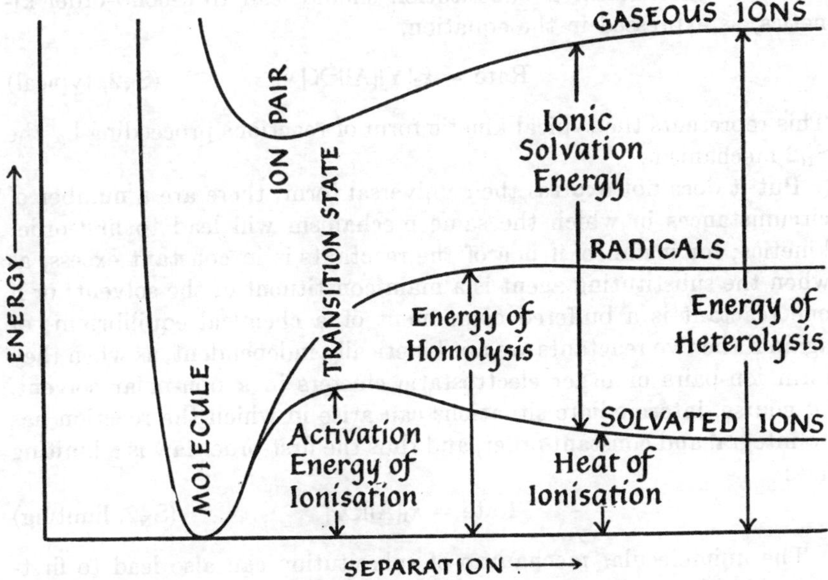

FIG. 27-1.—Schematic energy diagram for the ionisation of a covalent molecule in a polar solvent.

The ionisation is assumed to proceed through a transition state, that is, a state of maximal energy involving a stretched partial bond and a partial charge transfer, as might be represented by the symbol

$$(+\delta e)\text{Alk}\cdots\text{Br}(-\delta e)$$

It is implied that the normal molecule and the solvated ions are separated by such an energy barrier that there is not only an activation energy of ionisation, but also a finite activation energy of ionic recombination (Fig. 27-1). There is some experimental evidence for the existence of such a barrier (Section **32d**). Its theoretical interpretation is as follows. Some bond extension of the molecule, without any marked change in the electronic wave-function, is necessary before the electron transfer can begin; while thereafter the electronic wave-function will change strongly as the electron goes over with continuing atomic separation near the transition state. Then the transfer brings the solvation energy of the developing charges into the energy balance to a rapidly increasing degree, and eventually to such a degree that further separation involves a net decrease of energy.

(27d) The Kinetic Criterion of Mechanism.—Provided that both reacting species are in small and controllable concentration, the bimolecular mechanism of substitution should lead to second-order kinetics, as expressed in the equation,

$$\text{Rate} = k_2[\text{Y}][\text{AlkX}] \qquad (\text{S}_\text{N}2,\ \text{typical})$$

This represents the typical kinetic form of reactions proceeding by the S_N2 mechanism.

But it does not express their universal form: there are a number of circumstances in which the same mechanism will lead to first-order kinetics; for instance, if one of the reactants is in constant excess, as when the substituting agent is a main constituent of the solvent; or if one reactant is a buffered component of a chemical equilibrium; or again if the two reactants are not kinetically independent, as when they form ion-pairs or other electrostatic clusters in a non-polar solvent. Of course, intermediate situations can arise in which the reaction has no integral and constant order, and thus the first-order law is a limiting law:

$$\text{Rate} = k_1[\text{AlkX}] \qquad (\text{S}_\text{N}2,\ \text{limiting})$$

The unimolecular mechanism of substitution can also lead to first-order kinetics, with an overall rate equal to the heterolysis rate. However, this also is only a limiting law, which is obeyed to an approximation when the rate of reversal of the heterolysis is much smaller than the rate of co-ordination of the carbonium ion with the substituting agent. The approximation is often, though not always, a close one when the substituting agent is in large excess, as when it is an important constituent of the solvent:

$$\text{Rate} = k_1[\text{AlkX}] \qquad (\text{S}_\text{N}1,\ \text{limiting})$$

A more general situation arises when the rate of reversal of the heterolysis is comparable with that of combination of the carbonium ion with the substituting agent. The ratio of these specific rates being represented by some constant α, the kinetic equation takes the form

$$\text{Rate} = k[\text{AlkX}]\{1 + \alpha[\text{X}]/[\text{Y}]\}^{-1} \qquad (\text{S}_\text{N}1, \text{typical})$$

This equation expresses the typical kinetic form of reactions having the S_N1 mechanism: when it can be clearly distinguished from its simpler limiting forms, it is highly characteristic of the mechanism.

These equations illustrate the point that no uniform one-to-one correlation between mechanism and reaction order is to be expected. In judging the significance of reaction order, all the circumstances must be taken into account.

We possess several criteria of reaction mechanism. Each of them has a useful range of application, and each a "blind spot." The kinetic criterion is the most widely applicable single criterion. The chief area in which it leads to no conclusion is where the substituting agent is a major constituent of the solvent, if then the observed kinetics do not deviate appreciably from first-order kinetics. For then we do not know, by this evidence only, whether the kinetics represent a limit for the S_N2 mechanism due to the large excess of substituting agent, or a limit for the S_N1 mechanism due to lack of sufficient reversibility in the heterolysis. In practice one applies all possible criteria: there are but few cases which fail to respond to such treatment.

(27e) The Designation of Mechanism.—Already in the last chapter (Sections **23c** and **23d**), and again in this one, we have given names and symbols to a number of reaction mechanisms in accordance with the system now usual, referring to a "bimolecular" electrophilic substitution "S_E2," to a "unimolecular" nucleophilic substitution, "S_N1," and so on. This general method of designating mechanism was introduced[13] in 1928, and is worth a note here, since, in spite of subsequent reference to the point,[14] it has not been universally appreciated[15] that the numerical indication in the symbolic label, no less than in the verbal name, refers to the *molecularity* of the reaction, and not to its kinetic order. Clearly this must be so: for the designations are intended to distinguish mechanism, a molecular matter, and molecularity is a salient feature of mechanism, whereas kinetic order is merely one of a number of measurable macroscopic quantitites, which depend in part on mechanism and in part on circumstances other than mechanism.

[13] C. K. Ingold and E. Rothstein, *J. Chem. Soc.*, **1928,** 1217.

[14] L. C. Bateman, K. E. Cooper, and C. K. Ingold, *J. Chem. Soc.*, **1940,** 925.

[15] See for instance pp. 81 and 84 of "Principles of Ionic Organic Reactions," by E. R. Alexander, Wiley and Sons, New York, 1950.

In reckoning molecularity for purposes of nomenclature and notation, one has in mind the following convention and definition. A composite reaction is conventionally designated by the *molecularity of its rate-determining stage.* The molecularity of a reaction stage is defined as the *number of molecules necessarily undergoing covalency change.* This definition, which has been in consistent use[16] since 1933, is deliberately drawn more tightly than if it had referred to the number of molecules "necessarily participating," or to the number "involved" in reaction; and the reason, which, though subsequently emphasized,[17] has occasionally fallen out of sight,[18] may be restated. It is simply that we wish our definition to be general, and to be convenient for reactions in solution. In such reactions, unknown numbers of solvent molecules, especially of polar solvent molecules, and sometimes also polar solute molecules, are normally more or less deeply implicated as participants in reactions, through the electrostatic forces they exert on reacting ions and polar molecules, and on processes of heterolysis and co-ordination. If we should seek to include these electrostatically participating molecules in reckoning molecularity, then nearly all reactions in solution would have to be described as "multimolecular"; and that would be unfortunate, since useful possibilities of classification would be lost. Therefore it has become customary to take for granted, as its universality warrants, all such electrostatic participation, often summarised in the term "solvation," in reactions in solution, and to define molecularity in such a way that it takes account only of those molecules which necessarily change their bonds. This seems sound from another point of view. The bond changes must be considered to constitute a salient characteristic of reaction mechanism: therefore molecularity, defined as stated, provides a generally suitable basis for a primary classification of mechanism. But solvation changes are susceptible of many subtle variations, of most of which we know very little; and therefore solvation changes are better regarded as leading to variants of mechanisms fundamentally characterised by the covalency changes, that is, by molecularity in the sense defined.

(28) POLAR EFFECTS ON MECHANISM AND RATE OF NUCLEOPHILIC SUBSTITUTION

(28a) Constitutional Influences in the Radical Substituted: Alkyl Radicals.—Alkyl groups release electrons with an intensity dependent

[16] E. D. Hughes, C. K. Ingold, and C. S. Patel, *J. Chem. Soc.*, **1933**, 526.

[17] L. C. Bateman, M. G. Church, E. D. Hughes, C. K. Ingold, and N. A. Taher, *J. Chem. Soc.*, **1940**, 1008.

[18] For instance in certain papers by C. G. Swain, *J. Am. Chem. Soc.*, 1948, **70**, 119, and later.

on homology and branching. In many systems the inductive and hyperconjugative modes of electron release increase together with homology, and thus the order of intensity of the effect among the simpler normal and branched-chain homologues is as follows:

$$\text{Me} < \text{Et} \sim n\text{-Pr and higher normal}$$

$$\text{Me} < \text{Et} < i\text{-Pr} < t\text{-Bu}$$

Bimolecular nucleophilic substitutions (S_N2) involve simultaneous electron transfers from the substituting agent to the alkyl group and from the latter to the expelled group. In general these transfers will not be exactly balanced in the transition state of the reaction, so that a polar effect on rate is to be expected. Since it depends only on a lack of exact balance, it should be a small effect; and detailed consideration would be necessary in order to predict its direction. Those parts of an alkyl group which are close enough to the centre of substitution will also exert a steric effect, as will be described in Section **34**. But, except in special structures, this effect also is small in comparison with that next to be described.

In the rate-determining stage of unimolecular nucleophilic substitution (S_N1), there is an electron transfer from the alkyl group to the displaced group, without any compensating gain of electrons by the alkyl group. Hence a large kinetic polar effect is to be expected. And its direction is unambiguous: electron release must accelerate such substitutions.

Suppose that we examine the effect of different alkyl groups on rate and mechanism in a given kind of nucleophilic substitution in alkyl compounds, for example, the alkaline hydrolysis of alkyl bromides, the medium and the temperature being always the same. And suppose that we thus consider in turn the members of a series of alkyl groups arranged in order of increasing capacity for electron release. It would usually be true that, at the beginning of the series, that is, for the methyl group, the bimolecular mechanism of substitution (S_N2) would be in control. But as we pass along the series—so strong is the kinetic effect of electron release on the unimolecular mechanism (S_N1)—the facility of this mechanism becomes increased, until a point is reached at which it becomes the main route through which reaction proceeds.

Corresponding to this change in the molecular mechanism, there will be observable changes, first, in the absolute reaction rate, and secondly, in the kinetic form of the reaction, as can be understood with the aid of Fig. 28-1. Up to the point of mechanistic change, some slow change of rate, often a decrease, will be observed as we proceed along the series of alkyl groups. But from the point of mecha-

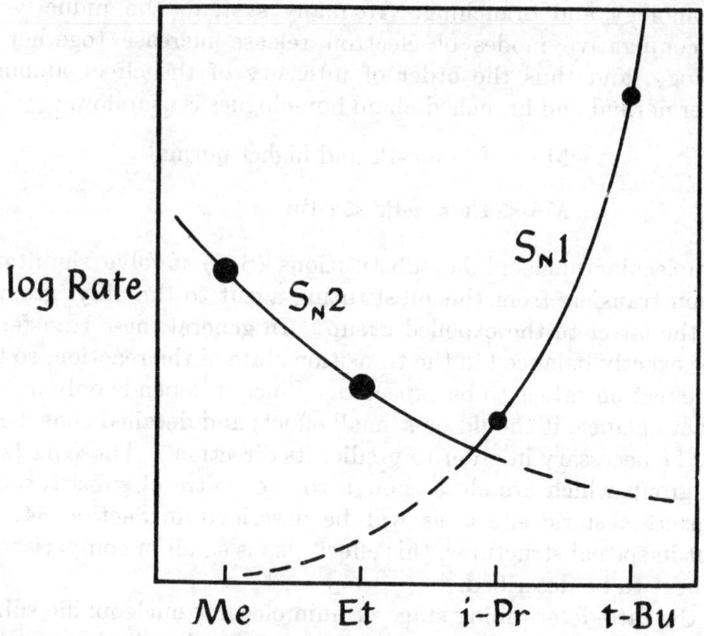

FIG. 28-1.—Schematic illustration of changes of mechanism, kinetic order, and rate, in a nucleophilic substitution, Y + AlkX = AlkY + X, with variable groups Alk arranged in order of increasing electropositivity. (The detailed placing of the points will depend on X, Y, and the solvent.)

nistic change onward, a great increase in reaction rate should be apparent. Again, up to the point of mechanistic change second-order kinetics should be found, if the concentrations are suitably chosen. But from the point of mechanistic change onward, the kinetic order with respect to the substituting agent should in general disappear, and we should find either the typical kinetic form of the unimolecular mechanism, or perhaps the limiting first-order form (Section **27d**).

These effects of constitution were predicted when only fragmentary indications were available,[19] but they have since been well established, in the first place, for the important series

Alk = Me, Et, *i*-Pr, *t*-Bu

with respect to such substitutions as the hydrolysis of alkyl bromides by dilute alkali hydroxide in aqueous alcohol,[20] and the substitu-

[19] E. D. Hughes, C. K. Ingold, and C. S. Patel, *J. Chem. Soc.*, **1933**, **526**.

[20] E. D. Hughes and C. K. Ingold, *J. Chem. Soc.*, **1935**, **244**; E. D. Hughes, *ibid.*, p. 255; E. D. Hughes, C. K. Ingold, and U. G. Shapiro, *ibid.*, **1936**, **255**; L. C. Bateman, K. A. Cooper, E. D. Hughes, and C. K. Ingold, *ibid.*, **1940**, 925.

tive Hofmann degradations of dilute sulphonium hydroxides in water:[21]

$$OH^- + Alk{\cdot}Br \rightarrow Alk{\cdot}OH + Br^-$$

$$OH^- + Alk{\cdot}\overset{+}{S}R_2 \rightarrow Alk{\cdot}OH + SR_2$$

And similar effects have been demonstrated for other alkyl series.

As to the two reactions and the alkyl series formulated, for fixed concentrations, solvent, and temperature, the absolute rates of both

TABLE 28-1.—RATES OF SUBSTITUTION OF ALKYL BROMIDES. (Medium: 80 vols. % EtOH+20% H_2O. Temperature: 55°)

	MeBr	EtBr	*i*-PrBr	*t*-BuBr	
Second-order rate constants[1] . .	2140	170	4.7	—	$\times 10^{-5}$
First-order rate constants[2]	—	—	0.24	1010	
Specific rates in 0.01 *N* NaOH[3]	21.4	1.7	0.29	1010	

[1] In $sec.^{-1}$ $mole^{-1}$ l.

[2] In $sec.^{-1}$.

[3] The specific rate is the fraction of surviving alkyl bromide converted per second.

were found to drop moderately from methyl to ethyl, either to drop or to rise somewhat, depending on alkali concentration, from ethyl to *iso*propyl, and to rise steeply from *iso*propyl to *t*-butyl. For both reactions, the kinetic order was second for methyl and ethyl; and it was first in suitably dilute solution for *iso*propyl, and first for *t*-butyl. These changes are illustrated by the figures[21] given in Table 28-1 for the hydrolysis of the alkyl bromides in "80%" aqueous ethyl alcohol and they could equally be illustrated by figures for alkyl oxy-esters, for example, nitrates.[22]

The four groups, methyl, ethyl, *iso*propyl, and *t*-butyl, exemplify all the more striking phenomena of nucleophilic substitution, as encountered in saturated alkyl compounds, except for some special effects, discussed later, which arise in more complex branched groups, such as the *neo*pentyl group, and the tri-*t*.-butylcarbinyl group, and in certain alicyclic groups. For the present we may note that the higher normal alkyl groups behave broadly like ethyl; there are differences of reaction rate, but by no more than small multiples (higher homologues reacting somewhat more slowly than ethyl compounds), and there are no differences of kinetic order for fixed physical conditions. Thus, the substitutions undergone by the primary alkyl bromides under attack

[21] E. D. Hughes and C. K. Ingold, *J. Chem. Soc.*, **1933**, 1571; J. L. Gleave, E. D. Hughes, and C. K. Ingold, *ibid.*, **1935**, 236.

[22] J. W. Baker and D. M. Easty, *J. Chem. Soc.*, **1952**, 1192, 1208.

by ethoxide ions in dry ethyl alcohol are all second-order processes; and their relative rates[23] at 55° (methyl being included for comparison) are as follows:

Me 17.6, Et 1.00, *n*-Pr 0.31, *n*-Bu 0.23, *n*-Amyl 0.21

The analogous reactions of alkyl iodides with phenoxide ions are also second-order substitutions. Segaller obtained the following relative rates[24] at 42.5°, and found these values to be but little dependent on temperature:

Me 4.84, Et 1.00, *n*-Pr 0.40, *n*-Bu 0.39, *n*-Hexyl 0.36,
n-Heptyl 0.35, *n*-Octyl 0.34, *n*-Cetyl 0.33

The higher secondary alkyl groups, 2-*n*-butyl, 2-*n*-amyl, 3-*n*-amyl, and 2-*n*-octyl, behave basically like the *iso*propyl group. Mechanistically, these groups are marginal; and substitutions either of second order or of first order can be observed. But the rates of corresponding substitutions of any one order are the same for all these groups to well within a factor of two, as the following figures[25] show. For the second-order reactions of the bromides with ethoxide ion in dry ethyl alcohol at 25°, the measured relative rates were as follows:

i-Pr 1.00, 2-Bu 1.29, 2-Amyl 1.16, 3-Amyl 0.93

For the first-order reactions of the bromides in "60%" aqueous ethyl alcohol at 80°, the relative rates were as below:

i-Pr 1.00, 2-Bu 1.04, 2-Amyl 0.79, 3-Amyl 0.85, 2-Octyl 0.99

Higher tertiary alkyl groups behave similarly to the *t*-butyl group, showing, like the latter, a strong tendency to unimolecular substitution.[26,27] Most of the measured rates are first-order rates. They differ from one tertiary group to another; but, except for quite highly branched or polycyclic groups, where factors enter which need not be

[23] I. Dostrovsky and E. D. Hughes, *J. Chem. Soc.*, **1946**, 157, *et seq.*; M. L Dhar, E. D. Hughes, C. K. Ingold, and S. Masterman, *ibid.*, **1948**, 2055.

[24] D. Segaller, *J. Chem. Soc.*, 1913, **103**, 1154; 1914, **105**, 106.

[25] E. D. Hughes, C. K. Ingold, and U. Shapiro, *J. Chem. Soc.*, **1936**, 225; E. D. Hughes and U. G. Shapiro, *ibid.*, **1937**, 1177, 1192; M. L. Dhar, E. D. Hughes, and C. K. Ingold, *ibid.*, **1948**, 2058.

[26] K. A. Cooper and E. D. Hughes, *J. Chem. Soc.*, **1937**, 1183; K. A. Cooper, E. D. Hughes, and C. K. Ingold, *ibid.*, p. 1280; E. D. Hughes and B. J. MacNulty, *ibid.*, p. 1283; M. L. Dhar, E. D. Hughes, and C. K. Ingold, *ibid.*, **1948**, 2065; E. D. Hughes, C. K. Ingold, and L. I. Woolf, *ibid.*, p. 2084; H. C. Brown and R. S. Fletcher, *J. Am. Chem. Soc.*, 1949, **71**, 1845; H. C. Brown and A. Stern, *ibid.*, 1950, **72**, 5068.

[27] J. Shorter and C. N. Hinshelwood, *J. Chem. Soc.*, **1949**, 2412.

considered now, they differ by no more than small multiples. This may be illustrated by Shorter and Hinshelwood's measurements[27] of the first-order rates of solvolysis of a number of tertiary alkyl chlorides and iodides in "80%" aqueous ethyl alcohol. The following figures represent relative rates at 35° for a series of tertiary groups with one growing branch (Am = amyl):

	$MeCMe_2$	$EtCMe_2$	n-$PrCMe_2$	n-$BuCMe_2$	n-$AmCMe_2$
Chlorides:	1.00	1.61	1.41	1.33	1.21
Iodides:	1.00	1.85	1.77	1.75	1.53

The following relative rates at 35° show the effect of successively building up the three branches of a tertiary alkyl group:

	CMe_3	$EtCMe_2$	Et_2CMe	Et_3C
Chlorides:	1.00	1.61	2.33	2.60
Iodides:	1.00	1.85	3.14	4.39

It is to be understood that these reactions must each give several products, in general, an alcohol, an ethyl ether, and one or more olefins; for the carbonium ion formed by the initial heterolysis can end its life either by the uptake of an anion or by the loss of a proton. However, the rates of these parallel reactions are collectively controlled by their common slow stage, the ionisation, and it is to the rate of this process that the measurements (of liberated halide ion) are considered to refer.

We have thus the situation that on passing along the series, methyl, any primary alkyl, any secondary alkyl, any tertiary alkyl, the mechanism of nucleophilic substitution changes from bimolecular to unimolecular at some point, which, in the reactions illustrated, is usually located between the primary and the secondary alkyl groups, and, for some reactions, notably those of alkyl halides in aqueous solvents, lies closely about the secondary groups. However, what for initial simplicity was called a "point" of mechanistic change would be better described as a "region." For the change is not sharp; and a sufficiently filled-in series would contain an interior band of groups for which both mechanisms can be realised in easily established conditions.

There are simple macrochemical, and probably also molecular, reasons for this. For first, rate of substitution by the bimolecular mechanism is proportional to the concentration of the substituting agent, while in general rate by the unimolecular mechanism is not. Therefore a change in the concentration of the substituting agent can alter the relative rates by the two mechanisms. Then, rate by the unimolecular mechanism is often much more critically dependent on the ionising power of the solvent than is rate by the bimolecular mechanism. This is notably true of the reactions of alkyl halides: for them, formic acid is outstanding as an ionising solvent, and will promote dominating unimolecular reactions even of primary alkyl halides: aqueous ethyl alcohol and aqueous acetone are successively less ionising, and dry alcohol and dry acetone are successively less ionising still. For the decompositions of 'onium salts, where both reactants are ions, a different situation obtains, as we shall see in Section **29a**: rate by the bimolecular mechanism is highly sensitive to the medium, as rate by the unimolecular mechanism is not. However, it is as true for these reactions as for those of alkyl halides, that the two mechanisms differ notably in their dependence upon solvent, a change in which can accordingly alter their relative importance. To the extent to which we can conveniently vary it, temperature has a somewhat weakly differential action on the two mechanisms; but the effect is broadly systematic, a raised temperature acting in the direction of a reduced solvent polarity. If then we are dealing, with respect to a given reaction, with an alkyl group situated somewhere near the "point" of mechanistic change, that is, a group whose tendencies to use the two mechanisms are not too highly unbalanced, it will evidently be possible to make either mechanism dominating by adjusting the conditions of the reaction, particularly with respect to the reagent concentrations and the solvent.

Such adjustments can readily be made, with the effect indicated, in the reactions of secondary alkyl halides. In poorly ionising solvents, such as alcohols, and with large concentrations of an active nucleophile, such as alkoxide, azide, or thiolate ions, bimolecular substitutions are observed; but, in a good ionising solvent, such as formic acid, and as the concentrations of active anions are reduced, the kinetic and other characteristics of the substitution go over into those of the unimolecular mechanism. In short, secondary alkyl halides belong to the border "region."

These considerations suggest means of making observations which could be illustrated by the broken portion of the S_N2 curve of Fig. 28-1. In the reactions of alkyl halides, for instance, one might employ such poorly ionising solvents that the secondary halides, and possibly even the tertiary halides, would be unable to ionise, and would be forced to react, if at all, by the S_N2 mechanism. One might consider the S_N1 curve to have been depressed by such means until it does not interfere with observation of the S_N2 curve. Of course, it helps to use a considerable concentration of a strongly nucleophilic reagent. Three examples of this effect will be given.

Dry ethyl alcohol is a poor ionising solvent for alkyl halides. Using it, Wisliscenus[28] studied their interaction with ethyl sodioacetoacetate:

$$\bar{C}H\begin{matrix}\diagup CO\cdot CH_3\\ \diagdown CO_2Et\end{matrix} + RHal \rightarrow RCH\begin{matrix}\diagup CO\cdot CH_3\\ \diagdown CO_2Et\end{matrix} + Hal^-$$

He established the rate series, Me > Et > *i*-Pr > *t*-Bu, the rate for the group *t*-Bu being unobservably small. Here we see the continuous fall of rate illustrated by the curve drawn for the S_N2 mechanism in Fig. 28-1.

Menschutkin[29] examined the second-order reactions between triethylamine and alkyl iodides in solvent acetone:

$$NEt_3 + RI \rightarrow R\overset{+}{N}Et_3 + \bar{I}$$

His relative rates at 100° were as follows:

Me 100, Et 8.8, *n*-Pr 1.7, *n*-Bu 1.2, *n*-Hept 0.9, *n*-Oct 0.9, *i*-Pr 0.18

The investigation of *t*-Bu was frustrated by olefin elimination, and part of the measured rate for *i*-Pr may have been due to this cause. However that may be, the results establish the S_N2 rate series, Me > Et > higher normal > *i*-Pr.

The effect of alkyl structure on the second-order rate of reaction of halide ions with alkyl halides, the Finkelstein reaction, as it is called, was first investigated by Conant and Kirner[30] in the example

$$I^- + RCl \rightarrow RI + Cl^-$$

with acetone as solvent. Subsequently, de la Mare, Fowden, Hughes, and others[31] examined six of the nine reactions

$$Y^- + RX \rightarrow RY + X^-$$

where X, Y = Cl, Br, I, examples in which X and Y are the same halogen being covered by isotopic labelling. The variation of rate with alkyl structure was qualitatively similar in all these reactions: the quantitative differences will be gone into later. For the present,

[28] J. Wisliscenus, *Ann.*, 1882, **212**, 232.

[29] N. Menschutkin, *Z. physik. Chem.*, 1890, **5**, 589.

[30] J. B. Conant and W. R. Kirner, *J. Am. Chem. Soc.*, 1924, **46**, 235.

[31] P. B. D. de la Mare, *J. Chem. Soc.*, **1955**, 3169; E. D. Hughes, C. K. Ingold, and J. D. H. Mackie, *ibid.*, pp. 3173, 3177; P. B. D. de la Mare, *ibid.*, p. 3180; L. H. Fowden, E. D. Hughes, and C. K. Ingold, *ibid.*, pp. 3187, 3193; P. B. D. de la Mare, *ibid.*, p. 3196; E. D. Hughes, C. K. Ingold, and A. J. Parker, *ibid.*, 1960, 4400.

the general rate pattern may be illustrated by the relative rates at 25° in acetone for the reaction between radiobromide and alkyl bromides:

Me 100, Et 1.31, *n*-Pr 0.81, *i*-Pr 0.015, *t*-Bu 0.004

These results establish the S_N2 rate series Me>Et>higher primary >*i*-Pr>*t*-Bu for Finkelstein substitutions.

The opposite procedure to that illustrated in these examples is to employ such good ionising solvents, and such poor nucleophilic reagents, that even primary alkyl halides react by the ionisation mechanism S_N1. We can imagine that the S_N1 curve in Fig. 28-1 might thus be raised so far that the whole of it could be observed without interference from the S_N2 curve.

An illustration of such an effect has been given by Bateman and Hughes. They developed the use of formic acid as a solvent for reactions of alkyl halides, showing in several ways that formic acid behaves as a better ionising solvent than water for these compounds.[32] They studied the hydrolysis of a number of alkyl bromides by water in formic acid:

$$H_2O + RBr \rightarrow ROH + H^+ + Br^-$$

Even for primary halides, this reaction is essentially a first-order one, its rate being at most only slightly dependent on the (small) concentration of the water. The observed relative rates[33] at 100°, namely,

MeBr 1.00, EtBr 1.71, *i*-PrBr 44.7, *t*-BuBr *ca.* 10^8

yield the rate series, Me<Et<*i*-Pr<*t*-Bu. Here we see the strong continuous rise in rate, corresponding to the curve drawn for the S_N1 mechanism in Fig. 28-1.

In special cases, the S_N1 mechanism of substitution can be observed for primary halides in aqueous alcoholic solvents: this happens when the alkyl structure has been so chosen that S_N2 substitution is sterically excluded. The simplest known example is that of *neo*pentyl bromide (Section **35**).

The molecular reason why we should not expect the change from a bimolecular to a unimolecular mechanism to be sharp, in other words, why we should not expect to classify every individual molecular act of substitution as either bimolecular or unimolecular, with nothing in between, follows from an elementary picture of the two processes. In one, the expelled group is liberated with help from the attacking reagent; in the other, the liberated group gets free without such help;

[32] L. C. Bateman and E. D. Hughes, *J. Chem. Soc.*, **1937,** 1187; **1940,** 935, 940, 945; I. Dostrovsky and E. D. Hughes, *ibid.*, **1946,** 171.

[33] L. C. Bateman and E. D. Hughes, *J. Chem. Soc.*, **1940,** 945

and yet there must be degrees of assistance which could be offered by the substituting agent and accepted by the heterolysing system.[34] This situation is discussed further in the next Section.

(28b) Constitutional Influences in the Radical Substituted: Alkyl Radicals Containing Substituents.—Just as alkyl groups are derived from methyl by the entrance of α-alkyl substituents, so aralphyl groups are derived by the introduction of α-aryl substituents. In alkyl compounds, the separation of a group with its shared electrons is assisted by the inductive effect: and any formed carbonium ion is stabilised at best by hyperconjugative mesomerism. In aralphyl compounds containing α-phenyl substituents, the more powerful mechanism of conjugative electron displacements is available to assist the separation of the displaced group; and a formed carbonium ion is stablised by conjugative mesomerism. It is therefore to be expected, and it is found, that α-phenyl substituents in aralphyl groups exert a facilitating polar effect on both the bimolecular and the unimolecular mechanism of nucleophilic substitution, and a particularly strong one on the unimolecular mechanism. It is a useful rough rule that one α-phenyl substituent is about as good as two α-alkyl substituents for the purpose of determining the relative importance of the mechanisms. Thus, for the reactions of aralphyl halides, the benzyl group, although primary, belongs to the mechanistic border region, like secondary alkyl groups; and the α-phenylethyl group, though secondary, tends strongly to promote unimolecular reactions, as do tertiary alkyl groups.

The two aralphyl series,

$$R = CH_3,\ CH_2Ph,\ CHPh_2,\ CPh_3$$
$$R = CH_2Ph,\ CHMePh,\ CMe_2Ph$$

have been studied sufficiently to locate the change of mechanism, the first series with respect to both of the aqueous reactions,

$$OH^- + R\cdot Hal \rightarrow R\cdot OH + Hal^-$$
$$OH^- + R\cdot NR_3'^+ \rightarrow R\cdot OH + NR_3'$$

and the second series with respect only to the halide substitution. In each case the change occurs at or about the benzyl group, members to the right, in either series, undergoing unimolecular reactions.

Olivier showed[35] that the hydrolysis of benzyl chloride, in "50%" aqueous acetone in the presence of alkali hydroxide, can be approximated as the sum of two reactions, one independent of the reagent

[34] J. L. Gleave, E. D. Hughes, and C. K. Ingold, *J. Chem. Soc.*, **1935,** 236.

[35] S. C. J. Olivier and A. P. Weber, *Rec. trav. chim.*, 1934, **53,** 869; S. C. J. Olivier, *ibid.*, p. 891.

hydroxide ion and the other proportional to its concentration; and he showed that on going over to water as solvent the reaction becomes much more nearly independent of hydroxide ion. The hydrolysis of benzhydryl chloride has been extensively investigated.[36] It proceeds, in aqueous alcohol containing hydroxide ion, independently of the hydroxide ion. Furthermore, a detailed study of the reaction in aqueous alcohol and in aqueous acetone has shown that the kinetics are first-order only in first approximation, the actual kinetic law agreeing with the general case of unimolecular solvolysis. The hydrolysis of α-phenylethyl chloride, in "80%" aqueous acetone containing hydroxide ion, proceeds independently of the hydroxide ion.[37] Triphenylmethyl chloride is hydrolysed in aqueous solvents at such a high rate that the reaction has not yet been studied accurately. But the high rate can be taken as evidence that the unimolecular mechanism is in operation.

In the ammonium hydroxide reactions, the change of mechanism appears between the benzyl and benzhydryl groups.[38] Methyl and benzyl substituents in ammonium ions are eliminated as alcohols at rates approximately proportional to the concentration of hydroxide ions, while benzhydryl groups are eliminated as benzhydrol at rates which are independent of the hydroxide ions. This is taken to mean that the first two groups use the bimolecular mechanism, and the third the unimolecular mechanism; while there are indirect indications that the triphenylmethyl group also uses the unimolecular mechanism.

The allyl group appears to resemble the benzyl group with respect to the hydrolysis and alcoholysis of its halides: it is another mechanistically marginal group for these reactions of halides in aqueous alcoholic solvents; but hydrolysis is unimolecular in formic acid.[39]

The effect of *p*-alkyl substituents in a benzyl compound on the rates of various bimolecular and one unimolecular substitution is shown in an investigation by Bevan, Hughes, and the writer,[40] covering, besides nucleophilic aliphatic substitution, some analogous reactions of nucle-

[36] A. M. Ward, *J. Chem. Soc.*, **1927,** 2285; N. T. Farinacci and L. P. Hammett, *J. Am. Chem. Soc.*, 1937, **59,** 2542; L. C. Bateman, E. D. Hughes, and C. K. Ingold, *ibid.*, 1938, **60,** 380; E. D. Hughes, C. K. Ingold, and N. A. Taher, *J. Chem. Soc.*, **1940,** 949; M. G. Church, E. D. Hughes, and C. K. Ingold, *ibid.*, p. 966.

[37] A. M. Ward, *J. Chem. Soc.*, **1927,** 445; E. D. Hughes, C. K. Ingold, and A. D Scott, *ibid.*, **1937,** 1201.

[38] E. D. Hughes and C. K. Ingold, *J. Chem. Soc.*, **1933,** 69; E. D. Hughes, *ibid.*, p. 75.

[39] C. A. Vernon, *J. Chem. Soc.*, **1954,** 423.

[40] C. W. L. Bevan, E. D. Hughes, and C. K. Ingold, *Nature*, 1953, **171,** 301,

TABLE 28-2.—RELATIVE RATES OF SOME NUCLEOPHILIC SUBSTITUTIONS OF ARALPHYL AND ARYL COMPOUNDS AND OF THEIR PARA-METHYL AND PARA-T-BUTYL DERIVATIVES (BEVAN AND HUGHES).

Reactants	Solvent	Temp.	Molecularity	Relative rates p-H	p-Me	p-Bu^t
—C₆H₄—$CH_2\cdot Br + C_5H_5N$	Me_2CO	20°	2	1	1.66	1.35
—C₆H₄—$CH_2\cdot Br + I^-$	Me_2CO	0	2	1	1.45	1.35
—C₆H₄—$CH_2\cdot Br + EtO^-$	EtOH	25	2	1	1.48	1.36
—C₆H₄—$CH_2\cdot Br + Bu^tO^-$	Bu^tOH	60	2	1	1.32	1.18
—C₆H₄—$CH_2Cl + EtO^-$	EtOH	25	2	1	1.58	1.47
—C₆H₄—$CH_2\cdot Br + H_2O$	HCO_2H	25	1	1	57.9	28.0
—C₆H₄—$CH_2\cdot \overset{+}{N}C_5H_5 + EtO^-$	EtOH	20	2	1	0.507	0.629
—C₆H₄—$CO\cdot OEt + HO^-$	85% aq-—EtOH	25	2	1	0.436	0.616
—C₆H₄—$CO\cdot Cl + HOEt$	EtOH	0	2	1	0.531	0.667
—C₆H₂(NO_2)₂—$Cl + EtO^-$	EtOH	50	2	1	0.173	0.310

The data for the reaction of benzyl bromides with pyridine (top line) are by J. W. Baker and W. S. Nathan (*J. Chem. Soc.*, **1935**, 1844).

ophilic substitution in the carboxyl group and the aromatic ring. Their relative rates are recorded in Table 28-2. They show that when, as in reactions requiring electron supply, a para-methyl substituent in the benzyl group increases reaction rate, a para-*t*-butyl substituent also increases it, but to a smaller extent; and that when, as in reactions requiring electron withdrawal, a *p*-Me substituent retards, a *p*-*t*-butyl substituent also retards, but less strongly. The relative magnitude of the effects of the two alkyl groups agrees with the theory that hyperconjugative interaction with the benzene ring becomes increased or decreased according to the alteration of polarity at the reaction site during the formation of the transition state. The sharp contrast in the magnitude of the kinetic effect when we pass over from any bimolecular substitution to the strongly electron-demanding unimolecular form of substitution, illustrates not only the different electrical situations created in the two mechanisms, but also the importance of the electromeric aspect $+E$ of the polar effect of alkyl groups.

The kinetic effects of hyperconjugation, as shown by a somewhat greater variety of alkyl groups with respect to a typical unimolecular reaction, may be illustrated by some data[41] for the hydrolysis of *p*-alkylbenzhydryl chlorides in "80%" aqueous acetone. As shown in Table 28-3, the rate series is as follows,

$$H < \{Me > Et > i\text{-}Pr > t\text{-}Bu\}$$

and to every rate inequality there corresponds an oppositely directed inequality in the Arrhenius energies of activation. Just the same rate sequence has been found[42] for the unimolecular solvolysis in aqueous ethanol of 1,1-dimethylpropargyl chloride and its 3-alkyl homologues, $R\cdot C\vdots C\cdot CMe_2\cdot Cl$, with R = H, Me, Et, *i*-Pr, *t*-Bu.

Table 28-3.—Rates and Arrhenius Activation Energies for the Hydrolysis of *p*-Alkylbenzhydryl Chlorides in 80% Aqueous Acetone.

p-Substituent	H	Me	Et	*i*-Pr	*t*-Bu
$10^6 k_1$ at 0°, with k_1 in sec.$^{-1}$	2.82	83.5	62.6	47.0	35.9
E (kcal./mole)	21.0	18.9	19.4	19.8	20.1

As we have noticed (Sections **7c** and **7d**), deuterium is inductively more electropositive than light hydrogen, but is less polarisable, and hence is less electropositive in a hyperconjugative electromeric effect. We should expect hyperconjugation appreciably to assist the ionisation of *t*-butyl halides and their simpler homologues,

$$H\!-\!C\!-\!C\!-\!Cl$$

Observed effects of substitution of light hydrogen by deuterium in *t*-alkyl halides on the rates of their unimolecular reactions lend some support to this presumption.

V. J. Shiner first showed[43] that the rates of unimolecular solvolysis of such halides are reduced, usually by some units per cent, by the introduction of deuterium, particularly at positions from which a hyperconjugative effect could be propagated to the ionisation centre. For the solvolysis of *t*-amyl chloride in "80%" aqueous ethanol, the relative rates at 0° were

[41] E. D. Hughes, C. K. Ingold, and N. A. Taher, *J. Chem. Soc.*, **1940,** 949

[42] A. Burowoy and E. Spicer, *J. Chem. Soc.*, **1954,** 3654.

[43] V. J. Shiner, *J. Am. Chem. Soc.*, 1953, **75,** 2925.

$$\underset{100}{CH_3\cdot CH_2\cdot \overset{Cl}{\overset{|}{C}}(CH_3)_2} \qquad \underset{71}{CH_3\cdot CD_2\cdot \overset{Cl}{\overset{|}{C}}(CH_3)_2}$$

$$\underset{56}{CH_3\cdot CH_2\cdot \overset{Cl}{\overset{|}{C}}(CD_3)_2} \qquad \underset{41}{CH_3\cdot CD_2\cdot \overset{Cl}{\overset{|}{C}}(CD_3)_2}$$

—figures which signify a reduction in rate by 16% for each D put into the methylene group, and by 9% for each put into the α-methyl groups. The requirement of an unbroken system capable of transmitting a hyperconjugative effect from source to reaction centre is illustrated in E. S. Lewis's demonstration[44] that the replacement of CH_3 by CD_3 in p-$CH_3\cdot C_6H_4\cdot CHMe\cdot Cl$ reduces by 10% the rate of solvolysis of the chloride in acetic acid, whilst the corresponding isotopic substitution in m-$CH_3\cdot C_6H_4\cdot CHMe\cdot Cl$ makes no difference to the rate. The expected stereochemical requirement for transmission of the hyperconjugative effect of a single hydrogen atom, *viz.*, that its bond should not lie in the plane of the carbonium ion being formed,[45] has been charmingly demonstrated by Shiner[46] in the example of the dibenzo*dicyclo*-octyl chloride formulated below. The plane of the eventual 2-carbonium ion is that of the bridge drawn with thickened bonds; and the 1- and 4-bridge-head hydrogen atoms lie in that plane. Shiner found that, whilst the introduction of two deuterium atoms to give a 3-CD_2 group reduced the rate of solvolysis in "60%" aqueous ethanol by 12%, such introduction to give 1-CD and 4-CD groups made no difference to the rate.

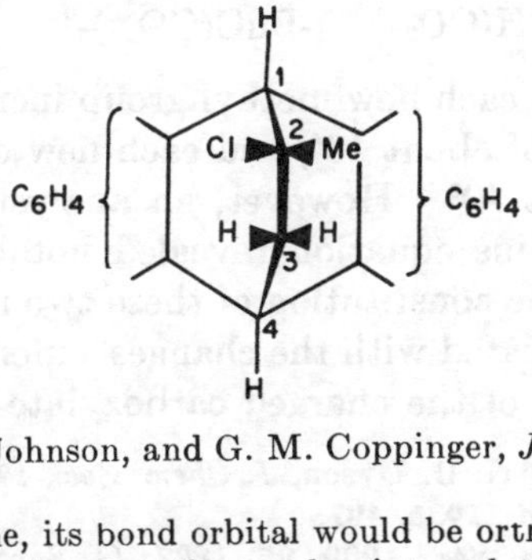

[44] E. S. Lewis, R. R. Johnson, and G. M. Coppinger, *J. Am. Chem. Soc.*, 1959' **81**, 3140.

[45] If it lay in the plane, its bond orbital would be ortnogonal to the "empty" orbital of the carbonium ion, *i.e.*, the overlap integral would be zero. Strictly, this condition for non-interaction should refer to the transition state of formation of the carbonium ion, rather than to the carbonium ion itself. But, as we shall see later, the electron is almost wholly transferred in this type of transition state, which therefore approximates in shape to the carbonium ion itself.

[46] V. J. Shiner, *J. Am. Chem. Soc.*, 1960, **82**, 2655.

As a first illustration of the production of a change of mechanism by the introduction of non-hydrocarbon substituents into an alkyl group, we may consider groups containing the inductively electron-repelling carboxylate-ion substituent, $-CO_2^-$, since this case has importance in connexion with the steric course of substitution, later to be discussed. The experimental material refers to the solvolysis in water, or in aqueous alcohol, of α-halogenoacylate ions. The bromoacetate ion was studied by Dawson and his coworkers,[47] the α-bromopropionate ion by Senter and Wood,[48] the bromomalonate ion by Madsen,[49] and this ion together with the α-bromomethylmalonate ion by Hughes and Taher.[50] The last-named authors established changes of mechanism in two series, as indicated below, the main evidence being that hydrolyses of the bromides of the residues written to the left of the dividing lines are accelerated by alkali, while the corresponding reactions of the radicals written to the right are not thus accelerated:

$$(S_N2)\left\{\begin{matrix} CH_3 & CH_2(CO_2^-) & | & CH(CO_2^-)_2 \\ CH_2Me & | \; CHMe(CO_2^-) & & CMe(CO_2^-)_2 \end{matrix}\right\}(S_N1)$$

The earlier location of the point of mechanistic change in the second series is consistent with the known facilitating effect of methyl substituents on the unimolecular mechanism: α-methyl- and α-carboxylate-ion substituents appear to act similarly in promoting unimolecular substitution. Gripenberg, Hughes, and the writer subsequently examined[51] two further series of carboxylated bromides, throughout which the unimolecular mechanism of solvolysis prevails:

$$\left.\begin{matrix} CMe_3 & CMe_2(CO_2^-) & CMe(CO_2^-)_2 \\ t\text{-}BuCH_2 & t\text{-}BuCH(CO_2^-) & t\text{-}BuC(CO_2^-)_2 \end{matrix}\right\}(S_N1 \text{ throughout})$$

They concluded that each new methyl group increased the unimolecular rate by a factor of about 10^4, and each new carboxylate-ion group by a factor of about 10^3. However, an analysis of the rate data in terms of the Arrhenius equation revealed notable differences in the energetic and entropic constitution of these two rate ratios, differences which could be associated with the changes suffered by the energy and entropy of solvation of the charged carboxylate-ion substituents.

[47] H. M. Dawson and N. B. Dyson, *J. Chem. Soc.*, **1933**, 49, 1133; H. Brooke and H. M. Dawson, *ibid.*, **1936**, 497.

[48] G. Senter, *J. Chem. Soc.*, **1909**, **95**, 1827; G. Senter and H. Wood, *ibid.*, **1915**, **107**, 1070; **1916**, **109**, 681; W. A. Cowdrey, E. D. Hughes, and C. K. Ingold, *ibid.*, **1937**, 1208.

[49] E. H. Madsen, *Z. physik. Chem.*, **1914**, **86**, 538.

[50] E. D. Hughes and N. A. Taher, *J. Chem. Soc.*, **1940**, 956.

[51] J. Gripenberg, E. D. Hughes, and C. K. Ingold, *Nature*, **1948**, **164**, 480.

The unimolecular mechanism would be expected to be still more prominent in the reactions of the halides of residues in which a carboxylate-ion substituent has been introduced into an aralphyl group, as in the radical $CHPh(CO_2^-)$. Actually, the work of Senter and Tucker establishes[52] that the unimolecular mechanism exclusively controls the aqueous hydrolysis of the α-chloro- and α-bromo-phenylacetate ion.

Turning from carboxylate-ion substituents to halogen substituents, which can release electrons towards a carbonium ionic centre by a conjugative mechanism, we may first consider Olivier and Weber's comparative study[53] of the hydrolysis of benzyl chloride, benzal chloride, and benzotrichloride in "50%" aqueous acetone containing alkali hydroxide. A number of successive chlorine displacements are, of course, involved in the last two cases, but the results show that the loss of the second and third chlorine atoms follows immediately on that of the first, to which, therefore, the rate measurements refer in every case. The hydrolysis of benzyl chloride, though mechanistically marginal, was predominantly bimolecular in the solvent used, the rate depending largely on the hydroxide-ion concentration. Benzal chloride underwent hydrolysis more rapidly, and at a rate which was independent of the hydroxide ions. Benzotrichloride was hydrolysed more rapidly still, again independently of hydroxide ions. The hydrolysis of benzhydryl chloride is of the same general form, as we have seen; and that of benzhydrylidene chloride is again of the same form, but faster. In all cases, as Bensley and Kohnstam have shown,[53] each extra chlorine atom decreases the Arrhenius activation energy of hydrolysis. These results lead us to assume that, in addition to the phenyl group, the second and third chlorine atoms, when present, supply electrons to the reaction centre, thereby promoting ionisation of the first chlorine atom, and an overall unimolecular hydrolysis. Each chlorine atom will contribute its effect in this direction; but when the first chlorine atom has, by its hydrolysis, become replaced by an oxygen atom, the latter will release electrons in the same electromeric manner, but very much more strongly:

$$Cl—C—Cl \qquad RO—C—Cl$$

So it comes about that second and third stages of hydrolysis follow instantly upon the first stage.

[52] G. Senter, *J. Chem. Soc.*, 1915, **107**, 908; G. Senter and S. H. Tucker, *ibid.*, 1916, **109**, 690.

[53] S. C. J. Olivier and A. P. Weber, *Rec. trav. chim.*, 1931, **53**, 869; J. S. Hine and D. E. Lee, *J. Am. Chem. Soc.*, 1951, **73**, 22; B. Bensley and G. Kohnstam, *J. Chem. Soc.*, 1956, 287.

In the absence of the phenyl group, the largest possible accumulation of α-chlorine atoms, that in carbon tetrachloride, does not suffice to promote the ionisation of one of them sufficiently to make that process the dominating mechanism of alkaline hydrolysis or alcoholysis in aqueous or alcoholic solvents. The polyhalogenomethanes can exhibit a quite different type of mechanism, as will be noted in Section **44**.

What several halogen substituents in a methyl halide cannot do, a single methoxyl substituent can: methoxymethyl chloride undergoes very rapid hydrolysis and alcoholysis, to give formaldehyde or formals, in aqueous and alcoholic solvents. It was inferred in 1935, simply from the high rates, that these reactions are unimolecular, and this has since been kinetically confirmed.[54] The rate-determining step, which is estimated to proceed at least 10^{14} times faster than that of the corresponding reaction of methyl chloride, is the ionisation of the chlorine atom to leave a mesomeric cation, which is partly an oxonium ion, but also partly a carbonium ion, and accordingly extracts a hydroxide or alkoxide ion very rapidly from a molecule of the solvent:

$$\mathrm{Me\ddot{O}{-}CH_2{-}Cl} \xrightarrow[\text{slow}]{} \mathrm{Me\overset{+}{O}{=}CH_2} + \overset{-}{\mathrm{Cl}}$$

$$\mathrm{EtOH} + \mathrm{Me\overset{+}{O}{:}CH_2} \xrightarrow[\text{fast}]{} \mathrm{MeO{\cdot}CH_2{\cdot}OEt} + \overset{+}{\mathrm{H}}$$

If the solvent is water, the product of the analogous unimolecular substitution is a semiacetal of formaldehyde:

$$\mathrm{Me\ddot{O}{-}CH_2{-}Cl} \xrightarrow[\text{slow}]{} \mathrm{Me\overset{+}{O}{=}CH_2} + \overset{-}{\mathrm{Cl}}$$

$$\mathrm{H_2O} + \mathrm{Me\overset{+}{O}{:}CH_2} \xrightarrow[\text{fast}]{} \mathrm{MeO{\cdot}CH_2{\cdot}OH} + \overset{+}{\mathrm{H}}$$

This undergoes a still more rapid second stage of hydrolysis to formaldehyde by an essentially similar mechanism, after the appropriate proton transfer:

$$\mathrm{{}^{-}O{-}CH_2{-}\overset{+}{O}HMe} \rightarrow \mathrm{O{=}CH_2} + \mathrm{OHMe}$$

A *p*-methoxyl group in benzyl or benzhydryl halides or arenesulphonates also promotes unimolecular solvolysis in solvents such as the lower alcohols and aqueous acetone; and it increases the reaction

[54] P. Ballinger, P. B. D. de la Mare, G. Kohnstam, and B. M. Prestt, *J. Chem. Soc.*, **1955**, 3641.

rate by factors around 10^4. A *p*-phenoxy-group has similar but weaker effects: the increases of rate are by factors of some hundreds. A *m*-methoxy group shows not the smallest vestige of any such effects. All this[55] is consistent with the idea that electromeric electron supply to the potential carbonium ion is dominating in the activation of the CX-ionisation. The weaker activation by the *p*-phenoxy- than by the *p*-methoxy-group is explained by the competing conjugation of the unsubstituted phenyl group in the former, with the lone electrons of the oxygen atom. The absence of any such effect of *m*-methoxyl is explained on the basis that an electromeric effect cannot be transmitted to the site of reaction in such a system.

Kohnstam has used the *p*-methoxy- and *p*-phenoxy-benzyl systems in order to examine the nature of mechanisms near the S_N1-S_N2 border region.[56] In Section **30** we shall consider his method, one of the better of the kinetic methods, for the diagnosis of S_N1 and S_N2 solvolytic mechanisms. By this and other tests, the hydrolysis of *p*-methoxy- and that of *p*-phenoxy-benzyl chlorides in "70%" aqueous dioxan are S_N1 processes. But they are sufficiently near the border region to allow observable intervention by a variety of anions, including quite weakly nucleophilic anions. All anions more nucleophilic than the tetrafluoroborate and perchlorate intervene to give added rates of second-order form, well beyond the range of normal salt effects, for which correction can be made. The question for consideration is that of the extent to which such anions, in their bimolecular participation, take over part of the task of supplying electrons in the transition state to that carbon atom which is losing an electron to the departing chlorine atom.

In unimolecular solvolysis this task is performed wholly internally by the polarisable *p*-oxybenzyl system. If we modify that system, as from *p*-methoxybenzyl to the less efficiently electron-supplying *p*-phenoxybenzyl system, we raise the free energy of activation of the carbon-chlorine ionisation, as is observed in a rate ratio, k_1(OMe)/k_1(OPh), equal to 135 at 20°. If the anion attacking in a bimolecular substitution took over only an insignificant part of the task of supplying the electrons to the heterolysing centre, leaving the internal electromeric system almost as completely responsible as before, then the activation energy should be raised by almost the same amount, and we

[55] S. Altscher, R. Baltzly, and S. W. Blenheim, *J. Am. Chem. Soc.*, 1952, **74**, 3649; J. K. Kochi and G. S. Hammond, *ibid.*, 1953, **75**, 3445; M. Simonetta and G. J. Farini, *J. Chem. Soc.*, **1954**, 1840; G. R. Cowie, J. R. Fox, M. J. H. Fitcher, K. A. Hooton, D. M. Hunt, G. Kohnstam, and B. Shillaker, *Proc. Chem. Soc.*, **1961**, 222; J. R. Fox and G. Kohnstam, *ibid.*, 1964, 115.

[56] G. Kohnstam, A. Queen, and T. Riber, *Chem. and Ind.*, **1962**, 1287.

should observe a bimolecular rate ratio, $k_2(\text{OMe})/k_2(\text{OPh})$, nearly equal to 135 at 20°. If, to go to the other extreme, the attacking anion supplied nearly all the electrons needed at the heterolysing centre in the transition state, making the latter almost independent of the internal electromeric system, then it should make but little difference whether this involves a methoxy- or a phenoxy-group, and the bimolecular rate ratio, $k_2(\text{OMe})/k_2(\text{OPh})$, should be close to unity. Thus we have in the rate ratios a scale with both ends fixed, a scale such as one cannot make with the rates themselves. By placing anions ranging from small to large nucleophilic strengths on that scale, one can rank them with respect to the proportions, from nothing, represented by the ratio 135, to all, expressed by the ratio unity, in which they contribute the electrons which the transition state needs.

This is Kohnstam's interpretation of the data in Table 28-4. The

TABLE 28-4.—RATE-CONSTANTS (SEC.$^{-1}$ MOL.$^{-1}$ L.) FOR SUBSTITUTION BY ANIONS IN *p*-METHOXY- AND *p*-PHENOXY-BENZYL CHLORIDES IN "70%" AQUEOUS ACETONE AT 20° (KOHNSTAM).

Anion	$10^4k_2(\text{OMe})$	$10^6k_2(\text{OPh})$	$k_2(\text{OMe})/k_2(\text{OPh})$
$Ph\cdot SO_3^-$	2.0	1.6	125
NO_3^-	3.2	2.3	139
F^-	4.2	4.9	86
radio-Cl^-	6.6	7.6	87
Br^-	7.9	50.9	15.5
N_3^-	34.5	710.3	4.9

benzenesulphonate and nitrate ions, although they react bimolecularly, contribute minimally, in the presence of the internal electromeric systems, to the supplying of the required electrons. The fluoride and chloride ions take on some sort of equitable share of that task. The strongly nucleophilic bromide and azide ions themselves provide almost the full supply of electrons that the reaction needs. All these substitutions are bimolecular. But they evidently cover a spectrum, leading, at one end, to the border region with the unimolecular mechanism.

An important group of nucleophilic substitutions involves preliminary protonation of the introduced substrate, but otherwise exhibits no differences of principle from the reactions of the neutral molecules and pre-formed ions already considered. Alcohols can be etherified by alcoholic strong acids; and ethers can be hydrolysed by strong aqueous acids: these are obviously substitutions of the ionic conjugate acids of the alcohols and ethers, Alk·OH_2^+ and Alk·OHR^+, the oxonium-ion groups being easily displaced in nucleophilic substitutions, as are the substituents SR_2^+ and NR_3^+. In the replacement reactions of such substrates, the introduced group need not be derived from the alcoholic or aqueous medium, if sufficient of another nucleophilic reagent, such as iodide ion, is present, as in Zeisel's process for estimating aromatically bound methoxyl groups by conversion with aqueous hydriodic acid into methyl iodide. For the simpler aliphatic alcohols, dialkyl ethers, and alkyl aryl ethers, these reactions are slow, requiring somewhat high temperatures in preparative experiments. It is often quite uncertain whether the bimolecular or unimolecular mechanism of substitution is being used, though we have indications (Section **28d**) that either may be used, according to the constitutional and environmental conditions. With *t*-butyl alcohol as substrate in sulphuric acid as solvent, the unimolecular mechanism must be employed, because, when the substituting agent is left out, the ultraviolet spectrum of the *t*-butylium ion (closely similar to that of isoelectronic trimethylboron) can be seen, and the rate of formation of this carbonium ion can thus be followed.[57] It would seem that *t*-butylium bisulphate is largely ionised in solvent sulphuric acid.

Acetals, while stable in alkaline solution, undergo a facile hydrogen-ion-catalysed hydrolysis in aqueous acid. These reactions of the simpler acetals go enormously faster than do the corresponding reactions of the simpler dialkyl ethers: from Skrabal's data[58] it is estimated that the extra ethoxyl group which diethyl acetal, CH(OEt)Me·O·C_2H_5, contains when compared with diethyl ether, CH_2Me·O·C_2H_5, increases the rate of hydrolysis by a factor of about 10^{11}. One might therefore rather safely presume that the acetal reactions at least are unimolecular substitutions of the appropriate conjugate acids (S_N1cA):

$$\mathrm{MeO{-}CH_2{-}\overset{+}{O}HMe} \xrightarrow[\text{slow}]{} \mathrm{Me\overset{+}{O}{=}CH_2 + HOMe}$$

$$\mathrm{H_2O + Me\overset{+}{O}{:}CH_2} \xrightarrow[\text{fast}]{} \mathrm{MeO{\cdot}CH_2{\cdot}OH + H^+}$$

The process is similar to that written above for the hydrolysis of methoxymethyl chloride, and, as in that case, the produced semiacetal is assumed to undergo a still more rapid second stage of hydrolysis to the aldehyde.

Brönsted and Wynne-Jones first drew the conclusion that the hy-

[57] J. Rosenbaum and M. C. R. Symons, *Proc. Chem. Soc.*, **1959**, 92.

[58] A. Skrabal and R. Skrabal, *Z. physik. Chem.*, 1938, **181**, 449.

drolysis of acetals is specific-hydrogen-ion catalysed, that is, that it depends on a pre-equilibrium proton uptake.[59] This has been confirmed by subsequent observations that, at acidities high enough to show the distinction, the rate follows Hammett's acidity function h_0 rather than the stoicheiometric acidity;[60] and that a change of solvent from H_2O to D_2O increases the rate by a factor of three.[61] That the point of carbon-oxygen fission is at the central carbon atom, and not at an alkyl group, was first deduced by O'Gorman and Lucas from their observation that formals of optically active secondary alcohols are hydrolysed without racemisation.[62] This has been confirmed by the observation that ^{18}O, if present, in the aqueous solvent used for the hydrolysis of acetals, does not appear in the produced alcohols.[63]

The effect of alkyl substitution on the rate of hydrolysis of acetals is consistent with the assumption of a unimolecular mechanism. For the acetals of pentaerythritol with formaldehyde, acetaldehyde, and acetone, the rates of hydrolysis[64] in aqueous hydrochloric acid at 25° have the following ratios:

$$H_2\ 1, \qquad HMe\ 6000, \qquad Me_2\ 10{,}000{,}000$$

That is, each methyl substituent at the seat of substitution increases the rate by a factor of approximately $10^{3.5}$. These large kinetic effects can be understood on the basis that the methyl substituents are bound directly to the carbon atom which becomes cationic in the unimolecular mechanism. They are consistent with other known effects of α-methyl substituents on rate by this mechanism, for instance, among the rates of α-carboxylato-alkyl halides described above.

(28c) Constitutional Influences in the Substituting Agent.—There is another group of constitutional effects, which can be used to distinguish the bimolecular and unimolecular mechanisms of substitution: rate by the bimolecular mechanism will depend on the nucleophilic strength of the substituting agent, while rate by the unimolecular mechanism may not: if it does not, we can be sure (apart from a special circumstance mentioned in Section **32h**), that the substituting agent is not even present in the transition state, and therefore is not covalently involved therein.

[59] J. N. Brönsted and W. F. K. Wynne-Jones, *Trans. Faraday Soc.*, 1929, **25**, 39.

[60] D. McIntyre and F. A. Long, *J. Am. Chem. Soc.*, 1954, **76**, 3240.

[61] W. J. C. Orr and J. A. V. Butler, *J. Chem. Soc.*, **1937**, 330.

[62] J. M. O'Gorman and H. J. Lucas, *J. Am. Chem. Soc.*, 1950, **72**, 5489.

[63] F. Stasink. W. A. Sheppard, and A. N. Bourns, *Canad. J. Chem.*, 1956, **34**, 123.

[64] A. Skrabal and M. Zlatewa, *Z. physik. Chem.*, 1926, **122**, 349.

The phenomenon that different substituting agents react at the same rate in unimolecular substitutions in the same substrate has been illustrated in many systems. Calcium formate and calcium chloroacetate, when present in formic acid in which *t*-butyl chloride is undergoing hydrolysis by added water, do not increase the rate of destruction of the chloride, even though much of what would otherwise have been *t*-butyl alcohol appears in the product as *t*-butyl formate or chloroacetate, which can be shown not to have been produced by esterification of first-formed alcohol.[65] Again, sodium azide, when dissolved in aqueous acetone, in which *pp'*-dimethylbenzhydryl chloride is undergoing hydrolysis, leaves the rate of disappearance of the chloride unaltered, except for a salt effect (Section **32**); yet much of what would otherwise have been *pp'*-dimethylbenzhydrol appears as *pp'*-dimethylbenzhydryl azide, which is certainly not formed by way of the alcohol.[66] This is a striking contrast to the reaction of sodium azide with *p*-methoxybenzyl chloride and with *p*-phenoxybenzyl chloride, where the mechanism of substitution, S_N1 with weak nucleophiles, goes over to S_N2 with azide ion, with the marked kinetic effects illustrated in Table 28-4. In solvent sulphur dioxide the three reagents, triethylamine, pyridine, and fluoride ion were found to substitute benzhydryl chloride at similar rates; and pyridine, iodide ion, and fluoride ion were found to substitute *m*-chlorobenzhydryl chloride at similar rates. In the last case, those special deviations from first-order kinetics which are expressed in the equation called "S_N1 typical" in Section **27d**, deviations which, when clearly observable, diagnose the unimolecular mechanism, were prominent.[67]

We have in these phenomena illustrations of the principle of another criterion of mechanism. When different substituting agents introduce different replacing groups at different rates, depending on the nucleophilic strength of the reagent, then we may usually infer (though not always, as we saw in the preceding Section) that the bimolecular mechanism of substitution is under observation. But when different substituting agents introduce different groups, or even the same group, at the same rate, then it is made probable that the unimolecular mechanism is at work.

During the earlier development of the theory of nucleophilic aliphatic substitution, this criterion was considerably employed in order

[65] L. C. Bateman and E. D. Hughes, *J. Chem. Soc.*, **1940,** 935.

[66] L. C. Bateman, E. D. Hughes, and C. K. Ingold, *J. Chem. Soc.*, **1940,** 974; L. C. Bateman, M. G. Church, E. D. Hughes, C. K. Ingold, and N. A. Taher, *ibid.*, pp. 995, 998.

[67] L. C. Bateman, E. D. Hughes, and C. K. Ingold, *J. Chem. Soc.*, **1940,** 1011, 1017.

to indicate a unimolecular mechanism in those hydrolytic reactions of halides which, even in alkaline solution, had first-order kinetics to within the accuracy of the measurements made up to that time. *t*-Butyl chloride and benzhydryl chloride, for example, were shown to be hydrolysed in aqueous acetone in an approximately first-order fashion, and at rates which remained substantially the same in acid, neutral, and alkaline solution: in particular, hydroxide ion produced no acceleration. It was concluded that the reactions are unimolecular, their rates being governed by the rates of ionisation of the halides. To the argument that the observed rates might represent rates of the bimolecular attack of a water molecule on the halides, the reply was that in that case the hydroxide ion, which is a much more powerful nucleophilic reagent, should, when present in quantity, produce a faster reaction, as we know it does with other halides, for instance methyl or ethyl halides.

We come now to the intricate question of what determines nucleophilic strength. The difficulty in making a precise statement about this is that the property in question is determined not only by the nucleophile, but also by the task before it, often to the extent that two nucleophiles will stand in opposite orders of efficiency before two alternative tasks, for instance, attack on two different types of substrate, or on the same substrate in two different types of solvent. The presence of a cationic charge in the substrate will favour anionic rather than neutral nucleophiles, although this effect is relatively small.[68,72] The significant property of a solvent is its absolute and relative power to solvate cations and anions.[69] It may make a difference also whether one is assessing nucleophilic strength by the equilibrium extent, or by the rate, of a reaction: obviously, we should express the method of assessment by referring to thermodynamic or kinetic nucleophilic strength, when the context does not make this distinction.

A nucleophile, when extracting a proton, is said to be behaving as a base: nucleophilic strength, in this specialisation, is basic strength, or "basicity." The broad validity of Brönsted's catalytic law shows that thermodynamic basicity and kinetic basicity run roughly parallel. But very different relations may appear when the task before the nucleophile is not proton extraction, but is one of attack on saturated or unsaturated carbon, or on some other element. For example, thermodynamic basicities in hydroxylic solvents stand in the order

[68] C. G. Swain, C. B. Scott, and K. H. Lohmann, *J. Am. Chem. Soc.*, 1953, **75**, 136.

[69] J. Miller and A. J. Parker, *J. Am. Chem. Soc.*, 1961, **83**, 117; A. J. Parker, *J. Chem. Soc.*, **1961**, 1328, 4398; *Quart. Rev. Chem. Soc.*, 1962, **16**, 163.

$F^- > Cl^-$, etc., and $RO^- > RS^-$, etc. (R = H, alkyl, aryl); but the reverse orders apply to rates of nucleophilic substitution at a saturated carbon atom of a neutral substrate in a hydroxylic solvent. In general, the basicity orders are also reversed for rates of substitution at aliphatic and aromatic but not carbonyl carbon in hydroxylic solvents. As far as is known, they are not reversed for rates of substitution in quadriligant boron, phosphorus, and sulphur.[70,73]

This general situation must mean that nucleophilic strength depends on a combination of several characters of the nucleophile, and that a particular combination of characters fits a nucleophile better for some tasks than others. The main internal characters are, of course, polarisation and polarisability, in their generalised connotation. The important external characters are solvation, and, frequently but not universally, steric interaction with the substrate.

As to polarisation, we must obviously take in Brönsted's teaching that nett electric charge is a small matter at the very close reaction-sites involved, relatively to the intense and highly local field at such a site, that is, in the orbital involved in the nucleophilic function. Such generalisation is automatically allowed for, if, following Edwards and others,[71,72] we use the empirical value of the thermodynamic basic strength of a nucleophile as the first component of all the nucleophilic strengths that that nucleophile can display in other reactions. The assumption is that, perhaps because of the moderate heat changes in acid-base equilibria, or because of the relative smallness of the hydrogen orbital offered for overlap with the nucleophilic orbital, polarisability makes a relatively small contribution to thermodynamic basic strengths. The problem is then to allow for the additional importance of polarisability in the activations, which we measure as rates, of other reactions of the nucleophiles.

Edwards proposed to allow for the added importance of polarisability in other reactions in a very simple way, *viz.*, by including in the calculated free energy of activation a term proportional to the logarithm of the molecular refraction of the nucleophile. His equation is[71]

$$\log (k_n/k_{aq}) = \beta(1.74 + pK_a) + \alpha \log (R_n/R_{aq})$$

where k_n/k_{aq} is the rate-constant of the reaction of the substrate with the nucleophile, relatively to that of its reaction with water taken as the standard nucleophile, pK_a refers to the conjugate acid of the

[70] J. F. Bunnett, *Ann. Rev. Phys. Chem.*, 1963, **14,** 271.

[71] J. O. Edwards, *J. Am. Chem. Soc.*, 1954, **76,** 1540; 1956, **78,** 1819.

[72] W. P. Jencks and J. Carriuolo, *J. Am. Chem. Soc.*, 1960, **82,** 1778.

nucleophile, R_n/R_{aq} is the molecular refraction of the nucleophile relatively to that of water, and β and α are constants measuring the importance of polarisation and polarisability, respectively, in the reactions of that substrate in the reaction conditions.

This equation has a sufficient semi-quantitative success to show that the approach is sound. If we use solution values of ionic refractions, it will make some allowance for the effect of anion solvation on polarisability.[69] One could not expect full quantitative success, because the polarisability allowed for is an overall isotropic average, whereas more important than this will be the inhomogeneous, directed polarisability in the nucleophilic orbital at the reaction site. In the absence of an independent source of such submolecular polarisability data, what has been done is to study the dependence on nucleophile structure of deviations from the Edwards equation.

An important result of such a study was the discovery by Jencks and Carriuolo[72] of a group of nucleophiles, including OCl^-, OOH^-, $OOMe^-$, N_3^-, SO_3^{2-}, $NH_2 \cdot OH$, $Me_2N \cdot OH$, *N*-hydroxy-piperidine, *N*-hydroxyphthalimide, acetoxime, salicylaldoxime, acethydroxamic acid, *iso*nitroso-acetone, *iso*nitroso-acetylacetone, and 4-aminopyridine-1-oxide, which had abnormally high nucleophilic strengths in the reactions studied, and, as Edwards and Pearson subsequently pointed out, in all reactions for which data have been recorded. Edwards and Pearson called this the "alpha" effect, ascribed it to the presence of unshared electrons on the atom, called the "alpha" atom, next the nucleophilic atom, and in explanation proposed an analogy with the effect of the oxygen electrons of methoxymethyl chloride in promoting chloride ionisation.[73]

The ascription of the effect to the unshared "alpha" electrons is not completely correct, as is shown by some of the examples, *e.g.*, azide ion and 4-aminopyridine-1-oxide; and the analogy is a poor one, because, unlike the carbon-chlorine bond electrons of methoxymethyl chloride, which vacate their carbon orbital in favour of the oxygen electrons, the nucleophilic electrons never leave their orbital to provide accommodation for the "alpha" electrons. We have here another of those fairly common situations (we encountered one in connexion with OH-hyperconjugation in Section **24j**) in which the valency-bond-approximation, even with mesomerism included, is an insufficient theoretical frame for a qualitative description. The reason is that

[73] J. O. Edwards and R. G. Pearson, *J. Am. Chem. Soc.*, 1962, **84**, 16. In privately published lectures, the writer has used the term "anticonjugation" to express energy-raising by interactions of antibonding electrons, in contrast to energy-lowering by interactions with bonding electrons, *i.e.*, conjugation.

electronic motion between contiguous, but non-conjugated, atomic and bond orbitals is comparably important to motion within the orbitals: when this happens we have no recourse but to go over to a molecular orbital outlook. The real condition for the "alpha" effect is that the highest occupied orbital centred largely on the nucleophilic atom is antibonding, with a node normal to the bond between that atom and the "alpha" atom. These electrons provide a special factor of inhomogeneous polarisability towards any substrate able to make large use of the polarisability of the nucleophile. Thus the hypochlorite ion has 14 valency shell electrons, *viz.*, two σ-bonding (the conventional bond), four σ-non-bonding (two lone pairs about the extended line of the bond), four π-bonding electrons, and, highest in energy, four π^*-antibonding electrons. These π^*-electrons "ask" nothing better than to be gathered, as two of them may be, by overlap into the empty or emptying orbital of an electrophilic substrate, so to become low-energy bonding electrons. The peroxide ions have two antibonding electrons. The azide ion has four centred jointly on the two terminal atoms. Most of the other examples in the list given above have two antibonding electrons, or, if more, two peculiarly relevant antibonding electrons, as in 4-amino-pyridine-1-oxide which has two centred mainly on oxygen, or in the sulphite ion which has two that are antibonding simultaneously in all three bonds. (It is an easy and instructive exercise to consider what stationary electron waves would "go" into a potential hollow of the symmetry of the sulphite ion, and how many of those with least nodes, and particularly least nodes cutting between adjacent atoms, would be occupied by the available electrons.)

(28d) Constitutional Influences of the Replaced Group.—The ease of expulsion of halogens from alkyl halides, alike in S_N2 and S_N1 substitutions, has the general order

$$F < Cl < Br < I$$

the inequalities becoming successively less important along the series. Thus in hydroxylic solvents the first inequality is typically represented by a rate ratio of some thousands, the second by one of some tens, and the third by one of some units. The tendency is towards higher ratios, for any given pair of halogens, as the mechanism moves from S_N2 to S_N1 with change of alkyl structure or of substituting agent. In S_N2 reactions the ratios are frequently higher in aprotic than in hydroxylic solvents: it is suggested[74] that the ratios are reduced in hydroxylic

[74] M. H. R. Hoffmann, *J. Chem. Soc.*, 1965, 6253, 6762.

solvents by halogen solvation, which preferentially favours the separation, as anions, of the lower halogens, for which incipient hydrogen-bonding in transition states would be more marked. Steric effects on the outgoing group appear to have small importance.

It is difficult to choose a solvent allowing fair comparison between these initially neutral expelled groups, and the initially cationic ammonium and sulphonium groups, because the conditions of solvation, and its variation through the initial, transition, and final states of reaction, are inevitably widely different for neutral and charged replaceable groups. As a matter of observation, in hydroxylic solvents, the order of ease of expulsion of the alkylated ammonium and sulphonium groups is

$$NR_3^+ < SR_2^+$$

The oxy-ester groups constitute a class of initially neutral departing groups which can be replaced in nucleophilic substitutions. The sulphonoxy-groups of arene- and alkane-sulphonic esters have been much investigated. Their substitutions closely parallel those of alkyl halides, *e.g.*,

$$Ar'S^- + R\cdot OSO_2Ar \rightarrow R\cdot SAr' + OSO_2Ar^-$$

$$EtOH + R\cdot OSO_2Ar \rightarrow R\cdot OEt + HOSO_2Ar$$

and, as with alkyl halides, olefin eliminations may concurrently occur. With alkyl sulphonates as with alkyl halides, the mechanism of substitution may be bimolecular or unimolecular; and the changes of mechanism with changes of alkyl structure, substituting agent, and solvent are very similar. However, the sulphonoxy-group cannot be given a unique place in the order of ease of expulsion of neutral outgoing groups, given above for the halogens. Hoffmann has shown[74] that the rate of expulsion of the sulphonoxy-group may be less than that of bromine, or much more than that of iodine, depending on the alkyl structure, substituting agent, and solvent, as illustrated in Table 28-5 by the ratios of rate-constants for the reactions of corresponding toluene-*p*-sulphonates (in one series benzenesulphonates) and bromides. These rate-constants are either second-order rate-constants of substitution by mechanism S_N2, or first-order, or approximate first-order, rate-constants of solvolyses, which may have mechanism S_N2, or mechanism S_N1. In the latter case the rate is allowed to be kinetically unseparated from those of the olefin elimination E1, the measured rate being the rate of the ionisation common to these two processes. In suitable structural conditions, the products of S_N1 and E1 reactions may be Wagner-Meerwein-rearranged.

TABLE 28-5.—RATIOS, k_{OTs}/k_{Br} (OR k_{OBs}/k_{Br}), OF THE RATE-CONSTANTS OF BIMOLECULAR SUBSTITUTION AND UNIMOLECULAR SUBSTITUTION AND ELIMINATION OF ALKYL TOLUENE-*p*- (OR BENZENE-)-SULPHONATES (ROTs OR ROBs) AND ALKYL BROMIDES, WITH VARIOUS NUCLEOPHILES IN VARIOUS SOLVENTS (HOFFMANN).

Alkyl	Kinetic order	Presumed mech.	Nucleophilic anion	Solvent	Temp.	k_{OTs}/k_{Br}
Me	2	S_N2	Cl^-	Me_2CO	25°	0.42
Me	2	S_N2	p-$MeC_6H_4S^-$	EtOH	0°	0.36
Et	2	S_N2	p-$MeC_6H_4S^-$	EtOH	0°	0.40
				50% aq.-EtOH	0°	0.39
s-Bu	2	S_N2	p-$MeC_6H_4S^-$	92% aq.-EtOH	0°	2.3
Me	2	S_N2	OEt^-	EtOH	0°	5.4
Me	2	S_N2	OH^-	H_2O	0°	6.3
Me	1	S_N2	—	EtOH	50°	16
Et	1	S_N2	—	EtOH	50°	15
i-Pr	1	mixed	—	EtOH	50°	73
t-Bu	~1	S_N1+E1	—	EtOH	50°	>3000
PhMeCH	1	S_N1	—	EtOH	50°	845
Me	1	S_N2	—	H_2O	50°	18[Bs]
Et	1	S_N2	—	H_2O	50°	17[Bs]
n-Pr	1	S_N2	—	H_2O	50°	17[Bs]
i-Bu	1	S_N2	—	H_2O	50°	12[Bs]
*neo*Pen	1	S_N1+E1[w]	—	H_2O	50°	5.6[Bs]
i-Pr		mixed	—	H_2O	50°	105[Bs]
Me	1	S_N2	—	HCO_2H	95°	24
Et	1	mixed	—	HCO_2H	95°	41
n-Pr	1	S_N2	—	HCO_2H	95°	47
i-Bu	1	S_N2	—	HCO_2H	95°	58
*neo*Pen	1	S_N1+E1	—	HCO_2H	95°	90
i-Pr	1	S_N2	—	HCO_2H	95°	360
t-Bu	1	E1	—	MeCN	0°	5130
PhMeCH	1	E1	—	MeCN	0°	470

[Bs] Ratios k_{OBs}/k_{Br}, determined by R. E. Robertson (refs. to original literature are given by Hoffmann[74]).

[w] Products of aqueous solvolysis are Wagner-Meerwein rearranged (β-to-α methyl shift).

The data in the table, only a sample of the many adduced by Hoffmann, show that the sulphonate/bromide rate-ratio can vary from less than 1 to more than 1000; and that the variation follows a definite pattern. Bimolecular substitutions with anionic reagents of high nucleophilic strength towards carbon (*e.g.*, RS^-) give ratios of order 0.5, with anions of markedly lower nucleophilic strength towards carbon (*e.g.*, OH^-), ratios of order 5, and with neutral hydroxylic solvent molecules (EtOH, H_2O, HCO_2H), ratios of order 20. For unimolecular solvolysis in the same solvents, and in acetonitrile which allows only elimination, the ratios start in this broad region and rise to some thousands, as the rates of the unimolecular reactions rise from low values to high ones. Compounds of the primary alkyl group, *neo*pentyl, whose slow unimolecular reactions can be observed at all only because their bimolecular substitutions are rendered still slower by steric hindrance (Section **34**), give the lowest ratio, 6 for reactions in water, in which the solvolysis products are Wagner-Meerwein-rearranged, to 90 in the much better ionising solvent, formic acid. Compounds of the secondary alkyl group, *iso*propyl, whose solvolysis rates in formic acid are considerably greater, gave a ratio 360 in that solvent. The still more rapidly reacting secondary compounds of the 1-phenylethyl group gave ratios around 500–800. And the even more rapidly reacting tertiary compounds represented in the table by those of the *t*-butyl group gave ratios above 3000.

Hoffmann's interpretation is that, when the substrate and the reaction conditions are such that a large fraction of an electron must be driven into the departing group before the latter can break away, that is, when a large electronic charge must be so transferred in the transition state, the sulphonoxy-group, which can distribute such a charge among its three oxygen atoms and the benzene ring with a mesomeric reduction of energy, can break away in a less activated and accordingly faster reaction than that of any monatomic leaving group such as a halogen atom, even a large one. Thus the theory is that the sulphonate/bromide rate-ratio indicates the fraction of an electron transfer, from the carbon atom which bears the departing group to the departing group, that has occurred in the transition state.

The pattern of the results can be understood on this basis. The "point of no return" of the electron being transferred from the carbon atom to the departing group will come early in the transfer process, if, in bimolecular reactions, the "return" of the electron is being resisted by an irreversible driving of electrons into the carbon atom from an attacking strong nucleophile. And the point of no return will be set progressively later as the nucleophilic strength of the reagent is progressively reduced. Unimolecular reactions, on the other hand, are activated mainly by polarisability involving electron delocalisation within the substrate; and the freer the delocalisation—the freer, that is, the electron transfer *and* the return—the faster the reaction will go, and the more nearly complete the transfer will have to be before the electron cannot return. So, the correlation between extent of transfer and rate is opposite in bimolecular and in unimolecular reactions. Some Wagner-Meerwein rearrangements may involve earlier points of no return than would be normal to this correlation, the condition for this being one of suitable timing in the advance of the shifting alkyl branch (which carries its bonding electrons with it—see Chapter X—somewhat in the manner of a nucleophile) on the carbon atom concerned in the electron transfer.

We shall see in Section **32** that a method is known by which, in favourable cases, the fraction of an electron transferred in the formation of the transition state of a unimolecular reaction can be quantitatively estimated, and that that fraction is about 0.6 electron for the aqueous solvolysis of *t*-butyl chloride. Given a few more such fixed points, it is conceivable that a calibration scale for Hoffmann's ratios might be established.

(29) SOLVENT EFFECTS IN NUCLEOPHILIC SUBSTITUTION

(29a) Solvent Effects on Rate.—It is established in the preceding Sections that a number of general reactions, such as the hydrolytic reactions of alkyl halides, and the decompositions of quaternary ammonium salts, which were at one time not considered to have any particular relation to each other, in fact show such resemblances as justify our classifying them all in the family of nucleophilic substitutions. Nevertheless, a sub-classification of such reactions, according to *charge-type*,[75] provides a useful way of signalising certain differences, which appear against the background of the general resemblance. In no respect do such differences appear more clearly than in relation to the role of solvents.

In a nucleophilic substitution, an electron is transferred from the substituting agent to the seat of substitution, and from the latter to the expelled group. The substituting agent, before reaction, may be negatively charged or neutral, becoming, respectively, formally neutral or positive, after reaction. The expelled group, before reaction, may be formally neutral or positive, becoming, as the case may be, negative or neutral, afterwards. These two dual possibilities are independent of each other; and so, nucleophilic substitutions can be divided into four charge-types. They are as shown in Table 29-1.

Solvation is essentially an electrostatic phenomenon. When an ion or polar molecule is put into a solvent having polar molecules, it orients and attracts the molecules of the solvent, thereby doing electrostatic work; and work done, means energy lost, so that the system becomes more stable. The energy of solvation of an ion in a polar solvent can be very large, often of the order of the strength of a covalent bond.[76]

[75] E. D. Hughes and C. K. Ingold, *J. Chem. Soc.*, **1935, 244.**

[76] For a charmingly simple semi-quantitative treatment, see R. W. Gurney, "Ions in Solution," Cambridge Univ. Press, 1936, especially Chap. 1.

It follows that a change from a less polar to a more polar solvent will increase or decrease the exothermicity of a reaction according as the products are more or less polar than the factors. There may be counteracting changes of entropy: for solvation, though it reduces energy, may increase the organisation of solvent molecules, thereby decreasing the probability of the solvated state. However, it is a generally valid assumption that the energy change will dominate the free-energy change, and that, accordingly, equilibria will shift towards more polar products in more polar solvents.

TABLE 29-1.—CHARGE-TYPES OF NUCLEOPHILIC SUBSTITUTION.

Type 1:—Initially, reagent negative, group neutral.

Examples
$$\begin{cases} H\bar{O} + RCl \rightarrow ROH + \bar{Cl} \\ \bar{I} + RCl \rightarrow RI + \bar{Cl} \end{cases}$$

Type 2:—Initially, reagent neutral, group neutral.

Examples
$$\begin{cases} R_3'N + RCl \rightarrow R\overset{+}{N}R_3' + \bar{Cl} \\ H_3N + RCl \rightarrow R\overset{+}{N}H_3 + \bar{Cl}\ (\rightarrow RNH_2) \\ H_2O + RCl \rightarrow R\overset{+}{O}H_2 + \bar{Cl}\ (\rightarrow ROH) \end{cases}$$

Type 3:—Initially, reagent negative, group positive.

Examples
$$\begin{cases} H\bar{O} + R\overset{+}{N}R_3' \rightarrow ROH + NR_3' \\ \bar{I} + R\overset{+}{N}R_3' \rightarrow RI + NR_3' \end{cases}$$

Type 4:—Initially, reagent neutral, group positive.

Examples
$$\begin{cases} R_3'N + R\overset{+}{S}R_2'' \rightarrow R\overset{+}{N}R_3' + SR_2'' \\ H_3N + R\overset{+}{S}R_2'' \rightarrow R\overset{+}{N}H_3 + SR_2''\ (\rightarrow RNH_2) \\ H_2O + R\overset{+}{S}R_2'' \rightarrow R\overset{+}{O}H_2 + SR_2''\ (\rightarrow ROH) \end{cases}$$

The corresponding theory[75] of solvent effects on reaction kinetics is that a change to a more polar solvent will decrease or increase the heat of activation (to which the Arrhenius energy of activation is the usual approximation) according as the transition state of reaction is more or less polar than the initial state of the reactants. There may be counteracting changes in the entropy of activation (approximately represented by the Arrhenius frequency factor); but the qualitative theory assumes that the energy change will dominate the rate change, and that therefore a more polar solvent will accelerate or retard reaction according as the transition state is more or less polar than the initial state. It is, of course, necessary, even for qualitative purposes, to have some idea as to the main factors summarised in the term "polarity." Concerning reactants and transition states, the following three assumptions have been made as to the amount of solvation to be expected in the presence of electric charges:

(1) Solvation will increase with the magnitude of the charge.
(2) Solvation will decrease with increasing dispersal of a given charge.
(3) The decrease of solvation due to the dispersal of a charge will be less than that due to its destruction.

Concerning solvents, it has been assumed that polarity, that is, power to solvate charges in solutes, will

(1) increase with the molecular dipole moment of the solvent;
(2) decrease with increased thickness of shielding of the dipole charges.

The "protic" solvents, those with the thinly shielded protons of hydroxyl or amide groups, as in sulphuric acid, water, methanol, and formamide, thus constitute the generally most strongly solvating class of solvents. They solvate anions particularly strongly, and small anions with great strength. The polar aprotic solvents, such as sulphur dioxide, dimethylsulphoxide, tetramethylenesulphone (sulpholane), formdimethylamide, nitromethane, and acetonitrile, are moderately solvating, but less specific, with a bias towards the solvation of cations. Acetone, acetic acid (which is mainly dimeric), benzene, and heptane illustrate further progressive decreases in polarity and solvating power.

These arguments and assumptions can be used for the purpose of making qualitative predictions about the effect of solvent polarity on the rates of all heterolytic reactions of known mechanism. In the application to nucleophilic substitution, the principal factors are charge-type and mechanism. Discussion of the bimolecular mechanism is straightforward. For the unimolecular mechanism, the initial and transition states of the rate-determining stage are the states relevant to the problem. These applications are illustrated in Table 29-2. The middle three columns show, for each charge-type and mechanism, what happens to the charges on converting the initial into the transition state. The last column shows the predicted kinetic effect. Here the terms "large" and "small" have a purely relative significance: they arise from the theory that the effect of the dispersal of a charge should be notably smaller than the effect of its creation or destruction.

There is much evidence of the correctness of these predictions. De Bruyn and Steger showed[77] that rates of alkaline hydrolysis of methyl and ethyl iodides in aqueous ethyl alcohol are decreased on in-

[77] C. A. L. de Bruyn and A. Steger, *Rec. trav. chim.*, 1899, **18**, 41, 311.

TABLE 29-2.—PREDICTED SOLVENT EFFECTS ON RATES OF NUCLEOPHILIC SUBSTITUTIONS.

Charge-type	Disposition of charges: Initial state	Disposition of charges: Transition state	Effect of activation on charges	Effect of increased solvent polarity on rate
Bimolecular Mechanism				
1	$\overset{-}{Y}+RX$	$\overset{\delta-}{Y}\cdots R\cdots\overset{\delta-}{X}$	Dispersed	Small decrease
2	$Y+RX$	$\overset{\delta+}{Y}\cdots R\cdots\overset{\delta-}{X}$	Increased	Large increase
3	$\overset{-}{Y}+R\overset{+}{X}$	$\overset{\delta-}{Y}\cdots R\cdots\overset{\delta+}{X}$	Reduced	Large decrease
4	$Y+R\overset{+}{X}$	$\overset{\delta+}{Y}\cdots R\cdots\overset{\delta+}{X}$	Dispersed	Small decrease
Unimolecular Mechanism (rate-controlling stage)				
1 and 2	RX	$\overset{\delta+}{R}\cdots\cdots\overset{\delta-}{X}$	Increased	Large increase
3 and 4	$R\overset{+}{X}$	$\overset{\delta+}{R}\cdots\cdots\overset{\delta+}{X}$	Dispersed	Small decrease

creasing the proportion of water. Hughes found[78] that the rate of hydrolysis of *t*-butyl chloride (which is unaffected by added alkali) in aqueous alcohol is increased on increasing the proportion of water. Le Roux and Sugden observed[79] that the rate of bromine exchange between bromide ion (introduced as lithium bromide) and *n*-butyl bromide in solvent acetone is reduced by adding 10% of water to the medium. Davies and Lewis noticed[80] that the rates of combination of diethylaniline and of several aryldiethylphosphines with ethyl iodide in solvent acetone is increased by adding 10% water to the medium. Menschutkin proved[81] that the combination of triethylamine with ethyl iodide proceeds more rapidly in alcohols than in hydrocarbons. He placed solvents in the rate series, $MeOH > EtOH > Me_2CO > C_6H_6 > C_6H_{14}$ for this reaction; and the same general sequence has been confirmed[82] for the reactions of other primary alkyl or methyl halides

[78] E. D. Hughes, *J. Chem. Soc.*, **1935,** 255.

[79] L. J. LeRoux and S. Sugden, *J. Chem. Soc.*, **1939,** 1279; L. J. LeRoux, S. Sugden, and R. H. K. Thompson, *ibid.*, **1945,** 586.

[80] W. C. Davies and W. P. G. Lewis, *J. Chem. Soc.*, **1934,** 1599.

[81] N. Menschutkin, *Z. physik. Chem.*, 1890, **5,** 589.

[82] G. Carrara, *Gazz. chim. ital.*, 1894, **24,** 180; A. Hemptinne and A. Bekaert, *Z. physik. Chem.*, 1899, **28,** 225; H. von Halban, *ibid.*, 1913, **84,** 128; H. E. Cox, *J. Chem. Soc.*, 1921, **119,** 142; J. A. Hawkins, *ibid.*, 1922, **121,** 1170; G. E. Muchin, R. Ginsberg, and C. Moissejera, *Ukrain. Chem. J.*, 1926, **2,** 136; H. Essex and O. Gelormini, *J. Am. Chem. Soc.*, 1926, **48,** 882; H. McCombie, H. A. Scarborough, and F. F. P. Smith, *J. Chem. Soc.*, **1927,** 802.

with other amines or with sulphides, by a number of subsequent investigators. Von Halban[83] established that the decomposition of triethylsulphonium bromide takes place more slowly in alcohols than in acetone. Gleave, Hughes, and the writer[84] showed that the rate of alkaline hydrolysis of the trimethylsulphonium cation is decreased by increasing the proportion of water in an aqueous alcoholic solvent; while Hughes and the writer found[85] that the rate of hydrolysis of the *t*-butyldimethylsulphonium ion (which is unaffected by added alkali) is also decreased by the same change of solvent.

All this was known in 1935, the date of promulgation of the theory. But no bimolecular reactions of charge-type 4 were then known; and their existence, and the kind of kinetic solvent effects they would exhibit, had to remain a prediction until 1960, when Hughes and Whittingham described some examples.[86] They showed, for instance, that the second-order reaction between trimethylamine and the trimethylsulphonium ion in four solvents gave the rate series $H_2O < MeOH < EtOH < MeNO_2$. Thus a rate increase attended a progressive reduction in solvent polarity. Evidently the initial state was being more strongly solvated than the transition state. The relative rates, and the parameters of the Arrhenius equation for this reaction in the four solvents, are set out in Table 29-3. The figures show that the solvation energies fall along the solvent series by more than enough to determine the rate series, notwithstanding the countervailing effect of solvation entropy.

TABLE 29-3.—RELATIVE RATES AND ARRHENIUS PARAMETERS OF THE REACTION $Me_3N + CH_3 \cdot SMe_2^+ \rightarrow Me_3N \cdot CH_3^+ + SMe_2$ IN FOUR SOLVENTS (HUGHES AND WHITTINGHAM).

Solvent	H_2O	MeOH	EtOH	$MeNO_2$
Rel. rate (45°)	1	6	10	119
$\log_{10} A$	4.90	3.05	0.94	0.19
E_A (kcal./mole)	23.1	21.6	20.6	18.0

The same general situation may be illustrated by the data[86,87] given in Table 29-4, for the dependence of substitution rate on the

[83] H. von Halban, *Z. physik. Chem.*, 1909, **67**, 129.

[84] J. L. Gleave, E. D. Hughes, and C. K. Ingold, *J. Chem. Soc.*, **1935**, 236; as to mechanism, see Y. Pocker and A. J. Parker, *J. Org. Chem.*, 1966, **31**, 1526.

[85] E. D. Hughes and C. K. Ingold, *J. Chem. Soc.*, **1933**, 1571.

[86] E. D. Hughes and D. J. Whittingham, *J. Chem. Soc.*, **1960**, 806.

[87] R. A. Cooper, M. L. Dhar, E. D. Hughes, C. K. Ingold, B. J. MacNulty, and L. D. Woolf, *J. Chem. Soc.*, **1948**, 2043.

TABLE 29-4.—OBSERVED SOLVENT EFFECTS ON RATES OF NUCLEOPHILIC SUBSTITUTIONS.

Type	Example[1]	Rate[2] constant	Vol. % H_2O in aqueous EtOH								Predicted effect
			0	10	20	30	40	50	60	100	
			Bimolecular Mechanism[3]								
1	i-PrBr+$\bar{O}H$	$10^5 k_2^{55°}$	6.0	—	4.9	—	3.0	—	—	—	Small decr.
2	i-PrBr+H_2O	$10^7 k_1^{55°}$	1.73	—	23.6	—	66.7	—	—	—	Large incr.
3	$Me_3\overset{+}{S}+\bar{O}H$	$10^4 k_2^{100°}$	7240	—	178	—	15.1	—	—	0.37	Large decr.
4	$Me_3\overset{+}{S}+NMe_3$	$10^5 k_2^{45°}$	6.67	—	—	—	—	—	—	0.65	Small decr.
			Unimolecular Mechanism[4]								
1 and 2	t-BuCl	$10^6 k_1^{25°}$	—	1.71	9.14	40.3	126	367	1294	—	Large incr.
	t-BuBr	$10^3 k_1^{55°}$	0.20	—	13.2	—	—	—	—	—	
	t-AmCl	$10^6 k_1^{25°}$	—	—	14.5	—	148	—	—	—	
	t-AmBr	$10^4 k_1^{25°}$	0.11	—	5.8	—	—	—	—	—	
3 and 4	t-Bu$\overset{+}{S}Me_2$	$10^5 k_1^{50°}$	1.90	—	1.24	—	—	—	—	0.60	Small decr.
	t-Am$\overset{+}{S}Me_2$	$10^3 k_1^{65°}$	—	—	0.62	—	—	0.45	—	—	

[1] The contraction Am signifies amyl (pentyl). The reagents entered as OH^- and H_2O will consist partly of OEt^- and EtOH, respectively.

[2] Second-order constants, k_2, are in sec.$^{-1}$ mole^{-1} l., and first-order constants, k_1, are in sec.$^{-1}$, the temperature being indicated by superscripts.

[3] The rate constants given for reaction by the bimolecular mechanism refer to substitution only (S_N2), accompanying olefin elimination (E2) having, where necessary, been measured and allowed for. The reason is that bimolecular elimination is a reaction which proceeds independently of bimolecular substitution: the reactions do not share any common process. It is assumed that the neutral or acid solvolytic reaction of *iso*propyl bromide is mainly bimolecular.

[4] The rate constants given for reactions by the unimolecular mechanism are overall first-order constants, covering both substitution and elimination (S_N1+E 1). This is because the first stage of unimolecular elimination is identical with the first stage of unimolecular substitution: it is the stage to which the measurements and the theoretical predictions refer.

composition of aqueous ethyl alcoholic solvents. For both the bimolecular and the unimolecular reactions of the various charge-types, the rates (fourth column) shift in the predicted directions (fifth column). Furthermore, corresponding to the predicted distinction between "small" and "large" effects, there are marked differences in the orders of magnitude of the observed effects, which may appear, in the one case, as rates varying by a few units-fold only, and, in the other, as rates varying by large factors such as 10^4, over the complete range of composition of the binary solvent series.

Parker has extensively illustrated the differing specificities of ion-solvation in protic and aprotic solvents.[69] Two of his examples are in Table 29-5. They are S_N2 substitutions, one aliphatic, and the other aromatic. (The latter is relevant, because the theory of kinetic solvent effects, though first illustrated in the field of nucleophilic aliphatic substitutions, is applicable to all heterolytic reactions in solution.) In both reactions, the initial state is more strongly solvated than the transition state; and the reagent anion is expected to be the more strongly solvated of the reactants, and to be particularly strongly solvated in protic solvents. Thus, as polarity progressively falls along the series of solvents, which runs from protic to aprotic in Table 29-5, the reactions should go successively faster, as indeed they do. The three middle solvents of the series are *N*-homologues, and, apart from specific effects, one might have expected the rates to rise smoothly over that part of the solvent series. In fact, we see a great jump in the rate of either reaction as the last labile, potentially hydrogen-bonding hydrogen atom becomes replaced by methyl between formmethylamide and formdimethylamide. Evidently anion solvation by the intense local field of such an exposed proton constitutes a major term in the solvation of the initial states of these reactions.

TABLE 29-5.—RELATIVE RATES OF THE REACTIONS
(A) $Cl^- + CH_3I \rightarrow CH_3Cl + I^-$
(B) $N_3^- + p\text{-}NO_2C_6H_4F \rightarrow p\text{-}NO_2 \cdot C_6H_4N_3 + F^-$
IN FIVE SOLVENTS AT 25° (PARKER).

Solvent	MeOH	$HCONH_2$	HCONHMe	$HCONMe_2$	$MeCONMe_2$
Reaction (A)	1	12.5	45.3	1,200,000	7,400,000
Reaction (B)	1	5.6	15.7	24,000	84,000

(29b) Solvent Effects on Product Proportions.—If two substituting agents Y_1 and Y_2 are competing for the same substrate RX, to form products RY_1 and RY_2 in the same solution, there are clearly two measurable kinetic quantities, the effect of the medium on which might be discussed. These two quantities can be chosen to be the total rate of destruction of RX, and the ratio RY_1/RY_2 in which the products appear. The point of this choice is that it is suitable for the demonstration of a significant difference between the bimolecular and unimolecular mechanisms of substitution. In the bimolecular mechanism, there is only one reaction stage, and therefore the overall rate and the product ratio must be together determined in that stage. In the unimolecular mechanism, the rate is determined in the common slow stage: it is, indeed, the rate of heterolysis of RX. But now the product ratio is determined in a completely independent way, namely, by the competition of succeeding fast stages. On this distinction one can base a criterion of mechanism, which makes use of kinetic solvent effects. It involves ascertaining whether the effects of medium changes on overall rates and on product proportions, in a competitive system such as that indicated, are linked together, or are independent of each other.

Such a criterion of mechanism is of chief value in relation to those first-order reactions in which a substituting agent inevitably retains a constant active-mass, because it is an important constituent of the solvent. The main applications have hitherto been to reactions of this kind, notably, the hydrolysis and alcoholysis of alkyl halides in initially neutral aqueous alcoholic solvents.

A simple illustration is furnished by the solvolysis of benzhydryl chloride in initially neutral aqueous ethyl alcohol to give benzhydryl ethyl ether and benzhydrol.[88] If one starts with dry ethyl alcohol as solvent, and then adds water, the overall rate goes up. But that is not because of an additional production of benzhydrol. In fact, only small amounts of benzhydrol are formed: the main effect of the added water is to accelerate the production of benzhydryl ethyl ether. Clearly rate and product composition are here being independently determined. This is consistent with the unimolecular mechanism, but not with the bimolecular mechanism.[89]

A more quantitative way of applying the same test involves using a mixture-law formula, by means of which, if the rate of the reaction is known at two extremes of solvent composition of a binary solvent system, it can be computed by interpolation for solvent mixtures of intermediate composition. One such formula[90] uses partial vapour pressures as parameters of composition, and takes the form,

$$\text{Rate} = (k_a p_a + k_w p_w) p_{\text{RX}} \tag{1}$$

where the k's are rate constants, the p's are vapour pressures, and the subscripts refer to alcohol, water, and the alkyl halide. Modified

[88] N. T. Farinacci and L. P. Hammett, *J. Am. Chem. Soc.*, 1937, 59, 2544.

[89] L. C. Bateman, E. D. Hughes, and C. K. Ingold, *J. Am. Chem. Soc.*, 1938, 60, 3080.

[90] A. R. Olson and R. S. Halford, *J. Am. Chem. Soc.*, 1937, 59, 2644.

interpolation formulae have been proposed;[91] however, all that is now asked of any such additive two-term expression is that, given the two rate constants, k_a and k_w, determined by rate measurements at two solvent compositions, it will reproduce measured rates at other solvent compositions. Supposing that it does so, that is, that the sum of the two terms does describe the total rate, then the test of mechanism consists in ascertaining whether the ratio of the two terms describes the product ratio, or, in other words, whether product composition can be calculated by a formula, such as the following, which is based upon the kinetically measured constants k_a and k_w:

$$\text{ROAlk}/(\text{ROH} + \text{ROAlk}) = k_a p_a/(k_a p_a + k_w p_w) \qquad (2)$$

If the reaction has the bimolecular mechanism, this should be possible. If it has the unimolecular mechanism, then the rate-measured constants k_a and k_w are irrelevant to the consideration of product composition.

This test has been applied to the solvolysis of a typical primary, and a typical tertiary halide, namely, *n*-butyl bromide and *t*-butyl chloride, in initially neutral, aqueous, methyl, and ethyl alcoholic media.[92] In each case, equation (1) was found accurately to reproduce the series of rate constants; however, as is shown in Table 29-6, equation (2) correctly reproduced the compositions of the products from *n*-butyl bromide, but showed no relation to the compositions of the products from *t*-butyl chloride. This agrees with other evidence that the simpler primary halides are solvolysed by the bimolecular mechanism, and tertiary halides by the unimolecular mechanism, in aqueous alcoholic solvents.

The method has also been used[93] when only one of the competing reagents is a constituent of the solvent. (It could also be used when neither reagent comes from the solvent; but then the problem of mechanism can usually be solved more simply.) It has been mentioned already (Section **28c**) that when sodium azide is added to aqueous acetone in which *pp'*-dimethylbenzhydryl chloride is undergoing hydrolysis, the rate is unchanged except for a salt effect (Section **32**), although much of what would have been *pp'*-dimethylbenzhydrol appears in the product as *pp'*-dimethylbenzhydryl azide. When one employs aqueous acetone of a fixed composition, and increases the concentration of dissolved azide ion in successive experiments, the propor-

[91] P. D. Bartlett has suggested using mole-fractions of the solvent components in place of vapour pressures: *J. Am. Chem. Soc.*, 1939, **61**, 1630

[92] L. C. Bateman, E. D. Hughes, and C. K. Ingold, *J. Chem. Soc.*, **1938**, 881; M. L. Bird, E. D. Hughes, and C. K. Ingold, *ibid.*, **1943**, 255

[93] L. C. Bateman, E. D. Hughes, and C. K. Ingold, *J. Chem Soc.*, **1940**, 974.

TABLE 29-6.—TEST OF SOLVOLYTIC MECHANISM BY SOLVENT VARIATION.

Percentage of ether, 100 ROAlk/(ROAlk+ROH), formed in the solvolysis of alkyl halides RHal in aqueous methyl or ethyl alcohol, as found, and as calculated from the variation of total solvolysis rate with solvent composition.

Solvent and temp.	Mols. % of H_2O	% ROAlk	
		Found	Calc.
n-Butyl Chloride			
$MeOH—H_2O$ mixtures at 59.4°	14.1	88	86
	26.3	74	75
	30.8	72	72
	48.3	61	61
	60.1	51	53
$EtOH—H_2O$ mixtures at 75.1°	25.8	63	63
	56.2	50	45
	73.7	35	39
t-Butyl Bromide			
$MeOH—H_2O$ mixtures at 25.0°	16.4	83	43
	28.4	68	29
	40.0	49	17
$EtOH—H_2O$ mixtures at 25.0°	26.4	53	18
	44.7	33	11
	68.3	18	8

TABLE 29-7.—TEST OF SOLVOLYTIC MECHANISM BY VARIATION OF THE SOLVENT AND OF A DISSOLVED SUBSTITUTING AGENT.

Rates and product proportions in the hydrolysis of *pp'*-dimethylbenzhydryl chloride in aqueous acetone containing sodium azide at 0°, the water content and the azide ion concentration being independently varied.

Vol. % H_2O	Conc. NaN_3	% RN_3 formed[1]		Vol. % H_2O	Conc. NaN_3	Total rate[2]	% RN_3 formed[1]
		Found	Calc.				
50	0.0512	60.3	60.3	10	0.051	1.59	60.3
50	0.1001	75.8	76.5	15	0.051	7.05	59.6
50	0.2002	85.8	87.7	20	0.054	22.4	61.2
50	0.4867	95.8	94.8	50	0.052	v. fast	60.0

[1] Defined as 100 $RN_3/(RN_3+ROH)$, where $R=(p\text{-}MeC_6H_4)_2CH$.

[2] Measured in the presence of the salt: 10^4k_1, with k_1 in sec.$^{-1}$

tion of formed alkyl azide increases as would be calculated from the hypothesis that the rate of production of the organic azide is proportional to the concentration of azide ions, while the rate of the competing hydrolysis remains constant. This is illustrated in the left-hand side of Table 29-7. When one fixes the concentration of azide ions, say, at 0.05 M, and increases the proportion of water in the aqueous acetone, from 10% to 50%, then the rate of total reaction increases greatly, but the proportion in which dimethylbenzhydryl azide is produced remains exactly the same. This is illustrated in the right-hand side of Table 29-7.

Since products may vary when rates are constant, and *vice versa*, one needs no calculation here in order to discern that rates and products are being independently determined, as they would be in the unimolecular mechanism:

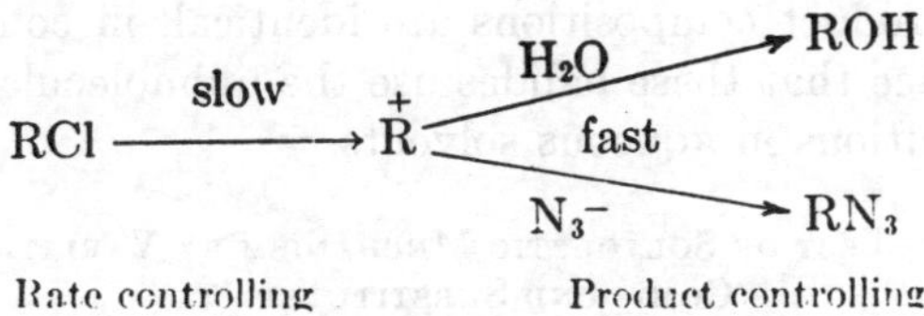

One can draw the further conclusion that, provided sufficient water is present for the purpose, the first-formed carbonium ion is solvated by a shell of fixed composition, so that the rate at which the ion covalently unites with one of the solvating water molecules is independent of the composition of the bulk of the medium.[94] On the other hand, the rate at which azide ions unite with the carbonium ion depends on the rate at which they break through the solvation water shell, and that depends in the normal way on the concentration of azide ions in the external medium.

This test of mechanism can be complemented with another. In the unimolecular mechanism, product composition is determined by competition for the carbonium ion, and not, as in the bimolecular mechanism, by competition for the original alkyl halide molecule. Therefore if we separately place two alkyl halides, containing the same alkyl group but a different halogen, say, an alkyl chloride and the related bromide, in the same competitive situation, for instance, an acetone-water mixture of fixed composition containing a fixed concentration of dissolved azide ion, then, assuming the unimolecular mechanism to be at work, the compositions of the products should be the same, even

[94] The original conclusion that the shell is of water only is not logically compulsory

though the rates of reaction might be very different

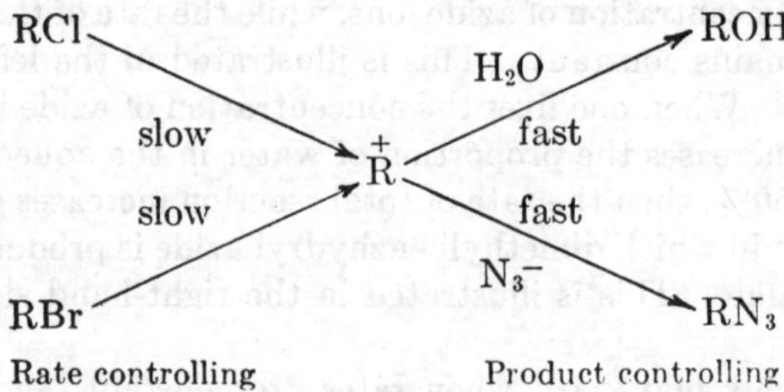

The test has been applied[95] to the hydrolysis of benzhydryl chloride and bromide in aqueous acetone containing dissolved sodium azide, with the results given in Table 29-8. Although the rates are markedly different, the product compositions are identical, in conformity with all other evidence that these halides use the unimolecular mechanism in their substitutions in aqueous solvents.

TABLE 29-8.—TEST OF SOLVOLYTIC MECHANISM BY VARIATION OF THE COMPOUND SUBSTITUTED.

Rates and product compositions in the hydrolysis of benzhydryl chloride and bromide in "90%" aqueous acetone containing 0.101 *M* sodium azide at 50°.

RHal	k_1 (sec.$^{-1}$)	ROH(%)	RN_3(%)
Ph_2CHCl	12.4×10^{-5}	66.0	34.0
Ph_2CHBr	416×10^{-5}	66.5	33.5

(29c) Mechanism in Polar Aprotic Solvents.—Following the earliest studies of dichotomy of nucleophilic mechanism in non-solvolytic and solvolytic substitutions in hydroxylic solvents, investigations were made in which the complications of solvolysis in the study of unimolecular substitutions were avoided by the use of aprotic solvents. Such solvents could not themselves react, but were polar enough to support the initial ionisations on which unimolecular substitutions and eliminations depend.

The first such solvent to be so employed was sulphur dioxide. Its dielectric constant is about 15 (the exact value depending on temperature). It is able to support the ionisations of *t*-butyl and benzhydryl halides to give low concentrations of carbonium ions, although it does introduce in a mild form complications of salt and polar solute effects, which we shall find it convenient to describe later. These complica-

[95] M. G. Church, E. D. Hughes, and C. K. Ingold, *J. Chem. Soc.*, **1940,** 966.

tions do not obscure the broad results that one does again find the dichotomy of S_N2 and S_N1 substitutions, and that one does observe the latter free from any accompanying solvolysis. The reaction between methyl iodide and pyridine had the kinetics of an S_N2 substitution. The reactions of *t*-butyl bromide, and of *m*-chlorobenzhydryl chloride, with fluoride ions supplied as tetraethylammonium fluoride, had the kinetics of S_N1 processes, incidentally with large salt effects of a form completely diagnostic of that mechanism (cf. Section **32f**). The reactions of the same two substrates with pyridine and with triethylamine gave kinetics which showed that these substitutions were at least mainly of S_N1 type, though there were deviations which seemed to arise from the long range of electrostatic forces in the medium.[96]

The use of nitromethane, as an aprotic medium of higher dielectric constant, about 40, largely eliminated the disturbances due to long-range forces, and led to observations in 1954 involving two new points of principle. In this medium, *t*-butyl bromide underwent reactions of substitution, with or without accompanying elimination, with radiobromide ion, with chloride ion, and with nitrite ion, all supplied, *e.g.*, as tetraethylammonium salts. The kinetics were of first order in the substrate, and zeroth order in the substituting agents. Salt effects of the right type for unimolecular reactions were observed, and, at low salt concentrations, the reactions with all three reagents had the same rate. The same substrate underwent similar substitutions with water, ethanol, and phenol, with first-order kinetics, and at the same rate, at low concentrations of these reagents, as the common rate of substitution with anions. All six reactions were evidently rate-dependent on the same ionisation rate. But at higher concentrations of the hydroxylic reagents the rate rose linearly with the reactant concentration, that is, there was a superposed second-order rate-term. Now this did not indicate the incursion of an S_N2 substitution at higher reactant concentrations, because the slope of the curve of rate versus reactant concentration, *i.e.*, the second-order rate coefficient, did not rise with the nucleophilic strength of the hydroxylic substituting agent, but rose with its acidity. The rate order was $PhOH > H_2O > EtOH$, the rate ratios being 5.5:2:1. This indicated general acid catalysis of an S_N1 substitution of an alkyl bromide, a process involving a transition state of the form

$$t\text{-}\overset{\delta+}{\text{Bu}} \cdots \overset{\delta-}{\text{Br}} \cdots \text{H} \cdots \text{OR}$$

[96] L. C. Bateman, E. D. Hughes, and C. K. Ingold, *J. Chem. Soc.*, **1940, 1011**, 1017; M. L. Bird, E. D. Hughes, and C. K. Ingold, *ibid.*, **1954**, 634; C. A. Bunton, C. H. Greenstreet, E. D. Hughes, and C. K. Ingold, *ibid.*, pp. 642, 647.

In hydroxylic solvents, as we shall see in Section **31b**, acid catalysis of the nucleophilic substitutions of alkyl fluorides is observed, but not of other alkyl halides. Presumably, acid catalysis is in principle possible in the nucleophilic substitutions of all alkyl halides, but depends on having a solvent which is sufficiently non-basic not to be competitive, as a base, with the alkyl halide.[97]

The second matter of principle disclosed in 1954 was a new mechanism of nucleophilic substitution—new to the extent that it consists of the same two chemical steps as mechanism S_N1, but with a reversed rate-order, and hence, according to our rules for the designation of mechanism (Section **27e**), is to be designated differently. It involves the slow bimolecular reaction of the substituting agent with a carbonium ion, rapidly formed from the substrate in a pre-equilibrium. The mechanism was designated $S_N2(C^+)$. Of course, it requires a very stable, easily formed, and somewhat slowly reacting, carbonium ion. The examples were of the reaction of triphenylmethyl chloride in nitromethane with hydroxylic substituting agents:

$$\left.\begin{array}{l} Ph_3C{-}Cl \underset{\text{fast}}{\rightleftharpoons} Ph_3C^+ + Cl^- \\ \\ Ph_3C^+ + ROH \underset{\text{slow}}{\rightleftharpoons} Ph_3C\cdot OR + H^+ \end{array}\right\} S_N2(C^+)$$

Triphenylmethyl chloride, on dissolution in nitromethane, shows the spectrum of the triphenylcarbonium ion immediately; and if radiochloride ion is introduced, chloride exchange to equilibrium is instantaneous. The reactions with water, ethanol, and phenol were investigated.[97] They are markedly reversible, running, in typical convenient conditions, to equilibria of 10–20% conversions. They can be run to 100% conversion, at the cost of elaborating the mechanism, by addition of pyridine to take up the formed hydrogen chloride, and the rate is then independent of the excess of pyridine. An instantaneous spectral change shows that the pyridine forms a complex with the carbonium ion, presumably a pyridinium ion, with charge divided between the nitrogen atom and the aralphyl group. One then observes second-order rates, which rise, not as before with the acidity of the substituting agent, but with its nucleophilic strength. The rate order is $EtOH > H_2O > PhOH$, the rate ratios being 20:5:1. Evidently the reagents are acting as nucleophiles; and they must be acting on the complex carbonium ion

We leave to Section **32g** and **32h** the consideration of mechanism

[97] E. Gelles, E. D. Hughes, and C. K. Ingold, *J. Chem. Soc.*, **1954**, 2918; P. B. D. de la Mare, E. D. Hughes, C. K. Ingold, and Y. Pocker, *ibid.*, p. 2930.

in weakly polar and non-polar solvents, because this is much bound up with the study of salt effects, with which we deal in Section **32**.

(30) TEMPERATURE EFFECTS IN NUCLEOPHILIC SUBSTITUTION

(30a) The Entropy of Activation.—By measuring the rate of a reaction over a range of temperature and applying the rate-equation of the transition-state theory (Section **6d**), we may determine the heat of activation $\Delta H^{\neq}$, and the entropy of activation $\Delta S^{\neq}$. These quantities are themselves functions of temperature, and the determined values should be taken to apply to the mean temperature of the range.

Many factors contribute to an entropy of activation. When, in a bimolecular reaction, two initial-state particles join together to make one transition-state particle, the translational and rotational entropies of two particles become reduced to those of one; there is a small additional entropy of vibration, but not nearly enough to compensate for the loss of entropy. These changes constitute a negative contribution to the entropy of activation. When, owing to the creation (or destruction) of charges during the formation of a transition state, the solvating molecules of the polar solvent become more tightly (or loosely) bound, the entropy of these solvating molecules will be reduced (or increased). This will constitute a negative (or positive) contribution to the entropy of activation. When, as is usual, certain bonds in the reactants become loosened in the transition state, the vibrations, to which they supply restoring forces, will gain entropy, and so make a positive contribution to the entropy of activation.

It was proposed by Long[98] that, on account of the first of the factors mentioned, that of molecularity, S_N2 reactions should generally possess smaller positive or greater negative entropies of activation than the most nearly analogous S_N1 reactions; and that this broad distinction could constitute a criterion of mechanism, one of particular utility in the difficult field of solvolytic reactions. Long illustrated the distinction in the domain of acid-catalysed hydrolyses, as of acetals and carboxylic esters, where conjugate acids are the effective substrates in the substitution processes of acid hydrolysis. He emphasised that the proposed criterion of mechanism must be used with circumspection, because within the same mechanism a great scatter of values of entropies of activation is found. We illustrate both the general principle and the scatter in the field of uncatalysed solvolysis of alkyl

[98] F. Long, J. G. Pritchard, and F. E. Stafford, *J. Am. Chem. Soc.*, 1957, **79**, 2362; F. A. Long and L. L. Schaleger, "Advances in Physical Organic Chemistry," Editor V. Gold, Academic Press, London and New York, 1963, Vol. 1, p. 1.

halides and sulphonates in Table 30-1, which summarises the teaching of the numerous data that have been provided by Kohnstam and Robertson and their respective collaborators. Notwithstanding the scatter, one sees that the entropies of activation of the bimolecular solvolyses run about 9–14 cal./deg. more negative than those of the most nearly comparable unimolecular solvolyses, in conformity with Long's general principle.

TABLE 30-1.—ENTROPIES OF ACTIVATION (CAL./MOLE/DEG.) AT 50° FOR THE SOLVOLYSIS OF ALKYL HALIDES AND SULPHONATES (KOHNSTAM, ROBERTSON).[1]

Replaced group	Range of Solvents	Presumed S_N1		Presumed S_N2	
		Examples of alkyl	Range $\Delta S^{\neq}$	Examples of alkyl	Range $\Delta S^{\neq}$
Cl or Br	H_2O	*t*-Bu, *neo*Pen	+ 3 to +9	Me, Et, *i*-Pr	− 9 to − 5
	50% aq-EtOH, 50–80% aq.-Me_2CO	*t*-Bu, Ph_2CH, *p*-MeO·C_7H_6, $PhCHCl$, $PhCCl_2$	−14 to −9	Et, *i*-Pr	−23 to −19
$MeSO_3$ or *p*-$TolSO_3$	H_2O	*i*-Pr, *neo*Pen	−5 to −3	Me, Et	−14 to −12

[1] The Table records the ranges covered by the many precise figures, given by Robertson for solvent water, and by Kohnstam for the aqueous organic solvents, in the publications cited in Kohnstam's review, "The Transition State," *Spec. Pubs. Chem. Soc.*, 1962, **16**, 179, and in the following subsequent publications: G. R. Cowie, H. J. M. Fitches, and G. Kohnstam, *J. Chem. Soc.*, **1963**, 1585; E. A. Moelwyn-Hughes, R. E. Robertson, and S. Sugamori, *ibid.*, **1965**, 1965.

The scatter will have many causes, but an important group of them will result from the second of the factors mentioned above, namely, solvation. The table shows that, in either the unimolecular or the bimolecular mechanism, the entropies of activation are higher, that is, more positive or less negative, in water than in aqueous-organic solvent mixtures. No doubt the entropy of the water which will solvate the polar transition states will start lower in solvent water than in the mixed solvents, to which an entropy of mixing has been added. But for each mechanism, and for each individual substrate, in a given solvent, the detailed geometry of the solvation shells in the initial and transition states will vary, and this is bound to cause case-to-case variation in the entropies of activation.

(30b) The Heat Capacity of Activation.—Precise measurements of the rate of a reaction over a temperature range allows a determination to be made of the temperature-gradient of the heat of activation, $d\Delta H^{\neq}/dT$, which is called the heat capacity of activation, $\Delta C^{\neq}$. This quantity is in principle a function of temperature; but it is already a first differential coefficient with respect to temperature, and its own variation with temperature has not yet been detected.

Kohnstam has proposed[99] that, for a given mechanism, and a given solvent, the dimensionless ratio $\Delta C^{\neq}/\Delta S^{\neq}$ should be less sensitive to variations of the substrate than is $\Delta S^{\neq}$ itself, or $\Delta C^{\neq}$ itself; and that therefore, for a given solvent, this ratio provides a sharper test of mechanism than any that could be based on either $\Delta S^{\neq}$ or $\Delta C^{\neq}$ alone. He has illustrated this proposition by data for the solvolyses of alkyl halides and sulphonates in "50%" aqueous ethanol, and in "50%," "70%," "80%," and "85%" aqueous acetone.[99] Some figures for "50%" aqueous acetone are reproduced in Table 30-2. The proposal does not work well for solvent water, wherein the values of $\Delta S^{\neq}$ for unimolecular substitutions are often close to zero, the ratios $\Delta C^{\neq}/\Delta S^{\neq}$ then becoming large and sensitive to substrate variation.

TABLE 30-2.—HEAT CAPACITIES AND ENTROPIES OF ACTIVATION FOR SOLVOLYSES AT 50° OF ALKYL HALIDES IN "50%" AQUEOUS ACETONE (KOHNSTAM)[1].

Alkyl halide	$-\Delta S^{\neq}$, cal./deg.	$-\Delta C^{\neq}$, cal./deg.	$\dfrac{\Delta C^{\neq}}{\Delta S^{\neq}}$	Mean
n-PrBr	26.8	23.4	1.13	
n-BuBr	20.8	27.6	1.32	1.13
$PhCH_2Cl$	22.4	21.6	0.95	
$PhCH_2Br$	20.8	23.6	1.13	
t-BuCl	11.3	29.7	2.63	
$Ph\cdot CHCl_2$	11.3	29.4	2.62	
p-$MeC_6H_4\cdot CHCl_2$	12.0	39.3	3.27	2.89
p-$NO_2C_6H_4\cdot CHPhCl$	10.8	33.5	3.10	
$PhCCl_3$	16.2	46.1	2.83	

[1] The data are from references cited in the note under Table 30-1. Further consistent data for alkyl toluene-*p*-sulphonates have been given by G. Kohnstam and D. Tidy, *Chem. and Ind.*, **1962**, 1193.

[99] B. Bensley and G. Kohnstam, *J. Chem. Soc.*, **1957**, 4747; G. Kohnstam, *ibid.*, **1960**, 2066; *idem*, "The Transition State," *Chem. Soc. Special Pubs.*, 1962, **16,** 179; G. R. Cowie, H. J. M. Fitches, and G. Kohnstam, *J. Chem. Soc.*, **1963,** 1585.

The typical result for aqueous organic solvents is that, as illustrated in Table 30-2, the ratios $\Delta C^{\neq}/\Delta S^{\neq}$ classify the substrates into two groups, exactly as they might have been classified according to their mechanisms of solvolysis presumed for other reasons: we believe that the first four substrates in Table 30-2 employ the bimolecular mechanism, and that the last five employ the unimolecular mechanism. A similar dichotomy of ratios has been demonstrated for other aqueous organic solvents. The ratios associated with the bimolecular and unimolecular mechanisms vary with the solvent, but always the ratio relating to the unimolecular mechanism is very considerably larger than that relating to the bimolecular mechanism.

This general difference in the ratios which characterise the bimolecular and unimolecular mechanisms may mean that, whilst the negative quantities, $\Delta C^{\neq}$ and $\Delta S^{\neq}$, both reflect restrictions of position and motion, placed in the transition states on the involved water molecules, they do so with a difference which itself reflects the different patterns of the two types of transition state. In a bimolecular transition state the loss of certain, initially classically energised, degrees of freedom of the one covalently involved water molecule will reduce both the entropy and the heat capacity. Additional reductions will arise from the electrostriction of solvation water; but, because bimolecular transition states are somewhat mildly polar, these reductions will be small in comparison with those next to be considered. In a unimolecular transition state there is no covalently involved water molecule. However, a strong electrostriction of the water molecules of the solvation shell of this highly polar transition state will reduce both the entropy and the heat capacity, though now, as will be explained, with an importance directed more towards the heat capacity. The reason for this expectation is that entropy is a temperature-average of heat capacity weighted for low temperatures,[100] and that solvation, involving hydrogen bonding, in a unimolecular transition state must largely restrict the hydrogen vibrations, which, because of their relatively high frequencies, are unexcited at low temperatures in both the initial and transition states, but are partly energised at the experimental temperature in both states. Therefore the effect of the entropic restrictions of solvation should be directed particularly towards the heat capacity at the experimental temperature. This leads to a high ratio $\Delta C^{\neq}/\Delta S^{\neq}$, when, as in S_N1 reactions, the restrictions of the transition state come mainly from electrostatic solvation by water, and do not, as they do in S_N2 reactions, come mainly from the covalent involve-

[100] More exactly: $S = \int_0^T \frac{C}{T} dT$.

ment of water. Of course, this rationalisation is tentative; but it does illustrate how the ratio $\Delta C^{\neq}/\Delta S^{\neq}$ might be more sensitive to the mechanism than to the substrate, and might have higher values for the unimolecular than for the bimolecular mechanism.

(31) CATALYTIC EFFECTS IN NUCLEOPHILIC SUBSTITUTION

(31a) Cosolvents as Catalysts.—The term catalysis is generally allowed to include accelerative effects on reactions by added substances which themselves suffer no permanent chemical change, independently of whether the mechanism of catalysis involves covalent or electrostatic intervention by the catalyst. Thus the acceleration of a reaction in a solvent in which it is slow, by the addition of a fairly small amount of one in which it is fast, can be described as a catalysis. However, the mechanism is here electrostatic, and consists in the better solvation of the polar transition state of reaction.

In no department of the study of nucleophilic substitution have greater difficulties arisen, through the mistaken idea that reaction order is synonymous with molecularity, than in relation to solvent effects. The matter was first raised[101] in 1937. Bateman and Hughes had just shown[102] that the rate of hydrolysis of *t*-butyl chloride to *t*-butyl alcohol by water in solvent formic acid is independent of the (small) water concentration. Their interpretation was that water, although the substituting agent, does not enter covalently into the rate-determining stage of the unimolecular mechanism assumed to be in operation; and does not even there enter electrostatically, because formic acid is a better solvating agent than water. In opposition, it was argued[101] that, because the hydrolysis of *t*-butyl bromide and of benzhydryl chloride in moist acetone is accelerated by added water in what was claimed to be an asymptotically linear manner (though linearity was never shown), therefore the substitution (and, by a strange generalisation, all alkyl halide substitutions) must be bimolecular. Now whether or not the reactions in moist acetone are in fact bimolecular (as they might be), the conclusion does not follow from the evidence.[103] As is shown in Table 29-2, *both* S_N2 and S_N1 substitutions of charge-type 2 are strongly accelerated by polar solvents: the factor of increase from acetone to water is probably 10^4-10^6. Therefore the curve of rate against solvent composition for any reaction, even a non-hydrolytic one, of charge-type 2 in this binary solvent system is likely to rise from the acetone end of the range so

[101] W. Taylor in several papers: for references and a discussion, see *J. Chem. Soc.*, **1940**, 899, *et seq.*

[102] L. C. Bateman and E. D. Hughes, *J. Chem. Soc.*, **1937**, 1187.

[103] L. C. Bateman, K. A. Cooper, and E. D. Hughes, *J. Chem. Soc.*, **1940**, 913; M. G. Church and E. D. Hughes, *ibid.*, p. 920.

steeply as to produce at least the effect of a unit of reaction order with respect to water. This can happen merely because water is so much more favourable as a solvent than acetone, that, in excess of the latter, the former behaves as a catalyst: in other words acetone cannot exclude water from participating in the (electrostatic) solvation of the polar transition state, whether of an S_N2 or of an S_N1 substitution.

Since 1948, the matter has been raised again in a slightly different form,[104] the proposition now being that "bimolecular" and "unimolecular" substitutions are alike in mechanism, in that all alkyl halide substitutions are actually termolecular. The field of previously presumed bimolecular substitutions was illustrated by the reaction between pyridine and methyl bromide to give *N*-methylpyridinium bromide in benzene containing methanol: the rate was said to be proportional to $[C_5H_5N][MeBr][MeOH]$. It would, of course, be possible for an S_N2 substitution to give approximately these kinetics over a certain concentration range, first, because the reaction, which is of charge-type 2, is strongly accelerated by polar solvents, and second because methanol is so very much more polar than benzene. Thus the factor [MeOH] could represent electrostatic cosolvent catalysis. The field of previously presumed unimolecular substitutions was exemplified by the reaction between methyl alcohol and triphenylmethyl chloride in solvent benzene containing an added pyridine base. The rate of methanolysis was at first stated to be proportional to $[MeOH]^2[Ph_3CCl]$, the pyridine base having no effect except to take up formed hydrogen chloride. Later, it was agreed[104,105] that the reaction, with or without pyridine base, had no firm quadratic dependence on methanol, but had an apparent order in methanol which rose smoothly from one or less to three or more, passing with no sign of arrest through the value of two with rising concentration of the methanol. This conceded, the case for universal termolecularity was dropped. The reaction of concern probably does go by a variant of the S_N1 mechanism. But the ions formed by the primary ionisation remain together; and, owing to the great range of electrostatic forces in solvent benzene, they attract to themselves, in various numbers, the most strongly polar cosolvent or solute species present, so to form multipolar aggregates, within which the nucleophilic substitution is completed.[106] We shall refer later (Section **32**) to evidence suggesting that the physical assembly of such an aggregate in a solvent of low

[104] C. G. Swain in several papers: for references and a discussion, see *J. Chem. Soc.*, **1957**, 1206, *et seq.*

[105] C. G. Swain and E. E. Pegues, *J. Am. Chem. Soc.*, 1958, **80**, 812.

[106] E. D. Hughes, C. K. Ingold, S. F. Mok, S. Patai, and Y. Pocker, *J. Chem. Soc.*, **1957**, 1265.

dielectric constant may be a faster process than the final covalency change within the aggregate. When a pyridine base is present, the substituting agent is likely to act on the triphenylmethyl-pyridinium complex, rather than on the carbonium ion, because the latter, when formed in other solvents in spectrally visible amounts, is seen to be instantly destroyed by pyridine bases (Section **29a**).

(31b) Acid Catalysis.—The solvolyses of primary, secondary, and tertiary alkyl chlorides, bromides, and iodides, in initially neutral, or in acidic, hydroxylic solvents, exhibit no sign of catalysis either by added acid, or by the acid formed. Alkyl fluorides are in a different case. Quite generally, their solvolyses in similar conditions exhibit, and may in practice depend on, acid catalysis. This was discovered by Miller and Bernstein for the solvolysis of variously substituted benzyl fluorides in "70%" aqueous ethanol.[107] The phenomenon was generalised to the solvolysis of aliphatic primary, secondary, and tertiary alkyl fluorides in aqueous ethanol by Chapman and Levy, who added some kinetic particulars of the catalysis.[108]

For primary and secondary alkyl fluorides, such as *n*-amyl, 2-methyl-*n*-butyl, and *cyclo*hexyl fluoride, the reactions are not only catalysed by initially added hydrogen chloride, but also are autocatalysed by the formed hydrogen fluoride. For tertiary alkyl fluorides, such as *t*-butyl and *t*-amyl fluorides, the autocatalysis disappears, and the relatively rapid catalysed solvolyses show first-order kinetics, with rate-constants proportional to the concentrations of the added strong acid.

As all the investigators recognised, these catalyses depend on the same forces as render the fluoride ion basic, readily hydrogen bonding, and outstandingly strongly solvated in protic solvents: similar properties in a weakened form will belong to the potential fluoride ion in the transition states of the solvolysing alkyl fluorides. We can perhaps understand the kinetic difference between the primary and secondary alkyl fluorides, on the one hand, and the tertiary fluorides, on the other, by assuming that the former use the S_N2 mechanism of solvolysis and the latter the S_N1 mechanism, and by then applying Hoffmann's principle that the electron transferred in carbon-halogen heterolysis is less extensively transferred in the transition state of an S_N2 substitution than in that of an S_N1 substitution. In an S_N2 transition state, the potential fluoride ion might be sufficiently negatively charged, and hence sufficiently basic, to hydrogen-bond with an acid, but not to extract a proton from an acid, the transition states

[107] W. T. Miller and J. Bernstein, *J. Am. Chem. Soc.*, 1948, **70**, 3600.
[108] N. B. Chapman and J. L. Levy, *J. Chem. Soc.*, **1952**, 1677.

therefore taking forms such as

$$H_2O \cdots R \cdots F \cdots H \cdots OH_2^+$$

$$H_2O \cdots R \cdots F \cdots H \cdots F$$

These are transition states of general-acid catalysis, including autocatalysis. In S_N1 transition states, on the other hand, the more negatively charged, and hence more basic, potential fluoride ion may take up a proton completely. These transition states will therefore assume the form

$$\overset{\delta+}{R} \cdots \overset{\delta-}{F} \cdots H^+$$

which represents specific hydrogen-ion catalysis. The autocatalysis would then disappear, and we should have first-order specific rates proportional to the hydrogen-ion concentration at low acidities (and to Hammett's h_0 at high ones—a point not yet tested).

The same difference in the reactions of fluoride and of other halides appears again among those of acyl halides.[109] The solvolyses of acyl fluorides in hydroxylic solvents are acid-catalysed, whilst those of acyl chlorides are not.

Acid catalysis in the aqueous hydrolysis of acetals was discussed in Section **28b**. Acid catalysis in the solvolysis of alkyl oxy-esters in hydroxylic solvents will be considered in Chapter XV.

It was noted in Section **29c** that acid catalysis in the reactions of alkyl halides other than fluorides can be observed in an aprotic solvent of low enough basicity not to be competitive, as a base, with the alkyl halide substrate. An investigation of the catalysis by hydrogen chloride of the isotopic chloride exchange reaction between 1-phenylethyl chloride and hydrogen radiochloride(^{36}Cl) in nitromethane solvent has been recorded by Pocker and his coworkers.[110] They show that the rate of substitution has two terms:

$$v = k_1[\mathrm{RCl}] + k_2[\mathrm{RCl}][\mathrm{HCl}]$$
$$(S_N1) \qquad (S_N1\text{-HCl})$$

They show also that the first term represents the uncatalysed rate of ionisation of 1-phenylethyl chloride, because it can be measured, with identical results, by other reactions. For example, it can be measured by the unimolecular elimination to give styrene, which 1-phenylethyl chloride undergoes in nitromethane when pyridine is added to stop

[109] C. W. L. Bevan and R. F. Hudson, *J. Chem. Soc.*, **1953**, 2187.

[110] Y. Pocker, W. A. Mueller, F. Naso, and G. Tocki, *J. Am. Chem. Soc.*, **1964**, **86**, 5011, 5012.

reversal of this reaction. This term, then, represents the unmodified mechanism S_N1. The investigations furthermore show, by a stereochemical method, the full explanation of which we must leave for Section **33**—but the method is sharply definitive—that the second term of the rate equation does not represent a superposed S_N2 substitution, but does represent the ionising extraction of chloride ion from 1-phenylethyl chloride by hydrogen chloride molecules; in other words, it represents general acid catalysis of the rate-controlling ionisation of an S_N1 process, through a transition state of the form

$$\overset{\delta+}{R} \cdots Cl \cdots H \cdots \overset{\delta-}{Cl}$$

This is a catalysed unimolecular mechanism, which we might symbolise S_N1-HCl.

(31c) Metal-Salt Catalysis.—A common method for converting a halide, AlkHal, into an alcohol, AlkOH, is to boil the former with water containing suspended silver oxide. If, as solvent, an alcohol ROH is used, instead of water, then the product is an ether, AlkOR, instead of the alcohol AlkOH. The same products are more quickly formed if, in place of silver oxide, a soluble silver salt, such as the nitrate or acetate, is employed; but then the corresponding alkyl ester, such as $Alk \cdot NO_3$ or AlkOAc, is usually formed, along with the alcohol or ether.

Kinetic investigations have shown[111] that the rate-determining stage of all these reactions involves the alkyl halide and the silver ion, and takes place largely on the surface of any insoluble silver salt present, including always the formed and precipitated silver halide, as well as any initially introduced insoluble salt, such as silver oxide.

These reactions are pictured as S_N1-like substitutions, initiated by the ionisation of the halogen compound on the surface of the silver salt with the aid of adsorbed silver ions, and completed through the uptake by the formed carbonium ion of an anion from the solution:

$$\text{AlkHal} + \text{Ag}^+ \xrightarrow[\text{surface}]{\text{AgX}} \text{Alk}^+ + \text{AgHal}$$

$$\begin{cases} \text{Alk}^+ + H_2O \longrightarrow \text{Alk} \cdot \text{OH} + H^+ \\ \text{Alk}^+ + \text{ROH} \longrightarrow \text{Alk} \cdot \text{OR} + H^+ \\ \text{Alk}^+ + Y^- \longrightarrow \text{Alk} \cdot Y \end{cases}$$

[111] G. Senter, *J. Chem. Soc.*, 1910, **97**, 346; 1911, **99**, 95; J. W. Baker, *ibid.*, **1934**, 987; A. N. Kappanna, *Proc. Indian Acad. Sci.*, 1935, **2**, 512; E. D. Hughes, C. K. Ingold, and S. Masterman, *J. Chem. Soc.*, **1937**, 1236; W. A. Cowdrey, E. D. Hughes, and C. K. Ingold, *ibid.*, **1937**, 1243.

This interpretation is further supported by observations of three kinds. One is that the effect of constitutional changes on reaction rate is qualitatively similar for silver-ion catalysed substitution and for unimolecular substitution: thus, for both reactions we have the alkyl rate series, tertiary > secondary > primary. The second type of observation is that the stereochemical course of silver-ion catalysed substitutions has been shown[112] to follow the rules applicable to S_N1 substitutions, and not the different rules of S_N2 substitutions (Section **33e**). The third is that, where S_N1 substitution leads (through isomerisation of Alk^+) to rearranged products, while S_N2 substitution gives normal products, the silver-ion reaction has been shown[113] to yield rearranged products (Chapter X).

In the catalysis of alkyl halide substitutions by mercuric salts[114] there need be no precipitate, and hence no surface catalysis. On the other hand, three types of homogeneous catalyst are conceivable, Hg^{++}, HgX^+, and HgX_2: the first and last of these have been claimed as sole effective catalysts in different cases, and there must, no doubt, be cases in which pairs of catalysts act concurrently.[114,115,116] Apart from the catalysis, the reactions are clearly of S_N1 type. For, first, the "mass-law effect," that is, deviations from first-order kinetic form, arising from the reversibility of the rate-controlling initial step (Section **32a**), have been observed.[115] Second, the stereochemical course of the catalysed reactions obeys the rules for S_N1 reactions.[115,116] And third, it has been observed that rearranged products are formed, under catalysis of mercuric nitrate, where the uncatalysed S_N1 reaction would give rearranged products.[113]

Many silver salts are soluble in acetonitrile. Pocker and Kevill have investigated the electrochemical condition, through the electrical conductance of tetraethylammonium and silver nitrate, nitrite, and perchlorate in acetonitrile, and have studied the kinetics, and products, including the stereochemistry, of their reactions of substitution

[112] E. D. Hughes, C. K. Ingold, and S. Masterman, *loc. cit.;* W. A. Cowdrey, E. D. Hughes, and C. K. Ingold, *loc. cit.*

[113] F. C. Whitmore, E. L. Whittle, and A. H. Popkin, *J. Am. Chem. Soc.*, 1939, **61**, 1586; I. Dostrovsky and E. D. Hughes, *J. Chem. Soc.*, **1946**, 166, 169.

[114] B. H. Nicholet and D. R. Stevens, *J. Am. Chem. Soc.*, 1928, **50**, 135, 212; I. Roberts and L. P. Hammett, *ibid.*, 1937, **59**, 1063; O. T. Benfey, *ibid.*, 1948, **70**, 2165.

[115] K. Saramma and R. I. AnantaRaman, *Proc. Indian Acad. Sci.*, 1959, **49**, 111; *J. Am. Chem. Soc.*, 1960, **82**, 1574; K. Saramma, Thesis, Kerala, 1965.

[116] K. Bodendorf and H. Böhme, *Ann.*, 1935, **516**, 1; R. I. AnantaRaman, C. A. Bunton, and E. D. Hughes, results personally communicated.

and olefin elimination with 2-octyl bromide and chloride.[117] All the salts were found to be somewhat weak electrolytes with ionic dissociation constants in the region of 10^{-2} mole/l. But the ionisation of silver nitrite was peculiar, in that the principal anion formed was a stable complex, $Ag(NO_2)_2^-$, and only a very small amount of the free nitrite ion, NO_2^-, was produced.

The reaction of tetraethylammonium nitrate with 2-octyl bromide was a reversible second-order reaction of nitrate ion with the substrate, going with inversion of configuration by mechanism S_N2 (cf. Section **33d**):

$$NO_3^- + RBr \rightleftharpoons RNO_3 + Br^- \qquad (S_N2)$$

In contrast to the reaction next to be discussed, there was no concurrent formation of octenes. The reaction of silver nitrate with 2-octyl bromide was much faster, and was of kinetic order 2.5, that is, 1.0 in substrate, and 1.5 in salt. With added tetraethylammonium nitrate the order in salt broke up into two parts, an order of 1.0 in silver nitrate and an order of 0.5 in total nitrate. Silver bromide was precipitated, and this carried the reaction to completion; but no heterogeneous catalysis by the precipitate could be detected in the presence of the dissolved silver salt. The reaction of silver nitrate with 2-octyl chloride exhibited all the same characteristics. In both reactions octenes were formed, but in different proportions, 7.9% at 45° from the bromide, and 3.3% at 45° from the chloride. The 2-octyl nitrate was largely inverted in configuration but was partly racemised, as would be expected from an S_N1-type reaction (cf. Section **33e**). Thus, 2-octyl bromide at 100° gave 16% octenes, and the 84% of 2-octyl nitrate was inverted, with a drop to 87% in optical purity: these figures were independent of the concentration of silver nitrate, and the presence or absence of tetraethylammonium nitrate.

The interpretation of the kinetics was as follows. The order one-half shows the presence in the transition state of nitrate ion deriving from salts stored mainly in ion-pair form, the total composition of the transition state being $NO_3^- + RHal + AgNO_3$. The products point to the intermediate formation of a carbonium ion R^+, which reacts while still under the influence of the halide ion. The overall rationalisation is that RHal ionises, but only when attacked at both ends, *i.e.*, by the electrophile $AgNO_3$ and by the nucleophile NO_3^-, in a mechanism which may be symbolised NO_3^--S_N1-$AgNO_3$. As it applies also to other silver salts, we write it below in a generalised form.

[117] Y. Pocker and D. N. Kevill, *J. Am. Chem. Soc.*, 1965, **87**, 4760, 4771, 4778.

In this example $X = NO_3$:

$$\left.\begin{array}{l} RHal + Ag^+X^- \rightleftharpoons RHal \cdots Ag^+X^- \\ X^- + RHal \cdots Ag^+X^- \xrightarrow[\text{slow}]{} X^-R^+Hal^-Ag^+ + X^- \\ X^-R^+Hal^-Ag^+ \longrightarrow \begin{cases} RX + AgHal \\ \text{Olefin} + HX + AgHal \end{cases} \end{array}\right\} (X^- - S_N1 - AgX)$$

This formulation shows the carbonium ion as a component of an ion quadruplet, an idea which we shall meet again in Sections **32g** and **32h**.

The reactions of 2-octyl bromide with tetraethylammonium nitrite and silver nitrite were similar to those with the corresponding nitrates in all respects, save as might have been anticipated from the special mode of ionisation of silver nitrite. Thus the reaction with silver nitrite was not faster, but was considerably slower than the reaction with tetraethylammonium nitrite, obviously because the proportion of free nitrite ion formed from silver nitrite is so very low; and the rate of the reaction with silver nitrite was not much increased by added tetraethylammonium nitrite if not in excess, plainly because the added nitrite ion is sequestered by the silver nitrite to form the stable complex anion, $Ag(NO_2)_2^-$. However, these details do not disturb the conclusion that the mechanism of the silver reaction is X^--S_N1-AgX, with $X = NO_2$.

Tetraethylammonium perchlorate had but little action on 2-octyl bromide at temperatures at which silver perchlorate reacted with it to produce initially 2-octyl perchlorate and octenes. This silver-salt reaction had simple kinetics only if the silver salt was in quite low concentration, when the kinetic order was 1.0 in substrate, and 1.0 (not 1.5) in salt. Added tetraethylammonium perchlorate only slightly raised the rate. Evidently the unpaired perchlorate ion cannot easily function as a nucleophile in assisting ionisation of the substrate, and the assumption was that an acetonitrile molecule takes over that function in an allied mechanism, MeCN-S_N1-$AgClO_4$.

Silver perchlorate is soluble in benzene, in which it reacts fairly rapidly with alkyl halides. Pocker and Kevill have studied the kinetics and products of the reaction with 2-octyl bromide.[118] The reaction was found to be of order 1.0 in substrate and 1.5 in salt, at low concentrations of the latter. Added tetra-*n*-butylammonium perchlorate markedly increased the rate. The initial products were 2-octyl perchlorate and octenes, formed in the respective proportions

[118] Y. Pocker and D. N. Kevill, *J. Am. Chem. Soc.*, 1965, **87**, 5060.

61% and 38% at 25°, proportions which were independent of the concentration of either salt. As was shown by back-conversion with bromide ions in S_N2 conditions (Section **33d**), the formed 2-octyl perchlorate was dominantly of inverted configuration, but was partly racemised, as for an S_N1-type mechanism (Section **33e**). All this is consistent with the general mechanism formulated above, which for this case would be symbolised ClO_4^--S_N1-$AgClO_4$. There is a problem of reconciling the high rate with the very low equilibrium concentration of unpaired perchlorate ions, and the mechanism may in fact be a derivative form of a mechanism of that general type.

(32) SALT EFFECTS ON NUCLEOPHILIC SUBSTITUTION

(32a) Predicted Mass-Law Effects on Kinetics.[119]—We noted in Section **27d** that the unimolecular mechanism has, typically, a somewhat complex kinetic form, which does not necessarily reduce to first-order form when the conditions become such that the bimolecular mechanism would have first-order form, for example, when the substituting agent is the solvent. The reason is the reversibility of the initial heterolysis in unimolecular reactions, as may be illustrated by the hydrolysis of an alkyl chloride in an aqueous solvent:

$$RCl \underset{(2)}{\overset{(1)}{\rightleftarrows}} R^+ + Cl^- \underset{(3)}{\overset{H_2O}{\longrightarrow}} ROH + H^+ + Cl^-$$

As larger chloride-ion concentrations are built up by reaction (3), reaction (2) gains in importance, so that the rate-determining ionisation becomes progressively retarded by its reversibility, without necessitating any reversal of the overall reaction, which may be a completely irreversible hydrolysis: the rate simply falls further and further behind the first-order rate as reaction proceeds. This can be expressed by specialising the typical equation of S_N1 reactions, suitably for a substituting agent in constant active mass. The result is as follows,

$$dx/dt = k_1(a - x)(1 + \alpha x)^{-1}$$

where a is the initial concentration of alkyl halide, and x is the concentration of chloride ion formed by hydrolysis. The factor $(1+\alpha x)^{-1}$ describes the progressive fall in the "specific rate" $(dx/dt)/(a-x)$; and the "mass-law constant" α, which is of the dimensions of reciprocal concentration, is the ratio of the rate of capture of the carbonium ion by chloride ion in unit concentration to the rate of its capture by the solvent water.

[119] L. C. Bateman, M. G. Church, E. D. Hughes, C. K. Ingold, and N. A. Taher, *J. Chem. Soc.*, **1940**, 979.

An analogous effect is obviously to be expected if, instead of relying on the formed hydrogen chloride, one initially introduces some hydrogen chloride, or sodium chloride, or any other ionising chloride. The difference is that the reaction rate will now be depressed from the beginning, according to the equation,

$$dx/dt = k_1(a - x)\{1 + \alpha(c + x)\}^{-1}$$

where *c* is the concentration of initially introduced chloride ion.

These mass-law constants α must in principle vary with the circumstances of the competition between the anions and the solvent for the carbonium ion. They vary strikingly with the substrate, rising with those structural changes that would increase the relative stability of the carbonium ion. They vary much less strongly with the medium.

These effects of salts on unimolecular reactions relate to "common-ion salts," that is, salts having an anion identical with that given by the alkyl compound: "non-common-ion salts," that is, salts with any other anion, for instance, sodium azide in the example of the hydrolysis of an alkyl chloride, cannot produce a like effect, for such salts intervene only after the rate-determining ionisation:

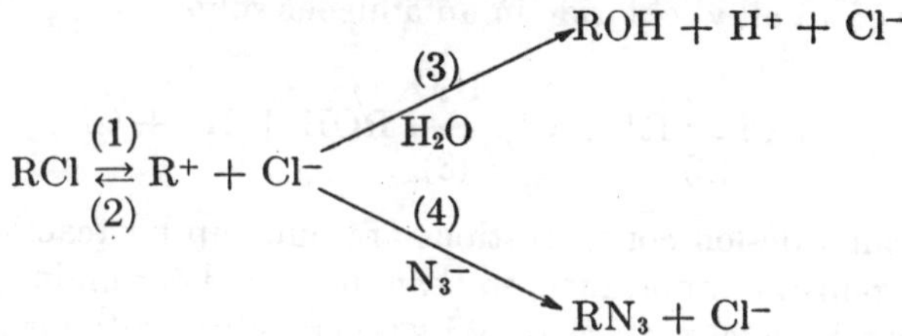

Thus, mass-action gives these salts no effect at all on the initial rate of destruction of the alkyl halide, although, by supplying new competition for the carbonium ion, they should weaken the growing retardation produced by the developing chloride ion.

Bimolecular substitution involves quite a different set of consequences. In the irreversible hydrolysis of a chloride by the mechanism,

$$H_2O + RCl \rightarrow ROH + H^+ + Cl^-$$

mass action can confer no kinetic effect either on the produced chloride ion or on any added "common-ion" salt. On the other hand, an added "non-common-ion" salt, such as sodium azide, if it intervenes at all, must accelerate the destruction of the alkyl halide from the outset, since it provides an extra mode of attack on that molecule:

$$N_3^- + RCl \rightarrow RN_3 + Cl^-$$

(32b) Predicted Ionic-Strength Effects.[119]—Superposed on the mass-law effects described above, there will always be electrostatic effects connected with the ionic strengths of the solutions. The theory of these effects is qualitatively analogous to that of solvent effects. Just as in the unimolecular ionisation of a neutral molecule, or in a bimolecular reaction between neutral molecules, a solvent of increased polarity accelerates, because the polar transition state can better stabilise itself by attracting solvent dipoles, so also, in the same reactions, inert salts will accelerate, because the transition state charges can better stabilise themselves by attracting suitable ionic atmospheres. Again, just as the solvent effect is greater in the unimolecular than in the bimolecular case, because of the greater diffusion of charge in the transition state of the latter, so also, and for the same reason, the accelerating effect of ionic strength should be more marked in the unimolecular case. These electrostatic effects of salts will naturally depend on the dielectric constant of the solvent: the smaller the dielectric constant, the stronger will be the electrostatic forces exerted on and by the ions, and the greater their kinetic effects.

Illustrating again by the unimolecular hydrolysis of an alkyl chloride, we may first note that the ionic strength rises during reaction. Hence the electrostatic effect of ionic strength should produce a progressive rise in the specific rate. If we should introduce initially any salt, either of the "common-ion" or of the "non-common-ion" type, the resulting electrostatic effect should be to increase rate from the commencement of reaction.

In case the bimolecular mechanism of hydrolysis is in operation, the various electrostatic effects would be qualitatively as described, but considerably weaker.

The ways in which the mass-law and ionic-strength effects are thus predicted to combine in the two mechanisms of solvolysis are sum-

TABLE 32-1.—PREDICTED MASS-LAW AND IONIC-STRENGTH EFFECTS ON THE UNIMOLECULAR AND BIMOLECULAR SOLVOLYSIS OF AN ALKYL HALIDE.

		MASS LAW	+	*IONIC STRENGTH*
S_N1	Formed ions	*Progressive fall in specific rate*	+	Progressive rise in specific rate
	Common-ion salt	*Retardation*	+	Acceleration
	Non-common-ion salt	No initial effect	+	Acceleration
S_N2	Formed ions	No effect	+	Small progressive rise in specific rate
	Common-ion salt	No effect	+	Small acceleration
	Non-common-ion salt	Acceleration	+	Small acceleration

marised in Table 32-1. The ionic-strength effects will be of chief concern to us when they occur along with mass-law effects. The most interesting of the predictions in the table are the two entered in italics. They are mass-law effects in the unimolecular mechanism, and are diagnostic of that mechanism. But they are overlaid by substantial, and qualitatively contrary, ionic-strength effects. We therefore must be able analytically to separate the mass-law and ionic-strength effects, so to isolate the diagnostic mass-law effect. We gave in Section **32a** a first-approximate quantitative theory of the mass-law effect. For the purposes of the analysis, we must match this with a first-approximate quantitative theory of the ionic-strength effect.

Such a theory[119] has been given, which is based on the supposition, to be critically examined later, that, the solutions being sufficiently dilute, we need take account only of long-range electrostatic forces. These cause the ambient ions to arrange themselves into a dilute "ionic atmosphere" around any central dipole taken to represent the charge transferred from carbon to halogen in the formation of the transition state of ionisation in the unimolecular mechanism. For a central univalent ion, contained in such a dilute ionic atmosphere, the Debye theory has already derived an activity coefficient, given by the "limiting law" as

$$-\ln f_i = \sqrt{\frac{2}{1000}} \cdot \boldsymbol{N}^{1/2} \boldsymbol{e}^3 \cdot \mu^{1/2} (D\boldsymbol{k}T)^{-3/2}$$

where $\boldsymbol{N}$ is Avogadro's number, $\boldsymbol{e}$ is the electronic charge, $\boldsymbol{k}$ is Boltzmann's constant, μ is the ionic strength of the solution, and D is the dielectric constant of the solvent. Similarly, we can calculate (just by picking out the right solution of Poisson's equation, as encountered in the Debye theory) that, for a central dipole of two point-charges $\pm z\boldsymbol{e}$ separated by a distance d, the activity coefficient would be given by

$$-\ln f_d = \frac{4\pi}{1000} \cdot \boldsymbol{N}\boldsymbol{e}^4 \cdot z^2 d \cdot \mu (D\boldsymbol{k}T)^{-2}$$

Thus, in order to calculate the kinetic effects of ionic strength, all we have to do is to put these activity coefficients into the Brönsted rate equation (Section **6d**). In particular for the reversible ionisation,

$$RX \underset{k_2}{\overset{k_1}{\rightleftharpoons}} R^+ + X^-$$

we must put f_d and f_i into the equations:

$$\text{Rate of dissociation} = k_1[\text{RX}]\cdot f_d$$

$$\text{Rate of ionic recombination} = k_2[\text{R}^+][\text{X}^-]\cdot\frac{f_i^2}{f_d}$$

These equations contain one disposable parameter, the so-called "ionic-strength constant," σ, defined by

$$\sigma = z^2d$$

Our calculation of the mass-law effect on the rate of a unimolecular reaction had one disposable constant, namely the "mass-law constant," α, defined as k_2/k_3. Thus, our calculations of ionic-strength effects involve the same, but not a greater, degree of arbitrariness, and should be satisfactory for analysis of the superposed effects.

The ionic-strength constant σ has the dimensions of length. Assuming that z, the fraction of an electron which is transferred from carbon to halogen on activation to the transition state of ionisation, is not a very small fraction, σ should be of the order of magnitude of a bond-length, as indeed it is: we can conveniently express it in Angstrom units. It does not vary with the solvent in the range "70%"–"90%" aqueous acetone, though it might vary over a wider range of solvents. It does vary with the constitution of the substrate, increasing markedly when increasing conjugation or hyperconjugation would further separate the centres of location of the developed dipole charges, or, in other words, would increase d.

The above-described treatment of ionic-strength effects, that is, of the long-range electrostatic effects of the nett charges of the ambient ions, is sufficient only provided that their local-field effects, as summarised in the term "specific" salt effects, with respect to which every ion is different, can be neglected. The thermodynamic outlook on overall salt effects, coulombic plus specific, is that the ambient ions, by increasing cohesion, increase the "internal pressure," and that that increase (unless a countervailing specific attraction between ambient ions and the solute is present and predominant) will tend to "squeeze" the organic solute out, *e.g.*, to salt it out, or volatilise it, and, quite generally, to increase its activity coefficient. We have been calculating the difference, from the initial to the transition state, of that part of the total salt effect which depends on the long-range coulombic field of the nett charges of the ambient ions. There remains the specific part of the effect, *i.e.*, that part which depends on local interactions, and accordingly on properties of the ions other than their nett charge, properties which therefore vary from one ion to another among ions of the same charge. Whether this specific effect is significant for the initial state, or for the transition state, or, as would really matter, for the difference between the two, are questions which should be investigated.

These questions have been definitively studied by Clarke and Taft.[120] Their example was the hydrolysis of *t*-butyl chloride in water, a reaction for which the mass-law effect on the kinetics is negligibly small. Their method was to examine the effect of added salts on the initial vapour pressure of the dissolved *t*-butyl chloride, and on the rate of its hydrolysis, so obtaining data which gave the effect of each salt on the initial state and on the transition state separately. Their results showed that the total effect of a salt on a single state, initial or transition, contained a considerable specific part differing from salt to salt, but that, for simple inorganic salts, the specific effect was almost identical in both states, and hence disappeared from the difference. This must mean that the specific effects of the salts are indeed due to local ion-solvent interaction, the resulting increment of internal pressure acting similarly on the initial and transition states, presumably because their volumes are sufficiently similar. Thus the difference of total salt effects, between the initial and transition states, is essentially the coulombic difference, calculated as discussed above. Clarke and Taft confirmed its non-specific nature, and its coulombic dependence on charge through, and only through, the macroscopic ionic strength, over a much larger variety of salts than had been used before, including, as is particularly significant, 2-1 and 1-1 electrolytes in the same comparison. We shall refer later to their conclusions concerning dipole development in the transition state of the unimolecular hydrolysis of *t*-butyl chloride.

The predictions in Table 32-1, which are entered in italics, arise from the mass-law effect on the unimolecular mechanism, and are the downward drift of specific rate during reaction in the absence of added salts, and the overall retardation produced by added "common-ion" salts, but not by other salts. We shall illustrate the observation of these effects in the following Sections.

(32c) Observed Effects of Produced Ions on Kinetic Form of Solvolysis.—We may first examine an example of unimolecular solvolysis, namely, the hydrolysis of *t*-butyl bromide in aqueous acetone,[121] in which the mass-law effect is sufficiently small to allow the ionic

[120] G. A. Clarke, T. R. Williams, and R. W. Taft, *J. Am. Chem. Soc.*, 1962, **84**, 2292; G. A. Clarke and R. W. Taft, *ibid.*, p. 2295.

[121] L. C. Bateman, E. D. Hughes, and C. K. Ingold, *J. Chem. Soc.*, **1940**, 960.

strength effect to be observed substantially in isolation. The specific rate then rises with the progress of reaction. This can be seen in Fig. 32-1, even though what is there plotted is the integrated first-order rate constant $t^{-1} \ln \{a/(a-x)\}$, which will rise only about half as steeply as the specific rate $(dx/dt)/(a-x)$, because of the averaging effect of integration. Two experiments in solvents of different water content, and therefore of markedly different dielectric constant, are shown. The curves are those given by the theory of the effect for dilute solutions. The required ionic-strength constant σ, for *t*-butyl bromide, may be obtained either from similar experiments under other conditions or from the observed kinetic effects of added "non-common-ion" salts (Section **32d**). Thus the theoretical curves owe nothing directly to the experimental data with which they are being compared in Fig. 32-1. The agreement confirms the applicability of the ionic-strength theory. In particular, it confirms the calculated dependence of the kinetic salt effect on the solvent only through the dielectric constant of the latter. This implies that the ionic-strength constant σ is not solvent-dependent over this range of solvents.

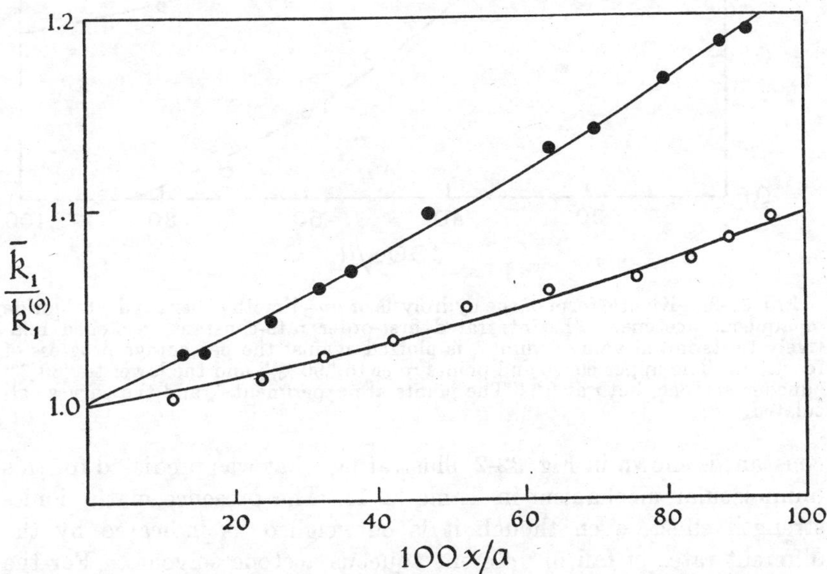

FIG. 32-1.—Kinetic form of the hydrolysis of *t*-butyl bromide in aqueous acetone. The integrated first-order rate-constant, reckoned relatively to its initial value as unity, is plotted against the percentage progress of reaction. The upper curve and associated points relate to "90%" and the lower to "70%" aqueous acetone, both at 25°. The points are observational, and the curves are calculated from the electrostatic theory of the ionic-strength effect, with the aid of an independently determined value of the ionic-strength constant σ.

As a complementary example, we may examine the kinetic form of the hydrolysis of *pp'*-dimethylbenzhydryl chloride in aqueous acetone. In this reaction, there is a large ionic-strength effect, but a still larger mass-law effect, with the result that the specific rate falls strongly with the progress of reaction. The fall in the integrated first-order rate-

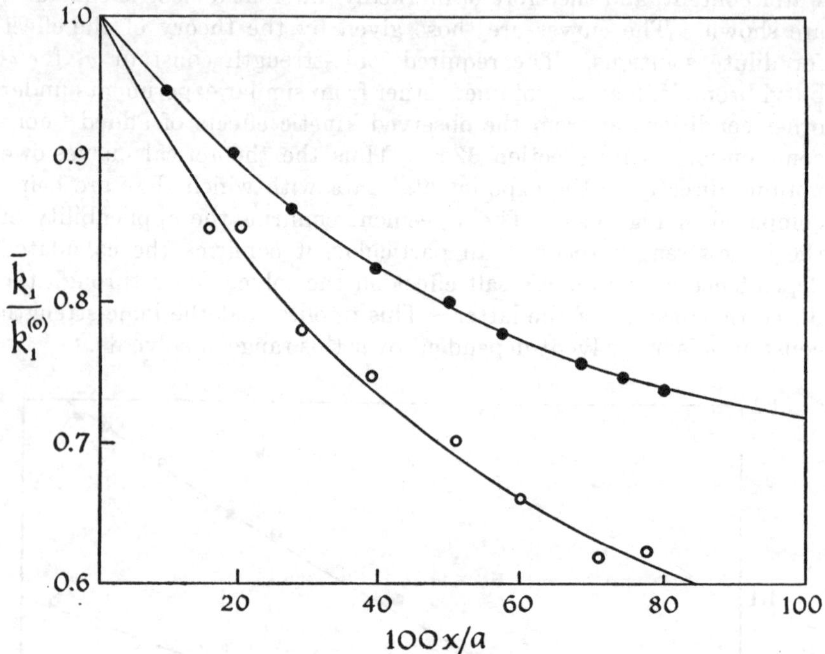

Fig. 32-2.—Kinetic form of the hydrolysis of *pp'*-dimethyl-benzhydryl chloride in aqueous acetone. The integrated first-order rate-constant, reckoned relatively to its initial value as unity, is plotted against the percentage progress of reaction. The upper curve and points refer to "90%," and the lower to "80%" aqueous acetone, both at 0°. The points are experimental, and the curves calculated.

constant is shown in Fig. 32-2, illustrating what was predicted for this unimolecular mechanism in Table 32-1. The presence of the ionic-strength effect, even though it is outweighed, is indicated by the different rates of fall in different aqueous acetone solvents. For the ionic-strength effect depends on the dielectric constant, and therefore on the water content, of the medium; while the mass-law effect is presumed to be independent of the water content, since azide intervention has been shown to be independent (Section **29b**); and the plausible assumption that chloride-ion intervention is likewise independent agrees with quantitative calculations on the kinetic form of the hydrolysis. The curves in Fig. 32-2 are theoretically calculated with the aid of values of the ionic-strength and mass-law constants, σ and α, for dimethylbenzhydryl chloride. The constant σ is evaluated from the kinetic effect of added "non-common-ion" salts (Section **32d**). The constant α may be deduced either from an experiment of the type of one of those illustrated, or from the kinetic effect of added "common-ion" salts (Section **32d**). It should be remarked that the

TABLE 32-2.—EFFECTS OF ADDED SALTS ON THE INITIAL RATES OF HYDROLYSIS OF ALKYL HALIDES IN AQUEOUS ACETONE.

Aqueous acetone	Temp.	Salt	Concn. of salt	% Change of rate
t-Butyl Bromide[1]				
"90%"	50°	NaN_3	0.10	+40%
"90%"	50°	LiCl	0.10	+39%
"90%"	50°	*LiBr	0.10	+42%
Benzhydryl Chloride[2]				
"80%"	25°	*LiCl	0.10	−13%
"80%"	25°	LiBr	0.10	+17%
Benzhydryl Bromide[2]				
"80%"	25°	LiCl	0.10	+27%
"80%"	25°	*LiBr	0.10	−13%
pp′-*Dimethylbenzhydryl Chloride*[3]				
"90%"	0°	NaN_3	0.05	+69%
"85%"	0°	NaN_3	0.05	+48%
"85%"	0°	*LiCl	0.05	−46%
"85%"	0°	LiBr	0.05	+46%
"85%"	0°	NMe_4NO_3	0.05	+52%
"80%"	0°	NaN_3	0.05	+36%

[1] L. C. Bateman, E. D. Hughes, and C. K. Ingold, *J. Chem. Soc.*, **1940,** 960.
[2] O. T. Benfey, E. D. Hughes, and C. K. Ingold, *J. Chem. Soc.* **1952,** 2488.
[3] L. C. Bateman, E. D. Hughes, and C. K. Ingold, *J. Chem. Soc.*, **1940,** 974.

agreement between the theoretical curves and the observational points depends critically on a certain assumption about the molecularity of the fast reaction between the carbonium ion and water; but we shall come to this point in Section **32e**.

(32d) Observed Effects of Added Salts on Initial Rate of Solvolysis.—Some observations on the effects of added salts on the initial rates of unimolecular hydrolysis of four alkyl halides in aqueous acetone are summarized in Table 32-2. What is measured is in all cases the rate of liberation of halide ions from the alkyl halide; for this will give the ionisation rate, whereas the rate of acid production will not do so, if the anion of the added salt intervenes in reaction to form a stable product. The salts are taken in either of two standard concentrations. It will be noticed that the "non-common-ion" salts (those without an asterisk) increase rate without exception, as they should according to the predictions of Table 32-1. But the "common-ion" salts (marked by an asterisk), except that used with *t*-butyl bromide, which is otherwise known to have a very small mass-law effect, depress the initial rate of hydrolysis, thereby establishing the mass-law retardation predicted for the unimolecular mechanism in Table 32-1.

From data of the type illustrated in Figs. 32-1 and 32-2, and in Table 32-2, the ionic-strength and mass-law constants, σ and α, have been computed[119] for the solvolysis of a number of tertiary butyl, benzhydryl, and alkyl-benzhydryl halides in aqueous organic solvents, mainly aqueous acetone. The obtained figures are in Table 32-3. For *t*-butyl bromide, α is of the order of 1 l./mol., and is too small either to affect the kinetic form of solvolysis, or to make any distinction between the kinetic effects of common-ion and non-common-ion salts. The kinetic form of solvolyses, and the kinetic effects of salts, thus provide values of σ. Bunton and Nayak have, however,

TABLE 32-3.—IONIC-STRENGTH CONSTANTS σ (IN A) AND MASS-LAW CONSTANTS α (IN l./MOL.) FOR THE SOLVOLYSIS OF ALKYL HALIDES IN AQUEOUS ACETONE.

Alkyl halide	Solvent v/v% aqueous acetone	Temp.	σ from		α from	
			Kinetic form	Non-common-ion salts	Kinetic form	Common-ion salts
t-BuCl	80%[a]	35°	—	—	—	0.25
t-BuBr	70–90%	25–50°	0.75	0.8	—	—
Ph_2CHCl	70–90%	25–50°	—	1.6	10	13
Ph_2CHBr	80–90%	25°	—	1.75	50	70
4-*t*-$BuC_6H_4\cdot CHPhCl$	80–90%	25–50°	—	2.2	20	—
4-$MeC_6H_4\cdot CHPhCl$	80%	25°	—	—	35[b]	31[b]
$(4\text{-}MeC_6H_4)_2CHCl$	80–90%	0°	—	2.75	70	90

[a] Solvent aqueous methanol: C. A. Bunton and B. Nayak, *J. Chem. Soc.*, **1959,** 3854. Further values by this method for substituted benzhydryl chlorides in "70%" aqueous acetone at 0° again show that electropositive substituents increase α; J. H. Bailey, J. R. Fox, E. Jackson, G. Kohnstam, and A. Queen, *Chem. Comm.*, **1966**, 122.

[b] Calculated assuming $\sigma = 2.2\ A$.

evaluated α for *t*-butyl chloride in aqueous methanol, as 0.2–0.3 l./mol., from the uptake of radioactivity from radiochloride ion. In the benzhydryl and alkyl-benzhydryl examples, the constants σ and α are comparably important, and the procedure has been, first, to determine σ from the non-common-ion salt effect, and then, with its help, to evaluate α from the kinetic form of solvolysis, and also from the common-ion salt effect.

Using the two-point-charge model, we can calculate, *e.g.*, for *t*-butyl bromide undergoing solvolysis in aqueous acetone, what charge would have to be transferred during activation through a distance estimated as the CBr bond length in the transition state, in order to give the observed constant, $\sigma = 0.8$ *A*. The estimated distance is taken as the Morse-curve stretched length, 2.4 *A*, at the activation energy. The answer is 0.6 electron. Clarke and Taft, using the same model, similarly derived from their study of salt effects in the separate initial and transition states of hydrolysis of *t*-butyl chloride in water the picture of 0.2 electron transferred from C to Cl in the initial state and 0.8 electron so transferred in the transition state.[120] As they remark, such estimates of electron transfer are somewhat artificial. If we make a similar calculation for the charge transfer accompanying activation to the transition state of solvolysis of 4,4′-dimethylbenzylhydryl chloride in aqueous acetone, using the observed constant, $\sigma = 2.75$ *A*, the answer is 1.1 electron, *i.e.*, more than enough fully to ionise the halogen. Of course, the centroid of the positive charge will not be at the α-carbon nucleus, but will be further back in the alkyl group. Also the Morse-curve stretched length is only a lower limit to the transition-state bond length (cf. Fig. 27-1, p. 425). Moreover, the two-point-charge model, which theoretically requires great dilution, may not be very good in the only moderately dilute solutions employed. Nevertheless, Table 32-3 does show the regularity that σ increases as, for constitutional reasons, the distance of the electron transfer accompanying activation would be expected to increase.

The mass-law constants α refer to the reactivity of the fully formed carbonium ion: they specify the rate of its reaction with the halide counter-ion relatively to the rate of its reaction with water. Table 32-3 shows that that rate-ratio increases strongly as the constitution of the substrate is so changed that the carbonium ionic charge would become increasingly stabilised by wider dispersal. The cause of this may be that, whilst dispersal reduces reactivity, it relatively favours reaction with the anion, because the latter can, better than a neutral molecule would, collect the dispersed charge; *i.e.*, the anion can make better use of the polarisability of the carbonium ion.

(32e) Molecularity of Fast Steps of the Unimolecular Mechanism.—Consider the formulated unimolecular solvolytic substitution, having the component processes (1), (2), and (3), with process (1) slow, and (2) and (3) fast:

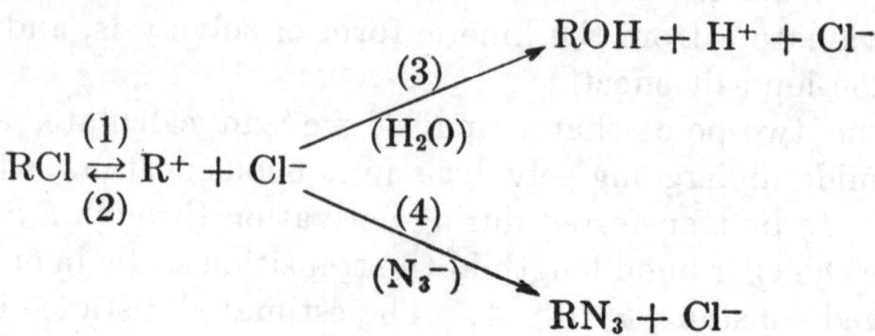

By taking into account the possible presence of the anionic reagent needed for the further fast process (4), we may consider simultaneously the non-solvolytic substitution involving processes (1), (2), and (4). The advantage of doing this is that we then have an observationally distinctive process (4), of the same general type as process (2), whose competition with the other fast processes can be studied.

A large amount of evidence that process (1) is unimolecular, in the sense of our general definition of molecularity (Section **27e**), has been reviewed in the preceding Sections.

We can now go a long way towards proving that process (2), and likewise process (4), are bimolecular. For, as described in Section **29b**, the proportion of alkyl azide formed has been found so to vary, when the concentration of azide ions is altered, as to show, first, that process (4) is unimolecular with respect to azide ions and, secondly, that process (4) has the same molecularity, presumably first, as have all the competing fast processes with respect to the carbonium ion. The conclusion is that process (4), and, by analogy, process (2), are bimolecular. As to process (2), this is confirmed, as we shall note below, by quantitative considerations concerning the kinetic form of the purely solvolytic substitution.

Furthermore, we can show that the ionic recombination processes (2) and (4) have a finite activation energy, as they should according to the theory of ionisation illustrated in Fig. 27-1 (p. 425), even though we cannot yet do better quantitatively than to secure lower limits to the actual values. It is necessary to measure the temperature coefficient of the degree of intervention of a non-common-ion in the reaction, or the temperature coefficient of the rate depression produced by an added common-ion. For example, Hawdon, Hughes, and the writer[122] have studied the hydrolysis of *pp'*-dimethylbenzhy-

[122] A. R. Hawdon, E. D. Hughes, and C. K. Ingold, *J. Chem. Soc.*, 1952, 2499.

dryl chloride in aqueous acetone, in the presence of sodium azide, over a temperature range, measuring the separate rates of production of the alcohol and of the alkyl azide. From the results one may calculate, using the Arrhenius equation, the energy of activation of process (1), and the difference $E_A^{(4)} - E_A^{(3)}$ between the energies of activation of processes (4) and (3). This difference was found to be a positive quantity (4.0 and 3.9 kcal./mole in "90%" and "85%" aqueous acetone, respectively). Thus, although we do not yet know whether process (3) has a finite activation energy, we can at least conclude that process (4) has one of not less than 4 kcal./mole. A similar conclusion is derived for process (2).

We may now consider[119] the molecularity of process (3). The basis of discussion is that any quantitative interpretation of the kinetics of unimolecular solvolysis, as influenced by both ionic-strength and mass-law effects, for instance, the kinetics illustrated in Fig. 32-2, must depend on the molecularities of *all* the component processes. This is so, because ionic strength alters overall rate, not only by changing the rate of the slow process (1), but also by so influencing the fast processes (2) and (3) as to affect the proportion in which formed carbonium ion is partitioned between them; and the ionic-strength effect on any process depends on the constitution of its transition state, and therefore on its molecularity. Now in view of what is stated above, we may take it that processes (1) and (2) are unimolecular and bimolecular, respectively, and that process (3) is unimolecular with respect to carbonium ion. What remains to be determined is the molecularity of process (3) with respect to water; and hence we may use the quantitative form of solvolysis kinetics in order to investigate this remaining character of the unimolecular mechanism of solvolysis.

The two most obvious hypotheses which present themselves for trial are (I) that process (3) is unimolecular with respect to water, and (II) that it is multimolecular with respect to water. Hypothesis (I) implies a transition state $(R \cdots OH_2)^+$, which, like R^+, will have an activity coefficient given by Debye's limiting law (Section **32b**). This leads to wholly incorrect kinetic forms, to which observational data, such as are illustrated in Fig. 32-2, could not possibly be fitted. Hypothesis (II) implies a transition state $[R \cdots (OH_2)_n]^+$ with n large: its most important kinetic feature is the large spatial (three-dimensional) diffusion of positive charge. This means that we cannot calculate its activity coefficient by Debye's limiting law. Because of the large diffusion of charge, the extra factor, which enters into the more general Debye-Hückel law applicable to it, will cause its activity coefficient to approximate more closely to unity. This assumption gives rate curves of the correct form; and it is in this approximation that the theoretical rate curves have been calculated with which the observations, such as are illustrated by the points in Fig. 32-2, have been compared.

The conclusion that process (3) is multimolecular with respect to water agrees with elementary intuition. It seems natural that a carbonium ion, formed within an aqueous solvation shell, should react with water by collapse of the shell, an occurrence needing little energy, but, because of its high molecularity, involving a large negative entropy. It does not seem reasonable that the carbonium ion should require a single high-energy water molecule, coming from without, as an attacking anion might, to break through the inner shell of already available water molecules.

The finding of multimolecularity in process (3) is also specifically supported by studies of the product compositions which result when a carbonium ion is attacked competitively by an anion and by water. It was mentioned in Section **29b** that the proportion of occasions in which the *pp′*-dimethylbenzhydryl cation, when present in various aqueous acetone solvents containing the same concentration of azide ions, will end its life to give alcohol, is independent of the concentration of the water. This shows that the reactive assembly is the carbonium ion with its aqueous solvation shell, not the carbonium ion and a kinetically independent water molecule.

(32f) Salt Effects on Unimolecular Substitutions in Solution in Sulphur Dioxide.—In this solvent, as we noted in Section **28c**, benzhydryl chloride undergoes substitution by triethylamine, pyridine, and fluoride ion, at similar rates; and *m*-chlorobenzhydryl chloride undergoes substitution by pyridine, iodide ion, and fluoride ion, at similar rates. The presumption is that all these substitutions are unimolecular. The kinetics of one of them, that of the reaction between fluoride ion, introduced as tetramethylammonium fluoride, and *m*-chlorobenzhydryl chloride, has been investigated in some detail.[123] It can be followed over a considerable proportion of its course without disturbance from reversibility. It shows a somewhat large accelerative, ionic-strength effect, and an enormous, retarding, mass-law effect. We may write the reaction,

$$\mathrm{RCl} \underset{(2)}{\overset{(1)}{\rightleftarrows}} \mathrm{R^+ + Cl^-} \xrightarrow[(3)]{\mathrm{F^-}} \mathrm{RF + Cl^-}$$

The accelerative effect of a non-common-ion salt may be illustrated

[123] L. C. Bateman, E. D. Hughes, and C. K. Ingold, *J. Chem. Soc.*, **1940**, 1017.

by the result that 0.05M tetraethylammonium fluoride substitutes at three times the limiting rate for low salt concentrations. As an example of the strong retarding effect of a common-ion salt, initially added tetraethylammonium chloride in 0.047M concentration reduced the initial rate of substitution by fluoride ion by a factor of 1/150. In the absence of an initially added saline chloride, the chloride ion formed by substitution retards that process so strongly that a reaction that starts rapidly is soon going very slowly. These very large mass-law effects measure the weakness of the competition which the solute substituting species presents to the common ion, relatively to the competition presented by a hydroxylic solvent, with which we see the common ion successfully coping in solvolytic substitutions. The main significance of these studies is to emphasize that the diagnostic characteristics of the unimolecular mechanism in solvolysis are by no means exclusively confined to solvolysis.

(32g) Salt Effects on Unimolecular-Type Solvolysis in Acetic Acid.—The key to the understanding of salt effects in acetic acid is the great range of electrostatic forces in that solvent. Its dielectric constant is about 6. In this solvent, two univalent counter-ions attract each other with an energy equal to the mean kinetic energy of either along a line at a separation of 150 A. At the usual practical salt concentrations, the ions, even if evenly distributed, would be closer together than that, and hence they must, for the most part, fall together as pairs or other aggregates of shorter force range. It has been known[124] since the 1930's that salts do exist in acetic acid essentially as ion pairs, in equilibrium with small proportions of simple ion and triplet ions, and perhaps also quadruplets.

The defining of an ion pair is a semi-semantic problem, rather like deciding at what point in the opening of a door it shall no longer be called "ajar." Bjerrum took, as a convenient separation at which to draw the boundary between ion pairs and dissociated ions, the separation, with a coulombic energy of $2\boldsymbol{k}T$, at which there are fewer pairs of counter-ions than at any other separation.[125] For a 1-1 electrolyte in acetic acid, this separation is 40 A: any two counter-ions closer together than that form an ion pair. For lower separations, down to touching, the number of ion pairs increases on a steepening curve. Thus the door of dissociation in acetic acid is not restricted to being closed or open, but can be ajar to a continuous distribution of extents, each Boltzmann-populated extent having its proper chemical

[124] I. M. Kolthoff and A. Willman, *J. Am. Chem. Soc.*, 1934, **56**, 1007; cf. M. M. Jones and E. Griswold, *ibid.*, 1954, **76**, 3247.

[125] N. Bjerrum, *Kgl. danske Vidensk. Selskab., Mat.-fys. Medd.*, 1926, **7**, No. 9.

and electrochemical activity, and all measurements being of appropriate averages.

Winstein and his associates have studied salt effects on the solvolysis in acetic acid of alkyl halides and arenesulphonates, for which there is stereochemical evidence (Section **33**) of a unimolecular type of mechanism, *i.e.*, one depending on preliminary ionisation of the substrate, irrespective of ionic dissociation.[126] They have described two kinds of salt effect. All substrates exhibited a "normal" salt effect, the rate rising linearly with salt concentration, often to quite high concentrations, *e.g.*, 0.1*M* of salt. Many substrates, *e.g.*, neophyl and pinacolyl halides or arenesulphonates, showed no other salt effect. A few substrates, *e.g.*, 1-*p*-anisyl-2-propyl toluene-*p*-sulphonate, showed additionally a "special" salt effect, *i.e.*, a sharp acceleration by the first $10^{-3}M$ of salt, curving off at about $3\times10^{-3}M$ into the "normal," much milder, and essentially linear effect. These phenomena and definitions are graphically illustrated in Figs. 32-3, 32-4, and 32-5, by reference to a subsequent detailed study of the special salt effect, by Topsom,[127] using the substrate cholesteryl toluene-*p*-sulphonate.

Winstein found that the "special" effect of lithium perchlorate on the solvolysis of an alkyl arenesulphonate was suppressed by introducing, in addition, the common-ion salt, lithium arenesulphonate, and that the latter salt, if used alone, could produce a rate lower than

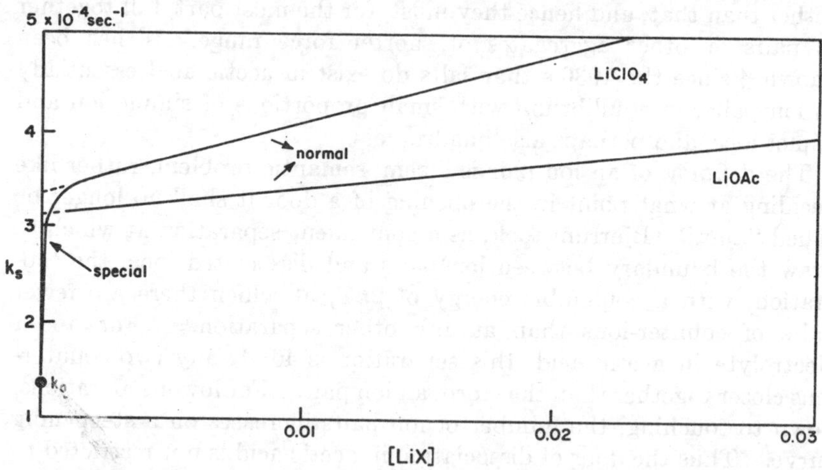

FIG. 32-3.—Rates of solvolysis of cholesteryl toluene-*p*-sulphonate at 50.2° in acetic acid containing salts.

[126] S. Winstein *et al.*, about twenty papers in *J. Am. Chem. Soc.*, since *ibid.*, 1954, **76**, 2597.

[127] R. D. Topsom, Thesis, London, 1959; A. D. Topsom, C. K. Ingold, and Y. Pocker, forthcoming paper.

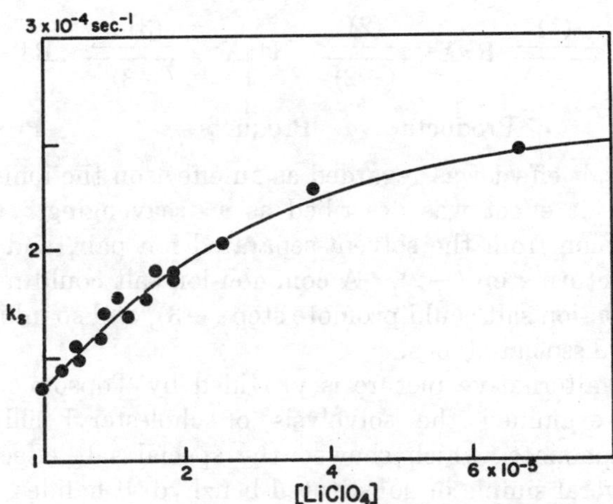

FIG. 32-4.—Left-hand part of the curve for $LiClO_4$ in Fig. 32-3 on a much expanded scale, *viz.*, ordinates ×2, and abscissae ×250.

the salt-free rate. His interpretation assumed the substrate to undergo ionic dissociation in separate steps to form, first, an "intimate" ion pair, written R^+X^-, then a "solvent-separated" ion pair, written $R^+\|X^-$ and assumed to have a monomolecular solvent layer between the ions, and finally, dissociated ions, three discrete species in equilibrium, any of which could be attacked by the solvent:

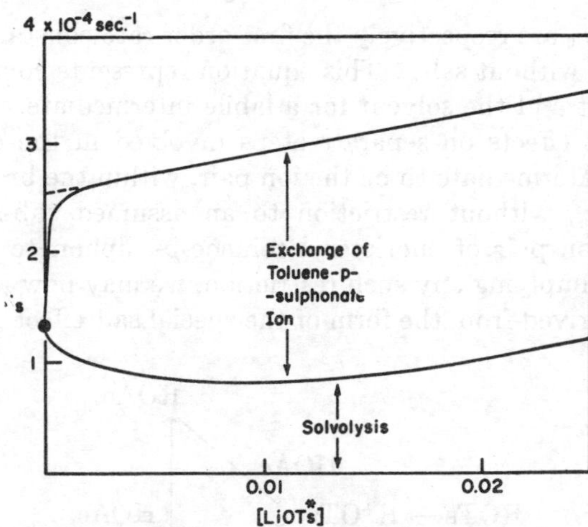

FIG. 32-5.—Rates of solvolysis and anion-exchange of cholesteryl toluene-*p*-sulphonate at 50.2° in acetic acid containing lithium radio-toluene-*p*-sulphonate.

$$\mathrm{RX} \underset{(-1)}{\overset{(1)}{\rightleftharpoons}} \mathrm{R^+}X^- \underset{(-2)}{\overset{(2)}{\rightleftharpoons}} \mathrm{R^+}\|X^- \underset{(-3)}{\overset{(3)}{\rightleftharpoons}} \mathrm{R^+} + X^-$$

$$\begin{array}{ccc} \downarrow & \downarrow & \downarrow \\ \text{Products} & \text{Products} & \text{Products} \end{array}$$

The normal salt effect was regarded as an effect on the ionisation (1). The special salt effect was described as a "scavenging," which displaced the anion from the solvent-separated ion pair, and thus suppressed the return step (−2). A common-ion salt could not do this. But a common-ion salt could promote step (−3), and so inhibit solvolysis through dissociated ions.

A possible alternative picture is provided by Topsom's investigation.[127] He examined the solvolysis of cholesteryl chloride and toluene-*p*-sulphonate, which showed the special salt effect, and he examined several simple or substituted benzhydryl halides, which did not do so. He studied four kinds of salts, non-common-ion salts which do not give a stable product different from the solvolysis product, non-common-ion salts which do give their own distinctive product, common-ion salts, and lyate-ion salts.

The form of the special salt effect of salts, such as lithium perchlorate, which do not give a distinctive product, was as illustrated for the solvolysis of cholesteryl toluene-*p*-sulphonate in Fig. 32-4. In the lower range of the special salt effect, the data fitted the equation

$$\frac{1}{k_s - k_0} = a + \frac{b}{[\text{salt}]}$$

where k_s and k_0 are respectively the first-order rate-constants of solvolysis with and without salt. This equation represents competition between the salt and the solvent for a labile intermediate. It does not allow for salt effects on separate steps involved in the competition. Taking this intermediate to be the ion pair, within the broad Bjerrum definition, *i.e.*, without restriction to an assumed sub-species, and writing the ion pair of cholesteryl toluene-*p*-sulphonate as R^+OTs^-, without now implying any such restriction, we may now represent the conclusion derived from the form of the special salt effect as follows:

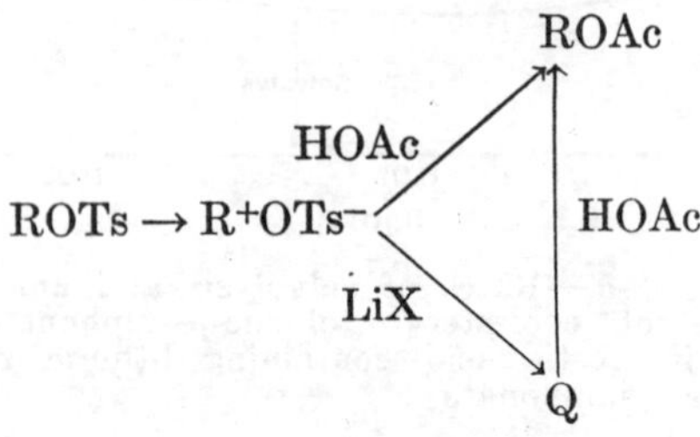

where Q is another labile intermediate, the nature of which has still to be considered.

The other classes of salts fell essentially into the same pattern. Non-common-ion salts giving a distinctive product, for example, lithium chloride in the solvolysis of cholesteryl toluene-*p*-sulphonate, fell into the pattern, if one reckoned with the total conversion of substrate, adding, in this example, the production of cholesteryl chloride to that of cholesteryl acetate. Common-ion salts, for example, lithium toluene-*p*-sulphonate in the same solvolyses, likewise conformed to the pattern, as is illustrated in Fig. 32-5, if one isotopically marked the toluene-*p*-sulphonate ion in the salt, and added the isotopic exchange rate to the solvolysis rate. The same kind of special salt effect was obtained with the lyate-ion salt, lithium acetate.

By examining the special salt effects of the salts added in pairs, Topsom was able to determine their relative rates of attack on the labile intermediate. He obtained, for instance, the following relative rates in the solvolysis of cholesteryl toluene-*p*-sulphonate:

LiOAc 70, LiBr 20, LiCl 10, $LiClO_4$ 4, LiOTs 1.

When the substrate was changed to cholesteryl chloride, the figures were different, and even the order of the salts was different. This is consistent with the identification of the labile intermediate as the carbonium ion pair; evidently it could not be the dissociated cholesterylium ion. In terms of the competition scheme, these experiments, in contrast to those next to be considered, bear on the formation (not the reactions) of the intermediate called Q.

By extrapolation of the linear normal salt effect, as illustrated in Fig. 32-3, Topsom could determine rates as they would be maximally accelerated by the special salt effect in the absence of the normal salt effect. Using the same illustration, that of cholesteryl toluene-*p*-sulphonate, the salt-free solvolysis rate of which (in 10^{-5} sec.$^{-1}$ at 50.2°) is 13.2, the extrapolated salt-accelerated rates were variously larger, *viz.*,

$LiClO_4$ 33.2, LiOAc 31.0, LiBr 28.5, LiCl 27.5, LiOTs 25.0

It will be understood that the extrapolations were of rates of total conversion of substrate, when more than one product was formed. The fact that all the figures are different shows that maximal special accelerations are not to be explained by total suppression of a common retrograde step, as in Winstein's scheme. The further fact that the maximal accelerations do not parallel the competitive efficiencies of the salts shows that the former are at least in part dependent on some other step than the formation of the intermediate Q. This must be a subsequent step, and it is taken to be the step of conversion of Q to products. Thus the idea is reached that that step may in some way share with the initial ionisation the task of rate control.

Topsom found that small additions of nitromethane to the acetic acid solvent selectively suppressed the special salt effects, so confirming that the latter arise as a special consequence of the low dielectric constant of acetic acid.

The idea that, in solvents admitting high penetration by electrostatic forces, a unimolecular-type mechanism can exist in which a further step of reaction participates in the overall rate-control, had been reached somewhat earlier, on quite different evidence, in reference to nucleophilic substitutions in the still less polar solvent, benzene.[128] Topsom used a similar scheme for solvent acetic acid, hypothetically identifying his intermediate Q as an ionic aggregate, termed a quadruplet, which has to undergo an activated geometrical reorganisation in order to admit a new path to final products. In the scheme,

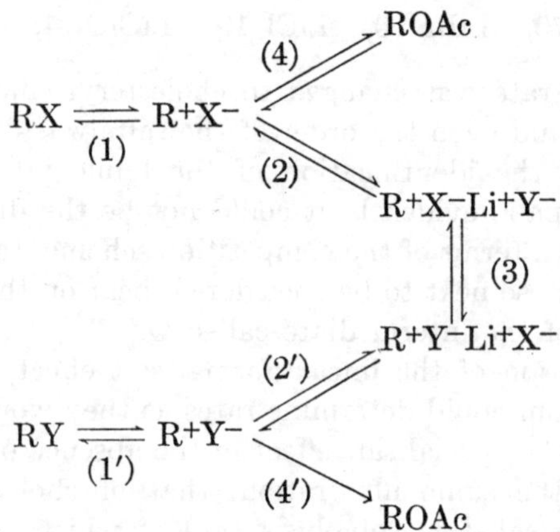

all steps may be significantly activated, except steps (2) and (2′), which are mainly diffusion-controlled, and are practically instantaneous by reason of the long range of electrostatic forces in the medium. In the circumstances in which we observe a special salt effect, the peaks A, B, and B' of the schematic free-energy diagram of Fig. 32-6 for the special salt effect of a common-ion salt are taken to be near enough to one another in height to allow them to be traversed comparably even though unequally. If B and therefore B' had been much lower than A, the mechanism would be S_N1 without any special

[128] E. D. Hughes, C. K. Ingold, S. F. Mok, S. Patai, and Y. Pocker, *J. Chem. Soc.*, **1957**, 1265; C. K. Ingold, *Proc. Chem. Soc.*, **1957**, 279.

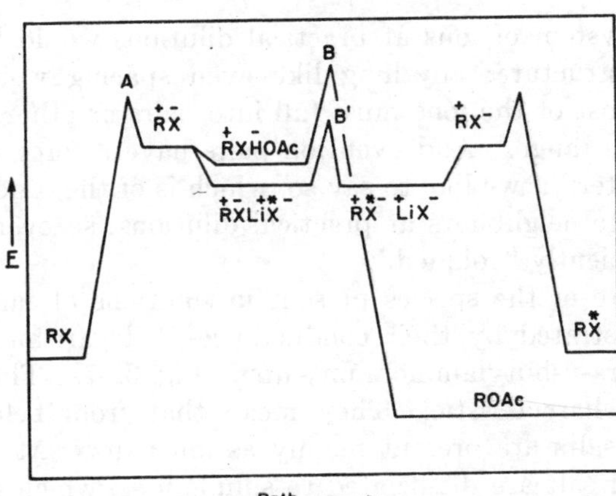

FIG. 32-6.—Schematic representation of free energy *versus* reaction co-ordinate, according to a theory of the special salt effect in S_N1-type solvolysis in acetic acid: the case of a common-ion salt.

salt effect. If *B′* and therefore *B* had been much higher than *A*, the mechanism would be $S_N2(C^+)$, as described for solvent nitromethane in Section **29c**. The special salt effect may therefore be described as a mechanism intermediate between S_N1 and $S_N2(C^+)$.

It is speculated that the resistance to the reorganisation (3) of the first-formed quadruplet, in order to bring it into the configuration that provides another path to products, arises from the electrostatic work needed to loosen the touching counter-ions sufficiently to permit their redisposition.

(32h) Salt Effects on Unimolecular-Type Substitution in Benzene.—In this solvent we have no solvolysis, and our reactions are of substitution by solute nucleophiles. Once again, the key to heterolytic mechanism is the great penetrating power of electrostatic forces in the solvent, the dielectric constant of which is 2.25. The mass-law of chemical kinetics depends on the statistics of encounters of independent particles, that is, of particles which, nearly all the time, are outside each other's force range. With highly polar solutes in benzene, this condition is rarely fulfilled. The interacting particles are frequently not independent, and in their regard our basic thinking on kinetics has to be changed.

Two univalent counter-ions attract each other in benzene with an energy equal to the mean kinetic energy of either along a line at a separation of 500 *A*. In the language of the collision theory of kinetics, their collision diameters are of the order of 500 *A*. The separations of solute neighbours at most practical dilutions are of order 50 *A*.

Clearly, a system of ions at practical dilutions would be an already "collided" structure: anything like even spacing would be highly unstable: most of the ions must fall into pairs or other aggregates of shorter force range. And even ion pairs have a force range, a "collision diameter" if we like to say so, which is of the order of the spacings of solute neighbours at practical dilutions: so even the ion-pair state is incipiently "collided."

The nature of the species present in solutions of salts in benzene may be illustrated by their conductances,[129] logarithmically plotted for some tetra-*n*-butylammonium salts in Fig. 32-7. The forms of the curves are characteristic. They mean that from below $10^{-5}M$ to $10^{-2}M$, the salts are present mainly as ion pairs. At $10^{-5}M$, a few millionths of salt are dissociated to simple ions, which carry most of the current: if they carried it all, the slope of the plot would be $-\frac{1}{2}$. At $10^{-4}M$, simple ions are adding to the pairs, to give triplet ions, again to the extent of a few millionths of the total salt; and now the triplet ions are carrying the greater part of the current: if they carried it all, the slope of the plot would be $+\frac{1}{2}$. (Lines of slopes $\pm\frac{1}{2}$ are included in the diagram.) But before this happens, the triplet ions themselves are becoming replaced by uncharged ion quadruplets; and so, near $10^{-3}M$, the gradient slackens. Finally, near $10^{-2}M$, charged aggregates higher than quadruplets are formed in increasing quantities. The small amounts of single and triplet ions create few notable kinetic effects. However, above $10^{-2}M$, when high aggregates become plentiful, simple kinetics in reactions of salts are not to be expected.

Two special kinetic situations can be envisaged as a result of working with a collided state.[128] The more interesting is this. When a substrate RX is ionised to an ion pair R^+X^- in benzene containing a reactive salt M^+Y^- in moderate concentration, the carbonium ion pair will not have to await a chance encounter as a condition for its reaction: the saline reagent will be already in its force range, present in effect from the moment of its birth. The encounter probability is unity, and an increase in reagent concentration cannot improve that. But if, as explained for the special salt effect in acetic acid (Section **32g**) the reactants, after first contact, have to undergo an activated redisposition of their constituent ions before the latter can covalently react, then the rate, without depending on the concentration of the reagent as we have seen, may depend on its identity, because the re-

[129] R. M. Fuoss and C. A. Krauss, *J. Am. Chem. Soc.*, 1933, **55**, 2387, 3614; 1935, **57**, 1; E. D. Hughes, C. K. Ingold, S. Patai, and Y. Pocker, *J. Chem. Soc.*, **1957**, 1206.

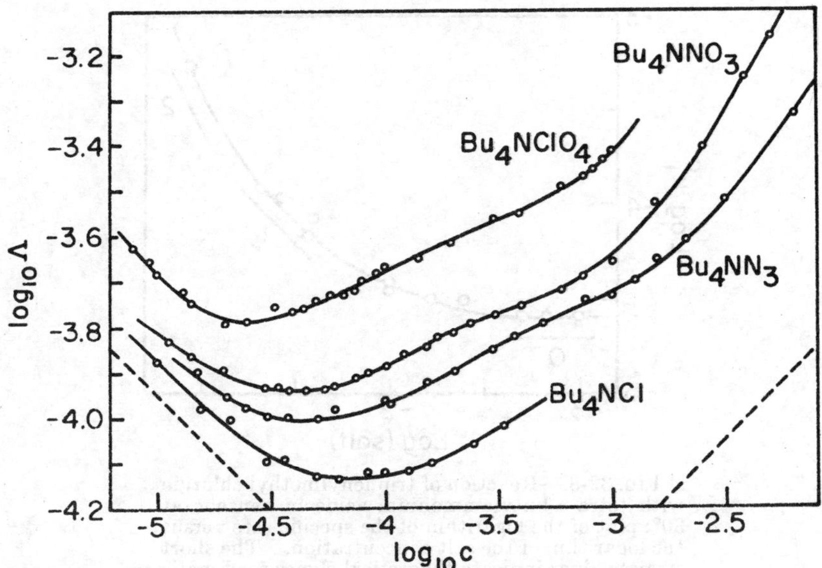

FIG. 32-7.—Electrical conductances of salts in benzene: plots of log Λ versus log *c*, and theoretical slopes for single and triple ions singly in equilibrium with a large excess of ion pairs. (Reproduced with permission from *J. Chem. Soc.*, **1957**, 1209.)

agent is present in what may be a kinetically significant second activation. It is a rider on this conclusion that, if we have a mixture of reactive salts, M^+Y^- and M^+Z^-, the rate of reaction with either will be reduced with its mole-fraction, and accordingly the total rate will change nearly linearly with salt composition (though it will not change with total salt concentration) from M^+Y^- to M^+Z^-. Such combinations of kinetic independence of reactant concentration with dependence on reactant identity are unknown among reactions in highly polar solvents. They could arise only in a collided state, and probably only then with reactants of suitable polarity and sterochemistry.

The second expected consequence of the great force range in benzene is widespread electrostatic catalysis, of no fixed kinetic order. Polar ambient species will exert their kinetic effect on a polar transition state, in various numbers, from various positions, including noncontiguous positions, which need not be specifically prescribed. It can be estimated that such catalysis by ambient ion pairs should become important at about $10^{-2}M$, and increasingly so at higher concentrations. We have, however, no quantitative theory of this form of catalysis.

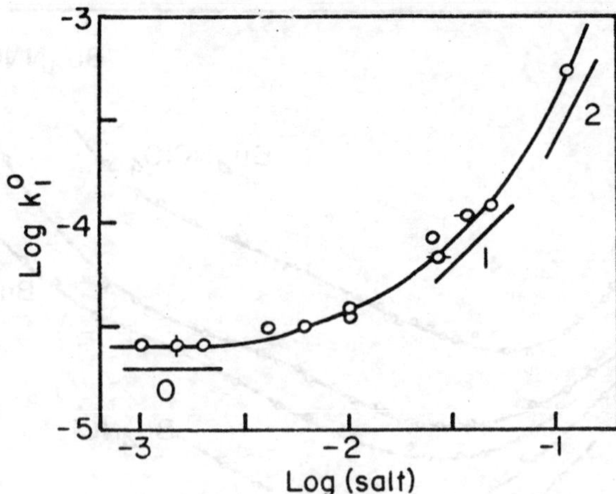

FIG. 32-8.—Reaction of triphenylmethyl chloride with tetra-*n*-butylammonium azide in benzene at 30°: plot of the logarithm of the specific rate versus the logarithm of the salt concentration. The short straight lines indicate theoretical slopes for kinetic orders of 0, 1, and 2 with respect to the saline reagent. (Reproduced with permission from *J. Chem. Soc.*, **1957**, 1232.)

Both these expectations may be illustrated by nucleophilic substitutions in triphenylmethyl chloride in benzene (a) by tetra-*n*-butylammonium radiochloride, and (b) by tetra-*n*-butylammonium azide.[130] At concentrations below $10^{-2}M$ in salt, the substitutions are of first order in substrate, but of zeroth order in salt. The saline azide is soluble enough to allow the rate to be followed above $10^{-2}M$, and then we see electrostatic catalysis, the effective kinetic order rising smoothly with concentration as illustrated in Fig. 32-8. Strikingly, the *rates of zeroth order in salt are different for the two salts:* they are as noted below in 10^{-5} sec.$^{-1}$, for 30°:

$$Ph_3C\cdot Cl + Bu_4N^+\overset{*}{Cl}^- \rightarrow Ph_3C\cdot\overset{*}{Cl} + Bu_4N^+Cl^- \qquad (k_1 = 0.50)$$
$$Ph_3C\cdot Cl + Bu_4N^+N_3^- \rightarrow Ph_3C\cdot N_3^- + Bu_4N^+Cl^- \qquad (k_1 = 2.50)$$

For mixtures of the two reactive salts, the rates, still of zeroth order in total salt, vary with salt *composition*. Thus, for a 50:50 mixture in the above conditions, the specific rate of chloride exchange is 0.25,

[130] C. G. Swain and M. M. Kreevoy, *J. Am. Chem. Soc.*, 1955, **77,** 1122; E. D. Hughes, C. K. Ingold, S. F. Mok, S. Patai, and Y. Pocker, *J. Chem. Soc.*, **1957,** 1220; E. D. Hughes, C. K. Ingold, S. Patai, and Y. Pocker, *ibid.*, p. 1230.

one-half of that shown above, and that of the azide substitution is 1.25, again one-half of that shown, the total rate of conversion of substrate being 1.50 in the above units. Yet to double (say) the concentrations of *both* salts makes no difference either to the rates or to the product composition. The addition of salts, such as tetra-*n*-butylammonium perchlorate, which give no product, has no kinetic effect.

The interpretation which has been offered[128] is essentially as explained for special salt effects in acetic acid (Section **32g**). In these S_N1-type reactions with salts, an activated ionisation of RX gives an ion pair R^+X^-, which instantaneously attaches to itself the nearest saline ion pair to give a quadruplet, $R^+X^-M^+Y^-$. Quadruplet formation is unactivated, and, with different 1-1 salts, is more or less similarly exothermic. But the first-formed quadruplets have to undergo activated reorganisation in order to provide a disposition of the component ions, $R^+Y^-M^+X^-$, which will allow the covalency changes necessary to give products.:

$$\begin{array}{ccccc} RX & \rightleftharpoons & R^+X^- & \rightleftharpoons & R^+X^-M^+Y^- \\ & & & & \downarrow\uparrow \\ RY & \rightleftharpoons & R^+Y^- & \rightleftharpoons & R^+Y^-M^+X^- \end{array}$$

The second activation barrier, that of the quadruplet redisposition, gives a free-energy peak either a little higher or a little lower than the ionisation peak, so allowing different salts to react with different zeroth-order rates, as schematically illustrated in Fig. 32-9.[131] If the reorganisation peak were much higher, we should observe the second-order mechanism $S_N2(C^+)$. If it were much lower, we should have a straightforward S_N1 reaction with equal zeroth-order rates, as in polar solvents. Thus the concept of a second activation barrier presumes a mechanism intermediate between S_N1 and $S_N2(C^+)$. As before, the resistance to quadruplet reorganisation is taken to arise from the electrostatic work needed sufficiently to loosen touching counter-ions. A rough coulomb-law calculation in the example of chloride exchange has given 4 kcal./mole for the difference in peak heights. One suspects that this is an overestimate.

[131] C. G. Swain has objected that he could not redescribe the results by applying stationary-state theory to the interpretation (*J. Am. Chem. Soc.*, 1958, **80**, 816). S. Winstein has repeated the objection (*ibid.*, 1961, **83**, 893). However, it was made plain originally (1957) that a collided state is assumed, in which the systems are not independent, and the applicability of stationary-state theory is therefore not expected.

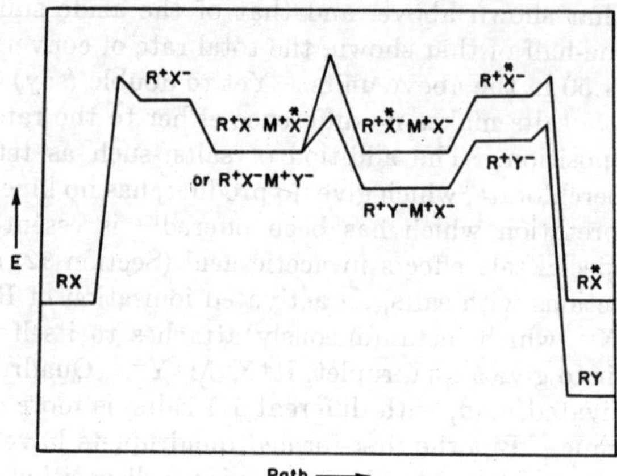

FIG. 32-9.—Schematic representation of free energy *versus* reaction co-ordinates, according to a theory of S_N1-type substitutions by saline reagents in benzene.

The observations are somewhat different with polar but molecular substituting agents, such as alcohols. Smoothly steepening logarithmic rate-curves are obtained, generally like that in Fig. 32-8, though there is some dubiety about the limiting slope at the lower extremity.[132] The non-common-ion non-product-forming salt, tetra-*n*-butylammonium perchlorate, accelerates these reactions. The common-ion salt, tetra-*n*-butylammonium chloride, represses this effect, and in the absence of the perchlorate, reduces the rate of alcoholysis below the salt-free rate. These phenomena are qualitatively similar to the special salt effect on solvolysis in acetic acid, though there seem to be some differences of functional form. It is nevertheless possible that they should be understood somewhat similarly.

[132] E. D. Hughes, C. K. Ingold, S. F. Mok, and Y. Pocker, *J. Chem. Soc.*, **1957**, 1238; E. D. Hughes, C. K. Ingold, S. Patai, and Y. Pocker, *ibid.*, p. 1256; C. G. Swain and E. E. Pegues, *J. Am. Chem. Soc.*, 1958, **80,** 812. The last-named authors showed that, in the presence of pyridine and other tertiary amines, and with methanol as the alcohol, the lower-limiting kinetic order in methanol is first. They regarded the methanol as attacking the free carbonium ion, but in view of the evidence (Section **29c**) that the latter, when spectrally visible, is instantly destroyed by pyridine, the attack may have been on the quaternary ammonium complex. On the other hand, the evidence for a lower order than first in methanol, in the absence of a tertiary amine, is not very strong, because the dilutions were so near the upper limit to which measurements could be made.

(33) STERIC ORIENTATION OF NUCLEOPHILIC SUBSTITUTION

(33a) The Problem of the Walden Inversion.[133]—In 1895 Walden[134] completed the following series of transformations, in which one optically active parent is converted by alternative genetic paths into either of two optical enantiomers:

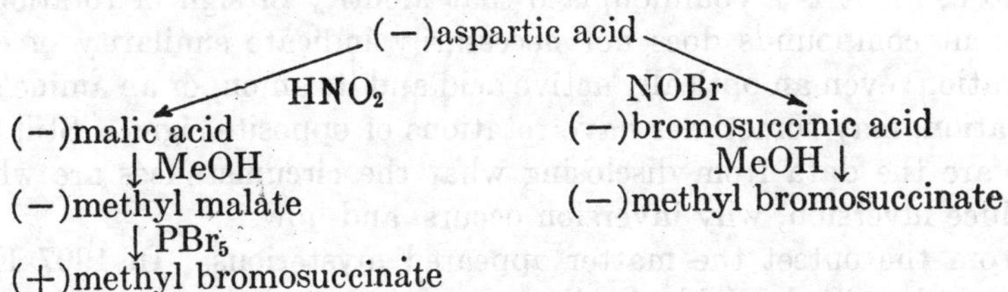

Soon afterwards he obtained, in the example formulated below, the same difference of result using alternative single processes of substitution; and he demonstrated, as the same scheme shows, the conversion of an optically active substance into its own enantiomer through two substitutions at the asymmetric centre:

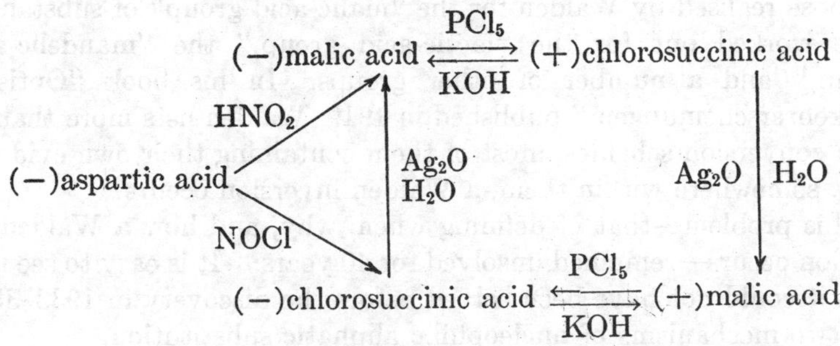

At least at one point in the first of these schemes, and at least at two in the second, a substitution must have occurred, during which the asymmetric atom and the three retained groups bound to it, go over into their enantiomeric configuration. Such an occurrence is called a *Walden inversion*, or an *optical inversion*. At least at two points in the second of the above schemes, a substitution at the asymmetric centre must have occurred in which the asymmetric atom and the three retained groups bound to it preserve their original configuration.

[133] Well-summarised accounts have been given by F. D. Chattaway and S. Smiles, *Ann. Repts. on Progress Chem.* (Chem. Soc. London), 1911, **8**, 60, by P. Frankland, *J. Chem. Soc.*, 1913, **103**, 717, and by P. Walden, "Optische Umkehrerscheinungen," Vieweg, Braunschweig, 1919.

[134] P. Walden, *Ber.*, 1895, **28**, 1287, 2766.

Thus inversion is not a universal concomitant of substitution. In fact, there are two kinds of substitution, those which invert configuration, and those which do not. A cyclic conversion scheme involving enantiomers is often called a *Walden cycle*.

Which of the above substitutions produce inversion, the data do not disclose; for it is a commonplace that identity of sign of rotation in different compounds does not necessarily indicate similarity of configuration: even an optically active acid and its anion, or an amine and its cation, may sometimes have rotations of opposite signs. Still further are the data from disclosing what the circumstances are which produce inversion, why inversion occurs, and how.

From the outset the matter appeared mysterious. In 1907 Emil Fischer described Walden's discovery as the most astonishing observation which had been made in the field of optical activity since the fundamental investigations of Pasteur. The mystery was not lessened by the discovery of many further examples during the succeeding decades, especially by Fischer himself and by McKenzie, mainly during the first decade of this century. Conversion schemes, similar to those realised by Walden for the "malic-acid group" of substances, were worked out for the "lactic-acid group," the "mandelic-acid group," and a number of other groups. In his book "Optische Umkehrerscheinungen," published in 1919, Walden lists more than 20 such conversion schemes, most of them containing their own evidence that, somewhere within them, a Walden inversion occurs.

This problem—that of defining when, why, and how a Walden inversion occurs—remained unsolved for 40 years. It is easy to see now that it could not have been solved before the discovery in 1933–35 of the two mechanisms of nucleophilic aliphatic substitution.

Ideally, the general problem can be broken down into two problems, demanding successive solution. First, one should rigorously correlate the configurations of the factors and products of substitutions at an asymmetric centre. Then, having the ability to identify Walden inversions, one ought to be able to discern the circumstances producing them, and hence to discover their mechanism. The following account is divided accordingly; but it should be explained that inevitably the two stages become a little mixed together, inasmuch as the most rigorous of the available methods of solving the correlation problem depends on knowing the solution of the mechanistic problem: therefore at the outset we have to proceed from a reasonably reliable, but not rigorous, method of handling the correlation question, only afterwards returning to add the safeguards which are necessary in order to elevate it to a rigorous procedure.

(33b) Correlation of Configuration.—The earliest attempts to assign relative configurations to the factor and product of a substitution were based on theories of the mechanism of substitution. Walden regarded the hydroxylation of a halogen compound by alkali hydroxide as a simpler reaction than hydroxylation by moist silver oxide, which he suspected of forming a molecular compound with the organic substance; and accordingly he assumed that the alkali hydroxide substitutes with retention of configuration, while silver oxide produces inversion.[135] Fischer, having noticed that some halogeno-acids give the same optical isomer when hydroxylated with alkali hydroxide, whether in the form of the halogeno-acids themselves or as their esters or amides, whereas when hydroxylated with silver oxide they give one enantiomer if the carboxyl group is free but the other if it is protected, likewise concluded that alkali hydroxide retains configuration, while silver oxide, when acting on a free halogeno-acid, produces inversion.[136] All these conclusions are now known to be erroneous.

Frankland based many assignments of relative configuration on observed regularities in the effect of particular reagents in yielding products with signs of rotation like or unlike those of their factors. He assumed that when a reagent nearly always gives a product with a retained or inverted sign of rotation, then it is a characteristic of that reagent respectively to retain or to invert configuration.[137] A high proportion of Frankland's assignments are now known to be correct.

Clough suggested the guiding idea that compounds of similar configuration might be expected to undergo similar changes in rotatory power with variations in physical conditions, for instance, in medium, concentration, temperature, and wave-length.[138] Applied without due circumspection, this method has led to many erroneous assignments; but Freudenberg, who has made a thorough study of its limitations, has employed it with marked success.[139] Of those of his assignments which have been subsequently checked, nearly all have been found correct.

All these methods, however high their percentage success as we now know it, depended on principles the reliability of which could not be

[135] P. Walden, *Ber.*, 1899, **32**, 1848.

[136] E. Fischer, *Ber.*, 1907, **40**, 489.

[137] P. Frankland, *J. Chem. Soc.*, 1913, **103**, 717.

[138] G. W. Clough, *J. Chem. Soc.*, 1914, **105**, 49; 1915, **107**, 96, 1059; 1918, **113**, 526; 1926, 1674.

[139] K. Freudenberg, F. Brauns, and H. Siegel, *Ber.*, 1923, **56**, 193; K. Freudenberg and L. Markert, *Ber.*, 1927, **60**, 2447; K. Freudenberg and A. Lux, *Ber.*, 1928, **61**, 1083; K. Freudenberg and W. Kuhn, *Ber.*, 1931, **64**, 703.

proved; and hence none of the conclusions reached carried any sense of certainty. On a different plane stands the method of Kenyon and Phillips,[140] which may be explained by means of the following example relating to 2-octyl compounds. Of the four reactions represented below, one. if not three, must involve inversion: this follows from the overall result. The only one which could do so is the extrusion of the sulphonate group by the attack of acetate ions in solvent ethyl alcohol (reaction I), since this is the only reaction of the four which exchanges a bond of the asymmetric carbon:

$$(+)C_8H_{17}\cdot OH \xrightarrow{RSOCl} (+)C_8H_{17}\cdot O\cdot SOR \qquad\qquad (-)C_8H_{17}\cdot OH$$

$$\downarrow \text{Oxd.} \qquad\qquad\qquad \downarrow Ac_2O$$

$$\text{(Reaction I)} \ldots\ldots\ldots\ldots (+)C_8H_{17}\cdot O\cdot SO_2R \xrightarrow{\bar{O}Ac} (-)C_8H_{17}\cdot OAc$$

It is now assumed that an attack on the organic sulphonate by chloride ions in ethyl alcohol (reaction II) would proceed by a similar mechanism, and would therefore, like the attack by acetate ions, produce an inversion of configuration. It is found that the alkyl chloride produced by the action of chloride ions on the alkyl sulphonate has a rotation of sign opposite to that of the alcohol which is the parent of the sulphonate:

$$\text{(Reaction II)} \qquad (+)C_8H_{17}\cdot O\cdot SO_2R \xrightarrow[Cl^-]{} (-)C_8H_{17}\cdot Cl$$

It follows that 2-octyl alcohol and 2-octyl chloride, when they have like signs of rotation, have like configurations.

The weakest part of this argument is not really very weak: it is the unproved assumption of an analogy of behaviour between acetate ion and chloride ion. If we take a further step of the same kind, and assume analogy of behaviour between the octyl sulphonate and the octyl halides, then we reach (see Section **33c**) a demonstrably correct conclusion concerning the attack of (radioactively labelled) iodide ion on 2-octyl iodide (reaction III): by comparing the rate of gain of radio-

[140] H. Phillips, *J. Chem. Soc.*, 1923, **123**, 44; J. Kenyon, H. Phillips, and H. G. Turley, *ibid.*, 1925, **127**, 399; A. J. H. Houssa, J. Kenyon, and H. Phillips, *ibid.*, **1929,** 1700; J. Kenyon and H. Phillips, *Trans. Faraday Soc.*, 1930, **26,** 451; J. Kenyon, H. Phillips, and F. M. H. Taylor, *J. Chem. Soc.*, **1933,** 173; J. Kenyon, H. Phillips, and V. P. Pittman, *ibid.*, **1935,** 1072; J. Kenyon, H. Phillips, and G. R. Shutt, *ibid.*, p. 1663; C. M. Bean, J. Kenyon, and H. Phillips, *ibid.*, **1936,** 303; E. D. Hughes, C. K. Ingold, and S. Masterman, *ibid.*, **1937,** 1196; E. D. Hughes, C. K. Ingold, and A. D. Scott, *ibid.*, p. 1201. Cf. A. H. J. Houssa and H. Phillips *J. Chem. Soc.*, **1932,** 108; M. B. Hayford, J. Kenyon and H. Phillips, *ibid.*, **1933,** 179.

activity with the rate of loss of optical activity by the organic halide, it has been shown (Section **33d**) that every molecular act of substitution inverts configuration:

$$\text{(Reaction III)} \qquad (+)C_8H_{17}\cdot I \xrightarrow[I^-]{} (-)C_8H_{17}\cdot I$$

As we shall see in the following Sections, what is required in order to render this method completely rigorous is something which it is quite easy to supply, namely, a kinetic proof that the reactions treated as analogous are all bimolecular processes.

In earlier times, before any absolute configurations were known, enantiomers had to be assigned space models relatively to an arbitrary assignment, made by Fischer, of space models to a standard substance, chosen by him to be glyceraldehyde. By this convention, the enantiomers of glyceraldehyde having (+)- and (−)-rotations are described as D- (dextro) and L- (laevo), respectively, and are given the configurations represented below by Fischer's method of projection (in which laterally projected groups are in front of, and others are behind, the plane of projection):

$$\begin{array}{ccc} & CHO & \\ & | & \\ H - & | & - OH \\ & | & \\ & CH_2OH & \end{array} \qquad\qquad \begin{array}{ccc} & CHO & \\ & | & \\ HO - & | & - H \\ & | & \\ & CH_2OH & \end{array}$$

$$(+) = \text{D} = (R) \qquad\qquad (-) = \text{L} = (S)$$

For the general asymmetric centre, a one-to-one correlation between the four groups about it and the four about the asymmetric centre of glyceraldehyde is assumed; and then the general asymmetric centre is described, irrespective of its optical rotation, as D or L according as the correlated glyceraldehyde would be D or L by the above convention.

Today, most of the well-known, optically active, organic compounds have been configuratively correlated with glyceraldehyde, and hence with one another. This has been done by the establishment of generic connections through chains of processes, in which either a group is changed without disturbing any bond of the asymmetric atom, or such a bond is exchanged in a reaction of known mechanism and known stereochemistry, as we shall explain in Section **33d**.[141]

[141] The first major step, taken in 1950, was to correlate the configurations of glyceraldehyde, which had up to then been essentially the reference substance for carbohydrates and their derivatives, with those of serine, which had been the

All that we need to know in order to specify the steric course of a reaction is the relative configurations of factor and product. We shall often in the sequel employ the symbols D and L, which signify relative configuration, for the purpose of describing the steric course of a substitution.

In fact, we usually know the absolute configurations of the substances involved. Fischer's assignment of configurations to glyceraldehyde was arbitrary, and had even chances of being right. But it *was* right. Bijvoet showed this[142] by an X-ray method in 1951. From this, it follows that, whenever we know a chain of correlations of configuration going back to glyceraldehyde, we know the absolute configurations.

It is often more convenient to specify absolute than to specify relative configurations. The difficulty about generalising the specification of relative configurations is that of prescribing the particular one-to-one correlation which is to be assumed between the four groups about a general asymmetric centre and the four about the asymmetric centre of glyceraldehyde. Absolute configurations are specified by the *sequence rule.*[143] For an asymmetric atom Cabcd, the groups abcd are set in order of decreasing atomic numbers of their first atoms, or, where this makes no distinction, of their second, and so on; and then the configuration is described as *R* (rectus) and *S* (sinister) according as the path a→b→c turns to right or left, as seen from the side of the model remote from d. In glyceraldehyde the sequence is OH, CHO, CH_2OH, H, the O of CHO counting twice because it is doubly bound. The absolute configurational symbols follow as sh own above. This system is extensible to all organic molecules which have the property of *chirality* (handedness), and hence the potentiality of optical activity, whether or not they contain an asymmetric atom, and whether or not the molecule is asymmetric as a whole. Chirality is compatible with a limited amount of symmetry, namely, with the possession of rotational axes of symmetry without restriction as to their multi-

---

independent reference substance for amino-acids and their derivatives. This link between the two standards brought great families of compounds within a single system of correlation (P. Brewster, E. D. Hughes, C. K. Ingold, and P. A. D. Rao, *Nature*, 1950, **166**, 178). Since then, most of the terpenes, the steroids, several groups of alkaloids, and a miscellany of other compounds have seen brought into the same unified correlation.

[142] B. J. Bijvoet, A. F. Peerdeman, and A. J. van Bommel, *Nature*, 1951, **168**, 271.

[143] R. S. Cahn and C. K. Ingold, *J. Chem. Soc.*, 1951, 612. R. S. Cahn, C. K. Ingold, and V. Prelog, *Experientia*, 1956, **12**, 81; *Angew. Chem. internat. Edit.*, 1966, **4**, 385.

plicity or number. A structure with chirality is called *chiral*, and one without it *achiral*.

(33c) Substitution Mechanism and Steric Orientation.—Most of the earlier theories of the steric course of substitution, notably those of Fischer,[144] Werner,[145] and Pfeiffer,[146] postulate the prior formation of an addition product, in which the entering group attaches itself to the asymmetric atom either on the side of the group to be replaced or on the opposite side. The theories of Gadamer[147] and Meisenheimer[148] are elaborated forms of the same type of view.

The idea that the attachment of the incoming group and the separation of the displaced group might be synchronous seems to have been first expressed by Le Bel.[149] But Lewis first explained how a Walden inversion might thus be effected.[150] This concept was developed by Olson and Long,[151] who concluded that every substitution in which only one bond is altered involves inversion; and by Meer and Polanyi,[152] who distinguished between substitutions dependent on attack by anions and cations, the former being supposed to produce inversion, and the latter retention of configuration.

The remaining mechanistic alternative, that of prior dissociation, was assumed by Lowry,[153] who suggested that substitution through an intermediate carbonium ion might proceed with predominating retention of form; and also by Kenyon and Phillips,[154] who supposed, on the contrary, that it would tend to produce inversion. Both interpretations assume that substitutions would be completed before the carbonium ion has had time to assume an effectively planar configuration.

When it became clear that duplexity of mechanism is general for nucleophilic aliphatic substitution, Hughes and the writer began employing the theory of synchronous addition and dissociation, and that of

[144] E. Fischer, *Ann.*, 1911, **381,** 126.

[145] A. Werner, *Ber.*, 1911, **44,** 873; *Ann.*, 1912, **386, 70.**

[146] P. Pfeiffer, *Ann.*, 1911, **383,** 123.

[147] J. Gadamer, *J. prakt. Chem.*, 1913, **87,** 372.

[148] J. Meisenheimer, *Ann.*, 1927, **456,** 126.

[149] J.-A. Le Bel, *J. chim. phys.*, 1911, **9,** 323.

[150] G. N. Lewis, "Valence and the Structure of Atoms and Molecules," p. 113.

[151] A. R. Olson, *J. Chem. Phys.*, 1933, **1,** 418; A. R. Olson and F. A. Long, *J. Am. Chem. Soc.*, 1934, **56,** 1294; 1936, **58,** 393.

[152] N. Meer and M. Polanyi, *Z. physik. Chem.*, 1932, **B, 19,** 164.

[153] T. M. Lowry, *Inst. intern. chim. Solvay, conseil chim.* (Brussels), **1925,** 130.

[154] J. Kenyon and H. Phillips, *Trans. Faraday Soc.*. 1930, **26,** 451; J. Kenyon, A. G. Lipscomb, and H. Phillips, *J. Chem. Soc.*, **1930,** 415.

prior dissociation, in combination, identifying the former mechanism with the bimolecular, and the latter with the unimolecular form of substitution. They assumed that, for physical reasons to be explained, bimolecular substitution will always produce inversion, while unimolecular substitution may involve inversion, racemisation, or retention of stereochemical form, depending on circumstances which have to be considered in detail.[155]

(33d) Steric Orientation in S_N2 Substitution.—For the bimolecular mechanism of substitution (S_N2), inversion was assumed to be the rule, because the transition state (I) leading to inversion must have much less internal energy than that (II) corresponding to retention of stereochemical form. The reason is that in state (I) the split bond X · · · C · · · Y, holding the incoming and outgoing groups, will have an approximately planar surface of zero electronic density (exactly planar if X = Y), in which the three bonds CR_3 can lie: this arrangement minimises the positive exchange energy between the altered and the preserved bonds and between the electron pairs whose bonding is being altered.[156] State (II) admits of no such stable arrangement.

The simplest demonstration of transition state (I) is that secured by Hughes and his colleagues by the isotopic tracer method for the halogen exchange reaction between halide ions and alkyl halide molecules. It was previously known that an optically active alkyl halide, in which the halogen-bearing carbon atom is the only centre of asymmetry, can usually be racemised by treatment in solution with an alkali metal halide having the identical kind of halogen. From this fact, the limited conclusion follows that, *if* the racemisation is due to replacement of the original alkyl halide halogen by a substituting halide ion, then *at least some* of the individual molecular acts of substitution involve inversion. However, a much more far-reaching conclusion can be secured by giving the halogen in the alkali-metal halide a radioactive label: for then, not only can the fact of substitution be estab-

[155] E. D. Hughes and C. K. Ingold, *J. Chem. Soc.*, 1935, 254; W. A. Cowdrey, E. D. Hughes, C. K. Ingold, S. Masterman, and A. D. Scott, *ibid.*, 1937, 1252.

[156] This assumes that higher carbon orbitals are not available to take care of the incoming electrons before the outgoing ones leave. It might not be true for nucleophilic substitutions at heavier elements.

lished, but also its kinetics can be determined, and its rate can be compared with the rate of loss of optical activity.

This has been done[157] in three examples, namely, the racemisation of 2-octyl iodide by sodium iodide, that of 1-phenylethyl bromide by lithium bromide, and that of α-bromopropionic acid by lithium bromide, dry acetone being the solvent in each case (the asterisk indicates radioactivity):

$$\overset{*}{I}^- + C_6H_{13}\cdot CHI\cdot CH_3 \rightarrow C_6H_{13}\cdot CH\overset{*}{I}\cdot CH_3 + I^-$$

$$\overset{*}{Br}^- + C_6H_5\cdot CHBr\cdot CH_3 \rightarrow C_6H_5\cdot CH\overset{*}{Br}\cdot CH_3 + Br^-$$

$$\overset{*}{Br}^- + CO_2H\cdot CHBr\cdot CH_3 \rightarrow CO_2H\cdot CH\overset{*}{Br}\cdot CH_3 + Br^-$$

In each example it was found, first, that substitution occurs with second-order kinetics, and therefore by the bimolecular mechanism; and, secondly, that the rate of loss of optical activity, being twice the rate of isotopic exchange, requires that *every* individual act of bimolecular substitution inverts configuration, and thus passes through transition state (I).

These examples all belong to charge-type 1 (negative reagent, neutral substrate), and this circumstance allowed an alternative proposal to be made, *viz.*, that the result depends, not on exchange forces, but on electrostatic forces: thus the carbon-halogen dipole in the alkyl halide could direct the anionic substituting agent towards its positive end, that is, towards that side of the carbon atom which is further from the halogen atom. However, it could be shown that this is not the true explanation; for by going over to charge-type 3 (negative reagent, positive substrate), we could reverse the direction of the dipole in the bond between the carbon atom and the outgoing substituent, and still observe substitution with an inverted configuration. When the general principle of bimolecular inversion was formulated, the literature contained an indication against the electrostatic explanation. It was a stereospecific substitution in the menthane series, and it is mentioned in the first edition of this book (p. 379). But it was less than conclusive, partly because asymmetric centres were present besides that at the seat of substitution, and still more because no kinetic proof of mechanism had been supplied. Much better examples have since been provided by Hughes and his collaborators.

[157] E. D. Hughes, F. Juliusberger, S. Masterman, B. Topley, and J. Weiss, *J. Chem. Soc.*, **1935**, 1525; E. D. Hughes, F. Juliusberger, A. D. Scott, B. Topley, and J. Weiss, *ibid.*, **1936**, 1173; W. A. Cowdrey, E. D. Hughes, T. P. Nevell, and C. L. Wilson, *ibid.*, **1938**, 209.

One example, which correlates the steric course of an S_N2 substitution of charge-type 3 with that of an S_N2 substitution of charge-type 1, runs as follows:[158]

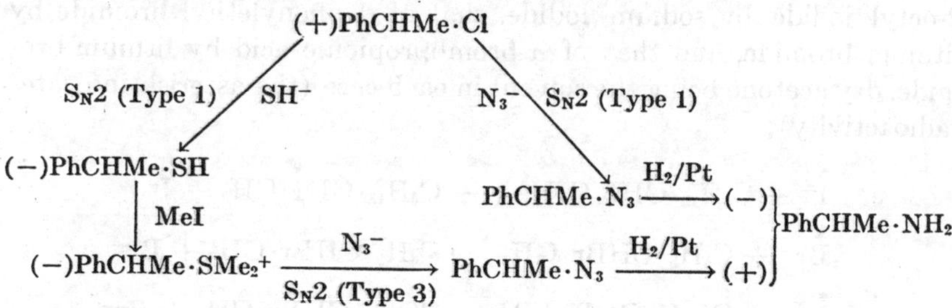

1-Phenylethyl chloride was converted, by kinetically controlled S_N2 processes of charge-type 1, (a) into a thiol, which was methylated, without touching the asymmetric centre, to a sulphonium ion, and (b) into an azide, which was reduced, again without touching the asymmetric centre, to an amine. The establishment by isotopic means of inversion in S_N2 substitutions of charge-type 1 carries the conclusion that the above sulphonium ion and amine are of like configuration. Then the sulphonium ion was converted by a kinetically controlled S_N2 substitution of charge-type 3 into an azide, which on reduction gave the other enantiomeric amine. This shows that the substitution of charge-type 3 proceeded with inversion of configuration, notwithstanding the countervailing electrostatic forces.

Another example correlates the steric course of an S_N2 substitution of charge-type 2 (neutral reagent, neutral substrate) with that of an S_N2 substitution of charge type 1. Hoffmann and Hughes's neutral reagent was now thiourea. Their scheme of correlation ran as follows:[159]

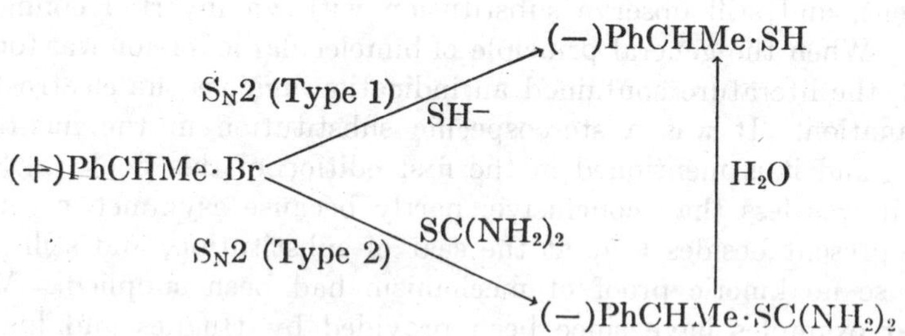

[158] P. Brewster, F. Hiron, E. D. Hughes, C. K. Ingold, and P. A. D. Rao, *Nature*, 1950, **166**, 178; F. Hiron and E. D. Hughes, *J. Chem. Soc.*, **1960**, 795; S. H. Harvey, P. A. T. Hoye, E. D. Hughes, and C. K. Ingold, *ibid.*, p. 800; cf. H. M. R. Hoffmann and E. D. Hughes, *ibid.*, **1964**, 1244; H. M. R. Hoffmann, *ibid.*, p. 1249.

[159] H. M. R. Hoffmann and E. D. Hughes, *J. Chem. Soc.*, **1964**, 1252.

1-Phenylethyl bromide was converted, by a kinetically controlled S_N2 process of charge-type 1, into a thiol of inverted configuration, and by a kinetically controlled S_N2 substitution of charge-type 2 into a thiouronium ion, which on hydrolysis without touching the asymmetric centre yielded the optically identical thiol. The substitution of charge-type 2 must therefore have proceeded with inversion of configuration.

The last of Hoffmann and Hughes's examples dealt with charge-type 4 (neutral reagent, positive substrate) on an independent basis. The scheme was as follows:[160]

$$(-)\text{PhCHMe}\cdot\text{SMe}_2^+ \xrightarrow[\text{SC(NH}_2)_2]{S_N2\ (\text{Type } 4)} (+)\text{PhCHMe}\cdot\text{SC(NH}_2)_2^+$$

$$\downarrow \text{H}_2\text{O}$$

$$(+)\text{PhCHMe}\cdot\text{SMe}_2^+ \xleftarrow[\text{MeOTs}]{} (+)\text{PhCHMe}\cdot\text{SH}$$

1-Phenylethyl-dimethylsulphonium ion was converted, by a kinetically controlled S_N2 substitution of charge-type 4, into a thiouronium ion, which, on hydrolysis to a thiol and methylation of the latter, processes which do not touch the asymmetric centre, gave back 1-phenylethyl-dimethylsulphonium ion with a rotation of the same magnitude but of opposite sign. This shows that the substitution of charge-type 4 proceeded with inversion of configuration.

Though much filling-in work has been done, the examples given in this Section constitute the framework of the case for the S_N2 Rule formulated below. The Rule was promulgated, with its theoretical basis in the Pauli principle, in 1937, and was the first valid rule which connected the steric course of a chemical reaction with its mechanism.[155] It is curious to reflect that it was accepted practically without question as from that date, and was widely and correctly applied for the correlation of configurations, long before the experimental proof of its validity was completed in 1964.

S_N2 Rule:—Substitution by mechanism S_N2 involves inversion of configuration, independently of all constitutional details.

This rule is so simple and definite, and so devoid of qualification, that it provides the most general and certain method we have for correlating configurations when one group replaces another at a singly-present asymmetric centre. When applying it, the chief experimental task is always to prove kinetically that the nucleophilic substitution is

[160] H. M. R. Hoffmann and E. D. Hughes, *J. Chem. Soc.*, **1964,** 1259.

indeed using the bimolecular mechanism. Many configurative relations have been established in this way.[161]

Bartlett's observation that halogen at a bridge-head is incapable of being replaced in an S_N2 process is consistent with the S_N2 Rule. Obviously, the bridged structure precludes a transition state of type (I). Quite a number of examples are now known, but Bartlett's original ones of 1-chloroapocamphane and 1-bromotriptycene, formulated below, adequately establish the point:[162]

```
CH2—CCl—CH2                    CBr
|    |    |                 /   |   \
|   CMe2  |           C6H4   o-C6H4   C6H4
|    |    |                 \   |   /
CH2—CH —CH2                    CH
```

(33e) Types of Steric Orientation in S_N1 Substitution.—The steric course of unimolecular nucleophilic substitutions is less simple to specify. In S_N2 substitutions, as has been shown, we observe universal inversion. In S_N1 substitutions, we find two classes of result. In what we might call the "normal" type of case, that is, in the absence of a special constitutional condition later to be specified, we find mixtures of inversion and racemisation in any proportion to both limits. The proportions depend on the substrate and the medium, in particular, on the stability of the carbonium ion given by the substrate, and the carbonium-ion-trapping efficiency of the medium. In the "abnormal" type of case, that is, in the presence of the constitutional condition, we find mixtures of retention of configuration and racemisation in any proportion to both limits. The proportions again depend on substrate constitution, and on the medium.

This breakdown of the sterochemical course of nucleophilic substitution into three cases spread over two mechanisms, one case belonging to mechanism S_N2, and two cases covering mechanism S_N1, to which one applies in the absence, and the other applies in the presence of a particular constitutional condition, was made in 1937, on the basis of the experimental data here summarised in Table 33-1. It was the answer to the 40-year-old problem of when a Walden inversion would occur.

The first two sections of Table 33-1 refer to aliphatic secondary alkyl halides.[163] They show that inversion is total when the mech-

[161] Many have been inferred without kinetic proof of mechanism, a dangerous proceeding.

[162] P. B. Bartlett and L. H. Knox, *J. Am. Chem. Soc.*, 1939, **61**, 3184; P. D. Bartlett and E. S. Lewis, *J. Am. Chem. Soc.*, 1950, **72**, 1005.

[163] E. D. Hughes, C. K. Ingold, and S. Masterman, *J. Chem. Soc.*, **1937**, 1196, 1236.

TABLE 33-1.—RELATION OF ROTATORY EFFECT TO MECHANISM OF SUBSTITUTION.

Halide substd.	Entrant group	Substituting agent	and Medium	Mech.	Config.	Optical purity
C_6H_{13} >CHCl CH_3	OEt	OEt^-	EtOH	S_N2	Inv	~100%
	OH	OH^-	60% aq · EtOH	S_N2	Inv	~100%
	OH	H_2O	60% aq · EtOH	S_N1	Rac, Inv	66%
	OEt	OEt^-	60% aq · EtOH	S_N2	Inv	~100%
	OEt	HOEt	60% aq · EtOH	S_N1	Rac, Inv	74%
C_6H_{13} >CHBr CH_3	OEt	OEt^-	EtOH	S_N2	Inv	~100%
	OH	Ag^+, AgBr	H_2O	Ag^+—S_N1	Rac, Inv	72%
	OEt	Ag^+, AgBr	EtOH	Ag^+—S_N1	Rac, Inv	94%
	OH	Ag^+, AgBr, Ag_2O	H_2O	Ag^+—S_N1	Rac, Inv	74%
	OEt	Ag^+, AgBr, Ag_2O	EtOH	Ag^+—S_N1	Rac, Inv	94%
	OH	H_2O	H_2O	S_N1	Rac, Inv	17%
	OH	H_2O	60% aq · Me_2CO	S_N1	Rac, Inv	5%
	OH	H_2O	80% aq · Me_2CO	S_N1	Rac, Inv	2%
C_6H_5 >CHCl CH_3	OMe	OMe^-	MeOH	S_N2	Inv	High
	OMe	HOMe	MeOH	S_N1	Rac, Inv	Low
	OEt	OEt^-	EtOH	S_N2	Inv	High
	OEt	HOEt	EtOH	S_N1	Rac, Inv	Low
	OH	Ag^+, AgCl, Ag_2O	H_2O	Ag^+—S_N1	Rac, Inv	3–29%
C_6H_5 >CHBr CH_3	OH	H_2O	H_2O	S_N1	Rac, Inv	Low
HO_2C >CHBr CH_3	OH	H_2O, H_2SO_4	H_2O	S_N2	Inv	~100%
MeO_2C >CHBr CH_3	OMe	OMe^-	MeOH	S_N2	Inv	~100%
	OMe	HOMe	MeOH	S_N2	Inv	~100%
	OMe	Ag^+, AgBr	MeOH	Ag^+—S_N1	Rac, Inv	89%
NHG · CO >CHBr[1] CH_3	OH	Ag^+ AgBr, Ag_2CO_3	H_2O	Ag^+—S_N1	Rac, Inv	73%
	OH	OH^-	H_2O	S_N2	Inv	~100%
	OH	H_2O, OH^-	H_2O	S_N1	Ret	~100%
	OMe	OMe^-	MeOH	S_N2	Inv	~100%
$\bar{O}_2C$ >CHBr CH_3	OMe	HOMe, OMe^-	MeOH	S_N1	Ret	~100%
	OH	Ag^+, AgBr	H_2O	Ag^+—S_N1	Rac, Ret	87%
	OH	Ag^+, AgBr, Ag_2O	H_2O	Ag^+—S_N1	Rac, Ret	28–58%
	OH	Ag^+, AgBr, Ag_2CO_3	H_2O	Ag^+—S_N1	Rac, Ret	36%

[1] G stands for the residue $CH_2 \cdot CO_2H$.

anism is known to be S_N2, and is accompanied by a minor amount of racemisation when the mechanism is or might be S_N1, or the silver-catalysed derivative-form of mechanism S_N1. The next two sections refer to secondary aralphyl halides, in which a formed carbonium ionic centre would be conjugated with the aryl group.[164] Here we find total inversion, when the mechanism is S_N2, and inversion accompanying extensive racemisation, when it is, or might be, S_N1, or a catalysed form of S_N1.

The definition of an S_N1 mechanism requires only that the substituting agent should not be covalently involved in the transition state of ionisation of the substrate. In this state, the outgoing anion has receded only by about 0.5 *A*. If the substituting agent were covalently to intervene when the anion had receded by only a little more than that, for instance, by 1.0 *A*, or by just far enough to make a touching ion pair, the substitution would still be unimolecular, but it would occur with inversion of configuration, because one side of the carbonium ion would be totally shielded by the outgoing anion. However, there must be a considerable range of greater counter-ion separations over which the receding anion will still shield one side of the carbonium ion to an appreciable degree, and, while allowing substitution with retention of configuration, will render it less probable than substitution with inversion. We shall then observe mixtures of inversion and racemisation. Only when the carbonium ion is so stable, and the trapping power of the medium is so low, that the receding anion has time to diffuse right out of the neighbourhood of the carbonium ion, before the substituting agent covalently attacks the latter, will substitution take place with total racemisation.[165] It is clear that the amount of racemisation in the mixture of inversion and racemisation will become greater as the stability of the carbonium ion increases, and as the trapping power of the medium decreases, that is, as the longevity of the carbonium ion in the medium increases.

When, as on passing from secondary alkyl to secondary aralphyl halides, mesomerism enters to increase the longevity of the carbonium ion, we find increased proportions of racemisation in the substitutions

[164] E. D. Hughes, C. K. Ingold, and A. D. Scott, *J. Chem. Soc.*, **1937**, 1201; E. D. Hughes, C. K. Ingold, and S. Masterman, *ibid.*, p. 1236.

[165] This concept of stereospecificity through shielding in S_N1 substitutions has occasionally been re-expressed as substitution in a carbonium ion pair. This statement will indeed cover many cases. But on any precise definition of an ion pair, it is too restrictive to constitute a specification of the conditions for complete or partial stereospecificity through shielding. One must, for instance, expect substantial shielding well beyond the Bjerrum distance in water.

as Table 33-1 shows. The same matter has been illustrated[166] by changing from the purely aliphatic secondary alkyl halides to aliphatic tertiary alkyl halides, such as methylethyl*iso*hexylcarbinyl chloride. For like media, the products from the tertiary compounds are, as they should be, much more extensively racemised.

The abnormal situation arises when a substituent is present which, before or after the heterolysing system has passed through its transition state, but before the separating group has receded to great distances, forms a weak bond, probably somewhat long and hence of largely electrostatic character, with the carbonium ionic centre on the side remote from the receding group. This side remains thereafter protected from attack by the substituting agent, until the separating group is far enough removed to permit an attack on its own side: this attack liberates the protecting group, and effects substitution with retention of configuration. If the protecting group is somewhat slow to intervene, a smaller or greater amount of racemisation may accompany a predominating retention of configuration. As to protecting groups, we take it at first as necessary (though in Chapter X the restriction will be removed) that they should be unsaturated, that is, that they should possess unshared or multiple-bond (p or π) electrons, which can combine weakly with the carbonium ionic centre. They might thus act either before or after the unimolecular heterolysis has passed through its transition state, reducing activation energy in the former case. However, the protecting group must not be so strongly nucleophilic or so favourably positioned that it will combine with sufficient strength to resist ejection, and hence resist entry of the eventual substituting agent. Thus the production of substitutions with retention of configuration is a delicate matter, involving a careful adjustment both of polar quality and stereochemical opportunity.

From a historical, as from other, points of view, the most important configuration-protecting group is the α-carboxylate-ion group, α-CO_2^-, as in the α-bromopropionate ion, $^-O_2C\cdot CHMe\cdot Br$. Part of the usefulness of the group for the purpose of producing substitution with retention of configuration arises from its electron-repelling nature: like an α-alkyl substituent, an α-carboxylate-ion substituent promotes S_N1 substitutions (Section **28b**), thereby providing one of the conditions needed to give retention of configuration. Then, the group, $—CO_2^-$, is nucleophilic, with the required unshared electrons. But its access is too limited stereochemically to allow it to form a strong bond: it

[166] E. D. Hughes, C. K. Ingold, R. J. L. Martin, and D. F. Meigh, *Nature*, 1950, **166**, 679; W. von E. Doering and H. H. Zeiss, *J. Am. Chem. Soc.*, 1953, **75**, 4733.

forms a weak bond, probably somewhat long and thus of largely electrostatic character, for pure covalencies lose strength very rapidly on extension. However, the weak bond will suffice to hold the configuration until the substituting agent enters the position from which the separating group departed. This is illustrated in the last four sections, particularly the last section, of Table 33-1. α-Bromopropionic acid, and its ester, and its amide, behave qualitatively like any other aliphatic secondary alkyl halides; but the α-bromopropionate ion brings in a qualitatively new situation.[167] It can be hydrolysed in alkaline solution by a mechanism kinetically identifiable as bimolecular, S_N2; and the produced lactic acid is formed, as it should be, with inversion. However, the α-bromopropionate ion can also be hydrolysed, even in dilute alkaline solution, by the kinetically identified unimolecular mechanism, S_N1; and then the lactic acid is formed with a strongly predominating retention of configuration. Schematically, this process may be represented as follows:

$$\mathrm{O{:}\overset{\displaystyle O^-}{\overset{|}{C}}\!-\!CHMe\!-\!Br} \rightarrow \mathrm{O{:}\overset{\displaystyle O^-}{\overset{|}{C}}\!-\!\overset{+}{C}HMe} \xrightarrow{H_2O} \mathrm{O{:}\overset{\displaystyle O^-}{\overset{|}{C}}\!-\!CHMe\!-\!OH}$$

In the example of the phenylbromoacetate ion, $\bar{O}_2C\cdot CHPh\cdot Br$, the derived carbonium ion has added stability on account of mesomerism; and therefore, even in strongly alkaline solution, the unimolecular mechanism prevails. However, much racemisation now accompanies the predominating retention of configuration arising from this mechanism.[168]

The importance of securing sufficiently weak binding by an intervening carboxylate-ion group can be illustrated by placing it in β-, γ-, and δ-positions with respect to the leaving halogen substituent. The reaction is then essentially an internal S_N2-type substitution. Halogen expulsion is accelerated by carboxyl intervention, and may be made so much faster than even a silver-ion catalysed S_N1 subsitution that the observed reaction is insensitive to silver ions. The product is a usually isolable β-, γ-, or δ-lactone, formed with inversion. Such lactones may be hydrolysed in various ways, but particularly easily in alkaline solution; and then the splitting occurs in the CO—O bond, not at the original seat of substitution, where necessarily the configuration of the lactone is preserved. Thus the original halogeno-acid is

[167] W. A. Cowdrey, E. D. Hughes, and C. K. Ingold, *J. Chem. Soc.*, **1937**, 1208.

[168] M. G. Church and E. D. Hughes, results personally communicated.

converted in alkaline solution into a hydroxy-acid with an overall inversion, as would not have happened in a unimolecular substitution in which configuration is held internally by a much weaker bond.

It is easily understood why the Walden inversion was discovered, and why almost all the early work on it was done, in the field of the reactions of α-substituted carboxylic acids. Although the point could not be appreciated at the time, the whole difficulty of observing a Walden inversion arose from its *prevalence*.[169] In order to "discover" it, one really had to discover the much less common phenomenon of substitution with retention of configuration, thereby demonstrating the existence of stereochemically contrasting processes. Now the α-situated carboxylate-ion group not only assists unimolecular substitutions, but also satisfies the somewhat restrictive conditions for producing a sufficient, but sufficiently weak, binding. And thus the reactions of the α-halogeno-acids provided a fertile field for demonstrating the existence of Walden inversions.

We may summarise the principles discussed in a second rule of spatial orientations in nucleophilic substitution. It is more equivocal than the S_N2 rule, and, in the form here given, applies only to the substitution at an acyclic carbon atom:

S_N1 Rule:—Substitution by mechanism S_N1 involves inversion of configuration mixed with racemisation in any proportions to both limits, unless weak internal binding of the carbonium ionic centre by a nucleophilic substituent temporarily occurs, when it involves retention of configuration mixed with racemisation in any proportions to both limits.

It will be seen that the conclusions that can be reached about mechanism solely from stereochemical results, without good kinetic evidence (for example, in solvolysis, for which significant kinetic evidence is often hard to obtain), are extremely restricted. Even if we may take it for granted (a) that a nucleophilic substitution is under observation and (b) that its mechanism is one of those already discussed (though others are known), we still have to beware of three non-sequiturs. An observation of total inversion of configuration does not by itself allow us to distinguish between mechanisms S_N1 and S_N2. An observation of total or partial racemisation does not allow us to conclude in favour of an S_N1 type of mechanism, unless it is shown that the observed stereochemical course is the result of a single irreversible step of substitution, with no concurrent, preceding, or succeeding processes. An observation of total or partial retention of configuration does not permit us to infer an S_N1 type of mechanism, unless the same stipula-

169 "If all the world were blue, we would not know what blueness was."

tions are fulfilled. In general, stereochemistry without kinetic support is a poor tool for the investigation of mechanism: to start with it, is to start at the wrong end.

(33f) Inversion of Configuration with Racemisation: Further Details.—We shall deal here with two extreme types of case. First we shall consider S_N1 solvolyses, in which the carbonium ion is so stable, and the solvent is such an inefficient trap for it, that, supposing the seat of substitution to be a sole asymmetric centre of optical activity, the solvolysis product is totally racemic. In some such cases, though not in all, the rate of loss of optical activity by the solvolysing solution is greater than the rate of appearance of the racemic solvolysis product. This means, of course, that substrate, if recovered from an incomplete solvolysis, would be found to be partly racemised.

Such an excess rate of racemisation can arise from any of several causes, with most of which we are not now concerned. For instance, the anions liberated by solvolysis may attack the still unsolvolysed substrate in a bimolecular way, so producing a certain proportion of inverted substrate molecules, and twice that proportion of "racemic" substrate. That occurrence can be detected kinetically: if the solvolysis is of first order, the racemisation will not be, because of the progressive accumulation of racemising anions. Again, dissociated anions, formed in the first step of unimolecular substitution, may recombine with the carbonium ion, so forming racemic substrate. This occurrence also can be detected kinetically: if the racemisation is of first order, the solvolysis will not be, because the build-up of anions will entail a growing proportion of ion-recombination, and hence a solvolysis rate falling increasingly with time behind the first-order rate (Section **32a**). If the product is racemic, the solvolysis rate is of first order, and the racemisation rate is of first order, an excessive racemisation rate can still arise because the solvolytic substitution is associated with a rearrangement, in which the intermediate carbonium ion passes through a symmetric configuration. This situation can be controlled by an examination of products. It will interest us in later Chapters, but not here.

An excessive first-order rate of racemisation, accompanying first-order solvolysis, to give a racemic but unrearranged product, was observed by Winstein and his co-workers in 1960.[170] They found, for example, that *p*-chlorobenzhydryl chloride, in solution in acetic acid

[170] S. Winstein, J. S. Gall, M. Hojo, and S. Smith, *J. Am. Chem. Soc.*, 1960, **82**, 1010.

containing lithium acetate at 25°, suffered racemisation some 30–70 times faster than it became converted to *p*-chlorobenzhydryl acetate. The same substrate in "80%" aqueous acetone underwent racemisation about 5 times faster than it became converted to benzhydrol.

These excesses of racemisation rate over solvolysis rate are, of course, to do with the reversibility of the rate-controlling step of ionisation, but, as the first-order kinetics show, with reversion before the counter-ions have attained kinetic independence:

$$RR'CHCl \rightleftharpoons RR'CH^+Cl^- \rightleftharpoons RR'CH^+ + Cl^- \xrightarrow[H_2O]{} RR'CH\cdot OH + HCl$$

Without necessarily assuming equilibria between a small number of discrete sub-species of ion pairs, we can say, quite generally, that, after the activation barrier of ionisation has been passed, and as the counter-ions diffuse apart, each separation will be associated with certain probabilities which we can measure only as integrals over all separations. There will be a finite probability, increasing with separation to an asymptote, that the solvent will react with the carbonium ion. There will be a finite probability, decreasing to a low value with increasing separation, that the ions will recombine. And then, beyond a small critical separation, there will be a finite probability, growing with separation, that a carbonium ion, destined to recombine with its counter-ion, will before it does so have undergone an average of a half-turn of rotation about an axis perpendicular to the interionic line. It is the product of the last two probabilities, integrated over all separations, that we measure as an excess of the first-order rate of racemisation over the first-order rate of solvolysis to a racemate.

Goering has devised a method of monitoring the separation of the counter-ions at smaller separations than those which would admit stereochemically notable amounts of rotation of the carbonium ion.[171] The method uses a carboxylic ester with isotopically distinguished carboxyl oxygen atoms. Then, any pair of counter-ions, recombining after such separation as will allow the anionic charge to spread between the oxygen atoms, will give a reconstituted ester with randomised oxygen isotopes. Thus when benzhydryl *p*-nitrobenzoate with carbonyl-^{18}O was hydrolysed in "90%" aqueous actone at 118.6°, oxygen randomisation in the unconverted ester proceeded at three times the rate of hydrolysis; and that means that, of the molecules

[171] H. L. Goering and J. F. Levy, *J. Am. Chem. Soc.*, 1962, **84**, 3853; *idem* and R. G. Brody, *ibid.*, 1964, **85**, 3059.

which become ionised to the relevant small separation, 25% become hydrolysed, while 75% become reconstituted. When optically active *p*-chlorobenzhydryl *p*-nitrobenzoate with carbonyl-^{18}O was hydrolysed in the same medium at 99.6°, of the molecules which became ionised to the separation detectable by oxygen randomisation, 28% suffered hydrolysis, while the rest became reconstituted, 56% with retention of the original configuration, and 16% after a half-turn of the carbonium ion to give an inverted configuration.

Fava and his coworkers have studied several reactions, each demonstrated to depend on ionisation, of variously substituted benzhydryl thiocyanates in acetonitrile. They have studied exchange with radiothiocyanate ion, $^{35}SCN^-$, which requires ionic dissociation; isomerisation to *iso*thiocyanates, which needs only a limited ion-pair separation; and the racemisation accompanying all these processes.[172] Isomerisation means that the anion turns end-for-end, and the inversion of configuration seen as racemisation means that the cation rotates by a half-turn before recombination. A pair of ions, separate enough to recombine without or with end-for-end reversal of the anion, or without or with rotation of the carbonium ion, has a better chance of recombining in any of these ways than of further dissociating to allow exchange, in the examples studied. In that of optically active *p*-chlorobenzhydryl thiocyanate in acetonitrile at 70°, the different courses open to the ion pair are pursued to the approximate extents noted below:

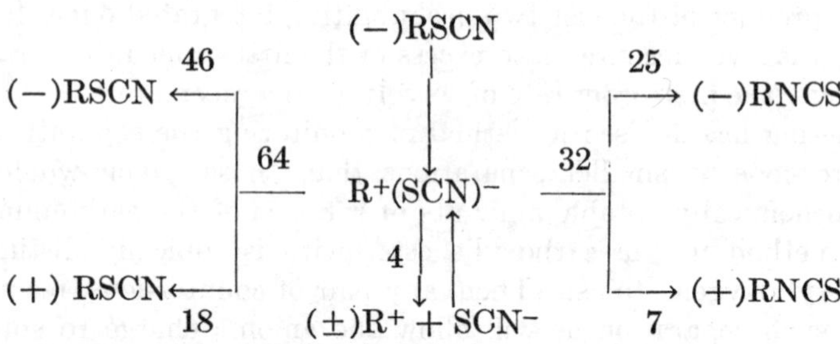

It is shown that the thiocyanate and *iso*thiocyanate with like signs of rotation have like configurations, and thus we see that reversal of the

[172] A. Iliceto, A. Fava, U. Mazzucato, and O. Rossetto, *J. Am. Chem. Soc.*, 1961, **83**, 2729; A. Fava, A. Iliceto, A. Ceccon, and P. Koch, *ibid.*, 1965, **87**, 1015; A. Ceccon, I. Papa, and A. Fava, *ibid.*, 1966, **88**, 4643; A. Fava, A. Iliceto, and A. Ceccon, *Tetrahedron Letters*, 1963, **11**, 685; A. Fava, U. Tonnelato, and L. Congiu, *ibid.*, 1965, **22**, 1657.

anion and rotation of the cation become permitted at about the same stage of separation of the counter-ions.

We now go to the other extreme of the range of S_N1 substitutions giving mixed inversion and racemisation, where the carbonium ion is so short-lived that it is hard to know if it is formed at all, *i.e.*, to distinguish mechanism S_N1 with perfect screening of the carbonium ion by its counter-ion, from mechanism S_N2. Grunwald, Heller, and Klein found that 1-phenylethyl alcohol, in ^{18}O-water containing 0.017*N* perchloric acid at 30°, underwent racemisation at 1.22 times the rate at which it exchanged oxygen with the solvent:[173]

$$H_2{}^{18}O + RR'CH \cdot OH_2^+ \rightarrow RR'CH \cdot {}^{18}OH_2^+ + H_2O$$

This does not illustrate an extreme situation. The rate ratio means that 61% of the acts of substitution invert configuration and 39% retain configuration; or, if we like to say so, 22% of the acts invert, and 78% racemise. There can be little doubt that in this example the main mechanism of substitution is S_N1, the substrate being taken as the conjugate acid of the alcohol. Consider now the same experiment with a purely aliphatic secondary alcohol. Bunton, Konasiewicz, and Llewellyn found that 2-butyl alcohol, in ^{18}O-water containing various small concentrations of perchloric acid at 100.8°, underwent racemisation at 2.00 times the rate at which it exchanged oxygen with the solvent.[174] Here, every act of substitution inverts configuration, and we have no way of telling whether the absence in this case of the carbonium-stabilising phenyl group has excluded S_N1 substitution in the conjugate acid, or has only reduced the life of the carbonium ion sufficiently to permit perfect screening. Competition experiments might resolve this dubiety.

Let us now consider a parallel contrast created by a change of medium. Weiner and Sheen noticed[175] that, when 2-octyl methanesulphonate is hydrolysed at 65° in "50%" aqueous dioxan, 94% of the 2-octanol formed had an inverted, and 6% a retained configuration. They also observed that, when the ester was hydrolysed in pure water, the formed 2-octanol was fully inverted. By no logical process does this tell us the mechanism of hydrolysis in pure water, but a plausible

[173] E. Grunwald, H. Heller, and F. S. Klein, *J. Chem. Soc.*, **1957**, 2604.

[174] C. A. Bunton, A. Konasiewicz, and D. R. Llewellyn, *J. Chem. Soc.*, **1955**, 604.

[175] H. Weiner and R. A. Sheen, *J. Am. Chem. Soc.*, 1965, **87**, 287, 292; R. A. Sheen and J. W. Larsen, *ibid.*, 1966, **88**, 2513. The investigators' own explanation cannot be entertained. It was that all retentions of configuration arise from two successive steps of configuration-inverting S_N2 substitution, the initial

surmise might be that the mechanism is S_N1 both in "50%" aqueous dioxan and in pure water, and that the stereochemical difference arises from the superior trapping power of pure water, which reacts with the carbonium ion before the counter-ion has receded to any distance.

This type of interpretation can consistently cover the other main stereochemical contrast disclosed by these workers, namely, that, when 2-octyl *p*-bromobenzenesulphonate was hydrolysed at 65° in "75%" aqueous dioxan, 88% of the formed 2-octanol had an inverted and 12% a retained configuration; whereas, when enough sodium azide was added to the solvent to change the products to 30% of 2-octanol and 70% of 2-octyl azide, both these substances were fully inverted. Again it is conceivable that the increase in the overall trapping power of the medium, now gained by the addition of azide ions, never allows the separating anion time to recede far enough to leave the carbonium ion seriously unshielded.[175]

So far in this Section we have dealt largely with solvolysis. Some of the same phenomena have been observed in non-solvolytic substitutions, in which, on the whole, kinetic investigations can more easily make mechanism more certain. Pocker and his coworkers have examined some substitutions of 1-phenylethyl chloride in nitromethane, and, through combined kinetic and stereochemical evidence, have distinguished three mechanisms, namely, the unimolecular, bimolecular, and acid-catalysed unimolecular mechanisms.[110]

At 99.8° the first-order rate of racemisation of 1-phenylethyl chloride in nitromethane, 1.2×10^{-5} sec.$^{-1}$, was 4.2 times the first-order rate of chloride exchange (S_N1), or, in the absence of an added source of chloride ions, the identical first-order rate of hydrogen-chloride

---

substituting agent being a dioxan molecule, which is subsequently expelled from combination; and that azide ions provide a diversion from the second step of the two-step configuration-retaining route to 2-octanol:

$$\mathrm{R{-}X} \xrightarrow{\mathrm{O(C_2H_4)_2O}} \mathrm{O(C_2H_4)_2\overset{+}{O}{-}R} \begin{cases} \xrightarrow{\mathrm{OH_2}} \mathrm{R{-}OH} \\ \xrightarrow{\mathrm{N_3^-}} \mathrm{R{-}N_3} \end{cases}$$

If this were so, the 2-octyl azide, formed in substitution for the 12% of 2-octanol of retained configuration, should have had a retained configuration. In fact, the formed 2-octyl azide was wholly inverted.

elimination to give styrene, 0.29×10^{-5} sec.$^{-1}$ (E1). The excess rate of racemisation measures, as before, that part of the ion-pair recombination for which the carbonium ion has rotated to give an inverted product.

With $NEt_4{}^{36}Cl$ as source of substituting chloride ions, a second-order exchange was superposed, the rate of which was 6.1×10^{-3} [RCl][$^{36}Cl^-$] mole l.$^{-1}$ sec.$^{-1}$. With this reaction was associated a second-order racemisation, the rate of which was 12.4×10^{-3} [RCl] [$^{36}Cl^-$] mole l.$^{-1}$ sec.$^{-1}$. This rate ratio, 1.97, in combination with the second-order kinetics, shows that mechanism S_N2 is here under observation.

With $H^{36}Cl$ to act as both a source of substituting chloride ion, and, as we shall see, a general-acid catalyst for ionisation of the substrate, a second-order chloride exchange was observed, the rate of which was 1.52×10^{-3}[RCl][$H^{36}Cl$] mole l.$^{-1}$ sec.$^{-1}$. With this exchange was associated a second-order racemisation, the rate of which was 1.50×10^{-3} [RCl][$H^{36}Cl$]. This rate ratio, 0.99, in combination with the second-order kinetics, shows that we are dealing here with the acid-molecule-catalysed derivative form of the unimolecular mechanism, HCl-S_N1; and furthermore that, with HCl to take away the ionised Cl^- (as the fairly stable complex anion, $ClHCl^-$), the carbonium ion R^+ becomes completely freed from shielding by its counter-ion, and therefore gives a totally racemic substitution product.

(33g) Retention of Configuration with Racemisation: Further Details.—As described in Section **33c**, the discovery of the Walden inversion depended on observation of the relatively uncommon substitutions, which, as was later shown, proceeded with a predominating retention of configuration. They had this stereochemical property, because they satisfied the two conditions of using the S_N1 mechanism, and of containing a substituent of such a nature and position as to provide a configuration-holding situation in the intermediate carbonium ion of the mechanism. The holding of an asymmetric configuration led to substitution with retention of configuration. The retention could be less than complete, when the structure also provided a conjugation, which could stabilise, and partly flatten, the carbonium ion.

All work on the Walden inversion in the first 42 years of its history, that is, from its discovery in 1895 to its rationalisation in 1937, depended on one substituent able to form a bond with the carbonium ion of the kind of strength that could carry an enantiomeric configuration from substrate to product in an S_N1 mechanism. This was the α-carboxylate ion substituent. From a wider point of view, this substituent provides a γ atom with unshared electrons. Since 1942,

Winstein has done great service in generalising the β-substituents (γ atoms) which will preserve configuration in an S_N1-type substitution. The list of them now includes α-CO_2^-, β-Cl, β-Br, β-OAc, β-OMe, and β-NHBz. Others have shown that β-SR groups belong to the same class.[176] Yet other γ-atoms with unshared electrons probably act similarly, for instance, carbonyl oxygen in the S_N1 substitutions of α-halogeno-carbonyl compounds; but the experimental evidence is not yet complete. We may notice a few of Winstein's examples.

Some of them function in solvolysis of organic halides in acetic acid under catalysis by silver salts. Substitution probably occurs by the catalytic mechanism Ag^+—S_N1. Thus the *erythro-* and *threo-*forms of 2-bromo-3-methoxy butane give, respectively, the *erythro-* and *threo-*forms of 2-acetoxy-3-methoxy butane.[177] Furthermore although the point was not established in this example, there can be no doubt, on account of an analogous investigation to be mentioned in the next Section, that, if the initial *threo-*compound had been a single optical isomer, say, D-*threo-*, then the product would have been the corresponding racemate, DL-*threo-*. This shows that the reaction must pass through an achiral configuration, and it is concluded that, on account of the symmetry of the system, the bonds of the methoxyl oxygen atom to the β- and α-carbon atoms pass through a state of equivalence, from which they can become non-equivalent and break on either side.

CH₃, OMe, H, C—C, H, Br (D or L) —Ag⁺→ [CH₃, CH₃, OMe, C—C, H, H]⁺ —HOAc→ { CH₃, CH₃, OMe, C—C, AcO, H, H ; CH₃, CH₃, OMe, C—C, AcO, H, H } (DL)

[176] A. R. Peters and E. Walker, *Biochem. J.*, 1923, **17**, 260; R. C. Fuson, C. C. Price, and D. M. Burness, *J. Org. Chem.*, 1946, **11**, 477; P. D. Bartlett and C. G. Swain, *J. Am. Chem. Soc.*, 1949, **71**, 1406.

[177] S. Winstein and R. E. Buckles, *J. Am. Chem. Soc.*, 1942, **64**, 2780, 2787; S. Winstein and R. R. Henderson, *ibid.*, 1943, **65**, 2096; S. Winstein and D. Seymour, *ibid.*, 1946, **68**, 118.

The substitution of OAc for OTs by solvolysis of an alkyl toluene-*p*-sulphonate in acetic acid without added reagents has given similar results. For this reaction, it is established by Winstein, McCasland, Lucas, and others,[178] that either a β-OAc or a β-NHBz group will cause replacement of α-OTs by OAc with retention of configuration. Thus, *trans*-1-acetoxy-2-toluene-*p*-sulphonyloxy*cyclo*hexane yields *trans*-1,2-diacetoxy*cyclo*hexane. The reaction is considered to proceed through a mesomeric, achiral, five-membered oxygen-ring cation, with pairs of equivalent, partly electrostatic bonds: it is represented by one asymmetric covalent structure below:

$$\underset{(\text{D or L})}{\begin{matrix} CH_2\cdot CH_2\cdot CH_2\cdot CH_2 \\ \text{AcO}\!-\!C\!-\!C\!-\!\text{H} \\ \text{H} \quad\quad \text{OTs}\end{matrix}} \rightarrow \left[\begin{matrix} CH_2\cdot CH_2\cdot CH_2\cdot CH_2 \\ C\!-\!C \\ \text{O}\!-\!\text{CMe}\!=\!\text{O} \\ \text{H} \quad\quad \text{H}\end{matrix}\right]^+$$

$$\rightarrow \underbrace{\begin{matrix} CH_2\cdot CH_2\cdot CH_2\cdot CH_2 \\ \text{OCMe}\cdots\text{O} \\ C\!-\!C \\ \text{O}\!-\!\text{MeCO} \\ \text{H} \quad\quad \text{H}\end{matrix} \qquad \begin{matrix} CH_2\cdot CH_2\cdot CH_2\cdot CH_2 \\ \text{O}\cdots\text{MeCO} \\ C\!-\!C \\ \text{OCMe}\!-\!\text{O} \\ \text{H} \quad\quad \text{H}\end{matrix}}_{(\text{DL})}$$

Up to 1946, all configuration-holding groups had unshared electrons which could be supposed to combine with the carbonium ion with partial charge transfer; but in that year Shoppee showed that similarly situated double-bond electrons could act likewise.[179] His discovery was that cholesteryl chloride and cholesterol undergo a number of

[178] S. Winstein, H. V. Hess, and R. E. Buckles, *J. Am. Chem. Soc.*, 1942, **64**, 2796; S. Winstein and R. E. Buckles, *ibid.*, 1943, **65**, 613; S. Winstein, C. Hanson, and E. Grunwald, *ibid.*, 1948, **70**, 812; S. Winstein, E. Grunwald, R. E. Buckles, and C. Hanson, *ibid.*, p. 816; S. Winstein, E. Grunwald, and L. L. Ingraham, *ibid.*, p. 821; S. Winstein, and E. Grunwald, *ibid.*, p. 828; G. E. McCasland, R. K. Clark jr., and H. E. Carter, *ibid.*, 1949, **71**, 638; H. J. Lucas, F. W. Mitchell jr., and H. K. Garner, *ibid.*, 1950, **72**, 2138.

[179] C. W. Shoppee, *J. Chem. Soc.*, **1946**, 1138, 1147.

substitutions, for example, acetolysis of the chloride to give cholesteryl acetate, with retention of configuration, whereas their dihydro-derivatives, the cholestanyl chlorides and cholestanol derivatives generally undergo all substitutions with inversion at the position substituted. It was concluded that the π electrons of the 5,6-double bond have configuration-holding properties for unimolecular substitution in the 3-position, the intermediate carbonium ion supposedly having its positive charge split between the 3- and the 6-positions. Soon afterwards, Winstein and Adams added the complementary kinetic evidence, *viz.*, that the acetolysis of cholesteryl toluene-*p*-sulphonate to give cholesteryl acetate also proceeds with retention of configuration, the rate of substitution in acetic acid being independent of acetate ions (apart from salt effects). The rate was sufficiently high to create the presumption that double-bond intervention occurs before the transition state of ionisation is reached, which therefore gains some of the stability that the ion gains from the splitting of its charge:[180]

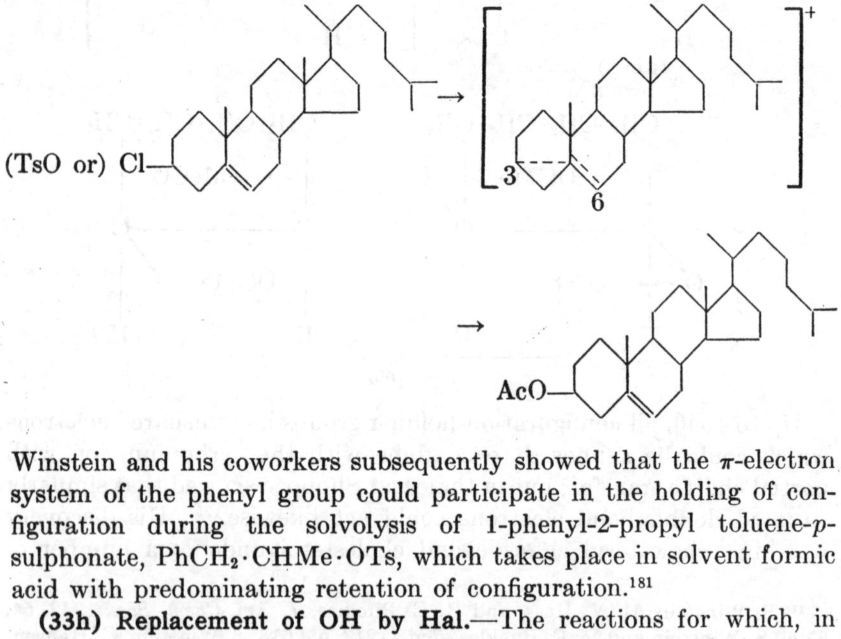

(TsO or) Cl— → [3 ---- 6]$^+$

→ AcO—

Winstein and his coworkers subsequently showed that the π-electron system of the phenyl group could participate in the holding of configuration during the solvolysis of 1-phenyl-2-propyl toluene-*p*-sulphonate, $PhCH_2 \cdot CHMe \cdot OTs$, which takes place in solvent formic acid with predominating retention of configuration.[181]

(33h) Replacement of OH by Hal.—The reactions for which, in 1937, mechanism could be kinetically determined, and relative configurations of factor and substitution product could therefore be de-

[180] S Winstein and R. Adams, *J. Am. Chem. Soc.*, 1948, **70**, 838

[181] S. Winstein, M. Brown, K. C. Schreider, and A. H. Schlesinger, *J. Am. Chem. Soc.*, 1952, **74**, 1140.

duced from polarimetric observations by means of the S_N2 Rule, were all replacements of halogen or oxy-ester groups by various halogen, oxygen, sulphur, and nitrogen substituents, including the substituents OH and NH_2. These configurational correlations at once gave the steric courses of certain reverse substitution processes, less amenable to direct kinetic determination of mechanism, in which the replaced group of the substrate was either OH or NH_2. So, part of the rationalising work of 1937[155] was to consider how far the deduced steric courses of these reactions could be accommodated to the S_N2 and S_N1 Rules, and thus to make deductions, often somewhat tentative, as to what mechanisms might be operative. As regards the reactions in which OH is replaced by Hal, one of the more definite results was the discovery that certain of these reactions were stereochemically inconsistent with both rules, and therefore must involve a new mechanism. This was assumed to consist of an internal transformation, through a cyclic transition state, in a complex formed from the substrate and reagent. This mechanism was called *internal nucleophilic substitution* and was labelled S_Ni.

A sample of the deduced steric courses of reactions of replacement of OH by Hal is given in Table 33-2, which relates to chlorination by the chlorides and oxychlorides of phosphorus and sulphur, and by hydrogen chloride. As far as the field could be covered, a generally similar series of results was obtained for bromination by the analogous brominating agents. Only the dominating stereochemical result, inversion (I) or retention (R) of configuration is indicated in the table: in

Table 33-2.—Steric Course of Replacement of OH by Cl.
Py = pyridine; A, E = acid and its esters;
OH-Ph-prop. = hydroxy-phenyl-propionic.

	PCl_3	PCl_3+Py	$POCl_3$	$POCl_3+Py$	PCl_5	PCl_5+Py	$SOCl_2$	$SOCl_2+Py$	HCl
2-*n*-Octyl alcohol	I	—	I	—	I	I	I	I	I
1-Phenylethyl alcohol	I	I	I	I	I	I	R	I	I
Lactic A, E	—	—	—	—	I	I	I	I	—
Malic A, E	—	—	—	—	I	—	I	—	—
Mandelic A, E	—	—	—	I	I	—	R	I	—
α-OH-α-Ph-prop. A, E	—	—	—	—	I	—	R	—	—
α-OH-β-Ph-prop. A, E	—	—	—	—	I	—	I	—	—
β-OH-β-Ph-prop. A, E	I	I	—	—	I	—	R	I	I

most of these reactions some racemisation occurs, but it is difficult to determine how much, if any, of this is inherent in the substitution process since the produced organic halide is in any case racemised by the simultaneously formed halide ions, or by the formed (or the used) hydrogen halide.

These results can be summarised in the statement that the halides of hydrogen and of phosphorus in all cases bring about a predominating inversion of configuration, and that thionyl chloride may or may not do so. In this case, retention of configuration is promoted by electron-releasing substituents at the seat of substitution (an early statement[182] that an α-phenyl substituent is necessary is too restrictive), and inhibited by reagents, such as tertiary bases, which produce chloride ions.[183]

The mechanisms which were suggested[155] in order to account for this general situation were as follows. It was assumed that the first step was always the formation of some kind of an ester-halide complex, if we may include in the term a hydrogen-bond complex with a hydrogen halide, $RO \cdot PCl_3^+$, $RO \cdot POCl_2$, $RO \cdot PCl_2$, $RO \cdot SOCl$, $RO \cdots HCl$, etc.; and that the complex may either ionise off a halogen atom, or undergo internal rearrangement (S_Ni). An ionisation of halogen would be followed either by an S_N2-type substitution by halide ion leading to inversion, or by an S_N1-type substitution involving predominating inversion in general, but predominating retention of configuration in the presence of a configuration-holding substituent. A rearrangement would involve a complete ionic severance of the CO-bond of the complex, but no separation of the formed ions, which would interact, with transference of a halide ion, retaining the original configuration. These ideas are represented below with reference to the thionyl chloride reaction.

It was assumed that the hydrogen halide and phosphorus halide complexes would have a greater tendency to lose a halide ion, and a smaller tendency towards heterolysis of the CO-bond and rearrangement, than would the thionyl halide esters; and that pyridine and other tertiary amines would promote the separation of halide ion by forming complex pyridinium or other ammonium halides; and also that the bonding of a strongly electron-releasing substituent, such as phenyl, o the seat of substitution would favour the CO-heterolysis, h—C—O-, and therefore promote the rearrangement.

[82] P. Frankland first drew this conclusion: *J. Chem. Soc.*, 1913, **103**, 717.

[183] J. Kenyon and H. Phillips first observed this effect of pyridine and of other ary amines: *J. Chem. Soc.*, **1930**, **415**, and several subsequent papers.

$$\begin{array}{c}{>}C{<}\overset{O}{}\!\!\!\underset{Cl}{}\!SO \longrightarrow {>}C\text{—}Cl + SO_2 \qquad (S_Ni)\\ \text{(retention)}\end{array}$$

$$\downarrow$$

$$\begin{array}{c}{>}C\cdot OSO^+ + Cl^- \longrightarrow Cl\text{—}C{<} + SO_2 \qquad (S_N2)\\ \text{(inversion)}\end{array}$$

$$\downarrow$$

$$ {>}C^+ + SO_2 + Cl^- \left\{\begin{array}{l} \rightarrow Cl\text{—}C{<} + SO_2 \\ \text{(inversion in general)} \\ \rightarrow {>}C\text{—}Cl + SO_2 \\ \text{(retention in special cases)}\end{array}\right\} \qquad (S_N1)$$

The above mechanisms of halogen introduction are more hypothetical and more of the nature of a rough outline than the well-established mechanisms S_N2 and S_N1 of halogen replacement. Modifications with added detail have been suggested by Lewis and Boozer,[184] but are not exclusively supported by the observations made; and thus the matter seems better left as a rough outline for the present. These workers isolated secondary alkyl chlorosulphites in optically active form, and showed that the transition states of their observed decompositions were highly polar—as is allowed, where not prescribed, in the general outline. The steric course of the decompositions depended in a complex way on the solvent.

The existence of the S_N1-type mechanism in these substitutions is strongly indicated by the experiments of Lucas and Winstein, who found in several examples that a β-situated halogen atom led to substitution of hydroxyl by halogen with retention of configuration.[185] Thus the *erythro*- and *threo*-forms of 2-bromobutan-3-ol, on treatment

[184] E. S. Lewis and C. E. Boozer, *J. Am. Chem. Soc.*, 1952, **74**, 308; 1953, **75**, 3182; 1954, **76**, 794.

[185] S. Winstein and H. J. Lucas, *J. Am. Chem. Soc.*, 1939, **61**, 1576, 2845; H. J. Lucas and C. W. Gould jr., *ibid.*, 1941, **63**, 2541; S. Winstein, *ibid.*, 1942, **64**, 2791.

with either hydrogen bromide or phosphorus tribromide, gave respectively the *meso*- and racemic forms of 2,3-dibromobutane. Furthermore, for the reaction of the bromo-alcohol with hydrogen bromide, it was established that a single optical *threo*-isomer of the alcohol gave a fully racemic *threo*-dibromide, thereby suggesting the mechanism represented below, which is entirely similar to that already given for unimolecular halogen displacement in the presence of a β-group with unshared electrons:

```
CH3    CH3          ┌CH3    CH3 ┐+       ⎧  CH3    CH3
 |  Br  |  H        |  |  Br   |  |       ⎪   | Br   |
 | /    | /         |  | /  \  |  |       ⎪   C ——— C
 C ———— C      →    |  C ———— C  |   →   ⎨   |   Br |
 |      |           |  |       |  |       ⎪   H      H          (DL)
 H     HO---HBr     └ H        H  ┘       ⎪  CH3    CH3
                                          ⎪   |      | Br
   (D or L)                               ⎪   C ——— C
                                          ⎩ Br|      |
                                              H      H
```

Shoppee has shown[179] that cholesterol is converted by phosphorus pentachloride and by thionyl chloride, without or with pyridine, into cholesteryl chloride with retention of configuration in the position substituted. The mechanism of these reactions doubtless bears a similarly close relation to that of the hydrolysis of the chloride, which, as already noted, proceeds with retention of configuration. We have here further evidence of the configuration-holding properties of the double bond of cholesterol.

Mechanism S_Ni has appeared in other reactions. An early example, due to Kenyon and Phillips,[140] is that the second step of the reaction of 2-octyl alcohol with phosgene goes with retention of configuration, evidently by an internal process:

```
C6H13—CH—CH3 → C6H13—CH—CH3 → C6H13—CH—CH3
       |               /  \              |
       OH             Cl   O             Cl        + CO2
                       \  /
                        CO
```

(33i) Replacement of NH_2 by OR or Hal.—These deaminations' which are effected by the action of nitrous acid, or of other nitrosyl compounds, on the primary amines, constitute the second group of reactions in which our knowledge of relative configurations, gained by application of the S_N2 Rule, was used in order to deduce the steric courses of reverse processes of substitution. From the steric courses, by comparison with the S_N2 and S_N1 Rules, the mechanisms of the deaminating reactions were provisionally inferred.[186] The main conclusion was that all deaminations were S_N1 substitutions of first-formed diazonium ions. The substitutions themselves were inaccessible to kinetic investigation, because they were fast relative to the formation of the diazonium ions. A concurrent study of the kinetics of formation of diazonium ions became definitive in 1950: as we shall see in Section **38c**, nitrosoamine formation, diazotisation, and deamination are all rate-controlled by *N*-nitrosation.

To return to the stereochemical evidence: some of the required polarimetric observations on reactions of deamination were already available in the early researches of Fischer and of McKenzie. Supplementing this, a polarimetric examination was made, for various groups R, of the following deamination processes:

$$RNH_2 + HNO_2 + \text{acid} + \text{solvent } H_2O \rightarrow ROH$$
$$RNH_2 + HNO_2 + \text{acid} + \text{solvent } EtOH \rightarrow ROEt$$
$$RNH_2 + NOCl + HCl + \text{solvent } H_2O \rightarrow RCl$$
$$RNH_2 + N_2O_3 \text{ or } NOCl + HBr + \text{solvent } H_2O \rightarrow RBr$$

When the polarimetric data were interpreted, by means of the already determined configurational correlations of the factors and products, so to give the steric courses of the reactions, a pattern of conclusions was obtained, which is illustrated in Table 33-3.

This table makes it quite clear that deamination in all its forms is

TABLE 33-3.—STERIC COURSE OF DEAMINATION.

Factor	Product			
RNH_2	ROH	ROEt	RCl	RBr
$C_2H_5 \cdot CH(NH_2) \cdot CH_3$	Rac +Inv	...	Rac +Inv	Rac +Inv
n-$C_6H_{13} \cdot CH(NH_2) \cdot CH_3$	Rac +Inv	Rac +Inv	Rac +Inv	Rac +Inv
$C_6H_5 \cdot CH(NH_2) \cdot CH_3$	Rac[1]+Inv	Rac[1]+Inv	Rac[1]+Inv	Rac[1]+Inv
$CH_3 \cdot CH(NH_2) \cdot CO_2H$	Ret	...	Ret	Ret
$CH_3 \cdot CH(NH_2) \cdot CO_2Et$	...	...	...	Rac +Inv
$C_6H_5 \cdot CH(NH_2) \cdot CO_2H$	Rac[1]+Ret	...	Rac[1]+Ret	Rac[1]+Ret

[1] Extensive racemisation in these reactions.

[186] P. Brewster, F. Hiron, E. D. Hughes, C. K. Ingold, and P. A. D. Rao *Nature*, 1950, **166**, 178.

obeying the S_N1 rule of steric orientation in substitution. It follows that the later steps of deamination must have the form of an S_N1 process, involving a carbonium-ionic intermediate. As stated, the reaction commences with an N-nitrosation, continues with rearrangement and ionisation of the primary nitrosamine to yield first the diazonium ion, and then the carbonium ion, and is completed by combination of the carbonium ion with either a solute anion, such as Cl^- or Br^-, or an anion such as OH^- or OEt^-, which has to be extracted from a molecule of the solvent:

$$RNH_2 \dashrightarrow RNH \cdot NO \rightarrow R \cdot N_2^+ \rightarrow \underbrace{R^+ \rightarrow RX}_{S_N1\text{-type}}$$

(33j) Orientation of Substitution in Alicyclic Systems.—In the strainless staggered ("chair") conformation of *cyclo*hexane, which is the stable conformation, six of the side-bonds are conformationally equivalent, and are described as *axial* (*a*, parallel to the trigonal axis), and the other six are also equivalent and are called *equatorial* (*e*, directed nearly radially outwards):

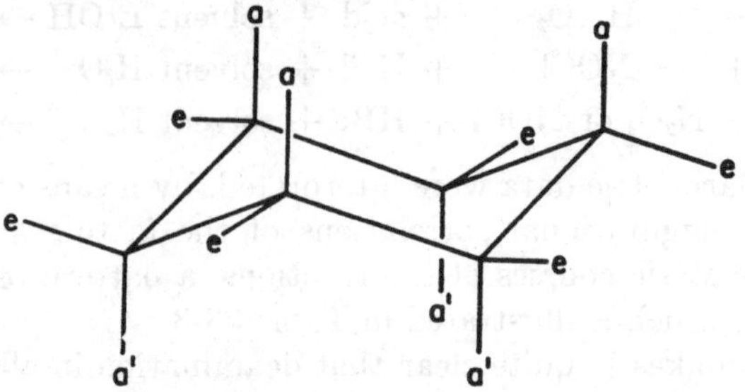

The most stable conformations of substituted *cyclo*hexanes will be those in which the substituent, or the largest substituent if there are several, occupies an equatorial position, so avoiding the steric 1,3-compressions (*aa* or *a′a′*) of axial substituents, or of one of them with axial hydrogen. When a displaceable substituent, such as a halogen or oxy-ester group, is axial, in the ground conformation, it can undergo an S_N2 replacement, with inversion, in that conformation. When, however, the displaceable group is equatorially situated, it cannot undergo an S_N2 replacement in that conformation, because of the shielding by the rest of the ring from a configuration-inverting attack by a nucleophile. The substrate must first change to a less stable conformation. The steric orientation of substitution will not be changed, because of the uncompromising definiteness of the S_N2 Rule; but the rate of substitution will be reduced.

This has been illustrated by Eliel and Ro,[187] in the example of the second-order substitution by phenylthiolate ion, PhS^-, in the *cis* and *trans* isomers of 4-*t*-butyl*cyclo*hexyl toluene-*p*-sulphonate:

$$t\text{-BuCH}\left\langle\begin{matrix}CH_2\cdot CH_2\\ \\ CH_2\cdot CH_2\end{matrix}\right\rangle CH\cdot OTs \rightarrow t\text{-BuCH}\left\langle\begin{matrix}CH_2\cdot CH_2\\ \\ CH_2\cdot CH_2\end{matrix}\right\rangle CH\cdot SPh$$

The reactions go with inversion: *trans*-ester gives *cis*-sulphide and *vice versa*; but in "95%" aqueous ethanol at 25°, the *trans*-ester reacts 19 times faster than the *cis*-ester. Eliel and Ro's interpretation is based on the plausible assumption that the *t*-butyl group will always occupy an equatorial position in a stable conformation. Then, in the *trans*-ester, the ester group will be axial, conformationally ready for S_N2 replacement. But in the *cis*-ester, the ester group will be equatorial in the ground conformation, and some energy will be needed to change the conformation before the S_N2 mechanism can operate.

Substitution in *cyclo*hexane derivatives by mechanism S_N1 is in a different case, inasmuch as the steric course is now determined by competitive shielding on the two sides of the carbonium ion; and we have here a built-in shielding by the rest of the ring, in competition with the usual shielding by the outgoing group. Furthermore, a purely aliphatic secondary carbonium ion, produced in a hydroxylic medium, is unlikely to have time enough to settle to an equilibrium conformation before it is trapped; and this entails that diastereoisomeric substrates, which would yield the same equilibrium carbonium ion, if the latter had time enough to reach equilibrium, will in fact give different S_N1 products or product-mixtures.

These matters have been illustrated particularly clearly for deamination. This, as we have seen, is an S_N1-type substitution. Its special features are that shielding by the departing nitrogen molecule is small, and that the latter releases its hydroxylic solvation shell early. In consequence, a purely aliphatic secondary carbonium ion, formed in this way, has no significant length of life, but reacts practically as soon as it is formed, and essentially as determined by the in-built shielding.

These deductions were first made by J. A. Mills,[188] from his analysis of observations by W. Hückel[189] and by Cornubert,[190] on the aqueous deamination of amino-derivatives of alkylated *cyclo*hexanes, and of

[187] E. E. Eliel and R. S. Ro, *J. Am. Chem. Soc.*, 1957, **79**, 5995.
[188] A. J. Mills, *J. Chem. Soc.*, **1953**, 280.
[189] W. Hückel, *Annalen*, 1938, **533**, 1.
[190] R. Cornubert, *Bull. Soc. chim.* (France), **1951**, C23.

cis- and *trans*-decalenes. Mills noticed that, of any pair of epimeric aminomenthanes, one gave almost exclusively an alcohol with retained configuration, whilst the other gave much menthene, together with alcohols formed with a predominating inversion of configuration. On examining the conformational situation, it appeared that the former behaviour was characteristic for an equatorial amino-group, and the latter for an axial one. Thus, menthylamine and *neo*menthylamine are taken to have the ground conformations shown below, in which the *iso*propyl group occupies an equatorial position. In menthylamine, the amino-group is therefore equatorial; and this is the epimer which gives menthol of like configuration. In *neo*menthylamine, the amino-group is axial; and it gives menthene, and more menthol than *neo*-menthol. Similar distinctions of behaviour were found in the decalene series, though there some of the conformational relations are more involved.

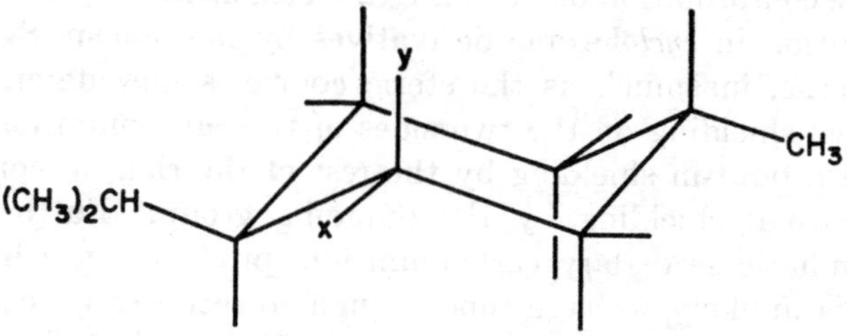

y

CH_3

$(CH_3)_2CH$

x

x = position of NH_2 in menthylamine and of OH in menthol
y = position of NH_2 in *neo*menthylamine and of OH in *neo*menthol

When we take the displaceable group from a secondary ring carbon to a bridge-head carbon, effects of the ring structure on its replacement become more dramatic. As we have already seen (Section **33c**), Bartlett showed, first in 1939, that the S_N2 mechanism becomes completely excluded. His examples were 1-chloroapocamphane and 1-bromotriptycene (formulae p. 520). His finding has since been confirmed in a number of other bridge-head systems, and there can be no doubt that it constitutes a general principle.

Substitution by mechanism S_N1 in bridge-head systems must proceed with total retention of configuration because of the total character of the built-in shielding. As to rates of substitution, Bartlett found in his examples that even S_N1 replacements were difficult. He concluded that the resistance presented by the rings to the flattening of the bridge-head carbonium ionic centre strongly impeded its formation. This finding also has been further illustrated; and Schleyer, in particular, has drawn attention to an interesting gradation of examples.[191] The rates of solvolysis in "80%" ethanol at 25° of the bridge-head bromides of *dicyclo*[1.2.2]heptane (norbornane), *dicyclo*[2.2.2]octane, and adamantane, relatively to that of *t*-butyl bromide, are as follows:

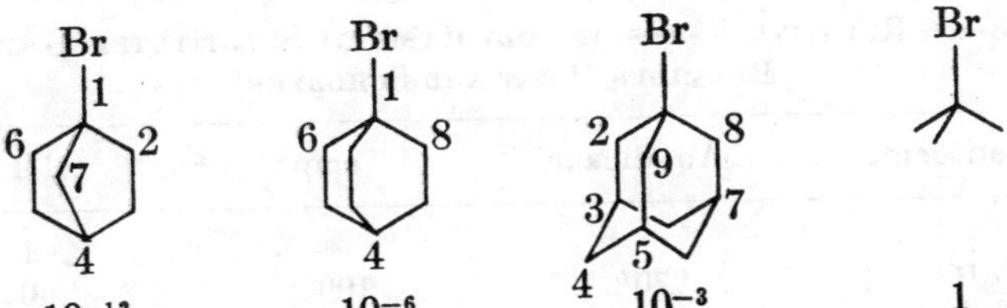

10^{-13} 10^{-6} 10^{-3} 1

These factors appear not to depend much on the out-going group: the exact values of (*t*-butyl)/(adamantyl) for halides in the above conditions are: chlorides, 1210; bromides, 817; and iodides, 1080. Nor do they seem to depend much on the solvolysing medium: the ratios (adamantyl)/(norbornyl) are 10^{10} for bromides in aqueous ethanol and 10^{11} for toluene-*p*-sulphonates in acetic acid.

As Schleyer points out,[191] Bartlett's concept of ring-strain resistance to carbonium-ion flattening would interpret these results. There is more resistance to bridge-head flattening in norbornane than in *dicyclo*[2.2.2]octane, and more in the latter than in adamantane. But there is more to say of the adamantylium ion, which can be studied, with hexafluoroantimonate as its counter-ion, in an SbF_5-SO_2 solvent. Schleyer and Olah and their coworkers[192] examined its proton magnetic resonance. The protons are not deshielded (deprived of electrons) to extents which, as usual, diminish with increasing distance from the positive charge: the tertiary protons of positions -3, -5, and -7 are deshielded somewhat more than the nearer protons of positions -2, -8, and -9. (The chemical shifts found for 2-H, 3-H, and 4-H were 4.50, 5.42, and 2.67 p.p.m., respectively.) And so the suggestion was made that the 1-cationic centre is appreciably stabilised by polarisable electrons from the tertiary 3-, 5-, and 7-CH bonds, which are attracted towards it within the adamantane cage. Consistently the solvolysis rates of 1-admantyl bromide have been found to be reduced by 3-substituents, markedly by electronegative 3-substituents, but mildly even by methyl groups, as illustrated in Table 33-4. The latter

[191] P. van R. Schleyer and R. D. Nicholas, *J. Am. Chem. Soc.*, 1961, **83**, 2700; R. C. Fort jr., and P. von R. Schleyer, *Chem. Rev.*, 1964, **64**, 277.

[192] P. von R. Schleyer, R. C. Fort jr., W. E. Watts, M. P. Comisarow, and G. A. Olah, *J. Am. Chem. Soc.*, 1964, **86**, 4195.

effect, though too small unequivocally to disclose its cause, is consistent, as Fort and Schleyer remark,[191] with the otherwise supported conclusion (Sections **7c** and **8d**) that methyl in an alkane is weakly electronegative.

TABLE 33-4.—RELATIVE RATES OF SOLVOLYSIS OF SUBSTITUTED 1-ADAMANTYL BROMIDES (FORT AND SCHLEYER).

Substituents	Aq.-dioxan	Temp.	Rel. rate
H			1
3-CO_2H	"70%"	100°	0.016
3-Br			2×0.0015
H			1
3-Me			0.69
3,5-Me_2	"80%"	70°	0.45
3,5,7-Me_3			0.31[a]

[a] Value by C. Grob, quoted by Fort and Schleyer.[191]

(34) STERIC EFFECTS ON RATE OF NUCLEOPHILIC SUBSTITUTION

(34a) The Concept of Steric Hindrance.—Although the general theory of organic chemical reactivity was given in its present form only since 1930, there have long existed certain more restricted theories directed to interpretations of anomalies or special effects. Such is the theory of steric hindrance, which was invented in the last century in order to explain why, in particular structural circumstances, certain general reactions do not take place with their accustomed ease. The interpretation given was very simple: it was that, in order to bring about a reaction in a complex molecule, one has to bring a reagent to an appropriate point; which may be difficult if the appropriate point lies in some well-shielded position among the branches of a branched structure.

Hofmann, who in the 1870's noticed[193] that highly methylated anilines, such as dimethylmesidine, seemed unable to react with methyl iodide, may have had a glimmering of this idea. It was certainly the guiding thought behind several planned researches in the 1890's. Claus illustrated it[194] by noting that aryl cyanides and benzamides having both ortho-positions substituted were exceptionally resistant to

[193] A. W. Hofmann, *Ber.*, 1872, **5**, 704; 1875, **8**, 61.

[194] A. Claus and J. Herbaborg, ***Ann.***, 1891, **265**, 364; A. Claus and R. Siebert, ***ibid.***, p. 378; A. Claus and C. Baysen, ***ibid.***, 1891, **266**, 223; A. Claus and L. Beck, ***ibid.***, 1892, **269**, 207; A. Claus and A. Weil, ***ibid.***, p. 216.

hydrolysis by the usual reagents. Kehrmann[195] demonstrated it by showing that the reactions of benzoquinones with hydroxylamine were restricted, at either carbonyl group, even by one, and very much by two, ortho-substituents, the effect apparently depending less on the chemical nature of the substituents than on their existence in proximity to the carbonyl group. Victor Meyer established the principle with particular thoroughness by showing[196] that ortho-disubstituted benzoic acids are more difficult to esterify, and their esters are harder to hydrolyse, than if the ortho-groups are absent; whereas the ortho-disubstituted phenylacetic acids, in which the site of reaction is removed one atom further out from the branched structure, are readily esterified, and their esters are easily hydrolysed. Again the chemical nature of the substituents seemed to matter less than their presence near the reaction site.

The classical theory of steric hindrance was simple, and its central idea was correct. Yet for 50 years, despite much additional illustration, it remained substantially undeveloped. The reason is fundamental. From about 1890 to 1940 steric hindrance was considered on a geometrical basis incorrectly restricted to that of normal molecules, in particular to the tetrahedral model of the carbon atom. Steric hindrance, as a kinetic phenomenon, should involve a differential consideration of the initial state of reactants and the transition state of reaction; and the latter is crucial, when a larger number of atoms have to be brought into an intimate geometrical relation in that state than in any normal molecule of the initial state. The geometry of transition states is not the same as that of normal molecules: a carbon atom at a reaction site does not, as we have seen, necessarily conform to the tetrahedral model. Only when the developing study of the Walden inversion had disclosed the configurations of transition states belonging to particular mechanisms, as explained in Section **33**, was it possible to consider steric hindrance from a geometrically correct viewpoint. Steric hindrance depends on the steric orientation of reaction; and steric orientation depends on reaction mechanism. It is easy to see why the study of steric hindrance, like that of steric orientation, could make no effective headway before 1935, when for the first time enough became known about reaction mechanism to enable these phenomena to be considered in proper relation to mechanism.

[195] F. Kehrmann, *Ber.*, 1888, **21**, 3315; F. Kehrmann and J. Messinger, *Ber.*, 1890, **23**, 3557; F. Kehrmann, *J. prakt. Chem.*, 1889, **40**, 257; *ibid.*, 1890, **42**, 134.

[196] V. Meyer, *Ber.*, 1894, **27**, 510; V. Meyer and J. J. Sudborough, *ibid.*, pp. 1580, 3146; V. Meyer, *Ber.*, 1895, **28**, 182, 1251, 2773, 3197; A. M. Kellas, *Z. physik. Chem.*, 1897, **24**, 221.

In 1937 the steric orientation problem was thus considered, as we have noticed. In 1941 Hughes extended the discussion to steric hindrance,[197] setting forth the principles stated above, and going on to show that the theory of steric hindrance, when given its correct geometrical basis, could be set on the road to quantitative dynamical development, progress at this stage being limited mainly by our (still) scanty knowledge (Section **5c**) of the repulsive forces between atoms not bonded to each other.

We do know that the forces between a pair of approaching non-bonded atoms remain weak, at first weakly attractive and later weakly repulsive, until a certain small separation is reached, within which the exchange forces of repulsion rapidly become strong. This it is which gives to steric hindrance its appearance of applying only to special situations. In principle non-bonding energy is present in every polyatomic molecule or transition state; but it very often remains slight enough not to have any qualitatively obvious effect on the reaction rate. When, however, owing to an increase, possibly quite a small increase, in the molecular complexity of a reactant, some non-bonded atoms in the transition state of reaction are forced to within a certain small and rather critical separation, then the non-bonding exchange energy may suddenly cease to be negligible in comparison with the energy involved in the bond changes. Qualitatively obvious kinetic effects then arise, which we describe by saying that steric hindrance is under observation.

Those steric effects on reactions which depend directly on differences of non-bonding compressional energy, we shall distinguish, when necessary, as *primary steric effects.* Throughout Section **34** we shall be concerned only with primary steric effects. The occasional need for a distinguishing adjective arises when reactions are subject, not only to these effects, but also to another group of steric effects, already mentioned in Chapters III and VI, in which non-bonding compression exerts its influence indirectly by interfering with the internal transmission of a conjugative polar effect. Effects of this latter group will be called *secondary steric effects.* We shall meet them again in later Chapters.

For the present, however, we are concerned only with primary steric effects, which depend directly on certain differences of non-bonding compressional energy. If, as envisaged above, the differences are between the initial and transition states of reaction, we shall observe *kinetic steric effects.* By far the most important group of such effects are those in which the compressional energy in the transition state is

[197] E. D. Hughes, *Trans. Faraday Soc.*, 1941, **37**, 603; A. G. Evans and M. Polanyi, *Nature*, 1942, **149**, 608, 653.

greater than that in the initial state. These are the kinetic effects summarised under the established term "steric hindrance," which we naturally retain because of its historical associations, though it will be convenient to be able to replace it by the more specific description *steric retardation*, when it becomes necessary to make it clear that the reference is to kinetic "hindrance," and not to thermodynamic "hindrance." It is believed that in some reactions, notably some dependent on a rate-controlling heterolysis, there is less non-bonding energy of compression in the transition state than in the initial state. This situation leads to the second possible type of kinetic steric effect, namely, *steric acceleration*.

(34b) Steric and Ponderal Retardation in Bimolecular Substitution.—A bimolecular nucleophilic substitution,

$$Y^- + CabcX \rightarrow YCabc + X^-$$

has a transition state, which in general approximates to the form shown in Fig. 34-1, and, when symmetry so determines, is exactly of that

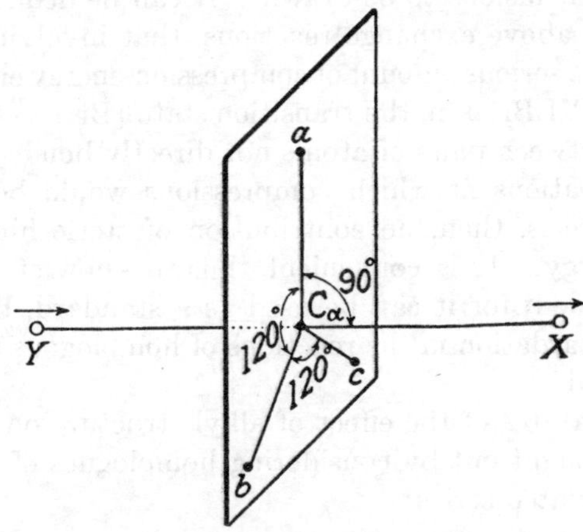

FIG. 34-1.—Model of the transition state in bimolecular nucleophilic substitution.

form.[198] We have to enquire to what extent pairs of atoms not directly bonded together have their energy raised by mutual compression, first, in the initial molecule CabcX, and then, as is especially important, in the transition state {Y · · · Cabc · · · X}⁻, since any excess of non-bonded energy of compression in the transition state will increase the activation energy of the reaction, and reduce its rate accordingly.

As an initial simplification, let us consider a symmetrical substitu-

[198] Two symmetrically off-plane transition states have been suggested, but for no compelling reason.

tion, such as the bromine exchange reaction, which can, of course, be studied by techniques of radioactivity:

$$Br^- + CabcBr \rightarrow BrCabc + Br^-$$

In the bimolecular transition state $\{Br \cdots Cabc \cdots Br\}^-$, the central carbon atom has the exact configuration of a triangular double pyramid; and the anionic charge is shared equally between the bromine atoms. Those bonds which are neither formed nor destroyed may be considered, for want of more exact information, to have their normal lengths. The half-formed and half-broken bonds to the bromine atoms have lengths which can be estimated in several approximate ways to be about 0.35 *A* greater than the length of a fully formed CBr bond.[199]

Our empirical knowledge concerning equilibrium distances between non-bonded atoms is derived mainly from X-ray-measured distances between molecules in crystals. As information applicable outside the solid state, it is not at all detailed or exact; but it does allow certain semi-quantitative conclusions to be drawn. It can be deduced that in the simplest of the above exchange reactions, that involving methyl bromide, there is no serious amount of compression energy either in the normal molecule, CH_3Br, or in the transition state $\{Br \cdots CH_3 \cdots Br\}^-$, all distances between pairs of atoms not directly bonded being greater than the separations at which compressions would begin to be important. There is, then, no contribution of steric hindrance to the activation energy. It is convenient thus to know of a reaction not sterically retarded; for it can be used as a standard, by reference to which steric retardation in the reactions of homologous alkyl bromides may be assessed.

The main features of the effect of alkyl structure on steric retardation can be brought out by considering homologues of two series, the α- and β-methylated series:

methyl, ethyl, *iso*propyl, *t*-butyl (α-series)

ethyl, *n*-propyl, *iso*butyl, *neo*pentyl (β-series)

When we are considering experimental data, it will be necessary to remember that, in the reactions of groups of the α-series, an appreciable polar effect may be expected, while in those of the β-series, but little of the polar effect of the variable part of the group should get through to the site of reaction.

[199] This is essentially the Morse-curve stretched-length at the energy of activation. It should be an underestimate, but can be computed without heavy guesswork, and provides a uniform basis for the comparative treatment of a number of substitutions.

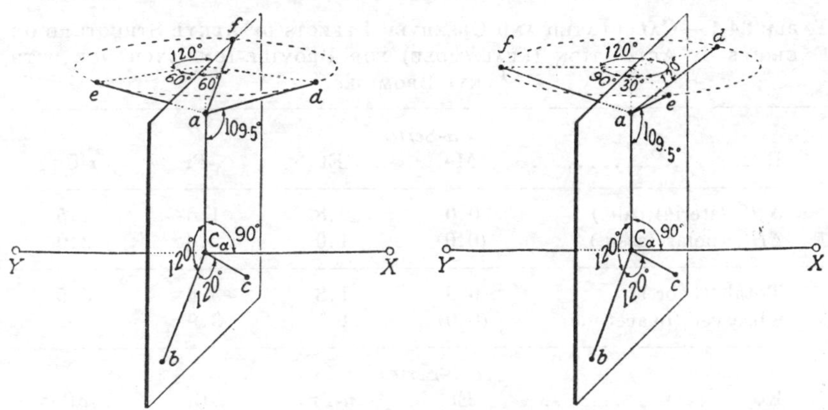

FIG. 34-2.—Configurations of alkyl groups in the transition states of bimolecular substitutions.

The significant forms of transition state for the reactions of these groups are shown in Fig. 34-2. In the methyl group, *a*, *b*, and *c*, are hydrogen atoms, which along the α-series are successively replaced by methyl groups. In the ethyl group, *d*, *e*, and *f*, are hydrogen atoms, which along the β-series become replaced by methyl groups. Whichever of the forms shown has the less compression energy is assumed to be the effective form: if we place hydrogen atoms at *d* and *e* when possible, the left-hand form would be effective for all the groups named, excepting the *iso*butyl group, which would use the other form, with methyl groups at *d* and *e*.

An estimate, first, from the geometry of the molecules and transition states, of the non-bonded compression distances, and then, from force-law formulae of the type given in Section **5c**, of the corresponding compression energies, and finally of the reductions of compression energy which follow when the entering and leaving halogens are allowed so to adjust their positions as to minimise their total (bonding+non-bonding) energies, gives the calculated steric contribution to the activation energy of the substitution. Such figures are illustrated for the bromide-ion exchange reaction in the lines labelled "$\Delta H^{\neq}$ (steric) (calc.)" in Table 34-1.

Owing to the approximations made, these figures have only semi-quantitative significance; so let us consider first their qualitative indications. First, in the α-series, the ethyl group provides a small steric energy of activation, which in the *iso*propyl and *t*-butyl groups becomes duplicated and triplicated, respectively. This is due to essentially independent compressions between each α-methyl substituent and each bromine atom in the transition state of reaction. Secondly, along the β-series, steric energy shows a strikingly accelerated growth

TABLE 34-1.—CALCULATED AND OBSERVED EFFECTS OF ALKYL STRUCTURE ON ENERGIES OF ACTIVATION (KCAL./MOLE) FOR BROMIDE-ION EXCHANGE WITH ALKYL BROMIDES.

		α-Series		
R....................	Me	Et	*i*-Pr	*t*-Bu
$\Delta H^{\neq}$ (steric)(calc.)	0.0	0.8	1.6	2.5
$\Delta H^{\neq}$ (polar)(assd.)	(0.0)	1.0	2.0	3.0
Total (theor.)	0.0	1.8	3.6	5.5
Observed (in acetone)	(0.0)	1.7	3.9	—
		β-Series		
R....................	Et	*n*-Pr	*i*-Bu	*neo*Pen
$\Delta H^{\neq}$ (steric)(calc.)	0.8	0.8	2.3	7.3
$\Delta H^{\neq}$ (polar)(assd.)	1.0	1.0	1.0	1.0
Total (theor.)	1.8	1.8	3.3	8.3
Observed (in acetone)	1.7	1.7	3.1	6.2

to an outstanding value in the *neo*pentyl group, which is thereby indicated as providing one of the special situations characteristic of the phenomenon of steric hindrance. The reason is that while the single β-methyl substituent of *n*-propyl can be turned to avoid the bromine atoms in the transition state, and the two of *iso*butyl can be turned partly to avoid them, of the three in *neo*pentyl, two necessarily lie closer to bromine atoms than the limit below which compressions become energetically serious. In general, compressions in initial states, while not insignificant absolutely, can be neglected in comparison with the compressions of transition states.

An argument of analogy, based on Victor Meyer's finding that steric hindrance is present in the carboxyl reactions of ortho-disubstituted benzoic acids, but not in those of the homologous phenylacetic acids, might have suggested more steric hindrance in bimolecular reactions of *t*-butyl halides, containing their halogen close to the branched structure, than in the corresponding reactions of *neo*pentyl halides, in which the halogen is moved one atom out from the branching point. However, the argument is misleading. The opposite conclusion indicated above results from recognising that the geometry of transition states, and not only that of normal molecular states, is significant for the consideration of steric retardation.

Similar calculations have been made for other incoming and outgoing pairs of halogens, with the result that, strange as it seems at first, calculated steric compressions are not very greatly affected by the sizes of the entering and displaced groups, which need not be identical, though calculations are made easier when they are the same. The reason is that there are compensating factors. Thus, if we replace the bromide ion in the bromine exchange reaction by an iodide ion, the larger halogen will set itself further from the central carbon atom in the transition state, so that all non-bonded distances from the iodine atom will be increased. But because of the larger size of iodine the various limits of separation below which compressions become important also become increased. The result is that the compressions remain similar, and their energies remain of the same order. Thus the value of $\Delta H^{\neq}$ (steric)(calc.), 7.3 kcal./mole for the exchange $Br^- + RBr$, as we have seen, is only 7.8 kcal./mole for the exchange $I^- + RI$.

For bimolecular substitutions in general, the extent to which steric compression in the transition state is sensitive to the size of the entering and displaced groups depends on the geometry of the transition state. In aliphatic nucleophilic substitution, the degree of compression, as explained above, is much more sensitive to the sizes of the permanently present groups involved in the compression, than to those of the displacing and displaced groups. In electrophilic aromatic substitution (Chapter VI), on the other hand, the amount of compression, as may easily be calculated assuming approximately tetrahedral bonding at the point of substitution in the transition state (Section **23d**), is only a little more sensitive to the size of an ortho-group than to that of the entering group; and the comparable importance of these two size factors in this form of substitution appears to be borne out by the recorded observations (Section **22b**). Yet other relations apply to effects of ortho-substituents in bimolecular nucleophilic substitutions in a benzyl halide. These effects again can be correlated with the specific geometry of the initial and of the transition states of substitution, as has been shown in detail by Charlton and Hughes.[200]

To return to reactions in simple alkyl systems—the above-described theoretical situation concerning bimolecular substitution was first explained in 1941 by Hughes,[197] who also recorded an experimental kinetic comparison, later amplified by Dostrovsky and himself,[201] of most of the above alkyl groups with respect to several substitution processes, thereby interpreting previously known facts in the qualitative chemistry of *neo*pentyl halides, which had been thought anomalous up to that time.

[200] M. L. Crossley, R. H. Kienle, and C. H. Benbrook, *J. Am. Chem. Soc.*, 1940, **62**, 1400; H. Cohn, E. D. Hughes, M. H. Jones, and M. G. Peeling, *Nature*, 1952, **169**, 291; J. C. Charlton and E. D. Hughes, *J. Chem. Soc.*, **1956**, 855.

[201] I. Dostrovsky and E. D. Hughes, *J. Chem. Soc.*, **1946**, 157, 161, 164, 166, 169, 171; I. Dostrovsky, E. D. Hughes, and C. K. Ingold, *ibid.*, p. 173.

Whitmore had directed attention to the remarkable inactivity of *neo*pentyl halides.[202] Except for its reactions with sodium and magnesium, *neo*pentyl chloride failed to undergo any of the common reactions of alkyl chlorides. Even *neo*pentyl iodide showed little or no tendency to react with ethoxide, hydroxide, or cyanide ions. Analogy with the classical examples of steric hindrance, analogy without reference to mechanism, made it difficult to hold steric hindrance responsible for these effects.

Dostrovsky and Hughes found[201] that the differences were quantitative rather than qualitative: thus *neo*pentyl bromide reacted with ethoxide ions in ethyl alcohol, and with iodide ions in acetone, about 10^4–10^5 times more slowly than do the simplest primary alkyl bromides. They also found that these marked distinctions of reactivity were peculiar to the bimolecular mechanism, and that, in several forms of unimolecular substitution, *neo*pentyl bromide was quite similar in reactivity to other primary alkyl bromides, as we shall note more fully

TABLE 34-2.—SECOND ORDER REACTIONS OF METHYL AND PRIMARY ALKYL BROMIDES WITH SODIUM ETHOXIDE IN ETHYL ALCOHOL.

	Me	Et	*n*-Pr	*i*-Bu	*neo*P
$10^3 k_2$ at 55°	34.4	1.95	0.547	0.058	0.00000826
$10^{-11} A$	7.2	2.1	—	0.95	0.0023
E (kcal./mole)	20.0	21.0	—	22.8	26.2

The units of k_2 and of A are sec.$^{-1}$ mole^{-1} l.

in the next Section. The observed second-order rates for the reactions of methyl and primary alkyl bromides with ethoxide ions in ethyl alcohol at 55° will serve to illustrate the special quantitative position of *neo*pentyl bromide in bimolecular substitution. The greater part, though not the whole, of each distinction of rate was found to be reflected in the Arrhenius energies of activation, as indicated by the figures in Table 34-2.

We have referred so far only to the calculated steric increments of activation energy, called "$\Delta H^{\neq}$ (steric)(calc.)" in Table 34-1. To this, we should add the polar increments, that is, the increments that arise from the inductive effect, when the parent methyl group of the homologous series is elaborated to the various higher alkyl groups. All that we can really say about this on theoretical grounds is that the

[202] F. C. Whitmore and G. H. Fleming, *J. Am. Chem. Soc.*, 1933, 55, 4161; F. C. Whitmore, E. L. Whittle, and A. H. Popkin, *ibid.*, 1939, 61, 1586; F. C. Whitmore, A. H. Popkin, H. I. Bernstein, and J. P. Wilkins, *ibid.*, 1941, 63, 124.

contributions of α-methyl substituents should be equal, and those of β-methyl substituents negligible, in first approximation. Taking the increments as 1 kcal./mole per α-methyl, and zero for β-methyl, we can set down the figures called "$\Delta H^{\neq}$ (polar)(assd.)" in Table 34-1. As will be seen from the table, the sum of these theoretical steric and polar energies, these constitutional increments of activation energy, follow the observed values fairly closely. The main discrepancy is found in the values for the *neo*pentyl group, which has considerable flexibility that is not allowed for in the calculations, a flexibility to neglect which makes steric compression appear more important than it is. Similar calculations and experimental data have been provided for other incoming and outgoing halogens. They are monotonously like those illustrated in the example of bromide exchange.

The theoretical and experimental energy data, already cited in Table 34-1, come from a later investigation of Finkelstein substitutions by Hughes and his colleagues.[203] They also concerned themselves with the calculation and observation of entropies of activation, as will now be explained.

In the calculation of steric energies of activation, one is required, as remarked already, to minimise bonding plus non-bonding energy under variations of halogen positions in the transition state: in geometrical language, one has to calculate an energy surface. Such a surface has the form of a basin: the height of its bottom represents the energy of the transition state, and the openness of its sides controls the entropy of the state. From the shape of the basin, one can calculate, by standard formulae, the steric increments of entropy of activation.

An unforeseen effect emerged in these calculations. The entropy of an energy basin depends, not only on the shape of the basin, but also on the masses and moments of inertia of the kinetic systems using it: the greater these inertial characters are, the more closely packed will be the relevant energy levels in the basin, and the greater therefore will be its receiving capacity, which we express in logarithmic form as its entropy. This simple consideration requires recognition of a class of structural effect, which had not before been comprehensively considered. It is neither steric nor polar; *i.e.*, it does not depend on distributions of bulk or charge. It has been termed *ponderal*, because it depends on the distribution of mass, independently of bulk or charge. Neutrons, having mass, but no bulk, and no charge, added as they could be, by an isotopic substitution, should produce a ponderal

203 P. B. D. de la Mare, B. D. England, L. Fowden, E. D. Hughes, and C. K. Ingold, *J. Chim. Phys.*, 1948, 45, 236; P. B. D. de la Mare, L. Fowden, E. D. Hughes, C. K. Ingold, and J. D. H. Mackie, *J. Chem. Soc.*, 1955, 3169 *et seq.* (8 papers); C. K. Ingold, *Quart. Rev. Chem. Soc.*, 1957, 11, 1.

kinetic effect. It cannot be doubted that ponderal effects on reaction rate have frequently passed unnoticed in admixtures with steric and polar effects.

The ponderal increment of activation entropy was computed as the effect on entropy of activation of a change of alkyl structure, in case such change had made no difference to the energy surface. The total entropy effect results from the combined changes of mass and of surface. The steric increment of activation entropy was thus computed by difference. The results are illustrated for the bromide exchange reaction in Table 34-3. One sees that all ponderal effects are negative (rate-reducing), and that they increase in magnitude with alkyl mass, and with the distance of the added mass from the halogen mass. The entropic steric effects are also all negative, except for the *t*-butyl group.

TABLE 34-3.—CALCULATED AND OBSERVED EFFECTS OF ALKYL STRUCTURE ON ENTROPIES OF ACTIVATION (IN CAL. DEG.$^{-1}$ MOLE^{-1}) OF BROMIDE-ION EXCHANGE WITH ALKYL BROMIDES.

	α-Series			
R....................	Me	Et	*i*-Pr	*t*-Bu
$\Delta S^{\neq}$ (ponderal)(calc.)	(0.0)	−1.45	−2.30	−1.95
$\Delta S^{\neq}$ (steric)(cal.)	(0.0)	−0.66	−1.52	+0.83
Total (theor.)	(0.0)	−2.11	−3.82	−1.12
Observed (in acetone)	(0.0)	−2.7	−4.7	—
	β-Series			
R....................	Et	*n*-Pr	*i*-Bu	*neo*Pen
$\Delta S^{\neq}$ (ponderal)(calc.)	−1.45	−2.64	−3.66	−4.39
$\Delta S^{\neq}$ (steric)(calc.)	−0.66	−0.67	−1.06	−1.86
Total (theor.)	−2.11	−3.31	−4.72	−6.25
Observed (in acetone)	−2.7	−4.1	−5.0	−9.6

Table 34-3 also contains the comparison with the observed effects of alkyl homology on entropy of activation. The observational values are simply the differences of the common logarithms of the Arrhenius pre-exponential factors, these differences having been multiplied by 4.575 for conversion to thermal units. The calculated entropic effects follow the pattern of the observations, but are always underestimated. The most likely source of error is the neglect of solvent effects. The hope was that, because two subtractions are involved in each figure, an initial state from a transition state, and a methyl group from a higher alkyl group, energies and entropies of solvation would cancel out in the difference of differences; but this may not be true. It is unlikely that error arises from the omission to calculate ponderal energies, which would be insignificant; this is because of the large mass of the kinetic particles. It is unlikely that the omission to allow for polar entropies would cause appreciable error; they must be very small because of the weakness of alkyl polarity. It should be remarked that the energy surfaces, and hence the steric energies, and the steric and ponderal entropies, are all calculated without any disposable constants: all the constants needed are given by experimental measurements of other kinds, of bond lengths, bond strengths, vibration frequencies, compressibilities, and the like.

Combination of the calculated energetic and entropic factors gives relative reaction rate which may be directly compared with observed values. Such a comparison is given in Table 34-4 for the bromide-ion exchange in acetone at 25°. It will be seen that there is general consistency to a factor of 5 over a rate range of 5,000,000.

TABLE 34-4.—OBSERVED AND CALCULATED STRUCTURAL EFFECTS ON THE RATES OF REACTIONS $Br^- + RBr \rightarrow RBr + Br^-$ IN ACETONE AT 25°.

α-Series				
R..................	Me	Et	*i*-Pr	*t*-Bu[1]
Relative rates (calc.)	1	0.017	0.000,35	0.000,053
Relative rates (obsd.)	1	0.013	0.000,14	0.000,039

β-Series				
R..................	Et	*n*-Pr	*i*-Bu	*neo*Pen
Relative rates (calc.)	0.017	0.0090	0.000,35	0.000,000,037
Relative rates (obsd.)	0.013	0.0085	0.000,44	0.000,000,20

[1] D. Cook and A. J. Parker show in a paper (*J. Chem. Soc.*, 1968, *B*, 142) seen too late to be summarised here that apparent rates of Finkelstein substitutions of *t*-butyl halides (but not of the other halides) are rendered markedly too high by concurrent elimination with subsequent addition. The agreement with calculation is here notably worse than it appears.

(34c) Kinetic Steric Effects in Unimolecular Substitution.—Steric retardation may enter bimolecular substitutions because the atoms are more congested in the transition state than in the initial state, and in some structures may be congested enough to produce a heightened energy barrier. On the other hand, steric retardation plays no comparable part in unimolecular substitution, because its transition state is formed through the incursion of longer-range electrostatic forces of solvation, with the result that the atoms nearest the reaction site are not more congested than before.[204]

Hughes and Dostrovsky applied these ideas in their study of the substitutions of alkyl halides.[205] They showed that, although Whitmore had taken strong measures with limited success in his attempts to hydrolyse the *neo*pentyl halides with reagents such as concentrated alcoholic alkali, hydrolysis can in fact be rather easily effected, without any alkali, by simply adding water to the alcohol. The reason is that, while any alkyl halide in principle has available an S_N2 and an S_N1 mechanism of hydrolysis, most primary alkyl halides find the S_N2 mechanism the more facile; but when this mechanism is sterically much impeded in a particular case, then the alkyl halide may do better if ionising conditions for the S_N1 mechanism are provided, since this mechanism is not sensitive to steric hindrance.

The matter can be illustrated by the figures in the top two lines of Table 34-5: they are relative rates of hydrolysis or alcoholysis for the four primary alkyl bromides of the β-series. In this table, rates which are known or believed to relate to bimolecular reactions are distinguished by parentheses: the other rates are those of unimolecular substitutions. The top line, which is there for comparison, refers to the already-discussed second-order reaction with ethoxide ions in dry ethyl alcohol: these reactions are certainly bimolecular, and we note the initially gradual, and then sudden, onset of steric hindrance along the series. The second line relates to solvolysis in "50%" aqueous ethyl alcohol: one observes that the first three figures run parallel in order of magnitude to those above them, but that the fourth drops below the third by a factor of 10^1, instead of 10^4. The interpretation given is that the first three figures are rates of bimolecular reactions with solvent molecules, and that the fourth (about a thousand times too large to be thus understood) is the unimolecular rate for the primary halide. In confirmation it was observed that, while the reactions of ethyl, *n*-propyl, and *iso*butyl bromide in "50%" aqueous alcohol are strongly accelerated by added alkali, the reaction of *neo*pentyl bromide is insensitive to added alkali. It was also observed that, whereas the

[204] E. D. Hughes, *Trans. Faraday Soc.*, 1941, **37**, 620; J. N. E. Day and C. K. Ingold, *ibid.*, p. 699.

[205] E. D. Hughes, *loc. cit.;* I. Dostrovsky and E. D. Hughes, *J. Chem. Soc.*, **1946**, 166, 169, 171; I. Dostrovsky, E. D. Hughes, and C. K. Ingold, *ibid.*, p. 190.

second-order reaction between *neo*pentyl bromide and ethoxide ions gave the normal product, *neo*pentyl ethyl ether, the reaction of *neo*pentyl bromide in "50%" aqueous alcohol produced *t*-amyl alcohol and its ethyl ether, as well as amylenes, a rearrangement having occurred, which, as we shall note in Chapter X, is diagnostic of the unimolecular mechanism for this particular alkyl group.

TABLE 34-5.—RELATIVE RATES OF BIMOLECULAR OR UNIMOLECULAR SUBSTITUTIONS OF PRIMARY AND TERTIARY ALKYL BROMIDES.

Primary R	$CH_3\cdot CH_2\cdot$	$CH_3\cdot CH\cdot CH_2\cdot$	$(CH_3)_2CH\cdot CH_2\cdot$	$(CH_3)_3C\cdot CH_2\cdot$
RBr + OEt^- in EtOH, 55°	(1)	(0.28)	(0.030)	(0.0000042)
RBr + "50%" aq-EtOH, 95°	(1)	(0.58)	(0.080)	0.0064
RBr + H_2O in HCO_2H, 95°	1	0.69	—	0.57
Tertiary R	$CH_3\cdot CMe_2\cdot$	$CH_3\cdot CH_2\cdot CMe_2\cdot$	$(CH_3)_2\cdot CH\cdot CMe_2\cdot$	$(CH_3)_3C\cdot CMe_2\cdot$
RCl + "80%" aq-EtOH, 25°	1	1.68	0.87	1.16
RBr + "80%" aq-EtOH, 25°	1	1.78	1.22	1.68
RI + "80%" aq-EtOH, 25°	1	2.00	1.62	2.84

The best known solvent for unimolecular substitutions in alkyl halides is formic acid, which ionises even primary alkyl bromides with sufficient freedom. Dostrovsky and Hughes used it as a solvent for their hydrolyses, obtaining the relative rates indicated by the third line of figures in Table 34-5; they are all of the same order of magnitude, as would be expected if all are unimolecular rates, steric hindrance and the polar effect of β-substitution being negligible.

The lower part of Table 34-5 refers to reactions in aqueous alcohol of three series of tertiary alkyl halides, having the same growing chain as that of the primary alkyl bromides.[206] There is a great weight of evidence that all these reactions are unimolecular; and it is significant that all the rates in each series are of the same order of magnitude, as they should be according to the hypothesis that unimolecular reactions are insensitive to steric hindrance, and that the polar effect of β-alkylation is negligible. There could be no clearer indication than that obtained by comparing any of these lines of figures with the top line of Table 34-5, that bimolecular and unimolecular substitutions have differently constituted transition states, that is, that the distinction between the mechanisms is fundamental.

[206] E. D. Hughes, *J. Chem. Soc.*, **1935,** 255; K. A. Cooper, E. D. Hughes, and C. K. Ingold, *ibid.*, **1937,** 1280; E. D. Hughes and B. J. MacNulty, *ibid.*, p. 1283; J. Shorter and C. N. Hinshelwood, *ibid.*, **1949,** 2412; H. C. Brown and R. S. Fletcher, *J. Am. Chem. Soc.*, 1949, **71,** 1845; H. C. Brown and A. Stern, *ibid.*, 1950, **72,** 5068; E. D. Hughes, C. K. Ingold, R. J. L. Martin, and D. F. Meigh, *Nature*, 1950, **166,** 679.

The S_N2-blocked primary, secondary, and tertiary alkyl halides of the structures, $Me_3C \cdot CH_2 \cdot X$, $Me_3C \cdot CHMe \cdot X$, $Me_3C \cdot CMe_2 \cdot X$, employ the S_N1 mechanism preferentially or exclusively, and with markedly increasing rates, and decreasing activation energies, along the homologous series. It has been estimated[207] that, for solvolysis of the bromides in "80%" aqueous ethanol, the activation energies are 30.0, 26.7, and 23.3 kcal./mole, respectively. Values reproducing the falls by 3–4 kcal./mole, as each α-methyl group is added to the system, follow for chlorides, and for other aqueous organic solvents.

Although steric retardation plays no part in the unimolecular nucleophilic substitutions of simple alkyl halides, it does enter mildly into those of secondary aralphyl halides having two ortho-substituents. This was established by Charlton and Hughes.[208] Their interpretation is illustrated by the following formulae for a di-ortho-substituted α-arylethyl chloride and the carbonium ion derived from it:

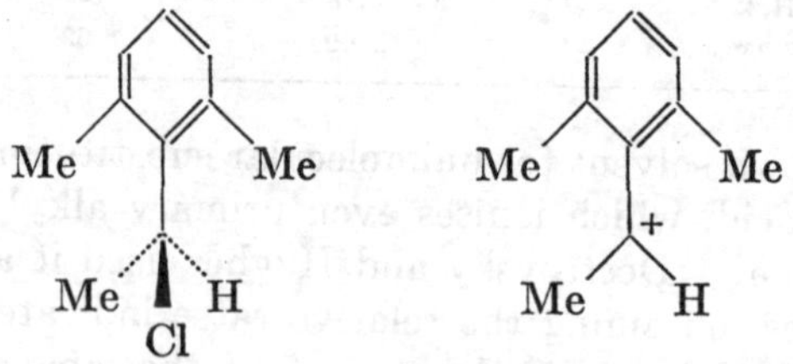

In the initial state, the reactive side-chain is tetrahedral, and all its substituents can be sufficiently off-plane to avoid significant pressure from the ortho-methyl groups. In the carbonium ion the bonding forces, if they could have their way, would bring all the bonds shown into a plane, so creating a maximum of pressure between the side-chain methyl group and one ortho-methyl group. The configuration of the transition state of the unimolecular mechanism, which is that of formation of the carbonium ion, will approach the configuration of the carbonium ion, and will contain a large part of the steric pressure in the latter. This excess of steric pressure produces steric retardation in this unimolecular reaction.

The nucleophilic substitutions of di-ortho-substituted α-arylethyl halides are predominantly unimolecular in polar solvents of polarity down at least to that of acetone. The solvolyses of α-mesitylethyl chloride, 2,4,6-$Me_3C_6H_2 \cdot CHMe \cdot Cl$, in aqueous ethanol and in ethanol, are demonstrably unimolecular. The aromatic methyl groups, of course, have a polar effect on these reactions. Charlton and Hughes estimated it by means of rate comparisons with isomers of

[207] E. D. Hughes *et al.*, *Nature*, 1950, **166**, 679.

[208] J. C. Charlton and E. D. Hughes, *J. Chem. Soc.*, **1954**, 2939; **1956**, 850.

lower homologues. They found no indication of a steric effect until the third of the three methyl groups shown in the graphic formulae above was introduced. Then the rates suddenly became smaller than polar effects alone should make them, to a degree corresponding to the presence, in the transition state of ionisation, of an excess of non-bonding energy amounting to about 1.0–1.5 kcal./mole.

The possibility of steric acceleration in unimolecular nucleophilic substitution, that is, of a situation in which non-bonding internal pressures of the initial state become appreciably relieved when the bond to be heterolysed becomes stretched in the transition state of ionisation, has been discussed by Brown and Hughes and their coworkers.[209] The idea is highly plausible, and may yet be convincingly illustrated for substitution, as it has been for elimination (Chapter IX); but the evidence adduced so far for substitution is not fully satisfactory. The difficulty is not to find an unexpectedly fast unimolecular substitution, but to find one in which the accelerating forces can only be non-bonding, and could not be bonding forces of the kind that we classify as cyclosynartesis (Section **33e**) or synartesis (Chapter X).

(35) NUCLEOPHILIC OLEFINIC SUBSTITUTION

(35a) Kinetic Character.—Nucleophilic olefinic substitutions of the form

$$Y^- + RR'CH{=}CR''{-}X \rightarrow RR'CH{=}CR''{-}Y + X^-$$

like nucleophilic aromatic substitutions, go very slowly in the absence of an electron-attracting substituent, such as a nitro-group, a sulphonyl group, or a carbonyl or carboxyl group. Thus, whereas Finkelstein substitutions by iodide ion in vinyl bromide or in ω-bromostyrene require temperatures above 200° in alcoholic solvents in order to achieve convenient rates, the corresponding reactions of iodide ion with *cis*- and *trans*-ω-bromo-*p*-nitrostyrene go relatively easily.[210]

All the detailed kinetic work on nucleophilic olefinic substitution has been done with substrates containing activating electronegative groups. Modena and his collaborators studied the substitutions[211]

[209] H. C. Brown and R. S. Fletcher, *J. Am. Chem. Soc.*, 1949, [illegible] 1845; H. C. Brown and A. Stern, *ibid.*, 1950, **72**, 5068; F. Brown, T. D. Davies, I. Dostrovsky, O. J. Evans, and E. D. Hughes, *Nature*, 1951, **167**, 987; E. D. Hughes, *Quart. Rev. Chem. Soc.*, 1951, **5**, 245.

[210] S. I. Miller and P. K. Yonan, *J. Am. Chem. Soc.*, 1957, **79**, 5031.

[211] F. Montenari, *Bull. Soc. Fac. Chim. ind.* (*Bologna*), 1958, **31**, 16; G. Modena, *Ricerca sci.*, 1958, **28**, 341; L. Maioli and G. Modena, *Gazz. Chim. Ital.*, 1959, **89**, 854; G. Modena and P. E. Todesco, *ibid.*, p. 866; *idem* and S. Tamti, *ibid.*, p. 878; S. Ghersetti, G. Lugli, G. Melloni, G. Modena, P. E. Todesco, and P. Vivarelli, *J. Chem. Soc.*, **1965**, 2227.

$$Y^- + PhSO_2 \cdot CH{=}CH{-}Cl \rightarrow PhSO_2 \cdot CH{=}CH{-}Y + Cl^-$$

$$Y^- + PhSO \cdot CH{=}CH{-}Cl \rightarrow PhSO \cdot CH{=}CH{-}Y + Cl^-$$

with $Y^- = MeO^-$, EtO^-, PhO^-, MeS^-, N_3^-. The kinetics were always of second order, first in each reactant. Vernon and his coworkers found the same for the substitutions[212]

$$Y^- + EtO_2C \cdot CH{=}CMe{-}Cl \rightarrow EtO_2C \cdot HC{=}CMe{-}Y + Cl^-$$

with $Y^- = EtO^-$, PhO^-, EtS^-, PhS^-.

These kinetics would be consistent with an S_N2 type of mechanism, perhaps analogous to the common mechanism of nucleophilic aromatic substitution in the presence of activating electronegative substituents (Section **26**). They would be equally consistent with the elimination-addition mechanism, proceeding by way of an intermediate acetylene, and analogous to the benzyne mechanism of nucleophilic aromatic substitution. However, this mechanism requires that *cis*- and *trans*-isomers of a substrate should give the same product, or the same mixture of products; and that, as we shall see, is not the observation. Moreover, Vernon carried out the reaction of ethylthiolate ion with the ethyl *cis*- and *trans*-β-chlorocrotonates in a deuterium ethoxide solvent, and found no deuterium in the substitution products. Thus the conclusion was that an S_N2 type of mechanism was under observation.

Modena and his coworkers[213] have shown, however, that the elimination-addition mechanism is concurrent with direct nucleophilic substitution when strongly basic nucleophiles, such as OMe^- in methanol, act on *cis*-β-arenesulphonylvinyl halides, though the *trans*-isomers use the direct mechanism exclusively:

$$\underset{\text{(ArSO}_2\text{, H / Cl, H)}}{\text{ArSO}_2(\text{H})C{=}C(\text{Cl})\text{H}} \xrightarrow[\text{HOMe}]{\text{OMe}^-} ArSO_2{-}C{\equiv}C{-}H \xrightarrow[\text{HOMe}]{\text{OMe}^-} \text{ArSO}_2(\text{H})C{=}C(\text{OMe})\text{H}$$

From *cis*-isomers, the formation of the acetylenic intermediate was followed spectrophotometrically. This mechanism was favoured by

[212] D. E. Jones and C. A. Vernon, *Nature*, 1955, **176**, 791; D. E. Jones, D. O. Morris, C. A. Vernon, and R. F. M. White, *J. Chem. Soc.*, **1960**, 2349.

[213] L. Di Nunno, G. Modena, G. Scorrazo, *J. Chem. Soc.*, **1966**, 1186.

raised temperatures: thus, in the reaction formulated, with Ar = p-C_6H_4Me, elimination-addition accounted for about half the total substitution at 0°, but three-quarters of it at 25°. Even the *cis*-isomers use only the direct S_N2 mechanism when much less strongly basic nucleophiles, such as primary and secondary amines, are employed.

Further evidence of the mechanism of direct substitution is of a stereochemical nature.

(35b) Steric Course.—In deciding the steric course of these substitutions one has to guard against error from pre- or post-isomerisation. Despite some trouble from the former cause, Miller and Yonan[210] were able to conclude that the substitutions by iodide ions in *cis*- and *trans*-ω-bromo-*p*-nitrostyrene went with substantially complete retentions of geometrical configuration. Modena found that his substitutions in sulphones and sulphoxides (formulae above) always proceeded with total retention of geometrical configuration.[211] Vernon could say nothing about the steric course of his substitutions by ethoxide ion in ethyl *cis*- and *trans*-β-chlorocrotonates (formulae above), because both gave the same ethoxy-product, and, its isomer being unknown, the possibility of post-isomerisation could not be checked. But the substitutions with thiolate ions in the same esters gave the result that, whilst the major part of each reaction proceeded with retention of geometrical configuration, a minor part went with geometrical inversion.[212] This is illustrated by the product compositions in Table 35-1. Thus, some geometrical inversion during these substitutions does occur, but the isomeric substrates do not give the identical mixture of products. Pre- and post-isomerisations were proved to be absent in these examples.

TABLE 35-1.—PRODUCTS OF SUBSTITUTION BY ETHYLTHIOLATE AND PHENYLTHIOLATE IONS IN ETHYL CIS- AND TRANS-β-CHLOROCROTONATE IN ETHANOL AT ABOUT 0° (VERNON).

Ethyl β-chlorocrotonate	Substituting agent	Substitution products *cis* (%)	*trans* (%)
cis	EtS^-	85	15
trans	EtS^-	9	91
cis	PhS^-	88	12
trans	PhS^-	36	64

From these data, following Vernon, we may try to infer the relative timing of the group-uptake and group-loss, and so try to particularise the S_N2-type mechanism here in operation. The spectrum of possibilities comprises two broad bands. In one, there is some overlap in time, from total to indefinitely small, between the uptake and the loss, so that the original double bond always remains above single in its multiplicity, and there is no discrete intermediate product. In the other band of possibilities, uptake and loss are separated in time, to leave between them a purely single-bonded intermediate adduct of finite free life, from indefinitely short to quite long. Of course, the two bands of possibilities merge into each other, because there will always be some statistical scatter of individual molecular reaction-paths, but reaction routes typical of each band would have the broad

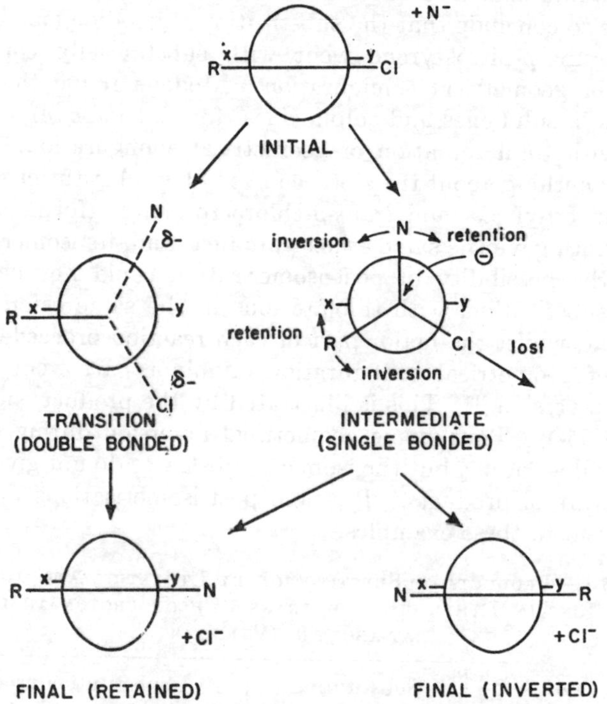

FIG. 35-1.—Stereochemistry of bimolecular nucleophilic substitution at an olefinic carbon atom in mechanisms without and with an addition intermediate.

In the examples discussed in the text, N, the nucleophilic anion, $=I^-$, RO^-, RS^-, or N_3^-, R = H or Me, and in *cis*-isomers x = *p*-$NO_2C_6H_4$, $PhSO_2$, PhSO, or EtO_2C, and y = H, whilst in *trans*-isomers, x = H, and y = *p*-$NO_2C_6H_4$, $PhSO_2$, PhSO, or EtO_2C. With the groups *p*-$NO_2C_6H_4$, $PhSO_2$, and PhSO, substitution proceeds with retention of geometrical configuration, whereas, with EtO_2C as the activating group, a minor proportion of geometrical inversion accompanies the predominating retention of geometrical configuration; and thus *cis*- and *trans*-substrates give mixtures, but not a common product mixture.

distinctions described. The two typical routes are shown in Fig. 35-1. If uptake and loss are overlapped in time, as in the route shown to the left, the product must have a totally retained geometrical configuration. This may be the type of mechanism operating in Miller and Yonan's substitution of *p*-nitrostyryl bromide, and in Modena's substitutions in olefinic sulphones and sulphoxides. If uptake and loss are time-separated, as in the reaction route shown towards the right of Fig. 35-1, the intervening single-bonded carbanion, which must at first be produced in a conformation corresponding to the *cis*- or *trans*-configuration of the substrate, will move from either such initial conformation towards its stable conformation; and so either or both substrates will substitute with a certain amount of geometrical inversion, and thus a certain approach towards a common product composition. This may be the situation in Vernon's thiolate-ion substitutions in the ethyl β-chlorocrotonates. If the intermediate, single-bonded carbanion should live long enough to attain its equilibrium conformation, then the *cis*- and *trans*-substrates should give a common product-mixture. This is not observed in the experiments cited. One suspects that the position of an individual mechanism in the range of mechanisms will depend on the electronegativity of the activating substituent, a substituent of high electron-absorbing power favouring the formation of an intermediate carbanion in a fast substitution.

The general analogy between these reactions and those of nucleophilic aromatic substitution will be clear, though analogy in itself is, of course, an untrustworthy guide to mechanism.

(36) ELECTROPHILIC ALIPHATIC SUBSTITUTION[214]

(36a) Scope and Expected Mechanisms.—Relatively to aromatic carbon, electrons are less available at saturated carbon, because they have to be drawn from a localised σ bond. And so it is not surprising that the usual reagents of electrophilic aromatic substitution fail to act similarly with corresponding alkane derivatives.

More positive expectations follow from attempting comparison between nucleophilic and electrophilic aliphatic substitution. In the one process, a space for an electron pair must be made by turning out the leaving group; and in the other, an electron pair must be supplied at the expense of the departing group. In the former reactions, the groups that enter and leave the substrate carry their bond electrons with them, and are commonly anions, such as oxy-anions, or halide ions; and in the latter reactions, the groups come and go without their

[214] O. A. Reutov, *Record Chem. Progress*, 1961, **22**, 1; C. K. Ingold, *ibid.*, 1964, **25**, 145; *Helv. Chim. Acta.*, 1964, **47**, 1191.

bond electrons, and so will commonly be cations, such as metal ions or hydrogen ions. Because so many of the simplest cations are metallic, we expect electrophilic aliphatic substitutions to occupy a central place in organo-metal chemistry, just as nucleophilic aliphatic substitution does occupy a central place in what, for contrast, we might call organo-non-metal chemistry. All metals, suitably co-ordinated, are potential participants in such reactions, and hence we might expect to find, or to see developed, as the main habitat of electrophilic aliphatic substitutions, the metal-for-metal substitutions of alkyl metals, substitutions of or by hydrogen constituting a special case.

The study of mechanism in electrophilic aliphatic substitution began its rapid advance only in the late 1950's. Mercury-for-mercury substitution was made, and has largely remained, the leading example, much as nitration became the leading example for the study of electrophilic aromatic substitution in the 1920's, '30's, and '40's. It was found in 1958 that one could optically resolve mercury alkyls, and could thus secure means to follow the stereochemical course of their substitutions. The first example of stable optical activity in a molecule containing a single asymmetric carbon atom, one of whose four attached atoms was a metal, was secondary-butylmercuric bromide, *s*-BuHgBr, which was optically resolved through the mandelate: other such resolutions of organo-mercury compounds have since been accomplished.[215] This stereochemical opening made substitutions in mercury alkyls an attractive starting point. The starting point could be made more attractive by specialising it to mercury-for-mercury substitutions, with labelling of the mercury atoms as necessary, because, when the in-coming and out-going atoms are of the same element, one avoids the necessity for an auxilliary research directed to correlating relative signs of rotation with relative configurations, a necessity which cannot be avoided when a different element is being introduced by the substitution. This was the device by which Hughes and his associates, 20 years earlier, had established the stereochemical S_N2 Rule (Section **33d**).

It was predicted at that time[216] that three, and only three, stoicheiometrically distinct electrophilic mercury-exchange reactions should

[215] H. B. Charman, E. D. Hughes, and C. K. Ingold, *Chem. and Ind.*, **1958**, 1517; *J. Chem. Soc.*, **1959**, 2523; O. A. Reutov and E. V. Uglova, *Izvest. Akad. Nauk, S.S.S.R., Otdel. khim. Nauk*, **1959**, 757; F. R. Jensen, L. D. Whipple, D. K. Keddergaertner, and J. A. Landgrebe, *J. Am. Chem. Soc.*, 1960, **82**, 2466; E. D. Hughes. C. K. Ingold and R. M. G. Roberts, *J. Chem. Soc.*, **1964**, 3900.

[216] H. B. Charman and C. K. Ingold, *J. Chem. Soc.*, **1959**, 2523.

exist, *viz.*, the one-, two-, and three-alkyl substitutions formulated below. The two-alkyl reaction was then known; and the others were soon discovered:

$$X_2Hg \; R\!-\!HgX \rightleftharpoons XHgR + HgX_2 \qquad \text{(one-alkyl)}$$
$$X_2Hg \; R\!-\!HgR \rightleftharpoons XHgR + XHgR \qquad \text{(two-alkyl)}$$
$$XRHg \; R\!-\!HgR \rightleftharpoons RHgR + HgRX \qquad \text{(three-alkyl)}$$

Three basic mechanisms of electrophilic aliphatic substitution were predicted at the same time, as counterparts to known mechanisms of nucleophilic substitution.[216] They were the "bimolecular" (S_E2), "unimolecular" (S_E1), and "internal" (S_Ei) mechanisms, formulated below for the stoicheiometric case of one-alkyl substitution. One of them, the bimolecular mechanism, was discovered and fully identified almost immediately. The others, along with several unanticipated variations of them, came to light within a few years:

$$X'\overset{+}{Hg} \; R\!-\!HgX'' \longrightarrow X'Hg\!-\!R + \overset{+}{Hg}X'' \qquad (S_E2)$$

$$\left.\begin{array}{l} R\!-\!HgX'' \xrightarrow[\text{slow}]{} \overset{-}{R} + \overset{+}{Hg}X'' \\ X'\overset{+}{Hg} + \overset{-}{R} \xrightarrow[\text{fast}]{} X'HgR \end{array}\right\} \qquad (S_E1)$$

$$\begin{array}{c} HgX'' \\ R \quad\quad Y \\ X'Hg \end{array} \longrightarrow \begin{array}{c} R \\ | \\ X'Hg \end{array} + \begin{array}{c} HgX'' \\ | \\ Y \end{array} \qquad (S_Ei)$$

These mechanisms can be kinetically diagnosed. The S_E2 mechanism requires second-order kinetics. It has an open transition state. The S_Ei mechanism also requires second-order kinetics. It has a closed transition state. The most obvious kinetic distinction between these mechanisms is that a substituting agent X'HgY' has first to ionise off Y' in order to engage in mechanism S_E2, wherefore rate along a series of mercuric salts of decreasing strength of co-ordination, *e.g.*, $HgBr_2$, $Hg(OAc)_2$, $Hg(NO_3)_2$, $Hg(ClO_4)_2$, should rise strongly; whereas rate by mechanism S_Ei would be zero if Y' were ionised off completely; and as the co-ordinating strength of Y' is needed to pull off the expelled mercury atom, rate along the same series should fall strongly. Mechanism S_E1 can be immediately diagnosed by its limiting kinetic form, of first order in substrate, and zeroth order in substituting agent.

As to stereochemical anticipations,[216] there can be no S_E2 rule theoretically based on the Pauli principle, because, in bimolecular electrophilic substitution, there are only two electrons in the changing atomic orbital; that is, there is no excess of electrons in competition for it, the circumstance which in nucleophilic substitution keeps the exchanging groups apart, and so leads to bimolecular substitution with inversion. Whatever the actual course of bimolecular substitution, it must result from a balance of forces which, *a priori*, we have no simple and certain way of weighting. As to the steric course of unimolecular electrophilic substitution, one is prejudiced to expect racemisation, though, in fact, we do not know with certainty the geometry of the carbanion, nor, in case it is pyramidal, do we know its inversion frequency. Internal electrophilic substitutions must proceed with total retention of configuration, because the transition states are cyclic, with rings too small to contain re-entrant angles.

(36b) The S_E2 Mechanism of Mercury Exchange.—In the period 1952–57, that is, before much had been done on the mechanism of mercury exchanges, reports by Wright, Nesmeyanov, Winstein, Reutov, and others[217] appeared on their stereochemistry. Conclusions were drawn, but they were not well proved, first, because the examples treated were mercury-substituted terpenes and other compounds possessing several centres of asymmetry in optically active form; so that every reaction involving mercury took place under a permanently present asymmetric influence. The second reason why one could not be satisfied with the conclusions was the fundamental one that the steric course of any reaction is a property of its mechanism, not of its stoicheiometry, and that therefore to prove a steric course apart from mechanism is like finding a lost hat without finding the owner. A kinetically known, kinetically single, reaction must first be found, and then stereochemical work, done in correlation with kinetics, is useful. Since 1958 the stereochemistry of mercury exchanges has been studied with singly-present centres of asymmetry, and in correlation with prior kinetic studies, by Reutov and his coworkers, and by Hughes and others.

[217] G. F. Wright, *Canad. J. Chem.*, 1952, **30**, 268; cf. A. G. Brook and G. F. Wright, *Acta Cryst.*, 1951, **4**, 50; G. F. Wright, *Ann. New York Acad. Sci.*, 1957, **65**, 436; A. N. Nesmeyanov, O. A. Reutov, and S. S. Poddubnaya, *Izvest. Akad. Nauk, S.S.S.R., Otdel. khim. Nauk*, **1953**, 649; S. Winstein, T. G. Traylor, and C. S. Garner, *J. Am. Chem. Soc.*, 1955, **77**, 3711; S. Winstein and T. G. Traylor, *ibid.*, 1956, **78**, 2597; O. A. Reutov, I. P. Beletskaya, and R. E. Mendelishvili, *Doklady Akad. Nauk, S.S.S.R.*, 1957, **116**, 617.

The first such work was with substitution of the two-alkyl stoicheiometric type,[218] for instance, substitution by mercuric salts in di-*s*-butylmercury in solvents such as acetone or ethanol:

$$s\text{-Bu}_2\text{Hg} + \text{HgX}_2 \rightarrow 2\ s\text{-BuHgX} \qquad (\text{S}_\text{E}2)$$

In acetone or ethanol, with the anions X = Br, OAc, NO_3, the reaction was of first order in each reactant, and thus second order overall. The rate of substitution rose so strongly along the anion series that the temperature had to be lowered at each step in order to establish kinetic form. In ethanol the rates were, with $HgBr_2$ at 25°, 0.39, with $Hg(OAc)_2$ at 0°, 5.3, and with $Hg(NO_3)_2$ at −47°, 7.6 sec.$^{-1}$ mole^{-1} l. With $Hg(ClO_4)_2$, the rate was so great at −50° that the kinetic form could not be ascertained. These findings diagnose mechanism S_E2.

It was then shown that this mechanism retains configuration. Optically active *s*-butylmercuric bromide was converted by means of an *s*-butyl Grignard compound (necessarily racemic, for Grignard compounds are optically unstable) into a di-*s*-butylmercury, which was thus labelled with optical activity in one only of its two otherwise equivalent alkyl groups. In the following equation, a degree-sign denotes the optical label:

$$s\text{-}\overset{\circ}{\text{Bu}}\text{HgBr} + s\text{-BuMgCl} \rightarrow s\text{-}\overset{\circ}{\text{Bu}}\text{HgBu-}s + \text{MgClBr}$$

This material then became the substrate for several mercury exchanges with mercuric salts, under the established kinetic conditions. With mercuric bromide, the exchange must give, as one sees from the equation,

$$s\text{-}\overset{\circ}{\text{Bu}}\text{HgBu-}s + \text{HgBr}_2 \rightarrow s\text{-}\overset{\circ}{\text{Bu}}\text{HgBr} + s\text{-BuHgBr}$$

an *s*-butylmercuric bromide with one-half of the specific activity of the material put into the Grignard reaction. To state this more carefully, the fraction should be one-half, provided that the label of optical activity sticks firmly to its alkyl group while the mercury atom bound to it is being replaced by a different one, or, in other words, provided that configuration is quantitatively retained in the substitution. In case the substitution should lead to racemisation, the individual molecular acts of substitution giving either enantiomer of the product with equal probability, the final specific activity would be one-quarter

[218] H. C. Charman, E. D. Hughes, and C. K. Ingold, *J. Chem. Soc.*, **1959**, 2530; O. A. Reutov and E. V. Uglova, *Izvest. Akad. Nauk, S.S.S.R., Otdel. khim. Nauk*, **1959**, 1691.

of the original. In case the substitution should involve inversion (like bimolecular nucleophilic substitution), the final activity would be zero. As shown in Table 36-1, the observed fraction of the original activity was one-half, for the second-order substitutions by $HgBr_2$, $Hg(OAc)_2$, and $Hg(NO_3)_2$, the anion in the product of the last two substitutions having been exchanged for bromide for the purpose of the polarimetric observation. Similar results have been obtained with 5-methyl-2-hexyl as the alkyl group having asymmetry at the mercury-bearing carbon atom.

TABLE 36-1.—STEREOCHEMISTRY OF THE S_E2 MECHANISM OF TWO-ALKYL MERCURY EXCHANGE BETWEEN MERCURIC SALTS AND DI-*s*-BUTYLMERCURY.

Initial *s*-BuHgBr......................., $[\alpha]_D^{20}$ −15.2°
therefore
Retention of configuration requires final *s*-BuHgBr, $[\alpha]_D^{20}$ −7.6°
Substitution with racemisation requires final *s*-BuHgBr, $[\alpha]_D^{20}$ −3.8°
Inversion of configuration requires final *s*-BuHgBr, $[\alpha]_D^{20}$ ±0.0°

Substituting agent	Solvent	Final *s*-BuHgBr
$HgBr_2$	EtOH	$[\alpha]_D^{20}$ −7.6°
$HgBr_2$+3LiBr	EtOH	$[\alpha]_D^{20}$ −7.8
$Hg(OAc)_2$	EtOH	$[\alpha]_D^{20}$ −7.5
$Hg(NO_3)_2$	EtOH	$[\alpha]_D^{20}$ −7.8
$Hg(NO_3)_2+HNO_3$	"50%" aq.-EtOH	$[\alpha]_D^{20}$ −7.2

When optically active *s*-butylmercuric bromide is mixed in ethanol with inactive di-*s*-butylmercury, the latter becomes active. When *s*-butylmercuric bromide containing radiomercury-203 is mixed in ethanol with ordinary di-*s*-butylmercury, the latter becomes radioactive. These label transfers are represented in the following equations, in which an asterisk denotes a label of radioactivity, as manifestations of the anticipated three-alkyl stoicheiometric form of mercury exchange:

$$\begin{aligned} RHgR + \mathring{R}HgBr &\rightarrow \mathring{R}HgR + RHgBr \\ RHgR + R\overset{*}{Hg}Br &\rightarrow R\overset{*}{Hg}R + RHgBr \end{aligned} \qquad (S_E2)$$

The equations show that the two label transfers should go at the same rate, as indeed they do.[219] The label transfers might conceivably have

[219] H. B. Charman, E. D. Hughes, C. K. Ingold, and F. G. Thorpe, *J. Chem. Soc.*, 1961, 1121.

resulted from two successive steps of the two-alkyl exchange, but in that case the optical label would go over twice as fast as the radioactive label, as is shown by the following equations:

$$\left.\begin{array}{l} \left\{\begin{array}{l} 2\overset{\circ}{R}HgBr \xrightarrow{\text{slow}} \overset{\circ}{R}Hg\overset{\circ}{R} + HgBr_2 \\ R_2Hg + HgBr_2 \xrightarrow[\text{fast}]{} 2RHgBr \end{array}\right. \\ \left\{\begin{array}{l} 2RH\overset{*}{g}Br \xrightarrow{\text{slow}} RH\overset{*}{g}R + H\overset{*}{g}Br_2 \\ R_2Hg + H\overset{*}{g}Br_2 \xrightarrow[\text{fast}]{} RH\overset{*}{g}Br + RHgBr \end{array}\right. \end{array}\right\} \text{(not found)}$$

The identical rates show that a simple three-alkyl exchange is under observation. Followed radiometrically in ethanol, it is of first order in each reactant, second overall. When the substituting agent is changed from *s*-BuHgBr to *s*-BuHgOAc and to *s*-BuHgNO$_3$, the rate rises strongly as before. Evidently the mechanism is again S$_E$2, as indicated above. Finally, a comparison of the radiometric and polarimetric kinetics shows that this mechanism, in three-alkyl substitution, is again characterised by total retention of configuration.

The one-alkyl mercury exchange in solvents such as ethanol:

$$RHgBr + H\overset{*}{g}Br_2 \rightarrow RH\overset{*}{g}Br + HgBr_2 \qquad (S_E2)$$

had been observed by the use of radiomercuric salts before its nature was recognised: it was originally taken for an overall result of two steps of two-alkyl substitution:[220]

$$\left.\begin{array}{l} 2RHgBr \xrightarrow{\text{slow}} R_2Hg + HgBr_2 \\ R_2Hg + H\overset{*}{g}Br_2 \xrightarrow[\text{fast}]{} RH\overset{*}{g}Br + RHgBr \end{array}\right\} \text{(not realised)}$$

A kinetic examination showed, however,[221] that the reaction was the one-alkyl stoicheiometric form of mercury exchange, going in one step, which, in ethanol, was of first order in each reactant, and thus of second order overall. This was established for methyl and *s*-butyl as alkyl groups (as it was subsequently for other alkyl groups), and for

[220] V. D. Nevedov and E. N. Sintova, *Zhur. fiz. Khim.*, 1956, **60**, 2356.

[221] E. D. Hughes, C. K. Ingold, F. G. Thorpe, and H. C. Volger, *J. Chem. Soc.*, **1961**, **1133**; cf. O. A. Reutov, *Angew. Chem.*, 1960, **72**, 198.

the anions I^-, Br^-, OAc^-, NO_3^- in the alkyl mercuric salt and in the mercuric salt. Again rate increased strongly along the anion series. Finally it was shown, by the use of optically active *s*-butylmercuric salts, that the exchange, followed radiometrically, could be run for many half-lives without any loss of optical activity. This showed that mechanism S_E2 is again in operation, and that it is still associated with total retention of configuration in the one-alkyl stoicheiometric form of exchange.

The effects of alkyl size and structure on bimolecular electrophilic mercury exchange between mercury-alkyls and mercuric ions can broadly be understood on the basis of primary steric effects. But the pattern of effects is quite different from that observed in nucleophilic aliphatic substitution (Section **34**). The reason is that the geometrical form of the configuration-retaining transition state in bimolecular electrophilic substitution is very different from that of the configuration-inverting transition state of bimolecular nucleophilic substitution. Relative to the latter group of reactions, steric retardations in bimolecular electrophilic substitutions are generally rather weak, as might be expected from the lesser concentration of electrons near the seat of substitution. In the reaction of alkyl-mercuric bromides with radiomercuric bromide, Hughes and Volger[222] found that α-methylation in the alkyl group reduced rate by a factor in the range 3–7, at each stage along the series methyl, primary alkyl, secondary alkyl; but that β-methylation made hardly any difference to the rate. In particular, the *neo*pentyl group did not occupy a special position, but was closely similar to any other primary alkyl group: *neo*pentyl mercuric bromide exchanged mercury at about three-quarters of the rate at which ethylmercuric bromide did so. We should expect something like this, because, in a configuration-retaining bimolecular electrophilic substitution, the two exchanging groups are on one side of the seat of substitution in the transition state, leaving free the whole of the other side for accommodation of the alkyl group.

Reutov and his coworkers have investigated polar effects in the second-order exchanges of aralphylmercuric salts with mercuric salts.[223] These effects also are quite small; and they are variable in direction with the example. In the exchanges of *p*-substituted benzylmercuric bromides with mercuric bromide in solvent quinoline, electropositive

[222] E. D. Hughes and H. C. Volger, *J. Chem. Soc.*, **1961**, 2389.

[223] O. A. Reutov, J. A. Smolina, and V. Kalyarin, *Doklady Akad. Nauk, S.S.S.R.*, 1961, **139**, 389; O. A. Reutov, V. I. Sokolov, I. P. Beletskaya, and Ya. S. Kyabokobylko, *Izvest. Akad. Nauk. S.S.S.R., Otdel. khim. Nauk*, **1963**, 965.

substituents slightly accelerate, and electronegative slightly retard. In the second-order exchanges of *p*-substituted α-carbethoxybenzylmercuric bromides with mercuric bromide in "80%" aqueous ethanol, the polar substituents again act mildly, but now in the opposite direction. Evidently there is a delicate balance between the import and export of electrons at the seat of substitution in the transition states of bimolecular electrophilic substitution.

(36c) The S_Ei Mechanism of Mercury Exchange.—During the kinetic study of mercury exchange between alkylmercuric and mercuric salts in ethanol and acetone, a catalysis by anions was observed.

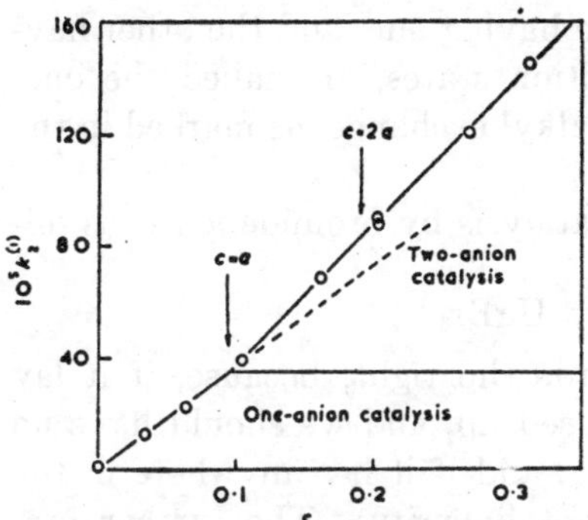

Fig. 36-1.—Effect of [LiBr] (c) on second-order substitution rate of MeHgBr+Hg*Br₂ (each 0.095) in ethanol at 0°. (Reproduced by permission from *J. Chem. Soc*., 1961, 1144.)

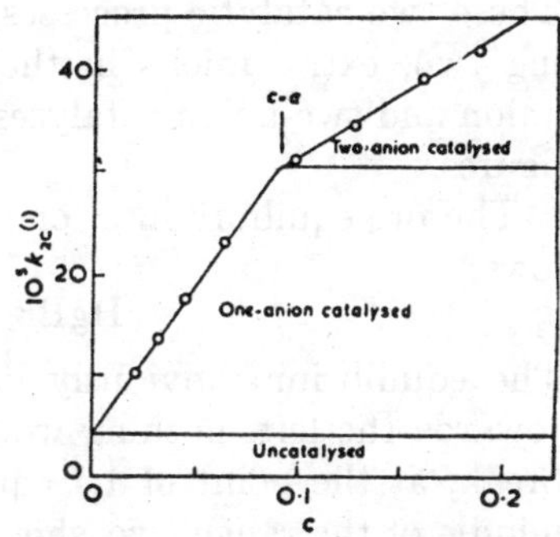

Fig. 36-2.—Effect of [LiBr] (c) on second-order substitution rate of $Me_3C \cdot CH_2HgBr + Hg^*Br_2$ (each 0.092) in ethanol at 100°. (Reproduced by permission from *J. Chem. Soc*., 1961, 2361.)

A catalysis implies a new mechanism. The order of catalytic effectiveness was $I^- > Br^- > Cl^- \gg OAc^- \gg NO_3^-$.[224] This is the order expected for a mechanism of type S_Ei (Section **36a**). The kinetic form of the catalysis is illustrated in Fig. 36-1 for the exchange between methylmercuric bromide and mercuric bromide under catalysis by lithium bromide in solvent acetone. The rate rises linearly with the concentration of lithium bromide, until this is equal to the concentration of mercuric bromide, when the curve suddenly takes a new direction, and then continues linearly as far as can be followed. The slope after the change of direction is not in all cases greater than before. With *neo*pentyl as the alkyl group, the second slope is less steep, as

[224] H. B. Charman, E. D. Hughes, C. K. Ingold, and H. C. Volger, *J. Chem. Soc.*, **1961**, 1142.

shown in Fig. 36-2. With *s*-butyl as the alkyl group, the second slope is the steeper when the catalytic anion is bromide, but much the less steep when it is acetate.[224] But, however the slopes may be related, the break is always present, and always at the point of 1:1 equivalence; and no second break has ever been found.

These kinetic characters define the mechanisms at work. We have two catalytic processes. At the lower catalyst concentrations, one catalytic anion, added to a reactant in pre-equilibrium, is thereby carried into the transition state of mercury exchange. At the higher catalyst concentrations, a second anion, taken up by one of the reactants in pre-equilibrium, is likewise carried into the transition state. These two catalytic processes, the one having one, and the other having two, extra anions in their transition states, are called the one-anion and two-anion catalyses of one-alkyl exchange, as marked in the figures.

The pre-equilibrium in one-anion catalysis by bromide ion is as follows:

$$HgBr_2 + Br^- \rightleftharpoons HgBr_3^-$$

The equilibrium obviously lies towards the right, because, if it lay towards the left, nothing would get used up, and we should have no break, at the point of 1,1-equivalence; and if it lay anywhere in the middle of the range, we should not get linearity. The further pre-equilibrium involved in two-anion catalyses could be

$$RHgBr + Br^- \rightleftharpoons RHgBr_2^-$$

Equally obviously, this lies to the left, because, if it lay to the right, we should get a second break at the point of 2:1 equivalence, as is not observed; and, if it lay in the middle of the range, we should not get linearity.

The ways in which these extra anions are taken to be included in the catalytic transition states are shown below:

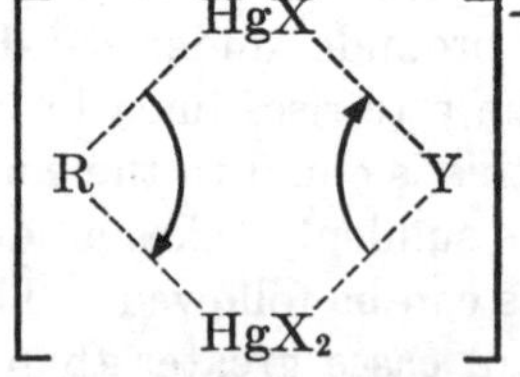

Transition state for S_Ei (one-anion catalysis)

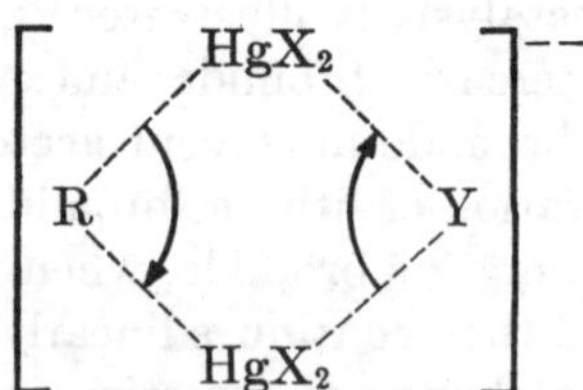

Transition state for S_Ei (two-anion catalysis)

The cyclic nature of these transition states again follows from the kinetic evidence. For, if we consider the case X = Y = Br, then, in the diagram of the transition state for one-anion catalysis, Y must, for reasons explained already, be brought in by the lower of the two mercury atoms, the entering atom. One has only to write down the chemical equation for the exchange to see that Y must be carried out by the upper of the two mercury atoms, the leaving atom. Therefore, in the transition state, it must be *on its way* from the one mercury atom to the other; that is, it must be bridging the two mercury atoms. Thus we have a cyclic transition state, and a mechanism of the general type which had been anticipated, and in advance of discovery had been labelled S_Ei. In two-anion catalysis, the additional anion has to go where mercury co-ordination is least complete. This mechanism is another particularisation of the general form of mechanism called internal, and labelled S_Ei.

It is an obvious requirement of these transition states that stereochemical configuration must be retained in the substitutions. The two forms of catalysis can be approximately isolated from each other by choosing conditions; and, with *s*-butyl as the alkyl group, each has been shown quantitatively to retain configuration.

These mechanisms also have been investigated with respect to kinetic effects of alkyl homology.[222] With simple alkyl groups up to *neo*pentyl, the pattern of effects qualitatively resembles that found in S_N2 exchanges. But the rate reductions in the higher homologues are generally stronger in the one-anion S_Ei exchanges, and stronger still in the two-anion S_Ei exchanges. This can be understood as arising from pressure on the out-of-plane anions in the cyclic transition states. Rough calculations of steric pressures, based on the assumed forms of the transition states, have given results consistent with the observations.

(36d) The S_E1 Mechanism of Mercury Exchange.—Kinetically diagnosed unimolecular mercury exchange was observed nearly concurrently by Reutov and his coworkers, and by Hughes, Roberts, and the writer, in the same example, that of the replacement of mercury in α-carbethoxybenzylmercuric bromide by the action of radiomercuric bromide in solvent dimethyl sulphoxide.[225] Hughes and his collaborators published the later, but their work included optical resolution of the substrate, and the stereochemistry of the substitution, as well as a study of catalysis.[226] The same thought underlay both investigations, *viz.*, to facilitate mechanism S_E1 by increasing the ease of formation

[225] O. A. Reutov, B. Praisnar, I. P. Beletskaya, and V. I. Sokolov, *Izvest. Akad. Nauk, S.S.S.R., Otdel. khim. Nauk*, **1963**, 970.

[226] E. D. Hughes, C. K. Ingold, and R. M. G. Roberts, *J. Chem. Soc.*, **1964**, **3900**.

of the carbanion on which it depends, as could be done by using, in place of simple alkyl groups, electronegatively substituted alkyl groups, and by employing a solvent that could solvate a carbanion without destroying it. (The solvent is very important for mechanism: the same substitution goes by mechanism S_E2 in aqueous acetone,[226] in aqueous ethanol,[227] and in pyridine.[228]) Reutov has since used the same principle with a second substrate, that is, in the reaction of *p*-nitrobenzylmercuric bromide with radiomercuric bromide in solvent dimethyl sulphoxide.[229] This also is an S_E1 substitution, but, of course, it does not permit easy stereochemical investigation.

The key observation is that the rate of substitution is of first order in the substrate and of zeroth order in the substituting agent. This, with all the collateral evidence, diagnoses mechanism S_E1 for these substrates in dimethyl sulphoxide, *e.g.*,

$$\left.\begin{array}{l} \text{Ph(EtO}_2\text{C)CH}\cdot\text{HgBr} \xrightarrow{\text{slow}} \text{Ph(EtO}_2\text{C)CH}^- + \text{HgBr}^+ \\ \text{Ph(EtO}_2\text{C)CH}^- + \overset{*}{\text{Hg}}\text{Br}_2 \longrightarrow \text{Ph(EtO}_2\text{C)CH}\cdot\overset{*}{\text{Hg}}\text{Br} + \text{Br}^- \end{array}\right\} \quad (S_E1)$$

After optical resolution of the substrate, the substitution represented was found to proceed with total racemisation; that is, the polarimetric rate of exchange was equal to the radiometric rate, and one had to conclude that each molecular act of substitution led with equal probability to either enantiomeric form of the substitution product.

(36e) The S_E1-$2X^-$ Mechanism of Mercury Exchange.—The substitution of α-carbethoxybenzylmercuric bromide by radiomercuric bromide in dimethyl sulphoxide is susceptible to a strong catalysis by bromide ion. This is a catalysis of the rate-controlling formation of the carbanion intermediate, and hence it is a derivative form of the unimolecular mechanism. However, a catalysis means a new mechanism,[226] and this one, the fourth known type of mechanism in mercury

[227] O. A. Reutov, V. I. Sokolov, I. P. Beletskaya, and Ya. S. Kyabokobylko, *Izvest. Akad. Nauk, S.S.S.R., Otdel. khim. Nauk*, **1963**, 965.

[228] O. A. Reutov, V. I. Sokolov, and I. P. Beletskaya, *Izvest. Akad. Nauk, S.S.S.R., Otdel. khim. Nauk*, **1961**, 1213.

[229] V. A. Kalyarin, T. A. Smolina, and O. A. Reutov, *Doklady Akad. Nauk, S.S.S.R.*, 1964, **156**, 95.

exchanges, was certainly not anticipated in 1958. A point of particular interest is that its rate in this example is proportional to the square of the bromide-ion concentration, and that, although in principle a rate term linear in bromide ion is possible, such a rate term was too small to be detected. So the catalytic mechanism, which we label S_E1-$2Br^-$, or, more generally, S_E1-$2X^-$, involves two bromide ions successively taken up by the substrate. Evidently, the adduct with one is not unstable enough to be a good catalytic intermediate, but the adduct with two is sufficiently unstable—presumably because a doubled negative charge can be split in the succeeding heterolysis to give two repelling anions, one of which is the critical carbanion intermediate of the mechanism. This mechanism also proceeds with total racemisation.

$$\left.\begin{array}{l} RHgBr \underset{}{\overset{\text{fast}}{\rightleftharpoons}} RHgBr_2^- \overset{\text{fast}}{\rightleftharpoons} RHgBr_3^{2-} \\ RHgBr_3^{2-} \xrightarrow[\text{slow}]{} R^- + HgBr_3^- \\ R^- + \overset{*}{Hg}Br_2 \xrightarrow[\text{fast}]{} R\overset{*}{Hg}Br + Br^- \end{array}\right\} \quad (S_E1\text{-}2X^-)$$

This catalytic mechanism has probably been found again by Reutov and his coworkers in their example of unimolecular exchange between *p*-nitrobenzylmercuric bromide and radiomercuric bromide in dimethyl sulphoxide.[230] There is a kinetic difference from the previous case, but only one that could be interpreted by assuming that, instead of both pre-equilibria lying on the left, as formulated above, the first now lies more centrally, whilst the second is still towards the left. The observation is that the first-order rate rises with bromide ion on a continuously steepening curve, but a curve whose rate of steepening becomes suddenly and very greatly increased when the rising bromide-ion concentration is near the mercuric bromide concentration.

(36f) Other Metal-for-Metal Substitutions.—Only the fringe of this large subject has yet been touched. We note here a few examples. One group of studies employs other Group B metals in combination with, or in place of, mercury. Another group employs metals of the first transition series.

Mercury(II)-for-gold(I) substitutions have been examined using phosphine-coordinated gold in the compounds substituted, and mer-

[230] V. A. Kalyarin, T. A. Smolina, and O. A. Reutov, *Doklady Akad. Nauk. S.S.S.R.*, 1964, 157, 919.

curic salts or alkylmercuric salts as the substituting agents. With simple alkyl groups in the alkyl-gold(I), second-order kinetics are observed, that is, first-order in each reagent, in solvents such as dioxan, aqueous dioxan, and dimethyl sulphoxide.[231] By changing the anion in the substituting agent to less covalent and more ionising types of anion, and by adding common anions, it has been made clear that the mechanism S_E2 is under observation, as in the examples,

$$Ph_3P\cdot Au\cdot CH_3 + HgBr_2 \xrightarrow{\text{dioxan}} Ph_3P\cdot AuBr + CH_3\cdot HgBr \quad (S_E2)$$

$$Ph_3P\cdot Au\cdot C_2H_5 + CH_3HgBr \xrightarrow[\text{sulphoxide}]{\text{dimethyl}} Ph_3P\cdot AuBr + C_2H_5\cdot Hg\cdot CH_3 \quad (S_E2)$$

Mercury(II)-for-gold(III) substitutions, using phosphine co-ordinated gold and simple alkyl groups in the alkyl-gold(III), seem remarkably similar to the corresponding gold(I) substitutions.[231] The common mechanism is again S_E2, as in the example,

$$Ph_3P\cdot Au(CH_3)_3 + HgBr_2 \xrightarrow[\text{dioxan}]{} Ph_3P\cdot Au(CH_3)_2Br + CH_3\cdot HgBr \quad (S_E2)$$

The unimolecular electrophilic mechanism S_E1 has been observed in mercury(II)-for-gold(I) substitutions involving electronegatively substituted alkyl groups in the gold-alkyl.[231] The reaction of $Ph_3P\cdot Au\cdot C(CN)(CO_2Et)\cdot(CH_2)_3\cdot CH_3$ with $CH_3\cdot HgCl$ is instantaneous in dimethyl sulphoxide at 0°. Though this does not prove anything, one can be fairly confident, on the grounds of the rate alone, that mechanism S_E1 is here under observation. By the use of a mixed solvent containing only 10% of dimethyl sulphoxide along with 90% of dioxan, the rate can be reduced sufficiently to permit an observation of kinetic form. The mechanism in this solvent is still S_E1, as is now proved by the kinetics. The rate is of first order in the 1-cyano-1-carbethoxy-*n*-amylgold and of zeroth order in the methylmercuric chloride. When the substituting agent is changed to ethylmercuric chloride, or to methylmercuric acetate, the absolute rate is exactly the same:

[231] B. J. Gregory and C. K. Ingold, *J. Chem. Soc.*, forthcoming.

$$\left.\begin{array}{l} Ph_3P\cdot Au\cdot \overset{CN}{\underset{CO_2Et}{C}}(CH_2)_3CH_3 \xrightarrow{\text{slow}} [Ph_3P\cdot Au]^+ + \left[\overset{CN}{\underset{CO_2Et}{C}}(CH_2)_3CH_3\right]^- \\ \left[\overset{CN}{\underset{CO_2Et}{C}}(CH_2)_3CH_3\right]^- + CH_3HgCl \xrightarrow{\text{fast}} CH_3Hg\cdot \overset{CN}{\underset{CO_2Et}{C}}(CH_2)_3CH_3 + Cl^- \\ [Ph_3P\cdot Au]^+ + Cl^- \xrightarrow{\text{fast}} Ph_3P\cdot AuCl \end{array}\right\} \quad (S_E1)$$

The tin(IV)-for-mercury(II) substitution in dimethylmercury as substrate, by trimethylstannic bromide as substituting agent, has second-order kinetics in acetonitrile, formdimethylamide, and dimethyl sulphoxide:[232]

$$MeHgMe + Me_3SnBr \rightarrow MeHgBr + Me_3SnMe \qquad (S_E2)$$

So has the radiometrically followed tin exchange tin(IV)-for-tin(IV), between tetramethyltin and the ionising salt, trimethylstannic trifluoroacetate, in acetonitrile:[232]

$$Me_3SnMe + Me_3\overset{*}{Sn}{}^+ \, CF_3CO_2^- \rightarrow Me_3\overset{*}{Sn}Me + Me_3Sn^+ \, CF_3CO_2^- \qquad (S_E2)$$

Salt effects show that these use the S_E2 mechanism.

Mercury(II)-for-thallium(III) substitutions in trialkylthalliums by alkylmercuric salts are too rapid in formdimethylamide to permit direct examination of their kinetics. Though their mechanism is not established, it is probable that these reactions use the S_N1 mechanism.[233] The slowest step in the sequence, the splitting off of a carbanion R^- from a trialkylthallium R_3Tl, is from a practical point of view inconveniently fast, but it nevertheless appears to be rate-controlling:

$$\left.\begin{array}{l} Et_3Tl \underset{\text{rate-controlling}}{\overset{\text{fast but}}{\rightleftharpoons}} Et^- + Et_2Tl^+ \\ s\text{-}BuHgNO_3 \xrightarrow[\text{very fast}]{} s\text{-}BuHg^+ + NO_3^- \\ Et^- + s\text{-}BuHg^+ \xrightarrow[\text{very fast}]{} s\text{-}BuHgEt \end{array}\right\} \quad (S_E1)$$

The radiometrically followed thallium(III)-for-thallium(III) substitu-

[232] C. K. Ingold and J. A. Keiner, *J. Chem. Soc.*, forthcoming.

[233] C. R. Hart and C. K. Ingold, *J. Chem. Soc.*, **1964**, 4372; F. R. Jensen and D. Heyman, *J. Am. Chem. Soc.*, 1966, **88**, 3438.

tion in a trialkylthalium by a dialkylthallic ion[234] is also very fast in formdimethylamide. Again, the mechanism is not proved, but it is probable that mechanism S_E1 is employed:

$$Et_3Tl \underset{\text{rate-controlling}}{\overset{\text{fast but}}{\rightleftharpoons}} Et^- + Et_2Tl^+ \qquad (S_E1)$$

$$Et^- + Et_2\overset{*}{Tl}^+ \xrightarrow[\text{very fast}]{} Et_3\overset{*}{Tl}$$

Despite a confused earlier literature concerning their molecular weight, it now seems clear that Grignard reagents, especially bromides, are monomeric in efficiently co-ordinating ether solvents, though they may dimerise, especially chlorides, probably by halogen-bridging, in less well co-ordinating solvents.[235] The Grignard reagents which have been crystallised carry two ether molecules per magnesium atom, and in those crystallised reagents which have been X-ray-examined, $EtMgBr(OEt_2)_2$ and $PhMgBr(OEt_2)_2$, the magnesium atom is tetrahedrally co-ordinated.[236] J. D. Roberts and his coworkers showed that Grignard reagents in ether are the stable components in the Schlenk equilibrium (the equilibrium of two-alkyl magnesium exchange, cf. Section **54c**), and that this equilibrium, in contrast to that of the analogous zinc exchange, is rapidly attained:

$$R_2Mg + MgX_2 \rightleftharpoons 2RMgX$$

Radiomagnesium, introduced into such a system, became statistically distributed faster than separation of components was effected.[237]

Although the mechanism of this reversible reaction is perhaps not strictly proved, an S_E1 mechanism, dependent on the rate-controlling, but rapid, formation of a carbanion, has been made probable by the stereochemical conclusions reached by Roberts and his collaborators, on the basis of their studies by the method of proton magnetic resonance.[237] In a solution of the *neo*pentyl Grignard compound $CMe_3 \cdot CH_2 \cdot MgCl$, in ether, the methylene hydrogen atoms were shown to

[234] The dialkylthallic ion R_2Tl^+ (which is isoelectronic with dialkylmercury) is very stable. Dialkylthallic salts of strong acids are strong electrolytes in water if soluble, and fairly strong in formdimethylamide.

[235] A. D. Vreugdenhil and C. Blomberg, *Rec. trav. chim.*, 1963, **82**, 453; E. C. Ashby and W. S. Becker, *J. Am. Chem. Soc.*, 1963, **85**, 118; E. C. Ashby and M. B. Smith, *ibid.*, 1964, **86**, 4363.

[236] G. D. Stucky and R. E. Rundle, *J. Am. Chem. Soc.*, 1963, **85**, 1002; L. J. Geggenberger and R. E. Rundle, *ibid.*, 1964, **86**, 5344; 1968, **90**, 5375.

[237] D. O. Cowan, J. Hsu, and J. D. Roberts, *J. Org. Chem.*, 1964, **29**, 3688; G. M. Whitesides, M. Witanowsky, and J. D. Roberts, *J. Am. Chem. Soc.*, 1965, **87**, 2854.

invert, in just the manner which, had the α-carbon atom been asymmetric and a centre of optical activity, would have been made manifest in a racemisation. The time of inversion was of the order of milliseconds at room temperature. By adding dioxan to the ether, magnesium chloride is precipitated, and so the equilibrium written above becomes pushed over to the left, thus providing a solution of the almost pure dialkylmagnesium, $(CMe_3CH_2)_2Mg$. In this material also, the methylene hydrogen atoms undergo stereochemical inversion, in a time which is now of the order of seconds at room temperature. The following mechanism for attainment of equilibrium in the two-alkyl magnesium-exchange would be consistent with these findings:

$$\left.\begin{array}{r} RMgCl \rightleftharpoons R^- + MgCl^+ \\ RMgCl \rightleftharpoons Cl^- + RMg^+ \\ Cl^- + MgCl^+ \rightleftharpoons MgCl_2 \\ R^- + RMg^+ \rightleftharpoons R_2Mg \end{array}\right\} \quad (S_E1)$$

A second group of studies of electrophilic metal-for-metal substitutions is characterised by the employment of octahedrally co-ordinating transition metals, such as chromium(III) and cobalt(III). This development is due to M. D. Johnson, who has introduced the use of cationically substituted, water-soluble alkyl groups, so permitting the use of solvent water, and the octahedral aquation of the transition-metal ions. Johnson's alkyl groups are of the pyridiomethyl type, such as the 4-picolinium groups

$H\overset{+}{N}C_5H_4$—CH_2— and $Me\overset{+}{N}C_5H_4$—CH_2—

and their 2- and 3-position isomers.

In this way, Coombes and Johnson[238] have, for example, examined a series of mercury(II)-for-chromium(III) substitutions in water. Writing Pym^+ for 4-pyridiomethyl, and X^- for Cl^-, Br^-, or NO_3^-, the following reactions have been kinetically studied:

$$\left.\begin{array}{l} Pym^+\text{—}Cr^{III}(H_2O)_5^{2+} + HgX_2 \\ \qquad \rightarrow Pym^+\text{—}HgX + Cr(H_2O)_6^{3+} + X^- \\ Pym^+\text{—}Cr^{III}(H_2O)_5^{2+} + HgX_3^- \\ \qquad \rightarrow Pym^+\text{—}HgX + Cr(H_2O)_6^{3+} + 2X^- \\ Pym^+\text{—}Cr^{III}(H_2O)_5^{2+} + HgX_4^{2-} \\ \qquad \rightarrow Pym^+\text{—}HgX + Cr(H_2O)_6^{3+} + 3X^- \end{array}\right\} \quad (S_E2)$$

[238] R. G. Coombes and M. D. Johnson, *J. Chem. Soc.*, **1966, A, 1805**.

According to the kinetic evidence, they all have mechanisms S_E2, even those by the complex anions of mercury(II) as substituting agents. None of the reactions is an S_Ei process, in which one of the mercury-borne anions combines with, and would be carried away by, the chromium atom. Apart from the kinetic evidence, this is made clear by the fact that the inorganic product is always $Cr(H_2O)_6^{3+}$, even when $Cr(H_2O)_5Cl^{2+}$, or $Cr(H_2O)_5Br^{2+}$, if formed, would be stable enough in the conditions to be found. The other striking point about the reactions formulated is that, with $X^- = Cl^-$, the three second-order rates are alike to within one power of ten, whilst with $X^- = Br^-$, the three rates are alike to within two powers of ten. Were the displaceable group neutral, we would expect, for electrochemical reasons, that the rates of electrophilic substitution would fall strongly as the substituting agent takes on negative charge. But apparently, the displaceable group being strongly positive, the coulombic attraction of the oppositely charged substrate and substituting agents approximately cancels the expected electrochemical kinetic effect.

(36g) Hydrogen-for-Metal Substitutions.—In this field, the mechanisms S_E2, S_E1, and S_E1-$2X^-$ have been recognised, together with some further mechanisms not yet encountered among metal-for-metal substitutions.

We note first some examples of acid protolyses of Group B metals. A number of acid protolyses of alkylmercuric salts,[239] and of dialkylmercury,[240] and tetra-alkyl-lead[241] compounds, that is, H(I)-for-Hg(II) and H(I)-for-Pb(IV) substitutions, have been described, which have second-order kinetics, and almost certainly take place by the S_E2 mechanism, for example:

$$\left.\begin{array}{l} CH_3HgI + HClO_4 \xrightarrow{\text{aq.-dioxan}} CH_4 + HgI^+ \\ (CH_2{:}CH\cdot CH_2)_2Hg + HClO_4 \\ \qquad \xrightarrow{\text{water}} CH_2{:}CHMe + CH_2{:}CH\cdot CH_2\cdot Hg^+ \\ (C_2H_5)_4Pb + HClO_4 \\ \qquad \xrightarrow[\text{acid}]{\text{acetic}} C_2H_6 + (C_2H_5)_3Pb^+ \end{array}\right\} (S_E2)$$

The evidence adduced by Roberts[237] that Grignard compounds and

239 M. M. Kreevoy, *J. Am. Chem. Soc.*, 1959, **79**, 5927.

240 S. Winstein and T. G. Traylor, *J. Am. Chem. Soc.*, 1955, **77**, 3747; M. M. Kreevoy, P. J. Steinwand, and W. W. Kayser, *ibid.*, 1964, **86**, 5013; 1966, **88**, 124.

241 G. C. Robinson, *J. Org. Chem.*, 1963, **38**, 843.

dialkylmagnesiums probably undergo magnesium exchange in ether or dioxan by the S_E1 mechanism makes it probable that these materials use that mechanism in their protolytic decompositions.

The mechanism S_E1-$2X^-$ has been found by Coad and Johnson[242] in the protolysis of 4-pyridiomethylmercuric chloride in the presence of chloride ions in water. A concurrent but less important mechanism, S_E1-X^-, involving only one chloride ion, a mechanism not previously realised in metal-for-metal substitutions, was also detected. The anions are taken up in pre-equilibrium, and then the formed complex ions spontaneously but slowly split off their chloromercuric groups to leave carbon as the carbanionic centre in a betaine, which becomes rapidly protonated. The two mechanisms may be written:

$$\mathrm{Pym^+HgCl} \rightleftharpoons \mathrm{Pym^+HgCl_2^-} \rightleftharpoons \mathrm{Pym^+HgCl_3^{2-}}$$

$$\left.\begin{aligned} &\mathrm{Pym^+HgCl_2^-} \xrightarrow[\text{slow}]{} \mathrm{Pym^\pm + HgCl_2} \\ &\mathrm{Pym^\pm + H^+} \longrightarrow \mathrm{HPym^+ (= 4\text{-picolinium})} \end{aligned}\right\} (\mathrm{S_E1\text{-}X^-})$$

$$\left.\begin{aligned} &\mathrm{Pym^+HgCl_3^{2-}} \xrightarrow{\text{slow}} \mathrm{Pym^\pm + HgCl_3^-} \\ &\mathrm{Pym^\pm + H^+} \longrightarrow \mathrm{HPym^+ (= 4\text{-picolinium})} \end{aligned}\right\} (\mathrm{S_E1\text{-}2X^-})$$

The rate is linear or quadratic in chloride-ion concentration, as the case may be, but in either case is independent of the acidity, provided that the picoline residue remains in cationic form.

A peculiar mechanism involving prototropic change applies to the protolysis of α-carbethoxybenzylmercuric chloride (or bromide) in aqueous organic solvents.[243] The pure substrate remains unchanged on boiling with dilute perchloric acid, but small concentrations of halide ions lead to rapid protolysis even at 0°. The rate is then quadratic in halide ions, and quadratic in hydrogen ions: and it has an inverse-first-power dependence on inorganic mercury(II). In the interpretation given, a pre-equilibrium uptake of two chloride ions is succeeded by a pre-equilibrium protolysis of the mercury substituent. This accounts for the second power in chloride ions, one power in hydrogen ions, and the one inverse power in mercury(II), in the rate expression. The organic product is automatically rearranged, having then the carbethoxyl group in enolic form. The reversion of this to the ordinary form is expected (Chapter XI) to require time, and to be catalysed by

[242] J. R. Coad and M. D. Johnson, *J. Chem. Soc.*, 1967, *B*, 635.
[243] J. R. Coad and C. K. Ingold, *J. Chem. Soc.*, 1968, *B*, 1455.

hydrogen ions. This is the explanation given for the second power in hydrogen ions in the rate equation. The reversion of the enol to the ordinary carboxyl form is taken to be the rate-controlling step in the whole chain of processes, which up to the formation of the enolic substance, that is, up to the stage at which the mercury has been acidolysed, is a two-anion catalysed bimolecular protolysis with rearrangement, S_E2'-$2X^-$, another mechanism so far unknown in metal-for-metal substitutions:

$$\left.\begin{array}{l} (EtO_2C)(Ph)CH\cdot HgCl \rightleftharpoons (EtO_2C)(Ph)CH\cdot HgCl_2^- \rightleftharpoons (EtO_2C)(Ph)CH\cdot HgCl_3^{2-} \\ H^+ + (EtO_2C)(Ph)CH\cdot HgCl_3^{2-} \rightleftharpoons (HO)(EtO)C{=}CH(Ph) + HgCl_3^- \end{array}\right\} (S_E2'\text{-}2X^-)$$

$$(HO)(EtO)C{=}CHPh \xrightarrow[\text{slow}]{H^+} EtO_2C\cdot CH_2Ph$$

As an example of acidolysis of a transition metal, we may note a protolysis of cobalt(III) by mechanism S_E1, as demonstrated by Johnson, Tobe, and Wong.[244] The 4-pyridiomethyl group is again written Pym^+. The preliminary equilibrium between the pentacyano- and the tetracyanoaquo-pyridiomethylcobalt complex can be set in any position by adjusting the acidity. The real substrate is the tetracyanoaquo-complex. This spontaneously but slowly loses a carbanion, which is actually a betaine, because the alkyl group contains a cationic substituent; and then the betaine rapidly becomes protonated:

$$\left.\begin{array}{l} Pym^+Co^{III}(CN)_5^{3-} \rightleftharpoons Pym^+Co^{III}(CN)_4(H_2O)^{2-} \\ Pym^+Co^{III}(CN)_4(H_2O)^{2-} \xrightarrow[\text{slow}]{} Pym^{\pm} + Co^{III}(CN)_4(H_2O)_2^- \\ Pym^{\pm} + H^+ \longrightarrow HPym^+(=\text{4-picolinium}) \end{array}\right\} (S_E1)$$

The rate is proportional to the equilibrium concentration of the tetracyanoaquo-pyridiomethyl complex, but is otherwise independent of the acidity, provided that the picoline residue remains in cationic form.

(36h) Substitution Adjacently to an Aromatic Ring.—Illuminati

[244] M. D. Johnson, M. L. Tobe, and L. Y. Wong, *J. Chem. Soc.*, **1967**, **A**, 491.

and his coworkers[246] have noted that, in the halogenation, by Cl_2 or Br_2 in acetic acid in the dark and without catalysts, of polysubstituted benzenes containing alkyl substituents, and also polar substituents, a minor proportion of side-chain α-halogenation in the alkyl groups accompanies the nuclear halogenation; and it does so over so wide a range of nuclear reactivities, as determined by the polar substituents, as to show that both reactions are similarly sensitive to polar influences: it is not possible that the nuclear reaction should be electrophilic, and the side-chain reaction homolytic. In hexa-substituted benzenes, the nuclear reaction is excluded, and in hexamethylbenzene, the absolute rate of side-chain halogenation was greater than that of nuclear substitution of pentamethylbenzene or any lower alkylbenzene; and it was enormously greater than could be contemplated for homolytic substitution in the conditions. Kinetically, the chlorination was of second order, first in substrate, and first in molecular chlorine. The rate-constants in Table 36-2 illustrate the polar sensitivity of this side-chain substitution.

Table 36-2.—Second-Order Rate-Constants of Side-Chain Monochlorination of Hexa-substituted Benzenes by Chlorine in Acetic Acid (Illuminati).

X in C_6Me_5X...	Me	Cl	Br	CN
k_2 at 18°...	3.90×10^6	—	—	1.06×10^2
k_2 at 30°...	—	1.27×10^5	7.90×10^4	2.64×10^2

Neither addition of halogen, nor loss of any side-chain, accompanied the side-chain substitutions. In chlorination, though not in bromination, the formed aralphyl halide was accompanied by a small proportion of the corresponding acetate, which was produced concurrently with, and not by a subsequent reaction of, the halide.

In the proposed mechanism,[245,246] the first step, the formation of a *cyclo*hexadienylium ion, ranks as a common first step for both nuclear and side-chain substitution when both occur, or a first step for either reaction when the other is excluded. The side-chain substitution is completed by a rearrangement, as illustrated below for the chlorination of hexamethylbenzene:

[245] G. Illuminati and F. Siegel, *Ric. Sci. Rend.*, 1964, **7**, 458; E. Baciocchi and G. Illuminati, *ibid.*, p. 462; *idem* and F. Siegel, *Spec. Pubs. Chem. Soc.*, 1965, **19**, 158; E. Baciocchi, A. Ciana, G. Illuminati, and C. Pasini, *J. Am. Chem. Soc.*, 1965, **87**, 3953.

[246] E. Baciocchi and G. Illuminati, *Tetrahedron Letters*, **1962**, 6371.

Me CH₂·Cl
Me
Me Me
Me

Me Cl Me Cl
CH₃ CH₂
Me Me
$C_6Me_6 \rightleftharpoons$ + $\rightleftharpoons$
Me Me Me Me
Me Me OAc⁻

Me
CH₂·OAc
Me

The details of the rearrangement are not proved, but the plausible proposal is that a proton loss (as from Doering's heptamethyl*cyclo*hexadienylium ion, cf. Section **24d**) is succeeded by an anionotropic rearrangement (cf. Chapter XI). This mechanism allows for the intervention of a lyate ion, as illustrated for acetate ion above.

(37) HOMOLYTIC ALIPHATIC SUBSTITUTION

(37a) Inorganic Prototype Reactions.—As noted in Section **18g**, a historical prototype for many homolytic substitutions in saturated organic molecules is the gaseous reaction between chlorine and hydrogen. It was for this reaction that, on the basis of experimental work by Bodenstein and others, Nernst in 1918 proposed the first specific chain mechanism, which all subsequent work has confirmed.

Chain initiation is through chlorine atoms, produced, initially in very small concentration, from the supplied molecular chlorine, either thermally, or photolytically, or by chemical reaction with some previously formed radical:

$$\mathrm{Cl{-}Cl} \rightarrow 2\dot{\mathrm{C}}\mathrm{l} \qquad (1)$$

The two steps, which by cyclic regeneration and repetition compose the chain, are themselves homolytic substitutions. The first of them (2) is a substitution by a chlorine atom on a hydrogen molecule:

$$\dot{\mathrm{C}}\mathrm{l} + \mathrm{H{-}H} \rightarrow \mathrm{Cl{-}H} + \dot{\mathrm{H}} \qquad (2)$$

As will be seen from the bond strengths in Table 18-3 (p. 253), this reaction is almost thermo-neutral. The rate of the overall reaction between chlorine and hydrogen has been measured, and the kinetics analysed in such detail, that the rate of this individual step is now well known; between 0° and 770°, the second-order rate constant is given[247] by

[247] P. G. Ashmore and J. Chanmugam, *Trans. Faraday Soc.*, 1953, **49**, 254.

$$k_2(\dot{Cl} + H_2) = 7.9 + 10^{10} \exp(-5500/RT)(\text{sec.}^{-1}\ \text{mole}^{-1}\ \text{l.})$$

The second step (3) of the cycle, which becomes repeated to form the reaction chain, is a substitution by a hydrogen atom in a chlorine molecule:

$$\dot{H} + Cl{-}Cl \rightarrow H{-}Cl + \dot{Cl} \tag{3}$$

As will be seen from Table 18-3, this process is exothermic by 45 kcal./mole. It is extremely fast, so fast that no reversion of the preceding thermo-neutral reaction can be detected.

It was made clear theoretically by London, Polanyi, and Eyring, many years ago, that the transition states of homolytic substitutions of the class to which reactions (2) and (3) belong must be linear.

Chain termination is by any process that can cause the chain-carrying radicals to disappear, such as their colligation (4), their reaction with a foreign substance, or their capture by a surface:

$$2\dot{Cl} \rightarrow Cl_2 \qquad 2\dot{H} \rightarrow H_2 \qquad \dot{H} + \dot{Cl} \rightarrow HCl \tag{4}$$

The overall reaction is strongly inhibited by oxygen, presumably because this material terminates chains by removing hydrogen atoms from participation in the propagation steps. It combines with the $\dot{H}$ atoms to form the $HO_2^{\cdot}$ radicals, and ultimately hydrogen peroxide.

The rate of the overall reaction of homolytic chlorination of molecular hydrogen is determined jointly by the frequency with which chains are started, the rate of the rate-controlling step (2) of a chain cycle, and the number of cycles contained in the chain, which itself depends on the rate of the totality of chain-terminating processes. The chains of the uninhibited reaction are long, usually running to many thousands of cycles. The kinetics of the overall process therefore depend not only on the kinetics of the rate-controlling chain step, but also on those of chain initiation and chain termination, even though only a very small proportion of converted material may have been stoicheiometrically involved in those processes.

(37b) Halogenation by Molecular Halogens.—The gaseous chlorination of alkanes and substituted alkanes by molecular chlorine kinetically resembles the gaseous chlorination of hydrogen so closely as to leave no doubt that it follows a like mechanism.[248] The kinetic chains are again long, often 10^4 cycles or more. As a first step, chlorine atoms

[248] N. N. Semenov, "Chemical Kinetics and Chain Reactions," Clarendon Press, Oxford, 1935, p. 122; E. W. R. Steacie, "Atom and Free Radical Reactions," Reinhold Publishing Corp., New York, 1934, p. 667; C. Walling, "Free Radicals in Solution," Wiley and Sons, New York, 1957, p. 352.

have to be produced. Thermally and photochemically initiated chlorinations have been studied.[249]

The first of the chain-carrying steps, which, for chlorination of the simpler alkanes at least, controls the rate of chain propagation, consists in attack by the chlorine atom on the alkane molecule, to extract a hydrogen atom, and produce an alkyl radical. This is illustrated in equation (5) for the reaction of methane:

$$\dot{Cl} + H—CH_3 \rightarrow Cl—H + \dot{C}H_3 \qquad (5)$$

This type of "hydrogen abstraction," as it is usually called, is very common as a chain-carrying step of homolytic substitutions in saturated compounds. It is in itself a homolytic substitution at hydrogen, and doubtless proceeds through a linear transition state. For the chlorination of methane, the reaction step is, as shown in Table 18-3 (p. 253), almost thermo-neutral; for homologous alkanes it will be slightly exothermic. The rate of attack of a chlorine atom on methane is of the same order of magnitude as the rate of its attack on hydrogen. This has enabled Trotman-Dickenson and his coworkers, by reference to the known absolute rate of the latter process, to obtain absolute rates for the attack of a chlorine atom on methane, by competitive chlorination of hydrogen and methane. The absolute rates for the attack of a chlorine atom on derivatives of methane were then obtained by competitive chlorinations of methane and the derivatives.[250] Some of these data are in Table 37-1.

TABLE 37-1.—ARRHENIUS PARAMETERS AND RATE CONSTANTS FOR CHLORINE ATOM ATTACK ON ALKANES.

Alkane	B sec.$^{-1}$ mole^{-1} l.	E_A kcal./mole	k_2 at 100° sec.$^{-1}$ mole^{-1} l.
CH_4	2.6×10^{10}	3.85	1.8×10^{8}
C_2H_6	12.0×10^{10}	1.00	310×10^{8}
$(CH_3)_2CH_2$	17.6×10^{10}	0.67	710×10^{8}
$(CH_3)_3CH$	19.6×10^{10}	0.86	613×10^{8}

The second step of the cyclic unit of the chain process consists in the attack by an alkyl radical on a chlorine molecule, as illustrated in equation (6) for the methyl radical. The products are the chlorine-

[249] R. N. Pease and G. F. Walz, *J. Am. Chem. Soc.*, 1931, 53, 3728; A. Coehn and H. Cordes, *Z. phys. Chem.*, 1930, *B*, 9, 1; L. T. Jones and J. R. Bates, *J. Am. Chem. Soc.*, 1934, 56, 2282; M. Tamura, *Rev. Phys. Chem. Japan*, 1941, 15, 86.

[250] H. O. Pritchard, J. B. Pyke, and A. F. Trotman-Dickenson, *J. Am. Chem. Soc.*, 1955, 77, 2629.

substitution product, methyl chloride, and a chlorine atom which will go back into step (5):

$$\dot{C}H_3 + Cl—Cl \rightarrow CH_3—Cl + \dot{C}l \qquad (6)$$

As Table 18-3 shows, this reaction is exothermic by 22 kcal./mole. It is very fast, so much so that no sign of reversion of the nearly thermoneutral reaction (5) has been detected.

Chain termination is, as before, by radical colligation, or by any other process which will remove chain-carrying radicals. Oxygen inhibits the chlorination of alkanes, presumably by capturing alkyl radicals to form $R\dot{O}_2$ radicals. By increasing the partial pressure of oxygen, one may pass from an oxygen-inhibited chlorination to a chlorine-catalysed oxidation of the alkane, and, over a range of partial pressures, may obtain products which are both oxidised and chlorinated, for instance, phosgene from methane.

The available evidence concerning the mechanism of homolytic chlorination by molecular chlorine in solution is less detailed, but, as far as it goes, points to the conclusion that the mechanism is essentially the same as in the gas phase, though the kinetic chains may often be shorter.

The first comprehensive survey of the products of homolytic chlorination, in the gaseous and liquid phases, of hydrocarbons was by Hass and his coworkers.[251] They noted that carbon skeletal rearrangements are not observed, though we shall notice an exception to this rule later. All the hydrogen atoms in an alkane suffer concurrent substitutions, at rates in the general order, primary < secondary < tertiary, the ratios moving towards unity as temperatures are raised. These workers introduced the very useful concept of "selectivity," which is defined by relative figures for the ratios of the rates of attack at the different types of hydrogen atom in a molecule to the number of hydrogens of each type. Thus, if propane underwent 60% of α-mono-substitution and 40% of β-mono-substitution, the selectivity ratio, secondary/primary, would be 2.

Because the mechanism starts with hydrogen abstraction, the relative rates of chlorination in the different positions of an alkane are controlled by the different rates of abstraction of the various hydrogen atoms by a chlorine atom in process (5) above. Hass's temperature effect must mean that rates of hydrogen abstraction are controlled in part by activation energies; and his rate order, as between primary, secondary, and tertiary hydrogen, must therefore mean that the corre-

[251] H. B. Hass, E. J. McBee, and P. Weber, *Ind. Eng. Chem.*, 1935, 27, 1190; 1936, 28, 333.

sponding activation energies are diminishing, as might have been expected, with the C—H bond strengths, that is, as the reaction becomes more exothermic. However, as Table 37-1 shows, apart from methane, for which the activation energy is 4 kcal./mole, the activation energies for the abstraction of a hydrogen atom by a chlorine atom in the homologous alkanes are all about 1 kcal./mole. This leaves little room for any great spread of rates. The relative rates of abstraction at 100° of a hydrogen atom from the groups CH_3, CH_2, and CH are approximately 1:4.3:7.0 in the gas phase and 1:2.0:3.0 in the liquid phase.[252,253] A hydrogen atom is abstracted from CH_4 with a relative rate of about 0.01.

Bromination at saturated carbon has close similarities with the more fully investigated chlorination. In general, brominations, in gas or solution, are chain reactions; but the chains are much shorter, grading down to a single-cycle, that is, a non-chain process. The main cause is energetic: short chains characterise the replacement of strongly bound hydrogen. At low temperatures it is difficult for the reactants to acquire the activation energy necessary to carry forward the chains in competition with non-activated chain-terminating colligation.

As reference to Table 18-3 will show, the rate-controlling step (7) in the bromination of methane by bromine atoms is endothermic by 14 kcal./mole: the activation energy must be greater than this. The activation energy was, indeed, determined by Kistiakowsky and his collaborators to be 17.8 kcal./mole:[254]

$$\dot{Br} + H{-}CH_3 \rightarrow BrH + \dot{C}H_3 \qquad (7)$$

As would be expected from such a figure, and as they found, the bromination of methane, at temperatures near 180°, is essentially a non-chain process.

As Table 18-3 shows, the succeeding step (8) is exothermic by 19 kcal./mole: this step will require but little activation energy:

$$\dot{C}H_3 + Br{-}Br \rightarrow CH_3Br + \dot{Br} \qquad (8)$$

It will therefore forestall any reversion of step (7), so rendering the overall bromination irreversible. This also is found experimentally.

With homologous alkanes, and with *cyclo*alkanes, the CH bonds initially to be broken are weaker, and kinetic chains appear. Jost[255] found

[252] C. Walling, "Free Radicals in Solution," Wiley and Sons, New York, 1957, Chap. 8.

[253] J. M. Tedder, *Quart. Revs. Chem. Soc.*, 1960, **14**, 336.

[254] H. C. Anderson, G. B. Kistiakowsky, and E. R. Van Artsdalen, *J. Chem. Phys.*, 1942, **10**, 305; 1943, **11**, 6; 1944, **12**, 469.

[255] W. Jost, *Z. phys. Chem. Bodenstein Festband*, **1931**, 291.

that the photochemical bromination of *cyclo*hexane was a chain reaction with an average chain-length near 2 at room temperature, but 12–37 at 100°.

With still weaker CH bonds to be broken, as in chloroform, reversibility appears. Sullivan and Davidson[256] found that for the bromination of chloroform in the gas-phase at 150–180° the equilibrium constant,

$$K = [BrCCl_3][HBr]/[HCCl_3][Br_2]$$

was about 2. They observed kinetics consistent with the scheme

$$Br_2 \rightleftharpoons 2\dot{Br}$$

$$Br + H{-}CCl_3 \underset{-9}{\overset{9}{\rightleftharpoons}} Br{-}H + \dot{C}Cl_3 \qquad (9)$$

$$\dot{C}Cl_3 + Br{-}Br \underset{-10}{\overset{10}{\rightleftharpoons}} BrCCl_3 + Br \qquad (10)$$

The forward reaction (10) was only about 25 times faster than the retrograde reaction (−9).

Homolytic bromination in alkanes is more selective than is chlorination in favour of secondary, and, still better, tertiary positions.[257] Thus the gaseous bromination of *iso*butane gives only the tertiary bromide, and of *iso*pentane gives about 20 times more tertiary than secondary bromide.

Iodination of alkanes by iodine is not observed, despite the easy thermal production of iodine atoms. The thermodynamics of the overall process are unfavourable: alkyl iodides would be more easily reduced by hydrogen iodide. The kinetics are likewise unfavourable, inasmuch as the step of attack by an iodine atom on the alkane would be prohibitively endothermic.

Fluorination with fluorine of alkanes and their derivatives is so rapid and so exothermic that detailed investigations of mechanism are difficult. Studies of products have been made, by Bigelow[258] and by Miller[259] particularly, working either with gases strongly diluted with nitrogen, or with solutions in a perfluorinated solvent. Methane gave all the

[256] J. H. Sullivan and N. Davidson, *J. Chem. Phys.*, 1951, 19, 143.

[257] M. S. Kharasch, W. Hered, and F. R. Mayo, *J. Org. Chem.*, 1941, 6, 818; B. H. Eckstein, H. A. Sheraga, and E. R. Van Artsdalen, *J. Chem. Phys.*, 1954, 22, 28; G. A. Russell and H. C. Brown, *J. Am. Chem. Soc.*, 1955, 77, 4025.

[258] L. A. Bigelow, *Chem. Revs.*, 1947, 40, 51.

[259] W. T. Miller jr., *J. Am. Chem. Soc.*, 1940, 62, 341; E. T. Hadly and W. T. Miller jr., *ibid.*, p. 3362; W. T. Miller jr., and A. L. Dittman, *ibid.*, 1956, 78, 2793; W. T. Miller jr., S. D. Koch, and F. W. McLafferty jr., *ibid.*, p. 4492.

possible fluorinated methanes, plus C_2F_6 and C_3F_8. Ethane gave as isolated products mono-, di-, tri-, penta-, and hexa-fluoroethanes, plus CF_4. Chloroform gave fluorochloroform, plus C_2Cl_6. Thus, besides normal substitution products, one obtains both dimeric products and fission products.

Fluorine can thermally generate atoms as easily as iodine can: the heats of atomisation are 37 and 36 kcal./mole, respectively. A chain reaction, propagated by attack of a fluorine atom to yield an alkyl radical which attacks a fluorine molecule, is energetically strongly favoured: the first and rate-controlling step in the case of methane would be exothermic by 34 kcal./mole. Even so, chain-ending radical colligations must be competitively important, because dimers are so commonly formed in isolable quantities. The conclusion that kinetic chains must thus be rendered short, coupled with the fact that, nevertheless, fluorinations proceed spontaneously and rapidly at $-80°$ in the dark and in the absence of chemical chain-initiators, makes one doubt whether chain initiation does depend on thermal fluorine atoms, and incline towards Miller's suggestion that chain initiation is accomplished directly by the plentiful fluorine molecules, which can produce both a fluorine atom and an alkyl radical by an attack of the form

$$RH + F_2 \rightarrow \dot{R} + HF + \dot{F}$$

which is nearly thermoneutral: ΔH for methane is $+3$, and for ethane -2 kcal./mole.

The formation of fission products, such as CF_4, has not been elucidated, but might result[260] from bimolecular homolytic substitutions S_H2, of the type

$$\dot{F} + CF_3{\cdot}CF_3 \rightarrow F{\cdot}CF_3 + \dot{C}F_3 \qquad (S_H2)$$

(cf. Section **18g**).

[260] An earlier prejudice against bimolecular homolytic substitution, except at terminal and univalent atoms, such as hydrogen, has been weakened by the discovery of a number of radical substitutions at interior and therefore multivalent atoms. Thus S—S bonds in disulphides (which are fairly strong—69 kcal./mole in dimethyl disulphide), and in thiosulphonates, have been broken by the attack of aryl or alkyl radicals, which are then recovered in combination with either fragment of the substrate, along with dimers of the accompanying radicals, *e.g.*,

$$ArS{-}SO_2{\cdot}Ar + Ph\dot{C}H_2 \rightarrow \begin{cases} ArS{-}CH_2Ph + \dot{S}O_2{\cdot}Ar \\ Ar\dot{S} + PhCH_2{-}SO_2{\cdot}Ar \end{cases}$$

(each radical $\rightarrow$ Dimer)

(J. Degani and A. Tundo, *Annali Chim.*, **1961, 51, 543**; *idem* and M. Tiecco, *ibid.*, p. 550; *idem*, *Gazz. Chim. ital.*, **1962, 92, 1204, 1213**.)

Hass's statement that skeletal rearrangements do not accompany chlorination has one known exception, but one so reasonable that it "proves the rule." A necessary condition for rearrangement in a reaction in a saturated structure is the formation of an intermediate with an incomplete electron shell, *i.e.*, either a carbonium ion or a neutral carbon radical. This mechanistic condition is fulfilled in the accepted mechanism of chlorination, which does involve a carbon radical. However, this condition, though necessary, is not sufficient. The thermodynamic condition that the free-energy change must be in the direction favourable to rearrangement, and the kinetic condition that the intermediate must live long enough to allow time for the group migration, have also to be satisfied. Now rearrangements by way of a carbonium ion have a very large literature, and are obviously much easier to realise than rearrangements by way of a carbon radical. Probably the kinetic condition, that the life of the intermediate must be longer than the time required for rearrangement, is much more easily satisfied in carbonium ions than it is in radicals; and non-fulfilment of this condition may be the reason why Hass never observed rearrangement. However, radicals can be produced which gain such stability by the internal migration of a sufficiently mobile group that an observable amount of rearrangement occurs, at least in some reactions. The simplest well-authenticated radical of this kind is the "neophyl" (2-phenyl*iso*butyl) radical, $PhMe_2C \cdot CH_2^{\cdot}$, which Urry and Kharasch produced by reduction of neophyl chloride with a Grignard reagent and cobaltous chloride.[261] They proved that they had made the radical by isolating its dimer; and they showed that part of it is rearranged in their conditions, by migration of the phenyl group, to give the presumably more stable 2-benzyl*iso*propyl radical, $PhCH_2 \cdot CMe_2^{\cdot}$, by isolating the dimer of that also. The non-dimerised reaction products were simple redox disproportionation derivatives of the rearranged radical, ωω-dimethylstyrene and 2-benzylpropane:

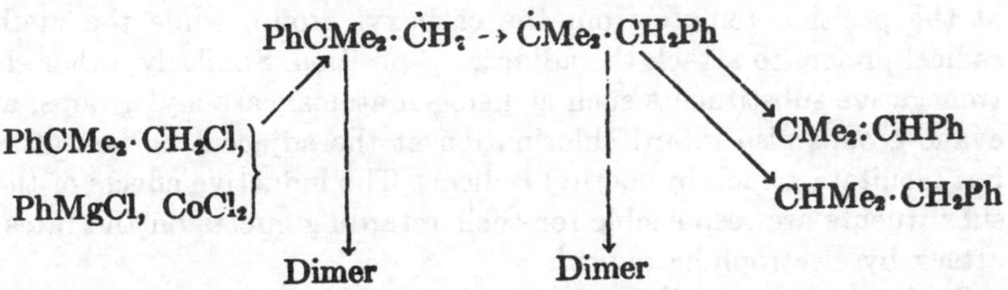

Now the neophyl radical is the radical, which, according to the radical-chain mechanism of chlorination, would be an essential intermediate in

[261] W. H. Urry and M. S. Kharasch, *J. Am. Chem. Soc.*, 1944, 66, 1438.

the homolytic chlorination of *t*-butylbenzene. It is therefore confirmatory of the mechanism that in the gaseous chlorination of this hydrocarbon at 190–245° by chlorine in light,[262] the products consist, not only of unrearranged 2-phenyl*iso*butyl (neophyl) chloride, as well as products of its further chlorination in the side-chain without rearrangement, but also of rearrangement products, such as 2-benzyl*iso*propyl chloride and the related rearranged olefins:

$$\left.\begin{matrix}Ph\cdot CMe_3,\\ Cl_2,\ h\nu\end{matrix}\right\} \nearrow Ph\cdot CMe_2\cdot\dot{C}H_2 \rightarrow \dot{C}Me_2CH_2Ph \searrow CMe_2{:}CHPh$$

$$Ph\cdot CMe_2\cdot\dot{C}H_2 \downarrow Ph\cdot CMe_2\cdot CH_2Cl \qquad \dot{C}Me_2CH_2Ph \downarrow Cl\cdot CMe_2\cdot CH_2Ph$$

Many radical reagents show a vestigial polarity, and this is particularly marked in the halogen atoms. As might be deduced from the difference of stability of Cl^- and Cl^+, the reagent $Cl^\cdot$ is markedly electrophilic: it abstracts a neutral hydrogen atom, but does so the more

TABLE 37-2.—SELECTIVITIES FOR HYDROGEN ABSTRACTION FROM PROPIONIC ACID.

Radical	CH_3—	—CH_2—	—CO_2H
$CH_3^\cdot$	1	7.8	
$Cl^\cdot$	1	0.03	

readily the greater the electron density at that hydrogen atom. In contrast, alkyl and aryl radicals (*e.g.*, $CH_3^\cdot$ and $C_6H_5^\cdot$) are neither markedly electrophilic nor markedly nucleophilic. Substituents quite often affect hydrogen abstraction by radicals of high and of low electron affinity in different ways. This can be illustrated by reference to the figures collected by Tedder[253] for hydrogen abstraction from propionic acid by $Cl^\cdot$ and $CH_3^\cdot$ (Table 37-2). Thus chlorine preferentially attacks at the position remote from the carboxyl group, while the methyl radical prefers to attack the adjacent α-position. Similarly, other electronegative substituents such as halogen atoms, carbonyl groups, and cyano-groups also retard chlorination at the adjacent carbon atoms, but facilitate attack by methyl radicals. The inductive effects of these substituents are responsible for their retarding effects on the rates of attack by electrophilic radicals.

Similar phenomena have also been observed in hydrogen abstraction from the side-chain of toluene. Some typical data on the relative rates of hydrogen-atom abstraction from ring-substituted toluenes have

[262] J. D. Backhurst, E. D. Hughes, and C. K. Ingold, *J. Chem. Soc.*, 1959, 2742.

TABLE 37-3.—RELATIVE REACTIVITIES OF SUBSTITUTED TOLUENES TOWARDS SOME RADICALS.

4-Substituent	Cl· at 40°[263]	Br· at 80°[264]	C_6H_5· at 60°[266]
CH_3O	—	11.7	—
C_6H_5O	2.50	—	0.97
CH_3	1.57	2.56	1.47
H	1.00	1.00	1.00
Cl	0.79	0.80	1.07
CN	—	0.11[265]	—
NO_2	0.32	0.11	0.81

been collected in Table 37-3. It can be seen that electron-releasing substituents enhance, while electron-attracting substituents retard, the relative rates of halogenation, but that the substituents have comparatively little effect on hydrogen abstraction by the phenyl radical.

The inductive effect is not always the predominating influence when the substituent is on the same carbon atom as the hydrogen which is being removed: for example, methyl chloride is more rapidly chlorinated than methane. This can be further illustrated by reference to Tedder's data[253] on the halogenation of 1-fluorobutane (Table 37-4). Bromination, which is the most selective of the halogenation processes, is strongly retarded at position 2 relatively to position 3, because of the inductive effect of the fluorine atom. However, bromination proceeds more rapidly at position 1 than at position 4. This is because the relatively weak abstracting agent best operates through a transition state in which the H—C bond has been considerably stretched and weakened. Such weakening at position 1 arises from the ability of the fluorine atom to conjugate with the carbon atom, thus facilitating hydrogen abstraction, despite the oppositely acting inductive effect of the fluorine atom:

F—C·····H Br

The singly-barbed arrows signify one-electron transfers. The oxygen atom of ethers is particularly prone to conjugation in this form. The initial and outstandingly predominant attack of chlorine atoms on ethers is at their α-carbon atoms,[267] though the immediate products are usually unstable.

[263] G. A. Russell and R. C. Williamson jr., *J. Am. Chem. Soc.*, 1964, **86**, 2357.

[264] C. Walling, A. L. Rieger, and D. D. Tanner, *J. Am. Chem. Soc.*, 1963, **85**, 3129.

[265] R. E. Pearson and J. C. Martin, *J. Am. Chem. Soc.*, 1963, **85**, 354, 3142.

[266] R. F. Bridger and G. A. Russell, *J. Am. Chem. Soc.*, 1963, **85**, 3754.

[267] H. Singh and J. M. Tedder, *J. Chem. Soc.*, **1966, B**, 612.

TABLE 37-4.—SELECTIVITIES IN THE HALOGENATION OF 1-FLUOROBUTANE (TEDDER).

	CH_2F—	—CH_2—	—CH_2—	—CH_3
Fluorination at 20°	0.3	0.8	1.0	1
Chlorination at 78°	0.9	1.7	3.7	1
Bromination at 146°	10	9	88	1

The retarding effect of COF and COCl groups on the chlorination of methylene groups in an attacked alkyl chain is diminished by relay in the manner characteristic of the inductive effect, though it is not easy to understand why the attenuation with distance is so similar in a polar solvent, as well as a non-polar solvent, to what it is in the gas phase. The facts of the matter are illustrated by Table 37-5, giving results from a paper by Singh and Tedder.[268]

TABLE 37-5.—SELECTIVITIES IN CHLORINATION OF *n*-HEXANOYL FLUORIDE IN THE GAS PHASE AND OF *n*-HEXANOYL CHLORIDE IN SOLUTION AT 50–52° (SINGH AND TEDDER).

	FCO—	—CH_2—	—CH_2—	—CH_2—	—CH_2—	—CH_3
Gas		0.16	1.5	4.0	4.4	1
	ClCO—	—CH_2—	—CH_2—	—CH_2—	—CH_2—	—CH_3
In CCl_4		0.17	0.58	1.6	2.0	1
In MeCN		0.16	0.51	1.6	2.2	1

We may remark further on the role of the solvent in radical reactions, since profound effects have been observed in chlorinations with molecular chlorine. One of Hass's rules for chlorination was that the liquid phase gives relative rates comparable to those obtained at much higher temperatures in the vapour phase. That is, selectivity is less in the liquid than in the vapour, at the same temperature. This has been rationalised by assuming that a chlorine atom, colliding with any portion of a hydrocarbon molecule, will be held in contact by surrounding solvent so long that there is a good chance for reaction, even if more reactive sites are available elsewhere.[252,269]

[268] H. Singh and J. M. Tedder, *J. Chem. Soc.*, **1966, B**, 605.

[269] C. Walling and M. F. Mayahi, *J. Am. Chem. Soc.*, 1959, **81**, 1485. This explanation may be incomplete, but one may question whether it should be discounted by reason of small differences in the parameters of Arrhenius equations for gas- and liquid-phase chlorinations observed by I. Galiba, J. M. Tedder, and J. C. Walton (*J. Chem. Soc.*, **1966, B**, 604). The Arrhenius equation is a crude instrument for the analysis of constitutional kinetic effects, and in the writer's opinion such small differences have no simple meaning.

In 1957, Russell[270] reported a more dramatic solvent effect, inasmuch as selectivity in liquid-phase chlorination could be greatly affected by the solvent. For example, in the photochemical reaction with pure 2,3-dimethylbutane at 25°, a tertiary hydrogen atom is 4.2 times as rapidly removed as a primary hydrogen atom. This tertiary/primary selectivity ratio rises to 20 for the dimethylbutane in 4*M* solution in benzene, to 35 in 4*M* solution in *t*-butylbenzene, and to 225 in 12*M* solution in carbon disulphide. The change in selectivity was attributed to complexing of the chlorine atoms by the solvent. The solvents that will form complexes include certain aromatic compounds, carbon disulphide, and N,N-dimethylformamide. Aliphatic hydrocarbons, nitrobenzene, olefins, and esters show no such indication of the formation of chlorine-atom complexes. Hydrogen abstraction from an alkane by a strongly complexed chlorine atom is an endothermic rather than an exothermic process, so that selectivities move towards or beyond those of a gaseous bromine atom. The increase in the selectivity of chlorination in aromatic solvents can be related to the basicity of the solvent as measured by the equilibrium constant for its interaction with hydrogen chloride at −78°C.[270] Russell proposed that the predominant factor in the solvent effect is the formation of a charge-transfer complex between the electronegative chlorine atom and the solvent. Walling[271] has suggested that factors such as the polarity and polarizability of the solvent may also be important in liquid-phase chlorinations.

Russell and his coworkers[272] have reported some significant results on the photochlorination of the more basic aromatic hydrocarbons. These reactants act as specific complexing reagents for chlorine atoms. The high selectivities observed in the absence of added solvents are destroyed by dilution with an inert non-complexing solvent. For example, at 40° a tertiary/primary selectivity ratio of 42 was obtained in cumene without a solvent, whilst the selectivity ratio dropped to 10 for 3*M* cumene in nitrobenzene, to 5 for 1.5*M* cumene in nitrobenzene, and to an estimated 3.5 at infinite dilution in that solvent.

Less profound solvent effects have been observed in hydrogen atom abstractions by radicals other than chlorine atoms, *e.g.*, alkoxy radicals[271,272,273] and peroxy radicals.[274,275] In these cases the solvent polarity

[270] G. A. Russell, *J. Am. Chem. Soc.*, 1957, **79**, 2977; 1958, **80**, 4987, 4997, 5002; *Tetrahedron*, 1960, **8**, 101.

[271] C. Walling and P. J. Wagner, *J. Am. Chem. Soc.*, 1964, **86**, 3368.

[272] G. A. Russell, A. Ito, and D. G. Hendry, *J. Am. Chem. Soc.*, 1963, **85**, 2976.

[273] G. A. Russell, *J. Org. Chem.*, 1959, **24**, 300.

[274] J. A. Howard and K. U. Ingold, *Can. J. Chem.*, 1964, **42**, 1250.

[275] D. G. Hendry and G. A. Russell, *J. Am. Chem. Soc.*, 1964, **86**, 2368.

and polarizability are certainly more important than its basicity in determining the magnitude of the solvent effect.

(37c) Halogenation by Other Reagents.—The preparative utility of the radical-chain halogenations described in the previous section is strongly limited. Apart from minor variations effected by changes in temperature or solvent, the nature of the products is predetermined by the halogen used in the reaction. This limitation has been largely overcome by the introduction of many special halogen carriers (S—X) which give products different from those obtained with halogen molecules, because the hydrogen atom is abstracted by a different radical (S· rather than X·). A few of the more important of the halogen carriers are listed in Table 37-6. The chain propagation can be represented by the scheme,

$$S{-}X + R\cdot \rightarrow R{-}X + S\cdot$$
$$S\cdot + RH \rightarrow SH + R\cdot$$

TABLE 37-6.—HALOGENATION BY SPECIAL REAGENTS.

Halogen carrier	Abstracting radical	Product
Sulphuryl chloride[252,276]	$SO_2Cl\cdot$ and $Cl\cdot$	Chloride
t-Butyl hypochlorite[277]	$(CH_3)_3CO\cdot$	Chloride
Carbon tetrachloride[252]	$CCl_3\cdot$	Chloride
Cl_2-Br_2 mixture[252]	$Cl\cdot$	Bromide
Trichlorobromomethane[278]	$CCl_3\cdot$	Bromide
N-Bromosuccinimide[x]	$Br\cdot$	Bromide

[x] See text.

Since the composition of the products is determined solely by the abstracting radical, the same isomer distribution of halides should be obtained with different halogens on the same chain carrier. Walling and Padwa[279] have shown that this is true for the halogenation of a number of hydrocarbons with *t*-butyl hypochlorite and *t*-butyl hypobromite. Identity of product composition has also been used to prove that bromine atoms rather than succinimidyl radicals are the reactive intermediates in brominations with N-bromosuccinimide (see Table 37-6).

Russell and Ito[276] have examined the products formed in the photochlorination of chloro*cyclo*pentane by a number of chlorinating agents.

[276] G. A. Russell and A. Ito, *J. Am. Chem. Soc.*, 1963, **85**, 2983.

[277] C. Walling and B. B. Jacknow, *J. Am. Chem. Soc.*, 1960, **82**, 6108, 6113.

[278] E. S. Huyser, *J. Am. Chem. Soc.*, 1960, **82**, 391, 394; *J. Org. Chem.*, 1961, **26**, 3261.

[279] C. Walling and A. Padwa, *J. Org. Chem.*, 1962, **27**, 2976.

Their results are given in Table 37-7. The relative reactivity at the β- and γ-position (*i.e.*, k_β/k_γ) gives a measure of the sensitivity of the attacking radical to the inductive effect of the α-chlorine atom. Since these reactivities are more or less similar for all the radicals, it seems reasonable to suppose that the more variable relative reactivity at the α-position (*i.e.*, k_α/k_γ) measures the sensitivity of the attacking radical to the strength of the carbon-hydrogen bond that is being broken. That is, the weakest carbon-hydrogen bond in the molecule is at the α-position, so that the extent of reaction at this position increases as the attacking species becomes less reactive. It follows that the sensitivity to bond dissociation energy is least for the "free" chlorine atom and greatest for the *t*-butoxy radical, the solvent-complexed chlorine atoms having intermediate positions.

TABLE 37-7.—RELATIVE RATES OF CHLORINATION OF CHLORO*cyclo*PENTANE AT THE α, β, AND γ POSITIONS (RUSSELL AND ITO).

Halogen carrier	k_β/k_γ	k_α/k_γ[a]
Cl_2 in CCl_4	0.50	0.29
Cl_2 in C_6H_6	0.43	0.36
SO_2Cl_2	0.54	0.42[b]
Cl_2 in CS_2	0.48	0.61
CCl_3SO_2Cl	0.58	1.1[b]
$(CH_3)_3COCl$	0.81	2.4

[a] Per hydrogen atom at 40°.
[b] 80°.

Special mention must be made of *N*-bromosuccinimide, since this very useful brominating agent functions in quite a different manner from the halogenating agents listed in Table 37-6. The reaction of N-bromosuccinimide with olefins in boiling carbon tetrachloride yields mainly allylic bromides, rather than the dibromide addition products which are commonly formed when bromine itself is the halogenating agent. The mechanism which was first proposed postulated a free-radical chain involving the succinimidyl radical as the chain carrier:[280,281]

$$S{-}Br \rightarrow S\cdot + Br\cdot$$

$$S\cdot + {-}CH_2{\cdot}CH{=}CH{-} \rightarrow SH + {-}\dot{C}H{\cdot}CH{=}CH{-}$$

$$SBr + {-}\dot{C}H{\cdot}CH{=}CH{-} \rightarrow S\cdot + {-}CHBr{\cdot}CH{=}CH{-}$$

$$\left\{ \dot{S} = \begin{array}{c} CH_2{-}CO \\ | \qquad \searrow \\ | \qquad\quad \dot{N} \\ | \qquad \nearrow \\ CH_2{-}CO \end{array} \right\}$$

[280] G. F. Bloomfield, *J. Chem. Soc.*, **1944**, 114.

[281] C. Walling, "Free Radicals in Solution," Wiley and Sons, New York, 1957, p. 381–386.

The radical-chain character of the reaction was well established by later studies.[282] However, work by Goldfinger[283] on allylic chlorination with N-chlorosuccinimide led him to suggest that halogen atoms rather than succinimidyl radicals were the chain carriers. He developed kinetic arguments to show that low halogen concentrations would favour substitution rather than addition. The function of the N-bromosuccinimide is to maintain a low, constant concentration of molecular bromine by a rapid heterolytic reaction with HBr:

$$\text{S—Br} + \text{HBr} \rightarrow \text{SH} + \text{Br}_2$$

The simple chain sequence

$$\text{Br}^{\cdot} + \text{—CH}_2\text{—CH=CH—} \rightarrow \text{HBr} + \text{—}\dot{\text{C}}\text{H}\cdot\text{CH=CH—}$$

$$\text{Br}_2 + \text{—}\dot{\text{C}}\text{H}\cdot\text{CH=CH—} \rightarrow \text{Br}^{\cdot} + \text{—CHBr}\cdot\text{CH=CH—}$$

will then occur with little interference from the homolytic process by which bromine adds to the double bond, because the first step of this addition is reversible:

$$\text{Br}^{\cdot} + \text{—CH}_2\text{—CH=CH—} \rightleftharpoons \text{—CH}_2\cdot\dot{\text{C}}\text{H}\cdot\text{CHBr—}$$

$$\text{Br}_2 + \text{—CH}_2\cdot\dot{\text{C}}\text{H}\cdot\text{CHBr} \rightarrow \text{Br}^{\cdot} + \text{—CH}_2\text{—CHBr}\cdot\text{CHBr—}$$

That is, the low bromine concentration maintained by the N-bromosuccinimide will favour hydrogen abstraction over addition. The Goldfinger mechanism has now received overwhelming support, both for allylic substitution[284,285] and for benzylic substitution.[264,265,285,286] There can be little doubt that the succinimidyl radical is not involved to any important extent in these brominations.

(37d) Autoxidation.—This is the name given to oxidation by molecular oxygen, in particular, by that contained in air. In 1832, the autoxidation of benzaldehyde was discovered by Liebig and Wohler.[287] In 1897, Jorissen noticed that an oxidising agent was transiently produced, and that, in the presence of excess acetic anhydride, twice the usual amount of oxygen was taken up.[288] The explanation, given

[282] J. Dauben jr. and L. L. McCoy, *J. Am. Chem. Soc.*, 1959, **81**, 4863, 5404; *J. Org. Chem.*, 1959, **24**, 1577.

[283] J. Adam, P. A. Gosselain, and P. Goldfinger, *Nature*, 1953, **171**, 704; *Bull. Soc. chim. Belges*, 1956, **65**, 533.

[284] F. L. J. Sixma and R. H. Riem, *Koninkl. Ned. Akad. Wetenschap. Proc.*, 1958, **61B**, 183.

[285] B. P. McGrath and J. M. Tedder, *Proc. Chem. Soc.*, **1961**, 80.

[286] G. A. Russell, C. De Boer, and K. M. Desmond, *J. Am. Chem. Soc.*, 1963, **85**, 365; G. A. Russell and K. M. Desmond, *ibid.*, 1963, **85**, 3139.

[287] F. Wohler and J. Liebig, *Ann.*, 1832, **3**, 253.

[288] W. R. Jorissen, *Z. physik. Chem.*, 1897, **22**, 34.

by Baeyer and Villiger in 1900,[289] was that the then unknown substance, perbenzoic acid, was first formed, and was subsequently reduced to benzoic acid by another molecule of benzaldehyde. They assumed that, in the presence of excess of acetic anhydride, the perbenzoic acid was converted to the stable substance perbenzoic acetic anhydride. In the absence of such a trapping agent, perbenzoic acid is the first isolable product of the autoxidation of benzaldehyde, though not until 1926 was it isolated by Jorissen and Van der Beek.[290] Then, the same workers, and also Bäckström, noticed that a transient oxidising agent more powerful even than perbenzoic acid, one that could oxidise anthracene and even carbon tetrachloride, preceded the perbenzoic acid. The characteristics of a radical-carried chain reaction were now becoming evident: the autoxidation could be promoted by light and by radical-forming chemical initiators, such as perbenzoic acid, and could be inhibited by "antioxidants," such as hydroquinone and other easily oxidised phenols and aromatic amines. From the quantum yield obtained on photo-initiation, Bäckström established the occurrence of kinetic chains of 10,000–15,000 cycles.[291] In 1934, Bäckström kinetically established chain propagation in the following steps (R = Ph), of which the second is rate-controlling:[292]

$$\dot{R}CO + O_2 = RCO{\cdot}O\dot{O}$$
$$RCO{\cdot}O\dot{O} + RCHO = RCO{\cdot}OOH + R\dot{C}O$$

The autoxidation of acetaldehyde (R = Me), which had been discovered in 1835 by Liebig and Wohler,[293] reached, after a similar history, the same stage of elucidation in 1930 in a kinetic investigation by Bowen and Tietz.[294] The absolute rate of the propagation steps, and of the termination process, for the autoxidation of benzaldehyde and for that of decanal (decanaldehyde), were determined in 1952 by Melville,[295] using the technique of intermittent photo-initiation, which he, and P. D. Bartlett, had simultaneously invented a few years earlier. Both the propagation steps are exothermic in all cases; however, the second

[289] A. v. Baeyer and V. Villiger, *Ber.*, 1900, **33**, 1575.

[290] W. R. Jorissen and P. A. A. Van der Beek, *Rec. trav. chim.*, 1926, **45**, 245; 1927, **46**, 43; 1930, **49**, 139.

[291] H. L. J. Bäckström, *J. Am. Chem. Soc.*, 1927, **49**, 1460; H. L. J. Bäckström and H. A. Beatty, *J. Phys. Chem.*, 1931, **35**, 2530.

[292] H. L. J. Bäckström, *Z. physik. Chem.*, 1934, **B**, **25**, 99.

[293] J. Liebig and F. Wohler, *Ann.*, 1835, **14**, 139.

[294] E. J. Bowen and E. L. Tietz, *J. Chem. Soc.*, **1930**, 234.

[295] H. R. Cooper and H. W. Melville, *J. Chem. Soc.*, **1951**, 1994; T. A. Ingles and H. W. Melville, *Proc. Roy. Soc.* (London), 1952, **A 218**, 175.

of those written above has an appreciable activation energy (5–8 kcal./mole).

The study of autoxidisable unsaturated and arylated hydrocarbons, unsaturated esters, and alkyl and aralkyl ethers has pursued a generally similar course. The first isolable products are generally what used to be called the "moloxides," which in course of time came to be recognised as hydroperoxides. Some can be isolated in good yield, but some only in low yield, and preferably at low conversions, because the hydroperoxides themselves decompose. In 1928, the hydroperoxide from *cyclo*hexene was isolated,[296] and in 1932 that from tetralin was obtained;[297] and during the next decade both these substances were proved, largely by Criegee, Hock, and Farmer, to be hydroperoxides with the functional group in an allyl or benzyl position:[296]

OOH OOH

During the 1940's and 1950's, many other hydroperoxides were isolated. That from cumene is easily formed; and it decomposes so cleanly under acid conditions to give phenol and acetone, that these reactions were developed as a manufacturing process:[298]

$$\mathrm{PhCHMe_2} \rightarrow \mathrm{PhCMe_2{\cdot}OOH} \xrightarrow{(\mathrm{H^+})} \mathrm{PhOH} + \mathrm{CMe_2{:}O}$$

The peroxides from ethyl linoleate have been carefully studied.[299] Hydrogen is most readily abstracted from the methylene group between the double bonds; but the hydroperoxides found consisted mainly of the conjugated isomers formulated below, evidently formed by rearrangement. These structures were proved by their reduction to ethyl 9- and 13-hydroxystearate:

[296] H. N. Stephens, *J. Am. Chem. Soc.*, 1928, **50,** 558; R. Criegee, *Ann.*, 1935, **522,** 75; R. Criegee, H. Pilz, and H. Flygare, *Ber.*, 1939, **72,** 1799; H. Hock and O. Schrader, *Naturwiss.*, 1936, **24,** 159; *Angew. Chem.*, 1936, **39,** 565; H. Hock and K. Ganieke, *Ber.*, 1938, **71,** 1430; 1939, **72,** 2516; E. H. Farmer and A. Sundralingham, *J. Chem. Soc.*, **1942,** 121.

[297] M. Hartmann and M. Seiberth, *Helv. Chim. Acta*, 1932, **15,** 1390; H. Hock and W. Susemihl, *Ber.*, 1933, **66,** 61.

[298] H. Hock and S. Lang, *Ber.*, 1944, **77,** 257.

[299] J. L. Bolland and H. P. Koch, *J. Chem. Soc.*, **1945,** 445; N. A. Khan, *J. Chem. Phys.*, 1953, **21,** 952; N. A. Khan, W. O. Lundberg, and R. T. Holman, *J. Am. Chem. Soc.*, 1954, **76,** 1779.

$$CH_3\cdot(CH_2)_2\cdot CH{:}CH\cdot CH_2\cdot CH{:}CH\cdot(CH_2)_7\cdot CO_2Et$$

$$\downarrow$$

$$CH_3\cdot(CH_2)_2\cdot\underset{}{\overset{OOH}{\overset{|}{C}H}}\cdot CH{:}CH\cdot CH{:}CH\cdot(CH_2)_7\cdot CO_2Et$$

$$+$$

$$CH_3\cdot(CH_2)_2\cdot CH{:}CH\cdot CH{:}CH\cdot\overset{OOH}{\overset{|}{C}H}\cdot(CH_2)_7\cdot CO_2Et$$

Saturated compounds are, on the whole, autoxidised with greater difficulty than unsaturated: they are attacked preferentially in their tertiary positions. Thus the peroxides

[decalin hydroperoxide: OOH at ring junction] and $(CH_3)_2\overset{OOH}{\overset{|}{C}}\cdot CH_2\cdot CH_2\cdot\overset{HOO}{\overset{|}{C}}(CH_3)_2$

have been obtained from decalin[300] and di-*iso*butyl,[301] respectively. As examples of autoxidation at secondary hydrogen, a monohydroperoxide has been obtained from *cyclo*hexane,[302] and *n*-decane has yielded a mixture of secondary hydroperoxides.[303] Ethers with α-hydrogen are autoxidised with great ease in their α-positions. A bishydroperoxide

$$(CH_3)_2\overset{OOH}{\overset{|}{C}}—O—\overset{OOH}{\overset{|}{C}}(CH_3)_2$$

has been obtained from di-*iso*propyl ether.[304]

Compounds which contain olefinic double bonds do not necessarily form a hydroperoxide as the sole, or even as the main, initial product: such substitution may give place to addition.[305] Mayo and his co-workers[306] have shown that olefins which polymerise or copolymerise

[300] R. Criegee, *Ber.*, 1944, **77**, 22; K. I. Ivanov and V. K. Savinova, *Compt. rend. Acad. Sci. U. R. S. S.*, 1945, **48**, 31.

[301] J. P. Wibaut and A. Strang, *Konink. Ned. Akad. Wetens. Proc.*, 1951, **B, 5**, 102.

[302] A. Farkas and E. Passaglia, *J. Am. Chem. Soc.*, 1950, **72**, 3333.

[303] K. I. Ivanov and V. K. Savinova, *Doklady Akad. Nauk, S.S.S.R.*, 1948, **59**, 493.

[304] A. Rieche and K. Koch, *Ber.*, 1942, **75**, 1016; K. I. Ivanov, V. K. Savinova, and E. G. Mikhailova, *J. Gen. Chem. U.S.S.R.*, 1946, **16**, 65, 1003.

[305] G. H. Twigg, *Spec. Suppl. Chem. Eng. Science*, 1954, **3**, 5.

[306] F. R. Mayo, *J. Am. Chem. Soc.*, 1958, **80**, 2465, 2497; *idem* and A. A. Miller, *ibid.*, 1956, **78**, 1017, 1023; 1958, **80**, 2480, 2493; *idem* and G. A. Russell, *ibid.*, p. 2560; D. E. van Sickle, F. R. Mayo, and R. M. Arluck, *ibid.*, 1965, **87**. 4824, 4832.

readily can give an almost exclusive yield of a 1:1 copolymer of the olefinic monomer and oxygen, *i.e.*, a polyperoxide:

$$R'OO\cdot + RCH{=}CH_2 \rightarrow R\dot{C}H{-}CH_2{-}OOR'$$

$$R\dot{C}H{-}CH_2{-}OOR' + O_2 \rightarrow RCH(O{\cdot}O\cdot){-}CH_2{-}OOR'$$

$$RCH(O{-}O\cdot){-}CH_2{-}OOR' + RCH{=}CH_2 \rightarrow RCH(O{-}O{-}CH_2{-}\dot{C}HR){-}CH_2{-}OOR'$$

and so on. High yields of polyperoxides with compositions approximating 1:1 copolymers have been obtained from several olefins, for example, styrene, methyl methacrylate, and vinyl acetate. Olefins can also react with peroxy radicals to form epoxides by the process[305,306,307]

$$-C{=}C- + ROO\cdot \rightarrow -\overset{O}{C{-}\;{-}C}- + RO\cdot$$

This reaction has been identified in the autoxidation of many simple olefins, for example, propylene, 2-butene, 2,4,4-trimethyl-1-pentene, *cyclo*hexene, and *cyclo*-octene.

Kinetic investigation of the autoxidation of, for example, *cyclo*hexene,[308] tetralin,[309] cumene,[310] ethyl linoleate,[311] and dibenzyl ether[312] has followed the same lines as for the autoxidation of aldehydes. It was first established that, whether the reaction was initiated thermally, or by light, or by chemical initiators, such as dibenzoyl peroxide or $\alpha\alpha'$-azobis*iso*butyronitrile, the chain contains the propagation steps here labelled p and q, of which the second, q, is rate-controlling:

$$(p) \qquad \dot{R} + O_2 \rightarrow RO\dot{O}$$

$$(q) \qquad RO\dot{O} + RH \rightarrow ROOH + \dot{R}$$

The principle underlying all these kinetic demonstrations is as follows. The general rate equation for such a chain reaction is some-

[307] W. F. Brill, *J. Am. Chem. Soc.*, 1963, **85**, 141; W. F. Brill and N. Indictor, *J. Org. Chem.*, 1964, **29**, 710.

[308] L. Bateman and G. Gee, *Proc. Roy. Soc.* (London), 1948, **A 195**, 376.

[309] C. H. Bamford and M. J. S. Dewar, *Proc. Roy. Soc.* (London), 1949, **A 198**, 252; A. E. Woodward and R. B. Mesrobian, *J. Am. Chem. Soc.*, 1953, **75**, 6189.

[310] H. W. Melville and S. Richards, *J. Chem. Soc.*, **1954**, 944.

[311] L. Bateman, *Quart. Revs. Chem. Soc.*, 1954, **8**, 147.

[312] L. Debiais, M. Niclause, and M. Letort, *Compt. rend.*, 1954, **239**, 539; *idem* and P. Horstmann, *ibid.*, p. 587.

what complicated, because three termination steps, labelled r, s, and t below, have to be taken into account:

$$\left.\begin{array}{ll} (r) & 2\dot{R} \rightarrow \\ (s) & RO\dot{O} + \dot{R} \rightarrow \\ (t) & 2RO\dot{O} \rightarrow \end{array}\right\} \text{Inactive products}$$

The rates of these termination processes depend, in order, on the zeroth, first, and second powers of the oxygen pressure; and so, by raising the oxygen pressure above a certain value which differs from case to case, but is commonly not above about 100 mm., the process t can be made sufficiently dominant to allow the other termination processes r and s to be neglected. When this happens, the rate of the whole chain reaction becomes independent of the oxygen pressure, and proportional to the first power of the concentration of the substrate. It also has a square-root dependence on the rate of initiation, R_i, which can be independently measured, for instance, from carbon dioxide production in initiation by means of dibenzoyl peroxide. Thus the rate equation, specialised to "high" oxygen pressures, is so simple and so characteristic that, if verified, it is diagnostic of the mechanism. Writing k_q and k_t for the second-order rate-constants of the kinetically important propagation and termination steps, labelled q and t, respectively, above, the rate equation becomes:

$$\text{Rate} = k_q[\text{RH}]\sqrt{\frac{R_i}{2k_t}}$$

By the use of lower oxygen pressures, the rates of the termination processes r and s may be compared with that of process t. For those few cases that have been examined, the three rate-constants are about of the same order of magnitude.

The methods described up to this point yield the rates of the steps on a relative basis; that is, one obtains only ratios of rate-constants. Absolute rate-constants may be determined by Bartlett and Melville's method of intermittent photo-initiation; and this has been done in a number of examples already mentioned[295,309,310,311] amongst others. The rate-constant of the first propagation step p may, for example, be about a million times greater than that of the rate-controlling step q. That is, it is within about one or two orders of magnitude of a diffusion-controlled rate-constant. The rate-constants of the three termination steps may equally be about a million times greater than the rate-constant of step q. For example, the second-order rate-constants for the oxidation of ethyl linoleate at 25° are

$$k_p = 1 \times 10^7,\quad k_q = 5,\quad k_r = 2 \times 10^7,\quad k_s = 5 \times 10^7,$$

and $k_t = 2 \times 10^7$ sec.$^{-1}$ mol.$^{-1}$ l.

A comprehensive study of constitutional effects on the absolute rate-constants k_q for hydrogen abstraction by peroxy radicals from hydrocarbons, and on the rate-constants k_t for self-destruction of peroxy radicals, has been made by Howard and Keith Ingold.[313] Rates of abstraction of hydrogen atoms increase generally along the series primary, secondary, tertiary hydrogen atoms. The rates also increase with the number of π electron systems, ethylenic or aromatic, which are bound to the carbon atom bearing the hydrogen atom, so making it an allylic or benzylic hydrogen atom. It also appears that a π electron system labilises a hydrogen atom more strongly when the whole allylic or benzylic system is part of a ring than when it is an open-chain structure. The rate-constants for self-destruction of two peroxy radicals increase generally in the order: tertiary peroxy radicals $<$ open-chain allylic secondary $\leqslant$ cyclic secondary $\leqslant$ open-chain benzylic secondary $<$ primary peroxy radicals $<$ hydroperoxy radicals.

We have so far been considering only the first phase of autoxidation, which is generally the formation of a hydroperoxide. There is commonly a second phase, which involves the decomposition of this substance. Autoxidations in general are autocatalytic, because the first-formed hydroperoxides decompose, and in so doing produce radicals which start new oxidation chains. That is, autoxidation is generally a branching chain reaction. The decomposition of the hydroperoxide to radicals can occur by both unimolecular and bimolecular processes:[314]

$$\mathrm{ROOH} \rightarrow \mathrm{R\dot{O}} + \mathrm{\dot{O}H}$$
$$\mathrm{ROOH} + \mathrm{HOOR} \rightarrow \mathrm{R\dot{O}_2} + \mathrm{H_2O} + \mathrm{R\dot{O}}$$

Decomposition to radicals is accelerated by those metallic ions of variable valency which can undergo one-electron transfer reactions.[314,315] The metal ion may act either as a reducing agent, as ferrous ion does, or as an oxidising agent, as ceric ion does:

$$\mathrm{Fe^{2+}} + \mathrm{ROOH} \rightarrow \mathrm{Fe^{3+}} + \mathrm{R\dot{O}} + \mathrm{OH^-}$$
$$\mathrm{Ce^{4+}} + \mathrm{ROOH} \rightarrow \mathrm{Ce^{3+}} + \mathrm{R\dot{O}_2} + \mathrm{H^+}$$

The ions of cobalt and manganese can act in both ways. That is, as cobaltous and manganous ions they reduce the hydroperoxide, and as cobaltic and manganic ions they oxidise it. These metallic ions are

[313] J. A. Howard and K. U. Ingold, *Can. J. Chem.*, 1967, **45**, 703.

[314] K. U. Ingold, *Chem. Revs.*, 1961, **61**, 563.

[315] C. Walling, "Free Radicals in Solution," Wiley and Sons, New York, 1957, p. 427.

therefore true catalysts for the decomposition of hydroperoxides. The radicals generated in this decomposition promote further oxidation with the consequent formation of more hydroperoxide, which, in turn, is decomposed by the metal ions. In this way, the ions of several transition metals function as autoxidation catalysts.

The rate of autoxidation of an organic substance can usually be very largely reduced by the addition of small concentrations of compounds known as *antioxidants*. Antioxidants fall into two main categories: (i) primary antioxidants, which destroy the chain-carrying radicals, and which are therefore often called *radical inhibitors*; and (ii) secondary antioxidants, which destroy the chain-branching hydroperoxides, and which may therefore be called *peroxide decomposers*.

Radical inhibitors are generally phenols or secondary aromatic amines, which contain a readily abstractable hydrogen atom, after loss of which they form, by mesomeric distribution of the radical centre, a stabilized, comparatively unreactive radical. That is, if AH represents the inhibitor, the primary step of inhibition for both phenols[316] and amines[317] can be represented by

$$R\dot{O}_2 + AH \rightarrow ROOH + \dot{A}$$

When this reaction competes successfully with the normal propagation reaction for peroxy radicals, the concentration of peroxy radicals will be reduced. The overall rate of oxidation will therefore decline, provided that the radical $\dot{A}$ is less able to continue the chain than the peroxy radical it has replaced. The rate of this primary step of inhibition is increased by the addition of electron-donating substituents to the aromatic ring of the inhibitor.[316,317] For a strong inhibitor, the radical $\dot{A}$ will be destroyed by reaction with another radical, for example, by colligation with itself or with a second peroxy radical:

$$\dot{A} + \dot{A} \rightarrow A_2$$
$$R\dot{O}_2 + \dot{A} \rightarrow ROOA$$

Products of these types have been identified in several phenol-peroxy radical reactions.[318,319] With a weaker inhibitor, the radical $\dot{A}$ may continue the oxidation chain by abstracting a hydrogen atom from the substrate[320] or its hydroperoxide:[321]

[316] J. A. Howard and K. U. Ingold, *Can. J. Chem.*, 1962, **40**, 1851; 1963, **41**, 1744, 2800; 1964, **42**, 1044.

[317] I. T. Brownlie and K. U. Ingold, *Can. J. Chem.*, 1966, **44**, 861.

[318] A. F. Bickel and E. C. Kooyman, *J. Chem. Soc.*, **1953**, 3211.

[319] E. C. Horswill and K. U. Ingold, *Can. J. Chem.*, 1966, **44**, 263, 269.

[320] L. R. Mahoney and F. C. Ferris, *J. Am. Chem. Soc.*, 1963, **85**, 2345.

[321] J. R. Thomas, *J. Am. Chem. Soc.*, 1963, **85**, 2166; 1964, **86**, 4807.

$$\dot{A} + RH \rightarrow AH + \dot{R}$$
$$\dot{A} + ROOH \rightarrow AH + ROO\cdot$$

Such weaker inhibitors, that is, those which enter into chain-transfer reactions of this type, are sometimes called *autoxidation retarders*. Their reactions lead to much more complex kinetic behaviour than is observed with the strong inhibitors.[320,321,322]

Peroxide decomposers are generally compounds which contain sulphur, selenium, or phosphorus, in forms which can be converted to a sulphoxide, selenoxide, or phosphine oxide. The conversion of hydroperoxides to non-radical products can be represented by the general equation,

$$ROOH + De \rightarrow ROH + DeO$$

For example, the reaction between saturated sulphides and certain hydroperoxides yields a sulphoxide:

$$ROOH + R'R''S \rightarrow ROH + R'R''SO$$

The simplest mechanism that has been proposed is based on the fact that the reaction is of second order in hydroperoxide in hydrocarbon solvents, but of first order in hydroperoxide in alcoholic solvents.[323] The reaction is therefore believed to involve a hydrogen-bonded hydroperoxide:

```
R—O———O + SR'R"                          R—O      O—SR'R"
  ⋮    |          In hydrocarbon            |
  H    H         ————————————————→          H      H
   \  ⋰          second order in                  /
    O—OR         hydroperoxide                 O—OR

R—O———O + SR'R"                          R—O      O—SR'R"
  ⋮    |            In AlkOH                |
  H    H         ————————————————→          H      H
   \  ⋰          first order in                   /
    O—Alk        hydroperoxide                 O—Alk
```

This idea produces a very plausible path for the clean abstraction of an oxygen atom from the middle of the formally linear hydroperoxide.

By using both a radical inhibitor and a peroxide decomposer the resistance to oxidation of organic substrates can frequently be improved to an extent greater than would be predicted on the basis of simple additivity. The two antioxidants are then said to show a *synergistic*

[322] J. A. Howard and K. U. Ingold, *Can. J. Chem.*, 1964, **42**, 2324; 1965, **43**, 2724.

[323] L. Bateman and K. Hargrave, *Proc. Roy. Soc.* (London), 1954, **A 224**, 389, 399.

effect towards one another. The radical inhibitor prevents the formation of long reaction chains, but it cannot completely suppress the formation of hydroperoxide. Destruction of this hydroperoxide by reaction with a peroxide decomposer prevents it from initiating new reaction chains by its normal cleavage to radicals. The two antioxidants thus act to complement and reinforce each other.

(37e) Nitration.—The nitration of alkanes and *cyclo*alkanes by dilute nitric acid at its boiling point or at higher temperatures (concentrated nitric acid effecting only oxidation under such conditions) has been known[324] since 1880. It was at one time thought, or at least hoped, that the nitration of alkanes and derivatives by dilute nitric acid at raised temperatures might be developed into a synthetic starting point comparably important with that of the nitration of aromatic compounds at lower temperatures by concentrated nitric acid or mixed acid. In fact the synthetic development of alkane nitration has been disappointing, although that process has a limited synthetic value.

The first systematic study of the products of such alkane nitrations was initiated in 1936 by Hass,[325] who used vapour flow at temperatures above, sometimes much above, 150°, and concluded that reaction occurred in the gas phase, because silica gel had no effect. The products consisted of a mixture of all the mono-nitro-compounds that could be formed by introducing a nitro-group in place of any hydrogen atom or any lower alkyl radical in the original alkane; and also of all the aldehydes and ketones that could result from oxygen uptake where hydrogen or a lower alkyl group had been removed, together with further oxidation products of such aldehydes or ketones. The ease of replacement of the different types of hydrogen was in the order, tertiary > secondary > primary, with some movement towards equality at raised temperatures. Carbon skeletal rearrangements were not observed: Hass was so impressed by this, that he made it the first of 13 "rules" in which he summarised his findings.

[324] F. Beilstein and A. Kurbatov, *Ber.*, 1880, **13**, 1818, 2028; cf. C. Ellis "The Chemistry of Petroleum Hydrocarbons," Chemical Catalog Co., New York, 1937, Vol. 2, p. 1087.

[325] H. B. Hass, E. B. Hodge, and B. M. Vanderbilt, *Ind. Eng. Chem.*, 1936, **28**, 339; H. B. Hass and J. A. Paterson, *ibid.*, 1938, **30**, 67; L. W. Seigle and H. B. Hass, *ibid.*, 1939, **31**, 648; H. H. Hibsham, E. H. Pierson, and H. B. Hass, *ibid.*, 1940, **32**, 427; H. B. Hass, J. Dorsky and E. B. Hodge, *ibid.*, 1941, **33**, 1138; H. B. Hass and E. F. Riley, *Chem. Revs.*, 1943, **32**, 376; H. B. Hass, *Ind. Eng. Chem.*, 1943, **35**, 1146; H. B. Hass and A. P. Howe, *ibid.*, 1946, **38**, 251; H. B. Hass and H. Shechter, *ibid.*, 1947, **39**, 817; H. B. Hass and L. G. Alexander, *ibid.*, 1949, **41**, 2266.

A specialised study of products was carried out in 1959 by Hughes and his coworkers,[326] in order to test the idea that alkyl radicals might be involved in the mechanism. It was shown that Hass's non-rearrangement rule is broken in the side-chain nitration of *t*-butylbenzene, which distinguishingly produces a rearranging radical, the "neophyl" radical, $PhCMe_2 \cdot CH_2^{\cdot}$ (cf. Section **37b**). Aqueous nitric acid (4–7%) nitrated *t*-butylbenzene in the vapour phase at 325–350° only in the side-chain, which it concurrently degraded, to form not only unrearranged oxidation products, such as acetophenone, but also rearranged products, such as benzaldehyde and ωω-dimethylstyrene:

$$PhCMe_3 \longrightarrow PhCMe_2\cdot\dot{C}H_2 \longrightarrow \dot{C}Me_2\cdot CH_2Ph$$

$$PhCMe_2\cdot\dot{C}H_2 \to PhCMe_2\cdot CH_2\cdot NO_2 \quad \text{and} \quad PhCO\cdot Me; \qquad \dot{C}Me_2\cdot CH_2Ph \to O{:}CHPh \quad \text{and} \quad CMe_2{:}CHPh$$

The use of dilute acid was necessary for the observation of rearrangement, and it was inferred that the water vapour acts mainly as an inert diluent, extending the life of the radical long enough to permit rearrangement.

A quantitative study of the production of nitromethane from methane and nitric acid at 280–490° in excess of nitrogen as diluent was described by Schay and Giber[327] also in 1959. They found that nitration and oxidation occurred in the ratio 35:65, which remained constant as the reaction progressed. Nitromethane does decompose relatively slowly at these temperatures, but they could measure this subsequent reaction, and allow for it. The oxidation products were formaldehyde, formic acid, and carbon dioxide.

The first of the theories of mechanism entertained by Hass[328] was that radicals, thermally produced from the nitric acid or from unstable oxidation products, abstract hydrogen from the alkane to give alkyl radicals, which engage in a chain reaction:

$$\dot{R} + HNO_3 \rightarrow RNO_2 + \dot{O}H$$
$$RH + \dot{O}H \rightarrow H_2O + \dot{R}$$

It was found that the known radical initiators, oxygen and chlorine, promoted the nitrations, and that the known radical inhibitor, nitric oxide, retarded them.

[326] H. C. Duffin, E. D. Hughes, and C. K. Ingold, *J. Chem. Soc.*, **1959**, 2734.

[327] G. Schay, J. Giber, J. Tamas, and D. Soos, *Magyar Kem. Folyoirat*, 1959, **65**, 311; J. Giber and T. Meisel, *Acta Chim. Akad. Sci. Hungary*, 1960, **22**, 455.

[328] R. F. McCleary and E. F. Dagering, *Ind. Eng. Chem.*, 1938, **30**, 64; H. B. Hass and J. A. Paterson, *ibid.*, p. 67.

At a later time Hass, and also Bachman,[329] supported the idea of non-chain radical mechanism,

$$HNO_3 \rightarrow HO + NO_2$$
$$RH + \dot{O}H \rightarrow \dot{R} + H_2O$$
$$\dot{R} + NO_2 \rightarrow RNO_2$$

though allowing that additional steps are possible. The suggestion was made that some part of the nitrogen dioxide which combines with the alkyl radical does so to form an alkyl nitrite, which, by decomposing in the known way to form a lower alkyl radical and a carbonyl compound, becomes responsible for a proportion of the oxidative degradation:

$$R'_3C{\cdot}ONO \rightarrow \dot{R}' + R'_2CO + NO$$

The kinetics of the gaseous nitration of methane diluted with nitrogen to a total pressure of 1 atmosphere and at 350° has been studied by Hughes and his colleagues.[330] Their data pointed to the following representation:

			ΔE (kcal./mole)
(*i*)	$HNO_3 \rightarrow HO + NO_2$		+40
(*p*)	$H\dot{O} + CH_4 \rightarrow H_2O + \dot{C}H_3$	chain	−16
(*q*)	$\dot{C}H_3 + HNO_3 \rightarrow CH_3NO_2 + \dot{O}H$	chain	−17
(*t*)	$\dot{C}H_3 + HNO_3 \rightarrow CH_3OH + NO_2$		−50

The second, (*q*), of the two chain steps is rate-controlling for chain propagation. The rate equation for this first-order chain reaction is

$$-\frac{d[HNO_3]}{dt} = -\frac{d[CH_4]}{dt} + k_i[HNO_3] = k_i\left\{2 + \frac{k_q}{k_t}\right\}[HNO_3]$$

where k_i is the first-order rate-constant, and k_q and k_t are the second-order rate-constants of the steps indicated in the chemical equations written above. The value of k_i was determined by separate experiments in which nitric acid was pyrolyzed in the absence of methane. The measured rates were found to give $k_q/k_t = 0.8$, which requires that $\frac{4}{9}$, or 44%, of the methane which reacts shall be converted into nitro-

[329] G. B. Bachman, H. B. Hass, L. M. Addison, J. V. Hewett, L. Kohn, and A. Millikan, *J. Org. Chem.*, 1952, **17**, 906, *et seq.* (5 papers); G. B. Bachman, N. T. Atwood, and M. Pollack, *ibid.*, 1954, **19**, 312; G. B. Bachman and N. W. Standish, *ibid.*, 1961, **26**, 570.

[330] T. S. Godfrey, E. D. Hughes, and C. K. Ingold, *J. Chem. Soc.*, **1965**, 1063.

methane, while 56% is being converted to oxidation products. Schay and Giber determined these proportions as 35% and 65%, respectively, but what we have been calling "nitromethane" in this discussion of the kinetic observations includes concurrently formed methyl nitrite, which, being unstable at the temperature, would appear as extra oxidation products. Thus the calculated 44% of so-called nitromethane could represent 35% of real nitromethane and 9% of methyl nitrite, consistently with the observed product composition.

The conclusion that the alkyl radical attacks the nitric acid molecule at its weak *interior* bond, and combines to comparable extents with either the nitroxyl or the hydroxyl moiety, is in line with Degani and Tundo's demonstration[260] that alkyl and aryl radicals attack the S—S bonds of disulphides and thiosulphonates, combining in each case with either moiety of these substrates. It is implied that this mode of attack of alkyl radicals on the nitric acid molecule is a main cause why the homolytic nitration of alkanes is always accompanied by their oxidation. This proposal is consistent with Hass's occasional recovery of alcohols in small amounts from gaseous nitrations of alkanes. Kinetically, the chain reaction, initiated by the dissociation step (*i*), is terminated by the oxidation step (*t*). The large degree of oxidation keeps the chains quite short. In the case illustrated, the chain length averages $1+k_q/k_t=1.8$ cycles.

CHAPTER VIII

Substitution at Hetero-elements

(38) ELECTROPHILIC SUBSTITUTION AT NITROGEN AND OXYGEN

(38a) N-Nitration.—Electrophilic substitution was first recognised and studied in the form of aromatic substitution, where the attack of the substituting agent is on the unsaturated electron shell of the substrate, that is, on conjugated carbon $2p$ electrons. Since the unshared $2p$ electrons of nitrogen and oxygen in aromatic amines and phenols can participate quite strongly in such conjugation, one may deduce that the $2p$ electrons of terligant nitrogen and biligant oxygen sufficiently resemble the unsaturated $2p$ electrons of carbon to share a general vulnerability to electrophilic substituting agents, subject to possible specific kinetic and thermodynamic restrictions. For a given substitution of this class, *e.g.*, nitration or nitrosation, we should expect the pattern of available mechanisms to be much the same for C-, N-, and O-substitution.

Nitration has proved to be one of the simpler forms of electrophilic aromatic substitution, because it is dominated by one outstanding mechanism, that of the nitronium ion. It is a mechanism of four steps (Section **23d**), rewritten below with the aromatic substrate expressed by RH instead of ArH, in order to allow for the generalisation that we shall now make to other classes of substrate:

$$\left.\begin{array}{ll} HNO_3 + HNO_3 \underset{-1}{\overset{+1}{\rightleftharpoons}} H_2NO_3^+ + NO_3^- & \text{(fast)} \\ H_2NO_3^+ \underset{-2}{\overset{+2}{\rightleftharpoons}} NO_2^+ + H_2O & \text{(slow)} \\ NO_2^+ + RH \underset{3}{\rightarrow} NO_2{\cdot}RH^+ & \text{(slow)} \\ NO_2{\cdot}RH^+ + NO_3^- \underset{4}{\rightarrow} NO_2{\cdot}R + HNO_3 & \text{(fast)} \end{array}\right\} \text{(Standard mechanism)}$$

The proof of mechanism is kinetic. The first step, which in its forward direction $+1$ is a proton uptake, and the last step 4, which is the compensating proton loss, are normally fast. The pre-equilibrium ± 1 can be verified, because one of the two nitric acid molecules acts only as an acid, and its function can be taken over by an added stronger acid, and therefore small additions of a very strong acid, such as sulphuric acid, accelerate nitration in a predictable way. And likewise, small additions of nitrate ions retard nitration in a predictable way. The middle steps ± 2 and 3 are in principle slow, and which will be rate-controlling depends on the balance of competition, for the nitronium ion formed in step $+2$, between two nucleophiles which can add it to themselves, *viz.*, water in step -2, and the substrate in step 3. By changing the concentration of the water, or the concentration or the intrinsic reactivity of the substrate, we can either make step 3 so much faster than step -2 that the formation of the nitronium ion in step $+2$ controls the rate of nitration, which is then of zeroth order in the substrate; or we can make step 3 so much slower than step -2, that the nitronium ion is formed in the pre-equilibrium now constituted by steps ± 2, and so the rate of nitration, controlled by step 3, becomes of first order in substrate. With suitably chosen aromatic substrates, the mechanism has been verified by this kinetic pattern for a number of solvents, ranging from polar solvents, such as nitromethane, containing only a little water. to highly aqueous nitrating media (Section **23**).

All these kinetic tests may be applied, and the pattern of results reproduced, for the N-nitration of amines to give nitroamines, provided that complications due to the basicity or other forms of reactivity of the amine substrates are avoided. This was first done by Blackall and Hughes[1] in 1952. It simplified correlation with aromatic nitrations to avoid pre-protonation of those unshared nitrogen electrons which are required to capture the nitronium ion. The nitration of methyl picramide (2,4,6-trinitro-N-methylaniline) to tetryl (N,2,4,6-tetranitro-N-methylaniline),

$$2,4,6\text{-}(NO_2)_3C_6H_2\text{—}N(H)Me \rightarrow 2,4,6\text{-}(NO_2)_3C_6H_2\text{—}N(NO_2)Me$$

is an N-nitration, in which no subsequent reaction can take place in the conditions, and the pre-existing nitro-groups so reduce basicity that no substantial amount of pre-protonation occurs in nitrating media not more highly acidic than $3M$-nitric acid in solvent nitromethane. Under such conditions, the whole of the described range of kinetic phenomena can be reproduced, so confirming that the mechanism is the same as for aromatic nitration.[1] The absolute zeroth-order rates are the same for the compound and for ethyl, *n*-propyl, and

[1] E. L. Blackall and E. D. Hughes, *Nature*, 1952, **170**, 972; E. D. Hughes, C. K. Ingold, and R. B. Pearson, *J. Chem. Soc.*, **1958**, 4357.

n-butyl picramide; and these rates are the same as for benzene, toluene, and ethylbenzene, etc., in the same conditions: all these rates are just the rate of formation of the nitronium ion in step +2 of the standard mechanism written above. The first-order specific rates depend on the rate of step 3, and are accordingly different for each substrate: for example, for methyl picramide, the specific first-order rate of N-nitration is 1.4 times greater than that of C-nitration for benzene.

With more basic amine substrates in the same nitration media, and also with the same substrates in more acidic media, two other phenomena appear. The first is automatic: pre-protonation of the amine becomes substantial, and limits the proportion of amine that is present in the free-basic form with which the nitronium ion reacts. The second, discussed by Halevi, Ron, and Speiser,[2] teaches the need to extend the standard mechanism of nitronium-ion nitration, when attempting to cover the case of N-nitration. The needed extension may be understood as follows.

Unlike aromatic nitro-compounds, nitroamines are acidolysed by strong acids: in other words, whilst aromatic C-nitration is irreversible, the N-nitration of amines has a substantial reversibility. In order to cover N-nitration, therefore, we have to allow for the reversibility of step 3 of the standard mechanism; and we may not take it to be deducible from analogy with aromatic nitration that the retrograde step −3 will always be slow in comparison with step 4, the final proton loss. The required generalisation may then be written as follows:

$$\left.\begin{array}{ll} HA + HNO_3 \underset{-1}{\overset{+1}{\rightleftharpoons}} H_2NO_3^+ + A^- & \text{(fast)} \\ H_2NO_3^+ \underset{-2}{\overset{+2}{\rightleftharpoons}} NO_2^+ + H_2O & \text{(slow)} \\ NO_2^+ + RH \underset{-3}{\overset{+3}{\rightleftharpoons}} NO_2\cdot RH^+ & \text{(slow)} \\ NO_2\cdot RH^+ + A^- \underset{4}{\rightarrow} NO_2\cdot R + HA & \text{(slow)} \end{array}\right\} \text{(Halevi's mechanism)}$$

Halevi and his coworkers were experimentally concerned with the nitration of methyl picramide ($RH = 2,4,6\text{-}(NO_2)_3C_6H_2\cdot NMeH$) by nitric acid, both in low concentration, but still with the latter in con-

[2] E. A. Halevi, A. Ron, and S. Speiser, *J. Chem. Soc.*, **1965**, 2560.

stant excess, in aqueous sulphuric acid of more than 50% concentration of the acid. They showed in this example that, as the acidity of the medium was raised, so to interfere with the acceptance of a proton by the medium from the nitro-ammonium adduct-ion $NO_2 \cdot RH^+ = 2,4,6\text{-}(NO_2)_3C_6H_2 \cdot NMe(NO_2)H^+$, rate-control moves on from step 3 (where step -3 is slow compared to step 4), to step 4 (when step 4 has become slow relatively to step -3). The conclusion was that any of the steps 2, 3, and 4 of the nitronium-ion mechanism could become rate-controlling, if account is to be taken of all classes of substrate.

Halevi, Ron, and Speiser established this conclusion by observation of the primary isotope effect, the method by which Melander had proved that, in aromatic C-nitration, step 4 is fast, so that rate-control can occur no later than in step 3 (Section **23d**). The method involves observing the kinetic effect of substituting deuterium for the particular hydrogen atom that is to be transferred in step 4: Halevi and his co-workers had to compare the first-order rates of nitration of 2,4,6-$(NO_2)_3C_6H_2 \cdot NHMe$ and 2,4,6-$(NO_2)_3C_6H_2 \cdot NDMe$ in their aqueous sulphuric acid media. And they were confronted with a difficulty, which was not before Melander in his work on aromatic C-nitrations, namely that, unlike C-hydrogen, N-hydrogen is rapidly exchanged with the hydrogen of the medium. Therefore it was necessary to make measurements on the amine $Ar \cdot NHMe$ in H_2SO_4/H_2O, and on the amine $Ar \cdot NDMe$ in D_2SO_4/D_2O; and then, the kinetic isotope effect of the medium, which would get included in the observed isotope effect, had to be eliminated from the rate comparison in order that this should relate only to the hydrogen transfer in step 4. The investigators therefore made their comparisons using H_2SO_4/H_2O and D_2SO_4/D_2O solutions, not of precisely equivalent composition, but of equal nitrating power, as calibrated by the rate of C-nitration of an aromatic reference compound, chosen, for various practical reasons, to be toluene-ω-sulphonic acid.

The results were as follows. In aqueous sulphuric acid of acid concentrations up to 50%, there was no hydrogen isotope effect, *i.e.*, the ratio of the first-order rate constants k_{1H}/k_{1D} was unity. This is the result which Melander obtained (except that he used tritium) for aromatic C-nitration (Section **23d**). As the acid concentration was raised towards 56%, the rate ratio measuring the isotope effect rose smoothly from 1.0 to 4.8. Above that acid concentration, the ratio remained 4.8. The latter ratio is raised above unity by the difference of zero-point energy between the initial and transition states of hydrogen transfer in step 4; and such a difference indicates a weakened binding of the hydrogen atom in the transition state. The ratio becomes upper-limiting when the acidity of the medium has reached such a value that step 4 has been made fully rate-controlling. The whole series of measurements therefore traces the shift of rate control from step 3 (when step 4 is much faster than step −3) to step 4 (when the increased acidity has reduced the rate of step 4 to much below that of step −3).

(38b) O-Nitration.—The first evidence that the esterification of an alcohol by nitric acid was in fact an O-nitration was given, in the example of the conversion of cellulose to cellulose nitrate ("nitrocellulose"), by Klein and Mentser in 1951.[3] They used oxygen-18, and showed thus that, for each group CH·OH converted, the replacement was of H by NO_2 with two oxygen atoms from the nitrating medium, not of OH by NO_3 with three oxygen atoms from that source. The proof of mechanism, establishing the nitronium-ion mechanism for alcohols generally, monohydric and polyhydric, including the other industrially important example, the conversion of glycerol to glycerol trinitrate ("nitroglycerine"), was first given by Hughes and Blackall in 1952.[4]

Their method was like that used for N-nitrations, as of methyl picramide, namely, to reproduce for O-nitration the whole pattern of kinetic phenomena, originally established for aromatic C-nitration. For sufficiently reactive alcohols, the changes of kinetic order from zeroth to first in substrate were demonstrated. They signify shifts of rate control between step 2 and step 3 of the standard mechanism of nitronium-ion nitration. This was done for the nitration, by $2M$-$4M$ nitric acid in nitromethane, of methyl alcohol, *p*-nitrobenzyl alcohol, ethylene glycol, trimethylene glycol, and glycerol, the last with respect to its α- and α'-hydroxyl groups only. For all these alcohols, the zeroth-order rate-constants reckoned per hydroxyl group converted (*e.g.*, counting one mole of ethylene glycol as 2 moles of convertible hydroxyl group) were identical with one another, and with the zeroth-order rate-constants for nitration of alkyl picramides, or of benzene or any of its homologues, under the same conditions. The first-order rate-constants were, of course, different for each alcohol: that for methyl alcohol was 30 times that of benzene (1.25 times that of toluene).

Some alcohols, like some aromatic substrates, are insufficiently reactive to capture all the formed nitronium ion, and so to exhibit

[3] R. Klein and M. Mentser, *J. Am. Chem. Soc.*, 1951, **71**, 5888.

[4] E. L. Blackall and E. D. Hughes, *Nature*, 1952, **170**, 972; E. L. Blackall, E. D. Hughes, C. K. Ingold, and R. B. Pearson, *J. Chem. Soc.*, 1958, 4366.

kinetics which are accurately of zeroth order in substrate, in the nitromethane nitrating media mentioned above. For example, *neo*pentyl alcohol is nitrated more slowly than any of the already mentioned alcohols, and with kinetics intermediate between zeroth and first order in substrate. Its first-order rate-constant in a somewhat aqueous solution of nitric acid in nitromethane is indirectly estimated to be of the order of 10^{-1} of that of benzene in like conditions. The behaviour of *neo*pentyl alcohol is thus comparable to that of chlorobenzene. Glycerol $\alpha\alpha'$-dinitrate is nitrated more slowly still under such conditions, and the kinetics are now of first order in substrate. It can be estimated that the first-order rate-constant is of the order of 10^{-2} of that of benzene. This behaviour might then be compared to that of *p*-dichlorobenzene or ethyl benzoate. When glycerol itself is taken as the substrate for nitration, a relatively fast zeroth-order nitration of the α- and α'-hydroxyl groups is succeeded by a slow first-order nitration of the β-hydroxyl group.

A basic example of O-nitration is the nitration of water, which can be made manifest by exchange of isotopically labelled oxygen (as shown by the underlinings in the equation below) between nitric acid and water:

$$HO{-}NO_2 + H{-}\underline{O}H \rightarrow HO{-}H + NO_2{-}\underline{O}H$$

In aqueous nitric acid, oxygen exchange takes place, with rates that rise strongly with increasing concentrations of acid, and have conveniently measurable values for compositions in or near 35–40 mole % of nitric acid. Bunton, Halevi, and Llewellyn demonstrated this by the use of an oxygen-18 label; and they measured the exchange rates over a range of compositions of aqueous nitric acid.[5]

The nitronium-ion mechanism, if hypothetically applied to the nitration of water, involves specialising steps 3 and 4 of the mechanism to $RH = H_2O$, so making them identical with steps -2 and -1, respectively:

$$NO_2{\cdot}OH + HNO_3 \xrightarrow[1]{} NO_2{\cdot}OH_2^+ + NO_3^-$$

$$NO_2{\cdot}OH_2^+ \xrightarrow[2]{} NO_2^+ + OH_2 \quad \text{(slow)}$$

$$NO_2^+ + OH_2 \xrightarrow[-2]{} NO{\cdot}OH_2^+$$

$$NO_2{\cdot}OH_2^+ + NO_3^- \xrightarrow[-1]{} NO_2{\cdot}OH + HNO_3$$

Here, the rate-controlling step can only be step 2, because nothing

[5] C. A. Bunton, E. A. Halevi, and D. R. Llewellyn, *J. Chem. Soc.*, 1952, 4913

competes with water for the formed nitronium ion. If, therefore, the observed oxygen exchange is indeed manifesting nitration of water by the nitronium-ion mechanism, the rate of exchange should be equal to the rate of formation of the nitronium ion in step 2; and this rate has been independently determined as the common zeroth-order rates of nitration of aromatic compounds which are reactive enough to be nitrated in zeroth-order form in the aqueous acids for which the oxygen-exchange rate has been determined.

Largely for the purpose of making such rate comparisons, Bunton, Halevi, and Stedman[6] determined the zeroth-order nitration rates of some side-chain-sulphonated polyalkylbenzenes, which are soluble in the media, and sufficiently reactive to exhibit zeroth-order nitration kinetics in the relevant range of aqueous-acid compositions. The aromatic substrates were the anions of mesitylene-α-sulphonic acid, *iso*durene-2α-sulphonic acid, and 2-mesitylethanesulphonic acid. To within the experimental uncertainties, the zeroth-order nitration rates of the three substrates were equal to one another, and also equal to the isotopically measured rates of oxygen-exchange in the media. The medium compositions (36.4–39.4 mole % HNO_3) corresponded to a threefold range of rates. These experiments leave no doubt but that oxygen exchange between nitric acid and water in aqueous nitric acid is an O-nitration in substrate water by the nitronium-ion mechanism.

(38c) N-Nitrosation, Diazotisation, and Deamination.—It will shorten subsequent description to state, in advance of the evidence, two general conclusions to which the kinetic study of these reactions has led.

The first conclusion contains the reason for treating together, as we shall, the three reactions named above. It is that all the reactions consist of, or start with, a rate-controlling N-nitrosation. With secondary amine substrates, the reaction ends there. With primary aromatic amines, succeeding fast ionisations lead to the diazonium ion, which is stable enough to be considered as the stable product. With primary aliphatic amines, this product is unstable, inasmuch as fast nitrogen loss leads to the carbonium ion, and thence to all the products it can form with the available reactants. This has become increasingly clear during the kinetic study of all three reactions. However, the study which has taken the lead, both in point of time and in disclosing the most detailed conclusions, has been that of diazotisation. In surveying the evidence, we shall therefore look to diazotisation to provide the continuous thread, and to the other reactions mainly in order to note certain similarities and differences.

[6] C. A. Bunton and E. A. Halevi, *J. Chem. Soc.*, **1952**, 4917; C. A. Bunton and G. Stedman, *J. Chem. Soc.*, **1958**, 4240.

The second general conclusion which it is convenient to state ahead of proof concerns a respect in which nitrosation presents a strong theoretical contrast to nitration. Nitration might conceivably have occurred through any theoretical nitronium carrier, NO_2X, where X^- is a base of any basicity from nothing (when it is absent) upwards; *e.g.*,

$$NO_2^+,\ NO_2{\cdot}OH_2^+,\ NO_2Br,\ NO_2{\cdot}NO_3,\ NO_2{\cdot}NO_2,\ NO_2{\cdot}OAc,\ NO_2{\cdot}OH$$

In fact, nitration occurs almost solely through NO_2^+, the main function of any other nitryl compound being to generate NO_2^+. Similarly nitrosation might theoretically occur through any nitrosonium carrier, NOX, *e.g.*,

NO^+, $NO{\cdot}OH_2^+$, NOBr, $NO{\cdot}NO_3$,[7] $NO{\cdot}NO_2$, $NO{\cdot}OAc$, $NO{\cdot}OH$

The contrasting fact is that nitrosation *does* occur through nearly all of these carriers, which, in many cases, are mutually interconvertible.

Experimentally, one achieves maximal simplification by excluding as many as one can of those anions which form covalent nitrosyl compounds, for instance, by operating with a dilute aqueous solution of nitrite made weakly acid with perchloric acid. Under these conditions, the possible nitrosonium carriers are reduced to the following four: NO^+, $NO{\cdot}OH_2^+$, $NO{\cdot}NO_2$, $NO{\cdot}OH$. We may set down the forms of kinetics which might arise in nitrosation by each of these carriers.[8] In the general case, one must take into account the possibilities (1) that the carrier considered is freely and immediately available, its attack on the amine being rate-controlling, and (2) that the carrier is formed from the supplied substances in a slow and rate-controlling manner, its reaction with the amine following immediately. But for some carriers there can be no question of slow formation. Two such carriers, in the simplified conditions mentioned, are molecular nitrous acid, which is supplied in quantity, and the nitrous acidium ion, which we assume to be formed from it in instantaneous pre-equilibrium. For these carriers, the expected kinetic forms are as shown in equations (1) and (2) below:

HNO_2, slow attack:

$$\text{Rate} \propto [\text{amine}][HNO_2] \qquad (1)$$

$H_2NO_2^+$, slow attack:

$$\text{Rate} \propto [\text{amine}][HNO_2][H^+] \qquad (2)$$

It should be made clear that, in these and similar formulae, the entries in the brackets are literal, and are not stoicheiometric totals. Thus

[7] W. G. Fateley, H. A. Bent, and B. Crawford, *J. Chem. Phys.*, 1959, **31**, 204; L. Parts and J. T. Miller jr., *ibid.*, 1965, **43**, 136.

[8] C. K. Ingold, "Substitution at Elements other than Carbon," Weizmann Science Press, Jerusalem, 1959, Chapter 2.

"amine" means free-basic amine, and "HNO_2" means undissociated molecules of the acid. Solvation is the only feature of composition which is nowhere expressed; and accordingly the hydrogen ion is represented by "H^+."

With dinitrogen trioxide as the carrier, the possibilities of slow attack and slow formation must both be taken into account. The former possibility assumes the pre-equilibrium,

$$2HNO_2 \rightleftharpoons N_2O_3 + H_2O$$

The latter takes the forward reaction to be rate-controlling, and assumes that all the atoms shown in the equation are contained in the transition state. The rate expressions then take the forms (3) and (4) below:

N_2O_3, slow attack:

$$\text{Rate} \propto [\text{amine}][HNO_2]^2 \qquad (3)$$

N_2O_3, slow supply:

$$\text{Rate} \propto [HNO_2]^2 \qquad (4)$$

Finally, with NO^+ itself as nitrosating agent, slow attack will depend on the pre-equilibrium,

$$HNO_2 + H^+ \rightleftharpoons NO^+ + H_2O$$

whereas slow supply might depend either on slow loss of water from pre-equilibrium nitrous acidium ion, or on slow loss of nitrite ion from pre-equilibrium dinitrogen trioxide:

$$NO \mid\!\!-\!\!-OH_2^+ \qquad NO \mid\!\!-\!\!-NO_2$$

The possible kinetic forms are therefore as shown at (5), (6), and (7), below:

NO^+, slow attack:

$$\text{Rate} \propto [\text{amine}][HNO_2][H^+] \qquad (5)$$

NO^+, slow supply via $H_2NO_2^+$:

$$\text{Rate} \propto [HNO_2][H^+] \qquad (6)$$

NO^+, slow supply via N_2O_3:

$$\text{Rate} \propto [HNO_2]^2 \qquad (7)$$

It will be noticed that some of the equations recur: (2) and (5) are the same, and so are (4) and (7).

The kinetics of diazotisation were first described in 1899 by Hantzsch and Schumann.[9] They worked in 0.002*N* HCl. They obtained rate

[9] A. Hantzsch and M. Schumann, *Ber.*, 1899, **32,** 1691.

curves of second-order form, and, without further trial, assumed this order to consist of first order in each reactant, as had been true of every second-order reaction discovered up to that time. They also thought of the amine as reacting through its salt, but this means nothing for kinetics at a constant acidity, and so we may translate their interpretation by means of equation (1). Their observations led them to the conclusion, for which they were criticised later, that different aromatic amines react at the same rate. In 1913–20 Tassilly[10] and in 1920 Boeseken and his collaborators[11] reinvestigated the matter, and again concluded in favour of second-order kinetics, with first-order in each reactant, as in equation (1). But Boeseken, who used slightly stronger acid than Hantzsch had done, about 0.01*N*, observed differences in the diazotisation rates of different amines, and was critical of the earlier suggestion of identical rates. However, in 1935, Reilly and Drumm, again using quite dilute acid, about 0.002*N*, recorded identical second-order diazotisation rates of three amines specially selected to have different expected reactivities in the amino-group,[12] a result which stimulated Boeseken to repeat his statement of disbelief.[13]

But by this date, a new type of result was emerging. In 1928, T. W. J. Taylor observed the third-order kinetics of equation (3) for the deamination of primary aliphatic amines;[14] and in 1929, he and Price obtained the same result for the N-nitrosation of secondary aliphatic amines.[15] In 1931 Abel found the same third-order kinetics for the reaction of ammonia itself with nitrous acid.[16] And in 1936, Schmid again found these kinetics for the diazotisation of aniline, but in stronger acid than had been used before, namely, about 0.2*N*.[17] Schmid wrote as though he were unaware of the second-order form of diazotisation, which had been consistently reported from 1899 to 1935; and subsequent writers, up to 1950, maintained this "conspiracy of silence": even Hammett, who first saw in 1940 that equation (3)

[10] E. Tassilly, *Compt. rend.*, 1913, **157**, 1148; 1914, **158**, 335, 489; *Bull. soc. chim.* (France), 1920, **27**, 19.

[11] J. Boeseken, N. F. Brandsma, H. A. J. Schoutissen, *Proc. Acad. Sci., Amsterdam*, 1920, **23**, 249.

[12] J. Reilly and P. J. Drumm, *J. Chem. Soc.*, **1935**, 871.

[13] J. Boeseken and H. A. J. Schoutissen, *Rec. trav. chim.*, 1935, **54**, 956.

[14] T. W. J. Taylor, *J. Chem. Soc.*, **1928**, 1099, 1897.

[15] T. W. J. Taylor and L. S. Price, *J. Chem. Soc.*, **1929**, 2052.

[16] E. Abel, H. Schmid, J. Schraftrank, *Zeit. phys. Chem.*, *Bodenstein Festschrift*, **1931**, 510.

[17] H. Schmid, *Z. Elektrochem.*, 1936, **42**, 579; H. Schmid and G. Muhr, *Ber.*, 1937, **70**, 421.

might mean nitrosation by dinitrogen trioxide,[18] did not mention that a discrepancy required to be explained. Some writers claimed, up to 1951, that equation (3) is experimentally in error, by its inclusion of an "unnecessary" molecule of nitrous acid;[19] but it is not in error.[20]

The discrepancy was resolved in 1950 when it was shown by Hughes, Ridd, and the writer, first, that the kinetic order of diazotisation does indeed drop from three to two as the acidity is reduced from the decinormal to the millinormal region; and second, that, whilst the third-order rate law had been correctly formulated, as at (3), the second-order law is in fact constituted, not from an order of one in each reactant, but from an order of zero in the amine and two in the nitrous acid, as at (4).[21] This observation of a kinetic transition, from zeroth to first order in substrate, with maintenance of second order in nitrous acid, completely proves that dinitrogen trioxide is the nitrosonium carrier. The argument is the same as that first employed to show that nitronium ion is its own "carrier" in aromatic nitration: the change of kinetic form follows a change of fortune of the substrate, as a competitor against water, for the carrier. In the present case, at millinormal acidities, the free-basic form of the amine is so plentifully present as to make the substrate the overwhelmingly successful competitor; and hence the rate of diazotisation is the rate, given by equation (4), of the purely inorganic processes that lead to dinitrogen trioxide. One sees why Hantzsch and others found that all aniline derivatives diazotise at the same rate. One also sees why Boeseken did not observe this: he had not pure second-order kinetics: for at his centinormal acidities, he must have been working in the region of the kinetic transition. At decinormal acidities, however, the free-basic form of the amine is so sparsely present that water becomes the overwhelmingly successful competitor, with the result that a pre-equilibrium "pool" of dinitrogen trioxide is maintained, off from which, slowly, the substrate takes its requirements, at a rate given by equation (3). The "pool" is often visible as a pale green colour (dinitrogen trioxide is deep blue and nitrite ion pale yellow) in diazotisations in

[18] L. P. Hammett, "Physical Organic Chemistry," McGraw-Hill, New York and London, 1940, p. 294.

[19] J. C. Earl and N. G. Hills, *J. Chem. Soc.*, **1939**, 1089; J. H. Dusenbury and R. E. Powell, *J. Am. Chem. Soc.*, 1951, **73**, 3266, 3269.

[20] A. T. Austin, E. D. Hughes, C. K. Ingold, and J. H. Ridd, *J. Am. Chem. Soc.*, 1952, **74**, 555; G. J. Ewing and N. Bauer, *J. Phys. Chem.*, 1958, **62**, 1449; L. F. Larkworthy, *J. Chem. Soc.*, **1959**, 3116.

[21] E. D. Hughes, C. K. Ingold, and J. H. Ridd, *Nature*, 1950, **166**, 642; *idem.*, *J. Chem. Soc.*, **1958**, 58, 65, 77, 88; E. D. Hughes and J. H. Ridd, *ibid.*, pp. 70, 82; L. F. Larkworthy, *ibid.*, 1959, 3116.

these conditions. In this kinetic form, different aniline derivatives do not diazotise at the same rate, as will be clear from Table 38-1. The evidence for N_2O_3 as the effective nitrosonium carrier in these conditions is thus complete.[22]

TABLE 38-1.—THIRD-ORDER RATE CONSTANTS [EQUATION (3)] (IN SEC.$^{-1}$ MOLE^{-2} L.^{2}) OF DEAMINATION, NITROSATION, AND DIAZOTISATION THROUGH PRE-EQUILIBRIUM DINITROGEN TRIOXIDE, IN DILUTE AQUEOUS ACID.

Amine	Temp.	$10^{-5}k_3$	Amine	Temp.	$10^{-5}k_3$
Deamination			*Diazotisation*		
NH_3	25°	0.04	$C_6H_5\cdot NH_2$	25°	27
$MeNH_2$	25°	4.8		0°	3.11
n-$PrNH_2$	25°	2.8	p-$MeO\cdot C_6H_4\cdot NH_2$	0°	3.56
N-*Nitrosation*			p-$Cl\cdot C_6H_4\cdot NH_2$	0°	0.92
Me_2NH	25°	4.0	p-Me_3N^+-$C_6H_4\cdot NH_2$	0°	0.14

The same kinetic transition has been observed by Kalatzis and Ridd for the N-nitrosation of N-methylaniline.[23] Once again, the transition from the kinetics of equation (4) to those of equation (3) is complete by the time that the acidity has been raised to $0.1N$.

Further study of diazotisation in dilute aqueous perchloric acid disclosed the action of another of the available carriers.[24] Its effect appeared as an extra rate, for which equations (3) and (4) could not account, when a reduced nitrous acid concentration strongly reduced the importance of rate terms dependent on its square. The new process was also favoured, relatively to such rate terms, by higher acidities (within the dilute range), and by the use of somewhat weakly basic amine substrates, such as o-chloroaniline and p-nitroaniline. This is a hydrogen-ion-catalysed reaction, and its kinetic form is that expressed in the third-order equation which occurs twice above, and is numbered (2) and (5). The reaction is therefore one of nitrosation either by the nitrous acidium ion $H_2NO_2^+$, or by the nitrosonium ion NO^+, formed in pre-equilibrium. The decision between these alternatives was achieved by setting up a competition between this simple acid catalysis, and joint catalysis by acid and by halide ion, to which we next turn.

It had been long known that chloride ion is a mild catalyst for

[22] J. H. Ridd, *Quart. Rev. Chem. Soc.*, 1961, 15, 418.

[23] E. Kalatzis and J. H. Ridd, *J. Chem. Soc.*, 1966, B, 529.

[24] E. D. Hughes, C. K. Ingold, and J. H. Ridd, *J. Chem. Soc.*, 1958, 77; L. F. Larkworthy, *ibid.*, 1959, 3304.

diazotisation, that bromide ion is a considerably stronger one, and that iodide ion is a stronger one still. Schmid showed (for chloride and bromide) that the halide ions added rate terms of the form of equation (8) below ($X^- = Cl^-, Br^-, I^-$).[25] Hammett suggested that this equation might be signifying a nitrosyl halide as the carrier.[18] Hughes and Ridd, starting from diazotisations running according to this equation, were able (for bromide and iodide) so to increase the trapping power of the substrate, relatively to water, by using somewhat weak bases in fairly high concentration, that the nitrosonium carrier became wholly trapped by the substrate.[26] The rate now became independent of the substrate concentration, and controlled only by those inorganic processes by which the carrier was produced: a kinetic transition had occurred, the fourth-order equation (8) giving place to a third-order equation (9). The form of this kinetic transition proves that the carrier is indeed the nitrosyl halide, NOX:

NOX, slow attack:

$$\text{Rate} \propto [\text{amine}][HNO_2][H^+][X^-] \quad (8)$$

NOX, slow supply:

$$\text{Rate} \propto [HNO_2][H^+][X^-] \quad (9)$$

The argument is the same as in the identification of the carrier dinitrogen trioxide, *i.e.*, nitrosyl nitrite. Equations (3) and (4) can be put in the same form as (8) and (9), respectively, X^- in the latter equations being specialised to NO_2^-.

An unequivocal interpretation of the ambiguous equation (2)/(5) could now be made.[27] Since a pre-formed ion NO^+ and a co-ordinating anion, say, Br^-, would combine instantly to form NOBr, diazotisation according to equation (9), which measures the rate of production of NOBr, provides an upper limit to the rate at which any NO^+ could possibly be formed. If diazotisation according to equation (2)/(5) did depend on pre-equilibrium NO^+, the rate by that equation could never exceed the rate by equation (9). It was found, however, that equation (2)/(5) and equation (9) provided rate terms quite independently of each other, and that either rate term could be arranged to exceed the other by suitable choices of concentrations. This showed that the nitrosonium ion was not involved in the determination either of equation (2)/(5) or of equation (9). The former, as observed, is therefore to be taken as equation (2), representing nitrosa-

[25] H. Schmid, *Z. Elektrochem.*, 1937, **43**, 626; H. Schmid and G. Muhr, *Ber.*, 1937, **70**, 421.

[26] E. D. Hughes and J. H. Ridd, *J. Chem. Soc.*, **1958**, 82.

[27] E. D. Hughes, C. K. Ingold, and J. H. Ridd, *J. Chem. Soc.*, **1958**, 88; cf. H. W. Lucien, *J. Am. Chem. Soc.*, 1958, **80**, 4458.

tion by the nitrous acidium ion. The latter represents formation of a nitrosyl halide by way of the nitrous acidium ion.

There is another way in which anions other than nitrite ion, "foreign" anions, as we might call them, can intervene in nitrosation: they may catalyse the formation of dinitrogen trioxide, which does the actual nitrosation. Anions of weak acids, buffer anions such as acetate or phthalate, can be most easily obsrved to act in this way. They may produce a nitrosyl compound, such as nitrosyl acetate, in a rate-controlling way, and then, whether this nitrosates the amine directly, or attacks nitrite ion to give dinitrogen trioxide, which then nitrosates the amine, provided that all such subsequent reactions are rapid, we shall observe kinetics in accordance with equation (9). But if the attack of the first-formed nitrosyl compound is on nitrite ion, and if also, when nitrite-ion concentrations are reduced, the nitrosyl compound attains pre-equilibrium, and its attack on nitrite ion becomes rate-controlling, the subsequent nitrosation by dinitrogen trioxide still being fast, a transition will be observed to a form of kinetics expressed by equation (10):

N_2O_3, slow supply via NOX:

$$\left.\begin{aligned}\text{Rate} &\propto [HNO_2][H^+][X^-][NO_2^-]\\ &\propto [HNO_2]^2[X^-]\end{aligned}\right\} \qquad (10)$$

The kinetic transition between equations (9) and (10) has been observed with X^- = acetate or phthalate.[28] Rate by equation (10) is that of the reaction of a nitrosyl acetate or phthalate with nitrite ion to form dinitrogen trioxide.

If we take proton transfers among acids in water as pre-equilibrium processes, equation (9) can only signify the bimolecular attack of the nucleophile X^- on pre-equilibrium nitrous acidium ion: nitrosation rate according to equation (9) measures an inorganic S_N2 process (9a):

$$X^- + NO\text{—}OH_2^+ \xrightarrow[S_N2]{} X\text{—}NO + OH_2 \qquad (9a)$$

Equation (4) constitutes a special case: it represents the self-dehydration (4a) of nitrous acid by bimolecular nucleophilic substitution of the conjugate base of the acid in the conjugate acid of the acid:

$$NO_2^- + NO\text{—}OH_2^+ \xrightarrow[S_N2]{} NO_2\text{—}NO + OH_2 \qquad (4a)$$

[28] E. D. Hughes and J. H. Ridd, *J. Chem. Soc.*, **1958,** 70; J. O. Edwards, J. R. Abbott, H. R. Ellison, and J. Nyberg, *J. Phys. Chem.*, **1959, 63,** 359; G. Stedman, *J. Chem. Soc.*, **1960,** 1702. Concerning the interpretation given by J. O. Edwards *et al.*, cf. J. H. Ridd, *Quart. Rev.*, 1961, 15, 425.

Another special case, studied by Stedman,[29] is the attack by azide ions, which leads to nitrosyl azide, a material which is known at low temperatures, but splits up to nitrogen and nitrous oxide instantaneously at room temperature:

$$N_3^- + NO\!-\!OH_2^+ \xrightarrow[S_N2]{} N_3\!-\!NO + OH_2 \rightarrow N_2 + N_2O + H_2O$$

Equation (2) for nitrosation by the nitrous acidium ion is another special case, in which the nucleophile is now the amine:

$$\begin{array}{l} RNH_2 + NO\!-\!OH_2^+ \xrightarrow[S_N2]{} RNH_2{\cdot}NO^+ + OH_2 \\ \qquad\qquad\qquad\qquad\qquad\quad \downarrow \\ \qquad\qquad\qquad\qquad\quad RNH{\cdot}NO + H^+ \end{array} \tag{2a}$$

Other special cases in which the nucleophile is a hydroxy-compound, which accordingly undergoes *O*-nitrosation, will be considered in the next section.

Equation (9) expresses the rate of conversion of a first-formed nitrosating agent, nitrous acidium ion, into a second nitrosating agent, *e.g.*, a nitrosyl halide or carboxylate. Equation (10) expresses the rate of conversion of such a second nitrosating agent into a third:

$$NO_2^- + NO\!-\!X \xrightarrow[S_N2]{} NO_2\!-\!NO + X^- \tag{10a}$$

Nitrosations by all such indirectly produced nitrosating agents, as represented in equations (8) and (3), are likewise inorganic S_N2 processes, as here written in the form (8a):

$$\begin{array}{l} RNH_2 + NO\!-\!X \xrightarrow[S_N2]{} R\overset{+}{N}H_2{\cdot}NO + X^- \\ \qquad\qquad\qquad\qquad\qquad\quad \downarrow \\ \qquad\qquad\qquad\qquad\quad RNH{\cdot}NO + H^+ \end{array} \tag{8a}$$

Such conversions by bimolecular nucleophilic substitutions appear to be a common property of nitrosyl compounds. We can summarise the whole of the kinetic evidence relating to diazotisation, or other N-nitrosations, in dilute aqueous acid, in the network shown in Fig. 38-1 of S_N2 interconversions of nitrosonium carriers, any of which can nitrosate the substrate.[8,21] Each link in this network, including each nitrosating attack on the substrate, has separately been made rate-controlling, and has been studied kinetically; and the numbers entered against the links in the network are the numbers given above to the equations which express the kinetics as each link controls the measured rate. The first step of all is, of course, the instantaneous proton uptake by nitrous acid to form pre-equilibrium nitrous acidium ion. In

[29] G. Stedman, *J. Chem. Soc.*, **1959,** 2943.

this ion, a water molecule occupies the place that has to become occupied by an amine molecule in order to secure a nitrosation. The replacement of water by amine may be direct. But a faster route may be provided by replacing the water by nitrite ion, and then replacing that by the amine. Again, some "foreign" anion, X^-, if present, might displace the water faster than nitrite ions can; and then it will itself subsequently have to be displaced by the amine, or perhaps by nitrite ion, which still later will become displaced by the amine.

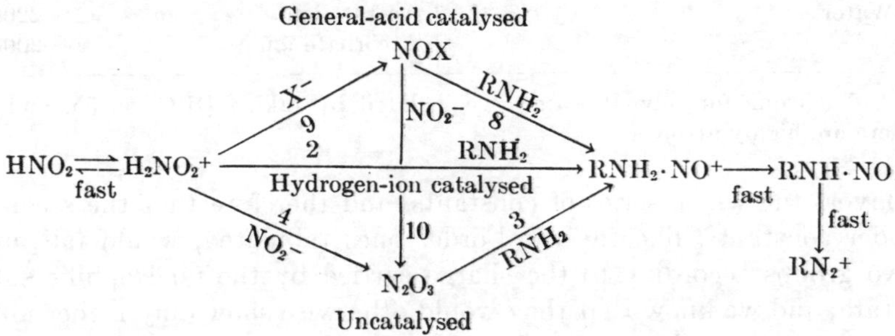

FIG. 38-1.—Nitrosation through a network of S_N2-type inorganic interconversions.

Ridd has rationalised[22] the empirically discovered fact that, although the nitrous-acidium-ion mechanism of nitrosation is the most direct, it is very easily displaced by the dinitrogen trioxide mechanism, in the absence of a "foreign" catalytic ion, or by a general acid-catalysed mechanism in the presence of such an ion. He has also rationalised the other empirically discovered fact that the nitrous-acidium-ion mechanism is most easily observed with aniline derivatives, such as *o*-chloro- or *p*-nitro-aniline, which have been weakened as bases and presumably as nucleophiles generally by electronegative substituents. Table 38-2 shows the third-order rate-constants, observed by himself and others, of reactions rate-controlled by N-nitrosation, O-nitrosation, and other forms of nitrosation, of a number of neutral and anionic nucleophiles (Nuc), according to the equation,

$$\text{Rate} = k_3[\text{Nuc}][\text{HNO}_2][\text{H}^+] \tag{2}$$

Now we do not know the basic strength of HNO_2, and therefore cannot convert these third-order constants into the second-order constants of the equation (2′),

$$\text{Rate} = k_2[\text{Nuc}][\text{H}_2\text{NO}_2^+] \tag{2′}$$

which represents the rate-controlling S_N2-type process. But we do know that multiplication by a single equilibrium constant would so

TABLE 38-2.—THIRD-ORDER RATE-CONSTANTS [EQUATION (2)] IN SEC.$^{-1}$ MOLE^{-2} L.^{2} OF REACTIONS RATE-CONTROLLED BY NITROSATION BY NITROUS ACIDIUM ION IN DILUTE AQUEOUS ACID AT 0° (RIDD).[22]

N-*Nitrosation*	k_3	*Nitrosation of Anions*	k_3
o-Chloroaniline	175	Nitrite ion	1893
o-Nitroaniline	145	Thiocyanate ion	1440
p-Nitroaniline	161	Azide ion	2340
2,4-Dinitroaniline	3.7	Chloride ion	975
O-*Nitrosation*		Bromide ion	1170
Ascorbic acid	63	Iodide ion	1370
Water	~4*	Acetate ion	2200
		Ascorbate ion	~2000

* The value for solvent water is calculated by taking [H_2O] as 55, and is therefore highly artificial.

convert the whole series of constants, and therefore that the second-order constants, like the third-order ones tabulated, would fall into two groups according to the charge carried by the nucleophilic substrate; and we know that they would otherwise show only rather mild constitutional influences. This suggests that the bimolecular rates are approaching that of a reaction that takes place whenever the reactants meet, and so have no activation energy beyond the 4–5 kcal./mole needed to part the solvent before the advancing reactant particles. The main constitutional effect would then be that of an anionic charge in increasing the cross section for the collisions with the cationic reagent, and hence increasing the encounter rate. Thus, in the network written above, the absolute rates of the reactions marked 4 and 9 will often be high, relative to those of the reaction marked 2.

It is possible approximately to translate the third-order rate-constants of the equation,

$$\text{Rate} = k_3[\text{Nuc}][\text{HNO}_3]^2 \tag{3}$$

as listed in Table 38-1, into second-order constants of the rate-controlling S_N2-type substitution, according to equation (3′):

$$\text{Rate} = k_2[\text{Nuc}][\text{N}_2\text{O}_3] \tag{3'}$$

The equilibrium constant $[N_2O_3]/[HNO_3]^2$ is approximately known. For the nitrosation of aniline by dinitrogen trioxide in water at 20°, k_2 has the value 0.9×10^7 sec.$^{-1}$ mole^{-1} l. This is smaller by several orders of magnitude than the rate-constant of a reaction that goes on encounter. So nitrosation by N_2O_3 must be a reaction which has a moderate activation energy, one that could be changed, as the nucleophilic power of the substrate will be changed, by polar substituents. Therefore, although the examples in Tables 38-1 and 38-2 overlap too little to allow of a direct check, it is inferred by Ridd that the reaction whose rate-equation is (3′) will be more sensitive to polar influences than is the reaction whose rate equation is (2′). So it can be understood why the latter reaction attains relative prominence when the former becomes the more strongly retarded by electronegative substituents, such as a nitro-group.

The general-acid-catalysed nitrosations which are dependent on pre-equilibrium nitrosyl halides must be rather closely similar to reactions that go on encounter. Schmid has converted[30] the fourth-order constants of hydrogen-chloride catalysed diazotisations, proceeding in accordance with equation (8),

$$\text{Rate} = k^4[\text{Nuc}][\text{HNO}_2][\text{H}^+][\text{Cl}^+] \qquad (8)$$

into second-order constants of the rate-controlling S_N2-step, whose equation is (8′),

$$\text{Rate} = k_2[\text{Nuc}][\text{NOCl}] \qquad (8')$$

by means of the known equilibrium constant $[\text{NOCl}]/[\text{HNO}_2][\text{H}^+][\text{Cl}^-]$. The rate constants in Table 38-3 are about one or two orders of magnitude smaller than rate-constants for bimolecular encounter.

TABLE 38-3.—SECOND-ORDER RATE-CONSTANTS [EQUATION (8a)] (IN SEC.$^{-1}$ MOLE^{-1} L.) OF DIAZOTISATIONS RATE-CONTROLLED BY NITROSATION BY NITROSYL CHLORIDE IN DILUTE AQUEOUS ACID AT 25° (SCHMID).[30]

Amine	k_2	Amine	k_2
Aniline	2.60×10^9	*o*-Chloroaniline	1.16×10^9
o-Toluidine	2.44×10^9	*m*-Chloroaniline	1.63×10^9
m-Toluidine	2.70×10^9	*p*-Chloroaniline	1.89×10^9
p-Toluidine	3.0×10^9		

In passing, let us notice the contrast between the picture, presented in Fig. 38-1, of nitrosation through many carriers, all interconvertible through inorganic S_N2-like substitutions, and the picture, schematised in Fig. 38-2, of nitration, where every possible carrier first undergoes heterolysis in an S_N1-like manner, to form a common effective carrier, the nitronium ion. It is evident that nitrosyl compounds, as a class, are less easily heterolysed to nitrosonium ion than nitryl compounds, as a class, are to nitronium ion. Lidstone has pointed out[31] that a

[30] H. Schmid and E. Hallaba, *Monatsh.*, 1956, **87**, 56; H. Schmid and M. G. Fouad, *ibid.*, 1957, **88**, 631; H. Schmid and C. Essler, *ibid.*, p. 1110.

[31] A. G. Lidstone, *Chem. and Ind.*, 1959, 1316.

similar difference appears between the ease of dehydration of formic acid and carbonic acid, with which the dehydration of nitrous acidium ion and nitric acidium ion are respectively isoelectronic, if we allow that the thermodynamically stable isomer of the former would be protonated on nitrogen, so that an endothermic proton shift $O:NH(OH)^+ \rightarrow O:N\cdot OH_2^+$ would be a necessary preliminary to, and its heat would become added to the activation energy of, the dehydration.

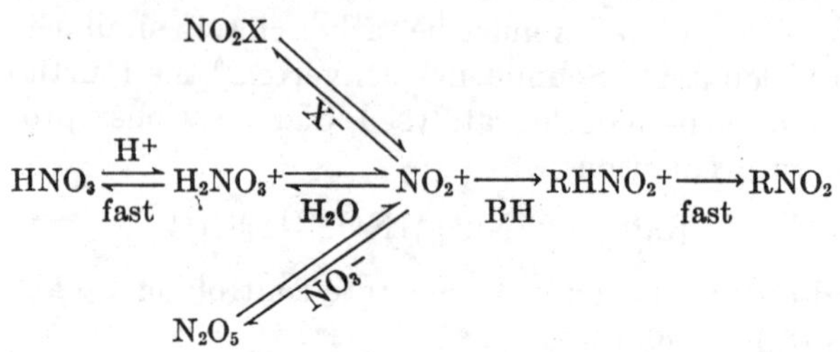

FIG. 38.-2.—Nitration by prior S_N1-type heterolysis of potential carriers to the nitronium ion.

All the above-described mechanisms of diazotisation or nitrosation apply to dilute aqueous acidic media. By extending these studies to more strongly acidic media, Ridd and his coworkers have uncovered two more mechanisms of N-nitrosation, in both of which the substrate is not the amine, but is the ammonium ion.

The previously described mechanisms of diazotisation may apply to any derivative of aniline at acidities below $0.5N$. But for weakly nucleophilic anilines, such as the nitro-anilines, the nitrous-acidium-ion mechanism of equation (2) remains in control up to $3N$ acid.[32] However, in diazotisations of more strongly nucleophilic anilines, such as aniline itself, and the toluidines, and in the N-nitrosation of N-methylaniline, a new mechanism takes control at acidities between $0.5N$ and $3N$ acid. With anilines of intermediate nucleophilic strength, such as the chloro-anilines, the new mechanism overlaps with the mechanism of equation (2) in this range of acidities. Due allowance being made for salt effects, the kinetic equation of the new mechanism[32] is

$$\text{Rate} \propto [ArNH_3^+][HNO_2]h_0 \qquad (11)$$

This equation is so written, because it applies to regions of acidity in which $[H^+]$, h_0, and j_0 differ. The product $[HNO_2]h_0$ is proportional to $[H_2NO_2^+]$, and signifies participation of the nitrous acidium ion,

[32] B. C. Challis and J. H. Ridd, *Proc. Chem. Soc.*, 1961, 173; *J. Chem. Soc.*, **1962,** 5197; *idem* and L. F. Larkworthy, *ibid.*, p. 5203.

formed in pre-equilibrium. (If the nitrosating agent had been NO^+, the corresponding product would have been $[HNO_2]j_0$.)[33] At the acidities in question, and with the amines to which equation (11) applies, the absolute rates are much too great, much too far above the relevant encounter rate, to allow it to be contemplated that nitrosation occurs through the free amine. Thus, equation (11) may be rewritten as (11′):

$$\text{Rate} \propto [ArNH_3^+][H_2NO_2^+] \qquad (11')$$

One's first thought is that this mechanism is rate-controlled by a one-step S_E2 nitrosation, by nitrous acidium ion, with expulsion of a proton, at the anilinium nitrogen atom; but a study of the effects of ring substituents in the aniline[34] has made it much more probable that the attack of the reagent is on the adjacent π-electron system, and that the substitution is completed by a rearrangement, as in Illuminati's mechanism (Section **36g**) for the side-chain chlorination and bromination of hexamethylbenzene and other polyalkyl benzenes by bromine in acetic acid. The following relative rates of diazotisation of some substituted anilines in 3*N* aqueous perchloric acid will bring out this point:

H	*p*-Me	*m*-Me	*p*-Cl	*m*-Cl	*p*-OMe	*m*-OMe
1	7.4	6.8	0.20	0.41	9.5	18.6

One sees that the strongest activation is by *m*-methoxyl, and that, in general, *m*-substituents have kinetic effects comparable with those of *p*-substituents. The suggestion is that the nitrosonium ion, conveyed by the nitrous acidium ion, adds at α- or ortho-carbon to give a nitroso-ammonio-*cyclo*hexadienylium ion, which, by a rearrangement the details of which are at present unsettled, transfers its nitroso-group to the ammonio-side-chain, with displacement therefrom of a proton:

$$Ar\cdot\overset{+}{NH_3} + NO\cdot\overset{+}{OH_2} \xrightarrow[\text{slow}]{} \overset{+}{Ar}\begin{smallmatrix}\diagup NO \\ \diagdown \overset{+}{N}H_3\end{smallmatrix} \rightarrow Ar\cdot\overset{+}{N}H_2\cdot NO + \overset{+}{H} \qquad (11a)$$

$$\downarrow$$

$$ArN_2^+ \leftarrow Ar\cdot NH\cdot NO + H^+$$

The second mechanism of the anilinium-ion substrate, also dis-

[33] N. C. Deno, H. E. Berkheimer, W. L. Evans, and J. H. Peterson, *J. Am. Chem. Soc.*, 1959, **81**, 2344.

[34] E. C. R. de Fabrizio, E. Kalatzis, and J. H. Ridd, *J. Chem. Soc.*, 1966, **B**, 533.

covered by Challis and Ridd,[35] was found at acidities of around 60% aqueous perchloric acid or 70% aqueous sulphuric acid. It has the special feature of rate-control by proton transfer from the nitrosated substrate to the reluctantly proton-accepting medium, much as in Halevi's N-nitrations at high acidities (Section **38a**).

The observations on nitrosation at these acidities are as follows. At any one acidity, the rates of diazotisation of aniline, *p*-toluidine, and *p*-nitroaniline are proportional to [stoicheiometric amine] [stoicheiometric nitrous acid]. At the acidities considered, the first factor represents completely formed $ArNH_3^+$, which must be the substrate, because the absolute rates are far too great to allow a free-basic substrate to be contemplated. Also at these acidities, the stoicheiometric nitrous acid is present essentially as nitrosonium ion;[36] and, as this not only is the most plentiful, but also should be specifically the most active nitrosating agent, it is practically certain that the second factor above, equivalent to $[NO^+]$, represents attack by NO^+ on the anilinium ion. When the acidity is raised, the rates of diazotisation fall, in approximate accord with the inverse second power of h_0, so that we may write the rate equation as at (12):

$$\text{Rate} \propto [ArNH_3^+][NO^+]h_0^{-2} \tag{12}$$

This suggests that two protons, corresponding to the two shown as being lost in mechanism (11a) above, are either both lost in pre-equilibria of strongly reversible processes, or, alternatively, the first of them is lost thus, whilst the second is lost in the rate-controlling step of the reaction, the more slowly at higher acidities because of the increasing reluctance of the medium to accept a proton. Challis and Ridd decided in favour of the second alternative, because they observed a tenfold rate reduction in solvents D_2SO_4/D_2O as compared with solvents H_2SO_4/H_2O. This large hydrogen-isotope effect clearly establishes the presence of a slow proton transfer, and the mechanism is therefore believed to be as follows:

$$\begin{array}{ccc} ArNH_3^+ + NO^+ & \underset{\text{fast}}{\rightleftharpoons} & ArNH_2 \cdot NO^+ + H^+ \\ & & \Big\downarrow \text{slow} \\ ArN_2^+ & \longleftarrow & ArNH \cdot NO + H^+ \end{array} \tag{12a}$$

The first step of equation (12a) may have to be developed in more detail, though the evidence is not yet forthcoming, somewhat in the

[35] B. C. Challis and J. H. Ridd, *Proc. Chem. Soc.*, **1960**, 245.

[36] N. S. Bayliss and D. W. Watts, *Austral. J. Chem.*, 1956, **9**, 319; K. Singer and P. A. Vamplew, *J. Chem. Soc.*, **1956**, 3971. Electronic spectrum of NO^+: B. Miescher, *Canad. J. Res.*, 1955, **33**, 355.

manner of mechanism (11a), to include an initial formation of a nitroso-*cyclo*hexadienylium ion, and a subsequent migration of the nitroso-group to the side-chain. It is probable that such a step of addition, which would be identical with the first step of an aromatic C-nitrosation, would be easily reversible.[37]

As to the fast reactions which succeed formation of the nitroso-derivatives of primary amines, our only evidence is from the nature, including the stereochemistry, of the isolable products. In the aromatic series, the diazonium ion is stable enough to be considered the end-product. As will be noted in Chapter XI, Hantzsch isolated aromatic primary nitrosoamines, and also diazo-hydroxides. Mainly as a result of his work, it is generally considered that conversions of nitrosoamines, through diazo-hydroxides, into diazonium ions, are rapid processes in acidic aqueous solvents, and that they occur by way of a prototropic isomerisation, through ions, followed by a pseudo-basic ionisation:

$$\mathrm{ArNH\cdot NO} \underset{\mathrm{H^+}}{\overset{-\mathrm{H^+}}{\rightleftharpoons}} \mathrm{Ar\bar{N}{-}N{=}O^-} \underset{-\mathrm{H^+}}{\overset{\mathrm{H^+}}{\rightleftharpoons}}$$

$$\mathrm{ArN{=}N{-}OH} \xrightarrow{\mathrm{H^+}} \mathrm{Ar\overset{+}{N}{\equiv}N} + \mathrm{H_2O}$$

In the aliphatic series, the diazonium ion is unstable. In aprotic solvents, it may not be formed, the end-product being the anhydro-base of the pseudo-base (Chapter XI), *viz.*, the diazo-alkane. Methyl nitrosoamine has been obtained in solvent ether at low temperatures, and has been shown to undergo conversion to diazomethane:[38]

$$\mathrm{CH_3\cdot NH\cdot NO} \rightarrow \mathrm{CH_3\cdot N{:}N\cdot OH} \rightarrow \mathrm{CH_2{:}N{:}N} + \mathrm{H_2O}$$

However, the final products of deamination of primary aliphatic amines in hydroxylic solvents cannot be formed by way of such a diazo-alkane, because Streitwieser and Schaeffer have shown that such reactions proceed without isotopic exchange between α-hydrogen and solvent hydrogen.[39] It was proposed by Baker, Cooper, and the writer in 1928,[40] and by Whitmore in 1932,[41] that deamination in the usual protic conditions proceeds by way of the diazonium ion and the carbonium ion:

$$\mathrm{RNH\cdot NO} \rightarrow \mathrm{RN{:}NOH} \rightarrow \mathrm{RN_2^+} \rightarrow \mathrm{R^+} \rightarrow \text{Products}$$

37 J. H. Ridd and E. A. Qureshi, *J. Chem. Soc.*, forthcoming.
38 E. Müller, H. Haiss, and W. Rundel, *Chem. Ber.*, 1960, **93**, 1541.
39 A. Streitwieser and W. D. Schaeffer, *J. Am. Chem. Soc.*, 1957, **79**, 2888.
40 J. W. Baker, K. E. Cooper, and C. K. Ingold, *J. Chem. Soc.*, **1928**, 426.
41 F. C. Whitmore, *J. Am. Chem. Soc.*, 1932, **54**, 3274.

This idea was not at first accepted, but was specifically supported in 1950[42] on stereochemical grounds, as already described in Section **33i,** and since that time seems not to have been seriously doubted, though there has been much discussion about the degree of solvation and length of life of the diazonium ion and the carbonium ion.

The products of the action of nitrous acid on methylamine in dilute aqueous acid, the simplest example of deamination, were described by Austin[43] in 1960. In one of his series of experiments, methylamine hydrochloride, 0.5 mole, and sodium nitrite, 1.5 mole, dissolved in water, 650 ml., gave, on slowly adding 0.3*N* sulphuric acid, 0.4–0.6 mole, the following products: methyl alcohol, 6–25%; methyl nitrite, 45–35%; nitromethane, 6%; methylnitrolic acid, 10–12%; methyl chloride, 13%; and the evolved nitrogen had a 3% excess volume, but contained a little carbon dioxide; also small amounts of hydrogen cyanide and of ammonia were produced. This work came curiously late in the history of organic chemistry, and the reason was that all early descriptions of the reaction were silent about its products, and inventive text-book writers had since filled that gap by guess-work, inaccurately as it happened, but plausibly enough to conceal that the gap existed. No one before Austin had found, or even guessed, that the main product is methyl nitrite, which, being a gas, goes away, like methyl chloride, with the nitrogen, unless steps are taken to condense it. A minor amount of the favourite "text-book product," methyl alcohol, is indeed found; and more would be found were it not further converted by O-nitrosation to methyl nitrite. A further amount of methyl nitrite, and some nitromethane, arise by direct capture of nitrite ion by the carbonium ion. More nitromethane would be found, were this not further converted by C-nitrosation to methylnitrolic acid. A certain proportion of this substance suffers decomposition to the expected hydrolysis products of its unknown dehydration product, nitryl cyanide, notably, HCN, and the products which would derive from HCNO, *viz.*, CO_2 and NH_3. Austin's explanatory scheme is as follows:

$$CH_3{\cdot}OH \xleftarrow{H_2O} (CH_3^+) \xrightarrow{Cl^-} CH_3Cl$$

$$CH_3{\cdot}OH \xrightarrow{HNO_2} CH_3{\cdot}ONO \qquad (CH_3^+) \xrightarrow{NO_2^-} CH_3{\cdot}ONO,\ CH_3{\cdot}NO_2$$

$$CH_3{\cdot}NO_2 \xrightarrow[HNO_2]{} HON{:}CH{\cdot}NO_2 \rightarrow HCN,\ CO_2,\ NH_3$$

[42] P. Brewster, F. Hiron, E. D. Hughes, C. K. Ingold and P. A. D. Rao, *Nature*, 1950, **166**, 178.

[43] A. T. Austin, *Nature*, 1960, **188**, 1086.

In deamination of higher primary aliphatic amines, wider opportunities open before the carbonium ion: it may not only complete a direct substitution (in various ways), but may also lose a proton, so completing an elimination; and it may rearrange with a migration of hydrogen or methyl, and only after that complete a substitution or an elimination. All these things do happen. Our concern will be with the eliminations in Chapter IX, and with the rearrangements in Chapter X. As to direct substitutions, the important result, that they take place with concurrent racemisation and inversion, has already been discussed (Section **33i**). As an additional example, *n*-butylamine[44,39] gives *n*-butyl products, *n*-butenes, and *s*-butyl products (hydrogen migration); and, with an α-deuterium atom, introduced to make an asymmetric α-carbon atom, the *n*-butyl products are comparably racemised and inverted.

(38d) O-Nitrosation and Dependent Oxidation.—The kinetics of the nitrosation of water has been investigated by Bunton, Llewellyn, Stedman, and others by the use of oxygen-18 as isotopic label (here indicated by an underline):

$$HNO_2 + H\underline{O}H \rightarrow NO\cdot\underline{O}H + H_2O$$

The various kinetic forms described above for diazotisation, nitrosation, and deamination of amines in dilute aqueous acid appear again in the oxygen exchange work, with only those modifications that would be expected from the change of substrate. Thus, those kinetic equations which do not contain the amine factor in the N-nitrosations reappear without modification, whilst those which do contain the amine factor reappear without it, because the new substrate, water, being the solvent, is in constant concentration.

At low acidities and at high concentrations (0.5–2.5*M*) of nitrous acid, the rate of exchange follows the kinetics of equation (4):

$$\text{Rate} \propto [HNO_2]^2 \qquad (4)$$

This rate is equal to the rate of diazotisation in this kinetic form in like conditions.[45] The meaning is that nitrosation of the solvent water, which is written with underlined oxygen symbols below, is by dinitrogen trioxide, and is rate-controlled by the formation of dinitrogen trioxide:

[44] F. C. Whitmore and D. P. Langlois, *J. Am. Chem. Soc.*, 1932, **54**, 3441.

[45] C. A. Bunton, D. R. Llewellyn, and G. Stedman, *Nature*, 1955, **175**, 83; *Spec. Pubs. Chem. Soc.*, 1959, **10**, 113; *J. Chem. Soc.*, **1959**, 568; C. A. Bunton, J. E. Burch, B. C. Challis, and J. H. Ridd, reported by J. H. Ridd, *Quart. Rev. Chem. Soc.*, 1960, **15**, 424.

$$\left.\begin{array}{c} NO\cdot OH + H^+ \rightleftharpoons NO{-}OH_2^+ \\ NO_2^- + NO{-}OH_2^+ \xrightarrow[\text{slow}]{} NO_2{-}NO + OH_2 \\ NO_2\cdot NO + \underline{O}H_2 \longrightarrow NO_2^- + NO{-}\underline{O}H_2^+ \\ NO{-}\underline{O}H_2^+ \longrightarrow NO{-}\underline{O}H + H^+ \end{array}\right\} \quad (4a)$$

Still at low acidities, but now at low concentrations of nitrous acid (near $10^{-3}M$), another form of kinetics takes charge:[46]

$$\text{Rate} \propto [HNO_2][H^+] \quad (2'')$$

This is what equation (2) degenerates to, when the substrate is the solvent, as it is in the oxygen exchange. It represents the nitrosation of water by nitrous acidium ion:

$$\left.\begin{array}{l} H_2\underline{O} + NO{-}OH_2^+ \rightarrow H_2\underline{O}{-}NO^+ + OH_2 \\ \qquad\qquad\qquad\qquad\qquad \downarrow \\ \qquad\qquad\qquad\qquad\quad H\underline{O}{-}NO + H^+ \end{array}\right\} \quad (2a'')$$

It was proved not to represent nitrosation by pre-equilibrium nitrosonium ion [equation (5)], by putting in azide ion, in competition with the water, and showing, by isotopic examination of the evolved nitrous oxide, that the azide ion is being nitrosated by an entity which has not exchanged its oxygen with water, as pre-equilibrium nitrosonium ion, if present, must have done.

A sufficiently active "foreign" anion in sufficient concentration may outdo both nitrite ion and water as substrate in nitrosation. Oxygen exchange then occurs in accordance with equation (9):

$$\text{Rate} \propto [HNO_2][H^+][X^-] \quad (9)$$

This has been demonstrated with acetate ion as the foreign anion.[47] The rate-controlling step is then (9a) with $X^- = OAc^-$, the exchange proceeding by way of nitrosyl acetate (= acetyl nitrite):

$$X^- + NO{-}OH_2^+ \rightarrow X{-}NO + OH_2 \quad (9a)$$

The subsequent steps are analogous to those set out above for oxygen exchange by way of dinitrogen trioxide.

The O-nitrosation of saturated alcohols appears to proceed simply: the nitrous esters are stable. However, the kinetics of their formation have not yet been investigated.

[46] C. A. Bunton and G. Stedman, *J. Chem. Soc.*, 1959, 3466.
[47] C. A. Bunton and M. Masui, *J. Chem. Soc.*, 1960, 304.

The O-nitrosation products from phenols and enols are unstable, and, when formed, lose nitric oxide. Overall, this is a one-electron oxidation. Its first product, from a monohydric phenol or enol, is an oxy-radical, $R\dot{O}$, and this initiates chain reactions, which may lead to polymeric products. However, a dihydric phenol, such as hydroquinone, or a conjugated enediol ("reductone"), such as ascorbic acid, will very rapidly undergo a second such step of one-electron oxidation, to give a diketone, such as quinone or dehydroascorbic acid, as the two-electron oxidation product. The stoicheiometry of such oxidations is as represented below in the example of ascorbic acid [R=$CH_2(OH)\cdot CH(OH)$—]:

$$\begin{array}{c}OH\quad OH\\ |\qquad\ |\\ C{=\!=}C\\ |\qquad\ |\\ RCH\cdot O\cdot CO\end{array} + 2HNO_2 \rightarrow \begin{array}{c}O\qquad O\\ \|\qquad\ \|\\ C{-\!-}C\\ |\qquad\ |\\ RCH\cdot O\cdot CO\end{array} + 2NO + 2H_2O$$

Bunton, Dahn, and Loewe and their coworkers have made a penetrating study of the kinetics of these oxidations, mainly of the oxidation of ascorbic acid by nitrous acid, in weakly acidic solutions of water or aqueous dioxan, without or with added "foreign" anions.[48] They have disclosed the following. Two substrates, which are often present in comparable amounts, are oxidised concurrently and independently, *viz.*, the ascorbic acid molecule, and the ascorbate ion, of which the latter is specifically the more reactive for oxidation. The oxidation of each of these substrates may be routed through any of the same set of nitrosonium-ion carriers, *viz.*, the nitrous acidium ion, dinitrogen trioxide, and, if the halide ions are supplied, nitrosyl chloride, and nitrosyl bromide, which provide known routes for N-nitrosation, diazotisation, deamination, and oxygen-exchange with water. From experiments in which the formation of dinitrogen trioxide, rather than its attack, was rate-controlling for the oxidation of either substrate, values for the rate of formation of dinitrogen trioxide were obtained which were in agreement with the values derived from the various N- and O-nitrosating reactions mentioned. Most of the network of Fig. 38-1 was encountered twice, once for each substrate, among the identified rate terms. The only steps *not* encountered were step 10, and, for the ascorbate ion only, step 2, as numbered in Fig. 38-1. Bunton, Dahn, and Loewe formulate the whole family of oxidation mechanisms as follows:

[48] C. A. Bunton, H. Dahn, and L. Loewe, *Nature*, 1959, **183**, 163; *Helv. Chim. Acta*, 1960, **43**, 320; H. Dahn, L. Loewe, E. Lüscher, and R. Menassé, *ibid.*, p. 287 *et seq.* (5 papers).

$R = CH_2(OH)\cdot CH(OH)$ $NOX = NO\cdot OH_2^+, NO\cdot NO_2, NOBr, NOCl$

$$\underset{RCH\cdot O\cdot CO}{HO{-}C{=}C{-}OH} \xrightarrow[\text{slow}]{NOX} \underset{RCH\cdot O\cdot CO}{ON\cdot O{-}C{=}C{-}OH} \xrightarrow[\text{fast}]{-NO} \underset{RCH\cdot O\cdot CO}{O\cdot{-}C{=}C{-}OH}$$

$$\underset{RCH\cdot O\cdot CO}{O\cdot{-}C{=}C{-}OH} \xrightarrow[\text{fast}]{NOX} \underset{RCH\cdot O\cdot CO}{O{-}C{=}C{-}O\cdot NO} \xrightarrow[\text{fast}]{-NO} \underset{RCH\cdot O\cdot CO}{O{=}C{-}C{=}O}$$

$$\underset{RCH\cdot O\cdot CO}{O^-{-}C{=}C{-}OH} \xrightarrow[\text{slow}]{NOX} \underset{RCH\cdot O\cdot CO}{ON\cdot O{-}C{=}C{-}OH}$$

(39) NUCLEOPHILIC SUBSTITUTION AT SECOND-ROW ELEMENTS

(39a) Substitution at Silicon.—Nucleophilic substitutions of trialkyl- or triaryl-silyl derivatives have been studied kinetically, stereochemically, and by both methods in correlation.

In 1957, Allen and Modena showed[49] that chlorine exchange between triphenylsilyl chloride and tetraethylammonium radio-chloride in dioxan proceeds by a second-order substitution, to which they assign the mechanism S_N2:

$$\overset{*}{Cl}^- + Ph_3Si\cdot Cl \rightarrow \overset{*}{Cl}\cdot SiPh_3 + Cl^- \qquad (S_N2)$$

Hydrolysis of the silyl chloride in aqueous dioxan was a first-order process, sensitive to anion catalysis; but the oxygen in the formed silyl hydroxide was not exchanged with isotopically distinguished oxygen from the solvent water: evidently there is no easy, reversible, additive reaction between the silyl derivative and water.

Since 1959, Sommer and Fyre have examined the stereochemistry of the products of various substitutions at silicon in methylphenyl-α-naphthylsilyl compounds (MePhNphSiX).[50] They described the "Walden cycle,"

[49] A. D. Allen and G. Modena, *J. Chem. Soc.*, **1957**, 3671.

[50] L. H. Sommer and C. L. Fyre, *J. Am. Chem. Soc.*, 1959, **81**, 1013; 1960, **82**, 3796; 1961, **83**, 220; L. H. Sommer, *Angew. Chem. internat. Edit.*, 1962, **1**, 143; L. H. Sommer, C. L. Fyre, G. A. Parker, and K. W. Michael, *J. Am. Chem. Soc.*, 1964, **86**, 3271, 3276; L. H. Sommer, G. A. Parker, and C. L. Fyre, *ibid.*, p. 3280; *idem* and N. C. Lloyd, *ibid.*, 1967, **89**, 857; L. H. Sommer and W. D. Korte, *ibid.*, p. 5802; L. H. Sommer, "Stereochemistry, Mechanism and Silicon," McGraw-Hill, New York, 1965.

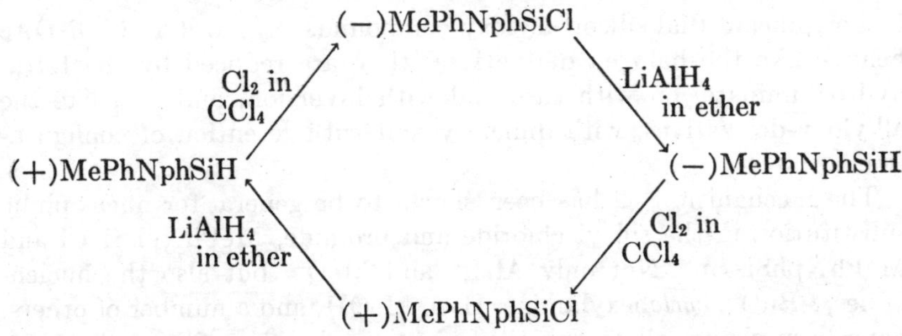

which they reasonably interpreted as alternate electrophilic chlorinations with retention of configuration, and nucleophilic replacements of chloride by hydride ion with inversion of configuration. More interesting is the absence of a Walden cycle, when the above nucleophilic replacement is set beside a process for accomplishing the same result in two steps, both of which are expected to be nucleophilic substitutions:

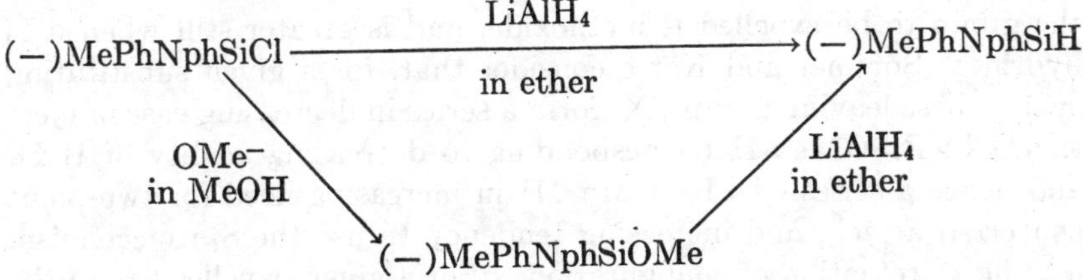

If the interpretation of the "Walden cycle" is right, one of these last steps must retain configuration. Sommer and Fyre, having assigned a number of relative configurations largely from considerations of isomorphism, concluded that the second of the successive steps has this property. This implies that the tetrahydroaluminate ion can act in two ways: it effects the easier nucleophilic replacements, as of halogens, as in the Walden cycle, by a one-point attack with inversion of configuration (S_N2); but it can accomplish the more difficult nucleophilic replacement of oxygen groups, such as methoxyl, only by a collaborative two-point interaction with the substrate, the reaction proceeding through a cyclic transition state with retention of configuration (S_Ni):

$$H_3Al\cdot H^- + MePhNphSi\cdot Cl \rightarrow H\cdot SiMePhNph + H_3Al\cdot Cl^- \qquad (S_N2)$$

$$MePhNphSi\begin{matrix} H^- \\ \\ OMe \end{matrix}AlH_3 \rightarrow MePhNphSi\cdot H + H_3Al\cdot OMe^- \qquad (S_Ni)$$

It is significant that silicon acyloxy-compounds, *e.g.*, MePhNPhSi·OAc behave like the halogen derivatives: they are reduced by the tetrahydroaluminate ion with ease and with inversion, and not, like the alkyloxy-derivatives, with difficulty and with retention of configuration.

The mechanism S_N2 has been shown to be general for nucleophilic substitution in the silicyl chloride and bromide, MePhNphSi·Cl and MePhNphSi·Br. Not only AlH_4^- and MeO^-, but also the nucleophiles, *t*-BuO^-, *cyclo*hexylamine, H_2O, MeOH, and a number of others, have been shown all to substitute in these halides with inversion of configuration.

The prevalence of stereochemical inversion, and therefore, it is deduced, of an S_N2 mechanism, in the replacement by nucleophilic substituting agents of halogen in the silicyl bromide and chloride, does not apply to the fluoride. Some reagents replace fluorine with retention of configuration, and hence, it is inferred, by a two-point attack of S_Ni type. The tendency to this type of substitution is greater when the group to be expelled is methoxide, and is greater still when it is hydride. Sommer and Korte consider that, for a given substituting agent, these leaving groups, X, form a series in decreasing ease of ejection, Cl>F>OMe>H (corresponding to decreasing acidity of HX), and hence a series Cl<F<OMe<H in increasing need for two-point concerted attack, and increasing tendency to use the S_Ni mechanism leading to retention of configuration. For a given expelled group the mechanism chosen will depend on the reagent, *e.g.*, how strongly nucleophilic it is, and, if it is an ionising molecule, how easily it liberates its anionic portion. For example, ionicity probably increases among the lithium derivatives of hydrocarbons along the series, simple alkyl<allyl or benzyl<benzhydryl. Among these, the simple alkyllithiums show the greatest tendency to substitute with retention of configuration, and hence, it is concluded, by a concerted S_Ni type of mechanism. Benzhydryl-lithium shows the greatest tendency to substitute with inversion, and therefore, presumably, by an S_N2 mechanism. The interaction of these two serial relations is shown below:

X =	Cl	F	OMe	H
Alkyl-lithium	inv.	ret.	ret.	ret.
Allyl-lithium	inv.	inv.	inv.	ret.
Benzyl-lithium	inv.	inv.	inv.	ret.
Benzhydryl-lithium	inv.	inv.	inv.	inv.

The stereochemistry of a reaction is, of course, a property of its mechanism, and it is therefore desirable that stereochemical observations should be correlated with independently based conclusions about mechanism. This is achieved in the kinetic investigation by Eaborn and his coworkers,[51] in which they paralleled the early research of Hughes on isotopically distinguished halide-ion replacements at carbon, the research which first established quantitatively inversion in S_N2 substitutions at carbon (Section **32d**). The newer work deals with the exchange of an isotopically labelled methoxyl group in optically active methylphenyl-α-naphthylsilyl methoxide for methoxyl from the methanolic solvent. The reaction was catalysed by acids, and by bases, and with great strength by sodium methoxide. The methoxyl group in the substrate was labelled by the radioactivity of tritium, and the rate of detritiation and of racemisation were compared. In all conditions, the rate of racemisation was just twice the rate of detritiation, that is, of methoxyl exchange. Thus, not only the substitution by preformed methoxide-ion, but also the solvolysis, and the acid-catalysed solvolysis, proceed with quantitative inversion of configuration, *e.g.*,

$$\text{MeO}^- + (-)\text{MePhNphSi}\cdot\text{O}\overset{*}{\text{Me}} \rightarrow (+)\text{MeO}\cdot\text{SiMePhNph} + \text{O}\overset{*}{\text{Me}}^- \qquad (S_N2)$$

Bearing in mind Allen and Modena's failure to detect either dissociative or additive mechanisms of nucleophilic substitution in a silyl halide, the conclusion would seem to be that not only second-order anion-exchange, but also the solvolyses, are forms of S_N2 substitution.

(39b) Substitution at Phosphorus.—Phosphorus was the first of the tetrahedral second-row elements to have its nucleophilic substitution definitively investigated. In 1953 and subsequently Dostrovsky and his collaborators examined the kinetics of the solvolyses in water, aqueous ethanol, and ethanol, and of substitution by anions, such as halide, ethoxide, and phenoxide ions, and by primary amines from methylamine to *t*-butylamine, in such hydroxylic solvents, of a number of ester-halides of phosphorus, *viz.*, phosphinyl chlorides and fluorides, $\text{Hal}\cdot\text{PO(R)}_2$, phosphonyl fluorides, $\text{F}\cdot\text{PO(R)(OR)}$, and phosphorochloridates and phosphorfluoridates, $\text{Hal}\cdot\text{PO(OR)}_2$, having groups R such as methyl, ethyl, *iso*propyl, benzyl, and phenyl.[52] The substitutions were of such types as the following examples illustrate, the products being alkyl phosphinates, phosphonates, or phosphates:

[51] R. Baker, R. W. Bott, C. Eaborn, and P. W. Jones, *J. Organometal. Chem.* 1963, **1**, 37.

[52] I. Dostrovsky and M. Halman, *J. Chem. Soc.*, **1953**, 502, 508, 511, 516; **1956**, 1004; M. Halman, *ibid.*, **1959**, 305; cf. R. S. Drago, V. A. Mode, J. G. Kay, and D. L. Lydy, *J. Am. Chem. Soc.*, 1965, **87**, 5010.

$$H_2O + Cl\cdot PO(Me)_2 \rightarrow HO\cdot PO(Me)_2 + HCl$$
$$OH^- + F\cdot PO(Et)(OEt) \rightarrow HO\cdot PO(Et)(OEt) + F^-$$
$$F^- + Cl\cdot PO(OPr^i)_2 \rightarrow F\cdot PO(OPr^i)_2 + Cl^-$$

The solvolyses were of first order, and all substitutions with solute nucleophiles were of second order, first in each reactant. Solvent and salt effects were inconsistent with ionisation mechanisms (S_N1), but were as might be expected for single-step bimolecular (S_N2) substitutions, throughout the examples examined. Substitution by solute nucleophiles in oxygen-18 water took place without oxygen exchange with the solvent. The evidence as a whole pointed to S_N2-type mechanisms, and was against both dissociation processes, and additive intermediates involving valency-shell expansion.

A number of "Walden schemes" have been developed among the phosphorus oxy-esters since 1959. The first, due to Green and Hudson,[53] led from a 3-phenanthrenylmethylphosphinyl chloride to enantiomeric phosphinates in one step and in two steps of substitution:

$$\begin{array}{ccc} (+)\text{PhenMePO}\cdot\text{Cl} & \xrightarrow{\text{OMe}^-} & (-)\text{PhenMePO}\cdot\text{OMe} \\ \downarrow{\scriptstyle \text{F}^-} & & \\ (-)\text{PhenMePO}\cdot\text{F} & \xrightarrow{\text{OMe}^-} & (+)\text{PhenMePO}\cdot\text{OMe} \end{array}$$

Either all these steps involve inversion of configuration, or one only of them does. Because of the formal similarity of the substitutions, it is more likely that they are all attended by inversion. A similar scheme in the phosphonate series was developed by Aaron and his coworkers.[54] The same argument applies:

$$\begin{array}{ccc} (-)\text{Me(OPr}^i\text{)PO}\cdot\text{Cl} & \xrightarrow{\text{OEt}^-} & (+)\text{Me(OPr}^i\text{)PO}\cdot\text{OEt} \\ \downarrow{\scriptstyle \text{MeS}^-} & & \\ (+)\text{Me(OPr}^i\text{)PO}\cdot\text{SMe} & \xrightarrow{\text{OEt}^-} & (-)\text{Me(OPr}^i\text{)PO}\cdot\text{OEt} \end{array}$$

A less usual type of example, due to Green and Hudson, shows that saponification of an alkyl phosphothionate breaks the oxygen-phosphorus bond with quantitative inversion of configuration at phosphorus. A pyrophosphothionate was built up, with optical activity centered on one only of two otherwise equivalent phosphorus atoms.[55]

[53] M. Green and R. F. Hudson, *Proc. Chem. Soc.*, **1959**, 227; *J. Chem. Soc.*, **1963**, 540; *Angew. Chem. internat. Edit.*, 1963, **2**, 11.

[54] H. S. Aaron, R. T. Oyeda, H. F. Frack, and J. H. Miller, *J. Am. Chem. Soc.*, 1962, **64**, 617.

[55] M. Green and R. F. Hudson, *J. Chem. Soc.*, **1963**, 3883.

The symmetry of the structure required that just one-half of the hydrolytic attack that would lead to the acid-ester must occur at the optically labelled phosphorus atom. But this was enough to make the product totally racemic, so proving that racemisation went at twice the rate of the substitution, which therefore entailed a quantitative inversion of configuration. The label of optical activity is denoted below by a degree sign:

$$(EtO)(Me)\overset{\circ}{P}S\cdot ONa + Cl\cdot PS(Me)(OEt)$$

$$\rightarrow (EtO)(Me)\overset{\circ}{P}S\cdot O\cdot PS(Me)(OEt)$$

$$\xrightarrow{OH^-} (HO)(Me)PS\cdot O\cdot PS(Me)(OEt)$$

Already in 1962, Green and Hudson had adapted, for substitution at phosphorus, Hughes's method of comparing the rate of an isotopic substitution of known kinetics at an asymmetric centre of optical activity with the rate of the concomitant racemisation. They showed that, in the replacement of a ^{14}C-labelled methoxyl group, in an optically active methyl phosphinate by entering unlabelled methoxide ion, the racemisation rate was twice the rate of the S_N2 substitution, and therefore that every molecular act of substitution inverted configuration.[56] This was the first firm demonstration of a stereochemical S_N2 rule in substitution at an element other than carbon. The label of radioactivity is denoted below by an asterisk:

$$OMe^- + (Ph)(Et)PO\cdot \overset{*}{O}Me \xrightarrow{MeOH} MeO\cdot PO(Et)(Ph) + \overset{*}{O}Me^-$$

The reason for the apparent absence of additive intermediates in substitutions of the oxy-esters of phosphorus may be that too much of the binding power of that element's empty $3d$ orbitals is used up by conjugation with the $2p$ electrons of the oxygen atoms. Certainly the situation is changed in the reactions of tetra-alkylphosphonium ions. Around 1930, Fenton, Hey, and the writer[57] examined the decompositions of tetra-alkylphosphonium hydroxides to trialkylphosphine-oxides and alkanes. They concluded from a study of constitutional effects on product proportions that a quinqueligant tetra-alkylhydroxyphosphane is formed, which ejects one alkyl group as a carbanion. In 1954, McEwen, VanderWerf, and their collaborators elaborated this mechanism, and established the whole concept more firmly,

[56] M. Green and R. F. Hudson, *Proc. Chem. Soc.*, **1962**, 307; *J. Chem. Soc.*, **1963**, 540.

[57] G. W. Fenton and C. K. Ingold, *J. Chem. Soc.*, 1929, 2342; L. Hey and C. K. Ingold, *ibid.*, **1933**, 531.

by showing that the reactions are kinetically of third order, first in the phosphonium ion, and second in hydroxide ion.[58] The conversion of tetrabenzylphosphonium hydroxide into tribenzylphosphine-oxide and toluene was therefore to be represented either by the following three-step mechanism:

$$(C_6H_5\cdot CH_2)_4P^+ + OH^- \rightleftharpoons (C_6H_5\cdot CH_2)_4P\cdot OH$$

$$(C_6H_5\cdot CH_2)_4P\cdot OH + OH^- \xrightarrow[\text{slow}]{} C_6H_5\cdot CH_2^- + (C_6H_5\cdot CH_2)_3PO + H_2O$$

$$C_6H_5\cdot CH_2^- + H_2O \longrightarrow C_6H_5\cdot CH_3 + OH^-$$

or by a four-step mechanism, as follows:

$$(C_6H_5\cdot CH_2)_4P^+ + OH^- \rightleftharpoons (C_6H_5\cdot CH_2)_4P\cdot OH$$

$$(C_6H_5\cdot CH_2)_4P\cdot OH + OH^- \rightleftharpoons (C_6H_5\cdot CH_2)_4P\cdot O^- + H_2O$$

$$(C_6H_5\cdot CH_2)_4P\cdot O^- \xrightarrow{\text{slow}} C_6H_5\cdot CH_2^- + (C_6H_5\cdot CH_2)_3PO$$

$$C_6H_5\cdot CH_2^- + H_2O \longrightarrow C_6H_5\cdot CH_3 + OH^-$$

Both mechanisms accommodate the result that the rate is increased when the group eliminated contains an electron-attracting *m*- or *p*-substituent, such as would be expected to accelerate the separation of a carbanion.

McEwen and VanderWerf's stereochemical work on this reaction disclosed yet another mechanism. They were able to conclude that the conversion of a phosphonium hydroxide into a phosphine-oxide and an alkane, by the mechanism two variants of which are written above, inverts configuration, because its product was enantiomeric with that given by a method which they developed for achieving the conversion by a mechanism involving a cyclic transition state, wherein configuration is almost certainly preserved. The details are that (+)benzylmethylethylphenylphosphonium hydroxide yields toluene and (−)methylethylphenylphosphine oxide; that the same (+)phosphonium ion loses a benzyl proton to *n*-butyl-lithium, so to give a a phosphonium-benzylide, which adds benzaldehyde, to yield a phosphonium-betaine; and that this decomposes to stilbene and the (+)phosphine-oxide:

[58] K. F. Kumli, W. E. McEwen, and C. A. VanderWerf, *J. Am. Chem. Soc.*, 1957, **79**, 3805 A. Bladé-Font, C. A. VanderWerf, and W. E. McEwen, *ibid.*, 1960, **80**, 2396, 2646; C. B. Parisek, W. E. McEwen, and C. A. VanderWerf, *ibid.*, p. 5503; W. E. McEwen, A. Bladé-Font, and C. A. VanderWerf, *ibid.*, 1962, **84**, 677; *idem*, K. F. Kumli and A. Zanger, *ibid.*, 1964, **86**, 2378; W. E. McEwen, G. Axelrad, M. Zanger, and C. A. VanderWerf, *ibid.*, 1965, **87**, 2948.

$$(+)\mathrm{PhCH_2\cdot\overset{+}{P}(Me)(Et)(Ph)} \xrightarrow{\mathrm{OH^-}} \mathrm{PhCH_2\cdot P(Me)(Et)(Ph)\cdot OH} \rightarrow \mathrm{PhCH_3} + (-)\mathrm{Et{-}PO(Me)(Ph)}$$

$$\downarrow \mathrm{BuLi}$$

$$\mathrm{PhCH{=}P(Me)(Et)(Ph)} \xrightarrow{\mathrm{PhCHO}} \mathrm{PhCH{-}\overset{+}{P}(Me)(Et)(Ph)},\ \mathrm{PhCH{-}O^-}\ (\text{ring-bonded}) \rightarrow \mathrm{PhCH{=}CHPh} + (+)\mathrm{OP(Me)(Et)(Ph)}$$

Asymmetric tertiary phosphines are optically stable. We should expect an electrophilic addendum having a sextet of electrons, such as an oxygen atom, or a sulphur atom, or a carbonium ion, to enter where the unshared valency electrons are, and therefore to add with retention of configuration. Certainly this assumption allows Horner's findings,[59] summarised below, to be interpreted consistently with McEwen and VanderWerf's diagnosis of inversion in the decompositions of phosphonium hydroxides. Horner obtained optically active methyl-*n*-propylphenylphosphine by electrolytic reduction of an optically resolved methyl-*n*-propylphenylbenzylphosphonium salt. He assumed this reaction to take place with predominating retention of configuration. He then converted the phosphine into a phosphine-oxide by direct oxidation, and into the enantiomeric phosphine-oxide by two different quaternisations, followed by decompositions of the resulting phosphonium hydroxides:

$$(-)\mathrm{Pr{-}\overset{+}{P}(Me)(Ph){-}CH_2Ph} \xrightarrow{\mathrm{OH^-}} (-)\mathrm{\overset{-}{O}{-}\overset{+}{P}(Me)(Ph){-}Pr}$$

$$(-)\mathrm{Pr{-}\overset{+}{P}(Me)(Ph){-}CH_2Ph} \underset{\mathrm{PhCH_2Br}}{\overset{2e}{\rightleftharpoons}} (+)\mathrm{Pr{-}P(Me)(Ph)}$$

$$(+)\mathrm{Pr{-}\overset{+}{P}(Me)(Ph){-}\overset{-}{O}} \xleftarrow{\mathrm{H_2O_2}} (+)\mathrm{Pr{-}P(Me)(Ph)}$$

$$(+)\mathrm{Pr{-}P(Me)(Ph)} \xrightarrow{\mathrm{S}} (+)\mathrm{Pr{-}\overset{+}{P}(Me)(Ph){-}\overset{-}{S}} \xrightarrow{\mathrm{MeI}} (+)\mathrm{Pr{-}\overset{+}{P}(Me)(Ph){-}SMe} \xrightarrow{\mathrm{OH^-}} (-)\mathrm{\overset{-}{O}{-}\overset{+}{P}(Me)(Ph){-}Pr}$$

[59] L. Horner, *Pure and Applied Chemistry*, 1964, 9, 225.

(39c) Substitution at Sulphur.—No kinetic studies, defining mechanisms of nucleophilic substitution at sulphur, are known to the writer, but it has been made clear since 1925 that such substitutions normally invert configuration. In that year, to the general surprise, Henry Phillips obtained *n*-alkyl sulphinates (*e.g.*, ethyl toluene-*p*-sulphinate) in optically active form.[60] In the course of this work, he showed that a single step of transesterification between such an ester and a normal primary alcohol (*e.g.*, *n*-butyl alcohol),

$$\mathrm{ArSO\cdot OR + R'OH \rightarrow ArSO\cdot OR' + ROH}$$

always inverted the sign of rotation. Phillips concluded that it inverted the configuration at the sulphur atom. No doubt, his conclusion was originally based on experience of effects of alkyl homology on optical rotation; but it became rationalised as a growing understanding of the physical mechanism of optical activity[61] made it plain that a homologous constitutional increment, whose own intrinsic optical absorption is of high energy, lying far in the ultraviolet, could not have any fundamental effect on the properties of the near-ultraviolet helical-type transition in the sulphinyl group, on which the optical activity with visible light of sulphinic esters depends. Following Phillips, we may formulate the transesterification in a way that amounts to assuming an S_N2 mechanism:

$$\mathrm{R'HO} + \mathrm{Ar(O^-)(\ddot{\ })S^{+}{-}OR} \rightarrow \mathrm{R'O{-}S(O^-)(Ar)(\ddot{\ })} + \mathrm{OHR}$$

Obviously one could build up a Walden cycle by similarly converting the formed R′-ester to an R″-ester, and thence to the enantiomeric R-ester, and then, with this as starting point, repeating the three conversions.

C. R. Johnson and his coworkers have developed Walden cycles based on the inversion that accompanies basic hydrolysis of an alkoxysulphonium ion to a sulphoxide. Their first example was effected with achiral materials, having planes of symmetry, the configurational inversion taking the form of a geometrical inversion about a ring.[62] Thus, *cis*-4-*p*-chlorophenylthian-oxide was ethylated with triethyloxonium tetrafluoroborate in solvent methylene chloride, and the

[60] H. Phillips, *J. Chem. Soc.*, **1925,** 2552.

[61] S. F. Mason, *Quart. Rev. Chem. Soc.*, 1963, **17,** 20; *Proc. Roy. Soc.* (London), 1967, **A, 297,** 3.

[62] C. R. Johnson, *J. Am. Chem. Soc.*, **1963, 85, 1020.**

formed ethoxysulphonium ion was then hydrolysed with aqueous sodium hydroxide to give the *trans*-thian-oxide, which, by a similar ethylation and subsequent hydrolysis, was reconverted to the *cis*-oxide:

$$\text{ClC}_6\text{H}_4\text{(ring)S}^+\text{–O}^- \xrightarrow{\text{Et}_3\text{O}^+\text{BF}_4^-} \text{ClC}_6\text{H}_4\text{(ring)S}^+\text{–OEt}$$

$$\downarrow \text{OH}^-$$

$$\text{ClC}_6\text{H}_4\text{(ring)S}^+\text{–OEt} \xleftarrow{\text{Et}_3\text{O}^+\text{BF}_4^-} \text{ClC}_6\text{H}_4\text{(ring)S}^+\text{–O}^-$$

$$\uparrow \text{OH}^- \text{ (back to the first compound)}$$

A chiral example has been reported,[63] in which optically active benzyl-*p*-tolylsulphoxide was, in four steps, alternately of ethylation and basic hydrolysis, converted to the enantiomer, and then recovered with 95% of its original optical rotation (rotations $[\alpha]_D^{25}$):

$$\underset{+94.6°,\ \text{back to } +89.9°}{CH_3C_6H_4\text{—}\overset{O^-}{S^+}\text{—}CH_2Ph} \xrightarrow{Et_3O^+BF_4^-} \underset{+203°}{CH_3C_6H_4\text{—}\overset{OEt}{S^+}\text{—}CH_2Ph}$$

$$\uparrow OH^- \qquad\qquad\qquad \downarrow OH^-$$

$$\underset{-208°}{CH_3C_6H_4\text{—}\underset{OEt}{S^+}\text{—}CH_2Ph} \xleftarrow{Et_3O^+BF_4^-} \underset{-92.4°}{CH_3C_6H_4\text{—}\underset{O^-}{S^+}\text{—}CH_2Ph}$$

Sulphinic esters are converted into sulphoxides by Grignard reagents. Whether the Grignard reagents act as such, or, as seems more probable, by prior ionisation (Section **36e**), such strong nucleophiles will almost certainly attack the sulphur atom in an S_N2-like manner, and, if we may extrapolate from the demonstrations of Henry Phillips and of Carl Johnson, will substitute with inversion of configuration:

$$EtMgBr \rightleftharpoons Et^- + MgBr^+$$

$$Et^- + (p\text{-}MeC_6H_4)(O^-)\ddot{S}^+\text{—}OC_{10}H_{19} \rightarrow Et\text{—}\ddot{S}(O^-)(C_6H_4Me\text{-}p) + OC_{10}H_{19}^-$$

[63] C. R. Johnson and J. B. Sapp, Am. Chem. Soc. Meeting, New York, Sept. 1963, abstracts p. 23Q, and personal communication from Dr. Carl R. Johnson

Mislow and his collaborators have shown definitely that this is so.[64] In several examples, including the reaction illustratively formulated between ethylmagnesium bromide and menthyl toluene-*p*-sulphinate, they have correlated the configurations of the chiral factor and product by comparative analysis of their rotatory dispersions in the ultraviolet, so demonstrating inversion.

The next problems in this area are obvious. It would be very desirable kinetically to establish the mechanisms assumed, and, by isotopic labelling, to test for reversibly formed additive intermediates.

[64] K. Mislow, M. M. Green, P. Laur, J. T. Melillo, T. Simmons, and A. L. Ternay jr., *J. Am. Chem. Soc.*, 1965, **87**, 1958.

CHAPTER IX

Olefin-, Acetylene-, and Carbene-forming Eliminations

(38) HETEROLYTIC MECHANISMS OF 1,2-ELIMINATION[1]

NUCLEOPHILIC substitution and olefin elimination occur side by side so frequently as to suggest that the duality of mechanism, which has proved the key to the interpretation of substitution, might have some parallel in the mechanism of elimination. Such has proved to be the case.

(38a) The Bimolecular Mechanism.—This was recognised as a general mechanism of olefin formation by Hanhart and the writer in 1927.[2] It is the most widespread of elimination mechanisms, and may be described as follows. A reagent Y, possessing nucleophilic, in particular, basic, properties, extracts the protonic part of a combined hydrogen atom, while an electron-attracting group X simultaneously separates in possession of its previously shared electrons. The hydrogen atom and the electron attractor being bound to adjacent carbon atoms in the original molecule, atomic electron shells can remain complete throughout the change; and thus a co-operative effect arises: two bonds are broken, but each fission assists the other, the two together constituting a single synchronised act. The mechanism may be formulated thus,

$$Y + H{-}CR_2{-}CR_2{-}X \rightarrow YH + CR_2{=}CR_2 + X \qquad (E2)$$

the arrows showing how the charges on Y and X become changed, though for the charges themselves there are several possibilities. Originally Y may be negatively charged or neutral, and X may be formally neutral or positive: all that the reaction necessitates is that, after the change, the formal charge of Y will be more positive by one unit, and that of X more negative by one unit, than before.

The consequences of the bimolecular mechanism have up to the present been illustrated with respect to the formation of olefins from tetra-alkylammonium salts,[2] certain tetra-alkyl phosphonium salts,[3]

[1] D. V. Banthorpe, "Reaction Mechanisms in Organic Chemistry," Editor E. D. Hughes, Vol. 2, "Elimination Reactions," Elsevier Publishing Co., London, 1962; "Studies in Chemical Structure and Reactivity," Editor J. H. Ridd, Methuen, London, 1966, Chap. 3.

[2] W. Hanhart and C. K. Ingold, *J. Chem. Soc.*, **1927**, 997; C. K. Ingold and C. C. N. Vass, *J. Chem. Soc.*, **1928**, 3125; J. v. Braun, W. Teuffert, and K. Weissbach, *Ann.*, 1929, **472**, 121; J. v. Braun and E. R. Buchmann, *Ber.*, 1931, **64**, 2610; J. v. Braun and K. Hamann, *Ber.*, 1932, **65**, 1580; C. K. Ingold and C. S. Patel, *J. Chem. Soc.*, **1933**, 68; E. D. Hughes and C. K. Ingold, *ibid.*, p. 523; *idem* and C. S. Patel, *ibid.*, p. 526; E. M. Hodnett and J. J. Flynn jr., *J. Am. Chem. Soc.*, 1957, **79**, 2300.

[3] G. W. Fenton and C. K. Ingold, *J. Chem. Soc.*, **1929**, **2342**; L. Hey and C. K. Ingold, *ibid.*, **1933**, **531**.

trialkylsulphonium salts,[4] sulphones,[5] nitroalkanes,[6] halides,[7] including fluorides,[8] sulphonates,[9] and carboxylates.[10] Nucleophilic reagents, neutral or negatively charged, have been employed, which range in basicity from water to alkoxide or amide ions. The following lists summarise the field of eliminations covered by the investigations mentioned:

$$X = \cdot NR_3^+,\ \cdot PR_3^+,\ \cdot SR_2^+,\ \cdot OH_2^+,\ SO_2R,\ \cdot NO_2,\ \cdot Hal,\ \cdot OSO_2R,\ \cdot OCOR$$
$$Y = OH_2,\ NMe_3,\ OH^-,\ OR^-,\ OAc^-,\ OAr^-,\ NH_2^-,\ CO_3^{2-}$$

The following reactions are typical of those studied in this connexion:

$$NMe_3 + ArCH_2\cdot CH_2\cdot \overset{+}{N}Me_3 \rightarrow H\overset{+}{N}Me_3 + ArCH{:}CH_2 + NMe_3$$

$$\overset{-}{O}H + CH_3\cdot CH_2\cdot \overset{+}{S}Me_2 \rightarrow OH_2 + CH_2{:}CH_2 + SMe_2$$

$$\overset{-}{O}H + CH_3\cdot CH_2\cdot SO_2\cdot Et \rightarrow OH_2 + CH_2{:}CH_2 + \overset{-}{S}O_2Et$$

$$\overset{-}{O}Et + ArCH_2\cdot CH_2\cdot Br \rightarrow HOEt + ArCH{:}CH_2 + \overset{-}{B}r$$

[4] L. Green and B. Sutherland, *J. Chem. Soc.*, 1911, **99**, 1174; C. K. Ingold, J. A. Jessop, K. I. Kuriyan, and A. M. M. Mandour, *ibid.*, **1933**, 533; C. K. Ingold and K. I. Kuriyan, *ibid.*, p. 991; E. D. Hughes and C. K. Ingold, *ibid.*, p. 1571; J. L. Gleave, E. D. Hughes, and C. K. Ingold, *ibid.*, **1935**, 236; K. A. Cooper, M. L. Dhar, E. D. Hughes, C. K. Ingold, B. J. MacNulty, and L. I. Woolf, *ibid.*, **1948**, 2043; K. A. Cooper, E. D. Hughes, C. K. Ingold, G. A. Maw, and B. J. MacNulty, *ibid.*, p. 2049; E. D. Hughes, C. K. Ingold, and G. A. Maw, *ibid.*, p. 2072; *idem* and L. I. Woolf, *ibid.*, p. 2077; E. D. Hughes, C. K. Ingold, and L. I. Woolf, *ibid.*, p. 2084; E. D. Hughes, C. K. Ingold, and A. M. M. Mandour, *ibid.*, p. 2090.

[5] G. W. Fenton and C. K. Ingold, *J. Chem. Soc.*, **1928**, 3127; *idem, ibid.*, **1929**, 2338; *idem, ibid.*, **1930**, 705.

[6] W. H. Jones, *Science*, 1953, **116**, 387.

[7] S. C. J. Olivier and A. P. Weber, *Rec. trav. chim.*, 1934, **53**, 1087; S. C. J. Olivier, *ibid.*, p. 1093; E. D. Hughes, *J. Am. Chem. Soc.*, 1935, **57**, 708; E. D. Hughes and C. K. Ingold, *J. Chem. Soc.*, **1935**, 244; *idem*, and U. G. Shapiro, *ibid.*, **1936**, 225; E. D. Hughes and U. G. Shapiro, *ibid.*, **1937**, 1177, 1192; E. D. Hughes, C. K. Ingold, S. Masterman, and B. J. MacNulty, *ibid.*, **1940**, 899; K. A. Cooper, M. L. Dhar, E. D. Hughes, C. K. Ingold, B. J. MacNulty, and L. I. Woolf, *ibid.*, **1948**, 2043; K. A. Cooper, E. D. Hughes, C. K. Ingold, G. A. Maw, and B. J. MacNulty, *ibid.*, p. 2049; M. L. Dhar, E. D. Hughes, C. K. Ingold, and S. Masterman, *ibid.*, p. 2055; M. L. Dhar, E. D. Hughes, and C. K. Ingold, *ibid.*, pp. 2058, 2065.

[8] W. H. Saunders jr., S. R. Fahrenholz, E. A. Caress, J. P. Lowe, and M. Schreiber, *J. Am. Chem. Soc.*, 1965, **87**, 3401; W. H. Saunders jr. and M. R. Schreiber, *Chem. Comm.*, **1966**, 145.

[9] W. Hückel, W. Tappe, and G. Legutke, *Ann.*, 1940, **543**, 191.

[10] C. R. Hauser, J. C. Shivers, and P. S. Skell, *J. Am. Chem. Soc.*, **1945**, **67**, **409**.

The evidence of mechanism has reference (1) to the need for a strong base, (2) to an isotopic demonstration of reaction in a single stage, (3) to the influence of constitutional factors, and (4) to that of environmental factors, on the ease and direction of reaction. We may consider items (1) and (2) here, leaving (3) and (4) to be discussed in later Sections.

The need for a strong base is qualitatively obvious throughout the investigated range of eliminations indicated above. It is expressed quantitatively by the second-order kinetics of the reaction:

$$\text{Rate} = k_2[\text{Y}][\text{HCR}_2\cdot\text{CR}_2\text{X}]$$

Second-order kinetics have, indeed, been formally established over practically the whole range of application illustrated above. The following reactions, the first taking place in water and the second in ethyl alcohol, are typical of those which have been shown to obey the second-order law:

$$\bar{\text{O}}\text{H} + \text{PhCH}_2\cdot\text{CH}_2\cdot\overset{+}{\text{N}}\text{Me}_3 \rightarrow \text{OH}_2 + \text{PhCH}{:}\text{CH}_2 + \text{NMe}_3$$

$$\bar{\text{O}}\text{Et} + \text{CH}_3\cdot\text{CHMe}\cdot\text{Br} \rightarrow \text{HOEt} + \text{CH}_2{:}\text{CHMe} + \bar{\text{Br}}$$

The need for a strongly basic reagent, as expressed in second-order kinetics, is consistent, not only with bimolecular elimination E2, but also with unimolecular elimination from the conjugate base of the substrate, E1cB. (Note that the numerical component, unity, in this symbol refers to the molecularity of the elimination from, not the formation of, the conjugate base.) This mechanism is dominant in eliminations which form a carbonyl double bond, or an olefinic double bond that is conjugated with a carbonyl group or a similarly electronegative unsaturated group (Chapter XIII); but it seems quite rare in eliminations to give simple olefins.

Skell and Hauser have shown[11] how bimolecular elimination, and unimolecular elimination from a conjugate base, may be distinguished by an isotopic test; and they have thus provided evidence that an entirely typical olefin elimination, namely, the production of styrene from 2-phenylethyl bromide and ethoxide ion, which has been shown to have second-order kinetics, actually proceeds by the bimolecular mechanism, E2:

[11] P. S. Skell and C. R. Hauser, *J. Am. Chem. Soc.*, 1945, **67**, 1661; D. G. Hill, B. Stewart, S. W. Kantor, W. A. Judge, and C. R. Hauser, *ibid.*, 1954 **76**, 5129.

$$\bar{O}Et + PhCH_2 \cdot CH_2 \cdot Br \rightarrow HOEt + PhCH{:}CH_2 + \bar{Br} \qquad (E2)$$

The alternative possibility would have involved the prior production of the conjugate base, a carbanion, and the unimolecular loss of bromide ion from the latter:

$$\left.\begin{array}{l} \bar{O}Et + PhCH_2 \cdot CH_2 \cdot Br \leftrightarrows HOEt + Ph\bar{C}H \cdot CH_2 \cdot Br \\ \qquad Ph \cdot \bar{C}H \cdot CH_2 \cdot Br \rightarrow PhCH{:}CH_2 + \bar{Br} \end{array}\right\} (E1cB)$$

However, in this mechanism, the first stage must be reversible; and therefore, if the reaction were conducted in a deuteroalcoholic solvent, such as DOEt, the original bromide should take up deuterium, and therefore unconverted material recovered after a partial transformation to styrene should be found to contain deuterium. In fact, Skell and Hauser found the bromide recovered after such partial conversion to be free from deuterium, a result which indicates against reaction through the conjugate base. We say "indicates," because, of course, negative evidence does not prove a negative in the strict sense; but one would want very clear positive evidence in order to accept an unusual mechanism. There has been quite a history of attempts to "discover" mechanism E1cB in the formation of simple olefins. The mechanism does seem very uncommon, though it possibly has a certain range of validity.[12]

(38b) The Unimolecular Mechanism.—This was first recognised as a general mechanism of olefin formation by Hughes in 1935.[13] Its main characteristic is that the electron-attracting group X breaks away, taking its previously shared electrons, under the influence of solvation forces, but without the co-operation of the proton-extracting reagent Y, thereby producing a carbonium ion, which subsequently loses a pro-

[12] An indication may have been provided by J. Hine, R. Miesback, and O. B. Ramsay, *J. Am. Chem. Soc.*, 1961, **83**, 1222; but the kinetics of the reaction studied were not simple, and the products were not examined. Again, T. I. Crowell, A. T. Hill, A. T. Kemp, and R. E. Lutz, *ibid.*, 1963, **85**, 2521, may have had the mechanism under observation; but their kinetics were involved, and needed several disposable constants for their representation. F. G. Bordwell, R. L. Arnold, and J. B. Banowski, *J. Org. Chem.*, 1963, **28**, 2496, probably did realise mechanism E1cB, when they observed easy *cis*-elimination of acetic acid from 1-nitro-2-acetoxy-2-phenyl*cyclo*hexane by the agency of piperidine in chloroform-ethanol. But they were producing, not a simple olefin, but an $\alpha\beta$-unsaturated nitro-compound. Mechanism E1cB is standard for the formation of $\alpha\beta$-unsaturated carbonyl compounds (Chapter XIII), and there can be little doubt that the same is true for $\alpha\beta$-unsaturated nitriles and nitro-compounds.

[13] E. D. Hughes, *J. Am. Chem. Soc.*, 1935, **57**, 708.

ton to the solvent or some other proton acceptor. The reaction thus has two stages, of which the first, the heterolytic separation of X, is rate-determining; so that the rate of the overall reaction is independent of any added base. The mechanism may be formulated thus,

$$\left.\begin{array}{l} H{-}CR_2{-}CR_2{-}X \xrightarrow[\text{slow}]{} H{-}CR_2{-}\overset{+}{C}R_2 + X \\ H{-}CR_2{-}\overset{+}{C}R_2 \xrightarrow[\text{fast}]{} \overset{+}{H} + CR_2{=}CR_2 \end{array}\right\} \quad (E1)$$

where the group X may be either formally neutral or positively charged before reaction, becoming, respectively, either negatively charged or neutral afterwards.

Up to the present this mechanism has been established, or made probable, in certain olefin eliminations of sulphonium salts,[14] halides,[15] and sulphonic esters,[16] that is, over the following range of electron-attracting groups:

$$\cdot X = \cdot\overset{+}{S}R_2, \cdot Cl, \cdot Br, \cdot I, \cdot O\cdot SO_2R$$

The following equations represent examples of elimination in which the unimolecular mechanism is certainly prominent:

$$CH_3\cdot CMe_2\cdot\overset{+}{S}Me_2 \rightarrow \overset{+}{H} + CH_2{:}CMe_2 + SMe_2$$

$$CH_3\cdot CMe_2\cdot Br \rightarrow \overset{+}{H} + CH_2{:}CMe_2 + \overset{-}{Br}$$

The evidence of this mechanism relates (1) to its insensitiveness to bases, (2) to its close correspondences with concurrent unimolecular

[14] K. A. Cooper, E. D. Hughes, C. K. Ingold, and B. J. MacNulty, *J. Chem. Soc.*, **1940,** 2038; K. A. Cooper, M. L. Dhar, E. D. Hughes, C. K. Ingold, B. J. MacNulty, and L. I. Woolf, *ibid.*, p. 2043; K. A. Cooper, E. D. Hughes, C. K. Ingold, G. A. Maw, and B J. MacNulty, *ibid.*, p. 2049; E. D. Hughes, C. K. Ingold, and L. I. Woolf, *ibid.*, p. 2084; E. D. Hughes, C. K. Ingold, and A. M. M. Mandour, *ibid.*, p. 2090.

[15] E. D. Hughes, *J. Am. Chem. Soc.*, 1935, **57,** 708; E. D. Hughes, C. K. Ingold, and A. D. Scott, *Nature*, 1936, **138,** 120; *J. Chem. Soc.*, **1937,** 1271; E. D. Hughes, C. K. Ingold, and U. G. Shapiro, *ibid.*, **1937,** 1277; K. A. Cooper, E. D. Hughes, and C. K. Ingold, *ibid.*, p. 1280; E. D. Hughes and B. J. MacNulty, *ibid.*, p. 1283; K. A. Cooper, E. D. Hughes, C. K. Ingold, G. A. Maw, and B. J. MacNulty, *ibid.*, **1940,** 2049; M. L. Dhar, E. D. Hughes, and C. K. Ingold, *ibid.*, pp. 2058, 2065; E. D. Hughes, C. K. Ingold, and A. M. M. Mandour, *ibid.*, p. 2090

[16] W. Hückel and W. Tappe, *Ann.*, 1939, **537,** 113; *idem* and G. Legutke, *ibid.*, 1940, **543,** 191.

substitution, (3) to the influence of constitutional factors, and (4) to that of environmental factors, on the rate and direction of reaction. We discuss effects (1) and (2) here, leaving (3) and (4) to be considered in later Sections.

The insensitiveness of unimolecular elimination to bases is reflected in the kinetic form of the reactions. In first approximation they are first-order processes,

$$\text{Rate} = k_1[HCR_2\cdot CR_2X]$$

in examples such as the following reaction, the rate of which in ethyl alcohol is nearly unaffected by added sodium ethoxide:

$$CH_3\cdot CMe_2\cdot Br \rightarrow \overset{+}{H} + CH_2{:}CMe_2 + \overset{-}{Br}$$

In second approximation, deviations from first-order kinetics occur, which are due to salt effects, as discussed in Section 32, and are highly characteristic of unimolecular processes. Such deviations as have been studied apply to the total processes of unimolecular substitution and elimination.

Unimolecular substitution and elimination S_N1 and E1 have a common slow step, stoicheiometry being determined by alternative subsequent fast steps:

$$HCR_2\cdot CR_2\text{—}X \xrightarrow[\text{slow}]{} HCR_2\cdot CR_2^+ \;\; \text{fast} \begin{cases} \xrightarrow{Y^-} HCR_2\cdot CR_2\text{—}Y & (S_N1) \\ \xrightarrow{Y^-} CR_2{:}CR_2 + HY & (E1) \end{cases}$$

The observed total rate, $k_1 = k(S_N1) + k(E1)$, is the rate of heterolysis of the substrate, but the proportion of olefin formed, $k(E1)k_1$, is determined by a partitioning of the cation among the paths open to it. If we could consider the anion as out of screening range, a series of substrates, with the same alkyl group but different removable groups X, could differ in any degree as to total rate, but should produce the same proportion of olefin. This was one of the arguments for the E1 mechanism of elimination from secondary and tertiary alkyl halides and sulphonium ions in aqueous ethanolic solvents, which was adduced in the later 1930's, though it was noted then that, since stereochemical studies of substitution were showing that screening had to be reckoned with, the constancy of olefinic proportion was expected to be only approximate. The illustrations given,[17] here reproduced in Table 38-1, showed that, with a fixed alkyl group, changes in the expelled group could change rate by factors of 100-fold or more without changing the olefin proportion by factors larger than 1.3.

TABLE 38-1.—EFFECT OF VARYING X IN UNIMOLECULAR REACTIONS OF AlkX ON THE OVERALL RATE (k, IN SEC.$^{-1}$) AND ON THE OLEFIN PROPORTION (k(E1)/k_1).

Solvent	Temp.	Alk.	X	$10^5 k_1$	$k(E_1)/k_1$
"60%" aq.-EtOH	100.0°	2-Octyl	Cl	0.805	0.13
			Br	26.8	0.14
"80%" aq.-EtOH	65.3	*t*-Butyl	$\overset{+}{S}Me_2$	11.8	0.357
			Cl	89.7	0.363
"60%" aq.-EtOH	25.0	*t*-Butyl	Cl	0.854	0.168
			Br	37.2	0.126
			I	90.1	0.129
"80%" aq.-EtOH	50.0	*t*-Amyl	$\overset{+}{S}Me_2$	6.66	0.478
			Cl	28.5	0.403
"80%" aq.-EtOH	25.2	*t*-Amyl	Cl	1.50	0.333
			Br	58.3	0.262
			I	174	0.260

When one passes to less dissociating solvents, such as dry ethanol, or to less dissociating and less basic solvents, such as anhydrous acetic acid, the above rule, which is a limiting rule, breaks down. Ion pairs are then more stable relative to dissociated ions, and so screening by the counter-ion becomes important, and different counter-ions will accordingly interfere with the completion of a substitution to different extents. Furthermore, the counter-ion may be a better receiver of the eliminated proton than is the solvent; and thus different counter-ions will promote completion of the elimination relative to the completion of substitution, to different extents. This second effect also has a stereochemical consequence, as we shall see in Section **41b**. In the meantime, let us illustrate with Winstein and Coicevera's finding[18] that *t*-butyl chloride, bromide, and dimethylsulphonium ion, in dry

[17] E. D. Hughes, C. K. Ingold, and U. G. Shapiro, *J. Chem. Soc.*, **1937**, 1277; K. A. Cooper, E. D. Hughes, and C.K. Ingold, *ibid.*, p. 1280; E. D. Hughes and B. J. MacNulty, *ibid.*, p. 1283; K. A. Cooper, E. D. Hughes, C. K. Ingold, and B. J. MacNulty, *ibid.*, **1940**, 2038.

[18] S. Winstein and M. Coicevera, *J. Am. Chem. Soc.*, 1963, 85, 1702.

ethanol at 75° gave 44%, 36%, and 18% of olefin, respectively, and in anhydrous acetic acid gave 73%, 69%, and 12% respectively. The chloride ion and bromide ion are, of course, much more basic than is the dimethyl sulphide eliminated from the sulphonium ion.

We know another carbonium-ion mechanism of olefin-forming elimination. We label it E2(C+), and think of it as related to mechanism E1, somewhat as mechanism E1cB is related to mechanism E2. Its characteristic is that the carbonium ion, instead of being formed slowly and losing its proton rapidly, is formed in rapid pre-equilibrium, so that the extraction of its proton by the attack of a base becomes the rate-controlling step:

$$\left.\begin{array}{l} H{-}CR_2{-}CR_2{-}X \underset{\text{fast}}{\rightleftharpoons} H{-}CR_2{-}CR_2^+ + X \\ Y + H{-}CR_2{-}CR_2^+ \xrightarrow[\text{slow}]{} YH + CR_2{=}CR_2 \end{array}\right\} E2(C^+)$$

In Section **29c** we noticed a carbonium-ion mechanism of nucleophilic substitution which was given the label $S_N2(C^+)$: it involved the pre-equilibrium formation of a carbonium ion followed by its rate-controlling combination with a base: the mechanism formulated above is the counterpart mechanism of elimination. Though it can be claimed as known, it appears to have lacked explicit discussion as an elimination mechanism. We mention it now in order to complete the central picture of 1,2-elimination mechanisms, but it will be convenient to defer discussion of the evidence concerning it to Sections **53a** and **54a** (Chapter XIII).

(39) CONSTITUTIONAL EFFECTS ON ORIENTATION AND RATE OF 1,2-ELIMINATION

(39a) The Orientation Rules and Their Significance.—The story of the analysis of constitutional effects on the direction and rate of eliminations starts in the last century, with observations made and summarising rules offered, for eliminations from particular classes of substrate, *viz.*, tetra-alkylammonium salts and alkyl halides. This was long before it was appreciated that such eliminations are members of a common family of reactions.

In 1851 Hofmann noticed[19] that quaternary ammonium hydroxides containing different primary alkyl groups decomposed to give mainly ethylene if an ethyl group was present. Much later, in 1927, Hanhart and the writer showed[2] that this rule can be generalised to a statement that quaternary ammonium hydroxides containing only primary alkyl

[19] A. W. Hofmann, *Ann.*, 1851, **78**, 253; **79**, 11

groups (an important qualification) give mainly that ethylene which carries the smallest number of alkyl substituents. We can call this the "generalised Hofmann rule."

In 1875 Saytzeff noticed[20] that secondary and tertiary alkyl halides which, when unsymmetrically branched, could give isomeric olefins by loss, along with halogen, of hydrogen from one or another of the branches, preferentially lost hydrogen from where there was least hydrogen. It amounts to the same to say that the alkyl halides give that ethylene which carries the largest number of alkyl substituents.

As long as no connexion was recognised between the reactions to which these rules applied, no one thought of comparing the rules. But after 1927, when eliminations became recognised as one family of reactions, the antithetical nature of the rules stood out, and it became a challenge to discover from what kind of constitutional influence each arose. The philosophy was, and is, that the respective influences must be general, that is, operative throughout organic chemistry, and not only in the limited field of simple alkyl substrates, within the confines of which the antithetical rules apply. Both influences must be present; and they must be independent, so that they can work either in conjunction or in opposition, and, where they work in opposition, give antithetical rules, according to which is dominant. The important problem was to identify the constitutional influences: the matter of how they could combine could then be expected to settle itself.

Half this question was answered in 1927, when it was proposed that the general influence, from which sprang the Hofmann rule for alkyl groups in 'onium decompositions, was one of the *polarity* of substituents on the *acidity* of the β-proton. However, the other half of the question could not be answered until after hyperconjugation was discovered in 1935.

(39b) Bimolecular Elimination, especially from Alkyl 'Onium Ions: Effects of Polarity, especially the Inductive Effect.—The operation of inductive polarisation in creating the situation summarised in the generalised Hofmann rule was described in 1927 as follows.[21] The substrate has to contain a strongly electron-attracting group, *viz.*, the group to be eliminated. This induces a positive charge on all the surrounding atoms, and so loosens the protons, a sufficient loosening of a β-proton permitting elimination by mechanism E2. A group which, by releasing electrons, tends to neutralise the induced positive charge on the β-carbon atom, and thus to tighten its hold on the β-protons,

[20] A. Saytzeff, *Ann.*, 1875, **179**, 296

[21] W. Hanhart and C. K. Ingold, *J. Chem. Soc.*, **1927**, 997.

will inhibit reaction. The terminal methyl of the n-propyl group acts in this way, and so determines that, in accordance with Hofmann's rule, the n-propyl group will show relatively little tendency to engage in an olefin-forming process, if an ethyl group is available to do so:

$$CH_3 \rightarrow \underset{|}{\overset{H}{C}}H-CH_2-\overset{+}{N}(Me)(Me) \;\vdots\; \underbrace{CH_2-\overset{H}{\underset{|}{C}}H-H}_{\text{eliminated}}$$

Similarly, an *iso*butyl group will not largely participate in elimination, if a n-propyl group, still more, if an ethyl group, is available; and, naturally, the terminal methyl residues in the n-propyl and *iso*butyl groups may be replaced by ethyl or higher homologous residues without changing these comparisons. This is the already stated generalisation of Hofmann's rule, namely, that of the preferential formation of the least alkylated ethylene.

Further generalisation follows from the consideration that the protective electron displacements can be relayed to the β-carbon atom from non-adjacent atoms, though only with considerable loss of intensity. Thus the protective effect to be observed in the n-propyl group will be increased in the n-butyl group, but not by so much as in the *iso*butyl group. In general, the effect will increase with homology, tending to a limit, but always subject to the condition that a branched-chain group is more effective than the isomeric normal-chain group.

Outside the range of hydrocarbon residues, one expects electron-attracting substituents to promote elimination, and to do so with best effect if they are directly bound to the β-carbon atom:

$$\underbrace{Cl \leftarrow \overset{H}{\underset{|}{C}}H-CH_2}_{\text{eliminated}} \;\vdots\; -\overset{+}{N}(Me)(Me)-CH_2-\overset{H}{\underset{|}{C}}H-H$$

These deductions from theory have been tested, first, for primary alkyl and substituted alkyl groups, in ammonium hydroxides and ethoxides, in sulphonium hydroxides and ethoxides, and in the alkali-promoted decompositions of sulphones; later, the observations were extended to cover secondary and tertiary alkyl groups.

To deal first with primary alkyl groups—for some years following 1927 the observations were wholly orientational. One form of this method was to place two olefin-forming alkyl groups in competition in the same 'onium ion or sulphone, as illustrated in the preceding formulae, and to measure the proportions in which the different olefins are present in the product of the completed reaction. Thus it has been shown[22] that, in the decompositions of sulphonium hydroxides, the first four primary alkyl groups stand in the following order with respect to the ease with which they split off as olefins:

ethyl > *n*-propyl > *n*-butyl > *iso*butyl

Another early method employed 'onium ions containing only one olefin-yielding alkyl group, and otherwise only methyl groups, the assumption being that changes in the olefin-forming group would not much affect the tendency of methyl to split off in a substitution process. This process thus provided a standard reaction against which one could measure the competing elimination. The decompositions of ammonium hydroxides were studied in this way,[21,23] and primary alkyl groups were placed in the following order with respect to the ease with which they yield olefins:

ethyl > *n*-propyl > *n*-butyl > *n*-amyl ~ *n*-octyl > *iso*amyl > *iso*butyl

Since these explanations and illustrations were given, a number of studies of product composition in 'onium eliminations have been recorded. One of the most impressive is that of 1952 by Smith and Frank,[24] who analysed mass-spectrometrically the olefin mixtures formed from quaternary ammonium hydroxides containing various olefin-forming alkyl groups. Some of their data are in Table 39-1. The second set of figures, in which the same two groups are present in various ratios, give olefin compositions which are different, but become identical after statistical correction for the varying initial abundances of the groups. This shows that the different alkyl groups in the ammonium ions act independently of one another. This being understood, the results in general show an orienting effect attenuated by relay in the way that is characteristic of the inductive effect. A γ-carbon, that is, the first carbon beyond the acidic β-proton, orients strongly, according to the Hofmann rule; a δ-carbon does so mildly; a second δ-carbon equally mildly. Now unlike inductive effects, primary steric effects do not attenuate: owing to the form of the non-bonding energy-distance curve, once they start, they mount rapidly with increasing material density around the reaction centre. We see that the third δ-carbon in the *neo*hexyl group does not orient as mildly as the first two, but orients much more strongly. As Smith and

[22] C. K. Ingold, J. A. Jessop, K. I. Kuriyan, and A. M. M. Mandour, *J. Chem. Soc.*, **1933**, 533.

[23] C. K. Ingold and C. C. N. Vass, *J. Chem. Soc.*, **1928**, 3125.

[24] P. A. S. Smith and S. Frank, *J. Am. Chem. Soc.*, 1952, **74**, 509.

TABLE 39-1.—PERCENTAGES OF OLEFINS FROM TETRA-ALKYLAMMONIUM HYDROXIDES (SMITH AND FRANK).

Alkyls in R_4N^+	Alkyl carbons beyond C_β		% Olefins found		For equal nos. groups	
	δ γ	δ γ	Lower	Higher	Lower	Higher
Et_2, n-Pr_2		C—	96	4	96	4
n-Pr_2, n-Bu_2	C—	C—C—	62	38	62	38
n-Pr, n-Bu_3	C—	C—C—	83	17	61	39
n-PR_3, n-Bu	C—	C—C—	36	64	62	38
n-Bu_2, i-$Amyl_2$	C—C—	(C)₂C—	67	33	67	33
n-Bu, i-Amyl, Me_2	C—C—	(C)₂C—	66	34	66	34
i-Amyl, *neo*Hex, Me_2	(C)₂C—	(C)₃C—C—	91	9	91	9

Frank point out, it is very probable that a primary steric effect first impinges at this point in the progressive ramification of the structure.

After 1935, when unimolecular elimination was discovered, it became necessary to confirm kinetically that the already studied eliminations from primary alkyl substrates were bimolecular, as in fact they were. Moreover, with the tool of kinetics, one could probe further than by product analysis alone; and, in particular, one could ascertain whether, not only those ratios of rates which constitute product composition, but also the rates themselves change with structural changes as is required by the theory of the Hofmann rule. Theory does require that alkyl extension beyond the β-carbon should reduce rate. The data, reproduced in the top section of Table 39-2, showed that this is indeed the case.[25]

New ground was broken in the study of secondary and tertiary alkyl

[25] D. V. Banthorpe, E. D. Hughes, and C. K. Ingold, *J. Chem. Soc.*, 1960, 4050.

'onium ions. It was known that the Hofmann rule applied to primary alkyl groups in 'onium ions, and the Saytzeff rule to secondary and tertiary alkyl groups in halides; but it was not known whether a different mechanism, or the type of the alkyl group, or the type of the expelled group was responsible for the difference. In conditions kinetically controlled to ensure bimolecular elimination, it was shown that eliminations from secondary and tertiary alkyl groups in sulphonium ions, as from primary alkyl groups, are governed by the generalised Hofmann rule. This is manifested in the secondary and tertiary groups by the fact that the double bond goes preferentially into the shorter of unequal branches of the groups, and that the rate differential, which determines this orientational result, is not caused by an enhanced rate of establishment of the double bond in the shorter branch, but is caused by a reduced rate of reaction in the longer branch of the alkyl group. This is illustrated in the lower two sections of Table 39-2. Thus, *s*-butyl-dimethylsulphonium ethoxide in the conditions indicated gives 26% of 2-butene and 74% of 1-butene, and, as the table shows, this is because the rate of establishment of the double bond in the longer branch of the *s*-butyl group is reduced below the rate of its establishment in one branch of the symmetrical lower-homologous *iso*propyl group.[26] Similarly, *t*-amyl-dimethylsulphonium

TABLE 39-2.—RATE CONSTANTS (k_2 IN SEC.$^{-1}$ MOLE^{-1} L.) OF BIMOLECULAR ELIMINATION FROM ALKYL 'ONIUM ETHOXIDES IN ETHANOL.

A: $RNMe_3{}^+OEt^- \rightarrow$ Olefin $+ HOEt + NMe_3$
B: $RSMe_2{}^+OEt^- \rightarrow$ Olefin $+ HOEt + SMe_2$

	R...		Et	*n*-Pr	*n*-Bu	*iso*-Bu
A	$10^5k_2(104°)$		71.3	5.16	2.82	1.68
B	$10^5k_2(64°)$		79	29	21	10
				R...	*i*-Pr	*s*-Bu
B	$10^5k_2(64°)$, total				1040	695
		longer branch			520	185
		shorter branch			520	510
				R...	*t*-Bu	*t*-Amyl
B	$10^5k_2(24°)$, total				80	56
		longer branch			27	8
		each shorter branch			27	24

[26] E. D. Hughes, C. K. Ingold, G. A. Maw, and L. I. Woolf, *J. Chem. Soc.*, **1948**, **2077**.

ethoxide gives 14% of 2-methyl-2-butene and 86% of 2-methyl-1-butene, and the essential reason is that the rate of reaction in the long branch is reduced relatively to the rate in one branch of the lower-homologous *t*-butyl group.[27]

A further study has been made of the effects of normal and branching homology in primary alkyl groups on the rates of decomposition of alkyl-dimethylsulphonium and alkyl-trimethylammonium ions under the action of ethoxide ions in ethanol, and of *t*-butoxide ions in *t*-butanol.[25] The object was to ascertain more quantitatively whether the expected attenuation by relay, characteristic of the inductive effect of alkyl extensions beyond the β-proton, shows in the rate data; and, if so, whether the rate of attenuation was as found in polar effects on other reactions, and whether the whole scale of the effect was what should be expected from the electronegativity of the polar end groups. The homologous series were also extended far enough to show at what stage of branching homology steric hindrance sets in.

The various series studied all teach the same lessons. The figures

TABLE 39-3.—SECOND-ORDER RATE-CONSTANTS OF ELIMINATION (k_2 IN SEC.$^{-1}$ MOLE^{-1} L.) FROM ALKYL-DIMETHYLSULPHONIUM ETHOXIDES IN ETHANOL AT 64°, AND DIFFERENCES IN FREE-ENERGY OF ACTIVATION.

R in $RSMe_2^+OEt^-$	10^5k_2 for E_2	$\Delta G^{\neq}$, kcal./mole	For last-added Me	$\Delta G^{\neq}$ calc.
$CH_3\cdot CH_2$—	79	0	—	0
$CH_3\cdot CH_2\cdot CH_2$—	29	0.67	0.67	0.70
$(CH_3)_2CH\cdot CH_2$—	10	1.38	0.71	1.60
$CH_3.CH_2\cdot CH_2\cdot CH_2$—	21	0.88	0.21	0.80
$(CH_3)_2CH.CH_2\cdot CH_2$—	16	1.06	0.18	0.83
$(CH_3)_3C\cdot CH_2\cdot CH_2$—	0.43	3.49	2.43	0.87

for one of them are in Table 39-3. The rate reductions produced by chain lengthening are conveniently expressed as increments in the free energy of activation $\Delta G^{\neq}$. One γ-carbon atom adds 0.7 kcal./mole to the free energy, and a second γ-carbon atom adds another 0.7 kcal./mole. A δ-carbon atom adds a further 0.2 kcal./mole, and a second δ-carbon atom adds another 0.2 kcal./mole. But the third δ-carbon of the *neo*hexyl group adds, not another 0.2, but 2.4 kcal./mole. This is evidently the stage of branching density at which steric hindrance, previously inoperative, abruptly sets in, just as Smith and Frank concluded from their study of compositions of olefins formed from ammonium ions with mixed alkyl groups.

Since electrostatic energy and charge should be proportional, the

[27] E. D. Hughes, C. K. Ingold, and L. I. Woolf, *J. Chem. Soc.*, **1948, 2084.**

indication is that the factor of attenuation of polarisation by transmission through a carbon atom is 3.5. Because of field effects (Sections **21e** and **22f**), the precise factor depends *inter alia* on the medium, which in these experiments was ethanol. A calculation, based on atom and bond polarisabilities, gives an approximate value of 5, but that applies to the gaseous ion. Many years ago, Branch and Calvin[28] deduced a value of 2.8 from the effects of homology on the strengths of carboxylic acids in water.

When we calculate from polarisability data how much charge the polar end-group should put on all the atoms in the alkyl structure, and then treat the energy of the charge induced on the β-hydrogen atom, in the field of the ethoxide ion in the transition state, as an electrostatic increment to free energy of activation, one obtains the values given in the last column of the table. Except for the *neo*hexyl group, they are of the order of magnitude of the values observed, and thus they show all that could be expected to be shown by so crude a calculation, namely, that inductive effects in the alkyl groups of terminal 'onium ions are of about the right size to produce the effects in rate, and hence on product composition, that we observe.

In the discrepant case, that of the *neo*hexyl group, we must assume the development of a steric compression of 2.2 kcal./mole in the transition state. There can be no doubt that this compression is developed between the β-*t*-butyl residue and the α-sulphonium group. We cannot calculate it by the methods illustrated in Section **34b**, because we do not know the geometry of the transition state precisely enough; but we can thus calculate that it must be less than 6.5 kcal./mole, and that it would be about 2 kcal./mole, if, in the transition state, the flattening of those groups about the forming double bond, which become coplanar with it when it is fully formed, had proceeded about half-way.[29]

In the figures already given, we have a warning that the theory of the Hofmann rule is not a complete theory of orientation and rate in bimolecular elimination, even for 'onium ions. Thus, the series, ethyl, *iso*propyl, *t*-butyl, is characterised by successively introduced

[28] G. E. K. Branch and M. Calvin, "The Theory of Organic Chemistry," Prentice-Hall, Englewood Cliffs, N. J., 1941, Chap. 6.

[29] In the period 1950–56, many suggestions appeared in the literature (see ref. 25) to the effect that the Hofmann pattern of orientation and rate in E2 substitutions in 'onium ions is due entirely to steric hindrance; but this idea, due to H. C. Brown, does not in fact reflect the known pattern of observations. After ten years, the same idea appeared again, without mention of the unanswered case against it (ref. 25), and with the new assumption that an undefined parameter called "steric requirements" runs contrary to size among the halogens (H. C. Brown and R. L. Klimisch, *J. Am. Chem. Soc.*, 1966, **88**, 1425).

TABLE 39-4.—RATES AND PROPORTIONS OF OLEFIN IN BIMOLECULAR REACTIONS OF ALKYLSULPHONIUM IONS.

Reactions with OEt^- in EtOH at 45°. Rates $k(S_N2)$ and $k(E2)$ in $sec.^{-1}$ $mole^{-1}$ l.

Alk in Alk$\cdot\overset{+}{S}Me_2$	Ethyl	*iso*Propyl	*t.*-Butyl
$10^5\,k(S_N2)$	37	73	≯90
$10^5\,k(E2)$	5.0	114	2930
Proportion of olefin, %	12	61	97–100

α-methyl substituents, which should exert a weak protecting effect on β-protons, and, if this were all, should reduce rate slightly along the series. Actually, as Table 39-4 shows, the rate rises considerably, even when allowance is made for the increasing numbers of β-protons. The accompanying S_N2 substitution does not show a corresponding rate increase, and hence the proportion of olefin rises along the series.

In β-extensions of the alkyl chains of 'onium ions, polarity, leading to the Hofmann pattern of constitutional effects on orientation and rate, dominates over unsaturation, which, as we shall see, is the generally dominant factor in eliminations from alkyl halides, and leads to the Saytzeff pattern of effects. But this dichotomy, as between 'onium ions and halides, is not absolute. As Saunders and his co-workers have shown,[8] one halogen, namely, fluorine, has such strong polarity that, in eliminations from alkyl fluorides, it produces a dominating Hofmann pattern. Thus, the 2-halogenopentanes, $CH_3\cdot CHX\cdot CH_2CH_2\cdot CH_3$, on treatment with potassium ethoxide in ethanol at the boiling point gave the following percentages of isomeric pentenes:

	F	Cl	Br	I
Pent-1-ene	82	36	25	20
Pent-2-ene	18	64	75	80

The same qualitative dichotomy and quantitative gradation were obtained for the 2-halo-2-methylpentanes, $(CH_3)_2CX\cdot CH_2\cdot CH_2\cdot CH_3$.

(39c) Bimolecular Elimination from Alkyl Halides: Effects of Unsaturation, especially the Electromeric Effect.—The identification of the polar mechanism underlying the Saytzeff rule as conjugative electron displacement, or, more particularly, hyperconjugative displacement, operating mainly during the course of reaction as an electromeric effect, was made[30] in 1941. The mechanism may be described for simple alkyl groups as follows. In the transition state of reaction, the electrons of a suitably situated CH bond, such as a γ-CH bond, become hyperconjugated with the unsaturation electrons of the partly

[30] E. D. Hughes and C. K. Ingold, *Trans. Faraday Soc.*, 1941, 37, 657.

formed $\alpha\beta$-double bond, as indicated below. This reduces the energy of the transition state, and so facilitates the reaction:

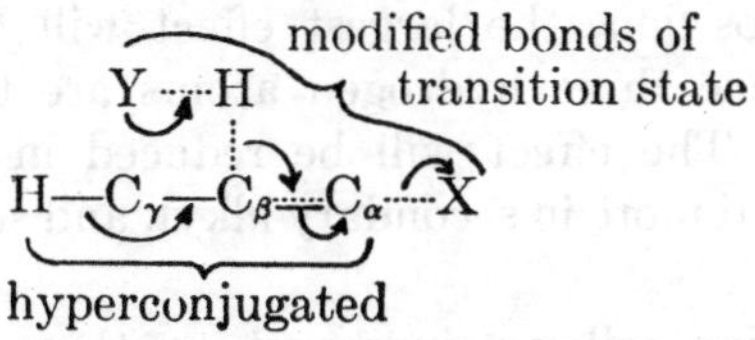

Just as in the preceding Section we followed the consequences of assuming the operation of the inductive effect, and found that they included the Hofmann rule, so now we shall do the same for the electromeric effect, and find that its very different consequences include the Saytzeff rule. In the present case, as in the former one, theoretical deduction is much more extensive than the original empirical rule. The expected consequences of the electromeric effect can be set down under four heads.

First on account of the electromeric effect, an alkyl residue, β-bound in the complete alkyl group, should stabilise the transition state of elimination of that group, and thus facilitate its separation as an olefin (contrary to the generalised Hofmann rule). This predicted effect might apply either to the reactions of different alkyl groups, or to those of unequal branches of the same alkyl group. Thus a *n*-propyl group should give propylene more easily than an ethyl group gives ethylene; and the symmetrical 3-amyl group should yield 2-pentene more easily than an *iso*propyl group yields propylene. Application to the branches of an unsymmetrical secondary or tertiary group gives Saytzeff's rule, namely, that the double bond prefers to set itself between most alkylated carbon atoms. Thus the 2-butyl group should give mainly 2-butene, and the *t*-amyl group mainly trimethylethylene.

Secondly, since either end of the developing double bond is equally available for hyperconjugation, α-bound residues in the complete alkyl group should have an electromeric effect generally similar to that of β-bound residues. Indeed, the effect of α-residues could be the greater, inasmuch as the electron-deficiency at the α-carbon atom may develop ahead of its being satisfied in double-bonding by the developing electron-excess at the β-carbon atom. It may be concluded that tertiary alkyl groups should suffer bimolecular elimination more readily then secondary, and these more readily than primary, provided that β-bound residues are exerting comparable effects in the cases compared. This should be true along series, such as, *t*-butyl > *iso*propyl > ethyl, and, *t*-amyl > *sec.*-butyl > *n*-propyl.

The third deduction is an extension of the first two, inasmuch as it defines the relative effects of different β-bound or α-bound alkyl residues. In either position, the largest effect will be exerted by the methyl residue, since three hydrogen atoms are there available for hyperconjugation. The effect will be reduced in homologous alkyl residues, and reduced more in secondary alkyl, and still more in tertiary alkyl residues.

A fourth deduction follows, inasmuch as there is nothing in the theory which restricts its application to alkyl groups. The relevant property of the influencing group is its unsaturation, and consequent ability to conjugate; and, if an α- or β-bound alkyl substituent can hyperconjugate with the incipient olefinic bond, thus assisting its production, a properly unsaturated substituent, such as vinyl or phenyl, similarly placed, must be able to conjugate with the developing double bond, thereby promoting its establishment much more strongly.

In this Section the above deductions will be illustrated by observations on rate and orientation in kinetically controlled bimolecular eliminations of alkyl halides. Tables 39-5 and 39-6 show the effect of β-bound residues and of α-bound residues on rate of olefin elimination,

TABLE 39-5.—BIMOLECULAR OLEFIN FORMATION FROM ALKYL BROMIDES WITH VARYING β-BOUND RESIDUES.

Reactions in ethyl alcohol. Rate constants k(E2) in sec.$^{-1}$ mole^{-1} l.

Series 1. $RCH_2 \cdot CH_2 \cdot Br + \bar{O}Et \rightarrow HOEt + RCH{:}CH_2 + Br^-$

$R_2CH \cdot CH_2 \cdot Br + \bar{O}Et \rightarrow HOEt + R_2C{:}CH_2 + Br^-$

Group	Ethyl	*n*-Propyl	*n*-Butyl	*n*-Amyl	*iso*Butyl	2-Phenylethyl
R or R_2	H	Me	Et	*n*-Pr	Me_2	C_6H_5
$10^5\,k$(E2), 55°	1.2	5.3	4.3	3.5	8.6	561

Series 2. $RCH_2 \cdot CHMe \cdot Br + \bar{O}Et \rightarrow HOEt + RCH{:}CHMe + Br^-$

Group	*iso*Propyl	*sec.*-Butyl	2-Amyl
R	H	Me	Et
$10^5\,k$(E2), 25°	0.118	0.282	0.196

Series 3. $RCH_2 \cdot CHEt \cdot Br + \bar{O}Et \rightarrow HOEt + RCH{:}CHEt + Br^-$

Group	*sec.*-Butyl	3-Amyl
R	H	Me
$10^5\,k$(E2), 25°	0.065	0.200

Series 4. $RCH_2 \cdot CMe_2 \cdot Br + \bar{O}Et \rightarrow HOEt + RCH{:}CMe_2 + Br^-$

Group	*t*-Butyl	*t*-Amyl
R	H	Me
$10^5\,k$(E2), 25°	1.00	4.20

TABLE 39-6.—BIMOLECULAR OLEFIN FORMATION FROM ALKYL BROMIDES WITH VARYING α-BOUND RESIDUES.

Reactions in ethyl alcohol at 25°. Rate constants k_2(E2) in sec.$^{-1}$ mole^{-1} l.

Series 1. $CH_3 \cdot CHR \cdot Br + \bar{O}Et \rightarrow HOEt + CH_2 : CHR + Br^-$

$CH_3 \cdot CR_2 \cdot Br + \bar{O}Et \rightarrow HOEt + CH_2 : CR_2 + Br^-$

Group	Ethyl	*iso*-Propyl	*sec.*-Butyl	2-Amyl	*t*-Butyl	*t*-Amyl	1-Phenyl-ethyl
R or R_2	H	Me	Et	*n*-Pr	Me_2	MeEt	C_6H_5
$10^5\,k$(E2)	0.025	0.118	0.065	0.080	1.00	0.85	0.79

Series 2. $CH_3 \cdot CH_2 \cdot CHR \cdot Br + \bar{O}Et \rightarrow HOEt + CH_3 \cdot CH : CHR + Br^-$

$CH_3 \cdot CH_2 \cdot CR_2 \cdot Br + \bar{O}Et \rightarrow HOEt + CH_3 \cdot CH : CR_2 + Br^-$

Group	*n*-Propyl	*sec.*-Butyl	3-Amyl	*t*-Amyl
R or R_2	H	Me	Et	Me_2
$10^5\,k$(E2)	0.083	0.282	0.200	4.20

in several series of primary, secondary, and tertiary alkyl bromides.[31] The rates entered relate to the establishment of the double bond in the *single* positions indicated; thus 10^5k for total formation of propylene from *iso*propyl bromide is 2×0.118, and for total butylenes from *sec.*-butyl bromide is $0.282 + 0.065$, in the units stated.

Table 39-5 shows that a single β-bound methyl radical increases the bimolecular rate of elimination, that two β-methyl residues do so more strongly, and that a single β-phenyl substituent does so more strongly still; and also that higher alkyl β-substituents increase the rate, but less strongly than does the β-methyl residue. Table 39-6 shows that a single α-methyl residue increases the bimolecular rate, that two α-methyl residues do so more strongly, as also does the α-phenyl substituent; while higher alkyl α-substituents also increase the rate, but less strongly than does the α-methyl residue. All this is in accord with the preceding theoretical deductions.

Nevertheless, some of the figures warn us that an interpretation on the basis of the electromeric effect only would not be accurate and complete. Thus the methyl residue exerts a larger effect from the α-position, while the phenyl residue acts much more strongly from the β-position. This could be the result of the simultaneous presence of the inductive effect, which becomes important only in the case of

[31] E. D. Hughes, C. K. Ingold, S. Masterman, and B. J. MacNulty, *J. Chem. Soc.*, **1940,** 899; M. L. Dhar, E. D. Hughes, C. K. Ingold, and S. Masterman, *ibid.*, **1948,** 2055; M. L. Dhar, E. D. Hughes, and C. K. Ingold, *ibid.*, pp. 2058, 2065; V. J. Shiner jr., M. J. Boskin, and M. L. Smith, *J. Am. Chem. Soc.*, 1955, **77,** 5515.

β-bound substituents, and for electron-repelling β-methyl would oppose the electromeric effect; but for electron-attracting β-phenyl would support it.

The way in which the rate effects in bimolecular elimination combine to produce orientational effects in secondary and tertiary alkyl halides can be understood from Table 39-7. There the already

TABLE 39-7.—ITEMISED RATES ILLUSTRATING THE DETERMINATION OF ORIENTATION IN BIMOLECULAR OLEFIN FORMATION FROM ALKYL BROMIDES.

Reactions with NaOEt in EtOH at 25°. Rate constants k(E2) in sec.$^{-1}$ mole^{-1} l.

	C=C—CH (β α) ←			$\overset{\alpha}{\text{CH}}$—$\overset{\alpha}{\text{C}}$Br—$\overset{\beta}{\text{CH}}$ (β α)	→ CH—$\overset{\alpha}{\text{C}}$=$\overset{\beta}{\text{C}}$		
No.	Substituents β	Substituents α	Rate per branch $10^5 k$(E2)		Rate per branch $10^5 k$(E2)	Substituents α	Substituents β
1	—	Me	0.118	$CH_3 \cdot CHBr \cdot CH_3$	0.118	Me	—
2	Me	Me	0.282	$CH_3 \cdot CH_2 \cdot CHBr \cdot CH_3$	0.065	Et	—
3	Et	Me	0.196	$CH_3 \cdot CH_2 \cdot CH_2 \cdot CHBr \cdot CH_3$	0.080	n-Pr	—
4	Me	Et	0.200	$CH_3 \cdot CH_2 \cdot CHBr \cdot CH_2 \cdot CH_3$	0.200	Et	Me
5	—	Me_2	1.00	$CH_3 \cdot CBr(CH_3)(CH_3)$	1.00	Me_2	—
					1.00	Me_2	—
6	Me	Me_2	4.20	$CH_3 \cdot CH_2 \cdot CBr(CH_3)(CH_3)$	0.85	MeEt	—
					0.85	MeEt	—

quoted second-order rate constants are reproduced as partial rates, corresponding to elimination along the different branches of the alkyl groups; and these partial rates are entered against the associated alkyl branches on either side of the chemical formulae; while adjacent to each figure is a note of the radicals bound to the α- and β-ends of the double bond formed.

Comparing entries 1 and 2, one observes (left-hand columns) that, in agreement with theory, the extra β-Me in example 2 accelerates the formation of 2-butene as compared with its lower homologue, but (right-hand columns) that the replacement of α-Me by α-Et retards, as it should, the formation of 1-butene. Both rate changes contribute to an orienting effect of the type required by the Saytzeff rule:

$$(81\%)\ CH_3{\cdot}CH{:}CH{\cdot}CH_3 \xleftarrow{E2} CH_3{\cdot}CH_2{\cdot}CHBr{\cdot}CH_3 \xrightarrow{E2} CH_3{\cdot}CH_2{\cdot}CH{:}CH_2\ (19\%)$$

By similarly comparing entries 2 and 3, one may understand how rate changes agreeing with theory combine to produce in example 3 a less extreme orientation of Saytzeff type, despite the increased dissymmetry of the original bromide:

$$(71\%)\ CH_3{\cdot}CH_2{\cdot}CH{:}CH{\cdot}CH_3 \xleftarrow{E2} CH_3{\cdot}CH_2{\cdot}CH_2{\cdot}CHBr{\cdot}CH_3 \xrightarrow{E2} CH_3{\cdot}CH_2{\cdot}CH_2{\cdot}CH{:}CH_2\ (29\%)$$

The comparison of examples 5 and 6 proceeds like that of 1 and 2, except that the doubled statistical weight of one of the olefins enters into the determination of the orientational proportions:

$$(71\%)\ CH_3{\cdot}CH{:}C(CH_3)_2 \xleftarrow{E2} CH_3{\cdot}CH_2{\cdot}CBr(CH_3)_2 \xrightarrow{E2} CH_3{\cdot}CH_2{\cdot}C(CH_3){:}CH_2\ (29\%)$$

Itemised analyses of E2 rates and product compositions, of the type illustrated in Table 39-7, have been carried further up the homologous series of secondary alkyl bromides by Shiner and his coworkers,[31] with results pointing to a continued dominating control by the electromeric effect.

It is convenient to refer here, since the point will be wanted later, to the differential effect of alkyl structure on substitution and elimination in the bimolecular reactions of alkyl halides, and on the resultant proportion of formed olefin. Illustrating by α-bound methyl radicals, it has been noticed that rate of bimolecular substitution decreases (Section 24a), and that rate of elimination increases (this Section), along the α-methylated series of alkyl groups: therefore the proportions of olefin must increase, as is exemplified in Table 39-8.

TABLE 39-8.—RATES AND PROPORTIONS OF OLEFIN IN BIMOLECULAR REACTIONS OF ALKYL BROMIDES.

Reactions with NaOEt in EtOH at 55°. Rates $k(S_N2)$ and $k(E2)$ in sec.$^{-1}$ mole^{-1} l.

α-Series	Ethyl	*iso*Propyl	*t*-Butyl
$10^5\,k(S_N2)$	118.2	2.1	Small
$10^5\,k(E2)$	1.2	7.6	50
Proportions of olefin, %	1.0	79	~100

Finally, let us recall that, as Saunders has shown,[8] alkyl fluorides are not like other halides. The polarity of the end-group is certainly stronger, and the α-unsaturation developed in the transition state may well be weaker. The observation is that the Hofmann pattern of effects dominates over the Saytzeff pattern in eliminations from alkyl fluorides.

(39d) Unimolecular Elimination from Alkyl 'Onium Ions and Halides: Electromeric Effect.—Unimolecular eliminations have been observed with secondary and tertiary alkyl 'onium ions, and with secondary and tertiary alkyl halides. It is found that the Saytzeff rule applies. One may conclude that the electromeric effect is the controlling influence.

It is not surprising that 'onium ions and halides show the same type of orientation in unimolecular elimination, though they show different types in bimolecular elimination. For in bimolecular reactions, the products are given by competing forms of attack on the 'onium ion or on the halide, that is, on different entities; whereas in unimolecular reactions, the products are formed by competing attacks on the same entity, namely, the carbonium ion, first produced from either the 'onium ion or the halide. However, it has been found that Saytzeff orientation is quantitatively more extreme in the unimolecular eliminations of 'onium ions or halides than in the bimolecular eliminations of halides.

Because of the two-stage nature of the unimolecular mechanism, the rate constant of elimination k(E1) is composite: it is the product of the rate of the primary heterolysis k_1, and the fraction of formed carbonium ion which completes the elimination process. In some ways this fraction, that is, the percentage of olefin formed in unimolecular reactions, is more simply related to structure than is the formal rate constant of the separate process of elimination.

As an example of structural effects on rate, and on the proportion of olefin formed in unimolecular reactions, Table 39-9, relating to secondary alkyl bromides, is given. From the figures[32] it is clear that a β-bound methyl radical facilitates the completion of an elimination, and a β-bound ethyl radical does the same, but not so strongly. This is the normal difference of hyperconjugation between the radicals, and is consistent with the theory of control by the electromeric effect.

The way in which the rates and proportions of unimolecular elimination along the different branches of an alkyl group combine to produce a structural effect on the overall elimination rate, on the olefin proportion, and on the orientation of elimination, is illustrated by the

[32] M. L. Dhar, E. D. Hughes, and C. K. Ingold, *J. Chem. Soc.*, **1948**, 2058.

TABLE 39-9.—UNIMOLECULAR OLEFIN FORMATION FROM SECONDARY ALKYL BROMIDES.

Reactions in "60%" aqueous ethyl alcohol at 80°. Rates k_1 and k(E1) in sec.$^{-1}$.

Alkyl group...	$(CH_3)(CH_3)CH\cdot$	$(CH_3\cdot CH_2)(CH_3)CH\cdot$	$(CH_3\cdot CH_2)(CH_3\cdot CH_2)CH\cdot$	$(CH_3\cdot CH_2\cdot CH_2)(CH_3)CH\cdot$
$10^5\, k_1$.........	7.06	7.41	5.97	5.61
$10^5\, k$(E1).....	0.32	0.63	0.90	0.38
Proportion of olefin, %....	4.6	8.5	15.1	6.8

analysis given in Table 39-10, for the unimolecular reactions of *t*-butyl and *t*-amyl bromides. The figures[33] may be compared with those of the similar analysis, given in entries 5 and 6 of Table 39-7, of the bimolecular reactions of these two halides. Corresponding data on the left of either table show a qualitatively similar structural influence: the extra β-Me residue in the amyl compound facilitates the establishment of the double bond in the alkyl branch which contains the residue. But the effect is larger for the unimolecular than for the bimolecular mechanism. This is true whether one fixes attention on the rate at which, or on the proportion in which, the double bond is established in the appropriate part of the molecule. However, the figures on the right of the two tables show a notable difference: the replacement of α-Me_2 by α-MeEt, which in the bimolecular reaction reduced the rate of introduction of the double bond into the relevant alkyl branch, as electromeric control would require, is now found to accelerate the same process in the unimolecular reaction. But this is easily explained by the mechanistic difference: the elimination rate, k(E1), contains, as a factor, the heterolysis rate k_1, which is greater for *t*-amyl than for *t*-butyl bromide: the molecules at this stage being saturated, the inductive effect dominates. We avoid this irrelevant consideration, if we pay attention to olefin proportions, rather than to rates, that is, to the final stages of the unimolecular process; and we then find that, in the completion of unimolecular elimination, the replacement of α-Me_2 by α-MeEt reduces the extent to which the double bond is established in the relevant branch, in agreement with the theory of electromeric control. The manner in which the itemised rates combine to produce overall rates, and olefin proportions, as well as the Saytzeff type of orientation, is shown at the foot of the table.

[33] M. L. Dhar, E. D. Hughes, and C. K. Ingold, *J. Chem. Soc.*, **1948**, 2065.

Table 39-10.—Itemised Rates Illustrating the Determination of Overall Results in Unimolecular Olefin Formation from Alkyl Bromides.

Reactions in ethyl alcohol at 25°. Rate constants k_1 and $k(\text{E1})$ in sec.$^{-1}$.

$C{=}C{-}CH \leftarrow$ (β, α) Substituents β	Substituents α	Per branch % Olefin	Per branch $k(\text{E1}) \times 10^5$	$CH{-}\overset{\alpha}{C}Br{-}\overset{\beta}{C}H$	Per branch $k(\text{E1}) \times 10^5$	Per branch % Olefin	Substituents α	Substituents β
—	Me_2	6.3	0.029	$CH_3{-}CBr(CH_3)_2$	0.029	6.3	Me_2	—
					0.029	6.3	Me_2	—
Me	Me_2	29.6	0.323	$CH_3{\cdot}CH_2{\cdot}CBr(CH_3)_2$	0.036	3.3	MeEt	—
					0.036	3.3	MeEt	—

Overall Rates and Proportions of Olefin Elimination

	$10^5\,k_1$	$10^5\,k(\text{E1})$	% Olefin
t-Butyl	0.45	0.086	19.0
t-Amyl	1.09	0.396	36.3

Overall Orientation of Olefin Elimination

	$CH_3{\cdot}CH{:}C(CH_3)_2$	$CH_3{\cdot}CH_2{\cdot}C(CH_3){:}CH_2$
t-Amyl	82%	18%

This type of itemised analysis of rates and product proportions in E1 eliminations has been extended considerably further up the series of tertiary alkyl chlorides, *i.e.*, from *t*-butyl chloride upwards, with results pointing to continued dominating control by the electromeric effect.[34]

We noted in Section **39b** that steric hindrance plays only a restricted role in E2 eliminations. It has been shown[34] that steric hindrance takes no clearly discernible part in controlling olefin proportions in E1 eliminations. This unimportance of steric hindrance in elimination, relative to substitution, is doubtless due to the exposed situation of the proton which becomes lost from the system in eliminations.

A comparison of the proportions in which olefins are formed in the unimolecular reactions of secondary and tertiary alkyl halides or sulphonium ions shows, as Table 39-11 illustrates, that an extra α-bound methyl substituent strongly directs the completion of unimolecular processes towards elimination.[35]

[34] E. D. Hughes, C. K. Ingold, and V. J. Shiner jr., *J. Chem. Soc.*, **1953**, 3827.

[35] M. L. Dhar, E. D. Hughes, C. K. Ingold, A. M. M. Mandour, G. A. Maw, and L. I. Woolf, *J. Chem. Soc.*, **1948**, 2109.

TABLE 39-11.—PROPORTIONS OF OLEFIN FORMED IN UNIMOLECULAR REACTIONS OF SECONDARY AND TERTIARY ALKYL COMPOUNDS IN AQUEOUS ALCOHOL.

	Alkyl compound	Solvent	Temp.	Olefin
sec.-	Propyl bromide	"80%" aq.-EtOH	80°	4.6%
	Butyl bromide	"60%" aq.-EtOH	80°	8.5%
t-	Butyl chloride	"80%" aq.-EtOH	65°	36.3%
	Butyl dimethylsulphonium	"80%" aq.-EtOH	65°	35.7%
	Amyl chloride	"80%" aq.-EtOH	50°	40.3%
	Amyl dimethylsulphonium	"60%" aq.-EtOH	65°	39.8%
	Amyl dimethylsulphonium	"80%" aq.-EtOH	65°	49.4%
	Amyl dimethylsulphonium	"80%" aq.-EtOH	83°	53.4%

(39e) Dichotomy in Elimination: Combination of the Inductive and Electromeric Effects.—Originally, the Hofmann rule applied to eliminations from primary alkyl groups in ammonium ions, and the Saytzeff rule to eliminations from secondary and tertiary alkyl groups in halides, in all cases without reference to mechanism. It was not clear at first what determined the boundaries of the fields of application of the two rules, whether the alkyl structure, the displaced group, or the mechanism. As shown in the preceding Sections, it is not the alkyl structure, but it is the displaced group and the mechanism in conjunction: in bimolecular elimination 'onium ions follow the Hofmann rule and halides, except fluorides, the Saytzeff rule, while in unimolecular elimination all follow the Saytzeff rule.

The remarkable changes which can take place in the influence of structure on reaction rate, olefin proportion, and the orientation of elimination, when we cross the boundary between the domains of these two rules, are illustrated in Tables 39-12 and 39-13. They are concerned with the same two compounds, the *t*-butyl- and the *t*-amyl-dimethylsulphonium ions: all that changes from one table to the other is the reaction mechanism.[35,36] Table 39-12 refers to the bimolecular mechanism: although both the rates and the olefin proportions are given for elimination along the various alkyl branches, it is the rates which, in this mechanism, have the simpler relation to structure (so the proportions are put in parenthesis). One observes that the extra methyl residue in the higher homologue decreases rate of elimination in the long branch of the *t*-amyl group, but has little influence on rate in the shorter branches, as should be the case if the inductive effect is in control. The overall results of these individual changes are indicated at the foot of Table 39-12. Table 39-13 refers to the same reactions by the unimolecular mechanism: again both rates and olefin

[36] E. D. Hughes, C. K. Ingold, and L. I. Woolf, *J. Chem. Soc.*, 1948, 2084.

proportions are given, but now it is the proportions which bear the simpler relation to structure (so the rates are put in parenthesis). One now finds that the extra methyl residue increases the proportion of elimination in the long branch of the *t*-amyl group, and decreases the proportion in the shorter branches, as should happen if the electromeric effect is in control. In the final outcome of these changes, indicated at the foot of Table 39-13, one observes a qualitative reversal of every one of the structural effects found for the bimolecular mechanism.

TABLE 39-12.—ITEMISED RATES ILLUSTRATING THE DETERMINATION OF OVERALL RESULTS IN BIMOLECULAR OLEFIN FORMATION FROM ALKYLSULPHONIUM IONS.

Reactions of sulphonium ethoxides in "97%" ethyl alcohol at 24°. Rate constants k_2 and k(E2) in sec.$^{-1}$ mole^{-1} l.

$\underset{\beta}{C}{=}\underset{\alpha}{C}{-}CH \longleftarrow \underset{\beta}{CH}{-}\overset{\alpha}{\underset{|\ \overset{+}{S}Me_2}{C}}{-}\overset{\beta}{CH} \longrightarrow CH{-}\overset{\alpha}{C}{=}\overset{\beta}{C}$

Substituents β	Substituents α	Per branch % Olefin	Per branch k(E2) $\times 10^5$			Per branch k(E2) $\times 10^5$	Per branch % Olefin	Substituents α	Substituents β
					CH_3	27	(33)	Me_2	—
—	Me_2	(33)	27	$CH_3\cdot C(\overset{+}{S}Me_2)$					
					CH_3	27	(33)	Me_2	—
					CH_3	24	(41)	MeEt	—
Me	Me_2	(14)	8	$CH_3\cdot CH_2\cdot C(\overset{+}{S}Me_2)$					
					CH_3	24	(41)	MeEt	—

Overall Rates and Proportions (Bimolecular)

	$10^5\,k_2$	$10^5\,k$(E2)	% Olefin
t-Butyl....................	80	80	100
t-Amyl....................	58	56	96

Overall Orientation (Bimolecular)

	$CH_3\cdot CH{:}C(CH_3)_2$	$CH_3\cdot CH_2\cdot C(CH_3){:}CH_2$
t-Amyl....................	14%	86%

Olefin elimination from alkyl compounds, other than sulphonium ions and halides, have been classified, though on less secure experimental grounds, with respect to mechanism and orientation; and thus the conclusion has been generalised that either the inductive or the electromeric effect may secure a dominating influence over rate and orientation, depending on the elimination mechanism and the dis-

TABLE 39-13.—ITEMISED RATES ILLUSTRATING THE DETERMINATION OF OVERALL RESULTS IN UNIMOLECULAR OLEFIN FORMATION FROM ALKYLSULPHONIUM IONS.

Reactions of sulphonium iodides in "97%" ethyl alcohol at 50°. Rate constants k_1 and k(E1) in sec.$^{-1}$.

C=C—CH (β, α) ←				CH—C—CH (β, α, β); $\overset{+}{S}Me_2$ on α	→ CH—C=C (α, β)			
Substituents β	Substituents α	Per branch % Olefin	Per branch k(E1) ×10^5		Per branch k(E1) ×10^5	Per branch % Olefin	Substituents α	Substituents β
				CH_3	(0.30)	17	Me_2	—
—	Me_2	17	(0.30)	$CH_3 \cdot C(\overset{+}{S}Me_2)$				
				CH_3	(0.30)	17	Me_2	—
				CH_3	(0.63)	4	MeEt	—
Me	Me_2	56	(8.41)	$CH_3 \cdot CH_2 \cdot C(\overset{+}{S}Me_2)$				
				CH_3	(0.63)	4	MeEt	—

Overall Rates and Proportions (Unimolecular)

	$10^5\, k_1$	$10^5\, k$(E1)	% Olefin
t-Butyl..................................	1.8	0.9	51
t-Amyl..................................	15.0	9.7	64

Overall Orientation (Unimolecular)

	$CH_3 \cdot CH{:}C(CH_3)_2$	$CH_3 \cdot CH_2 \cdot C(CH_3){:}CH_2$
t-Amyl..................................	87%	13%

placed group in conjunction. The dichotomy[30,35] is apparently as follows:

Inductive control............. mechanism E2; X = $\overset{+}{N}R_3$, $\overset{+}{S}R_2$, $\overset{+}{O}H_2$, $\overset{+-}{S}O_2R$, $\overset{+-}{N}O_2$, F

Electromeric control.........
- mechanism E2; X = Cl, Br, I, OSO_2R, OCOR
- mechanism E1; X = $\overset{+}{S}R_2$, $\overset{+}{O}H_2$, Cl, Br, I, OSO_2R

Alkyl structure does not directly come into the matter, though it enters indirectly, because it affects rate by either mechanism, and therefore the relative importance of the mechanisms.

The observation of separate fields of control by the inductive and electromeric effects must mean that in general both effects are present, but that, owing to circumstances still to be discussed, either one or the other dominates. Some apparent indications of the modifying influence of a minor effect on a broad result determined by a major one were noticed in Sections **39b** and **39c.** However, in order to obtain decisive effects, it is better to go outside the field of alkyl groups, and examine, on the one hand, more polar groups, and, on the other, more unsaturated groups; for then one finds that, in the first case, inductive effects, and in the second, electromeric effects, which would have been masked in the corresponding alkyl compounds, secure a clear control.

A good example of polar control by definitely polar groups is provided by Saunders and Williams' measurements of the rates of bimolecular elimination E2, under the agency of ethoxide ions in ethanol, of some para-substituted 2-phenylethylsulphonium ions and bromides.[37] Some of these rate constants are in Table 39-14. Qualitatively, it is obvious from the series, starting with methoxyl and ending with nitroxyl, of groups in order of their influence on rate, that a polar effect is under observation. As follows from the spread of the figures for each series of substrates, the reactions of the sulphonium ions are more sensitive to polar effects than are the reactions of the bromides. Saunders and Williams made quantitative their test for a polar origin of these kinetic effects by comparing them with the thermodynamic effects of the same para-substituents on the acidity constants of phenols. For both inductively and hyperconjugatively transmitted polar effects, the kinetically acidic β-proton of the 2-arylethyl sulphonium ions and bromides has almost the same structural relation to the para-substituents as that of the thermodynamically acidic proton of phenols. This method of comparing polar effects in different reactions will be considered in a general way in Chapter XVI, but it will be enough to say here that an identical type of polar effect is well proved if the logarithms of the rate or equilibrium constants for one of the reactions compared plot linearly against the logarithms of the rate or equilibrium constants of the other. By this test, the para-substituents certainly influence the rates of the bimolecular eliminations by

TABLE 39-14.—RATE-CONSTANTS (k_2 IN SEC.$^{-1}$ MOL.$^{-1}$ L.) OF THE BIMOLECULAR ELIMINATIONS,

$$p\text{-R}\cdot C_6H_4\cdot CH_2\cdot CH_2\cdot X \xrightarrow{OEt^-} p\text{-R}\cdot C_6H_4\cdot CH{:}CH_2$$

WHEN $X = SMe_2^+$ AND Br, IN ETHANOL AT 30° (SAUNDERS AND WILLIAMS).

R	MeO	Me	H	Cl	CO·Me	NO$_2$
$X = SMe_2^+ (10^4k_2)$	11	23	50	244	—	—
$X = Br (10^5k_2)$	16	23	42	191	1720	75,200

[37] C. H. DePuy and D. H. Froemsdorf, *J. Am. Chem. Soc.*, 1957, **79,** 3710; W. H. Saunders jr. and R. A. Williams, *ibid.*, p. 3712.

just the same polar mechanisms as those by which they change the equilibrium acidity of a phenol.

As a complementary example, consider bimolecular eliminations from alkyl 'onium ions. With simple alkyl groups, they obey the Hofmann rule. But if we introduce, either into the α- or into the β-position of such an alkyl group, a substituent of low polarity and high unsaturation, such as phenyl, then the Hofmann rule becomes abrogated: thus styrene is formed in preference to ethylene.[21] And this is not essentially an inductive effect, due to polarity in the aromatic side-bond, because it works from either the α- or the β-position with qualitatively similar results: the second-order elimination rates[26,38] for ethyl-, 1-phenylethyl-, and 2-phenylethyl-dimethylsulphonium ethoxides in ethyl alcohol at 64° stand in the ratios:

ethyl = 1, 1-phenylethyl = 100, 2-phenylethyl = 430

The high rates for both phenyl compounds show that the strongly unsaturated phenyl substituent is giving control to the electromeric effect—as would certainly not have happened if the substituent had been an alkyl radical. Much the same occurs in bimolecular eliminations from alkyl bromides, though one might be more ready to expect a dominating influence of unsaturation in this series. The rates of bimolecular elimination from ethyl, 1-phenylethyl, and 2-phenylethyl bromides by reaction with ethoxide ions in ethanol at 55° are approximately[34] in the ratios,

ethyl 1, 1-phenylethyl 35, 2-phenylethyl 350

One sees that, in olefin-forming elimination, as in any other heterolytic reaction, polarity and unsaturation play their roles, and do so by the inductive and conjugative modes of electron displacement, as the structure of the system allows. One sees also that the polarisation and polarisability of the system co-operate, but that, since unsaturation is being created in the reaction, the conjugative mode of electron displacement becomes more freely permitted during the formation of the transition state, and therefore takes the form of a polarisability effect, *viz.*, an electromeric effect. Thus it is clear that, when the influencing groups have a definite polarity or a definite unsaturation, they will exert an inductive or an electromeric effect, according to their nature, and that to speak of Hofmann-Saytzeff dichotomy in these circumstances is meaningless.

The Hofmann and Saytzeff rules, even in generalised form, apply only to simple, unsubstituted, saturated, alkyl groups—a very small

[38] E. D. Hughes, C. K. Ingold, and G. A. Maw, *J. Chem. Soc.*, **1948**, 2072.

sector of the range of groups in whose influence on elimination we are interested. They apply in this restricted area, because alkyl groups are unique among organic groups in being inherently destitute of those general properties of polarity and unsaturation on which the orientation and rate of elimination depend. They have practically no inherent polarity, but only a potential polarity actualised by induction from some polar group. They have no inherent unsaturation, but only a latent unsaturation activated by hyperconjugation with some unsaturated group. The antithetical rules apply to alkyl groups, because they have no properties with which to influence the elimination system, apart from the properties induced in them by the system itself. That is why it is the system which determines what they do. Polarity and the Hofmann rule will dominate when the end-group is an ionic centre or is otherwise very strongly electronegative, and when not too much unsaturation is developed too early in an E2 mechanism. Hyperconjugation and the Saytzeff rule will dominate, when the end-group is less polar, and when a large fraction of one electron is lost to the departing group in the transition state of an E2 mechanism. Hyperconjugation and the Saytzeff rule will dominate still more, when the whole of one electron is lost, before product formation begins, as it is in any E1 mechanism.

(40) ENVIRONMENTAL EFFECTS ON RATES AND PRODUCTS OF 1,2-ELIMINATION

(40a) Environmental Effects on Mechanism.—The early literature of olefin elimination is very confused, essentially for the reason that duality of mechanism was not understood. One of the questions to which considerable attention was paid was that of the proportions in which a basic reagent, acting on different alkyl halides, produces olefins. Nef obtained[39] more olefin in fixed conditions from tertiary alkyl halides than from secondary, and more from these than from primary: the order was *prim.* < *sec.* < *tert.* Brussoff's nearly simultaneous investigation[40] gave the contrary result that olefins were produced in greater proportion from secondary than from tertiary halides: *sec.* > *tert.* Segaller[41] subsequently reproduced the sequence, *sec.* < *tert.* Much later, one investigator set himself to decide between the two sequences, having assumed unjustifiably that both could not be right. Still later[30,42] the apparent discrepancies were reconciled, as follows.

[39] J. U. Nef, *Ann.*, 1899, **309**, 126; 1901, **318**, 1.

[40] S. Brussoff, *Z. physik. Chem.*, 1900, **34**, 129.

[41] D. Segaller, *J. Chem. Soc.*, 1913, **103**, 1421.

[42] E. D. Hughes, C. K. Ingold, S. Masterman, and B. J. MacNulty, *J. Chem. Soc.*, 1940, 899.

We have already noticed that, for any one mechanism of elimination, either E2 or E1, the proportion of olefin formed from simple alkyl compounds rises along the series *prim.*<*sec.*<*tert.* (because of the accelerating effect of an α-alkyl branch on αβ-double-bond formation). It is also apparent in the figures that for any type of alkyl group the proportion of olefin rises from the E1 to the E2 mechanism. Again it is true, and should be expected, that within the E2 mechanism the proportion of olefin rises with the basic strength of the reagent which extracts the β-proton. When, as we either increase the concentration of the reagent, or increase the basicity of the reagent, or decrease the ionising power of the solvent for an alkyl halide, the mechanism goes over from E1 to E2, it will do so at different points in these progressive changes for primary, secondary, and tertiary alkyl halides. With primary halides the mechanism may be already E2 before the progressive change begins, with secondary halides the change to E2 will occur at a relatively early stage, and with tertiary halides it will occur at a later stage. So there will be a certain range of any one of these environmental variables in which the secondary halide is using the E2 mechanism, while the tertiary is using the E1 mechanism. If the reagent is a strong base, such as hydroxide or ethoxide ions, the secondary halide will be giving more olefin than the tertiary halide. These were the conditions in Brussoff's work in aqueous ethanol. Nef's reagent was ethoxide ions in dry ethanol, towards which all his substrates act by the E2 mechanism. Segaller, and also Mereshkowsky,[43] employed the relatively weakly basic reagents, phenoxide ion, and acetate ion.

(40b) Solvent Effects on Rates and Products for Fixed Reaction Mechanisms.[30,44]—In Section **29a**, a theoretical treatment of kinetic solvent effects was outlined, and the results of its application to bimolecular and unimolecular nucleophilic substitution were compared with observational data. In this Section, we shall apply the same theory to bimolecular and unimolecular olefin elimination, and compare the conclusions with experiment.

As observed in Section **38**, nucleophilic substitutions and eliminations are closely parallel in mechanism. In the two bimolecular reactions, the electron transfers from reagent to expelled group are similar, but pass through a longer chain of atoms in elimination than in substitution. The two unimolecular reactions have a common rate-controlling stage; and the succeeding fast stages are similar, except

[43] B. K. Mereshkowsky, *Ann.*, 1923, **431**, 231.

[44] K. A. Cooper, M. L. Dhar, E. D. Hughes, C. K. Ingold, B. J. MacNulty, and L. I. Woolf, *J. Chem. Soc.*, **1948**, 2043.

TABLE 40-1.—CHARGE-TYPES OF OLEFIN ELIMINATION.

Type 1:—Initially, proton-acceptor negative, displaced group neutral.

Example:—$\bar{O}H + H \cdot CH_2 \cdot CHMe \cdot Br \rightarrow H_2O + CH_2{:}CHMe + \bar{B}r$

Type 2:—Initially, proton-acceptor neutral, displaced group neutral.

Example:—$HOEt + H \cdot CH_2 \cdot CMe_2 \cdot Cl \rightarrow H_2\overset{+}{O}Et + CH_2{:}CMe_2 + \bar{C}l$

Type 3:—Initially, proton-acceptor negative, displaced group positive.

Example:—$\bar{O}Et + H \cdot CHMe \cdot CMe_2 \cdot \overset{+}{S}Me_2 \rightarrow HOEt + CHMe{:}CMe_2 + SMe_2$

Type 4:—Initially, proton-acceptor neutral, displaced group positive.

Example:—$H_2O + H \cdot CHAr \cdot CH_2 \cdot \overset{+}{N}Me_3 \rightarrow H_3\overset{+}{O} + CHAr{:}CH_2 + NMe_3$

that the electron transfer involves a larger number of atoms in elimination than in substitution.

As before, we commence by classifying the reactions to be considered into four charge-types, as shown in Table 40-1. It is true of eliminations and substitutions alike, that the similarities between the four types are much more important than their differences; but kinetic behaviour with respect to solvent changes happens to be one of the ways in which, for either reaction, the four types differ.

The theory to be applied assumes that kinetic solvent effects arise mainly from differences in the solvation energy of the initial and transition states, such differences influencing the activation energy. It assumes also that the solvation of any state depends on the electric charges in that state, increasing with the amount of any charge, and decreasing with the wider distribution of a charge, all effects of charge magnitude being more important than those of distribution. Finally, it assumes that the solvating power of any solvent increases with its electric dipole moment, but decreases with increased shielding of the dipole charges, so that, for instance, the solvents, H_2O, EtOH, Me_2CO, C_6H_6, are in order of diminishing solvating power.

The application of these arguments to the bimolecular reactions is indicated in the uppermost part of Table 40-2. What happens to the charges on activation is shown in the middle three columns, while the kinetic deductions are in the last column but one. For the purpose of predicting solvent effects on the rate only of bimolecular elimination, only the entries against reaction E2 are needed. But in order to predict, as far as may be, how solvent changes affect the proportion in which the total bimolecular reaction gives olefin, one must consider the

TABLE 40-2.—PREDICTED SOLVENT EFFECTS ON RATES AND PROPORTIONS OF OLEFIN FORMED IN BIMOLECULAR AND UNIMOLECULAR ELIMINATIONS.

Charge-type	Reac.	Disposition of charges: Initial state	Disposition of charges: Transition state	Effect of activation on charges	Effect of more solvation: On rate	Effect of more solvation: Olefin propn.
			Bimolecular Mechanism: Rates and Proportions			
1	S_N2	$\bar{Y}+RX$	$\overset{\delta-}{Y}\cdots R\cdots\overset{\delta-}{X}$	Dispersed	Small decrease	Small decrease
	E2	$\bar{Y}+RX$	$\overset{\delta-}{Y}\cdots H\cdots C{=}C\cdots\overset{\delta-}{X}$			
2	S_N2	$Y+RX$	$\overset{\delta+}{Y}\cdots R\cdots\overset{\delta-}{X}$	Increased	Large increase	?
	E2	$Y+RX$	$\overset{\delta+}{Y}\cdots H\cdots C{=}C\cdots\overset{\delta-}{X}$			
3	S_N2	$\bar{Y}+R\overset{+}{X}$	$\overset{\delta-}{Y}\cdots R\cdots\overset{\delta+}{X}$	Reduced	Large decrease	?
	E2	$\bar{Y}+R\overset{+}{X}$	$\overset{\delta-}{Y}\cdots H\cdots C{=}C\cdots\overset{\delta+}{X}$			
4	S_N2	$Y+R\overset{+}{X}$	$\overset{\delta+}{Y}\cdots R\cdots\overset{\delta+}{X}$	Dispersed	Small decrease	Small decrease
	E2	$Y+R\overset{+}{X}$	$\overset{\delta+}{Y}\cdots H\cdots C{=}C\cdots\overset{\delta+}{X}$			
			Unimolecular Mechanism: Rates			
1, 2	S_N1 +E1	RX	$\overset{\delta+}{R}\cdots\overset{\delta-}{X}$	Increased	Large increase	—
3, 4	S_N1 +E1	$R\overset{+}{X}$	$\overset{\delta+}{R}\cdots\overset{\delta+}{X}$	Dispersed	Small decrease	—
			Unimolecular Mechanism: Proportions			
1, 3	S_N1	$\bar{Y}+\overset{+}{R}$	$\overset{\delta-}{Y}\cdots\overset{\delta+}{R}$	Reduced	—	?
	E1	$\bar{Y}+\overset{+}{R}$	$\overset{\delta-}{Y}\cdots H\cdots C{=}\overset{\delta+}{C}$			
2, 4	S_N1	$Y+\overset{+}{R}$	$\overset{\delta+}{Y}\cdots\overset{\delta+}{R}$	Dispersed	—	Small decrease
	E1	$Y+\overset{+}{R}$	$\overset{\delta+}{Y}\cdots H\cdots C{=}\overset{\delta+}{C}$			

kinetic deductions for the reactions S_N2 and E2 differentially; and this is why the entries for reaction S_N2 are included in the table. The theoretical difference is always that a charge is more widely dispersed in the transition state of elimination than in that of substitution. From this it follows, provided that the magnitude of the charges on the two transition states can be shown to be the same, as in reactions of charge-types 1 and 4, that the difference of dispersal will cause the predicted kinetic effect to be quantitatively greater for elimination than for substitution. This deduction leads finally to a conclusion about solvent effect on the proportion in which olefin is formed, as shown in the last column of the table. The words "large" and "small" in the last two columns reflect the argument that effects due to charge magnitude are likely to be more important than those due to charge distribution.

The corresponding argument for unimolecular reactions is outlined in the lower two parts of the table. The first of these refers to solvent effects on the rate of the total unimolecular reaction, S_N1+E1, that is, on the rate of the primary heterolysis. Thus it is the transition state of this process which here has to be considered. Discussion of solvent effects on the proportion of formed olefin proceeds, as is indicated in the last part of the table, by a differential consideration of solvent effects on the rates of the immeasurably fast processes, which complete the reactions S_N1 and E1. Thus it is the transition states of these fast processes which now are relevant. Their important differential feature is the greater dispersal of charge in the transition state of the fast stage of elimination. Provided that the magnitudes of the charges on these two transition states are identical, as in reactions of charge-types 2 and 4, this difference of charge dispersal, will, as before, permit a deduction to be made concerning solvent effects on the proportions in which olefin is produced.

TABLE 40-3.—OBSERVED SOLVENT EFFECTS ON RATES OF BIMOLECULAR ELIMINATION (E2).

Type	Example[1]	Rate[2] const.	Vol. % H_2O						Predicted effect
			0	10	20	30	40	100	
1	$\bar{O}H + i\text{-}PrBr$	$10^4\ k_2^{55°}$	1.46	—	0.71	—	0.47	—	Small decrease
3	$\bar{O}H + Et_2\overset{+}{S}$	$10^5\ k_2^{100°}$	—	—	2050	—	210	2.4	Large decrease
4	$H_2O + Ar(CH_2)_2\overset{+}{N}Me_3$	$10^4\ k_1^{100°}$	—	2.10	—	1.40	—	0.39	Small decrease

[1] The reactions of types 1 and 3 were conducted in aqueous ethyl alcohol and that of type 4, where $Ar = p\text{-}NO_2 \cdot C_6H_4$, in aqueous n-propyl alcohol.

[2] Second-order rate constants k_2 are in sec.$^{-1}$ mole^{-1} l., and first-order constants, k_1, are in sec.$^{-1}$. The figures are taken from tables in reference 44.

Some observed effects of solvent changes on rates of bimolecular eliminations, E2, are given in Table 40-3. The solvents are mixtures of either ethyl, or *n*-propyl alcohol, and water, mixtures in which water is, of course, the more polar solvent-component. The reactions of charge-types 1 and 3 are proved to be bimolecular by their kinetic order, and the figures tabulated are second-order rate constants. The reaction of charge-type 4 is solvolytic, and therefore the figures tabulated are first-order rate constants; but the reaction was believed to be bimolecular, because of the great sensitivity of the rate to weak bases, and this conclusion has been confirmed by the large reduction of rate which is observed when tritium is the hydrogen that has to be attacked.[45] In the last column of the table, the qualitative predictions are repeated for comparison with the data. The observed effects are in the expected directions; and corresponding to the predicted distinction between "large" and "small" effects, the figures either change by factors ranging over thousands, or alter by a few units-fold only, over the complete range of solvent composition.

The results of a similar test of the theoretically predicted solvent

TABLE 40-4.—OBSERVED SOLVENT EFFECTS ON THE PROPORTION OF OLEFIN FORMED IN BIMOLECULAR AND UNIMOLECULAR ELIMINATIONS.

Type	Example[1]	% H_2O in aqueous EtOH				Predicted effect
		0	20	40	100	
		Bimolecular Mechanism				
1	$\bar{O}H + i\text{-}PrBr$ (55°)	71%	59%	54%	—	Small decrease
3	$\bar{O}H + Et_3\overset{+}{S}$ (100°)	—	100%	100%	86%	?
		Unimolecular Mechanism				
2	*t*-ButylBr (25°)	19.0%	12.6%	—	—	Small decrease
	t-AmylCl (25°)	—	33.0%	25.7%	—	
	t-AmylBr (25°)	36.3%	26.2%	—	—	
4	*t*-Amyl$\overset{+}{S}Me_2$ (50°)	64.4%	47.8%	—	—	Small decrease
	t-Amyl$\overset{+}{S}Me_2$ (65°)	—	49.4%	39.8%	—	

1 The figures are from tables given in reference 44.

45 E. M. Hodnett and J. J. Flynn jr., *J. Am. Chem Soc.*, 1957, **79**, 2300.

effects on total rate by the unimolecular mechanism, that is, on the total rate, S_N1+E1, have already been included in Table 29-4 (p. 262). Again the direction of the effect is always correct; and again predicted "large" increases of rate from alcohol to water are realised as increases by factors of thousands, while predicted "small" decreases appear as decreases by factors of a few units.

The available evidence concerning the effect of the composition of alcohol-water mixtures on the proportions of olefin in bimolecular and unimolecular reactions of alkyl halides and 'onium ions is assembled in Table 40-4. The universal effect appears to be that of a moderate drop in proportion of olefin as the solvent becomes more aqueous. This agrees with theoretical predictions where these are definite. For comparison with the data, the theoretical predictions are reproduced in the last column of the table.

(40c) Effects of Temperature on Rates and Olefin Proportions.[46]— The known activation energies of bimolecular eliminations from alkyl chlorides, bromides, and iodides, by reaction with hydroxide or ethoxide ions in aqueous or dry ethanol are mostly in the range 20–24 kcal./mole, whilst for alkyl-dimethylsulphonium ions, the corresponding figures are somewhat higher, usually around 24–26 kcal./mole. With remarkable regularity, the activation energy of an E2-elimination, for any substrate in any solvent within the range described, is 2 ± 1 kcal./mole greater than the activation energy of the accompanying S_N2 substitution. This means that the higher the temperature, the higher is the proportion of olefin formed. Thus *iso*propyl bromide, in its bimolecular reactions with the lyate ions of "60%" aqueous ethanol, gives 53% of propylene at 45°, but 64% of propylene at 100°: this is a typical effect of temperature.

As a tentative interpretation, we can say for the reactions of the alkyl halides, as we did say in explanation of the solvent effect in their product proportions, that the unit of charge in the transition state of E2 elimination is spread over a greater number of atoms than in the transition state of the accompanying S_N2 substitution, wherefore the transition state of elimination will be the less strongly solvated, and a larger activation energy will be required to reach it, than to reach the transition state of the substitution. We cannot apply a corresponding argument to the reactions of alkyl sulphonium ions, because the amounts of charge retained in the transition states of elimination and substitution may not be the same. But we know empirically that the solvent effect on olefin proportion is qualitatively similar for halides

[46] K. A. Cooper, E. D. Hughes, C. K. Ingold, G. A. Maw, and B. J. MacNulty, *J. Chem. Soc.*, 1948, 2049.

and sulphonium ions, and so, if temperature effects on product proportions really are controlled by solvation, we might reasonably expect again to find, as indeed we do, qualitatively similar effects in the reactions of alkyl halides and sulphonium ions.

In unimolecular eliminations and substitutions, measured activation energies are of the initial slow step, common to the two reactions. For *t*-alkyl chlorides and bromides in dry or aqueous ethanol, the known unimolecular activation energies are mostly in the range 22–24 kcal./mole. For *t*-alkyl sulphonium ions they are strikingly larger, about 31–33 kcal./mole. This is almost certainly due to strong solvation of the ionic centre in the initial state of the sulphonium ions. The reason why so large a difference does not appear in the activation energies for either bimolecular elimination, or bimolecular substitution, of alkyl halides and sulphonium ions may well be that, in the bimolecular reactions, a large part of the extra de-solvation energy needed by the sulphonium ions is supplied by the coulombic energy of approach of the anionic reagent. Support for an interpretation based on solvation can be found in the circumstance that, in the unimolecular substitution discussed in Section **28b**, of alkyl bromides containing α-carboxylate-ion substituents, in water or aqueous ethanol solvents, activation energies, which would be 22–24 kcal./mole if the α-carboxylate-ion substituent were replaced by α-methyl substituents, are raised to about 29–33 kcal./mole.[47]

In unimolecular reactions, the proportions of olefin are determined by the relative rates of the alternative fast steps of decomposition of the carbonium ion. The observation is that, for all substrates which undergo concurrent unimolecular elimination and substitution, a rise of temperature increases the proportion in which olefin is formed. Thus, *t*-butyl bromide, on solvolysis in dry ethanol, gives 19% of *iso*butylene at 25°, but 28% at 55°, and the *t*-amyl-dimethylsulphonium ion, on solvolysis in "80%" aqueous ethanol, gives 48% of amylenes at 50°, but 54% at 83°. Though we cannot measure the activation energies of the fast processes which determine these product ratios, a survey of the ratios, in their dependence on temperature, shows that the activation energy of the process which completes an elimination must always be higher by 2 ± 1 kcal/mole than that of the process which completes the concurrent substitution.

These are fast reactions of the pre-formed carbonium ion, and the tentative interpretation of the differential temperature effect is that, in the transition state of the reaction that completes an elimination,

[47] E. D. Hughes, and N. A. Taher, *J. Chem. Soc.*, **1940**, 956; J. Gripenberg, E. D. Hughes, and C. K. Ingold, *Nature*, **1948**, **161**, 480.

the unit of positive charge is spread over a greater number of atoms, so leading to an energy less reduced by solvation, than in the transition state of the reaction that completes the concurrent substitution.

(41) STERIC COURSE OF 1,2-ELIMINATIONS

(41a) Steric Course of Acetylene-forming Eliminations.—The older literature of elimination contains several observations indicating the existence of stereo-chemically favourable and unfavourable situations for elimination in olefinic compounds. Michael[48] found that chlorofumaric acid is converted by alkali about 50 times faster than is chloromaleic acid into acetylene-dicarboxylic acid; and Chavanne[49] observed that *cis*-dichloroethylene is transformed about 20 times faster than is the *trans*-isomer by alkali into chloroacetylene:

$$\begin{array}{c} {}^-O_2C-C-Cl \\ \| \\ H-C-CO_2^- \end{array} \xrightarrow[50]{OH^-} {}^-CO_2\cdot C{\vdots}C\cdot CO_2^- \xleftarrow[1]{OH^-} \begin{array}{c} Cl-C-CO_2^- \\ \| \\ H-C-CO_2^- \end{array}$$

$$\begin{array}{c} H-C-Cl \\ \| \\ H-C-Cl \end{array} \xrightarrow[20]{OH^-} HC{\vdots}CCl \xleftarrow[1]{OH^-} \begin{array}{c} Cl-C-H \\ \| \\ H-C-Cl \end{array}$$

Further examples have more recently been provided by Cristol and his coworkers.[50] One of them is that *cis*-*p*-nitrostyryl bromide, in the presence of ethanolic sodium ethoxide, undergoes elimination 2300 times faster than the *trans*-isomer undergoes an alternative reaction of addition:

$$\begin{array}{r} p\text{-}NO_2\cdot C_6H_4-C-H \\ \| \\ Br-C-H \end{array} \xrightarrow{OEt^-} p\text{-}NO_2\cdot C_6H_4-C{\equiv}C-H$$

$$\begin{array}{r} p\text{-}NO_2\cdot C_6H_4-C-H \\ \| \\ H-C-Br \end{array} \xrightarrow{OEt^-} p\text{-}NO_2\cdot C_6H_4-CH_2-CH(OEt)_2$$

Evidently, *trans*-elimination, that is, elimination of *trans*-situated hydrogen and halogen, is favoured over *cis*-elimination, sometimes relatively slightly, but sometimes in a practically extensive way. We may recall Modena's demonstration (Section **35a**) that *cis*-β-arene-

[48] A. Michael, *J. prakt. Chem.*, 1895, **52**, 308.

[49] G. Chavanne, *Bull. soc. chim.* (Belges), 1912, **26**, 287.

[50] S. J. Cristol, A. Begoon, W. P. Norris, and P. S. Ranly, *J. Am. Chem. Soc.*, 1954, **76**, 4558.

sulphonylvinyl chlorides undergo nucleophilic substitution of the halogen by methoxide ion by way of an E2 *trans*-elimination to an acetylene derivative, followed by a *trans*-addition,

$$\begin{matrix} ArSO_2\text{—C—H} \\ \| \\ \text{Cl—C—H} \end{matrix} \rightarrow ArSO_2\text{—C}\equiv\text{C—H} \rightarrow \begin{matrix} ArSO_2\text{—C—H} \\ \| \\ \text{MeO—C—H} \end{matrix}$$

whereas the corresponding group replacement in *trans*-β-arenesulphonylvinyl chlorides can proceed only as a direct S_N2 substitution.

All these reactions make clear that *trans*-elimination is stereochemically favoured, although it appears that *cis*-elimination can occur. It was pointed out in 1948 that a heterolytic elimination involves[34] an internal S_N2-type substitution at the α-carbon atom, which will be restricted by the exclusion principle to receiving the new electron-pair on the side remote from that from which the old electron-pair becomes expelled (Section **33**). Concerted with this process, there is an S_E2-type substitution at the β-carbon atom. Such a substitution is not expected to be stereochemically restricted by any adamantine principle. However, the changing electron-pair in substitutions of this type is usually observed to exchange nuclei with retention of configuration (Section **36**), a behaviour which, in the concerted reaction, leads to *trans*-elimination, as shown below. If, however, in the transition state, the changing electrons were sufficiently released by the departing proton to allow their passage through the α-carbon atom, then their entry by substitution into the β-carbon atom would produce a *cis*-elimination as illustrated:[51]

trans-Elimination

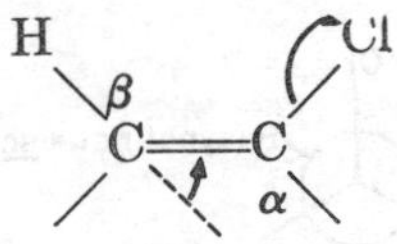

cis-Elimination

(41b) Steric Course of Olefin-forming Eliminations.—The stereochemical dependence of elimination from an alkyl derivative will be one on conformation. We shall now have either antiperiplanar (*ap*) elimination as the norm when the bond changes of the E2 mechanism are so synchronised that the proton transfer is not excessively advanced in the transition state, or synperiplanar (*sp*) elimination when the

[51] C. K. Ingold, *Proc. Chem. Soc.*, 1962, 265; cf. H. B. Charman, E. D. Hughes, and C. K. Ingold, *J. Chem. Soc.*, 1959, 1523, 1530.

proton transfer of the E2 mechanism is sufficiently far advanced in the transition state:[51]

ap-Elimination

sp-Elimination

In the normal staggered conformation of atoms about an alkane bond, an antiperiplanar (*ap*) conformation of the atoms to be eliminated allows an antiperiplanar elimination. And it is expected to be favoured, because it combines the normal stereochemical course of an S_E2 substitution with the inevitable stereochemical course of an S_N2 substitution.[34,51] The alternative possible conformation of the groups to be eliminated is the synclinal (*sc*) conformation. This is poorly adjusted even to that synperiplanar (*sp*) conformation which would allow normally the less favoured synperiplanar elimination. We therefore expect that a staggered overall conformation will lead to a strong preference for antiperiplanar elimination. In case the overall conformation were eclipsed (owing to some special cause), the eliminated atoms either would be anticlinal (*ac*), poorly adjusted to the normally stereochemically best *ap*-form of elimination, or they would be synperiplanar (*sp*), well adjusted to the normally stereochemically second-best *sp*-form of elimination. We therefore expect only a small preference (either way) between these two forms of elimination:

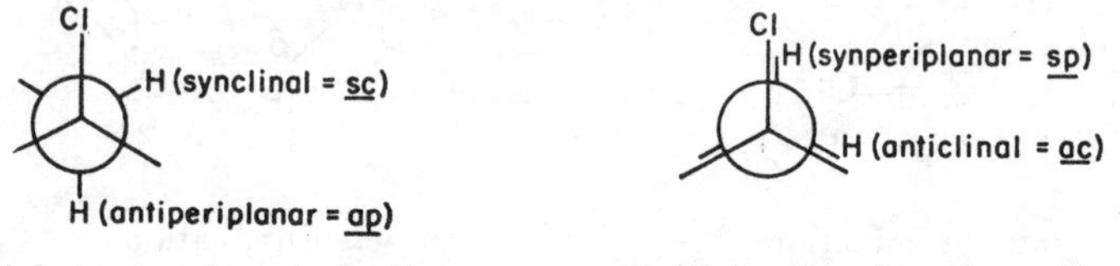

Cl
H (synclinal = sc)
H (antiperiplanar = ap)

Initial staggered conformations

Cl
H (synperiplanar = sp)
H (anticlinal = ac)

Initial eclipsed conformations

In *cyclo*alkanes, conformational and geometrical specifications are interlinked. In simple *cyclo*hexanes, in which the chair form is the most stable overall conformation, all ring bonds have staggered conformations, the exocyclic bonds therefore comprising two sets, *viz.*, the axial bonds (*a*) and equatorial bonds (*e*). A 1,2-*trans*-pair of such bonds may be either antiperiplanar (*ap*), or synclinal (*sc*), the former if both bonds are axial (*a*), and the latter if both are equatorial (*e*), as shown below. A 1,2-*cis*-pair must have one bond axial and the other equatorial, and therefore will inevitably be synclinal (*sc*), as shown. In a simple *cyclo*pentane ring, on the other hand, to the extent to which it may be taken as approximately planar, the ring bonds will have approximately eclipsed conformations, and a 1,2-*trans*-pair of bonds will therefore be anticlinal (*ac*), whilst a 1,2-*cis*-pair will be approximately synperiplanar (*sp*). And so, whereas in simple *cyclo*hexane derivatives we expect strongly favoured *trans*-elimination, provided that the eliminated atoms are in, or can easily get into, axial position, in simple *cyclo*pentane derivatives we expect small preferences between *trans*- and *cis*-elimination.

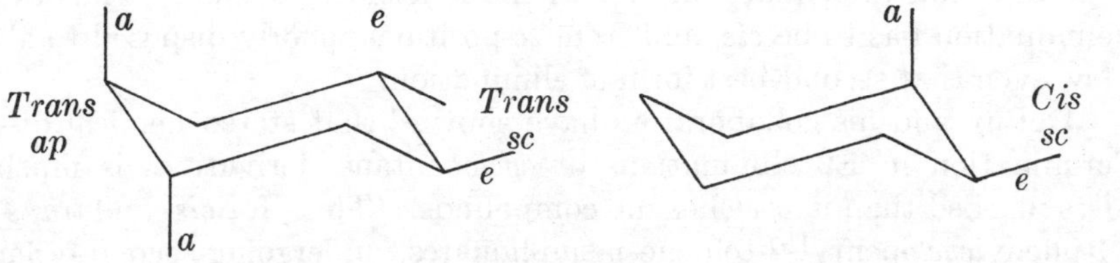

a *e* *a*
Trans *ap* *Trans* *sc* *e* *Cis* *sc* *e*
a

Two *trans*-conformations of *cyclo*hexane A *cis*-conformation of *cyclo*hexane

One of the simplest available illustrations of the great difference in the ease of E2 eliminations of *cis*- and *trans*-related pairs of atoms in *cyclo*hexane derivatives is presented by the benzenehexachlorides. They are known in several stereoisomeric forms, all of which undergo alkaline dehydrochlorination in three stages to form trichlorobenzenes.[52] For some of the isomers, the first step of dehydrochlorination is the only one which is measurably slow, whilst for others, the first two steps are both measurably slow. All the measured reaction steps of elimination have second-order kinetics, and, as Table 41-1 shows, all have activation energies in the region 19–21 kcal./mole except one. This is the first step of reaction of the β-isomer, whose much slower reaction has an activation energy of 32 kcal./mole. When this was observed in 1947, the first thought was that a different mechanism was in operation; but it has not proved possible to demonstrate any such change of mechanism, and the phenomenon has a stereochemical explanation. The configurations of the various stereoisomers of benzenehexachlorides are indicated, under their Greek-letter names in Table 41-1, by numbering the *cis*-assembly of chlorine atoms occupying one side of the *cyclo*hexane ring. One sees that the trigonal β-isomer

[52] S. J. Cristol, *J. Am. Chem. Soc.*, 1947, **69**, 338; E. D. Hughes, C. K. Ingold, and R. Pasternak, *J. Chem. Soc.*, **1953**, 3832.

TABLE 41-1.—ARRHENIUS ENERGIES OF ACTIVATION (IN KCAL./MOLE) OF THE SECOND-ORDER ALKALINE DEHYDROCHLORINATIONS OF BENZENE HEXACHLORIDES IN AQUEOUS ETHYL ALCOHOL.

Isomer	α	β	γ		δ		ε
Structure: *cis*-Cl's	1:2:4	1:3:5	1:4		1:3		1:2:3
Reaction stage	1st	1st	1st	2nd	1st	2nd	1st
90% EtOH (Pasternak)	19.0	32.3	20.4	20.1	21.6	21.1	—
80% EtOH (Cristol)	18.5	31.0	(20.6)		—	—	21.4

is the only one with all 1,2-HCl atom-pairs *cis*. Conformationally, all the Cl atoms are equatorial and all the H atoms are axial. Thus the elimination has to be *cis*, and from *sc*-positions, poorly disposed to allow even that second-best form of elimination.

DePuy and his collaborators have shown[53] that stereochemical discrimination in E2 eliminations of *cyclo*pentane derivatives is much less marked than in *cyclo*hexane compounds. Thus, for *cis*- and *trans*-1-phenyl*cyclo*pentyl 2-toluene-*p*-sulphonates, undergoing second-order reactions with *t*-butoxide ion in *t*-butyl alcohol,

H, Ph / OTs, H —(t-Bu⁻, 1)→ [1-Ph, 2] ←(t-Bu⁻, 14)— H, Ph / H, OTs

trans-elimination from the *cis*-isomer is only about 14 times faster than *cis*-elimination from the *trans*-isomer. The rate ratio for corresponding reactions of *cyclo*hexane substrates would be about 10^4. Such a difference of specificity would be expected for the E2 mechanism from the conformational considerations outlined above. DePuy and his coworkers have made it clear that both the *trans*- and the *cis*-eliminations use the E2 mechanism.

Sicher and his collaborators[54] have described examples in the *cyclo*decane series in which *anti*-elimination, that is, some approximation to the theoretically best *ap*-elimination, and *syn*-elimination, again

[53] C. H. DePuy, R. D. Thurn, and G. F. Morris, *J. Am. Chem. Soc.*, 1962, **84**, 1314; C. H. DePuy, G. F. Morris, J. S. Smith, and R. J. Stuart, *ibid.*, 1965, **87**, 242.

[54] J. Závada and J. Sicher, *Proc. Chem. Soc.*, **1963**, 96; J. Závada, M. Svoboda, and J. Sicher, *Tetrahedron Letters*, **1966**, 1627; J. Závada, J. Krupička, and J. Sicher, *Chem. Comm.*, **1967**, 66; M. Pánková, J. Sicher, and J. Závada, *ibid.*, p. 394.

some approximation to *sp*-elimination, occur side by side, and either to a comparable degree, or with *syn*-elimination proponderating over *anti*- by factors up to ten. The examples were the reactions of 1,1,4,4,-tetramethyl*cyclo*decane 7-toluene-*p*-sulphonate with potassium *t*-butoxide in dimethylformamide, which gave comparable amounts of the two forms of elimination, and that of the corresponding 7-trimethylammonium ion with methoxide ions in methanol, the reaction which gave an excess of *syn*-elimination. The products of either reaction were the *cis*- and *trans*-6,7-olefins and the *cis*-and *trans*-7,8-olefins:

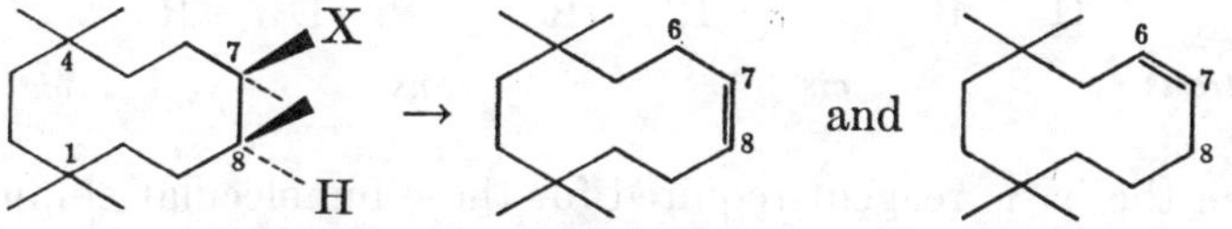

4 7 X 1 8 H → 6 7 8 and 6 7 8

cis and *trans* *cis* and *trans*

By deuterium-labelling alternatively in the *cis*- and *trans*-8-positions, it was shown that the hydrogen atom eliminated to form the 7,8-ene was always *trans* to the eliminated group X, *i.e.*, it was the hydrogen atom written as H above. It follows that the *cis*-olefin is formed by *anti*-elimination, and that the *trans*-olefin is formed, after a conformational twist, by *syn*-elimination. And from the ammonium ion, *syn*-elimination to form the *trans*-7,8-olefin is preferred by a rate factor of about ten over *anti*-elimination to give the *cis*-7,8-olefin.

Sicher and his coworkers have extended this demonstration to the acyclic series, as is important, because the already-mentioned demonstrations of the steric course of olefin-forming eliminations have all been in the alicyclic series.[54] The questions to be answered were whether, in bimolecular elimination from RHC(X)—C(H)HR′, the atoms (H) and (X) eliminated are conformationally *syn* or *anti*, and, in either case, which olefin, *cis* or *trans*, is formed. In the example studied, X was NMe_3^+, R was *neo*pentyl, and R′ was *n*-butyl; and either of the individually expressed hydrogen atoms of the group —C(H)HR′ was stereospecifically replaced by deuterium, to give the *threo*- and *erythro*-monodeutero-derivatives, which were the substrates for the elimination experiments. It can be followed from the formulae below that, if it is true that *trans*-olefin arises by *syn*-elimination and *cis*-olefin by *anti*-elimination, then the *threo*-isomer should lose deuterium when forming both the *cis*- and the *trans*-olefin, whilst the erythro-isomer should retain deuterium when forming both the *cis*- and the *trans*-olefin. This is essentially what happened:

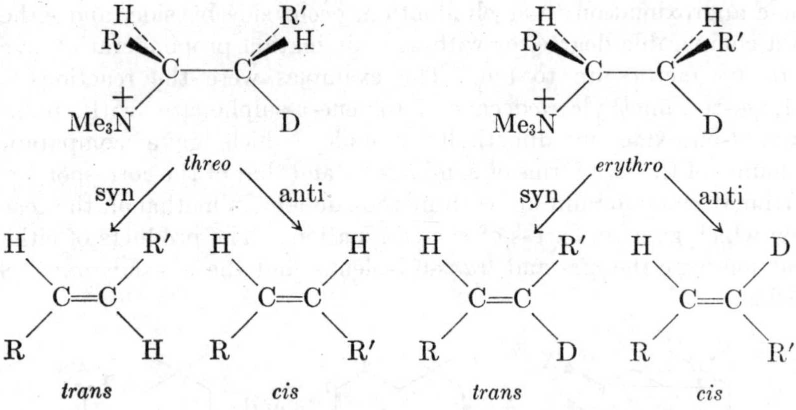

threo: syn → trans; anti → cis

erythro: syn → trans; anti → cis

When the basic reagent required for these bimolecular eliminations was methoxide ion in methyl alcohol, the quantities of *syn*-elimination to give *trans*-olefin and of *anti*-elimination to give *cis*-olefin were comparable, their ratio being about 5:4 from the *threo*-ammonium ion, and about 3:4 from the *erythro*-ion. When, however, the reagent was *t*-butoxide ion in either *t*-butyl alcohol or dimethylformamide, more than 90% of the reaction consisted of *syn*-elimination to give *trans*-olefin. The investigators concluded that *syn*-elimination is a common stereochemical form of elimination in Hofmann degradations. They pointed out, moreover, that the fact that in these experiments *syn*-elimination is particularly favoured by the more strongly basic reagent is consistent with the idea that *syn*-elimination is promoted by advancement of the proton transfer in the transition state of the bimolecular mechanism.[25,51]

Further support for this conclusion was provided. Banthorpe, Hughes, and the writer had concluded[25] that proton transfer was more advanced in E2 eliminations from ammonium ions than from sulphonium ions in like conditions, and for either kind of ion, more advanced when the base and medium were *t*-butoxide ions in *t*-butanol than when they were ethoxide ion in ethanol. Závada and Sicher found [54] that the same rules controlled the formation of *cis*- in place of *trans*-4-nonene from *n*-Pr·CH_2·CHX·Bu-*n*. They obtained mainly the *cis*-ene in ethanol or methanol, and more of it from the 4-nonyltrimethylammonium ion than from the -dimethylsulphonium ion: but they obtained mainly *trans*-ene from both ions in *t*-butanol:

Medium	*t*-BuO⁻/*t*-BuOH	EtO⁻/EtOH	MeO⁻/MeOH
X = NMe_3^+, % *cis*	26	74	81
X = SMe_2^+, % *cis*	9	64	—

There is thus good support from many sources for the view that *syn*-elimination is favoured (a) by advancement of the β-proton-transfer relatively to the α-electron-transfer in the E2 mechanism, and (b) by the degree to which the conformation of the alkyl compound approximates to that which would allow an exact *sp*-elimination. These are the factors which are theoretically expected thus to act.[51]

In a forthcoming paper (kindly shown in draft by Dr. Sicher to the writer), Sicher and Závada will point out that the correlation of *syn*-elimination with a *trans*-olefinic product and of *anti*-elimination with a *cis*-product means that the same individual hydrogen atom of the β-CH_2 group is preferentially lost in both forms of elimination. The two hydrogen atoms are initially rendered non-equivalent by induction from the asymmetric α-carbon atom. Why the non-equivalence correlates process with product in the particular manner found, and not in the other possible way, is not yet clear.

The stereochemical effect of auxiliary unsaturated or polar substituents has been investigated in the *cyclo*hexane series. Bordwell, Cristol, and others have shown[55] that in base-promoted eliminations from *cyclo*hexane substrates, the unsaturation of a β-phenyl substituent, in co-operation with the polar effect of an α-ammonium pole, can secure *cis*-elimination, which in this series is necessarily synclinal elimination; and, furthermore, that the strongly acidifying β-sulphone substituent, replacing the β-phenyl group, can exert a like effect, as in the following examples:

H—Ph, Me_3N^+—H $\xrightarrow{OH^-}$ —Ph   H—SO_2Ar, TsO—H $\xrightarrow{OR^-}$ —SO_2Ar

It was at one time supposed that the mechanism might have changed from concerted E2 to stepwise E1cB in such examples; but Shiner showed that that was not so.[56] On the other hand, one does receive a strong impression from the data that a sufficient acidification of the β-proton favours *syn*-elimination, as indeed, it should, within the scope of the E2 mechanism, by allowing the component electrophilic substitution at the β-carbon atom to proceed with inversion of configuration.

[55] R. T. Arnold and P. N. Richardson, *J. Am. Chem. Soc.*, 1954, **76**, 3649; J. Weinstock, R. G. Pearson, and F. G. Bordwell, *ibid.*, 1954, **76**, 4748; 1955, **77**, 6706; 1956, **78**, 3468, 3473; F. G. Bordwell and R. J. Kern, *ibid.*, 1955, **77**, 1141.

[56] V. J. Shiner jr. and M. L. Smith, *J. Am. Chem. Soc.*, 1958, 80, 4093; J. Weinstock, J. L. Bernardi, and R. G. Pearson, *ibid.*, p. 4961.

Antidating the above theory and illustrations of stereospecificity in E2 eliminations, W. Hückel, in 1940, made and substantially supported the first definite suggestion that the stereochemistry of elimination depends on the mechanism of elimination.[9] From studies of isomer ratios in products of eliminations from stereoisomeric alicyclic substrates, first in strongly basic conditions, and then in nearly neutral conditions, he deduced, first, that eliminations by mechanism E2 are stereospecific in the sense that *trans*-eliminations from *cyclo*hexane derivatives are strongly favoured, and second, that corresponding eliminations by mechanism E1 are not stereospecific. He did not institute any kinetic control of the assumed mechanisms, but he took it that eliminations in strongly basic conditions were likely to use the bimolecular mechanism, and that eliminations in nearly neutral conditions in highly ionising solvents were likely to employ the unimolecular mechanism.

Hückel's most extensive and informative group of studies related to menthyl and *neo*menthyl chlorides and trimethylammonium ions. This work has been revised and completed by Hughes and his collaborators, with the addition of kinetic control, and sometimes with adjustments of conditions for the purpose of separating the two mechanisms when they tend to run concurrently. The results are in Table 41-2.[57,58]

In all cases a group X, either Cl or NMe_3^+, leaves from position-3, along with a proton either from position-2, where there are two of them, one *cis* and one *trans* to X, or from position-4, where there is only one; and whether this is *cis* or *trans* to X is shown immediately under the name of the substrate in Table 41-2.

Entry 1 refers to E2 eliminations from *neo*menthyl chloride, for which stereospecific *trans*-elimination is possible in either of the alternative directions. The actual directions are therefore controlled by the factors which determine that E2 eliminations from alkyl chlorides normally follow the Saytzeff rule. In fact, the orientation of elimination does follow the Saytzeff rule. In entry 2, the substrate is menthyl chloride, in which the lone proton is *cis*. Therefore the elimination is forced by the stereospecificity of the E2 mechanism to take a direction contrary to that which should be predominating under the Saytzeff rule.[57]

Entry 3 deals with E2 elimination from the *neo*menthyl-trimethylammonium ion, which has a *trans*-proton on each side of the ammonium ion and hence is stereochemically unrestricted with respect to the direction of elimination. Bimolecular eliminations from alkyl

[57] E. D. Hughes, C. K. Ingold, and J. B. Rose, *J. Chem. Soc.*, **1953**, 3839.
[58] E. D. Hughes and J. Wilby, *J. Chem. Soc.*, **1960**, 4094.

TABLE 41-2.—COMBINED STERIC AND POLAR ORIENTATION OF ELIMINATION IN MENTHYL CHLORIDES AND -TRIMETHYLAMMONIUM IONS.

CH_2—CH_2—CHMe / *i*-PrC(H)·CH(X)·CH_2 (4) (3) (2) → CH_2—CH_2—CHMe / *i*-PrC═CH—CH_2 (4) (3) + CH_2—CH_2—CHMe / *i*-PrCH—CH═CH (3) (2)

Bimolecular Elimination; X = Cl (*solvent* EtOH)

	Reaction		3-Menthene	2-Menthene
1	*neo*Menthyl chloride + OEt^- [*trans*-(H)(X)]	E2	~78%	~22%
	Orientation:—Saytzeff			
2	Menthyl chloride + OEt^- [*cis*-(H)(X)]	E2	0%	100%
	Orientation:—"antiSaytzeff"			

Bimolecular Elimination; X = NMe_3^+ (*solvent* H_2O)

	Reaction		3-Menthene	2-Menthene
3	*neo*Menthyl-NMe_3^+ + OH^- [*trans*-(H)(X)]	E2	~88%	~12%
	Orientation:—Saytzeff (anomalous)			
4	Menthyl-NMe_3^+ + OH^- [*cis*-(H)(X)]	E2	0%	100%
	Orientation:—"superHofmann"			

Bimolecular Elimination; X = NMe_3^+ (*solvent* EtOH)

	Reaction		3-Menthene	2-Menthene
3′	*neo*Menthyl-NMe_3^+ + OEt^- [*trans*-(H)(X)]	E2	65%	35%
	Orientation:—Saytzeff (anomalous)			
4′	Menthyl-NMe_3^+ + OEt^- [*cis*-(H)(X)]	E2	0%	100%
	Orientation:—"superHofmann"			

Unimolecular Elimination; X = Cl (*solvent* "80%" aq.-EtOH)

	Reaction		3-Menthene	2-Menthene
5	*neo*Menthyl chloride [*trans*-(H)(X)]	E1	98.8%	1.2%
6	Menthyl chloride [*cis*-(H)(X)]	E1	68%	32%
	Orientation:—Saytzeff			

Unimolecular Elimination; X = NMe_3^+ (*solvent* H_2O)

	Reaction		3-Menthene	2-Menthene
7	*neo*Menthyl-NMe_3^+ [*trans*-(H)(X)]	E1	98.1%	1.9%
	Orientation:—Saytzeff			
8	Menthyl-NMe_3^+ [*cis*-(H)(X)]	E1	68%	32%
	Orientation:—Saytzeff			

ammonium ions usually follow the generalised Hofmann rule, so giving predominantly the least alkylated ethylene; but this one follows the Saytzeff rule of giving predominantly the most alkylated ethylene. We have here a real anomaly, inexplicable by theory as expounded up to this point; and we shall defer discussion of it to Section 41-3. In the meantime, let us continue to read the table. Entry 4 refers to E2 elimination from the menthyl-trimethylammonium ion, in which the stereochemical restriction works in the same direction as the Hofmann rule, but is much more demanding, with the result that the Hofmann olefin is formed, not merely predominantly, but exclusively. Entries 3′ and 4′ are like entries 3 and 4, respectively, except that the solvent water is replaced by solvent ethanol. The main point of interest is that the anomaly of entry 3 is reduced in entry 3′, but not eliminated.[58]

The rest of the Table deals with elimination from the same substrates by the unimolecular mechanism E1. Hückel's preconception was that this mechanism, since it goes by way of a carbonium ion, should have no dominant stereospecificity. His work was incomplete in this area, but had he had before him results corresponding to those of entries 5–8, he would doubtless have discussed them on the basis that corresponding chlorides and trimethylammonium ions should give the same carbonium ion, perhaps even that menthyl and *neo*menthyl derivatives should give the same carbonium ion, and that all olefin compositions, from whatever substrate, should accord with the Saytzeff rule. In fact, they all do accord with the Saytzeff rule.[57,58] Those from *neo*menthyl chloride and *neo*menthyl-trimethylammonium ion are practically identical, and are strongly unbalanced in the Saytzeff sense, as shown in entries 5 and 7. Those from menthyl chloride and menthyl-trimethylammonium ion are again identical, though more mildly unbalanced in the same sense, as appears from entries 5 and 8. It would seem that the carbonium ions retain no "memory" of what went away, but do retain a "memory" of where it went from, at the moment of their destruction by proton loss. In other words, though screening by the leaving group is unimportant, the carbonium ions fail to attain full conformational equilibrium.

When, in unimolecular elimination E1, the leaving group is a counter-ion, and the solvent has a very low basicity, the counter-ion may be the best available receiver of the proton from the carbonium ion; and if also the solvent has a low dielectric constant, so that ion pairs have some stability, then the unimolecular mechanism may acquire stereospecificity, inasmuch as the proton will tend to an orientation adjacent to the formed, but not yet departed, counter-ion; and so synperiplanar or synclinal elimination, *syn*-elimination, we may say, will be favoured, relatively to antiperiplanar or anticlinal, that is, *anti*-elimination. This has been made clear by Skell and his coworkers,[59] by measurement of the deuterium content of the *cis*- and *trans*-2-butenes formed from *erythro*- and *threo*-3-deuterobutyl 2-toluene-*p*-sulphonates. As is shown in the formulae below, *syn*-elimination from the *erythro*-substrate leads to deuterated *trans*-butene, or (after a conformational rotation in the model depicted) to undeuterated *cis*-butene; whereas *syn*-elimination from the *threo*-substrate would put the deuterium into the *cis*-butene. Of course, *anti*-eliminations give the opposite results.

OTs; CH_3, H; H, CH_3; D — *erythro-*

OTs; CH_3, D; H, CH_3; H — *threo-*

Some of the experimental results of these workers are reproduced in Table 41-3. An E2 elimination is included for comparison. The "solvolytic" eliminations are marked E1, and one sees the relative stereochemical indifference of these reactions largely disappearing as we pass towards solvent nitrobenzene. It is an indirect inference that the "solvolytic" reactions are of E1 type in the dry solvents, but the results themselves suggest that they are, as does the evidence (Section **42**) for E1 mechanisms in the gas phase, where the "solvent," empty space, represents the limit of low basicity and low dielectric constant, where ions are very stably paired, and where there is nothing except the counter-ion to take away the proton.

TABLE 41-3.—PROPORTIONS OF *syn*-ELIMINATION BY WHICH *cis* AND *trans*-2-BUTENE ARE FORMED FROM THE STEREOISOMERIC 3-DEUTEROBUTYL 2-TOLUENE-*p*-SULPHONATES, AS DEDUCED FROM THE DEUTERIUM CONTENT OF THE OLEFINS (SKELL).

Mechanism and conditions	Substrate	% *syn*-Elimination in formation of	
		trans-2-Butene	*cis*-2-Butene
E2-OEt^- in EtOH	*erythro-*	0	0
E1 "80%" aq. EtOH	*erythro-*	34	16
E1 Acetic acid	*erythro-*	82	65
E1 Nitrobenzene	*erythro-*	98	95
E1 Nitrobenzene	*threo-*	89	99

[59] P. S. Skell and W. L. Hall, *J. Am. Chem. Soc.*, 1963, **65**, 2851.

(41c) Stereochemistry and the Timing of E2 Bond Changes.—We now return to eliminations in dissociating solvents, such as aqueous solvents, and in particular to bimolecular eliminations.

We have dealt in part in the preceding section with the subject of the relative timing of the E2 bond changes, because it is impossible to discuss the stereochemistry of the E2 process without alluding to it. All we need do here, therefore, is to add some complementing remarks.

In E2 eliminations, the loss of the β-proton and the transfer of the α-electron, though concerted, will not keep exactly in step: their unbalance will control the charge, and the degree of unsaturation, in the transition state. This idea was adumbrated by Hanhart and the writer[2] in 1927, but it has been developed only more recently, and most comprehensively reviewed by Bunnett[60] in 1962. It has stereochemical implications, because the stereospecificity of E2 reactions depends on the coupling of the bond changes: their coupling will be strongest when they are nearly synchronous, and coupling will be weakened when either bond change runs strongly ahead of the other. The two limits of asynchronism, and hence of uncoupling, are in mechanism E1cB, in which the proton transfer constitutes a separate preliminary step, and in mechanism E1, in which the electron transfer is similarly completed first. One can picture, between these limits, a band of E2 mechanisms, in which the bond changes remain concerted, but may "lean" away from exact synchronisation in either direction, with losses of stereospecificity, and, of course, modifications in polar effects on rate.

We noticed in the preceding Section the evidence that a constitutional influence tending to acidify the β-proton, if sufficient, will allow *cis*-elimination in *cyclo*hexane and other compounds, in reactions which retain their E2 character. In these examples, we can reasonably assume that the E2 mechanism "leans" towards mechanism E1cB, with proton loss in the lead, to an extent which permits *cis*-elimination, and hence synclinal elimination, if the acidified proton is in the *cis*-position.

Unbalance in the other direction is thought to be involved in Hughes and Wilby's findings,[58] recorded in entries 3 and 3′ of Table 41-2, concerning E2 elimination from the *neo*menthyl-trimethylammonium ion. The striking thing about this reaction is the difficulty of observing it in a pure form, even in quite strongly alkaline aqueous solution: one observes it in admixture with the exceptionally facile E1 elimination. Now this E1 reaction, like all of those in Table 41-2, follows the Saytzeff rule. But the accompanying E2 reaction, which, as one of an

[60] J. F. Bunnett, *Angew. Chem. internat. Edit.*, 1962, 1, 225; C. K. Ingold, *Proc. Chem. Soc.*, **1962**, 265.

ammonium ion, might have been expected to follow the Hofmann rule, also follows the Saytzeff rule, though in a less decided way. Hughes and Wilby take it that the ease of the E1 reaction argues facile separation of the NMe_3^+ group (perhaps because it is axial, and under conformational pressure), and that this character will be carried into the E2 reaction, so allowing the separation of the trimethylammonium group to run ahead of the proton transfer. There will result a partial development of carbonium-ion character in the transition state of the E2 mechanism, and this factor, if dominant, will produce orientation according to the Saytzeff rule.

(42) UNIMOLECULAR 1,2-ELIMINATION IN THE GAS PHASE[61]

(42a) Constitutional Kinetic Effects.—It is attractive to study eliminations in the gas phase, that is, with abolition of the solvent. One must also abolish surface catalysis, but this can usually be done by suitably coating the containing surface. The homogeneous reaction then observable may consist of or contain a radical-carried process, which, if present, and not too important, can usually be suppressed by the addition of radical-trapping inhibitors. The residual reaction will then be a gaseous molecular reaction.

Gaseous molecular eliminations, mainly from alkyl chlorides, have been studied by Barton and his collaborators since 1949,[62] and from alkyl bromides and other halides, as well as from alkyl acetates and other esters, by Maccoll and his coworkers in many papers since 1953.[63] The reactions proceed at convenient rates in various temperature ranges, mostly comprised between 250° and 500°. They are all unimolecular processes, showing first-order kinetics, with, where tested,

[61] A. Maccoll, "The Chemistry of Alkenes," Editor S. Patai, Interscience Publishers, London, 1964, Chap. 3; "Gas-phase Heterolysis" in "Advances in Organic Chemistry," Editor V. Gold, Academic Press, London, Vol. 3, 1965, p. 91; "Studies in Chemical Structure and Reactivity," Editor J. H. Ridd, Methuen, London, 1966, Chap. 4.

[62] D. H. R. Barton and K. H. Howlett, *J. Chem. Soc.*, **1949**, 155, 165; D. H. R. Barton and P. F. Onyon, *Trans. Faraday Soc.*, 1949, **45**, 725; D. H. R. Barton and A. T. Head, *ibid.*, 1950, **46**, 114; *idem* and R. J. W. Williams, *J. Chem. Soc.*, **1952**, 453; **1953**, 1715.

[63] J. H. S. Green, A. Maccoll, and P. J. Thomas, *J. Chem. Phys.*, 1953, **21**, 178; and the subsequent papers cited in reference 61. The first important discussion of mechanism was by A. Maccoll and P. J. Thomas, *Nature*, 1955, **176**, 392. The subject was surveyed with further discussions of mechanism by A. Maccoll in "Theoretical Organic Chemistry—Kekulé Symposium," Butterworths Scientific Pubs., 1959, p. 230, in *Spec. Pubs. Chem. Soc.*, 1962, **16**, 158, and in the books of reference 61; cf. C. K. Ingold, *Proc. Chem. Soc.*, **1957**, 297.

the Lindemann fall-off at low pressures.[64] Their Arrhenius frequency factors are all about the theoretical, *viz.*, 10^{13} sec.$^{-1}$, for unimolecular gas reactions. Thus, the differences of rate between one reaction and another reflect fairly closely the difference in activation energy.

The first observations by Maccoll and his collaborators on the gaseous unimolecular dehydrobromination of alkyl bromides[63] showed that, energetically, these reactions depend almost wholly on the breaking of the CBr bond, and hardly at all on the breaking of the CH bond. If, in ethyl bromide as parent, successive methyl groups are introduced to make the CBr and CH centres primary, secondary, and tertiary, independently, relative rates are found which are shown in the upper part of Table 42-1. Evidently rate is determined essentially by the immediate environment of the CBr centre. The effect of the groups flanking the CH centre is relatively so trivial that it is hard to know whether it is really exerted there, or, after relay, still at the CBr centre. The matter can as easily be demonstrated in terms of the activation energies of the reactions, as given in the lower part of Table 42-1.

The next point, which was brought out by Maccoll and Thomas[63] in 1955, was that these and similar activation energies for gaseous unimolecular dehydrohalogenations do not follow the homolytic dis-

TABLE 42-1.—UNIMOLECULAR GASEOUS DEHYDROBROMINATIONS OF ALKYL BROMIDES $R_2C(H)\text{—}C(Br)R_2$ WHERE R = H OR Me.

Relative Rates at 380°	CBr primary	CBr secondary	CBr tertiary
CH primary	1	170	32,000
CH secondary	3.5	380	46,000
CH tertiary	6.3	—	130,000

Arrhenius Activation Energies, kcal./mole	CBr primary	CBr secondary	CBr tertiary
CH primary	53.9	47.8	42.2
CH secondary	50.7	46.5	40.5
CH tertiary	50.4	—	39.0

[64] This is a well-known phenomenon, *viz.*, a fall-off in rate, accompanying a change to second-order kinetic form, which occurs when the reduction in pressure reduces collision frequencies below what is needed to maintain Maxwellian distribution under the loss of high-energy substrate molecules by reaction.

TABLE 42-2.—ACTIVATION ENERGIES OF GASEOUS UNIMOLECULAR DEHYDROHALOGENATIONS COMPARED WITH HOMOLYTIC AND HETEROLYTIC CARBON-HALOGEN DISSOCIATION ENERGIES (KCAL,/MOLE).

Substrate	EtBr	*i*-PrBr	*t*-BuBr
Arrhenius E_A	53.9	47.8	42.2
$D(R\cdot + Br\cdot)$	67.2	67.6	63.8
$D(R^+ + Br^-)$	183.7	153.6	140.3
Substrate	EtCl	*i*-PrCl	*t*-BuCl
Arrhenius E_A	60.2	50.5	41.4
$D(R\cdot + Cl\cdot)$	80.9	82.2	78.3
$D(R^+ + Cl^-)$	192.8	166.3	150.2

sociation energies of the carbon-halogen bonds, but do follow the corresponding heterolytic dissociation energies. This is illustrated in Table 42-2, in which the activation energies for the dehydrobrominations are from Table 42-1, whilst those for the dehydrochlorinations are from the earlier work of Barton.[62]

Maccoll and Thomas then went on to demonstrate the close and detailed analogy between constitutional effects on the rates of gaseous unimolecular eliminations from alkyl halides, and on the rates of their heterolytic unimolecular reactions of substitution or elimination, S_N1 or E1, in aqueous or other highly polar solvents. And in every extension of the field of comparison which these workers, separately or together, have subsequently explored, this correspondence has been found to hold. We may here notice two examples, both due to Thomas.

One of the clearest of possible ways for telling to what extent CH-bond fission is involved in the unimolecular transition state of gaseous elimination is to weaken that bond strongly by making it an allyl or a benzyl CH bond. This involves introducing a β-vinyl or β-phenyl group into the alkyl halide. Thomas put β-vinyl into an alkyl bromide.[65] A comparison with the corresponding β-methyl compound then isolated the effect of the unsaturation in the vinyl group. As can be seen from the results in Table 42-3, it had no effect. It is clear that nothing has happened to the CH bond in the transition state of the unimolecular reaction. It is equally clear that no carbon-carbon double bonding could have developed in the transition state, which cannot "know" that it is on the way to becoming a conjugated diene. Similar results have been obtained by Maccoll and Stevenson with a β-phenyl substituent.[66]

[65] P. J. Thomas, *J. Chem. Soc.*, **1959**, 1192; **1961**, 136.

[66] B. Stephenson, Thesis, University of London, 1959; A. Maccoll, "Kekulé Symposium" (ref. 63), p. 237.

TABLE 42-3.—EFFECT OF A β-VINYL GROUP ON RATE OF GASEOUS UNIMOLECULAR DEHYDROBROMINATION.

Substrate	$\overset{\beta}{CH_3—\underset{H}{\underset{\vert}{CH}}}—\overset{\alpha}{\underset{Br}{\underset{\vert}{CH}}}—CH_3$	$CH_2{=}CH—\overset{\beta}{\underset{H}{\underset{\vert}{CH}}}—\overset{\alpha}{\underset{Br}{\underset{\vert}{CH}}}—CH_3$
Arrhenius A (sec.$^{-1}$)	$10^{13.53}$	$10^{12.94}$
Arrhenius E_A (kcal./mole)	46.5	44.7
Rel. rate at 380°	1.00	1.05

One of the most striking effects of substituents in promoting S_N1 or E1 reactions of alkyl halides in aqueous or other ionising solvents, as in unimolecular solvolysis, is the effect of an α-methoxy-group. The rate enhancements are so large that we can only estimate them indirectly. The accepted reason is that the α-methoxyl group is well adapted to conjugate with the carbonium ion first formed by heterolysis:

$$\left.\begin{array}{l} CH_3—\overset{\curvearrowright}{O}—CH_2—\overset{\curvearrowright}{Cl} \xrightarrow[\text{slow}]{} CH_3—\overset{+}{O}{=}CH_2 \\ \xrightarrow[\text{fast}]{H_2O} CH_3—O—CH_2\cdot OH \end{array}\right\} (S_N1)$$

The second of Thomas's examples is a test of the deduction that, if gaseous unimolecular elimination is really a heterolytic reaction E1, involving a first-formed carbonium ion, it should exhibit a similarly dramatic rate-enhancement:

$$\left.\begin{array}{l} CH_3—O—\underset{CH_2—H}{\underset{\vert}{CH}}—Cl \xrightarrow[\text{slow}]{} CH_3—\overset{+}{O}{=}\underset{CH_2—H}{\underset{\vert}{CH}} \\ \xrightarrow[\text{fast}]{} CH_3—O—\underset{CH_2}{\underset{\Vert}{CH}} \end{array}\right\} (E1)$$

Thomas measured the rate of the gas reaction of α-methoxy-ethyl chloride,[65] and found it measurable at temperatures 200° lower than those used for alkyl chlorides containing H or Me in place of MeO, *viz.*, ethyl and *iso*propyl chlorides. The latter is included in the comparison, because Me is a group which might hyperconjugate,

TABLE 42-4.—EFFECT OF AN α-METHOXYL GROUP ON RATE OF GASEOUS UNIMOLECULAR DEHYDROCHLORINATION: COMPARISON WITH SOLVOLYSIS.

Substrate	$CH_2(H)-CH(Cl)-H$	$CH_2(H)-CH(Cl)-CH_3$	$CH_2(H)-CH(Cl)-OCH_3$
A (sec.$^{-1}$)	$10^{14.6}$	$10^{13.40}$	$10^{11.46}$
E_A (kcal./mole)	60.8	50.5	33.3
Rel. rate, 330°	1	—	$10^{6.8}$
	—	1	$10^{4.3}$
Rel. rate, 0°	1	—	$10^{18.9}$
	—	1	$10^{11.9}$
S_N1 Solvolysis: Estimated Relative Rates			
Rel. rate, 0°	1	—	$\sim 10^{17}$
	—	1	10^{11}–10^{12}

rather than conjugate, with an electron-depleted α-carbon atom. The comparison of rates and Arrhenius parameters for these three chlorides is in Table 42-4. Relative rates are calculated in the first place for 330°, a temperature between the ranges used for the least and most reactive chlorides, and chosen to minimise the larger extrapolations. They are then calculated, less reliably because of the length of the extrapolations, for 0°, in order to allow comparison with relative solvolytic rates at 0°, as given at the bottom of the table. These values are indirectly estimated, and are accordingly only rough. But notwithstanding the approximate nature of the figures for 0°, the comparisons leave no doubt that the same type of process is being asisted by the methoxyl group in these two very different sets of conditions.

We need not pursue such detailed exemplification any further, but it should be mentioned that Maccoll and his coworkers have applied tests of this kind to nearly all the simple substituents in alkyl halides for which characteristic effects on S_N1 or E1 rates in solution are known. For example, although, as we have seen, a β-vinyl or a β-phenyl group has no significant effect on the gas reaction, an α-phenyl group, in gaseous unimolecular elimination, as in solvolytic S_N1 or E1 reactions, has a strong accelerating effect, stronger than one, if not quite as strong as two, α-methyl groups. The factors of increase are comparable in the gaseous and solution reactions, if we allow for the difference in the temperatures used in the two kinds of observation. Again, a β-chlorine atom has a mild retarding effect, and an α-chlorine atom a mild accelerating effect—much milder than the effect of an α-methyl group—on the gaseous reaction; and all these effects are parallel to and comparable with those well known in the area of unimolecular solvolytic reactions.[67]

Gaseous dehydrohalogenations and similar eliminations used to be considered on the basis of an assumed "four-centre transition state":

$$\begin{array}{ccc} R_2C & \overset{\cdots\cdots}{=\!=} & CR_2 \\ \vdots & & \vdots \\ H & \text{------} & X \end{array}$$

The implication was that all four bonds become changed simultaneously, and that no strong local polarities are anywhere developed. The teaching of Maccoll and Thomas, that gaseous dehydrohalogenation is a two-stage heterolytic process of type E1, the first, and the activated stage being an ionisation,

$$\begin{array}{c} R_2C{-}CR_2 \\ | \quad\;\; | \\ H \quad\; X \end{array} \xrightarrow{\text{slow}} \left\{\begin{array}{c} R_2C{-}\overset{+}{C}R_2 \\ | \\ H \end{array}\right\} X^- \xrightarrow{\text{fast}} R_2C{=}CR_2 + HX \qquad \text{(E1)}$$

came as a surprise to those brought up in the tradition that gas-phase processes are always homolytic, that heterolytic energies are inaccessible to gas reactions, and that ions do not occur in gases below flame temperatures. What is forgotten in the traditional outlook is that, although heterolytic energies of 140–190 kcal./mole, as listed in Table 42-2, really are inaccessible at the reaction temperatures, the greater part of any of these dissociation energies is the energy needed to dissociate the formed ions, which have not to be dissociated in order to complete an E1 elimination.[63]

It has to be considered whether the anion in the freshly formed ion-pair is attracted by, and rests against, the carbonium ionic centre and the hydrogen atom whose proton it will eventually extract, or whether it is attracted also by all the other hydrogen atoms which gain positive charges by supplying electrons hyperconjugatively to the carbonium ionic centre. Maccoll has advanced the latter view as a matter of principle, but of course would agree that differences of stereochemical opportunity must create great differences of action among the hydrogen atoms. What he has shown with C. J. Harding and R. A. Ross[68] is that, in the homogeneous gaseous dehydrochlorination of optically active 2-octyl chloride at 327–358°, the first-order rate of loss of optical activity from the reacting system is equal to, not greater than, the first-order rate of dehydrochlorination. This shows that an ion-paired chloride ion cannot migrate to the other side of the carbonium ion, and gives some support to the idea that the chloride ion is held by

[67] H. M. R. Hoffmann and A. Maccoll, *J. Am. Chem. Soc.*, 1965, **87**, 3774.
[68] C. J. Harding, A. Maccoll, and R. A. Ross, *Chem. Comm.*, 1967, **289**.

the protonic field of a next-neighbouring hydrogen atom. One of the examples given in Section **42c** again points in this direction.

Although dehydrohalogenations constitute the most fully studied examples of gaseous unimolecular eliminations, other such reactions have to some extent been examined, particularly the dehydrocarboxylations of acetates, and some other esters. From the recorded rate data for acetates one may construct Table 42-5, on the same pattern as Table 42-1 for bromides. It shows the same thing, namely, that rate is determined almost wholly by the immediate surroundings of the acetate-bearing carbon atom, and not by those of the carbon atom bearing the eliminated hydrogen atom. This is consistent with the idea of two steps, the first and the activated step being concerned essentially with acetate separation. Of course, other types of investigation would be needed to support any presumption of heterolytic dissociation, and to ascertain whether the second oxygen atom of the ester group is concerned in the bond changes which are in progress in the transition state. The smaller spread of the figures in Table 42-5 than in Table 42-1 indicates that the transition state of elimination from acetates is less polar than that of elimination from bromides. But whether the mechanism is the same or not, such a difference could be caused by the smaller electronegativity of the acetate group than of the bromide atom.

(42b) Orientation and Stereochemistry.—Barton first pointed out the predisposition of gaseous unimolecular eliminations from *cyclo*hexane compounds towards *cis*-elimination.[69] From menthyl chloride,

TABLE 42-5.—UNIMOLECULAR GASEOUS DEHYDROCARBOXYLATION OF ALKYL ACETATES $R_2C(H)$—$C(OAc)R_2$ WHERE R = H OR Me.

Relative Rates at ~400°

	C—OAc primary	secondary		tertiary	
CH primary	1	24	*(25)*	2000	*(1660)*
CH secondary	0.91	38	*(24)*	5000	*(2490)*
CH tertiary	0.46	—		6800	

NOTE.—The roman figures are from J. E. Scheer, E. C. Kooyman, and F. L. J. Sixma, *Rec. trav. chim.*, 1963, **82**, 1123; whilst the italic figures are from A. Maccoll, *J. Chem. Soc.*, **1958**, 3398, and E. U. Emovon and A. Maccoll, *ibid.*, **1962**, 335.

[69] D. H. R. Barton, *J. Chem. Soc.*, **1949**, 2197; D. H. R. Barton, A. J. Head, and R. J. Williams, *ibid.*, **1952**, 453; **1953**, 1715.

he obtained about 73% of elimination with the tertiary 4-hydrogen atom, which is *cis*, and necessarily synclinal, with respect to the chlorine atom. Maccoll and Bamkole[70] confirmed this result, and added the finding that *neo*menthyl chloride, in which the 4-hydrogen atom is *trans*, and conformationally antiperiplanar, with respect to the chlorine atom, gives 85% of elimination with one of the secondary 2-hydrogen atoms. The stable conformations of menthyl and *neo*menthyl chlorides, having all side-groups, or, if that is impossible, the largest of them, equatorial, are as shown below:

H, 4, CHMe$_2$, Me, 2, Cl, 1, 3

Menthyl chloride
(gives 27% 2-ene + 73% 3-ene)

H, 4, CHMe$_2$, Me, 2, 1, 3, Cl

*neo*Menthyl chloride
(gives 85% 2-ene + 15% 3-ene)

It may be deduced that these homogeneous dehydrochlorinations, as E1 processes, tend to direct double-bond formation according to the Saytzeff rule, unless an over-riding stereochemical preference for synclinal elimination determines otherwise. This stereochemical preference may be envisaged as a continuation into the gas phase of Skell's principle (preceding Section) that, in E1 eliminations in solution, the usual lack of any strong stereospecificity in basic and ion-dissociating solvents becomes changed, as the solvent becomes less basic and less disociating, to a preference for a synclinal form of elimination. In non-basic and non-dissociating solvents, as in the gas phase, the formed but not dissociated anion becomes attracted towards, and tends to take, the most accessible proton; and in *cyclo*hexane systems this will always be a synclinal proton.[71]

(42c) Elimination with Rearrangement.—One of the most definite and concise pieces of evidence that one can ever obtain of a unimolecular process involving a carbonium-ion intermediate is the observation of its association with a Wagner rearrangement. A Wagner rearrangement depends on the prior formation of an electron-deficient centre, and, except in a very few special cases in which this can be a radical centre, it has to be a carbonium ionic centre. The rearrangement consists in the movement of a group, usually a hydrogen

[70] T. Bamkole, Thesis, University of London, 1964; A. Maccoll, "Gas-phase Heterolysis" (ref. 61), p. 111.

[71] Barton, Head, and Williams noticed (ref. 69) that surface catalysis may change the direction of elimination. Therefore we make no attempt to discuss the orientation and stereochemistry of eliminations not known to be homogeneous.

atom or an alkyl group, with its bonding electrons, into the original carbonium ionic centre, so shifting that centre to some adjacent more stable position, before the carbonium ion becomes destroyed, as the unimolecular nucleophilic substitution or elimination becomes completed.

In 1961, Maccoll and Swinbourne demonstrated the first gaseous unimolecular Wagner rearrangement, in the dehydrochlorination of *neo*pentyl chloride.[72] This alkyl chloride has no β-hydrogen atom, but the decomposition proceeded at 444° at about one-quarter of the rate of that of ethyl chloride. Some 25% of the total reaction comprised fragmentations, in which methyl chloride and methane were split off to leave *iso*butene and the isomeric chloro*iso*butenes. But 75% of it consisted of dehydrochlorinations, characterised by the Wagner shift of a methyl group, that would convert a first-formed primary carbonium ion into a more stable tertiary carbonium ion, which could then lose one or another of its protons to give a mixture of *iso*amylenes. The composition, noted below, of the mixture of *iso*-amylenes obtained, tells us nothing of the relative rates of loss of the protons, because it is the equilibrium composition: though the hydrogen chloride, formed with the *iso*-amylenes, does not add to them to any measurable extent at the temperature, that must be a thermodynamic matter, because it does catalyse their rapid interconversion at that temperature. One can say, however, that the relative stabilities of the fully formed olefins are as hyperconjugation would make them, and it is a reasonable assumption that the transition states of formation of any two of them from the same carbonium ion and the same proton acceptor would reflect these stability relations:

$$(CH_3)_3C{-}CH_2{-}Cl \xrightarrow[\text{slow}]{} (CH_3)_2C{-}\overset{+}{C}H_2 \xrightarrow[\text{fast}]{} (CH_3)_2\overset{+}{C}{-}CH_2{-}CH_3$$

$$\xrightarrow{\text{fast}} \underset{30\%}{CH_2{=}C(CH_3){-}CH_2{-}CH_3} \quad + \quad \underset{65\%}{(CH_3)_2C{=}CH{-}CH_3} \quad + \quad \underset{5\%}{(CH_3)_2CH{-}CH{=}CH_2}$$

The eliminations, without and with rearrangement, from bornyl

[72] A. Maccoll and E. S. Swinbourne, *Proc. Chem. Soc.*, **1960,** 409; *J. Chem. Soc.*, **1964,** 149; R. C. Bicknell, Thesis, University of London, 1962; A. Maccoll "Gas-phase Heterolysis" (ref. 61), p. 110.

and *iso*bornyl chlorides, so well known as reactions in solution, have been realised as unimolecular gas reactions by Maccoll and Bicknell.[72] They present a picture of product control by stereochemical opportunity, and in particular of the partition of a formed but undissociated chloride ion between the possible neighbouring and next-to-neighbouring hydrogen atoms on the same side of the ring system as the chloride ion. The ring system has three sides, but we are concerned only with two of them, called *endo* and *exo*. The *endo*-2-chloride ion, from bornyl chloride, has three possibilities, *viz.*, to attack *endo*-3-hydrogen, *endo*-6-hydrogen, and a conformationally *endo*-directed hydrogen atom of the bridge-head methyl group, the last possibility involving a Wagner 1,2-shift of the 6-methylene group (which transforms a secondary 2-carbonium ion to a more stable tertiary 1-carbonium ion); and the *endo*-chloride ion uses all three of these possibilities, so giving bornylene, tricyclene, and camphene in the proportions shown below. The *exo*-2-chloride ion, from *iso*bornyl chloride, has before it only two alternatives, *viz.*, to attack either *exo*-3-hydrogen or a conformationally *exo*-directed hydrogen atom of the bridge-head methyl group, the latter possibility involving the same Wagner rearrangement; and the *exo*-chloride ion uses both the alternatives open to it, so producing bornylene and camphene in the proportions shown:

camphene
25%
75%
exo
3
1
6
2
H
Cl
H
H
55%
tricyclene
H
Cl
H
endo
bornyl chloride
20%
25%
isobornyl chloride
bornylene

1
2
6
+
+

Wagner change in carbonium ion
(The Cl takes out only H's on its own side of the three-sided structure.)

(42d) Homogeneous Acid Catalysis.—No examples of the catalysis of gaseous unimolecular elimination from alkyl halides or esters have been reported. However, the hydrogen halides strongly catalyse such elimination from alcohols and ethers. The first report on this subject was by Maccoll and Stimson in 1960, and further investigation of the phenomenon is due very largely to Stimson.[73]

The investigated reactions proceed in various temperature ranges, between the overall limits of about 240° and 520°. They have second-order kinetics, Rate $\propto$ [ROH or ROMe][HX]; but the hydrogen halide, HX, though it appears in the kinetic equation, is not consumed. In their catalytic power, the hydrogen halides stand in the order HI > HBr > HCl, typical approximate relative rates being 150:25:1, at, say, 380°. This suggests that the catalysing behaviour is connected with the acidity of the catalysts. The kinetic effect of structural changes in the alkyl group on the catalysed reactions is qualitatively like that observed in the dehydrohalogenation of alkyl halides, and is closely similar to that found in the dehydrocarboxylation of alkyl esters. The introduction of successive methyl groups adjacently to the eliminated hydroxyl group increases the rate by substantial factors, for instance, 1:25:1600 along the series ethyl, *iso*propyl, *t*-butyl alcohol at 440°; and yet the introduction of successive methyl groups adjacently to the eliminated hydrogen atom leaves all rates unchanged to within a factor of two. The suggestion is strong that activation is to do with the breaking of the carbon-oxygen bond, and not with the breaking of the carbon-hydrogen bond; and furthermore that, under catalysis by the gaseous acids, the carbon-oxygen bond is breaking as the C—Hal or C—OAc bond has been already concluded to break in the comparison reactions, that is, heterolytically. The mechanism may be formulated as in the following example:

$$(CH_3)_3C\text{—}OH \cdots H\text{—}Br \xrightarrow{\text{slow}} \left[(CH_3)_2\overset{+}{C}\text{—}CH_2\text{—}H \;\; Br^-\right] \longrightarrow (CH_3)_2C{=}CH_2 + HBr$$

Cross and Stimson have supported the general concept of the gaseous acid catalysis of elimination with the following example. It was al-

[73] A. Maccoll and V. R. Stimson, *J. Chem. Soc.*, **1960,** 2386; K. G. Lewis and V. R. Stimson, *ibid.*, 3087; R. A. Ross and V. R. Stimson, *ibid.*, p. 3090; R. E. Failes and V. R. Stimson, *ibid.*, **1962,** 653, V. R. Stimson and E. J. Watson, *ibid.*, **1960,** 3920; **1961,** 1392; **1963,** 1524; J. T. D. Cross and V. R. Stimson, *Chem. Comm.*, **1966,** 360; A. Maccoll "Gas-phase Heterolysis" (ref. 61), p. 117.

ready known that *iso*butylene, in the presence of an acid, such as sulphuric or tetrafluoroboric acid, strong enough to convert it to the *t*-butylium ion, would take up carbon monoxide to give the pivalylium ion, through which pivalic acid could be preparatively produced in a series of reversible steps as follows:

$$\mathrm{Me_2C{:}CH_2} \overset{\mathrm{H^+}}{\rightleftharpoons} \mathrm{Me_3C^+} \overset{\mathrm{CO}}{\rightleftharpoons} \mathrm{Me_3C\cdot CO^+} \overset{\mathrm{H_2O}}{\rightleftharpoons} \mathrm{Me_3C\cdot CO\cdot OH_2^+}$$
$$\rightleftharpoons \mathrm{Me_3C\cdot CO_2H + H^+}$$

The investigators reversed this overall result, and there can be no reasonable doubt that they reversed the path in outline, as a homogeneous gas reaction. For they found that, in the presence of hydrogen bromide at 340–460°, pivalic acid decomposed to *iso*butylene, carbon monoxide, and water, in a homogeneous gas reaction, which obeyed the kinetic equation

$$\text{Rate} \propto [\mathrm{Me_3C\cdot CO_2H}][\mathrm{HBr}]$$

although hydrogen bromide is not consumed. The mechanism corresponding to that given above would be as follows:

$$\mathrm{(CH_3)_3C{-}CO{-}OH \cdots Br{-}H} \xrightarrow{\text{slow}} \mathrm{(CH_3)_3C{-}CO^+ \quad Br^-} \longrightarrow \mathrm{(CH_3)_2\overset{+}{C}{-}CH_2{-}H \quad Br^-}$$
$$\longrightarrow \mathrm{(CH_3)_2C{:}CH_2 + HBr}$$

In the above interpretation of gaseous catalysed elimination, it is permissible to split the slow step into two by the inclusion of an oxonium ion-pair as an additional intermediate. But this elaboration seems not to be demanded by the present evidence.

(43) GROB'S FRAGMENTATIONS[74]

(43a) Incorporation of Fragmentation.—Basically, these reactions are eliminations in which a group of atoms, potentially having some stability as a cation, takes the place of the β-hydrogen atom in ordinary elimination, so that a substantial portion of the molecule may become split off. Grob pointed out, first in 1955, that reactions of

[74] C. A. Grob and W. Baumann, *Helv. Chim. Acta*, 1955, **38**, 594; C. A. Grob, *Experientia*, 1957, **13**, 126; *idem*, "Theoretical Organic Chemistry—Kekulé Symposium," Butterworths Scientific Pubs., London, 1959, p. 114.

this type are ubiquitous in organic chemistry. Some examples are given below.

The analogy is particularly easily seen when an alkyl halide having a β-t-butyl group splits off a t-butyl halide in place of (or in addition to) the usual eliminant, hydrogen halide:[75]

$$Me_3C—CHMe—CMe_2—Cl \rightarrow CHMe{=}CMe_2 + Me_3C—Cl$$

In this case, the potentially cationic β-group may be considered as helped by hyperconjugation to develop cationic character and so to participate in the elimination. But more such help could be given by full conjugation, as in a γ-hydroxyalkyl halide. In the following example a glycollic acid side-chain is split off from a *cyclo*hexane derivative, along with halogen from another side-chain:[76]

$$H—O—CH(CO_2H)—C_6H_{10}—CH(CO_2H)—Br \xrightarrow{OH^-} C_6H_{10}{=}CH\cdot CO_2H + O{=}CH\cdot CO_2H + HBr$$

Of course, if the carbon-carbon bond which undergoes fission is part of a ring, no carbon-chain will be lost from the molecule, as may be illustrated in the following example from steroid chemistry:[77]

$$C_{16}H_{30}\text{(steroid, 5-OH, 3-OTs)} \xrightarrow{t\text{-BuO}^-} C_{16}H_{30}\text{(ring-opened ketone with vinyl group)}$$

5-Hydroxycoprostanyl 3-toluene-*p*-sulphonate

Similarly, the potential anion will not be lost from the molecule, if it is double bonded, as in a carbonyl group. Many decarboxylations thus come into the general scheme, for example, that of malonic acid:[78]

[75] F. Brown, T. D. Davies, I. Dostrovsky, O. J. Evans, and E. D. Hughes, *Nature*, 1951, **167**, 897. For other examples, see F. C. Whitmore and E. E. Stahly, *J. Am. Chem. Soc.*, 1933, **55**, 4153; 1945, **67**, 2158.

[76] R. M. Beesley, C. K. Ingold, and J. F. Thorpe, *J. Chem. Soc.*, 1915, **107**, 1080. For other examples, see S. Searles and M. J. Gostatowsky, *J. Am. Chem. Soc.*, 1953, **75**, 3030; R. Lukes and J. Plesek, *Chem. Listy*, 1955, **46**, 1826.

[77] R. B. Clayton, H. B. Henbest, and M. Smith, *J. Chem. Soc.*, 1957, 1982.

[78] C. Hentzel, *Ann.*, 1866, **139**, 132.

$$\text{H—O—CO—CH}_2\text{—C}(=\text{O})\text{OH} \rightarrow \text{CH}_2\text{=C(OH)}_2 + \text{O=CO}$$

$$\downarrow$$

$$\text{CH}_3\text{—CO}_2\text{H}$$

So also do other general reactions, including the retrograde aldol reaction, as of *iso*butyraldol to *iso*butyraldehyde,[79]

$$\text{H—O—CH(CHMe}_2\text{)—CMe}_2\text{—CH=O}$$

$$\rightarrow \text{CMe}_2\text{=CH—OH} + \text{O=CH}\cdot\text{CHMe}_2$$

$$\downarrow$$

$$\text{CHMe}_2\text{—CH=O}$$

and the retrograde Michael reaction, as of β-phenyl-α-carboxyglutaric ethyl ester to cinnamic and malonic esters:[80]

$$\text{H—CH(CO}_2\text{Et)—CHPh—CH(CO}_2\text{Et)—C(=O)OEt} \rightarrow \text{CH(CO}_2\text{Et)=C(OH)OEt} + \text{CH(CO}_2\text{Et)=CHPh}$$

$$\downarrow$$

$$\text{CH}_2\text{(CO}_2\text{Et)}_2$$

γ-Aminoalkyl halides are in the same case as the γ-hydroxy-halides. Alkaloid chemistry contains many examples of the effect of an amino-group in determining carbon-carbon bond fission. The substrate in the example formulated below is the hydrogen-bromide adduct of quinidine, which, on treatment with aqueous silver nitrate, gives niquidine, with ring-opening, and (what was not noticed at first) a loss of one carbon atom as formaldehyde:[81]

[79] E. H. Usherwood, *J. Chem. Soc.*, 1923, **123**, 1717. This was a first example, on which the generality of the reaction was proposed and subsequently demonstrated.

[80] C. K. Ingold and W. J. Powell, *J. Chem. Soc.*, 1921, **119**, 1976. This was one of two examples on which the generality of the reaction was proposed, but there existed in the literature a much earlier though forgotten example due to D. Vorländer, *Ber.*, 1900, **33**, 3185.

[81] E. M. Gibbs and T. A. Henry, *J. Chem. Soc.*, **1939**, 240.

$$\text{Quinuclidine}(\text{CH(CH}_3\text{)Br})(\text{OH})\text{CH—Q} \rightarrow \text{CH}_2{=}\text{N}^+\text{(piperidine)}(\text{CH=CH—CH}_3)(\text{OH})\text{CH—Q} \rightarrow \text{CH}_2\text{O} + \text{HN(piperidine)}(\text{CH=CH—CH}_3)(\text{OH})\text{CH—Q}$$

(Q = 6-methoxy-4-quinolyl) (hypothetical) niquidine

So many reactions, which had never before been thought of as related, are thus grouped together, that a family name is needed, and Grob has proposed the name *fragmentations*. He assumes that all these reactions will be linked together, not only in structural form, but also by the common pattern of mechanisms through which they operate. Grob had undertaken the elucidation of this pattern in the field of reactions of γ-amino-halides and -sulphonates.

(43b) Mechanisms of Fragmentation.[74]—Grob envisages two mechanisms. The first is analogous to an E2 elimination, except that the basic reagent is now "built in." By the definition of molecularity, the process is unimolecular; but it goes in one step, as the E2 mechanism does, all bond changes being concerted. We might label it F1(E2). Its expected characteristics are as follows:

(1) It will give a single product, because there is no intermediate at which the reaction path could branch.

(2) It will be stereochemically favoured, if the bond to the leaving group, and the fragmented bond, and also the "axis" (dotted) of the basic electrons are all parallel (thick lines):

$$\underset{\text{B}}{\ddot{}} \curvearrowright \overset{(\text{S}_\text{N}2)}{\text{C}_\gamma} \curvearrowright \underset{(\text{S}_\text{E}2)}{\text{C}_\beta} \curvearrowright \overset{(\text{S}_\text{N}2)}{\text{C}_\alpha} \curvearrowright \text{X} \rightarrow \text{B}{=}\text{C}_\gamma + \text{C}_\beta{=}\text{C}_\alpha + \text{X}^- \qquad [\text{F1(E2)}]$$

The argument is that the component nucleophilic substitutions at C_γ and C_α must invert configuration, whilst the component electrophilic substitution at C_β will preferably retain it, wherefore the preferred conformations about BC_γ and $C_\beta C_\alpha$ are antiperiplanar (*ap*). Conformation about $C_\gamma C_\beta$ is unimportant.

(3) Structural modifications of the basic group B, as well as to the immediate surroundings of C_α, will be important for the rate.

(4) The mechanism provides no opportunity for a Wagner rearrangement.

Grob's second mechanism is analogous to E1 elimination, and, like it, consists of two steps: a slow formation of a C_α-carbonium ion is succeeded by fast fragmentation of the latter. We can label this mechanism F1(E1):

$$\left.\begin{array}{l} B{-}C_\gamma{-}C_\beta{-}C_\alpha{-}X \xrightarrow[\text{slow}]{} B{-}C_\gamma{-}C_\beta{-}\overset{+}{C}_\alpha + X^- \\ B{-}C_\gamma{-}C_\beta{-}\overset{+}{C}_\alpha \xrightarrow[\text{fast}]{} B\overset{+}{C}_\gamma + C_\beta{=}C_\alpha \end{array}\right\} \text{[F1(E1)]}$$

Its expected properties are as follows:

(1) It can give various products according to the possibilities open to the intermediately formed carbonium ion. In general, products of nucleophilic substitution, elimination, and fragmentation would be formed side by side.

(2) Conformation about the BC_γ and $C_\beta C_\alpha$ bonds will be much less important.

(3) Structural modifications to the basic group B will make but little difference to the rate of the overall reaction, which will depend essentially on the immediate surroundings of C_α.

(4) The observation of a Wagner rearrangement should be possible.

Grob has observed all the more positive characteristics in these two lists in different groups of examples, and has assigned mechanisms accordingly, as will be illustrated.

(43c) Mechanism Allied to E2 Elimination.—Reactions (1)–(3) below are assigned this mechanism, because the fragmentations are total, are stereospecific, and are kinetically highly dependent on the basic γ-group:

Rel. rate

(1) 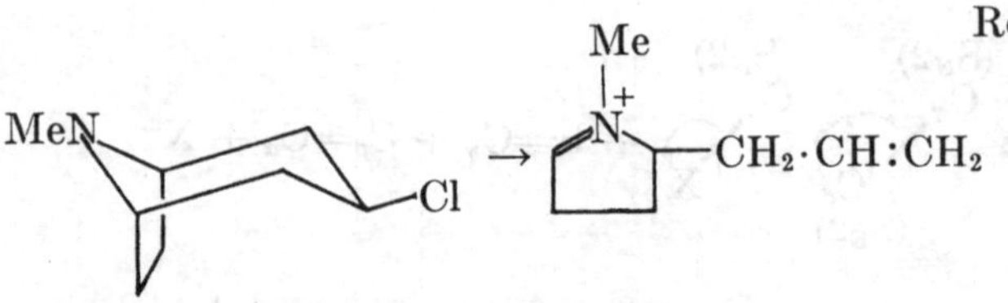 MeN ... Cl → (Me, N^+) ring —$CH_2 \cdot CH{:}CH_2$ 25,000[a]

3β-Tropanyl chloride

Rel. rate

(2) HN ... Cl → (H, N^+) ring —$CH_2 \cdot CH{:}CH_2$ 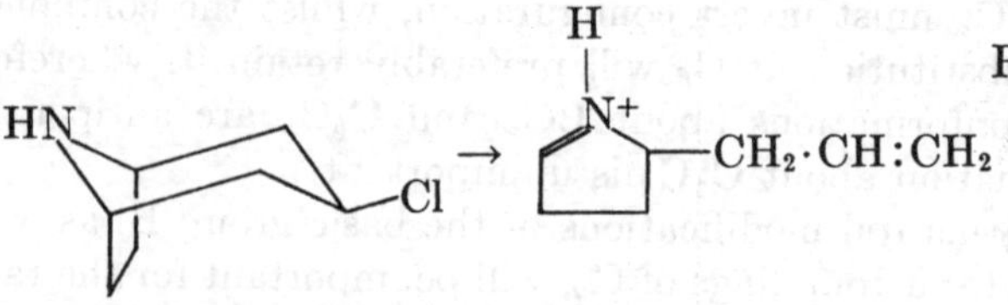 1400[a]

3β-Nortropanyl chloride

[a] Rates are relative to chloro*cyclo*hexane in "80%" aq.-EtOH at 82°. The last reaction is one of substitution and elimination only.

Rel. rate

(3) N(quinuclidine)—Cl → CH_2=N⁺(ring)=CH_2 53,000[b]

4-Chloroquinuclidine

[b] The rate is relative to that of 1-chloro*dicyclo*[2.2.2]octane in "80%" aq.-EtOH at 40°. The latter reaction is one of substitution only.

The reactions of the 3β-tropanyl and 3β-nortropanyl compounds depend on their stereochemistry. The geometrical isomer of substrate (1), *i.e.*, 3α-tropanyl chloride, in which Cl is *cis* with respect to the $CH_2 \cdot CH_2$ bridge, and the $C_\beta C_\alpha$ bond is conformationally synclinal in the chain $C_\gamma C_\beta C_\alpha X$, undergoes only nucleophilic substitution and elimination with no accompanying fragmentation.

(43d) Mechanism Allied to E1 Elimination.—Substrates (4) to (7) below, on hydrolysis in aqueous sodium hydroxide, give products of substitution, elimination, and fragmentation side by side. The basic γ-substituent is obviously important for product composition. So are the immediate surroundings of C_α; for the proportion of fragmentation falls to zero in these systems if C_α is made secondary or primary:

(4) $H_2N \cdot CH_2 \cdot CH_2 \cdot CMe_2$—Cl → 20% fragmentation

(5) $Me_2N \cdot CH_2 \cdot CH_2 \cdot CMe_2$—Cl → 45% fragmentation

(6) Me—N(piperidine ring)—CMe_2—Br → 60% fragmentation

(7) Me—N⁺(quinuclidine ring)—CMe_2—Br → 82% fragmentation

However, the basic γ-substituent and, even its replacement by an isoelectronic but non-basic hydrocarbon residue, makes no significant difference to the rates of the reactions. This is illustrated in examples (8) and (9):

Rel. rate

(8) $H_2N \cdot CH_2 \cdot CH_2 \cdot CMe_2 \cdot Cl \rightarrow$ 20% fragmentation 0.99[c]

Rel. rate

(9) $Me_2N \cdot CH_2 \cdot CH_2 \cdot CMe_2 \cdot Cl \rightarrow$ 50% fragmentation 0.75[c]

[c] Rates relative to that of $Me_2CH \cdot CH_2 \cdot CH_2 \cdot CMe_2 \cdot Cl$, taken as 1.00 in "80%" aq.-EtOH at 56°. This last reaction is one of substitution and elimination only.

A Wagner rearrangement arises in the solvolysis of quinuclidine-4-carbinyl toluene-*p*-sulphonate (example 10), which in "80%" aqueous ethanol undergoes enlargement of one ring with fragmentation of another:

(10) 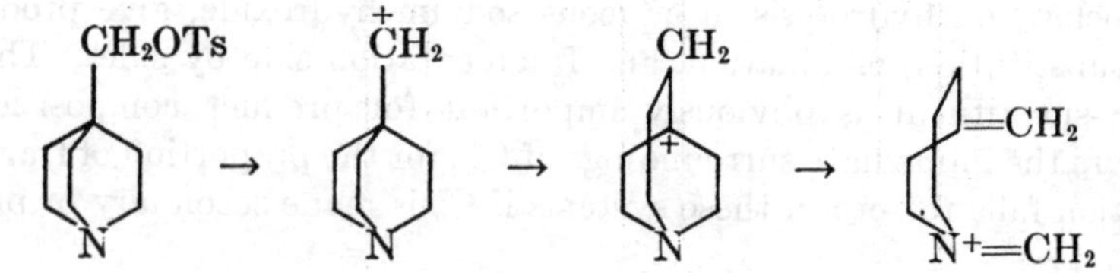 CH_2OTs → $\overset{+}{C}H_2$ → CH_2 → $=CH_2$, $N^+=CH_2$

(Rate = 0.22)

The reaction of the corresponding homocyclic substrate produces ring-enlargement with substitution only in the same conditions:

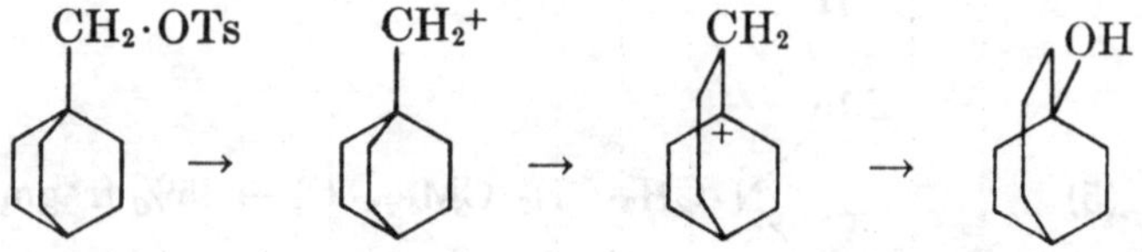

$CH_2 \cdot OTs$ → CH_2^+ → CH_2 → OH

(Rate = 1.00)

Relative to the rate of this reaction as unity, the rate of the quinuclidine fragmentation is only 0.22 in "80%" aqueous ethanol at 116°; and so, although the fragmentation product is formed in high yield, the nitrogen atom cannot be participating in the determination of the products until after a rate-controlling step is over. Therefore this reaction has mechanism F1(E1), consistently with its inclusion of a Wagner rearrangement.

(44) CARBENE-FORMING 1,1-ELIMINATIONS

The idea that the alkaline hydrolysis of chloroform to carbon monoxide and formate ion might proceed by way of "carbon dichloride" was first expressed by Geuther[82] in 1862. It was covered in a comprehensive scheme of such reactions advocated by Nef[83] in 1897. But it was not at any time generally considered probable until it was established by Hine[84] in 1950. He also established the detailed mechanism. And, generalising to related compounds, he and his co-workers identified the two known mechanisms of 1,1-elimination.

(44a) Unimolecular Elimination in a Conjugate Base.—It is known that an α-chlorine substituent, though it always increases the rate of an S_N1 substitution, usually reduces that of an S_N2 substitution. Consistently, the second-order alkaline hydrolysis of methylene chloride is considerably slower than that of methyl chloride. But the same reaction of chloroform is about 10^3 times faster than that of methylene chloride. It is also much faster than the reaction of carbon tetrachloride. This phenomenon of a rate maximum at haloforms is general among the halogenomethanes. Thus for all haloforms containing bromine, the second-order rate is of the order 10^3 times greater than for chlorobromomethane or for methylene bromide.

This phenomenon does not repeat itself in second-order substitutions by reagents such as the phenylthiolate ion, PhS^-, which are strongly nucleophilic for substitutions at a carbon atom, and are only mildly basic, that is, mildly nucleophilic towards hydrogen. For such substitutions, the haloforms are more slowly reacting than the dihalogenomethanes. However, these substitutions in haloforms are strongly catalysed by hydroxide ions.

Direct evidence that the relatively fast reactions of haloforms in the presence of strong bases depend on the acidity of the hydrogen atoms of the haloforms was provided by a study of alkali-catalysed hydrogen-deuterium exchange with the aqueous solvent. For chloroform, and, indeed, for all fluorine-free haloforms, hydrogen exchange is from 10 to 1000 times faster than hydrolysis. Evidently the first step of hydrolysis is that of hydrogen exchange, that is, the pre-equilibrium formation of the conjugate base of the haloform. In the example of chloroform, this is the trichloromethylide ion, CCl_3^-.

What happens to this carbanion was made clear by a study of salt effects on the alkaline hydrolysis of chloroform. The addition of

[82] A. Geuther, *Ann.*, 1862, **122**, 121.

[83] J. U. Nef. *Ann.*, 1897, **298**, 202.

[84] J. Hine, *J. Am. Chem. Soc.*, 1950, **72**, 2438; J. Hine, C. R. Peeks, and B. D. Oakes, *ibid.*, 1954, **76**, 827; J. Hine and A. M. Dowell, *ibid.*, p. 2688; J. Hine, C. H. Thomas, and S. J. Emerson, *ibid.*, 1955, **77**, 3886; J. Hine, A. M. Dowell, and J. E. Singley, *ibid.*, 1956, **78**, 479; J. Hine, S. J. Emerson, and W. H. Brader, *ibid.*, p. 2282; J. Hine and N. W. Burske, *ibid.*, p. 3337; *idem*, M. Hine, and P. B. Langford, *ibid.* 1957, **79**, 1406; J. Hine, R. Butterworth, and P. B. Langford, *ibid.*, 1958, **80**, 819.

sodium chloride repressed the rate, and control experiments with other salts, particularly the non-intervening salt sodium perchlorate, showed that the rate repression by chloride ion was a typical mass-law effect of a "common ion" in a unimolecular substitution (Section **32**). Analogous salt effects were observed with other haloforms.

These facts, all established by Hine and his collaborators,[84] compel acceptance of Hine's interpretation of 1950, namely, that for chloroform, and, as it turned out, for all haloforms containing not more than one fluorine atom, the conjugate base, trihalomethylide ion, formed in pre-equilibrium, undergoes a unimolecular reaction, the first and slowest step of which is the loss of a halide ion to give a dihalogenomethylene, that is a compound of bivalent carbon of the general class now known as carbenes. The carbene is then rapidly trapped by something, in aqueous solvents by water, to give carbon monoxide, and, in the presence of hydroxide ions, formate ions. This is a 1,1-elimination by unimolecular reaction of a conjugate base of the substrate, a description which one can conveniently contract in the symbol 1,1-E1cB:

$$\left.\begin{array}{l} CHX_3 + OH^- \underset{(-1)}{\overset{(1)}{\rightleftharpoons}} CX_3^- + H_2O \\ CX_3^- \underset{(-2)}{\overset{(2)\text{ slow}}{\rightleftharpoons}} CX_2 + X^- \\ CX_2 + H_2O \underset{OH^-}{\overset{(3)}{\longrightarrow}} CO,\ HCO_2,\ \text{and } X^- \end{array}\right\} \quad (1,1\text{-E1cB})$$

This mechanism of 1,1-elimination applies outside the field of the haloforms. One halogen atom is left out in the following example, in which the loss of a sulphone group, from a first-formed conjugate base, leads to a carbene and thence to the products:[85]

$$PhSO_2\cdot CHF_2 + MeO^- \rightleftharpoons PhSO_2\cdot CF_2^- + MeOH$$
$$PhSO_2\cdot CF_2^- \longrightarrow CF_2 + PhSO_2^-$$
$$CF_2 + MeOH \longrightarrow MeO\cdot CHF_2$$

In the example formulated below, a halogen-free sulphonium ion is rapidly and reversibly converted by aqueous alkali into its conjugate base, which slowly loses dimethyl sulphide to form an aromatic carbene, finally recovered as its stilbene dimer:[86]

[85] J. Hine and J. J. Porter, *J. Am. Chem. Soc.*, **1960, 82,** 6178.
[86] C. G. Swain and E. R. Thornton, *J. Am. Chem. Soc.*, **1961, 83,** 4033.

$$p\text{-}NO_2\cdot C_6H_4\cdot CH_2\cdot SMe_2^+ + OH^- \rightleftharpoons p\text{-}NO_2\cdot C_6H_4\cdot \bar{C}H\cdot SMe_2^+$$
$$\rightarrow p\text{-}NO_2\cdot C_6H_4\cdot CH$$
$$\rightarrow p\text{-}NO_2\cdot C_6H_4\cdot CH{:}CH\cdot C_6H_4\cdot NO_2\text{-}p$$

As Dr. W. T. Miller pointed out to the writer in 1954, there are a number of claimed carbene reactions, based on 1,1-elimination, in which it is not clearly shown that the first-formed carbanion ($CXYZ^-$) is not attacked in a bimolecular nucleophilic substitution, in the course of which an anion (X^-) is expelled, rather than in a unimolecular type of process depending on prior loss of the anion to give a carbene. In his early examples, Hine took care of the point, as described above. But this has not always been done, and, since processes of the bimolecular type do occur, it seems possible that carbene reactions have been claimed too widely.

It was discovered by Doering and Hoffmann that carbenes add to olefins very readily to form *cyclo*propane derivatives.[87] This reaction is highly diagnostic of the formation of carbenes by any stoicheiometric process, and, if by 1,1-elimination, it is a diagnostic of mechanism 1,1-E1cB. This method of trapping a carbene naturally works best when other "traps" are absent, that is, in an inert solvent containing the olefin, or in the olefin itself as solvent, as is illustrated by the following reaction in solvent tetramethylethylene:[88]

$$CHBr(CN)_2 + Et_3N \rightleftharpoons CBr(CN)_2^- + Et_3NH^+$$
$$CBr(CN)_2^- \longrightarrow C(CN)_2 + Br^-$$

$$C(CN)_2 + Me_2C{:}CMe_2 \longrightarrow \begin{matrix} Me_2C \\ | \quad \diagdown \\ | \quad\; C(CN)_2 \\ | \quad \diagup \\ Me_2C \end{matrix}$$

(44b) Bimolecular Elimination.—Hine found that the introduction of a single fluorine atom into a haloform, as in $CHFCl_2$, $CHFClBr$, or $CHFBr_2$, had a marked kinetic effect. For fluorine-free haloforms basic hydrolysis had second-order kinetics with a rate-constant equal to the second-order rate-constant k_1 of step (1) of mechanism 1,1-E1cB, multiplied by the small fraction $k_2/(k_{-1}+k_2) \approx k_2/k_{-1}$, in which formed conjugate base goes on to give the carbene rather than back to restore the haloform. The introduction of a single fluorine atom reduced the rate-constant k_1, but so increased the rate-constant k_2 that it became comparable to k_{-1}, and in particular cases somewhat larger

[87] W. v. E. Doering and A. K. Hoffmann, *J. Am. Chem. Soc.*, 1954, **76**, 6162.
[88] J. S. Swenson and R. Rapoport, *J. Am. Chem. Soc.*, 1965, **87**, 1397.

than k_{-1}, with the result that the fraction $k_2/(k_{-1}+k_2)$ became increased so strongly as to produce an increase in the overall rate, despite the reduction in k_1. This implies the beginning of a shift of rate control from step (2) to step (1); and so one might expect that the introduction of a second fluorine atom would complete this shift, and that the overall rate, now determined wholly by step (1), would decrease along with the individual rate-constant k_1.

Experiments showed, however,[89] that the difluoro compounds CHF_2Cl, CHF_2Br, and CHF_2I underwent alkaline hydrolysis much more rapidly than could have been expected on this basis. The reactions were much too fast to be understood as bimolecular nucleophilic substitutions, S_N2, and could be shown to depend specifically on the basicity of the reagent, rather than on its nucleophilic strength towards carbon. Furthermore, unlike the alkaline hydrolyses of other haloforms, the reactions took place with negligible hydrogen exchange between the substrate and the medium. The interpretation, given by Hine and his collaborators, is that the conjugate base is never formed, and that one is dealing with a one-step bimolecular 1,1-elimination, the mechanism here labelled 1,1-E2:

$$\left.\begin{array}{l} HO^- + H\text{—}CF_2\text{—}X \longrightarrow H_2O + CF_2 + X^- \\ CF_2 + H_2O \xrightarrow[OH^-]{} CO, HCO_2^-, \text{ and } F^- \end{array}\right\} \quad (1,1\text{-E2})$$

The possibility of producing carbenes by mechanism 1,1-E1 is theoretically obvious, but seems not yet to have been demonstrably realised.

[89] J. Hine and P. B. Langford, *J. Am. Chem. Soc.*, 1957, **79**, 5497; J. Hine and J. D. Porter, *ibid.*, p. 5493; J. Hine and A. D. Ketley, *J. Org. Chem.*, **25**, 606.

CHAPTER X

Saturated Rearrangements

(45) NUCLEOPHILIC REARRANGEMENTS IN SATURATED SYSTEMS

WE are to review the rearrangements involved in the reactions of isomerisation, substitution, or elimination undergone by saturated carbon, carbon-nitrogen, and carbon-oxygen systems. The term "saturated system" is not intended to imply that the rearranging molecule is always strictly saturated: rather it means that, if any multiple-bond or aromatic unsaturation is present, the rearrangement process, though it may take advantage of the unsaturation, is of a type that could proceed without it. For brevity, we call these processes *saturated rearrangements*.

Rearrangements that involve the shift of a group carrying an excess of electrons to an electron-deficient centre are termed *nucleophilic rearrangements*. Our concern in this Section will be with *saturated nucleophilic rearrangements*.

Several groups of rearrangements here come under consideration. We shall start with a general survey of two such groups (**45a, 45b**), then proceed to discuss the processes involved (**45c**), then refer to other rearrangements in which similar processes operate (**45d**), and lastly go into the finer details of mechanism (**45e–45h**).

(45a) Rearrangements in Carbonyl-forming Eliminations: Pinacol-Pinacolone and Allied Changes.—In 1859 Fittig discovered pinacol and in 1860 he recorded its conversion by sulphuric acid to a ketone, pinacolone:[1]

$$Me_2C(OH) \cdot CMe_2(OH) \rightarrow MeCO \cdot CMe_3$$

The striking feature of this change is the shifting of a methyl group from one of the glycol carbon atoms to the other. Numerous conversions of this pattern have since been discovered, and it has thus been made clear that Fittig's reaction typifies a very general transformation of substituted 1,2-glycols. By means of strong acids such as aqueous sulphuric acid, they may be converted into carbonyl compounds, with the shift of a substituent from the carbon atom which is increasing its binding with oxygen to give the carbonyl group, to the carbon atom which is losing its oxygen. Conversions of this general type are known as *pinacol-pinacolone* rearrangements.

As to the scope of the process, it is not necessary that the migrating radical shall be methyl or some other alkyl group: it may be phenyl or

[1] R. Fittig, *Ann.*, 1859, **110**, 17; 1860, **114**, 54.

another aryl group. Moreover, with these migrating groups it is not necessary that the glycol shall be ditertiary: it can at least be tertiary-secondary or disecondary. The following examples illustrate these points:

$$Ph_2C(OH) \cdot CPh_2(OH) \rightarrow PhCO \cdot CPh_3 \qquad \text{(Ref. 2)}$$

$$Me_2C(OH) \cdot CPh_2(OH) \rightarrow MeCO \cdot CMePh_2 \qquad \text{(Ref. 3)}$$

$$PhCH(OH) \cdot CMePh(OH) \rightarrow CHO \cdot CMePh_2 \qquad \text{(Ref. 4)}$$

$$PhCH(OH) \cdot CHPh(OH) \rightarrow CHO \cdot CHPh_2 \qquad \text{(Ref. 5)}$$

Other transformations, those of some tertiary-secondary and some disecondary glycols, and of most tertiary-primary and secondary-primary glycols, conform to the same pattern, provided that the shifting group is taken to be a hydrogen atom, as in the following examples (An = *p*-anisyl; Tol = p-tolyl):

$$MeCH(OH) \cdot CPh_2(OH) \rightarrow MeCO \cdot CHPh_2 \qquad \text{(Ref. 6)}$$

$$PhCH(OH) \cdot CPh_2(OH) \rightarrow PhCO \cdot CHPh_2 \qquad \text{(Ref. 7)}$$

$$PhCH(OH) \cdot CHAn(OH) \rightarrow PhCO \cdot CH_2An \qquad \text{(Ref. 8)}$$

$$MeCH(OH) \cdot CHPh(OH) \rightarrow MeCO \cdot CH_2Ph \qquad \text{(Ref. 9)}$$

$$CH_2(OH) \cdot CPh_2(OH) \rightarrow CHO \cdot CHPh_2 \qquad \text{(Ref. 10)}$$

$$CH_2(OH) \cdot CHMe(OH) \rightarrow CHO \cdot CH_2Me \qquad \text{(Ref. 11)}$$

$$CH_2(OH) \cdot CPhTol(OH) \rightarrow CHO \cdot CHPhTol \qquad \text{(Ref. 12)}$$

In the last example, Mislow and Siegel showed that an optically active factor gave an optically active product, thus proving that a carbon-bound hydrogen of the primary alcohol group is transferred in a stereospecific way to the carbon atom which loses its hydroxyl group; that is, the primary hydrogen is not lost with the tertiary hydroxyl group as water, to leave a vinyl alcohol, which rearranges.

The pinacol-pinacolone rearrangement has been extensively investigated, notably by Danilov and Venus-Danilova, by Tiffeneau, Orék-

[2] W. Thörner and T. Zincke, *Ber.*, 1877, **10**, 1473.
[3] W. Parry, *J. Chem. Soc.*, 1915, **107**, 108.
[4] M. Tiffeneau and Dorlencourt, *Ann. chim. phys.*, 1909, **16**, 237.
[5] A. Breuner and T. Zincke, *Ann.*, 1879, **198**, 141.
[6] R. Stoermer, *Ber.*, 1906, **39**, 2288.
[7] M. Tiffeneau, *Compt. rend.*, 1908, **148**, 29.
[8] A. Orékhov and M. Tiffeneau, *Bull soc. chim.* (France), 1925, **37**, 1410
[9] M. Tiffeneau, *Ann. chim. phys.*, 1907, **10**, 328.
[10] R. Stoermer, *loc. cit.;* M. Tiffeneau, *Ann. chim. phys.*, 1907, **10**, 328.
[11] A. Kötz and K. Richter, *J. prakt. Chem.*, 1925, **111**, 373.
[12] K. Mislow and M. Siegel, *J. Am. Chem. Soc.*, 1952, **74**, 1060.

hov, and Levy, and by Bachmann and his collaborators, with the general object of discovering which group migrates, or which is the principal one to migrate, when the structure admits several possibilities. The idea was to throw light on the firmness of binding of groups by determining their "relative migratory aptitudes." Actually the results of such experiments have to be considered in close relation to the mechanism of the rearrangement.

In the general case of a glycol,

$$R_1R_2C(OH)\cdot C(OH)R_3R_4$$

the direction of rearrangement will depend on two matters, which have to be taken in order. The first is that of which hydroxyl group will be lost: for this determines which of the two pairs of R's will supply an R to replace it. The rule on this question[13] is very well supported by experiment: hydroxyl loss from RR′C(OH) is facilitated by inductive and conjugative electron release ($+I$ and $+K$) from RR′, just as in ordinary unimolecular substitutions or eliminations (S_N1 and E1). It is clear that we have to think of the acid catalysis of the hydroxyl loss as a carbonium-ion forming heterolysis, similar to those undergone by the conjugate acids of alcohols in unimolecular reactions generally:

$$RR'C{-}OH_2^+ \rightarrow RR'C^+ + OH_2$$

Thus, an order of facilitation, such as,

$$(R, R' =)\ p\text{-anisyl} > \text{phenyl} > \text{alkyl} > H$$

each inequality in which is illustrated among the already given examples of pinacol-pinacolone changes, can readily be understood.

Supposing that the identity of the eliminated hydroxyl group is determined, the question remains as to which of two groups will shift from the adjacent position to take its place. As to this, we shall have to neglect migrating hydrogen, because of the ambiguity of mechanism already explained. As to other groups, the main principle is that that group will be the more mobile from which electron release ($+I$ and $+K$) is the stronger. Thus, when a structure could supply either an aryl or an alkyl group, it is the aryl group which actually migrates, as in the example,[14]

[13] C. K. Ingold, *Ann. Repts. on Progress Chem.* (Chem. Soc. London), 1928 25, 133.

[14] W. Thörner and T. Zincke, *Ber.*, 1880, 13, 641.

$$MePhC(OH)\cdot C(OH)MePh \rightarrow MeCO\cdot CMePh_2$$

When a structure could supply alternative aryl groups, as in Bachmann's symmetrical pinacols,

$$ArAr'C(OH)\cdot C(OH)ArAr'$$

it is the one more activated towards electrophilic agents which in fact migrates, as illustrated by the mobility series,[15]

p-anisyl > *p*-tolyl > *m*-tolyl > *m*-anisyl > phenyl
> *p*-chlorophenyl > *o*-anisyl > *m*-chlorophenyl

except for the anomalous position of the *o*-anisyl group which may be of steric origin.

The significance of the mobility rule as an indication of mechanism is that the migrating group uses its electrons to initiate binding with the neighbouring electron-deficient centre; and that it does this before the electrons of the eventually broken bond become adequately available.

It has been shown that the rate of the conversion of pinacol to pinacolone follows Hammett's h_0, as it should if it is specific-hydrogen-ion rather than general-acid catalysed, that is, if the first step is a pre-equilibrium formation of the conjugate acid of the glycol.[16,17] It has been shown further, from a comparison of the rate of the conversion in ^{18}O-water with the rate of ^{18}O-uptake, that the dehydration of the conjugate acid is reversed by addition of water to the carbonium ion at a rate which is competitive with the rate of the methyl migration in the carbonium ion.[17]

There are a number of rearrangements which are closely analogous to the pinacol-pinacolone change. One is the *rearrangement of substituted ethylene oxides* to carbonyl compounds under the influence of acids. The rules about which carbon atom parts company from the oxygen atom, and which group takes the place of the lost oxygen, seem to be quite the same as for the pinacol-pinacolone change. To cite one investigation as an example, it has been shown[18] that ethylene oxides of the type formulated below, give benzhydryl ketones, the oxygen atom parting from the Ph_2C group, when R = Me, Et, *n*-Pr, *i*-Pr,

[15] W. E. Bachmann and F. H. Moser, *J. Am. Chem. Soc.*, 1932, **54**, 1124; W. E. Bachmann and H. R. Sternberger, *ibid.*, 1933, **55**, 3821; 1934, **56**, 170; W. E. Bachmann and J. W. Ferguson, *ibid.*, p. 2081.

[16] J. F. Duncan and K. R. Lynn, *J. Chem. Soc.*, **1956**, 3512, 3519, 3674.

[17] C. A. Bunton, T. Hadwick, D. R. Llewellyn, and Y. Pocker, *J. Chem. Soc.*, 1958, 403; C. A. Bunton and M. D. Carr, *ibid.*, **1963**, 5854.

[18] R. Lagrave, *Ann. chim.*, 1927, **8**, 363.

n-Bu, *sec.*-Bu, Benzyl, or Phenyl; but that, when R = *p*-Anisyl, the other oxygen bond is severed, and the product is a phenyl ketone:

$$\overset{\text{O}}{\overbrace{Ph_2C\text{——}CHR}} \rightarrow Ph_2CH\cdot CO\cdot R \qquad (R = \text{alkyl or phenyl})$$

$$\overset{\text{O}}{\overbrace{Ph_2C\text{——}CHR}} \rightarrow PhCO\cdot CHPhR \qquad (R = p\text{-anisyl})$$

Another such rearrangement, sometimes called the *acyloin rearrangement*, consists in the conversion, usually effected by means of alcoholic sulphuric acid, of α-hydroxy-ketones or α-hydroxy-aldehydes into isomeric α-hydroxy-ketones, with the oxygen functions interchanged and a group displaced, as in the examples,

$$i\text{-Pr—}\overset{\text{O}}{\overset{\|}{C}}\text{—}\underset{\text{Me}}{\overset{\text{OH}}{C}}\text{—Me} \rightarrow i\text{-Pr—}\underset{\text{Me}}{\overset{\text{OH}}{C}}\text{—}\overset{\text{O}}{\overset{\|}{C}}\text{—Me} \qquad \text{(Ref. 19)}$$

$$\text{H—}\overset{\text{O}}{\overset{\|}{C}}\text{—}\underset{\text{Ph}}{\overset{\text{OH}}{C}}\text{—Ph} \rightarrow \text{H—}\underset{\text{Ph}}{\overset{\text{OH}}{C}}\text{—}\overset{\text{O}}{\overset{\|}{C}}\text{—Ph} \qquad \text{(Ref. 20)}$$

The *benzil-benzilic acid conversion*, first observed by Liebig, is usually effected by means of aqueous-alcoholic alkali hydroxide.[21] An addition compound, PhCO·COPh,KOH, has been isolated, and has been shown to undergo rearrangement to $Ph_2C(OH)\cdot CO_2K$, potassium benzilate.[22] A compound, PhCO·COPh,NaOEt, has also been obtained: it does not rearrange until water is added, when it gives sodium benzilate.[23] The rate of the conversion of benzil to benzilic acid in aqueous alkaline media is proportional to [benzil] $[OH^-]$; and this expression represents a catalysis specific to hydroxide ion, and not a particular case of general basic catalysis.[24] All these observations agree with the theory[25] that rearrangement proceeds through a hydroxide-ion addition complex by an electronic change similar to that formulated

[19] A. I. Oumnov, *Bull. soc. chim.* (France), 1928, **43**, 568.

[20] S. Danilov, *Ber.*, 1927, **60**, 2390.

[21] J. Liebig, *Ann.*, 1838, **25**, 27; N. Zenin, *ibid.*, 1839, **31**, 329; A. Jena, *ibid.*, 1870, **155**, 77.

[22] G. Scheuing, *Ber.*, 1923, **56**, 252.

[23] A. Lachmann, *J. Am. Chem. Soc.*, 1923, **45**, 1509.

[24] F. H. Westheimer, *J. Am. Chem. Soc.*, 1936, **58**, 2209.

[25] C. K. Ingold and C. W. Shoppee, *J. Chem. Soc.*, 1928, 371.

above for the acyloin rearrangement:

$$\mathrm{O{=}C(Ph){-}C({=}O){-}Ph} \xrightarrow{(\mathrm{OH^-})} \bar{\mathrm{O}}\mathrm{{-}C(OH)(Ph){-}C({=}O){-}Ph} \rightarrow \bar{\mathrm{O}}\mathrm{{-}C({=}O){-}C(O^-)(Ph){-}Ph}$$

$$\xrightarrow{(\mathrm{H^+})} \bar{\mathrm{O}}\mathrm{{-}C({=}O){-}C(OH)(Ph){-}Ph}$$

Carbonyl-forming rearrangements are known, which depend on positive carbon produced by the separation of elements other than oxygen, for example, halogens or nitrogen. An illustration is afforded by Tiffeneau's *iodohydrin rearrangements*, that is, the reactions of tertiary β-iodo-alcohols with silver or mercuric salts, which, as we know, catalyse forms of halogen separation having the general characteristics of unimolecular heterolysis (Section **31c**). He has shown that suitably substituted iodohydrins can be thus converted into carbonyl compounds with the shifting of a substituent, as in the following examples:

$$\mathrm{H{-}O{-}CMe(Ph){\cdot}CH_2{-}I} \rightarrow \mathrm{O{=}CMe{\cdot}CH_2Ph} \qquad \text{(Ref. 26)}$$

$$\mathrm{H{-}O{-}C(Me)} \text{ [ring: } \mathrm{C(Me)(OH){-}CH(I){-}CH_2{-}CH_2{-}CH_2{-}CH_2} \text{]} \rightarrow \mathrm{O{=}C(Me){-}CH} \text{ [ring: } \mathrm{CH{-}CH_2{-}CH_2{-}CH_2{-}CH_2} \text{]} \qquad \text{(Ref. 27)}$$

In these cases the direction of the rearrangement is not what it would have been, had the iodine atom been a hydroxyl group, and the reagent aqueous sulphuric acid: for in this situation the tertiary, not the secondary or primary, hydroxyl would be lost. Otherwise, the reactions exhibit the usual mobility orders, Ph > alkyl, and higher alkyl > Me.

Analogous rearrangements, called *pinacolic deaminations*, occur, as McKenzie showed, when tertiary β-amino-alcohols are deaminated by nitrous acid, a process believed to take place by loss of nitrogen from an initially formed diazonium ion, and known to exhibit unimolecular characteristics (Section **32i**). Some examples are formulated below

[26] M. Tiffeneau, *Compt. rend.*, **1907**, **145**, **593**.
[27] M. Le Brazidec, *Compt. rend.*, **1914**, **159**, **774**.

(An = *p*-anisyl):

$$HO\cdot CMe_2\cdot CHPh\cdot NH_2 \rightarrow MeCO\cdot CHMePh \qquad \text{(Ref. 28)}$$

$$HO\cdot CMePh\cdot CHPh\cdot NH_2 \rightarrow MeCO\cdot CHPh_2 \qquad \text{(Ref. 29)}$$

$$HO\cdot CPh_2\cdot CHPh\cdot NH_2 \rightarrow PhCO\cdot CHPh_2 \qquad \text{(Ref. 30)}$$

$$HO\cdot CPhAn\cdot CH_2\cdot NH_2 \rightarrow PhCO\cdot CH_2An \qquad \text{(Ref. 31)}$$

Here again, the direction of migration would have been different, at least in the last three examples, if the amino-group had been hydroxyl and the reagent had been a strong acid; for then the tertiary hydroxyl group would have left the molecule. Apart from this, the reactions illustrate the usual mobility series, An > Ph > Me.

(45b) Rearrangements in Olefin Elimination, Nucleophilic Substitution, and Olefin Addition: Wagner-Meerwein and Allied Changes.— Rearrangements of this class were first elucidated by Wagner in 1899, who recognised them as essential for an interpretation of the relationships between different members of the dicyclic terpene series. He perceived such rearrangements in the conversions of pinene into bornyl compounds. In proposing the formula now accepted for camphene, he assumed such rearrangements in its formation from, and conversion to, bornyl compounds. Meerwein made further interpretations of the same nature: he broadened the field of recognition and application of the rearrangement, so that it became accepted as one of the general phenomena of organic chemistry, no longer to be regarded as the peculiar and exclusive preserve of terpene chemistry. Moreover, Meerwein made a major contribution—undoubtedly the largest single one—to the elucidation of the mechanism of the change, as we shall notice later.

The dicyclic terpene field is rich in examples of the Wagner-Meerwein rearrangement, and some instances are represented below. Many rearrangements involve a change of ring structure by the shifting of one of the loops of a bridgehead over to an adjoining position, where originally there was either an electronegative substituent, or else a double bond by acid addition to which such a substituent could have been there acquired. However, other rearrangements involve only the shift of a methyl group to an adjoining position, which satisfies one of the conditions just stated. In either case the essential form of the change is the same.

[28] A. McKenzie and M. S. Lesslie, *Ber.*, 1929, 62, 288.
[29] A. McKenzie and R. Roger, *J. Chem. Soc.*, 1924, 125, 844.
[30] A. McKenzie and A. C. Richardson, *J. Chem. Soc.*, 1923, 123, 79.
[31] A. Orékhov and R. Roger, *Compt. rend.*, 1925, 180, 70.

The rearrangements could also be classified into groups according to the overall stoicheiometric result. Some are olefin-forming eliminations; others are nucleophilic substitutions, with isomerisation as a special case, and racemisation as a still more special case; and yet others involve addition to an olefin. In spite of that, the rearrangements conform to a common pattern, as we can show if, following Meerwein's lead, we represent them all as proceeding through a carbonium ion, first formed either by anion loss or proton uptake:

H_2C—H Cl → H_2C—H + → H_2C

*iso*Bornyl chloride → Camphene
(Refs. 32, 33)

Me Cl Me → Me + Me → Me Me

Camphenilyl chloride → Santene
(Ref. 34)

OMe

Camphene methyl ether

Cl

Camphene hydrochloride

→ + → Cl

*iso*Bornyl chloride
(Refs. 33, 35)

[32] G. Wagner, *J. Russ. Phys. Chem. Soc.*, 1899, **31**, 680.

[33] H. Meerwein and K. van Emster, *Ber.*, 1920, **53**, 1815; 1922, **55**, 2500.

[34] H. Meerwein, *Ann.*, 1914, **405**, 129; G. Komppa and S. V. Hintikka, *Bull. soc. chim.* (France), 1917, **21**, 13.

[35] H. Meerwein and L. Gérard, *Ann.*, 1923, **435**, 174; H. Meerwein, O. Hammel, A. Serini, and J. Vörster, *ibid.*, 1927, **453**, 16.

Pinene hydrochloride Bornyl chloride
(Ref. 33)

Racemisation of camphene hydrochloride (and hence of camphene, or of *iso*bornyl chloride)[36] (Ref. 37)

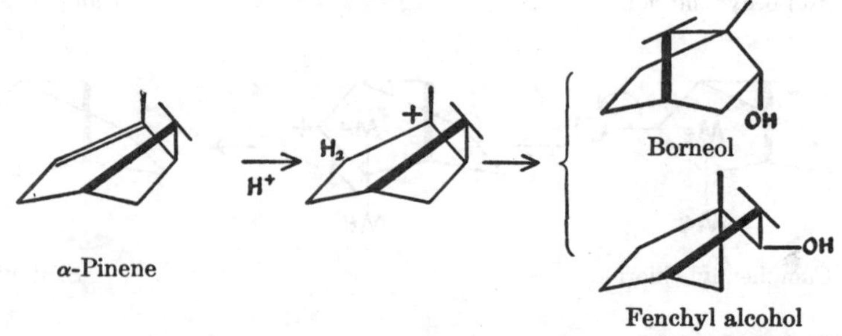

(Ref. 32, 33, 38)

The elimination with rearrangement from *iso*bornyl chloride to give camphene has been studied as a homogeneous gas reaction, as already recounted in Section **42c**.

Meerwein extended the application of the rearrangements outside the field of dicyclic terpenes.[39] He showed, for instance, that 2,2-dimethyl*cyclo*hexanol is converted by acidic dehydration into a mixture of *iso*propylidene*cyclo*pentane and 1,2-dimethyl*cyclo*hexene. These reactions are monocyclic models, the first for the conversion of

[36] In the dicyclic terpene series, such migrations of a methyl group (rather than of a cyclic member of the carbon frame) are known to us as Nemetkin rearrangements.

[37] The racemisation of camphane was interpreted on the basis of a Nemetkin methyl shift by J. L. Simonsen and L. N. Owen, in "The Terpenes," 2nd Edn., Cambridge Univ. Press, 1949, 2, 290. This has since been established by ^{14}C labelling as the main mechanism, by J. D. Roberts and J. A. Vining, *J. Am. Chem. Soc.*, 1953, **75**, 3165, and J. D. Roberts and R. Perry jr., *ibid.*, p. 3168.

[38] G. Wagner and W. Brickner, *Ber.*, 1899, **32**, 2302.

[39] H. Meerwein and W. Unkel, *Ann.*, 1910, **376**, 152; H. Meerwein, *ibid.* 1913, **396**, 200; 1914, **405**, 129; 1918, **417**, 255.

*iso*borneol into camphene, and the second for that of camphenilol into santene:

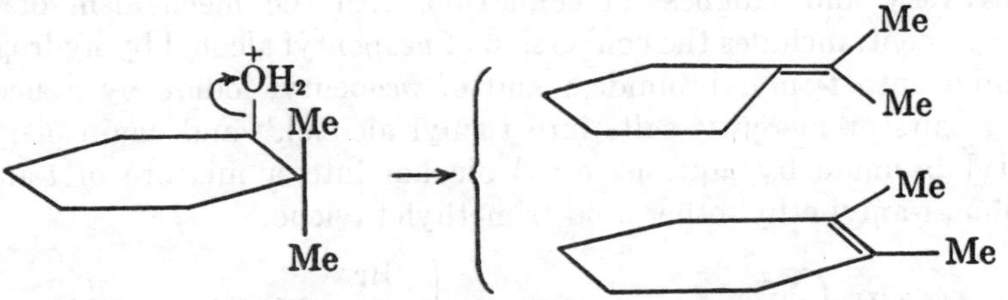

A monocyclic model for rearrangements initiated by proton co-ordination at an olefinic bond, rather than by anion loss (or a similar heterolysis) from a saturated molecule, is recognised[40] in the long-known conversion of α-campholytic acid by means of dilute sulphuric acid into *iso*lauronolic acid:

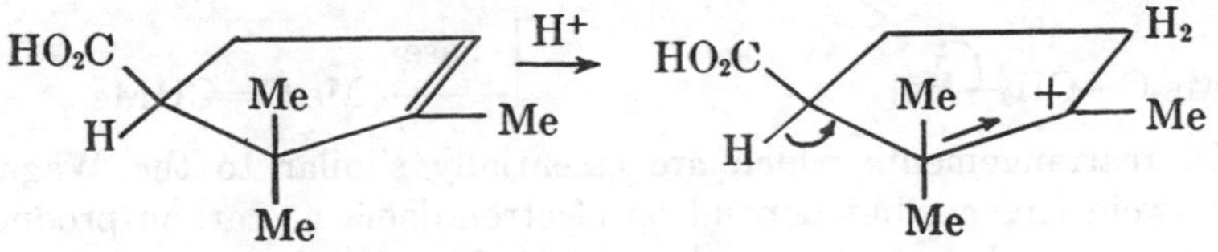

α-Campholytic acid

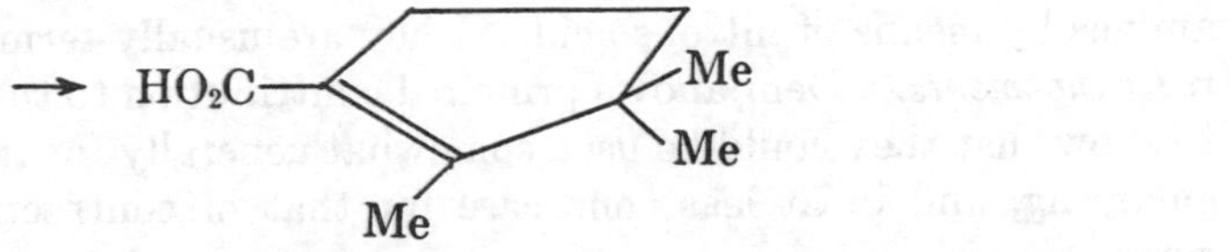

*iso*Lauronolic acid

As to simple acyclic models, the oldest is the conversion of pinacolyl alcohol by acid dehydration into tetramethyl-ethylene:[41] this is the main product, though later work has shown that 1-methyl-1-*iso*-propylethylene is also formed:[42]

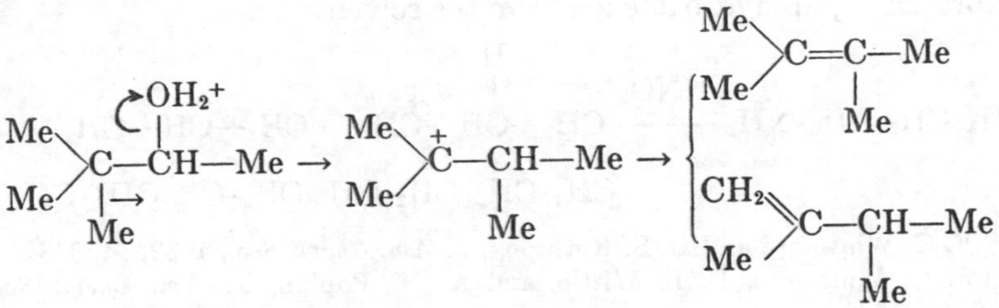

[40] C. W. Shoppee, *Proc. Leeds Phil. Soc.*, Sci. Sect., 1928, **1**, 301.

[41] N. Zelinsky and J. Zelikov, *Ber.*, 1901, **34**, 3249.

[42] F. C. Whitmore and H. S. Rothrock, *J. Am. Chem. Soc.*, 1933, **55**, 1100.

A still simpler group of examples, one which, moreover, derives importance from its study by Whitmore and his collaborators and by Dostrovsky and Hughes, in connexion with the mechanism of rearrangement, includes the conversion of *neo*pentyl alcohol by hydrogen bromide into *t*-amyl bromide,[43] and of *neo*pentyl iodide by aqueous silver salts or mercuric salts into *t*-amyl alcohol,[44] and again of *neo*pentyl bromide by aqueous ethyl alcohol into a mixture of *t*-amyl alcohol, *t*-amyl ethyl ether, and trimethylethylene:[45]

$$Me_3C—CH_2—\overset{+}{O}H_2 \searrow \qquad \qquad \begin{cases} \xrightarrow{Br^-} Me_2CBr\cdot CH_2Me \\ \xrightarrow{H_2O} Me_2C(OH)\cdot CH_2Me \\ \xrightarrow{EtOH} Me_2C(OEt)\cdot CH_2Me \\ \xrightarrow{base} Me_2C{=}CHMe \end{cases}$$

$$\begin{matrix} Me \\ Me \end{matrix}\!\!>\overset{+}{C}—\underset{\displaystyle Me}{\underset{|}{CH_2}}$$

$$Me_3C—CH_2—Hal \nearrow$$

Of rearrangements which are essentially similar to the Wagner-Meerwein change, but depend on electron-deficient carbon produced by the separation of groups other than halogens or oxygen groups, the most important are those associated with the deamination of primary amines by means of nitrous acid. They are usually termed *Demjanov rearrangements*. Demjanov's principal contribution to their study was to show that they could be used somewhat generally for the purpose of enlarging, and in at least one case for that of contracting, alicyclic rings.

It has been known for a long time that *n*-propylamine, on treatment with nitrous acid, yields some *n*-propyl alcohol together with a major proportion of *iso*propyl alcohol.[46] This shows that a high proportion of the carbonium ion, formed by loss of nitrogen from the first-produced diazonium ion (Section **38c**), suffers a 2→1 hydrogen shift, before taking up hydroxide ion from the solvent:

$$CH_3\cdot CH_2\cdot CH_2\cdot NH_2 \xrightarrow{HNO_2} CH_3—\overset{\displaystyle H}{\overset{|}{CH}}—\overset{+}{C}H_2 \rightarrow CH_3—\overset{+}{C}H—\overset{\displaystyle H}{\overset{|}{C}H_2}$$

$$\downarrow \qquad\qquad\qquad \downarrow$$

$$CH_3\cdot CH_2\cdot CH_2\cdot OH \qquad CH_3\cdot CH(OH)\cdot CH_3$$

[43] F. C. Whitmore and H. S. Rothrock, *J. Am. Chem. Soc.*, 1932, **54**, 3431.

[44] F. C. Whitmore, E. L. Wittle, and A. H. Popkin, *J. Am. Chem. Soc.*, 1939, **61**, 1586.

[45] I. Dostrovsky and E. D. Hughes, *J. Chem. Soc.*, **1946**, 166.

[46] E. Linnemann and A. Siersch, *Ann.*, 1867, **144**, 129; E. Linnemann, *ibid.*, 1872, **161**, 15.

Roberts has shown by ^{14}C-labelling that ethylamine is deaminated with a little 2→1 hydrogen shift: about 1.5% of the ethanol produced has the carbon atoms reversed.[47]

Roberts also showed that, of that part of the deamination of *n*-propylamine which leads to *n*-propyl alcohol, a small fraction involves rearrangement. The indication was that a ^{14}C label, originally in position-1 of the amine, had suffered some loss from the 1-position in the alcohol. Reutov identified some of the lost label in the 3-position of the alcohol, so disclosing a 3→1 hydrogen shift, such as we shall meet with again later:[48]

$$\overset{\displaystyle H}{\underset{\displaystyle CH_2}{|}}\cdot CH_2\cdot \overset{+}{C}H_2 \rightarrow \overset{+}{C}H_2\cdot CH_2\cdot \overset{\displaystyle H}{\underset{\displaystyle CH_2}{|}}$$

However, later work by Karabatsos and Orzech and by Lee, Kruger, and Wong makes evident that more than this is going on in the 3–4% of rearrangement contained in that part of the deamination process which ends in *n*-propyl alcohol.[49] For a ^{14}C label, or a tritium label, which is lost in part from position-1 during deamination, is recovered in the *n*-propyl alcohol partly in position-2, as well as partly in position-3. This might signify a 3→1 hydrogen shift accompanying a 2→1 methyl shift, another pattern of events with which we shall meet later.[50]

$$\overset{+}{C}H_2\!-\!\!\!\overset{\displaystyle CH_3}{\diagdown}\!\!\!-CH_2 \;\leftarrow\; CH_2\!-\!\!\!\overset{\displaystyle CH_3}{\diagup}\!\!\!-\overset{+}{C}H_2 \;\rightarrow\; CH_2\!-\!\!\!\overset{\displaystyle CH_2^+}{\diagup}\!\!\!-CH_3$$

(In these diagrams, the identity of the atoms is indicated by position,

[47] J. D. Roberts and J. A. Vancey, *J. Am. Chem. Soc.*, 1952, **74**, 5943; J. D. Roberts and C. M. Regan, *ibid.*, 1953, **75**, 2069; J. D. Roberts and M. Halmann, *ibid.*, p. 5759.

[48] O. A. Reutov and T. N. Shatkina, *Doklady Akad. Nauk S.S.S.R.*, 1960, **133**, 606; *Tetrahedron*, 1962, **18**, 237.

[49] G. J. Karabatsos and C. E. Orzech jr., *J. Am. Chem. Soc.*, 1962, **84**, 2839; *ibid.*, 1965, **87**, 4394; C. C. Lee, J. E. Kruger, and E. W. C. Wong, *ibid.*, pp. 3986, 3987.

[50] The investigators assume the intermediacy of a "protonated *cyclo*propane ring" (see p. 781), indeed, three such, interconvertible by shift of the supernumerary proton from bond to bond round the ring. The writer feels that the available data do not firmly pin-point either this type of explanation or that in the text. For instance, it is difficult on any view to understand why, as reported, the D atoms of a CD_2 group remain together in rearrangements accompanying the deamination of $CH_3\cdot CD_2\cdot CD_2\cdot NH_2$, but separate considerably in rearrangements attending deaminations of $CH_3\cdot CH_2\cdot CD_2\cdot NH_2$ and $CH_3\cdot CD_2\cdot CH_2\cdot NH_2$. One should remind oneself that the experimental work is made very difficult by the smallness of the amount of rearrangement in that minor portion of the deaminations which leads to *n*-propyl alcohol.

though the numbers by which the atoms are distinguished in a chemical name become changed with the isomerisation.)

Hydrogen displacements over longer chains of carbon atoms have been established by Whiting and his coworkers by careful analysis of deamination products of normal-chain amines.[51] For example, the deamination of 1-octylamine in acetic acid gave the following isomeric octyl acetates:

1-, 46.0%; 2-, 18.5%; 3-, 2.8%; 4-, 0.19%

and the following octenes:

$$\text{1-, 19.5\%}\begin{cases}\textit{cis}\text{-2-, 2.1\%;} & \textit{cis}\text{-3-, 0.52\%;} & \textit{cis}\text{-4-, —}\\ \textit{trans}\text{-2-, 7.7\%;} & \textit{trans}\text{-3-, 0.95\%;} & \textit{trans}\text{-4-, 0.08\%}\end{cases}$$

To what extent the longer shifts are direct, or are the overall results of a succession of shorter shifts, is not yet known. However, Prelog's demonstration of 1,5-shifts in *cyclo*decylamine deamination shows that direct shifts over considerable numbers of carbon atoms may occur if the direct distance is short enough (Section **15a**).

Whiting was largely concerned with the question of whether the first-formed diazonium ion lives long enough to allow its counter-ion to diffuse away before it loses nitrogen to yield the carbonium ion. The answer appeared to depend on the stability of the eventual carbonium ion, the nucleophilic strength of the anion, and the ionising power of the medium. For deamination of saturated primary alkylamines, such as 1-octylamine, in solvents of polarity from water to acetic acid, the diazonium ion certainly lives long enough to attain equilibrium dissociation. But when the carbonium ion that it will produce is secondary, the products are such as to suggest that the parent diazonium ion passes into the carbonium ion in the very near presence of the counter-ion, the diazonium ion itself having scarcely any free life.

By treatment with nitrous acid, *neo*pentylamine is transformed into *t*-amyl alcohol.[52] Here we observe the shifting of a methyl group during deamination:

$$(CH_3)_2\overset{\overset{\displaystyle CH_3}{|}}{C}\text{—}CH_2\cdot NH_2 \xrightarrow{HNO_2} (CH_3)_2\overset{\overset{\displaystyle CH_3}{|\rightarrow}}{C}\text{—}\overset{+}{C}H_2 \rightarrow (CH_3)_2\overset{\overset{\displaystyle HO}{|}}{C}\text{—}\overset{\overset{\displaystyle CH_3}{|}}{C}H_2$$

This simple methyl shift does not involve any hydrogen shifts, as Karabatsos, Orzech, and Megerson proved, by showing with the aid of isotopic labels that the three atoms of the methylene group of

[51] H. Maskill, R. M. Southam, and M. C. Whiting, *Chem. Comm.*, 1965, 496.
[52] M. Freund and F. Lenze, *Ber.*, 1891, 24, 2150.

the *neo*pentylamine identically compos[illegible] methylene group of the formed *t*-amyl alcohol.[53]

Some of the ring changes which have been effected by deamination are formulated below: *cyclo*butylamine[54] yields both *cyclo*butanol and *cyclo*propylcarbinol; *cyclo*propylmethylamine[55] likewise yields both *cyclo*propylcarbinol and *cyclo*butanol; and *cyclo*butylmethylamine[56] gives *cyclo*butylcarbinol and methylene*cyclo*butane, and also *cyclo*pentanol and *cyclo*pentene:

$$\begin{matrix} CH_2 \\ | \;\rangle CH\cdot CH_2\cdot NH_2 \rightarrow \\ CH_2 \end{matrix} \left\{ \begin{matrix} CH_2 \\ | \;\rangle CH\cdot CH_2\cdot OH \\ CH_2 \\ \\ CH_2 \\ / \quad \backslash \\ CH_2 \quad CH\cdot OH \\ \backslash \quad / \\ CH_2 \end{matrix} \right\} \leftarrow \begin{matrix} CH_2 \\ / \quad \backslash \\ CH_2 \quad CH\cdot NH_2 \\ \backslash \quad / \\ CH_2 \end{matrix}$$

$$\begin{matrix} CH_2 \\ CH_2 \langle \rangle CH\cdot CH_2\cdot NH_2 \rightarrow \\ CH_2 \end{matrix} \left\{ \begin{matrix} CH_2 \\ CH_2 \quad CH\cdot CH_2\cdot OH \text{ and } CH_2 \quad C{:}CH_2 \\ CH_2 \qquad\qquad\qquad\qquad CH_2 \\ \\ CH_2\cdot CH\cdot OH \qquad\qquad CH_2\cdot CH \\ CH_2 \langle \quad | \qquad \text{and} \quad CH_2 \langle \quad \| \\ CH_2\cdot CH_2 \qquad\qquad CH_2\cdot CH \end{matrix} \right.$$

Similarly, *cyclo*pentylmethylamine,[57] *cyclo*hexylmethylamine,[58] *cyclo*heptylmethylamine[57] and *cyclo*-octylmethylamine[59] yield respectively *cyclo*hexanol, *cyclo*heptanol, *cyclo*-octanol, and *cyclo*nonanol, always with other products, which in the last case are known to include *cyclo*octylcarbinol and 1-methyl*cyclo*-octene.

One might regard, as a backward extension of the same series of Demjanov ring transformations, the conversion of *cyclo*propylamine to allyl alcohol: it is consistent with this that an α-deuterium atom in

[53] G. B. Karabatsos, C. E. Orzech jr., and F. S. Megerson, *J. Am. Chem. Soc.*, 1964, **86**, 1994.

[54] N. Zelinsky and J. Gutt, *Ber.*, 1907, **40**, 4744; N. Demjanov, *ibid.*, p. 4961; N. Demjanov and M. Dojarenko, *Ber.*, 1908, **41**, 43.

[55] N. Demjanov, *J. Russ. Phys. Chem. Soc.*, 1903, **35**, 375; *ibid.*, 1907, **39**, 1077; *Ber.*, 1907, **40**, 4393.

[56] N. Demjanov and M. Luschnikov, *J. Russ. Phys. Chem. Soc.*, 1903, **35**, 26.

[57] O. Wallach, *Ann.*, 1907, **353**, 318.

[58] N. Demjanov, *J. Russ. Phys. Chem. Soc.*, 1904, **36**, 166.

[59] L. Ruzicka and W. Brugger, *Helv. Chim. Acta*, 1926, **9**, 318.

the amine arrives where it should, namely, in the β-position of the allyl residue:

$$\begin{matrix} CH_2 \\ | \quad \diagdown \\ | \quad CD\cdot NH_2 \\ | \quad \diagup \\ CH_2 \end{matrix} \xrightarrow{HNO_2} \begin{matrix} CH_2 \\ | \quad \diagdown \\ | \quad CD^+ \\ | \quad \diagup \\ CH_2 \end{matrix} \longrightarrow \begin{matrix} CH_2 \\ \diagdown\!\diagdown \\ CD \\ \diagup \\ HO\cdot CH_2 \end{matrix}$$

It has been noticed repeatedly that the carbonium ion formed from a diazonium ion is more prone to rearrangement than one formed from an alkyl sulphonate or other ester or halide by loss of an anion. Thus *n*-butyl *p*-bromobenzenesulphonate, on solvolysis in acetic acid, gives *n*-butyl acetate as the only butyl ester, whereas *n*-butylamine, when deaminated in the same solvent, gives 70% of *n*-butyl acetate plus 30% of *s*-butyl acetate.[60] The prevalent idea about this, which has stereochemical support as we shall see later, is that a carbonium ion derived by loss of an anion more completely attains such stability as is lent it by equilibrium solvation, than when formed by loss of a neutral nitrogen molecule. In a carbonium ion formed by the latter route, rearrangement may be competitive with the closing up of the solvation shell, and with the attainment of an equilibrium conformation within it.

(45c) Theories of the Pinacol-Pinacolone and Wagner-Meerwein Rearrangements.—The earliest ideas about the mechanism of the pinacol-pinacolone and allied rearrangements involved the assumption of three-membered-ring intermediates in these reactions. Around 1880, Breuer and Zincke suggested ethylene oxides,[61] and Erlenmeyer *cyclo*propanes,[62] as intermediates in pinacol-pinacolone conversions, for instance,

$$\underset{\diagdown\ O\ \diagup}{(CH_3)_2C\text{——}C(CH_3)_2} \quad \text{and} \quad \underset{\diagdown\ CH_2\ \diagup}{CH_3\cdot C(OH)\cdot C(CH_3)_2}$$

as applying to the original example of the change. Too little was known at the time of the properties of either type of compound to provide immediately any critical test of these suggestions.

The ethylene oxide hypothesis has been disproved, mainly in the period 1907–1924, by Tiffeneau and McKenzie and their coworkers, on evidence of two main kinds. The first is that, in the rearrangements accompanying the dehydration of glycols, or the dehydrohalogenation of β-iodo-alcohols, or the deamination of β-amino-alcohols, ethylene oxides cannot be isolated from the products of an incomplete reaction; and yet, when prepared by independent methods, they are found

[60] A. Streitwieser jr. and W. D. Schaeffer, *J. Am. Chem. Soc.*, 1957, **79**, 2888.

[61] A. Breuer and T. Zincke, *Ann.*, 1879, **198**, 141.

[62] E. Erlenmeyer, *Ber.*, 1881, **14**, 322 (footnote).

to be sufficiently stable to ensure that, if they were formed at all, they would be capable of being isolated. The other line of evidence is that in the dehydrohalogenations of β-iodo-alcohols, and in the deaminations of β-amino-alcohols, the whole direction of the group shift is frequently different from what it would be were an ethylene oxide first produced (Section 45a).

The *cyclo*propane hypothesis was disproved, first in 1905 by Montagne, and by Acree, in a somewhat specialised type of application, and then again in 1920 by Meerwein and van Emster in a more general way. Erlenmeyer's hypothesis requires the loss of a hydrogen atom from the migrating group in order to provide accommodation for its new bond. Montagne,[63] and likewise Acree,[64] showed that at least it is wrong to assume that, when an aryl group migrates, the hydrogen is lost from the ortho-position, which thus becomes the new point of attachment of the group; for if this were so, an original para-substituent would become a meta-substituent as a result of the group shift,

$$(p\text{-ClC}_6\text{H}_4)\text{C(OH)}\cdot\text{C(OH)(C}_6\text{H}_4\text{Cl-}p)_2 \rightarrow (p\text{-ClC}_6\text{H}_4)\text{CO}\cdot\text{C(C}_6\text{H}_4\text{Cl-}p)_2$$

whereas experiment showed that it remained a para-substituent.

One of the originally attractive points about the *cyclo*propane hypothesis was that it could be applied alike to pinacol-pinacolone and to Wagner-Meerwein changes, the latter applications being, indeed, slightly simpler than the former. A typical example of application to the Wagner-Meerwein rearrangement consists in the once widely credited assumption that the known hydrocarbon, tricyclene, is an intermediate in the interconversions of *iso*bornyl esters with camphene esters or camphene. However, Meerwein and van Emster showed[65] that this cannot be true, for two reasons. One is that, although tricyclene can be converted into camphene or its derivatives, it cannot be so converted by treatment with 33% sulphuric acid in conditions in which *iso*borneol yields camphene smoothly:

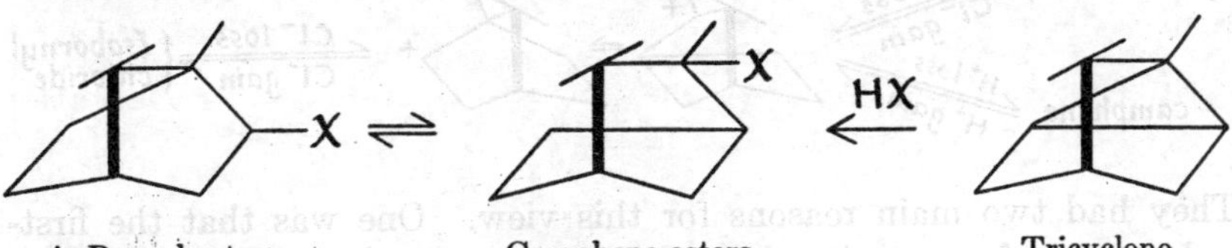

*iso*Bornyl esters   Camphene esters   Tricyclene

[63] P. S. Montagne, *Rec. trav. chim.*, 1905, 24, 105; 1906, 25, 411.
[64] S. F. Acree, *Am. Chem. J.*, 1905, 33, 180.
[65] H. Meerwein and K. van Emster, *Ber.*, 1920, 53, 1815.

The other reason is that, although racemisation accompanies acid-catalysed interconversions of *iso*bornyl with camphene esters under the conditions usually employed to effect these reactions, it is really the result of an independent process (a methyl shift, as explained in Section **45b**), which can be controlled by using somewhat mildly acidic catalysts such as formic acid, with the result, for instance, that optically active camphene yields active *iso*bornyl esters: this could not happen if achiral tricyclene were an intermediate.

Another discarded mechanistic hypothesis, introduced by Tiffeneau[66] in 1907, and used considerably by McKenzie in the 1920's, assumed free-radical intermediates, for example, diradicals of the form,

$$R_2C(O)\cdot CR_2$$

in the pinacol-pinacolone change. The inception of this theory belongs to a time when too little was known about the properties of free radicals to provide at once a crucial test of the idea. However, since then, although no-one has been concerned formally to disprove it, the theory has gradually fallen out of use. This was partly because, in 1922, Meerwein and van Emster offered a much better theory. And it was partly because our growing knowledge of the behaviour of radicals showed that, if Tiffeneau's theory were true, chain reactions, polymerisations, the homolysis of solvents, and many other characteristic phenomena should, contrary to observation, in general accompany the rearrangements.

Meerwein and van Emster's second paper,[67] that of 1922, marks the starting point of the modern theory of these rearrangements. They had made a kinetic study of certain rearrangements, notably the conversion of camphene hydrochloride into *iso*bornyl chloride; and they built up a convincing case for the view that these rearrangements depend on ionisation, the alteration to the carbon framework occurring in an initially formed carbonium ion:

camphene hydrochloride ⇌ (Cl^- loss / Cl^- gain); camphene ⇌ (H^+ loss / H^+ gain) → [carbonium ion] ⇌ [carbonium ion] ⇌ (Cl^- loss / Cl^- gain) *iso*bornyl chloride

They had two main reasons for this view. One was that the first-order rates of conversion depended on the solvent in a way that was

[66] M. Tiffeneau, *Bull. soc. chim.* (France), 1907, 1, 1221.
[67] H. Meerwein and K. van Emster, *Ber.*, 1922, 55, 2500

clearly to do with ionising power. The rate order for a number of solvents was as follows:

$$SO_2 > MeNO_2 > MeCN > PhNO_2 > PhCN > PhOMe > PhBr > EtBr > PhCl > C_6H_6 > \text{light petroleum} > \text{ether}$$

This order was substantially the same as that in which the solvents stood in relation to the ionising capacity of triphenylmethyl chloride. The other reason was that what we now call electrophilic catalysts, for instance, the hydrogen halides in non-basic solvents (Section **31b**), were catalysts for the rearrangement. The co-ordinating metal halides, $HgCl_2$, $FeCl_3$, $SbCl_3$, $SnCl_4$, and $SbCl_5$, all of which form additive compounds with triphenylmethyl chloride, were powerful catalysts for rearrangement, while the halides PCl_3 and $SiCl_4$, which do not yield such additive compounds, had no catalytic activity.

Somewhat later, Meerwein with other collaborators[68] added a third reason, which was that a series of camphene esters underwent conversion to *iso*bornyl esters at a rate which increased with the stability as an anion of the ester radical, as indicated by the strengths of the corresponding acids. The rate order,

2-chlorocymene-5-sulphonate > bromide > chloride > trichloroacetate > *m*-nitrobenzoate

can be understood as the order in which the different ester groups tend to pass into anionic form. Somewhat later still, the writer supplied a fourth argument,[69] namely, that structural changes which should increase the electron supply to the point from which the anion is required to separate, in fact facilitate rearrangement. The supporting data, drawn mainly from the literature of the pinacol-pinacolone group of rearrangements, were of the type set down in Section **45a**. Yet other arguments were adduced subsequently, as will be noted below.

Meerwein's theory, well established by 1928, identifies the primary indispensable step in these rearrangements. The total electronic change was explicitly formulated[70] at that time by Shoppee and the writer as below; who thus correlated the various types of rearrangements, essentially as we have done in the two preceding Sections, and also discussed the direction of rearrangement and the problem of migratory mobility, on the lines we have followed:

[68] H. Meerwein, O. Hammel, A. Serini, and J. Vörster, *Ann.*, 1927, **453**, 16.

[69] C. K. Ingold, *Ann. Repts. on Progress Chem.* (Chem. Soc. London), 1928, **25**, 133.

[70] C. K. Ingold and C. W. Shoppee, *J. Chem. Soc.*, 1928, 365; C. W. Shoppee, *Proc. Leeds Phil. Lit. Soc.*, Sci. Sect., 1928, **1**, 301; C. K. Ingold, *Ann. Rept. on Progress Chem.* (Chem. Soc. London), 1928, **25**, 124, 133.

$$^{-}O-\overset{\overset{R}{|\rightarrow}}{C}-C=O \qquad H-O-\overset{\overset{R}{|\rightarrow}}{C}-C-X$$

$$H-C-\overset{\overset{R}{|\rightarrow}}{C}-C-X \qquad H-C-\overset{\overset{R}{|\rightarrow}}{C}-C-X$$

During the 1930's Whitmore and his coworkers extended our acquaintance with the Wagner-Meerwein change in the acyclic series. They investigated especially the structurally simple conversion of *neo*pentyl into *t*-amyl compounds.[71] They found that *neo*pentyl alcohol and *neo*pentyl halides would undergo certain standard forms of nucleophilic substitution only with great reluctance; but that such substitutions, along with eliminations, could be effected easily by certain special methods, for instance, by treatment of the halides with aqueous silver or mercuric salts, and that then the products were rearranged *t*-amyl compounds or *iso*amylenes. In 1947 Dostrovsky and Hughes carried this demonstration to a conclusion.[72] They showed kinetically that the substitutions which proceeded tardily were S_N2 substitutions, and that the products were unrearranged, as in the example,

$$(CH_3)_3C\cdot CH_2\cdot Br \xrightarrow[S_N2]{OEt^- \text{ in EtOH}} (CH_3)_3C\cdot CH_2\cdot OEt$$

They showed also that the facile nucleophilic substitutions or eliminations were unimolecular or catalysed unimolecular processes, and that when this type of mechanism could be established the products were rearranged:

$$(CH_3)_3C\cdot CH_2\cdot Br \xrightarrow[S_N1\,+\,E1]{50\%\text{ aq.-EtOH}} \begin{cases}(CH_3)_2C(OH)\cdot CH_2(CH_3)\\(CH_3)_2C(OEt)\cdot CH_2(CH_3)\\(CH_3)_2C{:}CH(CH_3)\end{cases}$$

This kinetic work at once linked the study of rearrangements with that of unimolecular reactions of substitution and elimination in general, and thus brought to bear on the rearrangement problem the whole weight of the accumulated evidence of the mechanism of unimolecular reactions, as outlined in Chapters VII and IX.

The protolysis of *neo*pentyl Grignard compounds gives only *neo*pentane, and no *iso*pentane. This and similar substitutions of Grignard compounds almost certainly proceed through carbanions

[71] F. C. Whitmore and H. S. Rothrock, *J. Am. Chem. Soc.*, 1932, **54**, 3431; F. C. Whitmore, and G. H. Fleming, *ibid.*, 1933, **55**, 4161; F. C. Whitmore, E. L. Wittle, and A. H. Popkin, *ibid.*, 1939, **61**, 1586.

[72] I. Dostrovsky and E. D. Hughes, *J. Chem. Soc.*, **1946**, 157, 161, 164, 166, 169, 171.

(Section **26f**). Whitmore examined these and other *neo*pentyl-metal reactions, which do or might proceed through carbanions, and in no case obtained any evidence of rearrangement.[73]

Kharasch, who had studied radicals extensively, and, in particular, had made considerable use of Grignard reagents in conjunction with cobaltous chloride for the reduction of alkyl halides to alkyl radicals, found, with Urry,[74] that "neophyl" chloride, under such treatment, gave rearranged hydrocarbons, together with certain dimers, the production of which forms part of the evidence that radical reactions are really involved:

$$\begin{array}{ccccc} & & \text{Dimer} & & \text{Dimer} \\ & & \uparrow & & \uparrow \\ CMe_2Ph\cdot CH_2Cl & \rightarrow & CMe_2Ph\cdot\dot{C}H_2 & \rightarrow & CMe_2\cdot CH_2Ph \\ & & & & \downarrow \\ & & & & CHMe_2\cdot CH_2Ph + CMe_2{:}CHPh \end{array}$$

Whitmore was the first to appreciate[75] that rearrangements in certain nitrogen systems, namely, the Hofmann, Lossen, and Curtius rearrangements, to which further reference will be made later, belong to the same class of processes as pinacol-pinacolone and Wagner-Meerwein rearrangements, involving like the latter the initial production, by heterolysis, of an electron-deficient centre with a sextet of electrons. Whitmore avoided calling the electron-deficient carbon centre a carbonium ion. Indeed, he explicitly repudiated[76] association with Meerwein's theory, and with ionic mechanisms of rearrangement. Yet we find him describing[77] *neo*pentyl rearrangements as proceeding by way of "a *neo*pentyl system with 30 electrons," a concept which, when we count the valency electrons, seems very similar to that of Meerwein's carbonium ion.[78]

In 1946 Dostrovsky, Hughes, and the writer restated the position in the following two propositions,[79] namely,

[73] F. C. Whitmore, E. L. Wittle, and B. R. Harriman, *J. Am. Chem. Soc.*, 1939, **61**, 1535; F. C. Whitmore, A. H. Popkin, H. I. Bernstein, and J. P. Wilkins, *ibid.*, 1941, **63**, 124; F. C. Whitmore and H. D. Zook, *ibid.*, 1942, **64**, 1783; F. C. Whitmore, C. A. Weisgerber, and A. C. Shabica, *ibid.*, 1943, **65**, 1469.

[74] W. H. Urry and M. S. Kharasch, *J. Am. Chem. Soc.*, 1944, **66**, 1438.

[75] F. C. Whitmore, *J. Am. Chem. Soc.*, 1932, **54**, 3274.

[76] F. C. Whitmore and G. H. Fleming, *J. Chem. Soc.*, **1934**, 1269.

[77] F. C. Whitmore, E. L. Wittle, and A. H. Popkin, *loc. cit.*

[78] Whitmore subsequently explained in a letter to Hughes that he was driven to such equivocation by the severe pressure he was experiencing from contemporary opposition to the idea of the carbonium ion as an intermediate in organic chemistry.

[79] I. Dostrovsky, E. D. Hughes, and C. K. Ingold, *J. Chem. Soc.*, **1946**, 192.

(1) that it is necessary for rearrangement that an initial bond fission shall yield an atom with an incomplete octet (kinetic condition);

(2) that, when a mechanism is thus provided, the system will take advantage of it only if the free-energy change is in the right direction (thermodynamic condition).

The kinetic condition is necessary, but not sufficient. The additional need of the thermodynamic condition was illustrated by a comparison of the following three systems:

$$CMe_3 \cdot CH_2(X) \rightarrow CMe_2(X') \cdot CH_2Me$$

$$CMe_3 \cdot CHPh(X) \rightarrow CMe_2(X') \cdot CHPhMe$$

$$CPh_3 \cdot CHPh(X) \rightarrow CPh_2(X') \cdot CHPh_2$$

Given, in each case, the conditions for a unimolecular heterolysis of X, the first rearrangement goes forward, the second does not, and the third does.[80]

The work thus far outlined marks the conclusion of a definite stage in the development of the theory of saturated rearrangements, namely the establishment, and the electronic completion, and generalisation, of the Meerwein mechanism. There remained for settlement various matters of geometrical and dynamical detail, as will be noted in Sections 45e–45h.

(45d) The Wolff, Beckmann, Hofmann, Lossen, Curtius, and Schmidt Rearrangements.—The general requirement, that an initial bond-fission must produce an atom with an incomplete octet, suggests possible intermediates in addition to the carbonium ion. Sextets in the 2-quantum shell are contained in terligant positive carbon, biligant neutral carbon, biligant positive nitrogen, and uniligant neutral nitrogen; while septets are possessed by tercovalent neutral carbon and biligant neutral nitrogen. Rearrangements are known which can be referred to nearly all these intermediates, though the evidence that they are correctly so referred rests in some cases on formal similarity to more fully investigated rearrangements. Table 45-1 summarises the matter. It will be understood that every saturated rearrangement to which a distinctive name has been given is not explicitly entered. For example, the Demjanov rearrangement is taken to be included under the Wagner-Meerwein change. We now proceed to survey the outstanding cases.

[80] P. Skell and C. R. Hauser, *J. Am. Chem. Soc.*, 1942, 64, 2633.

TABLE 45-1.—TYPES OF SATURATED REARRANGEMENT.

Assumed intermediate	Rearrangement	Ref. to discussion
$>$C$^+$ (sextet)	Pinacol-pinacolone, etc.	Section 45a
	Wagner-Meerwein, etc.	Section 45b
$>$C (sextet)	Wolff	Section 45d
$>$N$^+$ (sextet)	Beckmann	Section 45d
—N (sextet)	Hofmann, Lossen, Curtius	Section 45d
$>$C— (septet)	Urry-Kharasch	Section 45c

The *Wolff rearrangement* consists in the conversion of an α-diazo-ketone, by heating in solvents, with or without surface catalysts, into nitrogen and a ketene, or into those products that would be formed from the ketene by reaction with such hydroxy- or amino-compounds as are present in solution:

$$\underset{\displaystyle R}{O{=}\overset{|}{C}{-}CHN_2} \rightarrow \underset{\displaystyle R}{O{=}C{=}\overset{|}{CH}} \begin{cases} + H_2O & \rightarrow HO_2C\cdot CH_2\cdot R \\ + R'OH & \rightarrow R'O_2C\cdot CH_2\cdot R \\ + NH_3 & \rightarrow NH_2\cdot CO\cdot CH_2\cdot R \\ + R'NH_2 & \rightarrow NHR'\cdot CO\cdot CH_2\cdot R \end{cases}$$

Since α-diazo-ketones are usually prepared from acid chlorides and diazomethane, the Wolff rearrangement[81] becomes a stage in the Arndt-Eistert process[82] for converting an acid into its next higher homologue:

$$R\cdot CO_2H \rightarrow R\cdot CO\cdot Cl \rightarrow R\cdot CO\cdot CHN_2 \rightarrow HO_2C\cdot CH_2\cdot R$$

The assumed mechanism is as follows:

$$O{=}\overset{\displaystyle R}{\overset{|}{C}}{-}CH{=}\overset{+}{N}{=}\overset{-}{N} \rightarrow O{=}\overset{\displaystyle R}{\overset{|}{C}}{-}CH \rightarrow O{=}C{=}\overset{\displaystyle R}{\overset{|}{CH}} \xrightarrow{H_2O} O{=}\overset{\displaystyle HO}{\overset{|}{C}}{-}\overset{\displaystyle R}{\overset{|}{CH_2}}$$

The evidence is that the diazo-compound certainly loses nitrogen, and therefore presumably produces a carbene; that the group certainly shifts from an adjacent position to this carbon, as the products of the

[81] L. Wolff, *Ann.*, 1912, **394**, 23.
[82] F. Arndt and B. Eistert, *Ber.*, 1935, **68**, 200.

reactions show, and as has been confirmed[83] by isotopic labelling of the carbon atoms between which the group shifts; and that ketenes, which should be the first stable products of rearrangement, can be isolated under aprotic conditions.[84] Some confirmatory stereochemical evidence is mentioned in the next Section.

The *Beckmann rearrangement* of ketoximes,[85] under the catalytic influence of strong acids, of hydrogen halides, or of phosphorus pentachloride, can be similarly understood, provided it is realised that the rearrangement takes place, not in the oxime itself, but in an acyl derivative, which alone has the necessary capacity for ionisation:

$$\text{Oxime} \rightarrow \underset{\text{R}'\text{C}=\text{N}}{\overset{\text{R}\quad\text{OAcyl}}{|\qquad|}} \rightarrow \underset{\text{R}'\text{C}=\overset{+}{\text{N}}}{\overset{\text{R}}{|\rightarrow}} \rightarrow \underset{\text{R}'\overset{+}{\text{C}}=\text{N}}{\overset{\text{R}}{\quad|}} \rightarrow \underset{\text{R}'\text{C}=\text{N}}{\overset{\text{HO}\quad\text{R}}{|\qquad|}} \rightarrow \text{Amide}$$

Reaction through an acyl derivative was established by Kuhara, whose work has been extended by Chapman:[86] both investigators have provided evidence for a rate-controlling ionisation of the acyl compound. It was found by Kuhara and his coworkers that the sulphonyl derivatives of oximes, after thorough purification, underwent facile rearrangement in neutral solvents, without any acid catalyst, to give O-sulphonyl derivatives of amides. Thus the benzenesulphonic ester of benzophenone oxime passed into an isomeric compound, which was easily hydrolysed to benzanilide and benzenesulphonic acid.

$$\text{Ph—}\overset{\overset{\text{Ph}}{|}}{\text{C}}\text{=}\underset{\underset{\text{O}\cdot\text{SO}_2\text{Ph}}{|}}{\text{N}} \rightarrow \text{Ph—}\underset{\underset{\text{O}\cdot\text{SO}_2\text{Ph}}{|}}{\text{C}}\text{=}\overset{\overset{\text{Ph}}{|}}{\text{N}} \rightarrow \text{Ph}\cdot\text{CO}\cdot\overset{\overset{\text{Ph}}{|}}{\text{NH}} + \text{HO}\cdot\text{SO}_2\text{Ph}$$

Kuhara and Chapman studied the rates of Beckmann rearrangements. Kuhara observed that rates of isomerisation of isolated oxime esters increase with the strength of the esterifying acid. Thus, he established the rate series,

$$\text{Ph}\cdot\text{SO}_3\text{H} > \text{CH}_2\text{Cl}\cdot\text{CO}_2\text{H} > \text{Ph}\cdot\text{CO}_2\text{H} > \text{CH}_3\cdot\text{CO}_2\text{H}$$

[83] C. Huggett, R. T. Arnold, and T. I. Taylor, *J. Am. Chem. Soc.*, 1942, **64,** 3043.

[84] G. Schroeter, *Ber.*, 1909, **42,** 2326; 1916, **49,** 2704; H. Staudinger and H. Hirzel, *ibid.*, p. 2522.

[85] E. Beckmann, *Ber.*, 1886, **19,** 988.

[86] M. Kuhara, K. Matsumiya, and N. Matsumami, *Mem. Coll. Sci. Kyoto Imp. Univ.*, 1914, **1,** 105; M. Kuhara and H. Watanabe, *ibid.*, 1916, **1,** No. 9, p. 349. A. W. Chapman and C. C. Howis, *J. Chem. Soc.*, **1933,** 806; A. W. Chapman, *ibid.*, **1934,** 1550; **1935,** 1223; A. W. Chapman and F. A. Fidler, *ibid.*, **1936,** 448.

In an investigation of the isomerisation of the picryl esters of the oximes of benzophenone and acetophenone to the N-picryl derivatives of benzanilide and acetanilide, Chapman found that the rates had a high dependence on solvent polarity. By making small additions of polar substances to mainly non-polar media, such as carbon tetrachloride, he established the rate sequence

$$MeCN > MeNO_2 > Me_2CO > PhCl > \text{non-polar solvents}$$

All this is characteristic for a process rate-controlled by ionisation.

Huisgen and his coworkers have shown that the introduction of electron-releasing substituents into the migrating phenyl group of acetophenone oxime benzenesulphonate accelerates rearrangement, whilst the introduction of electron-withdrawing substituents retards it.[87] This effect is characteristic of aryl migrations to electron-deficient centres in all saturated nucleophilic rearrangements.

As to catalysis by hydrogen chloride, Chapman noted that N-chloroimines do not rearrange, and that hydrogen chloride is not, as are most strong acids, a simple catalyst: it requires the simultaneous presence of an amide in order to become effective. In the absence of an initially added amide, the catalysis by hydrogen chloride assumes autocatalytic character, the induction period presumably representing the time required to build up a small supply of amide by rearrangement under some adventitious catalysis. Chapman plausibly suggests that the oxime ester which actually suffers rearrangement in catalysis by hydrogen chloride, is the ionic conjugate acid, $R_2C{:}N{\cdot}O{\cdot}CR{:}NHR^+$, of the imidol derivative of the oxime, a substance which could be produced by reaction of the oxime with an imido-chloride, first-formed from hydrogen chloride and the rearranged amide:

$$RCO{\cdot}NHR \xrightarrow{HCl} Cl{\cdot}CR{:}NR \xrightarrow{\text{oxime}} R_2C{:}N{\cdot}O{\cdot}CR{:}NR \xrightarrow{H^+} \text{cation}$$

The catalytic effect of phosphorus pentachloride may have a similar explanation; or it may involve the intermediate production of some kind of chlorophosphate of the oxime. Brodskii and Miklukhin showed[88] that, when benzophenone oxime is treated successively with phosphorus pentachloride, and with water which has been isotopically labelled with respect to oxygen, the water oxygen appeared in the formed benzanilide, which itself did not exchange oxygen with water under the experimental conditions. This is in agreement with the

[87] R. Huisgen, J. Witte, H. Wilz, and W. Jira, *Ann.*, 1957, **609**, 191.

[88] A. I. Brodskii and G. P. Miklukhin, *Compt. rend. acad. sci. U.S.S.R.*, 1941, **32**, 558; G. P. Miklukhin and A. I. Brodskii, *Acta Physiochim. U.S.S.R.*, 1942 **16**, 63.

Kuhara-Chapman mechanism, which requires the complete loss from the molecule of the original oxime oxygen.

The *Hofmann rearrangement* of amides,[89] through the action of halogens and a base, into *iso*cyanates, or into such products as *iso*cyanates would give by interaction with components of the system, for example amines by interaction with water, can be brought under the general scheme applying to all these rearrangements, as Whitmore was the first to point out.[75] The process may be formulated as follows, though the details of the hydrogen halide elimination, which produces the uniligant nitrene intermediate by the loss first of a proton and then of a halide ion, are still somewhat hypothetical:

$$\underset{\text{R}}{\text{O=C—NH}_2} \rightarrow \underset{\text{R}}{\text{O=C—N}}\!\!\genfrac{}{}{0pt}{}{\text{H}}{\text{Hal}} \rightarrow \underset{\text{R}}{\text{O=C—}\dot{\text{N}}} \rightarrow \text{O=C=N—}\dot{\text{R}} \rightarrow \text{R·NH}_2 + \text{CO}_2$$

The chief evidence is that the reaction can be conducted by treatment of pre-formed N-haloamides with bases, and that *iso*cyanates can be isolated as the first stable products under aprotic conditions. It follows that the hydrogen halide elimination, which should, as it would seem, produce the uniligant nitrogen compound, must occur; and the group migration indubitably occurs. Prossner and Eliel have shown, by Hoffmann-rearranging mixtures of two amides, one with deuterium in the R residue, and the other with ^{15}N in the nitrogen atoms, that no crossing occurs, and hence that the group migration is intramolecular.[90] The reaction has been found[91] to be accelerated by the introduction of electron-releasing substituents into the meta- or para-positions of a migrating phenyl group ($\dot{\text{R}}$), and to be retarded by the introduction there of electron-attracting groups: this may indicate that migratory mobility is following rules identical with those which apply to the pinacol-pinacolone change, and to those allied rearrangements for which the matter has been tested. There is definite evidence, as we shall note later, that the group shift is intramolecular.

The *Lossen rearrangement* is a close variant of the Hofmann rearrangement: by decomposing acyl derivatives, for example, benzoyl derivatives, of hydroxamic acids, preferably with the catalytic help of added bases, *iso*cyanates are formed, or, alternatively, such products as *iso*cyanates yield by interaction with the reactive components of the system, for example, amines by interaction with water:

[89] A. W. Hofmann, *Ber.*, 1882, **15**, 762.

[90] T. J. Prosser and E. L. Eliel, *J. Am. Chem. Soc.*, 1957, **79**, 2544.

[91] C. R. Hauser and W. B. Renfrow jr., *J. Am. Chem. Soc.*, 1937, **59**, 121.

$$O{=}C(R){-}N(H)(OAcyl) \rightarrow O{=}C(R){-}N \rightarrow O{=}C{=}N{-}R \xrightarrow{H_2O} \begin{cases} R\cdot NH_2 \\ + CO_2 \end{cases}$$

The evidence of mechanism corresponds generally to that applying to the Hofmann rearrangement, but with an extension relative to one point.[92] Like Hofmann's reaction, Lossen's has been found to be accelerated by electron-releasing, and retarded by electron-withdrawing, substituents in meta- or para-positions in a migrating phenyl group (R): Lossen's rearrangement has been additionally found to be retarded by electron-repelling, and accelerated by electron-withdrawing, substitutents in meta- or para-positions in an eliminated benzoyloxy-group (OAcyl). This last result is further confirmation of the theory that the rate-determining process involves the heterolytic separation of OAcyl as OAcyl⁻.

The *Curtius rearrangement* is a slightly more distant variant of the Hofmann and Lossen rearrangements: an acyl azide is caused to lose nitrogen by heating in solvents (as acyl diazo-methanes are in the Wolff rearrangement): the product is an *iso*cyanate (instead of the ketene formed in the Wolff rearrangement), or at least such compounds as a first-formed *iso*cyanate would give under the experimental conditions:

$$O{=}C(R){-}N{=}\overset{+}{N}{=}\overset{-}{N} \rightarrow O{=}C(R){-}N \dashrightarrow O{=}C{=}N{-}R \xrightarrow{H_2O} \begin{cases} RNH_2 \\ + CO_2 \end{cases}$$

We take into account here Schmidt's modification of the reaction, in which a carboxylic acid and hydrazoic acid are condensed in the presence of sulphuric acid to give an acyl azide, which is not isolated, but is allowed to decompose and rearrange. The product normally obtained after dilution with water is an amine, which is what is formed when an *iso*cyanate is treated successively with sulphuric acid and water. The modification needed[93] in the above scheme is in recognition of the circumstance that the sulphuric acid considerably accelerates decomposition of the acyl azide. This suggests that the loss of nitrogen occurs more easily in the conjugate acid of the azide than in the azide itself. The product should be an aminylium ion, having, like

[92] W. B. Renfrow jr. and C. R. Hauser, *J. Am. Chem. Soc.*, 1937, **59**, 2308: R. D. Bright and C. R. Hauser, *ibid.*, 1939, **61**, 618.

[93] M. S. Newman and H. L. Gildenhorn, *J. Am. Chem. Soc.*, 1948, **70**, 317.

that assumed for the Beckmann rearrangement, a sextet of 2-quantum nitrogen electrons:

$$\underset{}{O{=}\overset{\overset{R}{|}}{C}{-}N{=}\overset{+}{N}{=}\overset{-}{N}} \xrightarrow{H^+} O{=}\overset{\overset{R}{|}}{C}{-}NH{-}\overset{+}{N}{\equiv}N \longrightarrow O{=}\overset{\overset{R}{|\rightarrow}}{C}{-}\overset{+}{N}H$$

$$\longrightarrow O{=}C{=}\overset{\overset{R}{|}}{N} \xrightarrow{H_2O} \begin{cases} RNH_2 \\ +\,CO_2 \end{cases}$$

The evidence of mechanism of the Curtius rearrangement, including Schmidt's modification of it, is again essentially the same as for the Hofmann and Lossen rearrangements. Bothner-By and Friedman have shown, by ^{15}N-labelling, that the nitrogen bonded to carbon in R·CO·N:N:N becomes bonded to R in the rearrangement product.[94] This carries the conclusion that the migration of R is intramolecular. The kinetic effect of substituents in Schmidt's reaction has been investigated[95] only with respect to meta-substituents in a migrating phenyl group; but the rate series, Me > H > OH > Cl > NO_2, clearly indicates a polar effect on migratory mobility similar to that found in the other rearrangements. Moreover, the reaction is stereochemically similar to the Hofmann and Lossen rearrangements, as will be noted below.

(45e) Steric Course of Saturated Nucleophilic Rearrangements.— It is apparent from the general expression for the electronic transfers involved in all these rearrangements,

$$Y \curvearrowleft \overset{\overset{R}{|\rightarrow}}{A}{-}B{-}X$$

that one may ask three questions about the stereochemical course of the total process, as follows: (1) What is the configurational effect *at R* of the replacement of its bond to A by a bond to B? (2) What configurational effect *at B* has the substitution of its bond to X by a bond to R? (3) What effect *at A* accompanies the exchange of its bond to R by a bond to Y? This puts the problem in an inclusive form, although, actually, these questions are not all chemically significant for all rearrangements. We will take up these questions in turn. For present convenience we will call R the *migrating group*, B either the *migration terminus*, or the *seat of dissociation*, and A either the *migration origin*, or the *seat of association*.

The stereochemical effect of rearrangement, as it influences the con-

[94] A. A. Bothner-By and L. Friedman, *J. Am. Chem. Soc.*, 1951, **73**, 5391.

[95] L. H. Briggs and J. W. Lyttleton, *J. Chem. Soc.*, **1943**, 421.

figuration *of the migrating group* R, is a question relevant to all rearrangements in which R is an alkyl or substituted alkyl group, though not, of course, to those in which R is an aryl group. The question has not yet been directly answered either for the pinacol-pinacolone rearrangement, or for the Wagner-Meerwein change, or their close relations. But it has been indirectly answered, because the evidence, to which we shall come in the next Section, in favour of *synartesis*, that is, the common binding of A and B by the electrons of the bond from R during migration, would make no sense unless configuration were preserved at R. It has also been answered permissively in that many rearrangements are known in dicyclic and polycyclic compounds which would be mechanically impossible unless configuration were retained by the migrating residue. The question has been answered directly, and in the same sense, for the other rearrangements, namely, the Wolff rearrangement, involving group shift from carbon to carbon, and the Beckmann, Hofmann, Lossen, Curtius, and Schmidt rearrangements, involving group migration from carbon to nitrogen. The migrations to nitrogen are all closely connected, and the evidence concerning them will be summarised first.

In 1926–33 Wallis and his collaborators observed retention of optical activity when the appropriate derivatives of α-benzylpropionic acid were converted by the Curtius,[96] the Hofmann,[97] and the Lossen[98] rearrangements, into α-benzylethylamine; and von Braun and Friehmelt noticed that the same was true, when the Schmidt reaction[99] was employed. The optical rotations made it immediately certain that the stereochemical effects on these four processes were identical. By 1935, when Kenyon and Phillips had established, and with Pittman had suitably applied,[100] their method of deducing relative configurations from signs of rotation (Section **33b**), it had become fully clear that the common stereochemical result, observed by Wallis and von Braun, was retention of configuration:

$$\begin{array}{c}PhCH_2\\ \diagdown\\ CH_3{-}C{-}CO\\ \diagup\quad\ |\\ H\qquad N\!<\end{array} \;-\left\{\begin{array}{l}\text{Hofmann}\\ \text{Lossen}\\ \text{Curtius}\\ \text{Schmidt}\end{array}\right\}\!\rightarrow\; \begin{array}{c}PhCH_2\\ \diagdown\\ CH_3{-}C{-}NH_2\\ \diagup\\ H\end{array} + CO_2$$

[96] L. W. Jones and E. S. Wallis, *J. Am. Chem. Soc.*, 1926, **48**, 169.
[97] E. S. Wallis and S. C. Nagel, *J. Am. Chem. Soc.*, 1931, 53, 2787.
[98] E. S. Wallis and R. D. Dripps, *J. Am. Chem. Soc.*, 1933, 55, 1701.
[99] J. v. Braun and E. Friehmelt, *Ber.*, 1933, **66**, 684.
[100] J. Kenyon, H. Phillips, and V. P. Pittman, *J. Chem. Soc.*, **1935**, 1072.

In 1940 this conclusion received further support from an argument[101] due to Archer, as follows. β-Camphoramic acid must be a *cis*-compound, because of its relation to camphoric acid and thence to camphor. The 1-aminodihydro-α-campholytic acid, which it yields under the Hofmann procedure, must also be a *cis*-compound, because of its facile conversion to a lactam. Therefore configuration must have been retained in the Hofmann reaction:

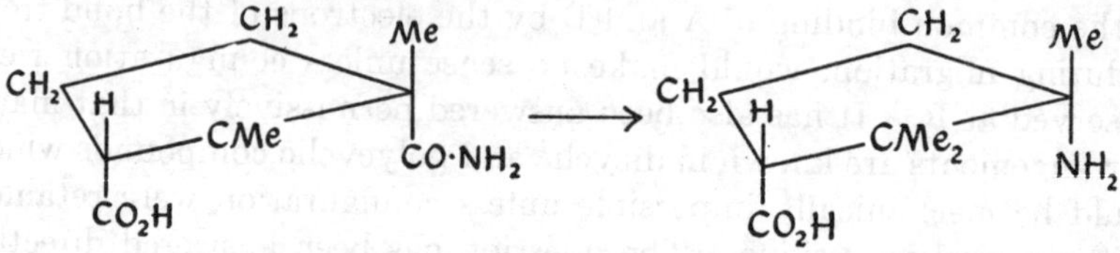

$$\text{CH}_2,\ \text{CH}_2,\ \text{H},\ \text{CMe},\ \text{Me},\ \text{CO·NH}_2,\ \text{CO}_2\text{H} \longrightarrow \text{CH}_2,\ \text{CH}_2,\ \text{H},\ \text{CMe}_2,\ \text{Me},\ \text{NH}_2,\ \text{CO}_2\text{H}$$

In 1941 Kenyon and Young included the Beckmann rearrangement in the above generalisation.[102] They converted optically active 3-heptylcarboxylic acid into 3-heptyl methyl ketone; and then they rearranged the amide of the acid by the Hofmann method, and the oxime of the ketone by the Beckmann method. The two procedures led to the same optical isomer of 3-heptylamine. Therefore, since the Hofmann rearrangement takes place with retention of configuration, so also does the Beckmann rearrangement:

$$\begin{array}{ccc}
(+)n\text{-BuEtCH·CO}_2\text{H} & \xrightarrow[\text{Hofmann}]{\text{amide, by}} & (+)n\text{-BuEtCH·NH}_2 \\
\downarrow \text{acid-bromide, reaction with CdMe}_2 & & \text{acetylation} \downarrow \uparrow \text{hydrolysis} \\
(+)n\text{-BuEtCH·CO·CH}_3 & \xrightarrow[\text{Beckmann}]{\text{oxime, by}} & (-)n\text{-BuEtCH·NH·CO·CH}_3
\end{array}$$

In 1946 Kenyon and his coworkers[102,103] concluded a study of the five allied rearrangement processes in the example of α-phenylethyl compounds, showing, by their figures (below) for the percentage retention of optical purity, how complete in each case[104] is the preservation of

[101] S. Archer, *J. Am. Chem. Soc.*, 1940, **62**, 1872.

[102] J. Kenyon and D. P. Young, *J. Chem. Soc.*, **1941**, 263.

[103] C. L. Arcus and J. Kenyon, *J. Chem. Soc.*, **1939**, 916; A. Campbell and J. Kenyon, *ibid.*, **1946**, 25.

[104] The observed small amount of the racemisation accompanying the Hofmann rearrangement of hydratropamide may be understood as arising from the employment here of aqueous alkali, a powerful racemising agent for prototropic compounds with mobile hydrogen at the centre of asymmetry, such as are the starting substances of all these rearrangements, as well as the intermediately formed *iso*cyanate. The other reactions do not involve strongly basic reagents.

configuration (R = PhMeCH throughout):

$$(+)R\cdot CO_2H \rightarrow \begin{cases} R\cdot C(:NOH)\cdot Me \text{—Beckmann} \rightarrow (-)R\cdot NHAc \ (99.6\%) \\ R\cdot CO\cdot NH_2 \text{ —Hofmann} \rightarrow (-)R\cdot NH_2 \ (95.8\%) \\ R\cdot CO\cdot NH\cdot OBz \text{ —Lossen} \rightarrow (-)R\cdot NH_2 \ (99.2\%) \\ R\cdot CO\cdot N_3 \text{ —Curtius} \rightarrow (-)R\cdot NH_2 \ (99.3\%) \\ R\cdot CO\cdot N_3 \text{ —Schmidt} \rightarrow (-)R\cdot NH_2 \ (99.6\%) \end{cases}$$

The one migration to carbon which has been similarly studied is the Wolff rearrangement. Lane and Wallis showed that this also proceeds with retention of configuration.[105] They converted α-n-butylhydratropic acid by the Arndt-Eistert procedure, which, as explained above, includes a Wolff rearrangement, into the next higher homologous acid, and then degraded the latter by the Barbier-Wieland method of acting on the ester with a Grignard reagent and oxidising the formed tertiary alcohol, back to the original lower homologue. The recovered acid was identical with the original (though the carboxyl group must have been a different one); and the retention of optical purity in the complete cycle was 99.5%:

$$n\text{-}C_4H_9\text{—}C(Ph)(Me)\cdot CO_2H \xrightarrow[+\ CH_2N_2]{\text{chloride}} n\text{-}C_4H_9\text{—}C(Ph)(Me)\cdot CO\cdot CHN_2 \xrightarrow{\text{Wolff}} n\text{-}C_4H_9\text{—}C(Ph)(Me)\cdot CH_2\cdot CO_2H$$

$$n\text{-}C_4H_9\text{—}C(Ph)(Me)\cdot CH_2\cdot CO_2H \xrightarrow{\text{Me-ester + PhMgBr}} n\text{-}C_4H_9\text{—}C(Ph)(Me)\cdot CH_2\cdot C(OH)Ph_2 \xrightarrow{CrO_3} n\text{-}C_4H_9\text{—}C(Ph)(Me)\cdot CO_2H$$

The high retentions of asymmetry obtained in the work of Kenyon and of Wallis strongly suggest that the migrating group never leaves the system. This has, indeed, been proved by arranging that, if it did so by as much as atomic distances for as long as collision durations, a blocked rotation would be released, and optical activity dependent on the blocking would be lost. Wallis and Moyer showed,[106] by the use of a substituted o-α-naphthylbenzamide, that this does not happen in the Hofmann rearrangement; and Bell,[107] employing a substituted o-phenylbenzamide and the corresponding benzoyl azide, established

[105] J. F. Lane and E. S. Wallis, *J. Am. Chem. Soc.*, 1941, **63**, 1674.
[106] E. S. Wallis and W. W. Moyer, *J. Am. Chem. Soc.*, 1933, **55**, 2598.
[107] F. Bell, *J. Chem. Soc.*, 1934, 835.

that it does not in either the Hofmann or the Curtius rearrangement; while Lane and Wallis,[108] using the related diazoacetophenone, proved that it does not in the Wolff rearrangement: the examples are formulated below:

Hofmann *Curtius* *Wolff*

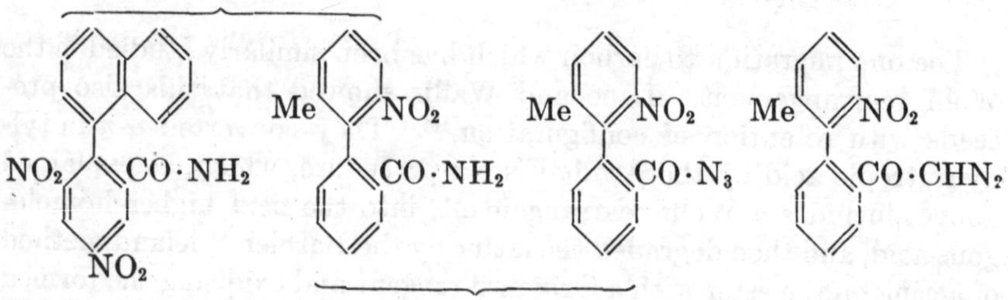

NO_2 $CO \cdot NH_2$ NO_2 (Wallis and Moyer)

Me NO_2 $CO \cdot NH_2$; Me NO_2 $CO \cdot N_3$ (Bell)

Me NO_2 $CO \cdot CHN_2$ (Lane and Wallis)

The second question on our programme relates to the configurational effect of the group shift *in the migration terminus*. This is a chemically significant matter only when, according to our representation of these changes, the ligancy of B could not at any time drop below three for carbon or two for nitrogen; and the three important cases are the pinacol-pinacolone change and its close analogues, the Wagner-Meerwein change and its near relations, and the Beckmann rearrangement (Table 45-1).

With reference to the pinacol-pinacolone and related changes, this problem has been attacked by two methods. Bartlett and his coworkers employ stereoisomeric ring compounds, which limit the migrating and eliminated groups to alternative characteristic orientations; and then they compare the ease of the reactions.[109] It was thus found that *cis*-1,2-dimethyl*cyclo*hexane-1,2-diol, on treatment with "20%" aqueous sulphuric acid, passed fairly smoothly into 2,2-dimethyl*cyclo*hexan-1-one, and that *cis*-1,2-dimethyl*cyclo*pentane-1,2-diol likewise gave 2,2-dimethyl*cyclo*pentan-1-one. But *trans*-1,2-dimethyl*cyclo*hexane-1,2-diol in similar conditions yielded 1-acetyl-1-methyl*cyclo*pentane, and *trans*-1,2-dimethyl*cyclo*pentane-1,2-diol gave only tars. Both *cis*- and *trans*-7,8-diphenylacenaphthene-7,8-diol, on treatment with aqueous sulphuric acid, yielded 8,8-diphenyl-

[108] J. F. Lane and E. S. Wallis, *J. Org. Chem.*, 1941, **6**, 443.

[109] P. D. Bartlett and I. Pöckel, *J. Am. Chem. Soc.*, 1937, **59**, 820; P. D. Bartlett and A. Bavley, *ibid.*, 1938, **60**, 2416; P. D. Bartlett and R. F. Brown, *ibid.*, 1940, **62**, 2927.

acenaphthene-7-one; but the *cis*-diol did it the more readily; and in the conditions in which the *trans*-diol underwent the conversion, it was also isomerised to the *cis*-diol:

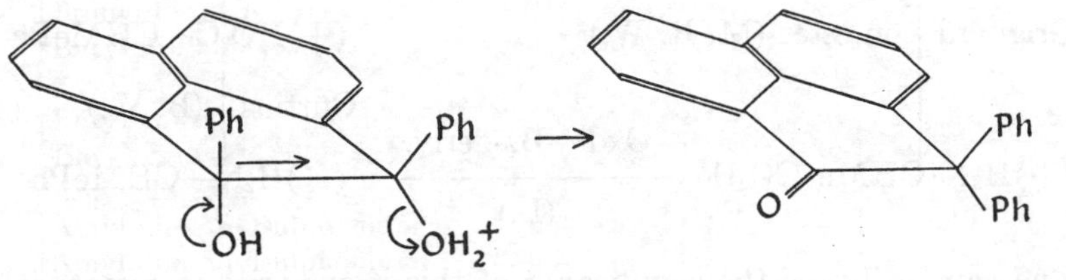

It is apparent from these results that the pinacol-pinacolone change proceeds more smoothly when the migrating group R is presented to the migration terminus B on the side opposite to that from which the eliminated radical X departs, than when it is presented on the same side. This would be unintelligible unless inversion at the migration terminus was the mode of reaction normally preferred.

The other method of examining the question is to permit attack on B from either direction, but to make B asymmetric, and to correlate its configurations before and after rearrangement. McKenzie and his coworkers laid a foundation on which Bernstein and Whitmore completed an application of this method to pinacolic deamination. Starting from optically active alanine, McKenzie, Roger, and Wills prepared by Grignard synthesis the optically active amino-alcohol written below; and this they deaminated by means of nitrous acid in an acetic acid solvent, to the optically active ketone indicated.[110] Their final product, the ketone, was subsequently obtained in optically active form by Conant and Carlson, by a Grignard synthesis from the chloride of hydrotropic acid.[111] McKenzie, Roger, and Wills's initial substance, alanine, was prepared by Leithe by oxidising the phenyl group of an optically active α-phenylethylamine, suitably protected at the amino-group.[112] And so it remained to complete the genetic cycle by linking hydrotropic acid with α-phenylethylamine: this Bernstein and Whitmore did by converting the acid into the amine through the Curtius reaction.[113] With optically active materials the genetic ring closed smoothly, as shown in the diagram. The initials indicate the investigators:

[110] A. McKenzie, R. Roger, and G. O. Wills, *J. Chem. Soc.*, **1926,** 779.
[111] J. B. Conant and G. H. Carlson, *J. Am. Chem. Soc.*, 1932, **54,** 4048.
[112] W. Leithe, *Ber.*, 1931, **64,** 2827.
[113] H. I. Bernstein and F. C. Whitmore, *J. Am. Chem. Soc.*, 1939, **61,** 1324

$$\begin{array}{ccc}
(-)Ph_2C\text{—}CHMe & \xrightarrow[\text{(M. R. W.)}]{HNO_2 \text{ in cold HOAc}} & (+)PhCO\text{—}CHMePh \\
\;\;| \quad\;\; | & & \uparrow \\
\;\;OH \;\; NH_2 & & \text{Grignard on } \big| \text{ chloride (C. C.)} \\
\uparrow & & \\
\text{Grignard } \big| \text{ on ester (M. R. W.)} & & (+)HO_2C\text{—}CHMePh \\
 & & \text{Curtius } \big| \text{ (B. W.)} \\
 & & \downarrow \\
(+)H_2N\cdot CHMe\cdot CO_2H & \xleftarrow[\text{(L.)}]{\text{Oxdn. Bz-deriv.}} & (-)H_2N\text{—}CHMePh
\end{array}$$

One can easily see the significance of this if one tries to restate it assuming that, on the only two occasions on which a bond at the asymmetric centre is changed, namely, the deamination and the Curtius reaction, the new group takes the precise position of the old one. Then, starting from alanine (1), and proceeding *via* the deamination (2)-(3), and the Curtius reaction (4)-(5), one comes round to alanine (6):

$$\begin{array}{lll}
(1) & CHMe(\;CO_2H\;)(\;NH_2\;) & \\
 & & \}\text{Grignard}\downarrow \\
(2) & CHMe(CPh_2OH)(\;NH_2\;) & \\
 & & \}\text{deamination}\downarrow \\
(3) & CHMe(\;COPh\;)(\;Ph\;) & \\
 & & \}\text{Grignard}\uparrow \\
(4) & CHMe(\;CO_2H\;)(\;Ph\;) & \\
 & & \}\text{Curtius}\downarrow \\
(5) & CHMe(\;NH_2\;)(\;Ph\;) & \\
 & & \}\text{oxidation}\downarrow \\
(6) & CHMe(\;NH_2\;)(CO_2H) &
\end{array}$$

Two groups have thus changed places, and this must produce an inversion: therefore the genetic ring should not close. The fact that it does, shows that either the deamination or the Curtius rearrangement has also produced an inversion; and since there is independent reason (above) for believing that the Curtius reaction does not behave thus, the conclusion is that the deamination is producing inversion. The further conclusion can be drawn from the record of McKenzie, Roger, and Wills that the inversion is not quantitative. They isolated the rearranged ketone in an almost quantitative yield, but it had only a 77% retention of optical purity, or, in other words, an 88% inversion of configuration. The reagent could not have racemised either the factor or the product, and so the racemisation must have occurred as part of the process. The total conclusion is, then, that the pinacolic deamination produces predominating inversion, along with some racemisation, at the migration terminus.

The cause of the partial racemisation, that is, of the minor amount of migration with retention of configuration at the migration terminus, has been made clear by a number of subsequent investigations. First, it was established in many examples that the stereospecificity of replacement at the migration terminus can lead to apparent abrogations of the rule for migratory mobility, in case the structure presents what should be the less mobile group in a stereochemically more favourable manner to the migration terminus. This is certainly the explanation of the deamination, formulated below, of McKenzie and Mills,[114] which has been cited as an exception to the polar rules; for phenyl migrated in preference to *p*-anisyl (An), as Pollak and Curtin[115] have confirmed:

$$\mathrm{Ph(An)C(OH)\!-\!CH(Ph)NH_2} \xrightarrow{\mathrm{HNO_2}} \mathrm{An\cdot CO\cdot CHPh_2}$$

The point to be noted is that, since there are two asymmetric centres, there exist two racemic diastereoisomeric amino-alcohols. This particular one was prepared from desylamine and anisyl magnesium bromide. Now McKenzie and Wood subsequently showed,[116] in the example formulated below, that two diastereoisomeric amino-alcohols, could, on deamination, rearrange in different ways, as indicated (Naph = 1-naphthyl):

$$\mathrm{Ph(Naph)C(OH)\!-\!CH(Ph)NH_2}\begin{cases}\alpha\text{-form} \xrightarrow{\mathrm{HNO_2}} \mathrm{Naph\cdot CO\cdot CHPh_2}\\ \beta\text{-form} \xrightarrow{\mathrm{HNO_2}} \mathrm{Ph\cdot CO\cdot CHPhNaph}\end{cases}$$

Such pairs of diastereoisomers are made by reversing Grignard reagents in the two steps of the Grignard synthesis from the amino-carboxylic ester, through the amino-ketone, to the amino-alcohol. The total synthesis has been estimated as 98–99% stereospecific. A. K. Mills, and Pollak and Curtin, have thus prepared a considerable number of diastereoisomeric pairs of amino-alcohols, and have shown that in every case the dominating migration is of the aryl group in-

[114] A. McKenzie and A. K. Mills, *Ber.*, 1929, **62**, 1784.
[115] P. I. Pollak and D. Y. Curtin, *J. Am. Chem. Soc.*, 1950, **72**, 961.
[116] A. McKenzie and A. D. Wood, *Ber.*, 1938, **71**, 358.

troduced by the first-used of the two aryl Grignard reagents.[117] Using this principle, Benjamin, Schaeffer, and Collins have built up, from each optical enantiomer of alanine, by two steps of Grignard synthesis with phenylmagnesium bromide, McKenzie, Roger, and Wills's diphenylcarbinol-amine (p. 756), but first with one of its phenyl groups, and then with the other one, labelled with ^{14}C. With either, they confirmed McKenzie, Roger, and Wills's finding that, on deamination, the phenyl migration proceeded with 88% of inversion and 12% of retention of configuration at the migration terminus. And then, by separating the inverted product from the racemic product, and, by degradation, locating the radioactivity in each, they were able to add the result that the 88% of product formed with inversion of configuration was produced only by migration of the phenyl of the first-used Grignard reagent, whereas the 12% formed with retention of configuration was derived only by migration of the other phenyl group.[118]

The rationalisation of this result brings together several conclusions already reached on independent grounds. First, according to the general electronic scheme, evolved as described in Section **45c**, and quoted at the beginning of this Section, the transaction by which the migration terminus B loses X and acquires R is a nucleophilic substitution; for the entering and separating groups both carry their bond electrons with them. If the bond changes are synchronised sufficiently to give the *local* transaction an S_N2-like character (though the overall substitution is S_N1), the stereochemical effect must be one of inversion at the migration terminus. If, however, X leaves sufficiently ahead to confer on the local transaction an S_N1-like nature, then racemisation will be permitted, to an extent depending on how far X^- diffuses (to total racemisation if X^- goes out of shielding range), before the migration occurs. Secondly, we saw in Sections **33i** and **38c** that the general stereochemical behaviour of deaminations points to an *overall* S_N1 character, that is, to a loss of X, in this case of N_2^+, before any foreign nucleophile can intervene. And we must take in the special conclusion, stated in Section **45b**, that the carbonium ion, formed by loss of N_2^+, is first formed in an incompletely solvated, highly reactive condition, in which it may function as the terminus of a group-shift, before conformational equilibrium has been attained.

The results of Benjamin, Schaeffer, and Collins sum up all this. A Newman projection of the diazonium ion from one of their isotopically

[117] The first edition of this book listed the known examples, but all are closely similar to the illustrations used above.

[118] B. M. Benjamin, H. J. Schaeffer, and C. J. Collins, *J. Am. Chem. Soc.*, 1957, **79**, 6160.

distinguished, diastereoisomeric amino-alcohols is on the left in the accompanying representation. The curved arrows attached to this formula show that, if ^{14}Ph migration follows N_2^+ loss closely enough, the product will be inverted, and that in such inverted material the only phenyl group which has undergone migration will be the labelled phenyl group. If, to go to the other extreme, the carbonium ion were formed and had a very long free life—in particular, long compared with the time required for conformational rotation—then the product would be racemic, and, moreover, each of its composing enantiomers would itself be an equlibrium mixture of two position-isomers, in one of which ordinary phenyl, and in the other labelled phenyl, has migrated. As Benjamin, Schaeffer, and Collins point out, the situation disclosed by their results is not this; on the contrary, it suggests a carbonium ion whose life is short in comparison with the time of a conformational rotation. It therefore reacts in conformations similar to that drawn here for the carbonium ion derived from the represented diazonium ion. The carbonium ion is drawn twice, in order to allow representation by curved arrows of the two things that can happen to it. One product, in general the main product, will have an inverted configuration, and will consist only of that position-isomer in which the labelled phenyl group has migrated. The second product will have a retained configuration, and this will consist only of the other position-isomer, namely, that in which ordinary phenyl has migrated.

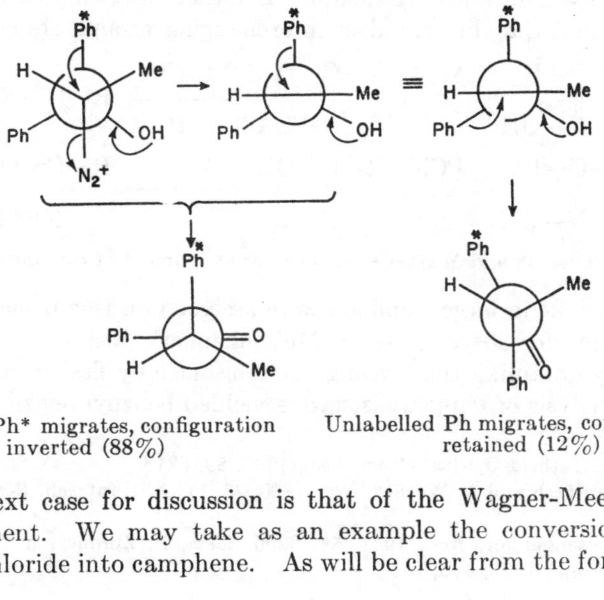

Labelled Ph* migrates, configuration inverted (88%)

Unlabelled Ph migrates, configuration retained (12%)

The next case for discussion is that of the Wagner-Meerwein rearrangement. We may take as an example the conversion of *iso*-bornyl chloride into camphene. As will be clear from the formulae on

p. 731, the carbon atom from which chlorine departs, forms its new bond on the side opposite to that previously occupied by chlorine. Actually, not only *iso*bornyl chloride, but also bornyl chloride is converted into camphene in ionising solvents, and in the presence of bases of strength from that of water upwards. But the reaction of *iso*bornyl chloride goes much more easily than does that of bornyl chloride, in which the new bond has to be established on the side of the carbon atom from which the chlorine leaves. Only in the reaction of *iso*bornyl chloride could the local transaction at the migration terminus have an S_N2-like character, and hence proceed necessarily with inversion. It has been shown by the use of optically active α-deutero*neo*pentylamine that the methyl migration accompanying its deamination gives inversion of configuration at the migration terminus.[119] We may infer that, in the Wagner-Meerwein rearrangement, inversion at the migration terminus is the preferred form of reaction.

The last case we have to consider, that of the Beckmann rearrangement of oximes, is a famous example of the fallibility of structural reasoning from reactions apart from their mechanism. Hantzsch and Werner, who in 1890 established the geometrical interpretation of the isomerism of oximes, had two methods of assigning configurations to the isomers.[120] For aldoximes, they relied on the observed facile conversion by bases of the acyl derivatives of one isomer only into the related nitrile. For ketoximes, they depended on the differing products of Beckmann rearrangements. In either case, the basic assumption was that the eliminated or interchanging groups are *cis*-related:

$$\begin{array}{c} \mathrm{R{-}C{-}H} \\ \| \\ \mathrm{N{-}OH} \end{array} \xrightarrow{Ac_2O} \begin{array}{c} \mathrm{R{-}C{-}H} \\ \| \\ \mathrm{N{-}OAc} \end{array} \xrightarrow[\text{etc.}]{K_2CO_3} \mathrm{R{-}C{\equiv}N}$$

$$\begin{array}{c} \mathrm{R{-}C{-}R'} \\ \| \\ \mathrm{N{-}OH} \end{array} \xrightarrow[\text{etc.}]{PCl_5} \begin{array}{c} \mathrm{R{-}C{-}OH} \\ \| \\ \mathrm{N{-}R'} \end{array} \rightleftarrows \begin{array}{c} \mathrm{R{-}C{=}O} \\ | \\ \mathrm{NH{\cdot}R'} \end{array}$$

Hantzsch and Werner's schemes for assignment of configurations

Configurations in large numbers were assigned on this principle without question for 30 years, when Meisenheimer[121] disproved it for ketoximes by obtaining the "wrong" stereoisomer by fission of an isoxazole: ozonolysis of triphenylisoxazole yielded benzoyl benzil β-monox-

[119] R. D. Guthrie, *J. Am. Chem. Soc.*, 1967, **89**, 6718.

[120] A. Hantzsch and A. Werner, *Ber.*, 1890, **23**, 11; A. Hantzsch, *Ber.*, 1891, **24**, 13.

[121] J. Meisenheimer, *Ber.*, 1921, **54**, 3206; *idem*, P. Zimmerman, and M. v. Kummer, *Ann.*, 1926, **446**, 205

ime; and the β-monoxime is that which undergoes Beckmann rearrangement to phenylglyoxanilide:

$$\begin{array}{c} \text{PhC}\text{——}\text{CPh} \\ \| \qquad \| \\ \text{PhC} \quad \text{N} \\ \diagdown \ \diagup \\ \text{O} \end{array} \xrightarrow{O_3} \begin{array}{c} \text{PhCO}\text{—}\text{CPh} \\ \| \\ \text{PhCO·O·N} \end{array} \underset{\text{KOH}}{\overset{\text{BzCl}}{\longleftarrow}} \begin{array}{c} \text{PhCO}\text{—}\text{CPh} \\ \| \\ \text{HO·N} \end{array}$$

$$\xrightarrow{PCl_5} \begin{array}{c} \text{PhCO}\text{—}\text{C·OH} \\ \| \\ \text{PhN} \end{array} \rightleftarrows \begin{array}{c} \text{PhCO}\text{—}\text{C=O} \\ | \\ \text{PhNH} \end{array}$$

A little later Brady and Bishop similarly upset the accepted configurations of aldoximes, by showing that the "wrong" member of a pair of isomers was the more easily converted to an isoxazole:[122] that form of 2-chloro-5-nitrobenzaldoxime whose acyl derivative yields a nitrile was smoothly converted by alkali, obviously by way of a nitrobenzisoxazole, into what the latter would give under the conditions, namely, the nitrosalicylonitrile:

$$\begin{array}{c} C_6H_4(NO_2)\cdot\text{C·H} \\ | \qquad \quad \| \\ \text{Cl} \qquad \text{HO·N} \end{array} \rightarrow \text{(nitrobenzisoxazole: } NO_2\text{-ring fused to CH=N–O)} \rightarrow \text{(benzene ring with } NO_2, \text{CN, OH)}$$

Also, Meisenheimer confirmed his reversal of previously accepted ketoxime configurations by a parallel cyclisation study:[121] that form of 2-chloro-5-nitrobenzophenone oxime, which by the Beckmann transformation gives a chloronitrobenzanilide (with a shift of C_6H_5), was the form which, with alkali, yielded a nitro-substituted phenylbenzisoxazole:

$$\begin{array}{c} C_6H_4(NO_2)\cdot\text{C}\cdot C_6H_5 \\ | \qquad \quad \| \\ \text{Cl} \qquad \text{HO·N} \end{array} \rightarrow \text{(benzisoxazole: } NO_2\text{-ring fused to } C\cdot C_6H_5\text{=N–O)}$$

These observations lead to two conclusions. The first is that the preferred form of elimination across the oxime double bond to give a nitrile, as across an ethylene double bond to give an acetylene (Section **41a**), is *trans*-elimination. The second, more directly relevant to the present discussion, is that in the Beckmann rearrangement the migrating group presents itself to the nitrogen atom on the side opposite to that from which the oxygen group leaves nitrogen.

Our third stereochemical query relates to the effect of rearrangement on configuration *at the migration origin* A. This is a significant ques-

[122] O. L. Brady and G. Bishop, *J. Chem. Soc.*, 1925, 127, 1357.

tion only when A is quadricoligant both before and after the change. The one important case is that of Wagner-Meerwein rearrangements in substitution, including the special case of substitution by the eliminated group, that is, isomerisation.

The answer is clear from the formulae already given for some of these changes (pp. 731, 732). Camphene methyl ether and camphene hydrochloride are directly converted into *iso*bornyl chloride: this is the *exo*-isomer, having its chlorine atom on the side of the ring opposite to that previously occupied by the displaced bond. Pinene hydrochloride is transformed directly into bornyl chloride: this is the *endo*-isomer, again having its halogen on the side of the ring opposite to that on which the displaced bond was originally located.

These examples indicate that inversion at the migration origin is the rule for Wagner-Meerwein rearrangements accompanying substitution and isomerisation. A further argument follows from the observation that the conversion of camphene hydrochloride into *iso*bornyl chloride is appreciably reversible.[67] One may therefore presume that Wagner-Meerwein isomerisations are in general reversible. Therefore, since the migration terminus in the forward process becomes the migration origin in its reversal, we must expect, by the principle of microscopic reversibility, identical stereochemical rules to apply to the migration terminus and migration origin. Consistently, the detailed evidence indicates that, at both centres, inversion is the favoured mode of reaction.

We may summarise the common outcome of the stereochemical studies of rearrangement described in this Section by the following general formula:

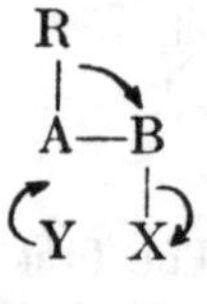

R
|
A—B
|
Y X

$\begin{cases} \text{at A, predominating inversion} \\ \text{at R, retention of configuration} \\ \text{at B, predominating inversion} \end{cases}$

(45f) Ionic Intermediates: Unsaturated Migrating Groups: Cyclisation.—The nature of the carbonium-ion intermediates in nucleophilic aliphatic rearrangements is a subject of considerable ramification,[123] and the present outline will be spread over this and the next two Sec-

[123] This area has been one of protracted controversy. Instead of pursuing its intricacies, the writer has simply taken a line through it, presenting the picture that he believes to be correct. He has derived much help from P. D. Bartlett's book, "Non-classical Ions" (W. A. Benjamin, Inc., New York, 1965), which contains reprints of some 75 of the original articles, and adds commentary which constitutes an important guide to the subject.

tions. We are conveniently introduced to it by our study of the Walden inversion in Section **33**, particularly Sections **33g** and **33h**. There we learned that nucleophilic substitutions with retention of configuration are S_N1 substitutions, in which a β-substituent, that is, a γ-atom, possesses p or π electrons with which it can co-ordinate with the formed or forming carbonium ion, to produce a three-membered ring, often with quite a weak new bond. If, in the final step of substitution, this ring opens at the new bond, we observe substitution without rearrangement, but with retention of configuration. However, some cyclic cations can attain, not necessarily as their most stable form, a symmetry of binding of the γ-atom by its old bond and by its new: and in that case the ring can be opened at either bond. Then we observe substitution without rearrangement and with predominating retention of configuration, and also substitution with rearrangement and a large degree of inversion of configuration at the migration terminus.

In one of the examples already given (Section **33h**), the conversion of an optically active *threo*-2-bromo-butan-3-ol by hydrogen bromide to racemic 2,3-dibromobutane was taken to indicate passage through an intermediate state in which the original 2-bromine atom lies on a plane of symmetry and consequently undergoes migration to the extent of 50%. It is more convenient here to start from the similar example, due to Cram, of 3-phenylbutane 2-toluene-*p*-sulphonate, an optically active *erythro*-form of which, on solvolysis in acetic acid, gave the active *erythro*-3-phenylbutane 2-acetate of like configuration, whereas an optically active *threo*-form of the toluenesulphonate yielded a racemic *threo*-form of the acetate. The interpretation assumes a cationic intermediate with the phenyl group on a two-fold rotational axis of symmetry in the *erythro*-conversion, but on a plane of symmetry in the *threo*-conversion, the phenyl group in each case undergoing 50% of migration:[124]

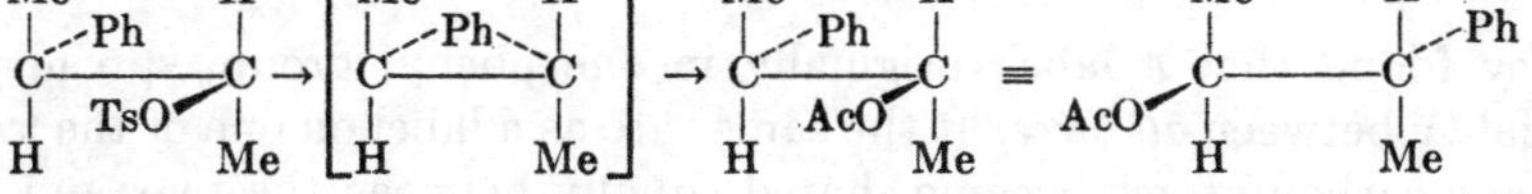

(2*S*)-*Erythro* → [bridged phenonium ion]$^+$ → (2*S*)-*Erythro* (acetate)

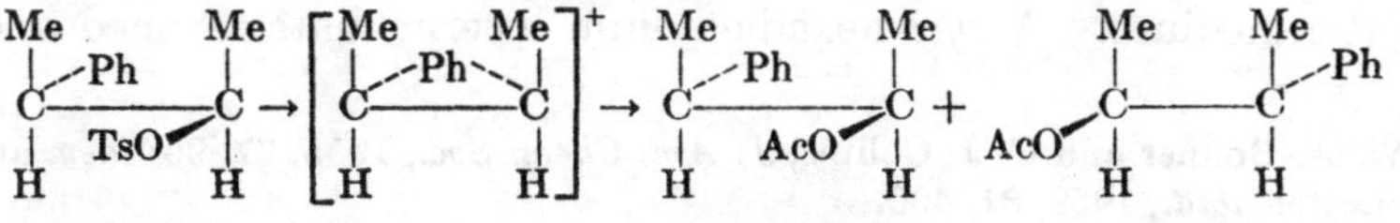

(2*R*)-*Threo* → [bridged phenonium ion]$^+$ → (2*R*)-*Threo* + (2*S*)-*Threo* (acetates)

[124] D. J. Cram, *J. Am. Chem. Soc.*, 1952, **74**, 2129.

The question now arises as to the status of these ionic structures here represented with three-membered rings. Are they, as shown on the left below, transition states of reversible interconversions of two position-isomeric carbonium ions, having charges localised the one on the migration origin and the other on the migration terminus? Or are they true intermediates, in which the charge is carried largely by, and distributed by mesomerism within, the migrating group? A classical formulation, as shown on the right below, for such an intermediate would be in order, because the phenyl migration is an internal electrophilic aromatic substitution by a formed or forming carbonium ion, and the first step of any such substitution is an addition to give a *cyclo*hexadienylium ion, so many of which have been isolated as salts, that one should expect a *cyclo*propane*spirocyclo*hexadienylium ion to be reasonably stable (cf. Sections **23c**, **24c**, **24d**):

$$\mathrm{RR'C(Ph)\!-\!\overset{+}{C}RR'} \rightleftharpoons \mathrm{RR'\overset{+}{C}\!-\!C(Ph)RR'} \qquad \text{cyclohexadienylium}(+)\text{ spiro to } \mathrm{RR'C\!-\!CRR'}$$

There is no generally applicable, single answer to the question: the answer depends on the case, in particular, on the degree to which the structure undergoing rearrangement favours residence of the carbonium ionic charge on the migration origin and migration terminus, on the one hand, and on the migrating group, on the other.

Bonner and Collins studied the acid-catalysed reversible isomerisation of 1,2,2-triphenylethyl acetate in acetic acid with triple isotopic labelling:[125]

$$\mathrm{Ph_2CH\!-\!CHPh(OAc)} \rightleftharpoons \mathrm{PhCH(OAc)\!-\!CHPh_2}$$

They found that a label, originally in one phenyl group, spread to equality between *all three*, at the same rate as a label on one of the two ethane carbon atoms became shared equally between the two, and as the isotopically distinguished acetate group became replaced by acetate from the medium. A *cyclo*hexadienylium intermediate, formed once

[125] W. A. Bonner and C. J. Collins, *J. Am. Chem. Soc.*, 1955, **77**, 99; *idem* and C. T. Lester, *ibid.*, 1959, **81**, 466.

per phenyl transfer, could not account for such a relatively high rate of label-spreading among the phenyl groups. Only many to-and-fro phenyl movements, while the acetate group is out of the way, that is, in the carbonium ion, can account for the observed relation between the rates of the three label transfers. Thus there are two carbonium-ion intermediates in this rearrangement, one with the charge on the migration terminus and the other with it on the migration origin; and they come into equilibrium with each other much more rapidly than either is destroyed by uptake of acetate ion. In this case the scales may be thought to be weighted in favour of retention of the charge on the migration terminus and migration origin, because these are both benzyl positions, and a charge, placed on either, is really spread by mesomerism in the attached phenyl groups, with stabilisation of the cation.

Caserio, Levin, and Roberts have arranged a "weighting" in the opposite sense, first, by having no unsaturated group except the single migrating aryl group, and then, by loading this with an oxy-substituent, in order to provide an extra location, of oxonium character, for the cationic charge; and they have proved the effectiveness of these arrangements in producing an intermediatc *cyclo*propane*spirocyclo*hexadiene ion of relatively long life, with the aid of a built-in tell-tale system.[126] Their substrate was 2-*p*-(ω-hydroxyphenetyl)ethylamine, which they deaminated with nitrous acid. The ethylamine residue was provided with two 1-deuterium atoms, whose transfer to the 2-position would diagnose a Wagner-Meerwein rearrangement. The ω-hydroxyethyl group was likewise provided with two ω-deuterium atoms, a distribution of which between the two hydroxyethyl carbon atoms would similarly diagnose a rearrangement in this group, by a reversible cyclic acetal formation, in the cation of the Wagner-Meerwein rearrangement. This could occur only if the Wagner-Meerwein cation should last long enough to permit rearrangement through the cyclic acetal during its lifetime. The observation was that both pairs of deuterium atoms became distributed over the relevant pairs of carbon atoms. This shows that the *cyclo*propane*spiro*-ion does last long enough to allow completion of another reaction, namely, the formation and rupture of the ethylene acetal. The *spiro*-ion is therefore a true intermediate in this case, and is not a representation of a symmetrical transition state between isomeric carbonium ions:

[126] M. C. Caserio, R. D. Levin, and J. D. Roberts, *J. Am. Chem. Soc.*, 1965, **87**, 5651.

The logically final step in this approach, that of using an O^--substituent, to the end that the usual intermediate cation becomes a neutral *cyclo*hexadienone, was achieved by Baird and Winstein.[127] Converting 2-*p*-hydroxyphenylethyl bromide into methyl ether in methyl alcoholic sodium methoxide, they were able spectroscopically to follow the rise and fall in concentration of the intermediate *cyclo*propane*spirocyclo*hexadienone, and also to isolate this substance. It had a stability maximum at about *p*H 12, but, above *p*H 14, rapidly added methoxide ion:

(45g) Ionic Intermediates: Saturated Migrating Groups: Synartesis. —A great part of the field of the Wagner-Meerwein and pinacol-pinacolone rearrangements is concerned with migrating groups without *p* or π electrons, saturated groups, such as methyl and higher alkyl residues, and hydrogen atoms, having only σ electrons. Since the late 1930's it has been appreciated that in such rearrangements, no less than in those involving unsaturated migrating groups, although the overall reaction is unimolecular, rate-controlled by an ionisation, the local transaction at the migration terminus can conform to either

[127] R. Baird and S. Winstein, *J. Am. Chem. Soc.*, 1963, 85, 567.

of two types. It may be of S_N1-type, the ionisation proceeding to beyond its transition state before the migrating group passes over:

$$\begin{matrix} R & & R & & R \\ | & \rightarrow & | & \rightarrow & | \\ A—B—X & & A—\overset{+}{B} & & \overset{+}{A}—B \end{matrix}$$

or it may be of S_N2-type, as formulated below, the migration and ionisation being concerted:

$$\begin{matrix} R & & R \\ | & \rightarrow & | \\ A—B—X & & \overset{+}{A}—B \end{matrix}$$

These processes allow of two observable distinctions. The first is stereochemical: the S_N1-type local process offers an opportunity for more or less racemisation, whereas the S_N2-type local process should produce stereospecific inversion at the migration terminus. The second distinction is kinetic: in the S_N1-type transaction, the rate-controlling heterolysis, not being internally pressed forward, should occur at about the same rate as if the heterolysing bond had the same local surroundings in simpler, non-rearranging, molecules; whereas in the S_N2-type transaction, the heterolysis will be accelerated by the concerted incursion of the migrating group. Examples of such abnormally fast rearrangements have long been known in the terpene series. The question arose as to why a *saturated* migrating group, such as methyl or a higher alkyl residue, should exert such a "driving force," as it is often called; and the hypothesis was offered that it was in order to form an ion rendered more stable than either

$$\begin{matrix} & R \\ & | \\ \overset{+}{A}— & B \end{matrix} \quad \text{or} \quad \begin{matrix} R & \\ | & \\ A— & \overset{+}{B} \end{matrix}$$

by a resonance between such canonical structures, that is, by a delocalisation of the migrating σ-electrons over the two atoms between which the cationic charge was assumed to be divided:

$$\begin{matrix} & R & \\ & \diagup \; \diagdown & \\ A & — & B \\ & + & \end{matrix}$$

The early notes on this idea belong to the period of 1940.[128] It was

[128] T. P. Nevell, E. de Salas, and C. L. Wilson, *J. Chem. Soc.*, **1939**, 1188; personal communications from C. K. Ingold cited by H. B. Watson in *Ann. Reports on Progress Chem.* (Chem. Soc. London), 1939, **36**, 197, and in H. B. Watson's book, "Modern Theories of Organic Chemistry," Oxford Univ. Press, 2nd Edn., 1941, p. 208.

used to good effect around 1950, particularly at the outset[129] of important developmental investigations by Winstein and by Roberts, to which we shall come. In this period, it was further discussed by Hughes,[130] by Winstein,[130] and by Hughes, Brown, Smith and the writer,[131] especially with respect to the kinetic effects of migration when concerted with an ionisation. The last-mentioned discussion pointed to boron chemistry as providing analogies for σ-bond delocalisation in carbonium-ion chemistry, and proposed to call such σ-bond delocalisation "synartesis" (fastening together), in contradistinction to π-bond delocalisation, already called "mesomerism."[132]

In order to illustrate the kinetic character of rearrangements involving S_N1-type transactions at the seat of dissociation, we may refer, first, to the solvolysis of *neo*pentyl bromide to yield *t*-amyl alcohol and other *t*-amyl products:

$$(CH_3)_3C\cdot CH_2Br \rightarrow (CH_3)_2C(OR)\cdot CH_2\cdot CH_3, \text{ etc.}$$

The first-order rates of separation of halide ion from this primary bromide are of the same order of magnitude as those applying to the unimolecular reactions, under like conditions, of quite simple primary bromides,[133] such as ethyl bromide, as is illustrated by the following comparison:

$$\text{Hydrolysis in wet } HCO_2H \text{ at } 95° \begin{cases} \text{ethyl bromide,} & k_1 = 2.70 \times 10^{-6} \text{ sec.}^{-1} \\ neo\text{pentyl bromide,} & k_1 = 1.53 \times 10^{-6} \text{ sec.}^{-1} \end{cases}$$

[129] S. Winstein and D. S. Trifan, *J. Am. Chem. Soc.*, 1949, **71**, 2953; J. D. Roberts, W. Bennett, and R. Armstrong, *ibid.*, 1950, **72**, 3329.

[130] E. D. Hughes, *Bull. soc. chim.* (France), 1951, **18**, p. C41; S. Winstein, *ibid.*, p. C55.

[131] F. Brown, E. D. Hughes, C. K. Ingold, and J. F. Smith, *Nature*, 1951, **168**, 65.

[132] Contemporaneously, Roberts and Lee introduced the term "non-classical" (J. D. Roberts and C. C. Lee, *J. Am. Chem. Soc.*, 1951, **73**, 5009), which has since been used to cover charge delocalisations of all kinds (mesomeric and synartetic) in carbonium ions. In the short run, this cannot be wrong, since it avoids positive description; but it will become wrong, in that any correct idea, when it has been accepted and used for a considerable time, becomes "classical." Mesomerism has reached that degree of seniority and acceptance. Synartesis may reach it.

[133] I. Dostrovsky and E. D. Hughes, *J. Chem. Soc.*, **1946**, 164, 166, 171. Chromatographic analyses of various *neo*pentyl solvolysis products have more recently been undertaken. H. M. R. Hoffmann and G. M. Fraser have given detailed analyses of the products from the toluene-*p*-sulphonate in the complete range of ethanol-water mixtures. They show that, along with the preponderating *t*-amyl and amylene products, *neo*pentyl products are found in the proportions 3–10%, and the unforseen by-product, 1,1-dimethyl*cyclo*propane, is formed in the proportions 0.0–0.3% (*Chem. Comm.*, **1967**, 561).

Evidently the migrating methyl group does not assist separation of the halogen, even though the migration must occur soon after the halogen has left, and before the solvent has had time to trap even the highly reactive primary carbonium ion. We draw this conclusion because so little unrearranged material has ever been recovered—none in the solvolysis mentioned, though that was done before chromatographic analysis became available.[133] The solvolysis of pinacolyl chloride, again to yield essentially rearranged products,

$$(CH_3)_3C \cdot CHCl \cdot CH_3 \rightarrow (CH_3)_2C(OR) \cdot CH(CH_3)_2, \text{ etc.}$$

illustrates the same situation in relation to a secondary halide. Heterolysis rates are now of the same order as those estimated for the unimolecular solvolysis of simple secondary chlorides,[134] such as *iso*propyl chloride:

$$\begin{matrix}\text{Solvolysis in 80\%} \\ \text{aq.-EtOH at } 80^\circ\end{matrix} \left\{\begin{matrix} \textit{iso}\text{propyl chloride,} & k_1 \sim 5 \times 10^{-7} \text{ sec.}^{-1} \\ \text{pinacolyl chloride,} & k_1 = 1.94 \times 10^{-7} \text{ sec.}^{-1} \end{matrix}\right.$$

Again the migration is not accelerating the heterolysis, even though it must occur soon after heterolysis has been determined.

A long known illustration, one which brings out stereochemical as well as kinetic aspects of the contrast between such rearrangements as involve an S_N1-type and those which involve an S_N2-type local transaction at the seat of dissociation, is that of the solvolysis of bornyl and *iso*bornyl halides or esters to rearranged products of the camphene series, camphene hydrate, camphene ethers, or camphene itself.[131] The first-order solvolysis of bornyl chloride takes place at rates which are of the same order of magnitude as those of the solvolysis of pinacolyl chloride, and therefore of the same order as those of unimolecular solvolysis of simple secondary chlorides, such as *iso*propyl chloride. However, the solvolysis of *iso*bornyl chloride, likewise to give camphene products, takes place at rates which are greater than any of the other rates mentioned by factors in the neighbourhood of 30,000–100,000. The following figures are illustrative:

$$\begin{matrix}\text{Solvolysis in 80\%} \\ \text{aq.-EtOH at } 80^\circ\end{matrix} \left\{\begin{matrix} \text{pinacolyl chloride,} & k_1 = 1.94 \times 10^{-7} \text{ sec.}^{-1} \\ \text{bornyl chloride,} & k_1 \sim 1.5 \times 10^{-7} \text{ sec.}^{-1} \\ \textit{iso}\text{bornyl chloride,} & k_1 \sim 1.4 \times 10^{-2} \text{ sec.}^{-1} \end{matrix}\right.$$

The large rate for *iso*bornyl is easily interpreted by the theory of synartesis. In this chloride, which has the *exo*-structure, the bond shift could be initiated before the chlorine atom has reached the sep-

[134] R. J. L. Martin, Thesis, London, 1949; E. D. Hughes, C. K. Ingold, R. J. L. Martin, and D. F. Meigh, *Nature*, 1950, **166**, 679.

aration of the transition state of its ionisation; and therefore the bond shift could have an accelerative effect on the reaction rate. In bornyl chloride, the *endo*-chloride, on the other hand, no bond shift can commence until the chlorine atom has moved out of the way, that is, to well beyond the transition-state separation; and therefore the bond shift cannot influence the reaction rate. In short, these chlorides provide the double illustration of rearrangements involving unaccelerated unimolecular and accelerated bimolecular "substitution" at the seat of dissociation:

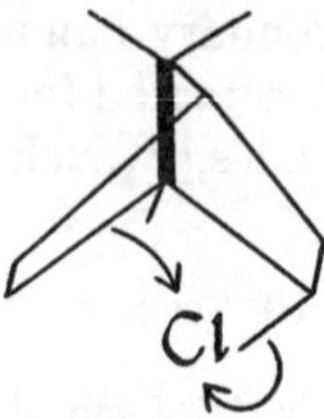

Bornyl chloride

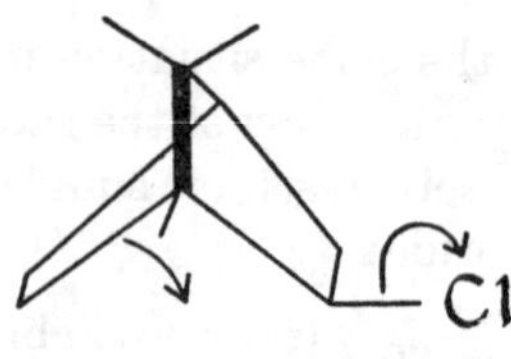

***iso*Bornyl chloride**

The concept of synartesis involves the consequence that even non-rearranging substitutions and eliminations may display accelerating effects, broadly similar to those accompanying rearrangements. For if a substitution or elimination is rate-controlled by an ionisation, and if the formed carbonium ion is rendered especially stable by synartesis, some part of that additional stability will belong to the transition state of its formation, wherefore the ion will be formed faster. But whether the ion, which in its synartetic constitution holds the potentiality of rearrangement, will actually complete a rearrangement, is a thermodynamic matter. If a rearrangement product would be less stable than its non-rearranged isomer, the latter will be formed; but it will be formed at an accelerated rate, because it is the formation, not the eventual reaction, of the synartetic ion which is rate-controlling.

Acceleration in non-rearranging reactions may be illustrated by the following example. The rate of hydrolysis of camphene hydrochloride in aqueous solvents to camphene hydrate and camphene is too great to be easily measured: it is obviously greater than the corresponding rate for simple tertiary alkyl chlorides. The rate of the analogous ethyl alcoholysis of camphene hydrochloride has been measured,[131] and has been found to be about 6000 times greater than the corresponding rate for *t*-butyl chloride:

Solvolysis in dry EtOH at 0°	*t*-butyl chloride,	$k_1 \sim 7 \times 10^{-9}$ sec.$^{-1}$
	camphene hydrochloride,	$k_1 = 4.0 \times 10^{-5}$ sec.$^{-1}$

The general principles governing the incidence of acceleration, due to synartesis in a carbonium ion, in non-rearranging and rearranging unimolecular substitutions and eliminations, rate-controlled by formation of the carbonium ion, have been illustrated by the schematic diagrams[131] reproduced as Figs. 45-1 and 45-2. We may refer first to the broken-line curves. Energy is here being schematically plotted as usual against a parameter of the reaction path. Initial and final states are not represented because they can stand in either order of energy, and their order does not influence mechanism, though it does determine whether or not the system will take advantage of an available mechanism. The representative points are assumed to enter either diagram from the left: they will leave mainly over which-

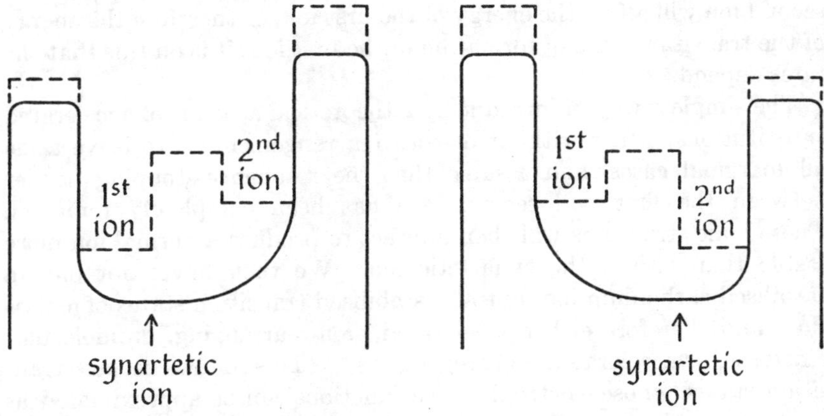

Fig. 45-1. Fig. 45-2.

(Schematic representation of non-rearranging and rearranging unimolecular reactions, without and with synartetic acceleration.)

Broken line.—Representative points entering and leaving by the left describe normal-rate non-rearranging, unimolecular reactions, such as the solvolysis of *t*-amyl bromide.

Full-line.—Points entering and leaving by the left describe accelerated non-rearranging reactions, such as the solvolysis of camphene hydrochloride. Of a maintained supply of points, those leaving by the right describe accelerated rearrangement, as of camphene hydrochloride to *iso*bornyl chloride.

Broken line.—Representative points entering by the left and leaving by the right describe normal-rate rearrangements, as in the unimolecular solvolysis of *neo*pentyl bromide.

Full-line.—Representative points entering by the left and leaving by the right describe accelerated rearrangements, as in the hydrolysis of *iso*bornyl chloride to camphene hydrate and camphene. Points returning over the left-hand barrier would describe an accelerated non-rearranging side-reaction.

ever of the bounding transition states lies the lower, and, in principle at least, to a minor extent over the boundary barrier which stands higher. The representative points therefore leave Fig. 45-1 mainly by the left: this means that the first carbonium ion is produced, and then recombines with some anion without rearrangement, as in the solvolysis of *t*-amyl bromide. The representative points leave Fig. 45-2 mainly by the right: the first carbonium ion is formed, and passes into the second carbonium ion, and thence into rearranged products, as in the unimolecular solvolysis of *neo*pentyl bromide. The central transition states appearing in the broken-line curves of Figs. 45-1 and 45-2 express the condition, which the examples mentioned fulfil, that both the non-rearranging substitution and the rearrangement shall be unaccelerated, that is, that they shall derive no extra rate from either the possibility or the actual occurrence of the group shift. For the central barrier is supposed to be adequate to preclude energetically significant resonance between the first and second ions. Hence, neither the potential existence nor the actual formation of the second ion will affect the energy of the first ion, or therefore the energy of the transition state of formation of the first ion: it is on this that the rates depend.

The simplest way of introducing a theoretical account of accelerated substitutions, either without or with rearrangement, is to leave aside all marginal cases, and assume that the resonance-stopping barrier between the first and second ions has been completely removed. These ionic structures will then interact to produce a normal ion more stable than either, the synartetic ion. We then have, not only a stabilised carbonium ion, but also stabilised transition states of ionisation, and therefore either accelerated, non-rearranging, unimolecular reactions, or accelerated rearrangements. (This follows because transition states, whose electronic wave-functions can be approximated as mixtures of those of the factors and products, thus reflect stability changes in the factors and products.)

A diagrammatic expression of this situation is given by the full-line curves in Figs. 45-1 and 45-2. Representative points which enter either diagram by the left and return by the left describe accelerated unimolecular reactions without rearrangement, such as the solvolysis of camphene hydrochloride. One sees how synartetic acceleration can arise on account of the possibility of a group shift, even in unimolecular reactions that involve no group shift. Representative points which pass right through either diagram from left to right describe accelerated rearrangements. Only a minor proportion of the points entering Fig. 45-1 from the left can pass through, but if the supply is maintained, and the thermodynamic relation of factor to product is suitable, an accelerated rearrangement will result. Most of the points which enter Fig. 45-2 from the left will pass through, and will describe an accelerated rearrangement, such as the hydrolysis of *iso*bornyl chloride to camphene hydrate.

The stalking-horse with which the closest view has been obtained of the structure and internal conversions of a synartetic carbonium ion of the class considered in this Section is the carbonium ion of norbornyl compounds. A conversion corresponding to that of *iso*bornyl chloride to camphene hydrochloride, but with the three methyl groups left out, is the conversion of an *exo*-2-norbornyl chloride into its enantiomer: such rearrangements, isomeric or otherwise, may thus be followed polarimetrically. In this system, we lose the methyl groups as markers of certain ring carbon atoms, but much more informative markers have been introduced by isotopic labelling, as we shall see. It is an important feature of the system that, if there is a synartetic ion, it has a plane of symmetry (C_s symmetry); and this, of course, has stereochemical consequences. In order that these relations can be followed easily, the structure of an *exo*-2-norbornyl halide or ester is drawn twice below, first in a familiar projection, and again after first turning the previous model round to bring position-1 to the front, and then rolling it over to bring the *exo*-side to the bottom. The further formulae show the Wagner-Meerwein conversion to the enantiomer, and the possible intermediate carbonium ion of C_s symmetry:

Wagner—Meerwein

exo-2-Norbornyl ester or halide — Enantiomer

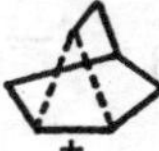

Structure of C_s symmetry for synartetic ion

Winstein and Trifan showed[135] that *exo*-2-norbornyl esters underwent solvolytic substitutions considerably more rapidly than their *endo*-isomers, though the rate differences were not so great as those of similar reactions of the bornyl series. Thus the *exo*-2-bromobenzene-*p*-sulphonate was converted in acetic acid to the *exo*-acetate about 350 times faster than the *endo*-sulphonate was so converted, the rate of the latter reaction being about the same as the rate of conversion of *cyclo*hexyl bromobenzene-*p*-sulphonate to *cyclo*hexyl acetate. Winstein and Trifan assumed that the reaction of the *exo*-sulphonate feels a "driving force," that is, that the group-shift becomes concerted with the ionisation before the transition state is reached. The product from

[135] S. Winstein and D. Trifan, *J. Am. Chem. Soc.*, 1949, **71**, 2953; 1952, **74**, **1147**, 1152.

both the *exo-* and *endo*-sulphonates was the pure *exo*-acetate. That from the *exo*-sulphonate was at least 99.95% racemised. That from the *endo*-sulphonate was 92% racemised, the remaining 8% being inverted. When the optically active bromobenzenesulphonate was undergoing solvolysis, it racemised substantially faster than it solvolysed (for example, about twice as fast). This shows that an optically inactive intermediate is reversibly formed, and can either go back into what it came from, with racemisation, or go on to give the product, with racemisation.

Roberts, Lee, and Saunders[136] built up norborneol (by Diels-Alder addition of vinyl acetate to *cyclo*pentadiene and subsequent steps) with ^{14}C labels in the 2- and 3-positions as marked in the formulae above. After acetolysis of the *exo*-2-bromobenzene-*p*-sulphonate, they took the formed *exo*-acetate to pieces by alternate oxidations and Curtius rearrangements, as follows, in order to find out where the labels had got to:

(norbornyl acetate, positions 7, 1, 2 OAc, 6, 5, 4, 3) → (dicarboxylic acid, CO_2H, CO_2H) → $2CO_2$ + (diamine, NH_2, NH_2)

$2CO_2$: 2,3; diamine: 1,7,4,5,6

→ CO_2 + (dicarboxylic acid, CO_2H, CO_2H) → $2CO_2$ + (diamine, NH_2, NH_2)

7   1,4,5,6   1,4   5,6

The results were as follows, the figures in parenthesis being those calculated on certain assumptions from the interpretation set out below:

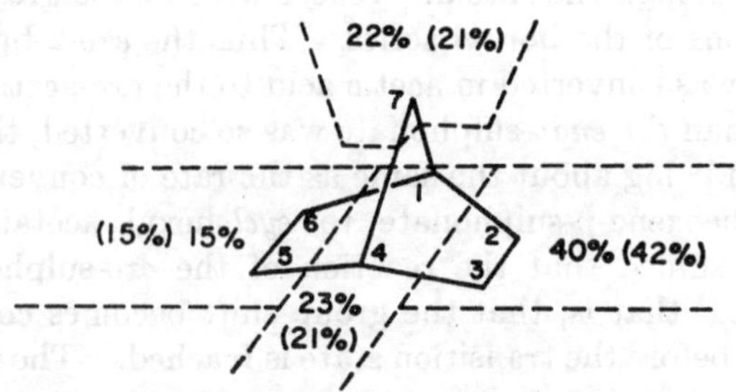

[136] J. D. Roberts and C. C. Lee, *J. Am. Chem. Soc.*, 1951, **73**, 5009; *idem* and W. H. Saunders jr., *ibid.*, 1954, **76**, 4501.

A Wagner-Meerwein rearrangement, through an intermediate structure having the plane of symmetry of the synartetic ion shown above, should cause sharing of the labels, originally in the 2,3-positions, equally with the 1,7-positions. If we may assume that the recovered 1,4-label was entirely a 1-label, then this expected distribution of labels does occur and does reach equilibrium within the lifetime of the carbonium ion. But a further spreading of labels to the 5,6-positions, a spreading which does not reach equilibrium in the lifetime of the carbonium ion, is also apparent in the observations. This finding requires the assumption of an $\alpha\gamma$-hydrogen shift, such as a 6→2 shift, of the general type established by Reutov in the deamination of *n*-propylamine (Section **45b**). In the present example, a shift of hydrogen from position-6 to position-2 or to position-1, in combination with the already considered shift of the 6-carbon atom from position-1 to position-2 and backwards, would allow labels from the 2,3,1,7-positions to spread to the 5,6-positions.

Two views regarding the intermediates involved in these changes have been considered. One view assumes that the carbonium ion of C_s symmetry formulated above, and redrawn as I below, passes by hydrogen shifts into two other, equivalent, carbonium ions, II and III, also of symmetry C_s. The rate of the cyclic interconversion of I to II and III has to be assumed to be comparable with, though less than, the rate at which I, indeed any of these equivalent carbonium ions, is destroyed by the nucleophilic substituting agents.

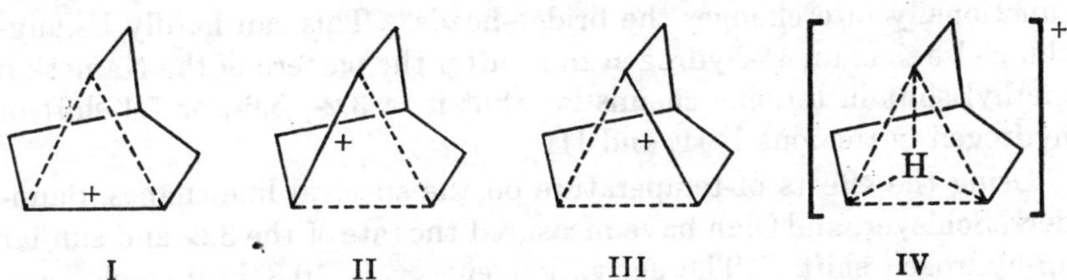

In equilibrium, the cyclicly interconvertible system I, II, III would be functionally trigonal, and the possibility of a single ion of the symmetry C_{3v} has been contemplated. It is formulated at IV and can be thought of as nortricyclene with an extra proton on the C_3 axis. In a bond picture, one has to have split bonds to the proton, as well as between the three carbon atoms that bind the proton. The positive charge is shared equally between the three carbon atoms, and to an undetermined extent by the bound proton. In order to interpret the observed label distribution, one has to assume that the C_s ion, I, is formed first, and that part of it reacts with the solvent or other nucleophile, while part passes into the C_{3v} ion, IV, which subsequently reacts with the nucleophile.

It seems probable that a distinction between these hypotheses, which have for some time been entertained in parallel, is provided by the study, by Schleyer and Olah and their collaborators,[137] of the proton magnetic resonance spectra of norbornyl halides dissolved in a mixture of antimony pentafluoride and sulphur dioxide. When *exo*-2-norbornyl fluoride is put into this solvent, it is completely converted into norbornylium hexafluoroantimonate, and the carbonium ion is long-lived, and stable enough to be studied spectrally up to 40°. Below $-60°$, the proton magnetic resonance spectrum shows three sharp peaks, with relative areas 6, 1, and 4; and there is no sign of further resolution at $-120°$. These are the requirements of the theory of three equivalent synartetic ions of C_s symmetry, cyclicly interconvertible by $\alpha\gamma$-hydrogen shifts, which must be faster, even at $-120°$, than the proton-spin transitions. The C_{3v} model IV for the carbonium ion requires four peaks of the relative areas 6, 1, 3, and 1, and the observations are therefore less simply interpreted on this basis.

Above $-60°$ a slower transformation in the norbornylium ion occurs, which simplifies the proton magnetic resonance spectrum: as the temperature is raised, the three peaks broaden and merge, and then the coalesced peak sharpens, until, above $-5°$, the spectrum consists of a single sharp peak. All the hydrogen atoms are now equivalent, and this can only mean that, superposed on the $\alpha\beta$-carbon and $\alpha\gamma$-hydrogen migrations already discussed, a slower rearrangement has set in, which functionally interchanges the bridge-heads. This can hardly be anything else than an $\alpha\beta$-hydrogen shift, after the pattern of the Nametkin methyl shift in terpene chemistry, that is, a 3,2-, 5,6-, or 7,1-shift of hydrogen in the ions I, II, and III.

Using the effects of temperature on the spectral line shapes, Saunders, Schleyer, and Olah have measured the rate of the 3,2- and similar $\alpha\beta$-hydrogen shifts. The activation energy is 10.8 kcal./mole; and the Arrhenius equation, $k=10^{12.3}\exp(-10{,}800/RT)$ sec.$^{-1}$, leads to a rate constant of 2.5×10^4 sec.$^{-1}$ at 25°.

Bartlett has made[138] an illuminating computation of the minimum

[137] P. von R. Schleyer, W. E. Watts, R. C. Fort jr., M. B. Comiserow and G. A. Olah, *J. Am. Chem. Soc.*, 1964, 86, 5679; M. Saunders, P. von R. Schleyer, and G. A. Olah, *ibid.*, p. 5680.

[138] P. D. Bartlett, "Non-classical Ions," W. A. Benjamin, Inc., New York, 1965, p. 525. The idea of synartetic acceleration has been formidably opposed by H. C. Brown (cf. *Special Pubs. Chem. Soc.*, 1962, 16, 140), with whom one may agree that some observed accelerations have been so accepted and credited to synartesis with apparently insufficient circumspection. However, as P. D.

rates of the two fast rearrangements, based on the fact that even the slower of them, the $\alpha\gamma$-hydrogen shift, cannot be frozen out in the nuclear magnetic resonance spectrometer at $-120°$. The specific rate must be at least 3×10^5 sec.$^{-1}$ at this temperature, and, assuming the above pre-exponential factor, $10^{12.3}$ sec.$^{-1}$, the activation energy is computed as unlikely to be much above 4.8 kcal./mole, a figure which leads to a rate of at least 6×10^8 sec.$^{-1}$ at 25°.

Continuing, Bartlett recalls that the rate of reaction of the norbornylium ion with acetic acid solvent in Roberts, Lee, and Saunders's work is 3.3 times the rate of the 6,2- and similar $\alpha\gamma$-hydrogen shifts; and also that the lower limit to the extent of racemisation in Winstein and Trifan's acetolysis of an *exo*-norbornyl ester shows that the rate of the carbon bond shift (if it has a separate rate) is at least 2000 times greater than that of the reaction of the ion with the solvent. By multiplying the factors, two of which are themselves lower limits, Bartlett calculates a minimum rate for the carbon bond shift (supposing that it has a separate rate), *viz.*, 4×10^{12} sec.$^{-1}$ at 25°. Such a rate obviously implies no activation energy, and is, indeed, meaningless except possibly as a vibration frequency.

It follows that, in the quiescent periods between the activated hydrogen shifts, the norbornylium ion has not to be pictured as an equilibrium system of a "first ion" and a "second ion," having charges differently localised, and separated by an intervening energy barrier. Rather we must regard it as one or another of the equivalent synartetic ions of C_s symmetry, such as might illustrate the schematic diagram in Fig. 45-3 (p. 778).

(45h) Ionic Intermediates: Mixed $\sigma\pi$-Delocalisation: Generalisation of Synartesis.—The first step of this extension of theory was taken in 1955 by Winstein, Shatavsky, Norton, and Woodward.[139] The background was that 7-norbornyl halides and esters were well known to be very slowly solvolysed, an effect commonly attributed to the difficulty of accommodating a carbonium ion to the small and rigidly held ring-angle at the 7-position: one knows that the ease of formation of bridge-head carbonium ions is an extremely sensitive function of their geometry and rigidity (Section **33g**). The new discovery was that *anti*-7-norbornenyl esters, which have a 2,3-double bond, are very rapidly solvolysed. It was subsequently found that 7-norbornadienyl esters, which have additionally a 5,6-double bond, are solvolysed

---

Bartlett makes clear in the book cited, this does not discredit the valid kinetic, stereochemical, spectroscopic, and isotopic-labelling evidence in favour of synartesis.

[139] S. Winstein, M. Shatavsky, C. Norton, and R. D. Woodward, *J. Am. Chem. Soc.*, 1955, **77**, 4183.

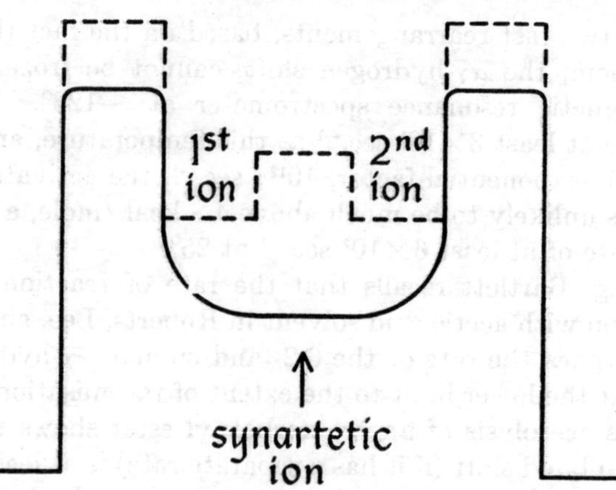

FIG. 45-3. Schematic representation of a carbonium ion with two symmetrically situated charge locations, and, arising from this situation, of a synartetic ion having a plane of symmetry. The norbornylium ion is an example.

more rapidly still.[140] The following approximate relative rates refer to the acetolysis of toluene-*p*-sulphonates:

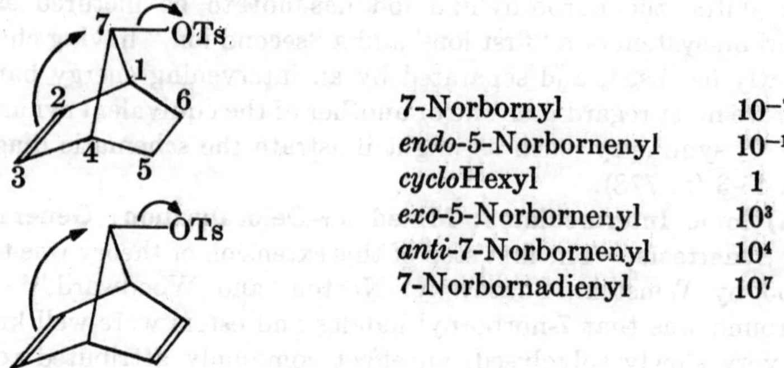

7-Norbornyl	10^{-7}
endo-5-Norbornenyl	10^{-1}
*cyclo*Hexyl	1
exo-5-Norbornenyl	10^{3}
anti-7-Norbornenyl	10^{4}
7-Norbornadienyl	10^{7}

These results gave birth to the idea that the lateral π electrons might move outwards, and thus accelerate the formation of, the 7-carbonium ionic centre.

To a suggestion that an integral covalency change places the charge in position-3 in a particularly stable "classical" ion with a 1,2,7-*cyclo*propane ring there were always several answers: but the simplest today may be that, as Story and Saunders showed,[141] the proton magnetic resonance spectrum of 7-norbornadienyl tetrafluoroborate in

[140] S. Winstein and C. Ordronneau, *J. Am. Chem. Soc.*, 1960, **82,** 2084.
[141] P. R. Story and M. Saunders, *J. Am. Chem. Soc.*, 1962. **84,** 4876.

sulphur dioxide, or in nitromethane, does not reveal 7 non-equivalent protons. Neither does it reveal three sets of 1, 2, and 4 protons, as equal involvement of the two double bonds, to give an ion with two planes of symmetry (C_{2v}), would require. It discloses four sets of 1, 2, 2, and 2 protons, and therefore points to the predominating involvement of one double bond, to give an ion with one plane of symmetry (C_s), at least as an effective symmetry over the life of proton-spin transitions. The above curved-arrow diagrams, which are written in explanation of the large accelerations, are consistent with the apparent symmetry.

We have seen already that synartesis can manifest itself, kinetically and stereochemically, either without rearrangement or with rearrangement: the type of product one gets depends on the thermodynamic situation. The Winstein-Woodward discovery illustrates synartesis in the generalised form which is to be described below, but without rearrangement. The generalised form of synartesis with rearrangement was first demonstrated by Le Ny in 1960.[142] She found that the double bond of Δ^4-*cyclo*heptenylmethyl bromobenzene-*p*-sulphonate increased the rate of its acetolysis to 30 times above that of the saturated analogue; and that the product from the unsaturated monocyclic ester was the saturated dicyclic ester, 2-*exo-dicyclo*[3.2.1]octyl acetate (OBrs means bromobenzene-*p*-sulphonate):

OBrs
|
CH_2
→ [ ]$^+$ → OAc

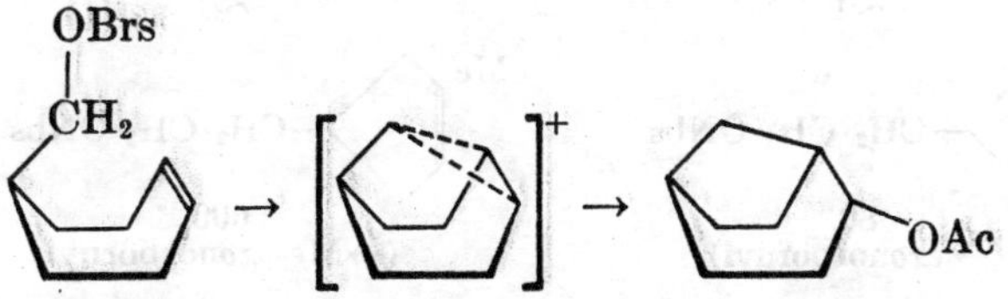

Analogous ring closures leading to norbornyl compounds have been described by Lawton and extensively by Bartlett and his coworkers.[143] The starting point is a β-(Δ^3-*cyclo*pentenyl)ethyl arenesulphonate: this is solvolysed in acetic acid containing sodium acetate at a first-order rate about 75–95 times greater than the rate of solvolysis of the corresponding saturated ester; and the unsaturated ester is solvolysed with ring closure to give *exo*-2-norbornyl acetate:

[142] G. Le Ny, *Compt. rend.*, 1960, **251**, 1526.

[143] R. G. Lawton, *J. Am. Chem. Soc.*, 1961, **83**, 2399; P. D. Bartlett and S. Bank, *ibid.*, p. 2591; *idem*, R. J. Crawford and G. H. Schmid, *ibid.*, 1965, **87**, 1288; P. D. Bartlett and G. D. Sargent, *ibid.*, p. 1277; P. D. Bartlett, W. D. Clossen, and T. J. Cogdell, *ibid.*, p. 1308; P. D. Bartlett, W. S. Trahanovsky, D. A. Boldon, and G. H. Schmid, *ibid.*, p. 1314.

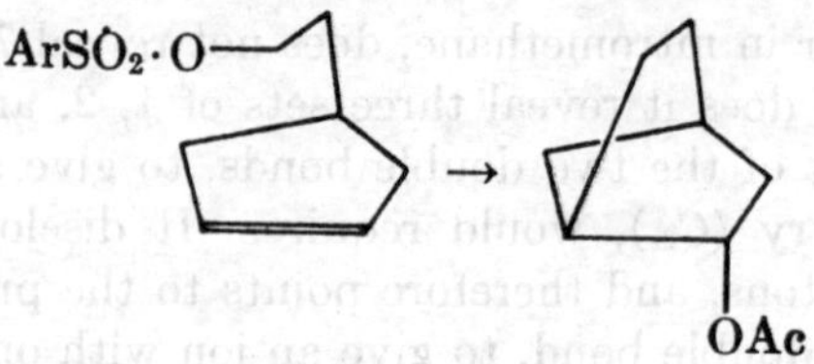

ArSO$_2$·O— → —OAc

Some approximate relative rates in Bartlett's examples, along with a a note of the type of product obtained, are given below (ONbs means nitrobenzene-*p*-sulphonate). The data bring out clearly the necessity for the double bond, and the importance of the ring and of the length of the side-chain, critical factors for the articulation involved in the synartesis manifested in accelerated cyclisation. They also show that the accelerating effect of a double bond is enhanced cumulatively and comparably by terminal methyl groups, as would be expected from the assumed nucleophilic function of the double-bond π electrons:

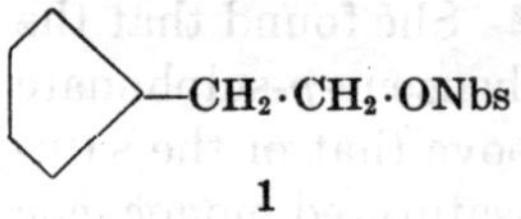

—CH$_2$·CH$_2$·ONbs 1

—CH$_2$·CH$_2$·ONbs 1.5

—CH$_2$·CH$_2$·ONbs ~1

—CH$_2$·CH$_2$·CH$_2$·ONbs ~1

Me, Me —CH$_2$·CH$_2$·CH$_2$·ONbs ~1

—CH$_2$·CH$_2$·ONbs 80 (→ *exo*norbornyl)

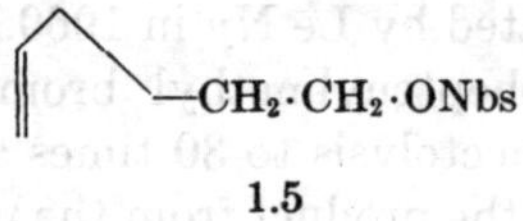

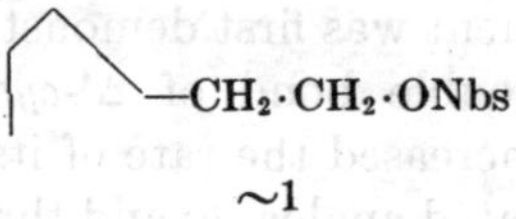

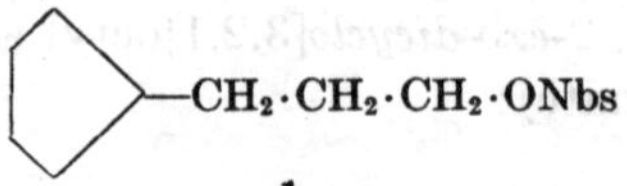

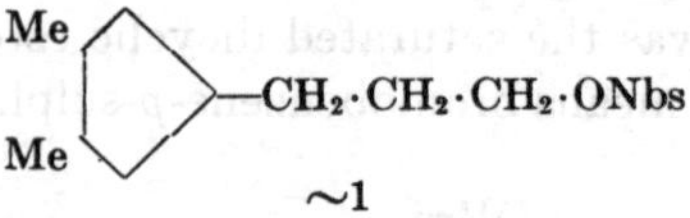

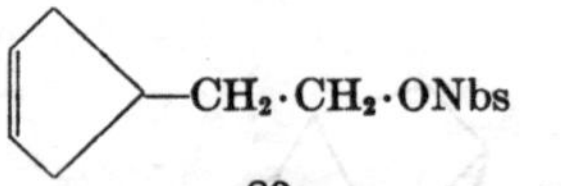

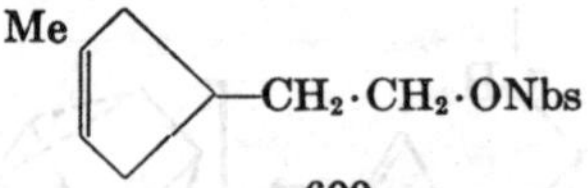

Me —CH$_2$·CH$_2$·ONbs 600 (→Me-*exo*norbornyl

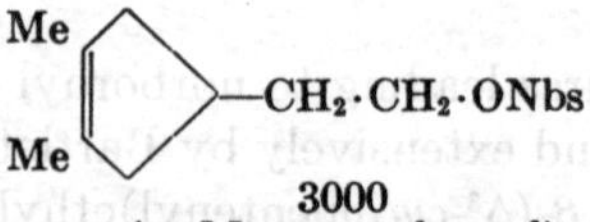

Me, Me —CH$_2$·CH$_2$·ONbs 3000 (→ Me$_2$-*exo*norbornyl)

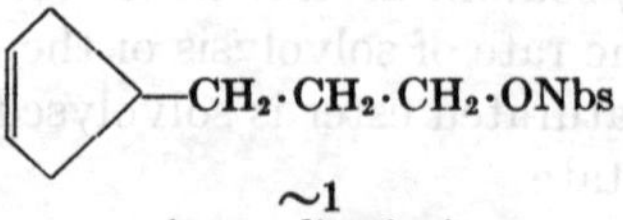

—CH$_2$·CH$_2$·CH$_2$·ONbs ~1 (no cyclisation)

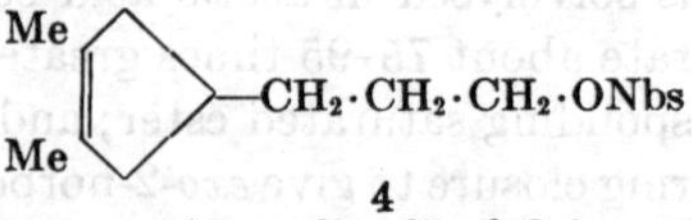

Me, Me —CH$_2$·CH$_2$·CH$_2$·ONbs 4 (some dicyclic olefin)

In 1959, when accelerations by Winstein and Woodward's laterally situated π electrons were known, but when no reports of conversions of such π electrons by rearrangement to σ electrons had yet appeared, J. D. Roberts and his associates, guided by an experimental study, to which we shall come, of a particularly self-contained nature, saw the need to widen the picture of synartesis.[144] Previously, the synartetic bond had been split into two partial bonds extending to the atoms which the migrating atom could bridge, and which would then share the carbonium ionic charge between them. This may often be a good first approximation; but in general and in principle, allowance should be made for partial detachment of the synartetic electron-pair from the bridging atom, in order to augment direct binding between the atoms bridged, and accordingly to allow some part of their charge to be passed back to the bridging atom. This amounts to adding a third canonical structure corresponding to the third starting point (used later by Le Ny, Lawton, and Bartlett) for the formation of a synartetic ion, *viz.*, that of π electrons lateral to an atomic carbonium-ion location. Therefore, following Robert's representation of "non-classical ions" in 1959, we make our three-centre binding by a synartetic electron-pair more nearly symmetrical than before by splitting the electron-pair into three partial bonds, rather than two. The three-centre two-electron bond is suitably represented by a dotted triangle:

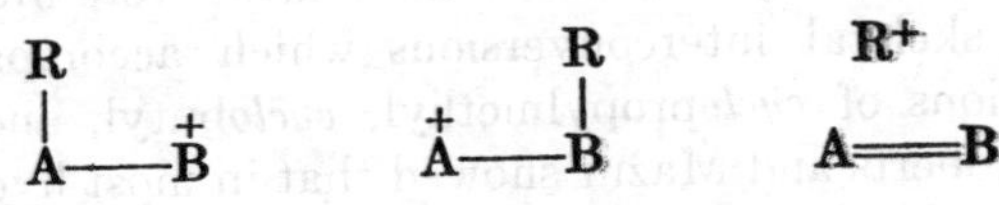

Canonical structures of a synartetic ion

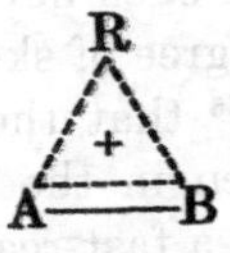

Synartetic ion

The simplest synartetic ion is, of course, the longest-known one,[145] J. J. Thomson's H_3^+; and it is probable that some other "non-classical" mass-sepectrometric ions, such as CH_5^+, may have a like constitution:

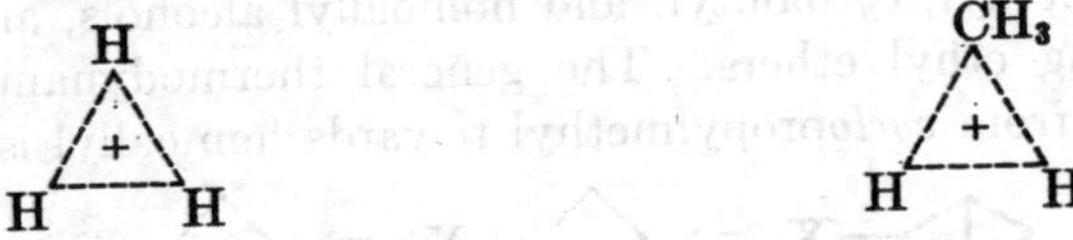

[144] J. D. Roberts and W. H. Mazur, *J. Am. Chem. Soc.*, 1951, **73**, 2509; W. H. Mazur, W. N. White, D. A. Semenov, C. C. Lee, M. S. Silver, and J. D. Roberts, *J. Am. Chem. Soc.*, 1959, **81**, 4390.

[145] J. J. Thomson, *Phil. Mag.*, 1911, **21**, 225; 1912, **24**, 209.

If a synartetic ion arises in any 1,2- or 1,3-hydrogen shift—as cannot be taken for granted, and is quite difficult to prove—it could be written as below. Such conceptual structures are sometimes described as a "protonated double bond" or a "protonated *cyclo*propane ring":

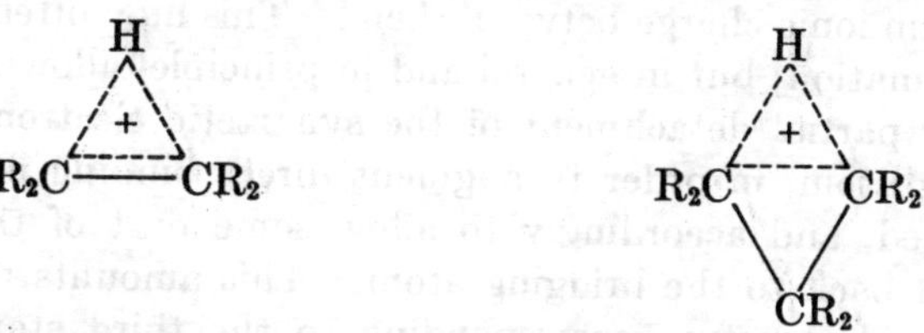

The vinylium ("protonated triple bond"), allylium, and *cyclo*propenylium ions are mass-spectrometrically well known, and the last two are to some extent known in more usual chemical situations. These ions are probably to be formulated thus:

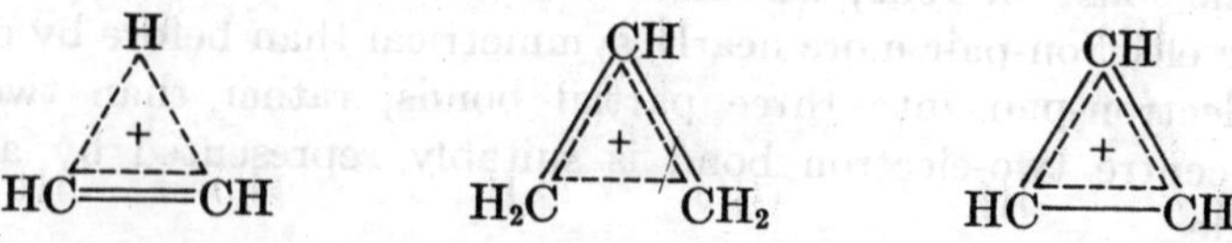

The experimental study[144] in which these ideas were first developed concerned the skeletal interconversions which accompany nucleophilic substitutions of *cyclo*propylmethyl, *cyclo*butyl, and homoallyl compounds. Roberts and Mazur showed that in most hydrolyses and acetolyses of the chlorides, most conversions of the alcohols to halides by means of phosphorus or hydrogen halides, and most nitrous deaminations of the amines, some degree of skeletal interconversion occurs. Bergstrom and Siegel showed[146] that the ethanolysis of *cyclo*propylmethyl benzenesulphonate, even in the presence of ethoxide ion, is kinetically of first order, and is a fast reaction, about ten times faster than the corresponding reaction of allyl benzenesulphonate. Caserio, Graham, and Roberts subsequently showed[147] that the aqueous ethanolysis of *cyclo*propylmethyl chloride and of *cyclo*butyl chloride give with comparable rapidity an identical mixture of six products, namely, *cyclo*propylmethyl, *cyclo*butyl, and homoallyl alcohols, and the three corresponding ethyl ethers. The general thermodynamic tendency seems to be from *cyclo*propylmethyl towards homoallyl isomers,

though the equilibrium constants are fairly moderate, for instance, 36 for *cyclo*propylmethyl and *cyclo*butyl chlorides at 25° (catalysis by

[146] C. G. Bergstrom and S. Siegel, *J. Am. Chem. Soc.*, 1952, **74**, 145.
[147] M. C. Caserio, W. H. Graham, and J. D. Roberts, *Tetrahedron*, 1960, **11**, 171.

zinc chloride). In general, the left-hand equilibrium seems to be attained more rapidly than the right-hand; thus *cyclo*propylmethanol is preparatively converted by dilute hydrochloric acid to *cyclo*butanol, and by concentrated hydrochloric acid and zinc chloride (Lucas's reagent) to homoallyl chloride. Of course, many products are not thermodynamically determined, inasmuch as an unstable intermediate may be trapped by the solvent faster than it can isomerise to a more stable intermediate.

Because of the strong bending of the bonds of the *cyclo*propane ring, they must have considerable π character, and even the bonds of the *cyclo*butane ring will have some π character. So our usually satisfactory division of bonds into σ and π types is somewhat indistinct in this system. The slightly greater accelerating effect of the *cyclo*propyl group than of the vinyl group on S_N1 reactions at an adjoining carbon atom shows, however, that conjugating ability is not wholly a matter of π content. Hart and his coworkers showed that such accelerating effects of simultaneously present *cyclo*propyl groups are cumulative;[148] on successively replacing the *iso*propyl residues in tris(*iso*propyl)carbinyl nitrobenzene-*p*-sulphonate by *cyclo*propyl residues, the relative rates of solvolysis in "80%" aqueous dioxan were increased as follows:

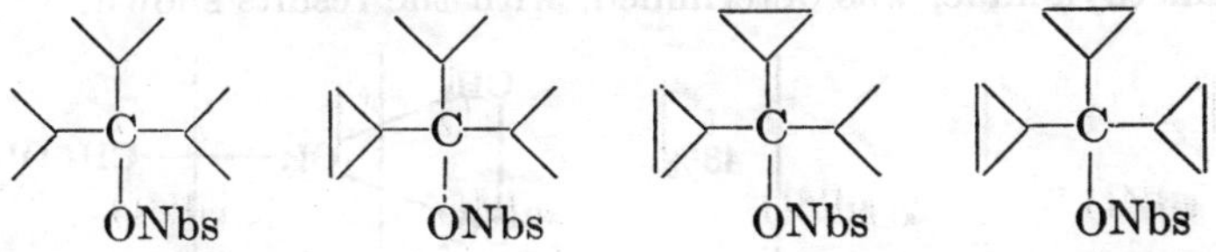

ONbs	ONbs	ONbs	ONbs
1	246	23,500	~30,000,000

In the work described by Roberts and his collaborators in 1959, a *cyclo*propylmethyl factor, having ^{14}C in the side-chain, was converted by nucleophilic substitutions into products, the distribution of the ^{14}C in which was determined by their degradation.[145] Two types of case were examined: the first is illustrated by the conversion of *cyclo*propylmethanol by Lucas's reagent into equilibrium products, the strongly preponderating component of which is homoallyl chloride. In this product the label distribution was observed to be as follows:

[148] H. Hart and J. M. Sandri, *J. Am. Chem. Soc.*, 1959, **81**, 320; H. Hart and P. A. Law, *ibid.*, 1962, **84**, 2462. The physical extent of the bond bending to which *cyclo*propane conjugation ($+K$) is credited, is well illustrated by an X-ray difference map of electron density of *cis*-1,2,3-tricyano-*cyclo*propane: prominent maxima appear 0.32*A* outside the midpoints of the sides of the triangle of internuclear lines defined by the ring atoms (A. Hartman and F. L. Hirshfeld, *Acta Cryst.*, 1966, **20**, 80).

$$\underset{\underset{100\%}{\uparrow}}{\overset{CH_2}{\underset{CH_2}{|}}\!\!>\!CH\cdot \overset{*}{C}H_2\cdot OH} \xrightarrow[ZnCl_2]{HCl} Cl-\underset{\underset{66.5\%}{\uparrow}}{\underbrace{CH_2\cdot CH_2}}-\underset{\underset{0.1\%}{\uparrow}}{CH}=\underset{\underset{33.4\%}{\uparrow}}{CH_2}$$

The inferred equal division of the label between the three methylene groups points *either* to one intermediate with a three-fold axis of symmetry (C_3) and perhaps with three planes of symmetry in addition (C_{3v}), *or* to three equivalent, cyclicly interconvertible intermediates, individually of lower symmetry (C_1 or perhaps C_s).

To go further, one must examine non-equilibrium products, derived by the trapping of a first-formed intermediate before it has had time to reach full equilibrium with other intermediates, if any. There is much evidence that the carbonium ion formed by loss of nitrogen from a diazonium ion in aqueous deamination is very rapidly trapped by the water (Section **45b**). The continued study was therefore of the aqueous deamination of *cyclo*propylmethylamine. Three alcohols were formed in the proportions given below, which are obviously far from equilibrium proportions. And in the two main products, the distribution of a ^{14}C label, originally in the side-chain of the *cyclo*propylmethylamine, was determined, with the results shown:

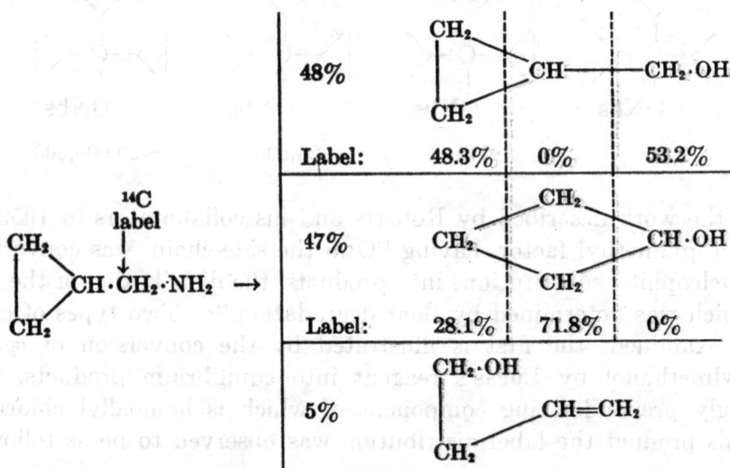

It is apparent that the highest concentration of the label is where it was originally put, that is, in the *cyclo*propyl side-chain. The only other positions having a label content above the equilibrium value are the 2- and 4-positions of *cyclo*butanol. The ring methylene groups of *cyclo*propylmethanol and the 3-methylene group of *cyclo*butanol have label contents below their equilibrium values. One sees here a picture of a succession of isomerisation processes of the carbonium ion, all with rates comparable with the rate of trapping of the ion by the solvent water; and of a wave or surge of reaction travelling along the successive processes. At the moment of trapping, the label content in the *cyclo*propyl side-chain has fallen from 100% a long way towards its equilibrium 33%, by transfer, presumably first, to the 2- and 4-methylene groups of *cyclo*butanol, where the content of label has risen from 0% to above the equilibrium value at the moment of trapping. This must mean that the succeeding label transfers have rates which are comparable with, and are not much larger than, the rate of these first label transfers, which therefore produce a temporary pile-up of label in the first transfer locations. In the products of the succeeding transfers the contents of label are still on the way up from 0% to these equilibrium values at the moment of trapping. Evidently one has to contemplate a series of intermediate carbonium ions, and not a single all-purpose intermediate ion.

An original *cyclo*propylmethylium ion[149] could be the starting point of three successive pairs of equivalent Wagner-Meerwein bond-shifts. In the projection in which they are represented below, one looks towards the tertiary carbon atom from a point on the backward extension of its CH bond line. It will be convenient to give letter-labels to the carbon atoms, as shown in the first formula. The interconversions are, of course, all reversible; but, for diagrammatic simplicity, the curved arrows marking bond changes, and also the reaction arrows, are given only those directions which correspond to the direction, left to right, of the nett reaction prior to equilibrium, *i.e.*, of the first surge. One sees that the radioactive label goes first, by simultaneous paths, into the 2- and 4-positions in the *cyclo*butylium ion; then, in parallel paths, into the ring-methylene positions in the *cyclo*propylmethylium ion; and finally, by converging paths, into the 3-position of the *cyclo*butylium ion. This makes good sense in relation to the observed radio-label distributions:[150]

[149] Its symmetry, C_s, as assumed, is that proved for its stable tertiary homologue, the *cyclo*propyldimethylcarbinylium ion, $(CH_2)_2CH \cdot CMe_2^+$, by the proton magnetic resonance spectrum of the latter in Olah's $FSO_3H/SbF_5/SO_2$ solvent (C. U. Pitman jr. and G. A. Olah, *J. Am. Chem. Soc.*, 1965, **87**, 5123). In this ion, the carbonium centre is, of course, stable in its tertiary location. The plane of symmetry bisects the ring and contains the side-chain carbon atoms. It contains even the methyl carbon atoms, because that conformation of the side-chain maximises its conjugation with the bent bonds of the ring.

[150] One can understand why, at the moment of trapping, the last-labelled 3-methylene group of the *cyclo*butylium ion has come up nearer to its equilibrium label content than have the earlier-labelled ring methylene groups of the *cyclo*propylmethylium ion, on the basis that the simultaneous first surges of reaction meet in the *cyclo*butylium ion on the extreme right of the diagram. It is possible to compute the observational figures quite closely from rate equations.

To each of the reaction arrows in this isomerisation scheme there corresponds a synartetic ion. These ions are written separately below. They are individually asymmetric (symmetry C_1), but, as formulated, they constitute three mirror-image pairs, the pairs being related by $(2\pi/3)$-rotations. Thus, *if* all these ions were always in equilibrium, their chemical behaviour would be indistinguishable from that of a single ion with a three-fold axis and three planes of symmetry (C_{3v}).[151]

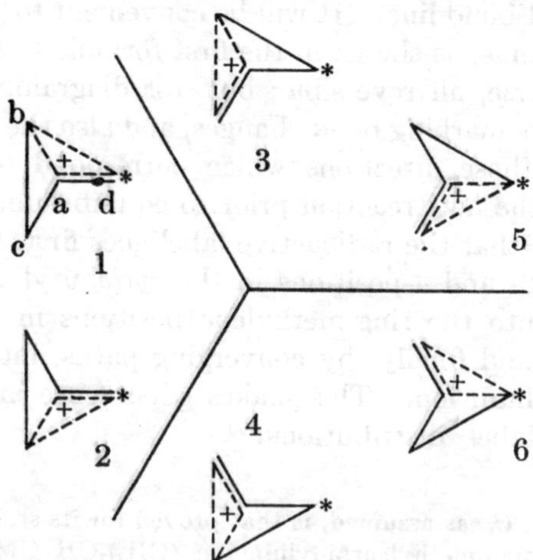

Two of the synartetic ions have their more-than-single bond in the position *ad*, two have it in the position *ac*, and two in the position *ab*.

[151] Roberts and his collaborators discuss the possible role of a C_{3v} ion, and conclude that it might be a "way point" in the interconversion of the C_1 ions, but could not itself be a genuine intermediate. Furthermore, they have introduced a methyl substituent into the side-chain of the *cyclo*propylmethylamine to give a chiral centre in optically active form, and have shown that this undergoes complete or almost complete racemisation in the formed homologue of *cyclo*propylcarbinol, so confirming that a single non-isomerising C_1 ion would be an insufficient intermediate (M. Vogel and J. D. Roberts, *J. Am. Chem. Soc.*, 1966, **88**, 2262).

If, in each case, the delocalised electron-pair were localised to form a double bond in the indicated position, homoallylium ions would be formed with various permutations of their carbon atoms. In assuming this, Roberts assumes the type of conversion later realised in reverse by Le Ny, Lawton, and Bartlett. The need for this assumption was doubtless a motive which led Roberts to his revised formulation of the synartetic carbonium ion.

The homoallylium ions are reached by branch paths at the points marked by spurs on the reaction-arrows of the cyclic isomerisation scheme written above. The synartetic ions, which could have been inserted at these points, are numbered to correspond. As can be seen from their structures, the homoallylium ions first formed, through synartetic ions 1 and 2, will have the radioactive label in position-4; those next formed, through synartetic ions 3 and 4, will have it in position-2; and those last formed, through synartetic ions 5 and 6, will have it in position-1. There will be no label in position-3. And so, in the general left-to-right reaction surge that precedes equilibrium, the radio-label should enter homoallylic products in the order 4, 2, 1. The label distribution in the 5% of formed homoallyl alcohol has not yet been determined.

(46) ELECTROPHILIC REARRANGEMENTS IN SATURATED SYSTEMS

It is obvious that one has to expect a class of heterolytic rearrangements which are in all respects the polar opposite of those reviewed in Section **45**: the loss of an anion or something equivalent to leave a carbonium ion or other electron-deficient centre, will be replaced in the expected class of rearrangement by the loss of a proton or other cation to leave a carbanion or other centre possessing an active unshared pair of electrons; and the migrating group, instead of shifting as a nucleophile with its full octet, will shift as an electrophile with a sextet, leaving the electrons of its old bond behind, and forming a new bond by co-ordination with the active unshared pair; while the electrons left behind may take up a proton. If this type of rearrangement, like the other, does not depend on multiple-bond unsaturation, we can term it *saturated electrophilic rearrangement*. The involved electronic changes would be as represented,

$$\begin{matrix} & & R & & \\ N & \curvearrowleft & A \text{---} & B & \text{---} M \end{matrix}$$

where M and N symbolise cationic species in general, though they would often be protons. Rearrangements of this nature are known, although they have not yet been studied as extensively as have saturated nucleophilic rearrangements.

(46a) The Stevens Rearrangement.—In this change, A is an 'onium atom, while B is carbon. Some examples will be given. The original example[152] is typical of those with which Stevens and his coworkers have carried out most of their subsequent investigations of the process: phenacylbenzyldimethylammonium hydroxide in water goes over smoothly into ω-dimethylamino-ω-benzylacetophenone, with a shift of the benzyl group from ammonium nitrogen to phenacyl carbon. Anticipating a discussion of the mechanism, we write the process on the assumption that a carbanion, actually the mesomeric anion of a keto-enol system (Chapter XI), is intermediately formed:

$$\underset{+}{Me_2N}(CH_2Ph)—CH(COPh)—H \xrightarrow{\bar{O}H} \underset{+}{Me_2N}(CH_2Ph)—\bar{C}H(COPh) \rightarrow Me_2\ddot{N}—CH(CH_2Ph)(CO\cdot Ph)$$

Within the field of carbonyl-ammonium compounds, the reaction has been considerably generalised. The group into which migration occurs, the phenacyl group in the above example, has been replaced by acetonyl. The migrating group, benzyl in the above case, has been replaced by allyl, 1-phenylethyl, benzhydryl, 9-fluorenyl, 3-phenylpropargyl, and phenacyl. The group from which the migration takes place, dimethylammonium in the original example, has been replaced by piperidinium. Moreover the analogous reaction of a carbonyl-sulphonium compound has been demonstrated:[153]

$$\underset{+}{MeS}(CH_2Ph)—CH(CO\cdot Ph)—H \xrightarrow{OH^-} \underset{+}{MeS}(CH_2Ph)—\bar{C}H(CO\cdot Ph) \rightarrow Me\ddot{S}—CH(CH_2Ph)(CO\cdot Ph)$$

It has been found that although the ketonic system present in all the above examples undoubtedly facilitates the reaction, it is not an essential factor: a group can migrate into a simple hydrocarbon residue, provided that the latter has sufficient stability in anionic form. Thus when benzhydryl-trimethylammonium bromide is treated with

[152] T. S. Stevens, E. M. Creighton, A. B. Gordon, and M. MacNicol, *J. Chem. Soc.*, **1928**, 3193; T. S. Stevens, *ibid.*, **1930**, 2107; T. S. Stevens, W. W. Sneddon, E. T. Stiller, and T. Thompson, *ibid.*, p. 2119; T. Thompson and T. S. Stevens, *ibid.*, **1932**, 55, 1932; J. L. Dunn and T. S. Stevens, *ibid.*, p. 1926; *ibid.*, **1934**, 279.

[153] T. Thompson and T. S. Stevens, *J. Chem. Soc.*, **1932**, 69.

lithium-phenyl, rearrangement occurs with migration of methyl into the benzhydryl group as follows:[154]

$$\mathrm{Me_2\overset{+}{N}(Me)\!-\!CPh(Ph)\!-\!H \xrightarrow{LiPh} Me_2\ddot{N}\!-\!C(Me)Ph(Ph)}$$

In this type of change, as conducted in aprotic solvents, there is probably no intermediate dipole. The stereochemical evidence indicates, as we shall see, synchronisation of the proton loss with the alkyl transfer from nitrogen to carbon.

The fact that, in all the more facile reactions, the migrating group shifts from an 'onium atom, that is, a centre predisposed to lose a cation, to a keto-enolic carbon atom, that is, a carbon centre notable for its ability to support a negative charge and react in anionic form (Chapter XI), provides a strong indication for the mechanism written.

A dependence of the process on hydroxide ions in aqueous solution, or on alkoxide ions in alcoholic solution, has been observed in all cases. In the phenacylbenzyldimethylammonium example, Thompson and Stevens found that the rate increased with the alkali concentration, tending, with excess of alkali, to a limit.[155] This indicates that, in the presence of a sufficient excess of alkali, the anionic centre is completely formed; and it supports the assumption of reaction in two stages, at least for this class of example.

Stevens established the intramolecular character of the migration by showing[156] that, when two rearrangements,

$$\mathrm{Me_2\overset{+}{N}G^1\cdot CH_2\cdot CO\cdot G^2 \rightarrow Me_2N\cdot CHG^1\cdot CO\cdot G^2}$$

$$\mathrm{Me_2\overset{+}{N}G^3\cdot CH_2\cdot CO\cdot G^4 \rightarrow Me_2N\cdot CHG^3\cdot CO\cdot G^4}$$

which separately took place at comparable rates, were carried out together in the same solution, only the above-written pure-bred products were formed, not the crossed products, $\mathrm{Me_2N\cdot CHG^3\cdot CO\cdot G^2}$ and $\mathrm{Me_2N\cdot CHG^1\cdot CO\cdot G^4}$. The groups G were as follows:

G^1 = *m*-bromobenzyl G^3 = benzyl

G^2 = phenyl G^4 = *p*-bromophenyl

[154] T. Thompson and T. S. Stevens, *J. Chem. Soc.*, 1932, 1932; E. D. Hughes and C. K. Ingold, *ibid.*, 1933, 71; G. Wittig, R. Mangold, and G. Felletschin, *Ann.*, 1948, 580, 116.

[155] T. Thompson and T. S. Stevens, *J. Chem. Soc.*, 1932, 55.

[156] T. S. Stevens, *J. Chem. Soc.*, 1930, 2107.

Much later, Johnson and Stevens repeated this test by the more sensitive method of employing a radioactive indicator. In one of the factors, a benzyl group had ^{14}C in its side-chain. The groups were now as follows:

G^1 = ^{14}C-benzyl G^3 = benzyl
G^2 = *p*-bromophenyl G^4 = phenyl

The rates of rearrangement of these substances, when they were rearranged individually, were $G^1G^2:G^3G^4 = 0.8:1.0$. When they were rearranged together, no radioactivity at all could be found in the G^3G^4 product.[157]

The effect of substitution in the migrating benzyl group of the phenacylbenzyldimethylammonium ion on the rate of rearrangement has been examined,[156,155] and the result is fairly clear-cut: electron-attracting substituents in this group accelerate its migration. The following order of rate holds for both meta- and para-substituents:

$$\mathrm{OMe} < \mathrm{H},\ \mathrm{Me} < \mathrm{Cl},\ \mathrm{Br},\ \mathrm{I} < \mathrm{NO_2}$$

This result led Stevens to suggest that the benzyl group migrates with its full octet, while a pair of electrons goes completely across from anionic carbon to nitrogen in compensation. Bennett and Chapman pointed out,[158] however, that the observed polar effect is equally consistent with the theory that the group migrates with a sextet only, since it may be supposed that the group has to commence forming its new bond before having freed itself from the electrons of the old one. The situation is the inverse, as it should be, of that obtaining in saturated nucleophilic rearrangements, where there is much evidence to show that the group goes over with its full octet, and that electron-releasing substituents facilitate its transfer.

The effect of substituents in the phenacyl group on rate of rearrangement has also been studied.[159] This effect is weaker; but now electron-attracting substituents retard the migrations. For para-substituents in the phenacyl ring the following rate sequence holds:

$$\mathrm{Me} > \mathrm{H} > \mathrm{OMe},\ \mathrm{Cl},\ \mathrm{Br},\ \mathrm{I} > \mathrm{NO_2}$$

Now the effect of these substituents on the formation of the anionic centre, and on its reactivity when formed, must be qualitatively opposite; and one must be observing the resultant of the two effects. If we assume, as the existence of a limit to alkali acceleration suggests, that the anionic centre is, in all the phenacyl examples, formed fairly

[157] R. A. W. Johnson and T. S. Stevens, *J. Chem. Soc.*, 1955, 4887.

[158] G. M. Bennett and A. W. Chapman, *Ann. Repts. on Progress Chem.* (Chem. Soc. London), 1930, **27**, 123. Cf. ref. 165.

[159] J. L. Dunn and T. S. Stevens, *J. Chem. Soc.*, 1932, 1926.

freely, so that the dominating polar effect should be that on its reactivity, then the above sequence can be understood.

As to the stereochemistry of the Stevens rearrangement in carbonyl compounds, it is known that the migrating group passes over with retention of configuration.[160] Campbell, Houston, and Kenyon found that, on using optically active phenacyl-(1-phenylethyl)dimethylammonium hydroxide, the 1-phenylethyl group was transferred without any racemisation at all. Subsequently Brewster and Kline degraded the product to an optically active γ-phenylbutyric acid of known configuration, thereby showing that the configuration of the 1-phenylethyl group had been preserved in the Stevens rearrangement.

As to the more difficult rearrangements in the absence of a carbonyl group, Hill and Chan were able to show that optical activity centred on ammonium nitrogen in allylbenzylmethylphenylammonium ion is retained in the Stevens rearrangement, in the product of which it must be centred on carbon.[161] This clearly indicates a single-step process:

$$\mathrm{Ph(Me)(PhCH_2)\overset{+}{N}{-}CH(H)(CH{=}CH_2)} \xrightarrow[\text{in } \mathrm{Me_2SO}]{\mathrm{KOBu}^t} \mathrm{Ph(Me)N{-}CH(CH_2Ph)(CH{=}CH_2)}$$

(46b) The Wittig Rearrangement.[162]—In this process atom A of the general scheme is neutral oxygen, while B is carbon: ethers, on metallation or by similar means, are isomerised to alcohols, with a migration of one alkyl group into the α-position of the other. Only a group, such as benzyl or allyl, which has enough stability as an anion to be fairly easily metallated, can act as the receiving end of this migration process, in the conditions hitherto used. Some examples are formulated below:

$$\mathrm{PhCH_2{\cdot}O{\cdot}CH_3 \rightarrow Ph{\cdot}CH(OH)CH_3} \qquad \text{(Ref. 163)}$$

$$\mathrm{(C_6H_4{-}C_6H_4)CH{\cdot}O{\cdot}CH_3 \rightarrow (C_6H_4{-}C_6H_4)C(OH)CH_3} \qquad \text{(Ref. 164)}$$

[160] A. Campbell, A. H. J. Houston, and J. Kenyon, *J. Chem. Soc.* **1947**, 93; J. H. Brewster and M. W. Kline, *J. Am. Chem. Soc.*, 1953, **75**, 5179.

[161] R. K. Hill and T.-K. Chan, *J. Am. Chem. Soc.*, 1966, **88**, 866.

[162] G. Wittig, *Experientia*, 1958, **14**, 389.

$$\begin{array}{l} CH_2{:}CH{\cdot}CH_2 \\ \qquad\diagdown \\ \qquad\quad O \rightarrow \\ \qquad\diagup \\ CH_2{:}CH{\cdot}CH_2 \end{array} \qquad \begin{array}{l} CH_2{:}CH{\cdot}CH{\cdot}OH \\ \qquad\qquad\quad | \\ \qquad\qquad\quad | \\ \qquad\qquad\quad | \\ CH_2{:}CH{\cdot}CH_2 \end{array} \qquad \text{(Ref. 165)}$$

Wittig's method of effecting the changes consisted in treating the ethers with lithium-phenyl. The first effect is to substitute a lithium atom for hydrogen in the α-position of the benzyl, or other reactive alkyl group. Rearrangement takes place in the metal derivative. Wittig assumes that this contains, or can easily give, a carbanion, to the negative centre of which the other alkyl group moves over as an electrophile, carrying with it only a sextet of its 2-quantum electrons:

$$\underset{\substack{|\\ Ph}}{\overset{\substack{CH_3\\ |}}{O{-}CH_2}} \xrightarrow{LiPh} \underset{\substack{|\\ Ph}}{\overset{\substack{CH_3\\ |}}{O{-}CH{-}Li}} \rightarrow \underset{\substack{|\\ Ph}}{\overset{\substack{CH_3\\ |}}{O{-}\bar{C}H}} \rightarrow \underset{\substack{|\\ Ph}}{\overset{\substack{CH_3\\ |}}{\bar{O}{-}CH}} \rightarrow \underset{\substack{|\\ Ph}}{\overset{\substack{CH_3\\ |}}{HO{-}CH}}$$

Hauser and Kantor brought about the same changes by treating the ethers with potassium amide in liquid ammonia, and then raising the temperature after the addition of ethyl ether. They are in agreement with Wittig's view of the mechanism, which certainly seems consistent with the structural and environmental conditions in which the reaction has been realised.

There is some qualitative evidence on the relative rates of migration of different alkyl groups. Among the 9-fluorényl ethers, Wittig and his collaborators observed the rate order, allyl, benzyl > methyl, ethyl > phenyl.[166] Hauser and Kantor, in the course of their investigation,[165] obtained the order *s*-butyl > *neo*pentyl. Wittig and Schlor established the order methyl > *t*-butyl.[167] The result that *neo*pentyl and *t*-butyl groups have relatively low rates of migration, within the range of simple saturated alkyl groups, indicates that the bond changes at the migration group are concerted, just as in the Stevens rearrangement.

[163] G. Wittig and L. Löhman, *Ann.*, 1942, **550**, 260.

[164] G. Wittig and W. Happe, *Ann.*, 1947, **557**, 205.

[165] C. R. Hauser and S. W. Kantor, *J. Am. Chem. Soc.*, 1951, **73**, 1437.

[166] G. Wittig and R. Clausnizer, *Ann.*, 1954, **588**, 145; G. Wittig and E. Stahnecker, *ibid.*, 1957, **605**, 69.

[167] G. Wittig and H. Schlor, *Suomen Kemistilehti*, 1958, **31**, 2.

CHAPTER XI

Unsaturated Rearrangements

(47) CATIONOTROPY

(47a) Growth of the Concept of Tautomerism.—In 1863 Geuther discovered ethyl acetoacetate;[1] and in the succeeding years a discussion arose between Geuther, on the one hand, and Edward Frankland and Duppa, on the other, concerning its constitution.[2] This question still remained open in 1877, when Johannes Wislicenus[3] established the separate steps in the processes of metal uptake and alkylation undergone by ethyl acetoacetate. A search for similar properties in other substances led in 1880 to their discovery by Conrad and Bischoff in ethyl malonate:[4] in later years such properties were found in many other alkylatable ketones and esters, each presenting its own form of the common constitutional ambiguity. The constitutional problem was generalised in another way when in 1887 Michael discovered[5] that O- as well as C-derivatives of ethyl acetoacetate could be produced through the same metal compound. It followed, and many analogies supported the idea, that such reactions did not locate the metal; and that, even if one could definitely ascertain the structure of the parent substance, those of its metal derivatives would remain ambiguous.

Contemporaneously with this development in the investigation of ketones and esters, observations over a wider field were disclosing other situations of a generally similar nature. In 1877 Butlerow[6] studied the isomerisation of the di*iso*butylenes, interpreting the double-bond shift by an assumed addition and elimination of water. He was clear that the ready occurrence of such reversible isomeric change would confer on a substance the power to undergo chemical reactions in accordance sometimes with one and sometimes with the other structure, depending on the reagent and conditions:

[1] A. Geuther, *Göttinger Anzeigen*, **1863**, 281; *Arch. Pharm.*, 1863, **106**, 97; *Jahresber.*, **1863**, 323.

[2] E. Frankland and B. F. Duppa, *Ann.*, 1865, **135**, 217; 1866, **138**, 204, 328; A. Geuther, *Z. Chem.*, **1868**, 58.

[3] J. Wislicenus, *Ann.*, 1877, **186**, **161**; **190**, 287.

[4] M. Conrad and C. A. Bischoff, *Ann.*, 1880, **204**, 121.

[5] A. Michael, *J. prakt. Chem.*, 1887, **37**, 473.

[6] A. Butlerow, *Ann.*, 1877, **189**, 44.

$$(CH_3)_3C{-}CH{=}C\begin{matrix}CH_3\\ \\ CH_3\end{matrix} \rightleftharpoons \left[(CH_3)_3C{-}CH_2{-}\overset{OH}{\underset{}{C}}\begin{matrix}CH_3\\ \\ CH_3\end{matrix}\right] \rightleftharpoons (CH_3)_3C{-}CH_2{-}C\begin{matrix}{=}CH_2\\ \\ CH_3\end{matrix}$$

In 1882 Baeyer and Oekonomides found[7] that the single substance isatin gave both O- and N-derivatives. Baeyer offered an interpretation of such observations in his principle of *pseudomerism*. This was that a substance might appear from its reactions to have more than one structure; that this was due to a facile interconversion of the structures; and that the reason why only one parent substance could be isolated was that one parent structure was more stable than the others. Baeyer somewhat arbitrarily assigned the imidol structure to isatin.

In 1874 Griess prepared[8] *p*-bromodiazoaminobenzene in two ways that would have been expected to give isomers. In 1884 Heinrich Goldschmidt found[9] that *p*-nitrosophenol, which had previously been prepared by Baeyer and Caro by the action of nitrous acid on phenol, could also be obtained by the action of hydroxylamine on *p*-benzoquinone.

In 1885–86 Conrad Laar[10] published his stimulating discussions of these phenomena. He noted that the known ambiguities of structure were of certain standard types referable to a small number of formal *systems*, and involving always an uncertainty in the position of one hydrogen atom and at least one double bond, as between the structures HX·Y:Z and X:Y·ZH, defining what he called a *triad* system. Laar's interpretation was that two such structures did not represent distinct and potentially separable species, but only the end-phases of an intramolecular oscillatory situation in a single chemical species. He called the phenomenon *tautomerism*, the name which has been most continuously used ever since, though without necessarily implying an acceptance of Laar's interpretation.

To most of Laar's contemporaries it was clear that he had not disposed of the alternative theory of Butlerow and Baeyer, namely, that one structure represented one substance, but that a facile isomeric change in either direction might allow either isomer to be synthesised by way of the other, or to undergo a reaction involving prior conversion to the other. And about a decade later this interpretation received very strong support through the isolation of separate, though

[7] A. v. Baeyer and S. Oekonomides, *Ber.*, 1882, **15**, 2093; A. v. Baeyer, *Ber*., 1883, **16**, 2188.

[8] P. Griess, *Ber.*, 1874, **7**, 1618.

[9] H. Goldschmidt, *Ber.*, 1884, **17**, 213.

[10] C. Laar, *Ber.*, 1885, **18**, 648; 1886, **19**, 730.

easily interconvertible, isomeric forms in a number of examples, including β-diketones, β-ketonic esters, β-aldo-esters, and a paraffinic nitro-compound.

In 1896 Claisen found that acetyldibenzoylmethane and tribenzoylmethane could each be isolated in two solid forms.[11] One form was a moderately *acid* substance, which gave a coloured ferric complex, a cupric complex, and a water-soluble sodium salt, instantly. The other was the sort of substance which Hantzsch classified as a *pseudo-acid:* it did not give salts instantly, but it yielded them after a time, which could be understood as the time required by the pseudo-acid to undergo conversion to its truly acid isomeride. The same distinction with respect to time applied to the reverse changes: from the salts, the acidic parent could be liberated instantly, and this substance required time in order to undergo further conversion to the pseudo-acid. Although it was not clear to Claisen, it was made clear in the contemporaneous investigations of Wilhelm Wisliscenus, and of Knorr, mentioned below, that such conversions in the fused or dissolved state show their reversibility by proceeding to an equilibrium, unless carried to completion by the crystallisation of one form; and also that such equilibria in solution depend on the solvent, and are generally more favourable to the pseudo-acid in more polar solvents. Claisen correctly regarded the pseudo-acidic substance as having the ketonic structure, and its acidic isomeride as having an enolic structure:

$Ph\cdot CO\cdot CH(CO\cdot Ph)_2$	$Ph\cdot C(OH):C(CO\cdot Ph)_2$
Pseudo-acid	Acid

Here then, it could be claimed, was a *keto-enol* tautomeric system reduced to its components: and the components were mutually convertible, but otherwise ordinary isolable substances having distinct structures, namely, the ketone and the enol.

In the same year, Wilhelm Wisliscenus began his investigation of the isomerism of methyl and of ethyl formylphenylacetate, each of which he obtained in a liquid and a solid modification.[12] Both forms were acidic, the solid the more so; yet only the less acidic liquid form gave a coloured iron complex. Originally Wisliscenus thought of the liquid as having the aldo-, and the solid a hydroxymethylene structure, though it was difficult thus to understand the formation of the iron complex from the liquid only. But further investigation[13] by him-

[11] L. Claisen, *Ann.*, 1896, **291**, 25.

[12] W. Wisliscenus, *Ann.*, 1896, **291**, 147; 1900, **312**, 34; *Ber.*, 1899, **32**, 2837.

[13] W. Wisliscenus, *Ann.*, 1912, **389**, 265; 1916, **413**, 206; 1920, **421**, 119; K. H. Meyer, *Ber.*, 1912, **45**, 2843; W. Dieckmann, *Ber.*, 1916, **49**, 2213; 1917, **50**, 1375.

self, by Kurt Meyer, and by Dieckmann in 1912–20 has shown that the liquid is actually a mixture of the aldo-form and one of the stereoisomeric hydroxymethylene forms. This is, without doubt, the internally hydrogen-bonded *cis*-isomeride, which would be the less acidic, but would be able to form a chelated iron complex (Section **7e**). The strongly acidic solid, which gave a ferric salt but not a co-ordinated iron compound, is, of course, the *trans*-hydroxymethylene isomeride:

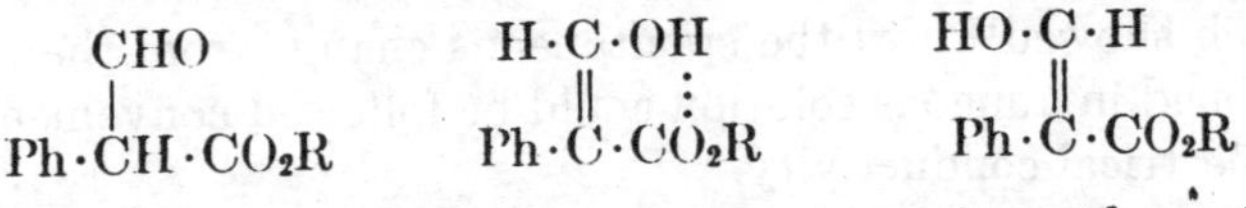

$$\begin{array}{c}CHO\\ |\\ Ph\cdot CH\cdot CO_2R\end{array}\qquad \begin{array}{c}H\cdot C\cdot OH\\ \| \quad \vdots\\ Ph\cdot C\cdot CO_2R\end{array}\qquad \begin{array}{c}HO\cdot C\cdot H\\ \|\\ Ph\cdot C\cdot CO_2R\end{array}$$

All these details were not correctly appreciated from the outset; but Wisliscenus was clear, even in 1896, as to the general tendency of such isomers towards reversible interconversion in solution.

In this year also, Knorr commenced his investigation of the isomerism of ethyl dibenzoylsuccinate and ethyl diacetylsuccinate, each of which he obtained in several forms, the latter in no less than five forms.[14] Two were recognised as the expected stereoisomeric diketones, two as the stereoisomeric mono-enols, and the remaining one as one of the three possible stereoisomeric di-enols, as was confirmed much later by Knorr and Kaufmann:[15]

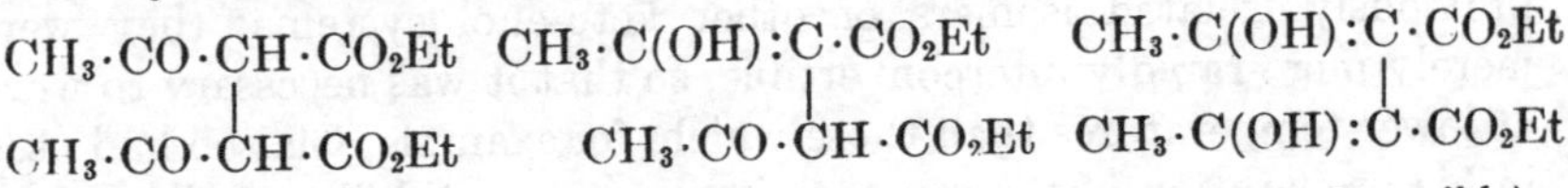

$$\begin{array}{c}CH_3\cdot CO\cdot CH\cdot CO_2Et\\ |\\ CH_3\cdot CO\cdot CH\cdot CO_2Et\\ \textit{meso- and rac.-}\end{array}\quad \begin{array}{c}CH_3\cdot C(OH){:}C\cdot CO_2Et\\ |\\ CH_3\cdot CO\cdot CH\cdot CO_2Et\\ \textit{cis- and trans-}\end{array}\quad \begin{array}{c}CH_3\cdot C(OH){:}C\cdot CO_2Et\\ |\\ CH_3\cdot C(OH){:}C\cdot CO_2Et\\ \text{(1 known, 3 possible)}\end{array}$$

In the course of his earlier work Knorr established that, when any of these forms was put into a solvent, a general interconversion of isomers took place, with the production of an equilibrium mixture. This again was subsequently confirmed by Kaufmann,[16] who was able to follow the conversion by analytical methods, and also quantitatively to determine the composition of the equilibrium mixture.

From the commencement of their work, both Wilhelm Wisliscenus and Knorr had some extremely shrewd ideas about the mechanism of isomerisation, believing the mobile hydrogen atom to shift as its ion, as we shall note in more detail later.

Still in 1896, Hantzsch and Schultz isolated a second form of phenylnitromethane.[17] In place of the well-known yellow oil, slowly soluble in aqueous alkali, they recovered, by careful acidification of an alkaline solution, a colourless, crystalline, more water-soluble, acid substance,

[14] L. Knorr, *Ann.*, 1896, **293**, 70; 1899, **306**, 322.
[15] L. Knorr and H. P. Kaufmann, *Ber.*, 1922, **55**, 232.
[16] H. P. Kaufmann, *Ber.*, 1922, 55, 2255; *Ann.*, 1922, **429**, 247.
[17] A. Hantzsch and O. W. Schultze, *Ber.*, 1896, **29**, 699, 2251.

which required time to revert to the yellow oil, though eventually this change became substantially complete. Here, the oily form was the pseudo-acid, while the crystalline isomeride, which Hantzsch called the *aci*-form, was an acid in the ordinary sense:

$$\underset{\text{Pseudo-acid}}{Ph\cdot CH_2\cdot NO_2} \qquad \underset{\text{Acid}}{Ph\cdot CH{:}NO\cdot OH}$$

Hantzsch showed[18] how the spontaneous change from the acid to the pseudo-acid in aqueous solution could be followed conveniently by the fall in electrical conductivity.

Strange as it seems in retrospect, Laar's hypothesis of intramolecular oscillation continued to be considered, and even elaborated, for more than a decade following these important experimental demonstrations. However, this line of speculation was seen to be unfruitful, and was abandoned somewhat before 1911, when Knorr, Rothe, and Averbeck[19] succeeded in separating the longest-known tautomeric substance, ethyl acetoacetate, into its ketonic and enolic components. Such a separation, in a substance universally accepted as a typical example of tautomerism, should have been impossible on Laar's theory of that phenomenon. The isomers were entirely analogous to the previously isolated isomers of other keto-enol systems: they were merely more rapidly interconvertible, so that it was necessary to work at lower temperatures than those which, for example, Claisen had used in his preparation of the separate isomers of acetyldibenzoylmethane. The keto-form of ethyl acetoacetate was crystallised from light petroleum at $-80°$; and the enol was obtained by treating the sodio-derivative, in suspension in light petroleum at $-80°$, with a deficit of hydrogen chloride, and pumping off the solvent from the filtered solution. It was shown that equilibria between the two forms are established in the liquid ester, and in solutions of the ester; and that the approach to equilibrium follows the kinetic law of first-order reversible interconversions, and is highly sensitive to catalysis by bases and acids.

Subsequently, Kurt Meyer and his coworkers[20] prepared the pure keto-ester and the pure enol by the more convenient method of distilling ethyl acetoacetate under reduced pressure with care to exclude catalysts. Quartz vessels were used in order to avoid the surface alkali on glass. The enol proved to be the more volatile isomer.

[18] A. Hantzsch, *Ber.*, 1899, **32**, 575, 3066; A. Hantzsch and A. Voit, *ibid.*, p. 607.

[19] L. Knorr, O. Rothe, and H. Averbeck, *Ber.*, 1911, **44**, 1138.

[20] K. H. Meyer and V. Schoeller, *Ber.*, 1920, **53**, 1410; K. H. Meyer and H. Hopff, *Ber.*, 1921, **54**, 579.

Since 1911 there has been no question but that the concept of tautomerism, in terms of which Conrad Laar had incorporated so many scattered observations into a phenomenon, has to be redefined, in the Butlerow-Baeyer way, as meaning *reversible isomeric change*. Problems of isolation and proof of identity of tautomers are dependent simply on temperature and the available techniques.

Kurt Meyer's discovery[21] in 1911 of a simple volumetric method of determining the enol content of keto-enol mixtures, added detail to the picture of equilibria between molecules of sharply distinguished structural types. The method was based on the observation that enols, but not keto-forms, rapidly react with bromine to give bromo-ketones. Any excess of bromine having been destroyed by an addition of 2-naphthol, the bromo-ketone was reduced by adding iodide, and the liberated halogen was titrated with thiosulphate:

$$\begin{matrix}-\mathrm{C}\cdot\mathrm{OH} \\ \| \\ -\mathrm{CH}\end{matrix} \xrightarrow[\mathrm{Br_2}]{} \begin{matrix}-\mathrm{C}{=}\mathrm{O} \\ | \\ -\mathrm{CHBr}\end{matrix} \xrightarrow[\mathrm{2HI}]{} \begin{matrix}-\mathrm{C}{=}\mathrm{O} \\ | \\ -\mathrm{CH_2}\end{matrix} + \mathrm{I_2}$$

Table 47-1 contains some equilibrium percentages of enol, as determined by Meyer in liquid keto-enols at ordinary temperature. Further data of a similar kind are given in Section **47d**.

TABLE 47-1.—ENOL CONTENTS OF LIQUID KETO-ENOLS (K. H. MEYER).

	% *Enol*		% *Enol*
Methyl acetoacetate	4.8	Ethyl acetonedicarboxylate	16.8
Ethyl acetoacetate	7.5	Acetylacetone	80.4
Methyl benzoylacetate	16.7	Benzoylacetone	98.0
Ethyl benzoylacetate	29.2		

Meyer also studied the enol contents of keto-enols in equilibrium in solution. Theoretically the more polar solvent should favour the more polar tautomer, because in this way solvation energy can be maximised. Meyer found that more polar solvents favoured the keto-forms of β-diketones and β-ketonic esters: some of his measurements on solutions of ethyl acetoacetate are given in Table 47-2. We must therefore conclude that Meyer's enols were less polar than the keto-forms. As far as is known, such enols are more volatile than the keto-forms. Both effects support the suggested relationship, which is generally understood (Section **2f**) as a consequence of the great loss of polarity which these enols suffer as a result of internal hydrogen bond-

[21] K. H. Meyer, *Ann.*, 1911, **380**, 212; K. H. Meyer and P. Koppelmeier, *Ber.*, 1911, **44**, 2718; K. H. Meyer, *Ber.*, 1912, **45**, 2843; 1914, **47**, 826.

TABLE 47-2.—ENOL CONTENT OF ETHYL ACETOACETATE IN VARIOUS SOLVENTS AT 18° (K. H. MEYER).

	% Enol		% Enol
Water	0.40	Acetone	7.3
25% Methyl alcohol	0.83	Chloroform	8.2
50% Methyl alcohol	1.52	Nitrobenzene	10.1
50% Ethyl alcohol	2.18	Ethyl acetate	12.9
Methyl alcohol	6.87	Benzene	16.2
Ethyl alcohol	10.52	Ether	27.1
Propyl alcohol	12.45	Carbon disulphide	32.4
Amyl alcohol	15.33	Hexane	46.4

ing.[22] However, as Wassermann has pointed out,[23] those keto-enols whose enolic forms cannot easily undergo internal hydrogen bonding are likely to exhibit the opposite solvent effect. His example was diketen ("dimeric keten"), which in non-hydroxylic solvents appears to be substantially ketonic, though it behaves as an enol in aqueous media:

$$\begin{array}{c} CH_2{:}C{-}CH_2 \\ \;\;|\quad\;\;| \\ \;\;O{-}C{:}O \end{array} \rightleftarrows \begin{array}{c} CH_2{:}C{-}CH \\ \;\;|\quad\;\;\| \\ \;\;O{-}C{\cdot}OH \end{array}$$

Some years before Meyer developed his technique for estimating equilibrium concentrations of enols, Lapworth had shown how bromination could be used to measure the rate of production of an enol from a carbonyl compound, which in equilibrium contained very little enol. His basic discovery, made in 1904, was that the rate of bromi-

[22] Meyer found that the equilibrium ratio, enol/ketone, for a number of keto-enols, in a number of solvents, could be approximated as the product of two factors, one depending only on the keto-enol, and the other only on the solvent. An equivalent statement is that the free-energy of isomerisation of any keto-enol in any solvent approximates to the sum of an isomerisation free-energy for the keto-enol in a standard solvent, and the solvation free-energy-difference between ketone and enol for the solvent with respect to a standard keto-enol. This was an early example of the now much-discussed additive-free-energy relation. It works in the case considered, because the solvation energy-differences must be nearly independent of those parts of the molecules that do not change in the reaction, solvation forces being highly localised on solute molecules. The experimental relation is consistent with the van't-Hoff-Dimroth law, which may be put in the form,

$$K_{\text{solution}} = K_{\text{gas}} \cdot r_{\text{Henry}}$$

where the K's are equilibrium constants for isomerisation in a solvent and as gas, and r is the ratio of solubilities (that is, of Henry's-law constants) of the gaseous isomers in the solvent.

[23] A. Wassermann, *J. Chem. Soc.*, **1948**, 1323.

nation of acetone in acidic aqueous solution is proportional to the concentration of acetone, and to that of hydrogen ions, but is independent of the concentration of bromine.[24] Lapworth's interpretation was that the measured process is the acid-catalysed enolisation of the acetone:

$$CH_3\cdot CO\cdot CH_3 \xrightarrow[\text{slow}]{H^+} CH_3\cdot C(OH):CH_2 \xrightarrow[\text{fast}]{Br_2} CH_3\cdot CO\cdot CH_2Br$$

In 1912 Kurt Meyer demonstrated a similar lack of dependence on the concentration of the halogen for the acid-catalysed aqueous bromination of malonic acid.[25] In 1926 Dawson examined the aqueous iodination of acetone, as catalysed by various acids and bases: for each catalyst the rate was independent of the concentration of halogen.[26] Bell and Longuet-Higgins have made similar observations for the hydroxide-ion-catalysed chlorination and bromination of acetone.[26] All these investigations have confirmed the essential correctness of Lapworth's interpretation: the only modification of it that would now be made is that, in basic catalysis, enolisation itself is a composite process, rate-controlled by ionisation, which is equally rate-controlling for halogenation:

$$CH_3\cdot CO\cdot CH_3 \xrightarrow[\text{slow}]{} CH_3\cdot C(\bar{O}):CH_2 \xrightarrow[\text{fast}]{} CH_3\cdot CO\cdot CH_2Br$$

In acid catalysis, however, and above some threshhold of acidity, the fast reaction may be a halogenation of the molecular enol. We may infer this from more recent work by R. P. Bell and his collaborators.[27]

They have shown, mainly in the examples of the chlorination or bromination of ethyl malonate and of acetone, that by reducing the concentration of the halogen to $10^{-4}M$ and less, the rate of its attack on anion or enol can be reduced to below the rate of the formation of anion or enol, so that the attack by the halogen becomes rate-controlling, and the overall rate becomes proportional to halogen concentration. In the example of the halogenation of ethyl malonate, they could then show, by following the rate in these conditions as a function of pH, that, in near-neutral and dilute acid solutions down to

[24] A. Lapworth, *J. Chem. Soc.*, 1904. **85**, 30.

[25] K. H. Meyer, *Ber.*, 1912, **45**, 2864.

[26] H. M. Dawson and J. S. Carter, *J. Chem. Soc.*, **1926**, 2282; H. M. Dawson and N. C. Dean, *ibid.*, p. 2872; H. M. Dawson and C. R. Hoskins, *ibid.*, p. 3166; R. P. Bell and H. C. Longuet-Higgins, *ibid.*, **1946**, 636; R. P. Bell and P. Jones, *ibid.*, **1953**, 88.

[27] R. P. Bell and M. Spiro, *J. Chem. Soc.*, **1953**, 429; R. P. Bell and K. Yates, *ibid.*, **1962**, 1927, 2285; R. P. Bell and G. G. Davis, *ibid.*, **1964**, 902.

pH 3, the entity attacked by the halogen is the anion, but that at higher acidities the halogenation proceeds mainly by attack on the molecular enol.

(47b) Analogy with Addition: Ring-Chain Tautomerism.—The decision that each tautomer has a separate existence, and that tautomerism is a form of chemical reaction, led in course of time to the proposal of analogies for tautomeric change among other chemical reactions. One such proposal, made by Hilda Ingold,[28] linked tautomeric changes with reversible additive reactions. This correlation was useful as a guide to the study, during the early 1920's, of what came to be called *ring-chain* tautomerism.

As an example of the argument, the general pattern of the aldol reaction may be considered: an addendum H—C, to which some "activating" group X, which might be a carbonyl group, must be bound, becomes added, H to O and C to C, to an unsaturated acceptor C=O:

$$\text{H—}\overset{|}{\underset{|}{\text{C}}}\text{X} + \overset{|}{\underset{|}{\text{C}}}\text{=O} \rightleftarrows \text{X}\overset{|}{\underset{|}{\text{C}}}\text{—}\overset{|}{\underset{|}{\text{C}}}\text{—O—H}$$

The equation is set up in reversible form, because Hilda Ingold formally established the general reversibility of aldol reactions. It was noted that the most condensed intramolecular form of this reaction that one could imagine is keto-enol change, the HC part of the keto-structure being "activated" as an addendum by the adjacent C=O part, which also acts as the acceptor:

$$\text{H—}\overset{|}{\underset{|}{\text{C}}}\text{—}\overset{|}{\text{C}}\text{=O} \rightleftarrows \overset{|}{\underset{|}{\text{C}}}\text{=}\overset{|}{\text{C}}\text{—O—H}$$

It was inferred by an interpolation, that less condensed forms of the same fundamental process would be capable of occurrence; and that they would involve reversible interchange between open-chain and cyclic isomers, a *keto-cyclol* tautomerism in the case illustrated:

$$\underbrace{\text{H—}\overset{|}{\text{C}}\text{X}\quad\overset{|}{\text{C}}\text{=O}}_{(\text{CR}_2)_n} \rightleftarrows \underbrace{\overset{|}{\text{C}}\text{X——}\overset{|}{\text{C}}\text{—O—H}}_{(\text{CR}_2)_n}$$

Thorpe and his coworkers studied a group of examples of this type.[29] The ketones were α-ketoglutaric acids having various open-chain or

[28] E. H. Ingold (*née* Usherwood), *Chem. & Ind.*, 1923, 1246; *J. Chem. Soc.*, 1923, **123**, 1717.

[29] S. S. Deshapande and J. F. Thorpe, *J. Chem. Soc.*, 1922, **121**, 1430; L. Bains and J. F. Thorpe, *ibid.*, 1923, **123**, 1206; J. W. Baker *ibid.*, 1925, **127**, 1678.

cyclic hydrocarbon substituents in the β-positions; and the cyclic isomerides were *cyclo*propanol acids:

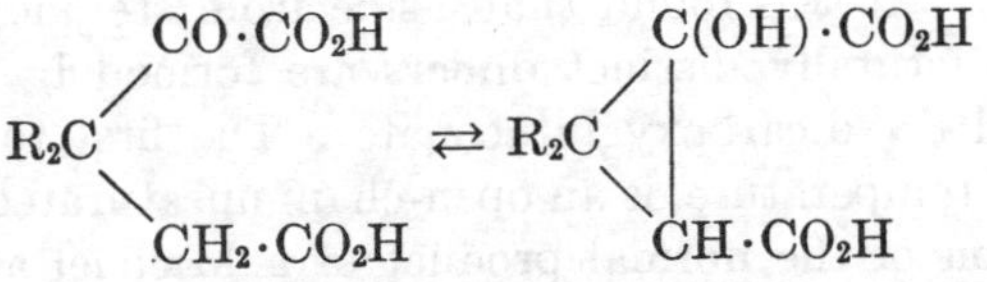

$$R_2C\begin{cases} CO\cdot CO_2H \\ CH_2\cdot CO_2H \end{cases} \rightleftarrows R_2C\begin{cases} C(OH)\cdot CO_2H \\ | \\ CH\cdot CO_2H \end{cases}$$

The systems were not very mobile, and alkali was added in order to effect interconversion at convenient speeds: thus the equilibria, set up in aqueous solution, were between the anions of the acids.

Michael's addition reaction is a starting point for the consideration of another such group of analogous processes: an addendum H-C, bearing an activating group X, adds to an acceptor C=C, which bears an activating group Y of similar type, H adding to the Y-end and C to the other end of the ethylenic bond:

$$H-\overset{|}{\underset{|}{C}}X + \overset{|}{\underset{|}{C}}=CY \rightleftarrows \overset{|}{\underset{|}{C}}X-\overset{|}{\underset{|}{C}}-\overset{|}{C}Y-H$$

The general reversibility of this reaction was established by Vorländer.[30] The most condensed intramolecular form of this reaction would involve the shifting of a hydrogen atom between the ends of a propene system flanked by activating groups:

$$H-\overset{|}{C}X-\overset{|}{C}=\overset{|}{C}Y \rightleftarrows \overset{|}{C}X=\overset{|}{C}-\overset{|}{C}Y-H$$

This is the so-called "three-carbon" triad system, which Thorpe extensively investigated in the example of the glutaconic acids and their esters, wherein the activating groups X and Y are carboxyl groups: he showed that, in dissymmetrically substituted glutaconic acids and esters, a hydrogen atom does shift very easily from end to end of the propene system. The corresponding *three-carbon ring-chain* system would be of the following general type:

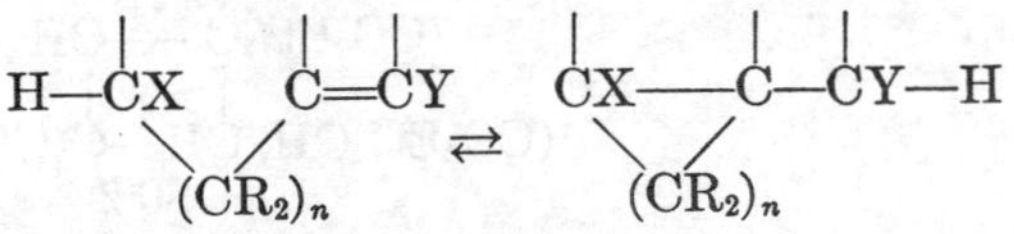

$$\begin{matrix} H-\overset{|}{C}X & & \overset{|}{C}=\overset{|}{C}Y \\ & \diagdown\;\diagup & \\ & (CR_2)_n & \end{matrix} \rightleftarrows \begin{matrix} \overset{|}{C}X & -\!-\!- & \overset{|}{C}-\overset{|}{C}Y-H \\ & \diagdown\;\diagup & \\ & (CR_2)_n & \end{matrix}$$

Thorpe[31] and his coworkers encountered an example of this type of tautomerism while investigating the steps in a process of dimerisation, which Guthzeit[32] had discovered in carboxyglutaconic esters, and

[30] D. Vorländer, *Ber.*, 1900, 33, 3185; C. K. Ingold and W. J. Powell, *J. Chem. Soc.*, 1921, **119**, **1976**; C. K. Ingold and E. A. Perren, *ibid.*, 1922, **121**, 1414.

[31] C. K. Ingold, E. A. Perren, and J. F. Thorpe, *J. Chem. Soc.*, 1922, **121**, 1765.

[32] M. Guthzeit, *Ber.*, 1898, **31**, 2753; *Ber.*, 1901, **34**, 675; M. Guthzeit, A. Weiss, and W. Schäffer, *J. prakt. Chem.*, 1909, **80**, 393.

Verkade[33] in cyanoglutaconic esters, and which, significantly, was catalysed by bases. It was found that, aside from stereoisomeric differences, two structurally distinct dimers are formed by the action of bases on ethyl $\alpha\alpha'$-dicarboxyglutaconate. The first to be formed, a liquid at room temperature, is an open-chain unsaturated ester, having the constitution of the normal product of a Michael addition of the α-CH group of one molecule of the glutaconic ester to the $C_\beta{:}C_\gamma$-double bond of another:

$$\begin{array}{ccc} (CO_2Et)_2CH\cdot \underbrace{CH{=}C}(CO_2Et)_2 & & (CO_2Et)_2CH\cdot CH\cdot CH(CO_2Et)_2 \\ + & \rightarrow & | \\ (CO_2Et)_2C{:}CH\cdot \overbrace{CH}(CO_2Et)_2 & & (CO_2Et)_2C{:}CH\cdot C(CO_2Et)_2 \end{array}$$

This was proved by hydrolysis, thermal decarboxylation, and subsequent oxidation, to methanetriacetic acid and oxalic acid. This liquid dimer underwent a fairly rapid, base-catalysed isomerisation to a solid dimer. The latter was saturated: and its constitution, as a *cyclo*-butane derivative, was established through that of its decarboxylated hydrolysis-product, the saturated tetracarboxylic acid, which was obtained in the five possible stereoisomeric forms, having, along with their various anhydrides, the genetic relations required by the assigned structure. If, during the isomerisation of the liquid dimeric ester, the solid isomer was allowed to crystallise, then conversion became complete. But in the absence of any such disturbance, a definite equilibrium was set up in the liquid phase, which ultimately contained the unsaturated and saturated isomers in the approximate proportions indicated below:

$$\begin{array}{c} (CO_2Et)_2CH \quad CH{=}C(CO_2Et)_2 \\ | \qquad\quad | \\ (CO_2Et)_2CH\cdot CH{-}C(CO_2Et)_2 \\ 20\% \end{array} \rightleftarrows \begin{array}{c} (CO_2Et)_2C{-}CH\cdot CH(CO_2Et)_2 \\ | \qquad\quad | \\ (CO_2Et)_2CH\cdot CH{-}C(CO_2Et)_2 \\ 80\% \end{array}$$

Special importance attaches to the ring-chain system allied to the reversible addition of water or alcohols to carbonyl compounds, as in semi-acetal formation:

$$H{-}OR + \overset{|}{\underset{|}{C}}{=}O \rightleftarrows RO{-}\overset{|}{\underset{|}{C}}{-}O{-}H$$

[33] P. E. Verkade, *Proc. Koninkl. Nederland. Akad. Wetenschap.*, 1919, **27**, 1133.

The analogous triad system is that of the presumed tautomerism of the carboxyl group:

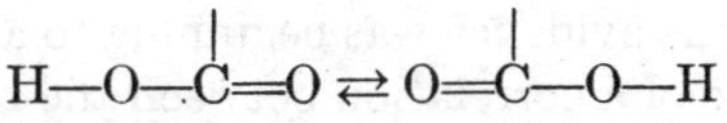

$$\mathrm{H{-}O{-}\overset{|}{C}{=}O \rightleftarrows O{=}\overset{|}{C}{-}O{-}H}$$

The ring-chain analogue is the *keto-lactol* system, which may be formulated as follows:

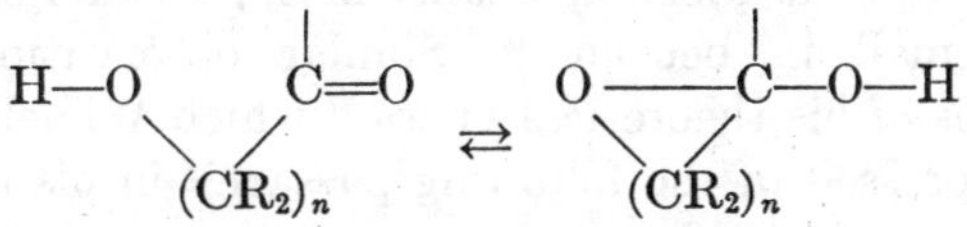

$$\begin{matrix} \mathrm{H{-}O} & & \mathrm{\overset{|}{C}{=}O} & \rightleftarrows & \mathrm{O} & \text{———} & \mathrm{\overset{|}{C}{-}O{-}H} \\ & \diagdown & \diagup & & & \diagdown \; \diagup & \\ & \mathrm{(CR_2)_n} & & & & \mathrm{(CR_2)_n} & \end{matrix}$$

Jacobson and Stelzner were the first to anticipate tautomerism of this type, essentially on the basis of the argument given; and they appreciated its importance for the chemistry of the sugars.[34] The fact that the reducing sugars have the typical properties of aldehydes and ketones, while their isomerism, and their relation to the glycosides, show them to be lactols, could be attributed to the occurrence of reversible changes of the type just formulated; while the conclusion that the two stereoisomeric lactol forms of a sugar, which should not be interconvertible directly, could come into equilibrium through their open-chain isomeride, would obviously explain the mutarotation displayed by freshly prepared solutions of practically all reducing sugars.

These ideas were advanced in 1913, but they received little attention until the case for them was restated in 1924. In the meantime, two suggestions of 1903 continued to be quoted, which could easily be shown to be inconsistent with the data. On the other hand, a survey[35] of carbohydrate compounds, including their nitrogen and sulphur derivatives, those which do, and those which do not, display mutarotation, showed that the constitutional conditions actually required were just what were needed in Jacobson and Stelzner's theory, namely, the system,

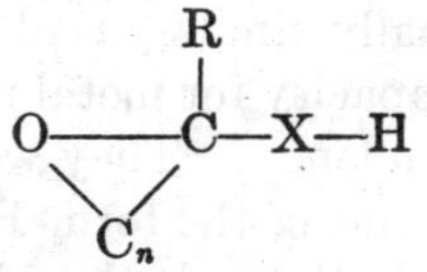

$$\begin{matrix} & & \mathrm{R} & \\ & & | & \\ \mathrm{O} & \text{———} & \mathrm{C{-}X{-}H} & \\ & \diagdown \; \diagup & & \\ & \mathrm{C_n} & & \end{matrix}$$

with an electronegative, but otherwise unrestricted, X and a wholly unrestricted R.

[34] P. Jacobson and R. Stelzner, in V. Meyer and P. Jacobson's "Lehrbuch der Organischen Chemie," Veit, Leipzig, 2nd Edn. 1913, I, 2, 886, 910, 915, 927.

[35] J. W. Baker, C. K. Ingold, and J. F. Thorpe, *J. Chem. Soc.*, 1924, 125, 268; R. Gilmour, *ibid.*, p. 705.

(47c) Development of the Concept of Prototropy.—The origin of the idea that the mobile hydrogen atom moves as its cation goes back to 1896. At that time evidence was beginning to accumulate which indicated the existence of a correlation between the rate of attainment of a tautomeric equilibrium and the dissociating power of the medium. Claisen found that the lability of the forms of acetyldibenzoylmethane was greatest in aqueous alcohol, smaller in dry alcohol or acetone, and undetectably small in benzene.[36] Similar observations by Knorr formed the basis of his theoretical views,[37] which Wilhelm Wisliscenus shared, and expressed in the following passage[38] in his review on tautomerism published in 1898:

> It is impossible to survey these phenomena without coming to the view that the interconversion of forms is connected with dissociation. One may assume that in these substances there is always some dissociation, setting free the mobile hydrogen atom, as cation, let us say forthwith, if only from a small number of molecules. In the anion the bond changes will take place all the more easily because they are no longer encumbered with the transport of the hydrogen atom.

Wisliscenus assumed that the slowness of tautomeric change arose from the circumstance that only a few molecules were dissociated at any one time.

The acceptance of these ideas outside the group of investigators in which they originated came slowly: their development came more slowly: indeed, there was scarcely any further development for a quarter of a century. The reason for this is fairly clear: if a hydrogen atom dissociates as a positive ion, to return to a different position, then the negative charge, which it left behind in the old position, must also move to the new one; and we cannot see in detail how that happens, until the electronic theory of valency teaches us that a bond shift *is* a shifting of an electric charge.

In 1922 Piggott and the writer commenced an investigation intended to relate mobility in formally similar triad systems to structure, and thence to alkylatability, capacity for metal uptake, and other chemical evidences of an ionising tendency. They worked with "symmetrical" triad systems, that is, systems of the form R·XH·Y:X·R′, since high mobility then showed itself through the identity of substances synthesised as written and with R and R′ interchanged, as well as through the double set of reactions of the individual produced by either route.

[36] L. Claisen, *Ann.*, 1896, **291**, 80, 86.

[37] L. Knorr, *Ann.*, 1896, **293**, 38.

[38] W. Wisliscenus, "Uber Tautomerie," Ahrens Sammlung, Stuttgart, 1898, **2**, 187.

The first comparison[39] was between the four formal systems, which can be constructed with either N or C for X and for Y, and with R and R′ as aryl groups:

$$\begin{array}{ll} Ar\cdot NH\cdot N{:}N\cdot Ar' & Ar\cdot CH_2\cdot N{:}CH\cdot Ar' \\ Ar\cdot NH\cdot CR{:}NAr' & Ar\cdot CH_2\cdot CR{:}CH\cdot Ar' \end{array}$$

Two of these systems had been examined much earlier.

Griess[40] was the original discoverer of tautomerism in the diazo-amino-system:

$$ArNH\cdot N{:}N\cdot Ar' \rightleftarrows Ar\cdot N{:}N\cdot NH\cdot Ar'$$

In 1874 he prepared *p*-bromodiazoaminobenzene, first, from the benzenediazonium ion and *p*-bromoaniline, and secondly, from the *p*-bromobenzenediazonium ion and aniline: the products were identical:

$$\left.\begin{array}{l} C_6H_5\cdot N_2^+ + C_6H_4Br\cdot NH_2 \rightarrow C_6H_5\cdot N{:}N\cdot NH\cdot C_6H_4Br \\ C_6H_4Br\cdot N_2^+ + C_6H_5\cdot NH_2 \rightarrow C_6H_4Br\cdot N{:}N\cdot NH\cdot C_6H_5 \end{array}\right\}\text{identical}$$

He did the same using a *p*-methyl in place of a *p*-bromo-substituent. Subsequently, Noelting and Binder[41] split the methyl compound, single as isolated, by the usual process of reduction to amine and hydrazine; and they obtained a mixture of two amines and two hydrazines:

$$C_6H_5\cdot NH_2,\quad C_6H_4Me\cdot NH_2,\quad C_6H_5\cdot NH\cdot NH_2,\quad C_6H_4Me\cdot NH\cdot NH_2$$

Finally, Meldola and Streatfield[42] studied the ethylation of a number of diazoamino-compounds by means of sodium ethoxide and ethyl iodide, thereby blocking any tautomeric system. From each unsymmetrically substituted diazoaminobenzene, Ar·NH·N:N·Ar′, a single individual as isolated, they obtained mixtures of two ethyl derivatives,

$$Ar\cdot NEt\cdot N{:}N\cdot Ar' \quad \text{and} \quad Ar\cdot N{:}N\cdot NEt\cdot Ar'$$

These could be separated, and identified each by synthesis from the appropriate diazonium ion and N-ethyl-arylamine.

The tautomerism of the amidine system was demonstrated by similar methods in 1895–99 through the researches of von Pechmann,[43]

[39] C. K. Ingold and H. A. Piggott, *J. Chem. Soc.*, 1922, **121**, 2381.

[40] P. Griess, *Ber.*, 1874, **7**, 1618; *Ann.*, 1886, **137**, 60.

[41] E. Noelting and F. Binder, *Ber.*, 1887, **20**, 3004.

[42] R. Meldola and F. W. Streatfield, *J. Chem. Soc.*, 1887, **51**, 102, 434; 1888, **53**, 664; 1889, **55**, 4122; 1890, **57**, 785; C. Smith and C. H. Watts, *ibid.*, 1910, **97**, 562.

[43] H. v. Pechmann, *Ber.*, 1895, **28**, 869, 2362; 1897, **30**, 1779.

Marckwald,[44] and Wheeler and Johnson:[45]

$$\mathrm{Ar\cdot NH\cdot CR{:}N\cdot Ar' \rightleftarrows Ar\cdot N{:}CR\cdot NH\cdot Ar'}$$

The identity of the N-phenyl-N′-*p*-tolyl-benzamidine, as prepared from N-phenyl-benzimidochloride and *p*-toluidine, and from N-*p*-tolyl-benzimidochloride and aniline, was established by von Pechmann:

$$\left.\begin{array}{l} \mathrm{C_6H_5\cdot N{:}CPh\cdot Cl + C_6H_4Me\cdot NH_2} \\ \qquad \rightarrow \mathrm{C_6H_5\cdot N{:}CPh\cdot NH\cdot C_6H_4Me} \\ \mathrm{C_6H_4Me\cdot N{:}CPh\cdot Cl + C_6H_5\cdot NH_2} \\ \qquad \rightarrow \mathrm{C_6H_4Me\cdot N{:}CPh\cdot NH\cdot C_6H_5} \end{array}\right\}\text{identical}$$

Marckwald split this compound by hydrolysis, and obtained two amines and two amides:

$$\mathrm{C_6H_5\cdot NH_2,\quad C_6H_4Me\cdot NH_2,\quad C_6H_5\cdot NH\cdot COPh,\quad C_6H_4Me\cdot NH\cdot COPh}$$

And von Pechmann blocked the tautomeric system by ethylation, obtaining separable ethyl derivatives,

$$\mathrm{C_6H_5\cdot N{:}CPh\cdot NEt\cdot C_6H_4Me} \quad \text{and} \quad \mathrm{C_6H_4Me\cdot N{:}CPh\cdot NEt\cdot C_6H_5}$$

whose structures he determined by synthesis from the appropriate imidochlorides and N-ethyl-arylamines. Wheeler and Johnson established essentially the same points in other cases, notably with formamidines, which they synthesised using imido-ethers and amines with permuted radicals, such as phenyl and *p*-tolyl:

$$\left.\begin{array}{l} \mathrm{C_6H_5\cdot N{:}CH\cdot OEt + C_6H_4Me\cdot NH_2} \\ \qquad \rightarrow \mathrm{C_6H_5\cdot N{:}CH\cdot NH\cdot C_6H_4Me} \\ \mathrm{C_6H_4Me\cdot N{:}CH\cdot OEt + C_6H_5\cdot NH_2} \\ \qquad \rightarrow \mathrm{C_6H_4Me\cdot N{:}CH\cdot NH\cdot C_6H_5} \end{array}\right\}\text{identical}$$

In contrast to the mobility of the diazoamino-system and of the amidine system, that of the terminally diarylated methyleneazomethine system was found to be extremely small.[39] By condensation between benzylamines and benzaldehydes with permuted substituents, isomers of the forms

$$\mathrm{Ar\cdot CH_2\cdot N{:}CH\cdot Ar'} \quad \text{and} \quad \mathrm{Ar'\cdot CH_2\cdot N{:}CH\cdot Ar}$$

could be separately prepared; and although, as was subsequently shown,[46] they can be interconverted, a strongly basic catalyst, such as

[44] W. Marckwald, *Ann.*, 1895, **286**, 343.

[45] L. H. Wheeler and T. B. Johnson, *Ber.*, 1899, **32**, 35; R. M. Roberts, *J. Am. Chem. Soc.*, 1950, **72**, 3603.

[46] C. K. Ingold and C. W. Shoppee, *J. Chem. Soc.*, **1929**, 1199.

ethoxide ions, is needed for the purpose; and then the reaction is slow. The terminally arylated three-carbon system was in just the same case:[39] by condensation between β-arylpropionates and araldehydes, isomers of the forms

$$Ar \cdot CH_2 \cdot CH{:}CH \cdot Ar' \quad \text{and} \quad Ar' \cdot CH_2 \cdot CH{:}CH \cdot Ar$$

could be produced; and they exhibited little tendency to change, although, as was shown later,[47] they can be slowly interconverted through the agency of sodium ethoxide

It was noted that, while diazoamino-compounds and amidines can readily be alkylated, the methyleneazomethine and propene compounds cannot: obviously mobility was correlated with alkylatability, and depended on the electronegativity of the atom from which, in either reaction, the hydrogen was required to separate: separation was easy when that atom was nitrogen, and difficult when it was carbon: the nature of the central atom of the triad system appeared to have little effect.

These conclusions were emphasized by going over from the three-carbon system terminated by two separate aryl groups, to the three-carbon system terminated by a single ortho-arylene group, as in indene.[48] Methoxy-indenes were synthesised by standard methods, proceeding through methoxy-1-hydrindamines, in the two forms written below; and they were found to be identical as isolated:

MeO-indene (CH_2, CH, CH) ⇄ MeO-indene (CH_2, CH, CH)

Fission of this single substance by oxidation gave a mixture of two methoxy-homophthalic acids:

MeO-C_6H_3($CH_2 \cdot CO_2H$)(CO_2H) and MeO-C_6H_3($CH_2 \cdot CO_2H$)(CO_2H)

On blocking the tautomeric system by condensation with piperonal, a mixture of two, separable, piperonylidene derivatives was obtained:

MeO-indene ($C{:}CH \cdot C_6H_3(O_2CH_2)$, CH, CH) and MeO-indene ($C{:}CH \cdot C_6H_3(O_2CH_2)$, CH, CH)

[47] C. K. Ingold and C. W. Shoppee, *J. Chem. Soc.*, **1929,** 447.

[48] C. K. Ingold and H. A. Piggott, *J. Chem. Soc.*, 1923, **123,** 1469.

Owing to the circumstances discussed in Section **13e**, indene belongs to one of the few types of hydrocarbon which easily form metal derivatives; and thus it was a significant item in the evidence which was being built up in favour of an ionisation theory of tautomerism, that the three-carbon system of indene had proved to be highly mobile. Evidently, tautomeric mobility followed alkylatability and ease of metal uptake, independently of other general chemical features, for example, whether the compound ordinarily functions as an acid, like most keto-enols, or as a base, like diazoaminobenzene, or is a hydrocarbon, like indene.

Soon after these observations were made, the ionic theory of mobile-hydrogen tautomerism, or *prototropy* (as Lowry named it, in the growing certainty that it depended on proton transfers), in principle a branch of *cationotropy*, was completed by the assumption of conjugative electron displacements accompanying the proton transfers. The theory was advanced in two forms. The first,[49] that proposed by Shoppee, Thorpe, and the writer, assumed the two-stage mechanism represented below:

$$\begin{matrix} B \; H \\ X\text{—}Y\text{=}Z \end{matrix} \rightleftarrows \begin{matrix} [B\text{—}H]^+ \\ [X\text{—}Y\text{—}Z]^- \end{matrix} \rightleftarrows \begin{matrix} H \; B \\ X\text{=}Y\text{—}Z \end{matrix} \qquad (B\text{–}S_E1')$$

This mechanism is here labelled B–S_E1', which means base-catalysed unimolecular electrophilic substitution with rearrangement. We shall often shorten this description, calling it the *unimolecular* mechanism of prototropic change, although a strict application of our general rule for assigning molecularities (Section **27e**) would make the above mechanism bimolecular. We have taken this kind of liberty before, for example, when we labelled some silver-ion-catalysed substitutions of alkyl halides Ag^+–S_N1, making a separate note of the catalyst, and thereby removing it from the numerically expressed reckoning of molecularity: we did this in order to preserve useful analogies with the uncatalysed reaction S_N1. The reasons for doing a similar thing now derive in part from the usual convenient, if inaccurate, fiction that a hydrogen ion, unlike other ions, is never produced or destroyed, but always transferred, that is, that it has no free life at all, but is always covalently bound to something. Yet one would like to recognise explicitly the analogy between the loss of a hydrogen ion from a rearranging system, in a case such as that formulated above, and the similar loss of a metal or other cation, which is believed to have some, and possibly an extensive, non-bound life. A related special

[49] C. K. Ingold, C. W. Shoppee, and J. F. Thorpe, *J. Chem. Soc.*, **1926**, 1477.

property of hydrogen is that of hydrogen-bonding, which often makes it uncertain how many molecules constitute the catalysing base. Thus the above equation could represent the ordinary aqueous ionisation of a carboxylic acid, in which a proton is lost from one oxygen atom, leaving a mesomeric carboxylate ion, to either oxygen atom of which the proton can be returned. The catalysing base might then be a water molecule; but it will much more frequently be a polymeric group of hydrogen-bonded water molecules, unknown as to number. And so, in order to avoid difficulty here, we prefer to keep the catalysing base out of the reckoning of molecularity. However, the main reason for so doing will only become apparent later: it is that our convention for prototropy preserves analogies with anionotropy (which is a form of nucleophilic substitution with rearrangement), and thus allows prototropy and anionotropy together to be treated as derivatives of ordinary non-rearranging, electrophilic, and nucleophilic substitution, with a useful degree of correspondence in the mechanisms utilised.

As the unimolecular mechanism is written above, the tautomeric system is given a triad form; but pentad and more extended conjugated systems, and also ring-chain systems, were included in the proposed mechanism. It was also envisaged that the original substance might, in some circumstances, undergo preliminary conversion to a modified form, for instance, to its conjugate acid, which then becomes the effective tautomeric substrate, and subsequently suffers deprotonation and rearrangement in successive steps, according to the mechanism as written.

It was pointed out that, in addition to the already noted factors of mobility, which were obviously consistent with mechanism $B\text{-}S_E1'$, certain others could be anticipated, which also seemed to agree with experience. One of these related to the catalysis of prototropy. The mechanism required a basic catalyst. Experience showed that, whenever mobility was sufficiently low to allow catalytic effects to be observed at all, bases were universal catalysts, and basicity was clearly the function that determined catalytic power. Furthermore, when mobility was very low, as with the diarylated methyleneazomethines and propenes, and with some of the ring-chain systems described in the preceding Section, then bases were the only effective catalysts. When mobility was so high that rates were unobservable, one could assume that the solvent, or the substance itself, was basic enough to accept the transferred proton. When acids showed catalytic activity (which occurs when the system contains unshared electrons), one could suppose that the original system, for example, the keto-enol, or the mutarotating sugar, was becoming converted, by a preliminary proton-uptake into its conjugate acid, which was essentially a new prototropic system, but so much more mobile than the old one, that the solvent, or some of the unprotonated original substance, could act as the base required by the mechanism. In more weakly ionising conditions, the original system could form with a covalent acid a hydrogen-bonded adduct of increased mobility.

This view of the mode of action of acid catalysts is a special case of another general consequence of the ionic theory of prototropy, namely that mobility should be increased by induced electronegativity, that is, by the inductive effect $-I$ of substituents: the attraction of electrons away from the seat of dissociation should accelerate isomeric

TABLE 47-3.—EFFECT OF SUBSTITUENTS ON RATE OF INTERCONVERSION OF ARYLATED TRIAD PROTOTROPIC SYSTEMS (SHOPPEE).

System I: $RC_6H_4\cdot CH_2\cdot N:CH\cdot C_6H_5 \underset{k_{-1}}{\overset{k_1}{\rightleftarrows}} RC_6H_4\cdot CH:N\cdot CH_2\cdot C_6H_5$ with $0.145N$ NaOEt in EtOH at 82°

System II: $RC_6H_4\cdot CH_2\cdot C(CO_2Et):CH\cdot C_6H_5 \underset{k_{-1}}{\overset{k_1}{\rightleftarrows}} RC_6H_4\cdot CH:C(CO_2Et)\cdot CH_2\cdot C_6H_5$ with 1.45 N NaOEt in EtOH at 85°.

	$10^5 (k_1+k_{-1})$ with (k_1+k_{-1}) in sec.$^{-1}$						
R............	NMe_2	Me	OMe	I	Br	Cl	NO_2
I, meta-R.....	16.8	30.6	69.6	204	263	296	4080
I, para-R.....	1.47	8.95	15.2	189	197	217	—
II, para-R.....	small	—	1.51	10.8	17.7	28.3	—

change, while electron repulsion towards that centre should retard it. In 1926 when the mechanism was proposed, this conclusion could be seen to agree with many scattered observations; but a more systematic illustration of it was subsequently given by Shoppee,[50] who examined the effect of meta- and para-substituents on the mobility of diarylated methyleneazomethines, and of para-substituents on that of an analogous three-carbon system. His values for the first-order rates of approach to equilibrium are in Table 47-3. Shoppee pointed out that, for each system, the rates form a monotonic series when arranged according to the dipole moments associated with the aromatic substituents.

A different type of example of the effect of induced electronegativity in conferring mobility on a three-carbon system is that furnished by

[50] C. W. Shoppee, *J. Chem. Soc.*, 1930, 968; 1931, 1225; 1932, 696.

flanking the system with ammonium-ion groups. Although salts of the cations

$$Me_3\overset{+}{N}\cdot CH_2\cdot CH{:}CH\cdot \overset{+}{N}Me_2Et \quad \text{and} \quad Me_3\overset{+}{N}\cdot CH{:}CH\cdot CH_2\cdot \overset{+}{N}Me_2Et$$

are separately isolable substances, they come readily into equilibrium in dilute alkaline aqueous or *iso*propyl alcoholic solution at room temperature.[51]

The summary of the position of the ionisation theory of mobile-hydrogen tautomerism, and, in particular, of the position of the unimolecular mechanism, around 1930 is that they agreed with a large body of general circumstances connected with prototropic mobility. The points may be recapitulated in order of the approximate date of their recognition:

(1) Mobility increases with the ionising power of the solvent (1896).
(2) Mobility is correlated with alkylatability and ease of metal uptake (1922).
(3) Mobility is highly dependent on the electronegativity of the atom from which hydrogen is required to separate (1922).
(4) Mobility is universally dependent on basic catalysis as far as can be observed, while some systems are also subject to acid catalysis (1926).
(5) Mobility is increased by electron-attracting substituents (1929).

Two further points were added in a review written about that time.[52] One was that Hilda Ingold's correlation with additive reactions created the presumption that similar mechanisms would apply to the reactions compared; and there was independent evidence that the additive reactions concerned are dependent on hydrogen ionisation. The other point was that some correspondence of mechanism was to be expected with anionotropy, which had recently been recognised as a general process, and was then beginning to yield evidence of having an ionic mechanism.

As mentioned already, the theory of prototropy was advanced in two forms: the second form of it was proposed in 1927 by Lowry.[53] This mechanism works in one stage, and requires, as a condition for the loss of a proton from one end of the system, the simultaneous supply of a proton to the other end:

[51] C. K. Ingold and E. Rothstein, *J. Chem. Soc.*, **1931**, 1666.
[52] C. K. Ingold and C. W. Shoppee, *J. Chem. Soc.*, **1929**, 1199.
[53] T. M. Lowry, *J. Chem. Soc.*, **1927**, 2554.

$$\begin{matrix} B_1 & H & & H{-}B_2^+ \\ & | & & \\ & X{-}Y{=}Z & & \end{matrix} \rightleftarrows \begin{matrix} B_1{-}H^+ & & H & B_2 \\ & & | & \\ & X{=}Y{-}Z & & \end{matrix} \qquad (B\text{–}S_E2')$$

In accordance with the explanation already given, this mechanism is labelled B–S_E2', which means base-catalysed bimolecular electrophilic substitution with rearrangement. For brevity we shall call it the *bimolecular* mechanism. For the forward reaction, base B_1 is denoted by B in the symbol, while acid HB_2^+ counts in the numerically expressed molecularity.

When the unimolecular and bimolecular mechanisms of prototropy were first put forward, it was widely assumed that they were mutually exclusive alternatives; and on several occasions a choice in favour of the unimolecular mechanism was proposed. Baker criticised the bimolecular mechanism on the grounds that polar substituents did not affect the rate of mutarotation of certain derivatives of sugars in the way which it seemed natural to expect on the basis of this mechanism.[54] But the bimolecular mechanism is complicated enough not to be wholly unequivocal in requirements of this nature. Pedersen objected[55] to the bimolecular mechanism on the basis of an analysis of the aqueous conversion rates of certain prototropic systems, namely, the mutarotation of glucose, and the enolisation, as measured by halogenation, of acetone. It was found that the rate of prototropic conversion of the system S in the presence of an acid HB and a base B^- contains terms in [S], in [S][HB], and in [S][B^-], each of which might represent either a unimolecular or a bimolecular prototropic isomerisation, since in aqueous reactions one may always include extra factors [H_2O] in the rate expressions; but that the rate does not contain a term of the expected magnitude[56] in [S][HB][B^-], as it should, if the mechanism in general is bimolecular. However, as Swain has pointed out,[57] this objection was over-pressed, because kinetic ambiguities, for example the impossibility of distinguishing[58] between a term in [S][HB][H_2O] and one in [S][H_3O^+][B^-], make it quite uncertain that the diagnostic term in [S][HB][B^-] should be as important as was supposed. Thus Pedersen's argument does not exclude the bimolecular mechanism of

[54] J. W. Baker, *J. Chem. Soc.*, **1928**, 1583, 1979; **1929**, 1205.

[55] K. J. Pedersen, *J. Phys. Chem.*, 1934, **38**, 581.

[56] The expectation is based on empirical regularities, of the nature of approximately additive free-energy relations, covering the kinetic effects of the various catalysts.

[57] C. G. Swain, *J. Am. Chem. Soc.*, 1950, **72**, 4578.

[58] The mass-law for proton transfer, $HB+H_2O=B^-+H_3O^+$, makes the product [HB][H_2O] proportional to [B^-][H_3O^+].

prototropy. Neither, of course, does Swain's argument exclude the unimolecular mechanism. Bell and Clunie[59] have underlined this point by applying Swain's argument to the hydration of acetaldehyde, a protolytic reversible addition reaction analogous to the ring-chain system of mutarotating glucose (Section **47b**). They examine the data for the rate terms,[60] and show that, with all allowances made for kinetic ambiguities, the bimolecular mechanism inevitably leads one to expect a much larger term in $[S][HB][B^-]$ than could be overlooked: yet no such term is found. It appears that, in this example at least, the bimolecular mechanism does not operate, and that therefore unimolecular mechanisms cannot be excluded from aqueous protolysis in general.

The summary of this piece of chemical history is that every attempt hitherto made to *exclude* either the unimolecular or the bimolecular mechanism of prototropy has failed. As we shall see (Section **47f**), the case has recently been reopened for excluding Lowry's bimolecular mechanism from even the limited range of validity that has been allowed to it. This issue is not yet resolved; but to prove a universal negative is always very difficult.

The acid catalysis of prototropy is conveniently regarded as involving a preliminary conversion of the original substance, by association with the acid catalyst, into a more mobile tautomer, in particular, the ionic conjugate acid, which will be much more acidic, and therefore more easily deprotonated in the effective position, than was the original substance. Probably most ionic conjugate acids are acidic enough to use the unimolecular mechanism of rearrangement, so that the total process can be described as base-catalysed unimolecular electrophilic substitution with rearrangement in the conjugate acid of the original tautomeric substrate, $B\text{–}S_E1'cA$.

(47d) Analogy with Elimination: Equilibrium and Rate.—In 1941 Hughes suggested a second scheme for correlating prototropic changes with other general reactions of which we have systematised knowledge. The original scheme of Hilda Ingold was to regard prototropic changes as internal forms of addition reactions: Hughes's proposal was the complementary one of regarding them as internal forms of elimination reactions. An illustrative comparison would be between

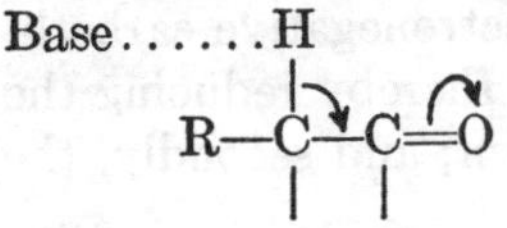

Base.....H Base.....H

R—C—C=O and R—C—C—X ($X = \overset{+}{N}, \overset{+}{S}$, Hal)

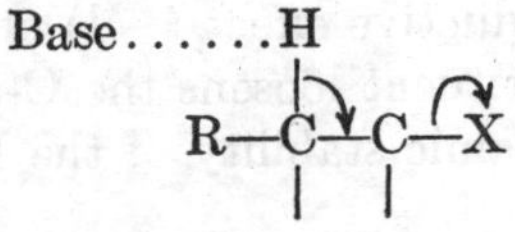

[59] R. P. Bell and J. C. Clunie, *Nature*, 1951, **167**, 363.

[60] R. P. Bell and B. de B. Darwent, *Trans. Faraday Soc.*, 1950, **46**, 34.

the first diagram, representing base-catalysed enolisation, and the second, an olefin elimination by mechanism E2. The formal difference is only that the group CO does not break up, while CX does. Now we saw in Chapter IX that substituents influence elimination by both the inductive and the conjugative modes of electron displacement; and that either may become dominant, and may lead to phenomena typified by Hofmann-type or by Saytzeff-type orientation, as determined by the polarity and unsaturation of the substituents, or, for alkyl substituents, by the polarity of the group X. The point of Hughes's comparison was that we have to expect the same two types of structural effect on prototropic change; and he showed, by examples of structural effects on both prototropic rates and equilibria, that this same concept of electronic dualism does indeed describe the pattern of constitutional influences on prototropy.[61] Let us now consider some thermodynamic and kinetic data from this point of view.

Our knowledge of *equilibria in keto-enol systems* is due mainly to the employment and development of the already-mentioned method of Kurt Meyer for determining enol contents by bromination. The method has been used extensively by Meyer himself, and by Dieckmann, Auwers, Conant, Schwarzenbach, and others. It has undergone a notable technical development in the hands of Schwarzenbach and his associates,[62] who by adapting a flow technique, and an electrometric device, have evolved a procedure permitting the measurement of much smaller concentrations of enol than can be determined with ordinary volumetric apparatus. A number of results, which have been obtained by the investigators mentioned, for the equilibrium percentages of enol at 25° or nearby temperatures, in the gas-phase, in the liquid keto-enol, in dilute solution in hexane, and in water, are assembled in Table 47-4, which is divided into labelled sections for convenience in reference.

Acetone, and other simple ketones, exist in equilibrium almost wholly in their keto-forms. As section A of Table 47-4 illustrates, the introduction of a carbethoxyl substituent increases the equilibrium percentage of enol; and, as the figures of sections A and B show, the acetyl group produces a similar but larger effect. We can regard these major effects on equilibrium as arising from a combination of two causes: first, the inductive effect ($-I$) of the electronegative carbethoxyl or acetyl substituent loosens the C-proton, thereby reducing the relative thermodynamic stability of the keto-form; and secondly, the

[61] E. D. Hughes, *Nature*, 1941, **147**, 812.

[62] G. Schwarzenbach and E. Felder, *Helv. Chim. Acta*, 1944, **27**, 1044; G Schwarzenbach and C. Witwer, *ibid.*, 1947, **30**, 656.

TABLE 47-4.—EQUILIBRIUM PERCENTAGES OF ENOL IN KETO-ENOL SYSTEMS.

		Gas	Liquid	Hexane	Water	Ref.
A	$CH_3\cdot CO\cdot CH_3$	—	0.00025	—	—	5
	$CH_3\cdot CO\cdot CH_2\cdot CO_2Et$	49	7.5	49	—	1, 4, 6
	$CO_2Et\cdot CH_2\cdot CO\cdot CH_2\cdot CO_2Et$	—	17	—	—	1
B	$CO_2Et\cdot CH_2\cdot CO_2Et$	—	0.0	—	—	1
	$CH_3\cdot CO\cdot CH_2\cdot CO\cdot CH_3$	92	80	92	15	1, 3, 4, 6
C	$CH_3\cdot CO\cdot CHMe\cdot CO_2Et$	14	4	12	—	4
	$CH_3\cdot CO\cdot CHEt\cdot CO_2Et$	10	3	14	—	4
	$CH_3\cdot CO\cdot CHPr^i\cdot CO_2Et$	6.1	5	6	—	4
	$CH_3\cdot CO\cdot CH(C_6H_5)\cdot CO_2Et$	80	30	67	—	4
	$C_6H_5\cdot CO\cdot CH_2\cdot CO_2Et$	—	21	—	—	2, 3
	$C_6H_5\cdot CO\cdot CHEt\cdot CO_2Et$	—	4	—	—	3
D	$HCO\cdot CH(CO_2Et)_2$	—	94	—	—	3
	$CH_3\cdot CO\cdot CH(CO_2Et)_2$	—	69	—	—	3
	$C_2H_5\cdot CO\cdot CH(CO_2Et)_2$	—	44	—	—	3
E	$C_2H_5\cdot CO\cdot CH_2\cdot CO\cdot CH_3$	—	72	—	—	3
	$CH_3\cdot CO\cdot CHMe\cdot CO\cdot CH_3$	44	33	59	2.8	3, 4, 5
	$CH_3\cdot CO\cdot CHEt\cdot CO\cdot CH_3$	35	28	26	—	3, 4
F	$CH_3\cdot CO\cdot CH_2\cdot CO\cdot C_6H_5$	—	99	—	—	1, 3
	$C_2H_5\cdot CO\cdot CH_2\cdot CO\cdot C_6H_5$	—	94	—	—	3
G	*cyclo*Pentanone	—	0.0048	—	—	5
	*cyclo*Pentanone-2-CO_2Et	27	4.6	—	—	2, 6
	*cyclo*Pentanone-2-$CO\cdot CH_3$	—	—	—	15	5
	*cyclo*Pentanone-2-CHO	—	—	—	41	5
H	*cyclo*Hexanone	—	0.020	—	—	5
	*cyclo*Hexanone-2-CO_2Et	91	74	—	—	2, 6
	*cyclo*Hexanone-2-$CO\cdot CH_3$	—	—	—	29	5
	*cyclo*Hexanone-2-CHO	—	100	—	48	3, 5
	Dimethyldihydroresorcinol	—	—	—	95	5

[1] K. H. Meyer, *Ann.*, 1911, **380**, 212; *Ber.*, 1912, **45**, 2843.

[2] W. Dieckmann, *Ber.*, 1922, **55**, 2470.

[3] K. v. Auwers and H. Jacobson, *Ann.*, 1922, **426**, 161.

[4] J. B. Conant and A. F. Thompson, *J. Am. Chem. Soc.*, 1932, **54**, 4039.

[5] G. Schwarzenbach and E. Felder, *Helv. Chim. Acta*, 1944, **27**, 1044; G. Schwarzenbach and C. Witwer, *ibid.*, 1947, **30**, 659, 669.

[6] R. Schreck, *J. Am. Chem. Soc.*, 1949, **71**, 1881.

conjugative effect ($-M$) of the unsaturated carbethoxyl or acetyl substituent demands a suitably situated double bond, and thus increases the relative thermodynamic stability of the enol. We may plausibly suppose that the difference between the effects of the carbethoxyl and acetyl groups is due at least mainly to the second of these causes, since the groups are strongly thus differentiated, and stand in the order acetyl > carbethoxyl, with respect to their $-M$-effects (Section **7e**).

Sections C, D, E, and F in the table illustrate in various ways the influence of simple alkyl groups, which is to reduce the equilibrium content of enol in β-ketonic esters and β-diketones. Here we must assume, with Hughes, that, for simple alkyl groups in such keto-enol systems, the inductive effect ($+I$) is dominant: it protects the C-proton, leading to increased thermodynamic stability of the ketone. Referring to the analogy with elimination, the carbonyl group seems to be comparable rather to 'onium groups than to halogen substituents in its capacity for bringing into the foreground the inductive effect of alkyl groups in β-keto-enol systems.

As follows from the comparison of acetone, *cyclo*pentanone, and *cyclo*hexanone, alkyl groups increase the equilibrium enol contents of simple ketones. This indicates a dominating hyperconjugative effect ($+M$). Presumably the enolic double bond, having no second carbonyl group with which to conjugate, as it has in β-keto-enols, is the more prone to hyperconjugate with alkyl residues.

As is shown by figures given in sections C and F, any effect of electropolar quality is overridden by that of unsaturation in the radical phenyl, whose tendency to participate in the longest possible conjugated system causes it to increase the relative thermodynamic stability of the enolic isomerides of β-diketones and β-ketonic esters.

Most of the discussed effects can be seen again in the data for *cyclo*pentane and *cyclo*hexane compounds, given in sections G and H, which illustrate the additional point that the larger ring is the more favourable for enol forms. The cause of this is not known; but it may involve the circumstance that the terminal hydrogen of the nearly strainless, puckered, residue —$(CH_2)_4$— in a *cyclo*hexene fulfils the stereochemical requirements for hyperconjugation with the cyclic C:C-group better than does the terminal hydrogen of the nearly strainless, nearly flat, residue —$(CH_2)_3$— in a *cyclo*pentene.

Turning to *kinetic effects on enolisation*, it is found that alkyl groups depress rate of base-catalysed enolisation, as measured by Lapworth's bromination method. This is apparent in Evans and Gordon's data for the rate of bromination of phenyl alkyl ketones, Ph·CO·CHRR', in 75% aqueous acetic acid containing acetate ions as the catalyst.[63]

[63] D. P. Evans, and J. J. Gordon, *J. Chem. Soc.*, **1938**, 1434.

The relative rates at 45° are as follows:

RR′.........	H, H	Me, H	Et, H	Pr^i, H	Me, Me
Rate.........	100	15.4	12.0	5.9	3.0

These values were quoted by Hughes[61] in support of his thesis that the inductive effect is the dominant part of the total kinetic polar effect of alkyl groups in simple keto-enol systems, just as it is in bimolecular elimination from ammonium and sulphonium ions.

Cardwell has recalled[64] that the base-catalysed iodination of primary alkyl methyl ketones, $R\cdot CH_2\cdot CO\cdot CH_3$, leads preparatively through $R\cdot CH_2\cdot CO\cdot CI_3$, to $R\cdot CH_2\cdot CO_2Et$, thereby indicating Hofmann-type orientation of the halogenation, and, as is inferred, of the rate-controlling enolisation, in agreement with the preceding kinetic evidence.

Cardwell and Kilner have noted[65] that in the acid-catalysed bromination of ketones quite other kinetic conditions arise: alkyl groups appear to exert a dominating hyperconjugative effect: for one observes Saytzeff-type orientation, and corresponding rate changes. Preparative observations are recalled which show that the ketones formulated below undergo acid-catalysed bromination mainly where marked with an asterisk, an indication that the enolic double bond is placed preferentially where it would be placed by the generalised Saytzeff rule:

$CH_3\cdot\overset{*}{C}H_2\cdot CO\cdot CH_3$ $\quad CH_3\cdot CH_2\cdot\overset{*}{C}H_2\cdot CO\cdot CH_3$ $\quad (CH_3)_2\overset{*}{C}H\cdot CO\cdot CH_3$

CH_3 $\quad CH_3$ $\quad CO\cdot CH_3$ $\quad CO\cdot\overset{*}{C}H(CH_3)_2$

Cardwell and Kilner have cited,[66] and have themselves made, some quantitative analyses of the proportions in which α- and α'-monobromination occurs under acid catalysis in unsymmetrical ketones; and they have combined the orientational ratios with Dawson's values[67] for the overall rates of acid-catalysed iodination of the ketones, in order to calculate (as is permissible, since bromination and iodination are equally rate-controlled by enolisation) the relative partial rates of establishment of the enolic double bond in the individual alkyl groups

[64] H. M. E. Cardwell, *J. Chem. Soc.*, **1951,** 2442.

[65] H. M. E. Cardwell and A. E. H. Kilner, *J. Chem. Soc.*, **1951,** 2430.

[66] J. R. Catch, D. F. Elliot, D. H. Hey, and E. R. H. Jones, *J. Chem. Soc.*, **1948,** 272; J. R. Catch, D. H. Hey, E. R. H. Jones, and W. Wilson, *ibid.*, p. 276.

[67] H. M. Dawson and R. Wheatley, *J. Chem. Soc.*, 1910, **97,** 2048; H. M. Dawson and H. Ark, *ibid.*, 1911, **99,** 1740.

of the various ketones. Their results are in Table 47-5, which is arranged to show what alkyl substituents flank the enolic double bond in either position. Taking the first two entries as an example, one sees that the extra β-methyl substituent in methyl ethyl ketone accelerates enolisation in the ethyl branch, while the change from α-methyl to α-ethyl retards enolisation in the methyl branch of methyl ethyl ketone. The other comparisons in the table can be followed through similarly: all consistently indicate hyperconjugative rate-control by the alkyl substituents. The relationships are, indeed, closely similar to those, shown in Table 39-7 of Chapter IX, for bimolecular olefin elimination from alkyl bromides, a reaction of typical hyperconjugative rate-control, as summarised in the generalised Saytzeff rule (p. 670).

TABLE 47-5.—RELATIVE PARTIAL RATES OF ACID-CATALYSED ENOLISATION OF KETONES, AS MEASURED BY HALOGENATION (CARDWELL AND KILNER).

$$\underset{\text{H}}{>}\overset{\beta}{\text{C}}{=}\overset{\alpha}{\underset{\text{OH}}{\text{C}}}{-}\text{CH}\underset{\text{H}}{<} \;\leftarrow\; \underset{\text{H}}{>}\text{CH}{-}\underset{\text{O}}{\overset{}{\text{C}}}{-}\text{CH}\underset{\text{H}}{<} \;\rightarrow\; \underset{\text{H}}{>}\text{CH}{-}\overset{\alpha}{\underset{\text{OH}}{\text{C}}}{=}\overset{\beta}{\text{C}}\underset{\text{H}}{<}$$

Substituents β	Substituents α	Rate for branch	Ketone	Rate for branch	Substituents α	Substituents β
—	Me	50	Me·CO·Me	50	Me	—
Me	Me	76	Et·CO·Me	28	Et	—
Et	Me	59	*n*-Pr·CO·Me	35	*n*-Pr	—
Me	Et	41	Et·CO·Et	41	Et	Me

Concerning the reason why hyperconjugation is dominating in the control by alkyl groups of acid-catalysed enolisation rate, although the inductive effect assumes this role for base-catalysed enolisation, Cardwell and Kilner plausibly suggest that much more unsaturation develops, through partial carbonium-ion formation, in the transition state of acid-catalysed enolisation, than in the base-catalysed reaction. In the specific case of hydrogen-ion catalysis, the effective initial tautomer is, not the ketone itself as in basic catalysis, but the conjugate acid of the ketone, a mesomeric ion[68] having the valency structures

$$>\text{CH}{-}\underset{|}{\text{C}}{=}\overset{+}{\text{O}}\text{H} \quad \text{and} \quad >\text{CH}{-}\underset{|}{\overset{+}{\text{C}}}{-}\text{OH}$$

Much as in unimolecular olefin elimination, which follows the generalised Saytzeff rule, such a development of carbonium-ion character

[68] In general acid catalysis, we have often to deal with a hydrogen-bonded salt-like complex, instead of a free cation.

would, as argued in Section **39e** of Chapter IX, excite strong hyperconjugation by alkyl groups in the transition state of formation of the carbon-carbon double bond.

We turn now to *equilibria in primary and secondary nitro-paraffins.* These substances exist permanently as normal nitro-compounds, in equilibrium with very small proportions of *aci*-isomerides. Turnbull and Maron measured the proportions of the isomerides in aqueous solutions of the simpler members of the series.[69] Their method was conductometrically to estimate, first, the acidity constant of the *aci*-compound (as is possible, because of the slowness of its conversion to the nitro-form), and then, the acidity constant of the nitro-isomeride (as can be done, because of the near-completeness of its ultimate formation). Since the ions are common, the ratio of the acidity constants gives the ratio of the isomers.

TABLE 47-6.—ACIDITY CONSTANTS AND EQUILIBRIUM PROPORTIONS OF THE NORMAL AND ACI-FORMS OF ALIPHATIC NITRO-COMPOUNDS IN WATER AT 25° (TURNBULL AND MARON).

Normal form	$CH_3 \cdot NO_2$	$MeCH_2 \cdot NO_2$	$Me_2CH \cdot NO_2$
pK_a of *aci*-form	3.25	4.41	5.11
pK_a of normal form	10.21	8.46	7.68
Proportion of *aci*-form	0.000011%	0.0089%	0.275%

From the results in Table 47-6 it is clear that methyl substituents increase the thermodynamic stability of the *aci*-isomeride, and also increase, though less strongly, that of the anion, with reference in either case to that of the normal nitro-isomeride. This must be due to a hyperconjugative $+M$-effect of methyl, acting on the fully formed CN-double bond in the *aci*-structure (formula below), and on that part of the double bond which is in the CN-location in the mesomeric anion. These effects contrast with those applying to β-ketonic esters and β-diketones: here, in the equilibrium problem, there is a fully formed CC-double bond available for hyperconjugation: yet the inductive effect of alkyl groups is dominating. We may perhaps attribute the greater significance of hyperconjugation than of the inductive effect of alkyl groups in the equilibrium problem of the nitro-*aci*-nitro-system, despite the opposite relation applying to the keto-enols, to the association of a positive charge with the unsaturation in the former, and to the already discussed, competing conjugation in the latter:

[69] D. Turnbull and S. H. Maron, *J. Am. Chem. Soc.*, 1943, **65**, 212.

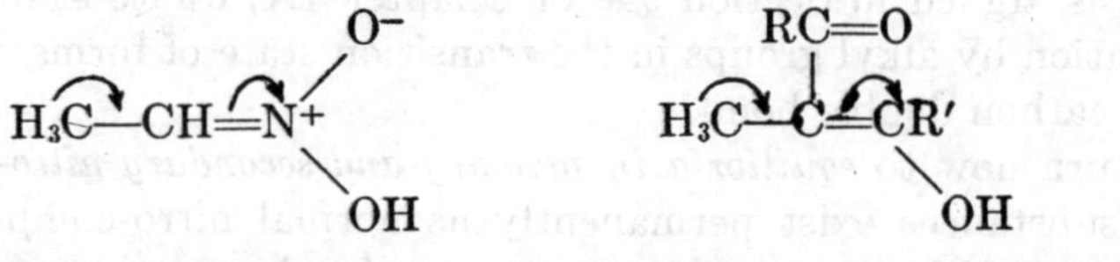

$$H_3C{-}CH{=}N^+(O^-)(OH) \qquad\qquad H_3C{-}C(COR){=}CR'(OH)$$

Strong hyperconjugation Weaker hyperconjugation

As to *kinetic effects on the isomerisation of nitro-paraffins*, Maron and LaMer have measured, by a conductometric method, the rate of neutralisation of some simple aliphatic nitro-compounds in aqueous solution.[70] This process is rate-controlling for the conversion of a nitro-compound into its *aci*-isomeride; and thus the rate of neutralisation has the same significance for the nitro-*aci*nitro-system as has the rate of base-catalysed bromination of ketones for the keto-enol system. The relative rates at 0° for some simple nitro-compounds, $RR'CH \cdot NO_2$, were as indicated:

R, R'.........	H, H	Me, H	Et, H	Me, Me
Rate..........	100	16.4	12.3	0.87

These figures show that alkyl substituents retard proton-loss from nitro-compounds, just as they do from ketones. We conclude that it is the inductive effect of the alkyl groups which is controlling the rate of proton-loss from the nitro-compounds, exactly as from ketones. And we explain why it is mainly the inductive effect which controls the rate, though it is chiefly the hyperconjugative effect of alkyl groups which controls the equilibrium in proton-loss from nitro-compounds, by assuming that, in the transition state of the proton transfer, there is not yet a sufficient growth of the CN-double bond to furnish the degree of unsaturation needed to excite a dominating hyperconjugative effect in alkyl substituents.

In the aldo-lactol ring-chain systems of the pyranose reducing sugars, aldehydic properties depend on high interconversion rates involving very small equilibrium proportions of the aldoforms:

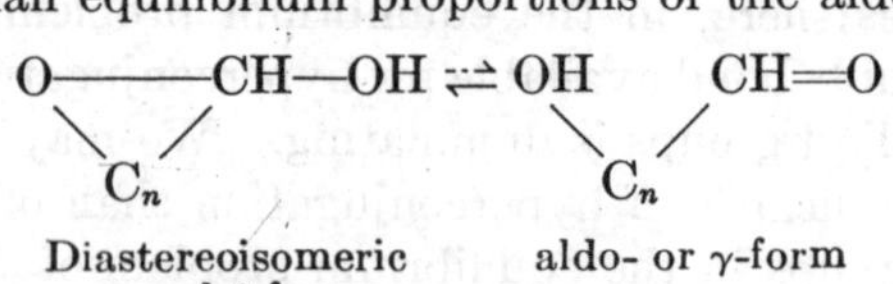

$$O{-}CH{-}OH \ (\text{ring through } C_n) \rightleftharpoons OH \quad CH{=}O \ (\text{open chain through } C_n)$$

Diastereoisomeric α- and β-forms aldo- or γ-form

The proportion of γ-glucose (aldo-form), present in equilibrium glucose in aqueous solution at *p*H 6.9 has been estimated[71] as 0.0026%.

[70] S. H. Maron and V. K. LaMer, *J. Am. Chem. Soc.*, 1938, **60**, 2588.

[71] J. M. Los, L. B. Simpson, and K. Weissner, *J. Am. Chem. Soc.*, 1956, **78**, 1564.

Equilibria among $\alpha\beta$- and $\beta\gamma$-unsaturated carboxylate ions, carboxylic esters, ketones, and nitriles have been studied extensively by Kon and Linstead and their coworkers.[72] The following systems are typical:

$$(\alpha\beta\text{-})\left\{\begin{array}{l} CH_3\cdot CH_2\cdot CH_2\cdot CH:CH\cdot CO_2^- \rightleftarrows CH_3\cdot CH_2\cdot CH:CH\cdot CH_2\cdot CO_2^- \\ CH_3\cdot CH_2\cdot CH_2\cdot CH:CH\cdot CO_2Et \rightleftarrows CH_3\cdot CH_2\cdot CH:CH\cdot CH_2\cdot CO_2Et \\ CH_3\cdot CH_2\cdot CEt:CH\cdot CO\cdot CH_3 \rightleftarrows CH_3\cdot CH:CEt\cdot CH_2\cdot CO\cdot CH_3 \\ (CH_3)_2CH\cdot CH:CH\cdot CN \rightleftarrows (CH_3)_2C:CH\cdot CH_2\cdot CN \end{array}\right\}(\beta\gamma\text{-})$$

The isomers involved in all these systems can be brought into equilibrium by means of basic catalysts: hydroxide ions in water form the usual conversion system for the carboxylate ions, and ethoxide ions in ethyl alcohol for the carboxylic esters, the methyl ketones, and the nitriles. The ketones are especially mobile, and a trace of adventitious base is often sufficient to bring about their isomerisation. The mobility of the systems is undoubtedly dependent fundamentally on the unsaturation of the oxygen and nitrogen atoms in the terminal groups; and thus the systems are more correctly regarded as *pentad keto-enol*, or *pentad cyano-imino-systems* than as three-carbon systems. But the enols and imines do not appear in the equilibria in more than quite minute proportions, which, in fact, have not yet been measured; and thus the equilibrium values available for discussion relate only to the proportions of alternative carboxyl, carbonyl, or cyano-forms, which differ simply with respect to the structure of a propene unit. For this reason the systems are often called "three-carbon" systems, the terminal group containing the unsaturated electronegative atom being separately designated the "activating group."

Kon and Linstead's observations may be summarised as follows. The equilibrium between the $\alpha\beta$- and $\beta\gamma$-unsaturated forms of any of these three-carbon systems is not particularly sensitive to the nature of the activating group, but is highly sensitive to substitution in certain positions in the propene unit. When the γ-position of the prototropic system, or every γ-position if there is more than one, is unsubstituted, as in the anions, esters, or nitriles of crotonic, $\beta\beta$-dimethylacrylic, and β-methylcinnamic acids, then the isomer almost exclusively present in equilibrium is the $\alpha\beta$-unsaturated substance:

[72] G. A. R. Kon and R. P. Linstead: their work was reviewed by the writer in *Ann. Repts. on Progress Chem.* (Chem. Soc. London), 1927, **24**, 109, and *ibid.*, 1928, **25**, 119; and, more extensively, by J. W. Baker in "Tautomerism," Routledge, London, 1934, Chap. 9. R. P. Linstead has contributed a table of data in H. Gilman's "Organic Chemistry," Wiley, New York, 1938, p. 819. These summaries give full references to the many original papers.

$$CH_3 \cdot CR:CH \cdot CO_2^- \rightleftarrows CH_2:CR \cdot CH_2 \cdot CO_2^-$$
$$(R = H, Me, Ph)$$

As the examples show, the replacement of β-hydrogen by β-methyl, or even by β-phenyl, makes no difference to this result. However, the introduction of one or two γ-methyl or other γ-alkyl groups shifts the balanced reaction towards the side of the βγ-unsaturated isomer, which now becomes usually an important, and often the preponderating form at equilibrium:

$$CH_3 \cdot CH_2 \cdot CR:CH \cdot CO_2^- \rightleftarrows CH_3 \cdot CH:CR \cdot CH_2 \cdot CO_2^-$$

A γ-phenyl group has a much larger effect in the same sense, the βγ-isomeride now being the exclusive form in equilibrium:

$$C_6H_5 \cdot CH_2 \cdot CR:CH \cdot CO_2^- \rightleftarrows C_6H_5 \cdot CH:CR \cdot CH_2 \cdot CO_2^-$$

Higher γ-alkyl groups are less effective than γ-methyl, as is shown for the system,

$$R \cdot CH_2 \cdot C(CH_2R):CH \cdot CO_2^- \rightleftarrows R \cdot CH:C(CH_2R) \cdot CH_2 \cdot CO_2^-$$

by the following data:

γ-Substituent (R)............	H	Me	Et	*i*-Pr
βγ-Form in equilibrium (%)....	0	79	67	51

β-Methyl substitution appears to favour βγ-unsaturated forms, but the examples are few, and the effect somewhat small, and possibly not consistent: the effect of even β-phenyl substitution is small, and is inconsistent in direction. Higher β-alkyl substituents involve γ-substitution of the system, and this has been considered. α-Methyl substitution favours αβ-unsaturated forms, as is illustrated for the system,

$$CH_3 \cdot CHR \cdot CH:CR' \cdot CO_2^- \rightleftarrows CH_3 \cdot CR:CH \cdot CHR' \cdot CO_2^-$$

by the following results:

Pentenoate ion....................	γ-Me	Parent	α-Me
βγ-Form in equilibrium (%).......	78	32	19

The following interpretation of these findings has been given.[73] The non-γ-substituted compounds exist in equilibrium practically entirely in their αβ-unsaturated forms, because conjugation between the propene double bond in this form and the unsaturated activating group increases the relative thermodynamic stability of the αβ-unsaturated

[73] P. B. D. de la Mare, E. D. Hughes, and C. K. Ingold, *J. Chem. Soc.*, 1948, 22.

isomers. β-Substituents conjugate or hyperconjugate with the propene double bond in either position, and therefore have only differential effects on the relative stabilities of the isomers. In the γ-methyl compounds, the energy of conjugation between the propene bond and the activating group in the $\alpha\beta$-unsaturated form is compensated to a considerable extent by the energy of hyperconjugation between the propene bond and the γ-methyl group in the $\beta\gamma$-unsaturated form. In the γ-phenyl compounds there is an over-compensation in the same direction by the larger mesomeric energy of conjugation between the propene double bond and the phenyl group in the $\beta\gamma$-unsaturated isomer. The weaker effects of higher γ-alkyl groups than of methyl, according to the sequence $H<\{Me>Et>i\text{-}Pr\}$, are normal consequences of hyperconjugation (Section **7i**). And finally, as γ-methyl hyperconjugates with the $\beta\gamma$-double bond, thereby favouring the $\beta\gamma$-unsaturated compounds, so α-methyl hyperconjugates with the $\alpha\beta$-double bond, thus favouring the $\alpha\beta$-unsaturated isomers.

The above explanation implies that, for equilibria, in systems of the type discussed, hyperconjugation by alkyl substituents is more important than induction: the analogy is with equilibria in nitro-*aci*nitro-systems, rather than with those in β-diketones. The probable reason is that, so long as the enol contents of these pentad keto-enol systems are not in question, inductive effects can be considered roughly to balance across the propene part of the system. A $+I$-effect exerted by R will protect the proton both in R—CH—C=C and in R—C=C—CH;[74] but if R is an unsaturated group, only the second system will experience the stabilising effect of conjugation; and if R is an alkyl group, only the second will experience its hyperconjugation.

Kon and Linstead have given figures for the influence of propene substituents on the rates of conversion of these systems; but the effects are complicated, and almost the only general statement that can be made is that alkyl substitution in all positions retards conversion. A complicated situation is theoretically expected, because mobility depends basically on the activating group, and substituents in the pro-

[74] The same is observed by Ossorio and his coworkers with respect to methyleneazomethines: when R is successively made Me, Et, *i*-Pr, *t*-Bu in the system

$$\underset{(I)}{\mathrm{R{-}\overset{H}{\overset{|}{C}}Ph{-}N{=}CHPh}} \underset{k_{-1}}{\overset{k_1}{\rightleftharpoons}} \underset{(II)}{\mathrm{R{-}CPh{=}N{-}\overset{H}{\overset{|}{C}}HPh}}$$

in ethanolic ethoxide, the rates k_1 and k_{-1} fall progressively and comparably by about 40-fold overall, while the equilibrium constants [(I)/(II)] move only over the range 1.22–1.47 (R. Perez Ossorio, F. G. Herrera, and A. Hidalgo, *Ann. Real Soc. Esp. Fis. Quim.*, 1956, **52,** 123; 1958, **54,** 471 *et seq.*, four papers).

pene unit will therefore influence mobility, not so much directly, as through effects transmitted to and relayed from the activating group.

Concerning the rates of formation of tautomers from a common anion, an analogy with simple pseudo-acids has been demonstrated. The equilibrium between ethyl *cyclo*pentylidenemalonate and ethyl *cyclo*pentenylmalonate is entirely in favour of the former:

$$\begin{array}{lcl}
\mathrm{CH_2\text{———}C\text{═══}C\cdot CO_2Et} & & \mathrm{CH\text{═══}C\text{———}CH\cdot CO_2Et} \\
\quad | \qquad\qquad | \qquad\quad | & \rightleftarrows & \quad | \qquad\qquad | \qquad\quad | \\
\mathrm{CH_2\cdot CH_2\cdot CH_2\quad CO_2Et} & & \mathrm{CH_2\cdot CH_2\cdot CH_2\quad CO_2Et}
\end{array}$$

However, Hugh and Kon found[75] that, if the sodium derivative of the ester is cautiously acidified (they used benzoic acid in a mixture of ethyl ether and light petroleum), then the unstable *cyclo*pentenyl ester, or at least a mixture rich in this isomeride, can be isolated, though eventually it passes into the stable *cyclo*pentylidene ester.

Thus, any of the systems discussed in this Section could be used to illustrate the rule given by Catchpole, Hughes, and the writer[76] for reactions through unstable intermediates, and thus for the unimolecular mechanism of prototropy. For this case it is that, *when a proton is supplied by acids to the mesomeric anion of weakly ionising tautomers of markedly unequal stability, then the tautomer which is most quickly formed is the thermodynamically least stable: it is also the tautomer from which the proton is lost most quickly to bases.* The properties of pseudo-acids provide a familiar illustration. When a salt of phenylnitromethane is acidified, the first-formed isomer is the thermodynamically unstable *aci*nitro-compound, which one may isolate by working quickly and with the avoidance of strong catalysts; but the ultimately formed isomer is, of course, the thermodynamically stable nitro-compound; and the *aci*-nitro-compound yields salts with bases much more quickly than does the nitro-compound.

The schematic energy diagram in Fig. 47-1 illustrates these relations. Kinetic control of the proportions in which tautomers are formed on supplying a proton to the mesomeric anion is regulated by the top two levels: thermodynamic control of their ultimate proportions is governed by the bottom two levels. And thus, from the ions, the less stable tautomer is first formed, though ultimately it must reionise and go over into the more stable tautomer. Therefore when, at the end of some sequence of reactions, tautomers are formed by an association of ions, the proportions of the tautomers will depend fundamentally on whether the control is kinetic or thermodynamic, that is, on whether the conditions do not or do permit fully formed tautomers

[75] W. E. Hugh and G. A. R. Kon, *J. Chem. Soc.*, **1930**, **775**.

[76] A. G. Catchpole, E. D. Hughes, and C. K. Ingold, *J. Chem. Soc.*, **1948**, **11**.

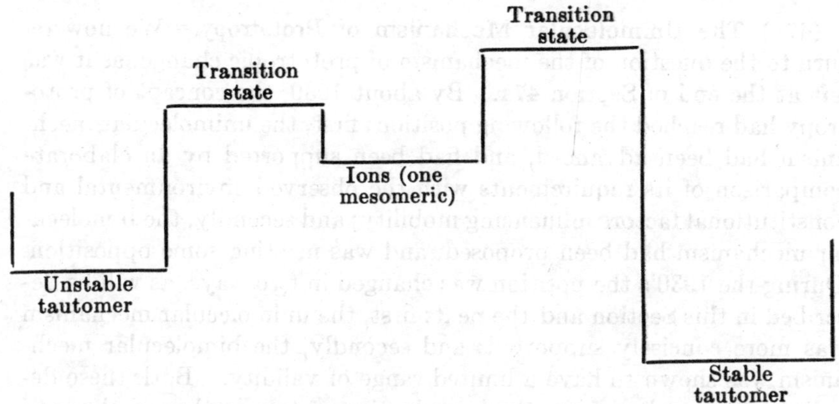

FIG. 47-1.—Schematic energy diagram, illustrating the distinction between the kinetic and thermodynamic control of the proportions of tautomers formed by ionic association; and also the distinction both of speed and of extent in the ionic dissociation of tautomers.

to come into equilibrium. As we shall see later, this is important for addition reactions. As to the ionic dissociation of tautomers, the diagram shows that the less stable tautomer will be ionised, not only to a greater equilibrium extent, but also more quickly, than the more stable tautomer.

These relations are intelligible on the general basis that the ionised form of the molecule is its least stable form, and that a less drastic electronic reorganisation, involving less activated energy, will be needed to convert it into the energetically less different unstable tautomer, than into the electronically and energetically very different stable tautomer. This type of rationalisation would apply to any reaction going through a highly energised intermediate state, *i.e.*, that the latter will pass with less electronic reorganisation, and therefore more quickly, into the markedly more energised of the end states. The deduction applies strictly only to electronic energy, but most of the energy of constitution of any state is electronic, so that the electronic energy will closely follow the total energy along a reaction co-ordinate.[77]

[77] Hammond has restated the principle in the looser form that the energised intermediate state will more closely resemble "in structure" the more energised end state (G. S. Hammond, *J. Am. Chem. Soc.*, 1955, **77**, 334). If "structure" is taken, as some have taken it, to mean configurational and conformational structure, the principle becomes untrue, because the relevant energies are quite minor parts of the total energy, and cannot be guaranteed to follow the latter on a reaction co-ordinate (*cf.* C. K. Ingold, "The Transition State," *Spec. Pubs. Chem. Soc.*, 1962, **16**, 119). The principle, as a paper by Hine reminds us (*J.*

(47e) The Unimolecular Mechanism of Prototropy.—We now return to the question of the mechanism of prototropic change, as it was left at the end of Section **47a**. By about 1930, the concept of prototropy had reached the following position: first, the unimolecular mechanism had been advanced, and had been supported by an elaborate comparison of its requirements with the observed environmental and constitutional factors influencing mobility; and secondly, the bimolecular mechanism had been proposed, and was meeting some opposition. During the 1930's the position was changed in two ways, as will be described in this Section and the next: first, the unimolecular mechanism was more concisely supported; and secondly, the bimolecular mechanism was shown to have a limited range of validity. Both these developments resulted from the introduction of two further methods of diagnosing prototropic mechanism, namely, through the study of changes of optical activity accompanying prototropic change, and through the study of accompanying hydrogen exchange, as disclosed by the use of the then newly available isotope deuterium.

In this Section we shall review that part of the work of the 1930's which was directed to the better establishment of the two-stage unimolecular mechanism of prototropy, B–S_E1'. It should be noted that the observations related to somewhat mobile prototropic systems, the main examples containing either the triad keto-enol systems, or the pentad cyano-imino-system. Two complementary types of case were studied, which will be considered in turn. In one, the investigated isomer was the thermodynamically stable member of its tautomeric system, for example, the ketonic member of the keto-enol system in a simple ketone. In the other, the main investigation was with the thermodynamically unstable tautomer, for example, a $\beta\gamma$-unsaturated nitrile susceptible of practically complete conversion to its $\alpha\beta$-unsaturated isomer.

In explanation of the principles involved in the examination of thermodynamically stable tautomers, let us consider the behaviour of a pseudo-acidic ketone, as predicted from the unimolecular mechanism. We have to take separate account of the catalysis of prototropy by bases and acids, and will first assume *basic catalysis*, which is the simpler form, and may be represented as follows:

$$\mathrm{B + H\cdot C{-}C{=}O \rightleftarrows \overset{+}{B}H + \left[C{-}C{-}O\right]^{-} \rightleftarrows B + C{=}C{-}O\cdot H}$$

Org. Chem., 1966, **31**, 1236), can be considered as derived from F. O. Rice and E. Teller's "principle of least motion" (*J. Chem. Phys.*, 1938, **6**, 489; 1939, **7**, 199).

In the case under discussion, the relative thermodynamic stabilities of the ketone, the ions, and the enol, will be as represented respectively, at the right, centre, and left of Fig. 47-1.

Lapworth had shown how the rate of enolisation of a pseudo-acidic ketone can, despite its thermodynamic stability, be measured indirectly by its rate of bromination, this rate being dependent on the catalyst, but independent of the halogen. The two-stage unimolecular mechanism describes the bromination and the enolisation as equally rate-controlled by the same initial proton-loss. In basic-catalysis, it regards the anion, not the enol, as the reactive entity towards electrophilic reagents, whether these be halogens, or acids supplying a proton. In bromination, it is presumed to be the anion which is trapped by the halogen; and, since the anion is rapidly and irreversibly brominated, the rate of bromination is equal to the rate of formation of the anion. As to enolisation, account is taken of the theory, which can be followed from Fig. 47-1, that the anion is protonated much more rapidly on oxygen than on carbon, so that the rate of production of enol will also be equal to the rate of formation of the anion, and therefore to the measurable rate of bromination.

Now these interpretations can be checked, because we have two other methods (and both are needed) of measuring the rate of formation of the anion. One depends on the circumstance that, if the carbon atom bearing mobile hydrogen is an asymmetric centre of optical activity, and is the only one present in the molecule, then optical activity must be lost in the mesomeric anion, in one of the valency structures of which this carbon atom is doubly bonded. Therefore, supposing the asymmetry condition to be fulfilled, the rate of formation of the anion should be measurable as a rate of racemisation, which should be equal to the measurable rate at which bromine, if added, would be taken up, all other conditions remaining the same: the relevant conditions are the temperature, the solvent, and the basic catalyst. It should be noted that the observation of such an equivalence of measured rates does not itself prove mechanism, because the enol, however produced, would be devoid of optical activity, and might be instantly brominated; so that if, for example, it were produced by an intramolecular jump of hydrogen, the rate of racemisation could still be equal to the rate at which added bromine would be taken up. However, as we shall see, a rate equality of the kind described forms a needed link in the evidential chain.

The remaining method of measuring the rate of formation of the anion is much less dependent on interpretation. The ketone, together with the basic catalyst, is dissolved in a deuteroxylic solvent, so that any anions formed by proton loss can take up only deuterons. From the relative thermodynamic stabilities of the ketone, the ions, and the enol, as illustrated in Fig. 47-1, it follows that, in stationary-state conditions, only a very small amount of the total keto-enol exists either as anion or as enol. Therefore, at all times after the brief initial period needed to set up stationary-state conditions, the rate of production of the anion will be equal to the rate of its conversion into the main product, namely, the deuteroketone; in other words, deuterons gained are at nearly all times kinetically equivalent to protons lost. Thus the measurable rate of deuteration should be equal to the other measurable rates, those of bromination and racemisation, provided that the foregoing interpretations of these latter processes are correct: equality would be a test of their correctness. The comparison requires, of course, that the conditions shall be the same, these conditions being the temperature, the solvent, and the catalyst. It is to be noted that the conditions include the solvent, which is necessarily a somewhat special solvent in the measurement of deuteration rate.[78]

The theory for the case of *acid catalysis* is somewhat more complicated, but the conclusions are similar. In general acid catalysis, the assumed first step is the conversion of the original prototropic system into a salt-like complex, which then suffers a rate-controlling deprotonation:

$$\mathrm{H\cdot C{-}C{=}O + HB \rightleftarrows H\cdot C{-}C{=}O,HB}$$

$$\mathrm{B' + H\cdot C{-}C{=}O,HB \rightleftarrows B'H^+ + [C{-}C{-}O]^-,HB}$$

$$\mathrm{\rightleftarrows B'H^+ + C{=}C{-}O\cdot H + B^-}$$

Here the entity instantly reactive towards halogens, or proton- or deuteron-donors, and also the first intermediate at which optical activity could be lost, is the deprotonated complex. The rate of its formation from the ketone is a composite quantity; but, because the ketone is the thermodynamically stable tautomer, it is just this rate which determines the measurable rates of bromination, of racemisation, and of deuterium uptake. In the special case of hydrogen-ion catalysis, the preliminary conversion is into the conjugate acid, and it is this

[78] The rates of reactions in general are not identical in hydroxylic and deuteroxylic solvents, because solvation energy depends in part on hydrogen zero-point energy.

which, under the unimolecular mechanism, suffers deprotonation at carbon, to give directly the enol:

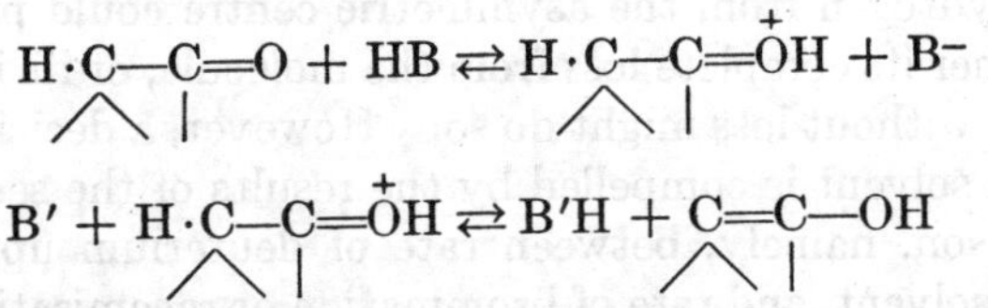

$$\mathrm{H\cdot \overset{|}{\underset{/\ \backslash}{C}}{-}\overset{}{\underset{|}{C}}{=}O + HB \rightleftarrows H\cdot \underset{/\ \backslash}{C}{-}\underset{|}{C}{=}\overset{+}{O}H + B^-}$$

$$\mathrm{B' + H\cdot \underset{/\ \backslash}{C}{-}\underset{|}{C}{=}\overset{+}{O}H \rightleftarrows B'H + \underset{/\ \backslash}{C}{=}\underset{|}{C}{-}OH}$$

The enol is now the deprotonated, and most active form, the rate of whose formation is the rate of bromination, racemisation, and deuterium exchange, under this specific type of catalysis.

The experimental rate comparisons were of two types. The first was between the rate of halogenation of a thermodynamically stable ketone or other such tautomer, and its rate of racemisation (the necessary circumstances of asymmetry being fulfilled), under common conditions as to temperature, solvent, and catalyst. The first such comparisons were made for acid-catalysed processes. Ramberg and Mellander[79] used the sulphone-acid (I), and compared bromination with racemisation in water containing hydrobromic acid as catalyst. Ramberg and Hedlund[80] examined the sulphone-acid (II) in similar conditions. Wilson and the writer[81] studied the ketone (III), comparing bromination with racemisation in aqueous acetic acid containing hydrobromic acid. Bartlett and Stauffer[82] employed the ketone (IV), comparing iodination with racemisation in acetic acid containing nitric acid. In all cases the halogenation rate equalled the racemisation rate. Then Hsü and Wilson[83] examined the theoretically simpler case of basic catalysis, using ketone (IV), aqueous acetic acid as solvent, and acetate ions as the basic catalyst, in a comparison of bromination with racemisation. Again the rates of the two processes were equal.

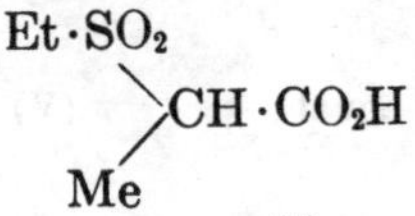

$\mathrm{(Et\cdot SO_2)(Me)CH\cdot CO_2H}$ (I)

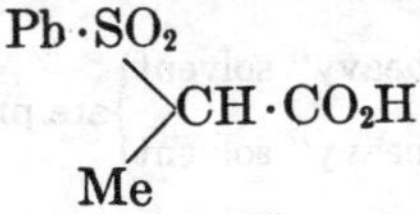

$\mathrm{(Pb\cdot SO_2)(Me)CH\cdot CO_2H}$ (II)

(III): indanone ring ($\mathrm{CH_2}$, CO) with $\mathrm{CH\cdot CH_2}$–$\mathrm{C_6H_4}$–$\mathrm{CO_2H}$

$\mathrm{(Et)(Me)CH\cdot CO\cdot Ph}$ (IV)

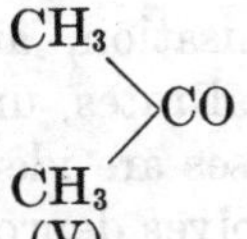

$\mathrm{(CH_3)_2CO}$ (V)

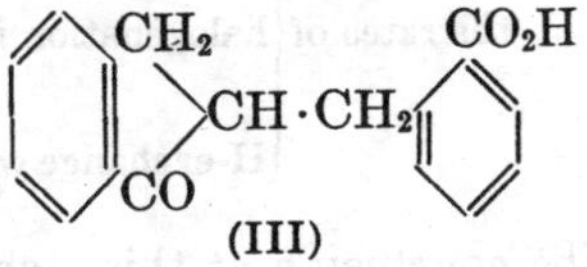

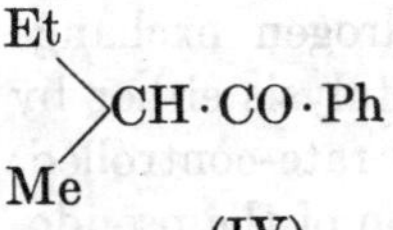

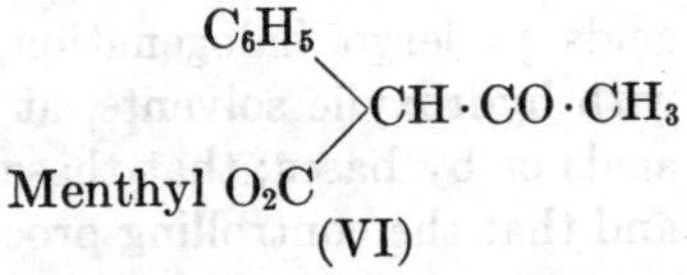

$\mathrm{(C_6H_5)(Menthyl\ O_2C)CH\cdot CO\cdot CH_3}$ (VI)

[79] L. Ramberg and A. Mellander, *Arkiv Kemi Mineral. Geol.*, 1934, **B**, **11**, No. 31.

[80] L. Ramberg and I. Hedlund, *Arkiv Kemi Mineral. Geol.*, 1934, **B**, **11**, No. 41.

[81] C. K. Ingold and C. L. Wilson, *J. Chem. Soc.*, **1934**, 773.

[82] P. D. Bartlett and C. H. Stauffer, *J. Am. Chem. Soc.*, 1935, **37**, 2580.

[83] S. K. Hsü and C. L. Wilson, *J. Chem. Soc.*, **1936**, 623.

As remarked above, such comparisons as these do not themselves identify the rate-controlling process. For any mode of removal of the mobile hydrogen from the asymmetric centre could produce racemisation: either its complete loss from the molecule, or its intramolecular migration without loss might do so. However, a decision in favour of loss to the solvent is compelled by the results of the second type of rate comparison, namely, between rate of deuterium uptake from a deuteroxylic solvent, and rate of bromination or racemisation, as measured in the same solvent, and under otherwise identical conditions. For acid-catalysed processes, the required comparison is contained in Reitz's demonstration[84] that the initial rate of bromination of "light" acetone, $CO(CH_3)_2$, in "heavy" water, D_2O, under catalysis by D_3O^+ is equal to the initial rate of uptake of deuterium by the acetone in the absence of the bromine. For base-catalysed processes, the comparison[85] was made by Hsü, Wilson, and the writer, who racemised and deuterated ketone (IV) in a D_2O-dioxan solvent with OD^- as catalyst: they found the rates of the processes equal.

The summary of these rate comparisons may be set out as follows:— For pseudo-acidic ketones under basic catalysis

the rates of:
- halogenation in "light" solvent } are proved equal (IV)
- racemisation in "light" solvent }
- racemisation in "heavy" solvent } are proved equal (IV)
- H-exchange with "heavy" solvent }

For pseudo-acidic ketones under acid catalysis,

the rates of:
- racemisation in "light" solvent } are proved equal (I–IV)
- halogenation in "light" solvent }
- halogenation in "heavy" solvent } are proved equal (V)
- H-exchange with "heavy" solvent }

The conclusion at this stage is that thermodynamically stable pseudo-acids undergo halogenation, racemisation, and hydrogen exchange with hydroxylic solvents, at identical rates, under catalysis either by acids or by bases; that these processes are identically rate-controlled; and that the controlling process involves deprotonation of the pseudo-acid.

In order directly to include isomerisation in the rate observations, it is necessary to go over to *thermodynamically balanced or unstable tau-*

[84] O. Reitz, *Z. physik. Chem.*, 1937, **179**, 119.
[85] S. K. Hsü, C. K. Ingold, and C. L. Wilson, *J. Chem. Soc.*, 1938, 78.

tomers. Comparisons of racemisation and isomerisation rates in a measurable balanced system were made by Kimball in example (VI): (−)menthyl (±)-α-phenylacetoacetate was crystallised from methanol in one diastereoisomeric form, which, in benzene containing a trace of piperidine, underwent mutarotation, representing racemisation in the phenylacetoacetate residue, at a rate of the order of twice that at which the ketonic ester underwent enolisation, as followed by the Kurt Meyer method, to give the equilibrium 71% of enol.[86] Evidently, optical activity was lost in the piperidine-deprotonated intermediate anion, which by re-protonation could go at comparable rates back to the ketone and on to the enol, with the result that the rate of the optical change was greater than the rate of enolisation.

Comparisons of hydrogen-exchange rates and isomerisation rates have been made in the unbalanced system of the unsaturated nitriles, *cyclo*hexenyl- and *cyclo*hexylidene-acetonitrile, formulated below. These are related analogously to the *cyclo*pentenyl- and *cyclo*pentylidene-malonic esters of Hugh and Kon, mentioned on p. 826: the βγ-unsaturated nitrile can be isolated, but it is thermodynamically quite unstable, passing with basic catalysts substantially completely into its αβ-unsaturated tautomer:

$$(\beta\gamma\text{-})\quad \begin{array}{l} CH_2\cdot CH{=}C{-}CH_2\cdot CN \\ \,| \qquad\qquad\;\; | \\ CH_2\cdot CH_2{-}CH_2 \end{array} \;\rightleftarrows\; \begin{array}{l} CH_2\cdot CH_2{-}C{=}CH\cdot CN \\ \,| \qquad\qquad\;\; | \\ CH_2\cdot CH_2{-}CH_2 \end{array}\quad (\alpha\beta\text{-})$$

The experimental comparison[87] was between the rate of base-catalysed isomerisation, and the rate of hydrogen exchange of either isomer with the medium. The isomerisation was catalysed by ethoxide ions in the deuteroxylic solvent EtOD; and the isomerisation rate was compared with the rate of uptake of deuterium by either tautomer. The result was that the rate of deuteration of the βγ-unsaturated nitrile was incomparably greater than its rate of isomerisation, and that this rate in turn was incomparably greater than the rate of deuteration of the αβ-unsaturated nitrile: H-exchange of βγ- ≫ conversion (βγ →αβ) ≫ H-exchange of αβ-.

Now if there were no intermediate product between the βγ- and αβ-unsaturated nitriles, that is, if the γ-hydrogen atom could be introduced only while the α-hydrogen atom was being withdrawn, then there should be agreement between the rate of hydrogen exchange and the rate of isomerisation. The very different relationship observed shows that there is an intermediate whose reversible formation involves hydrogen exchange with the medium, with the consequence that hy-

86 R. H. Kimball, *J. Am. Chem. Soc.*, 1936, **58**, 1963.
87 C. K. Ingold, E. de Salas, and C. L. Wilson, *J. Chem. Soc.*, **1936**, 1328.

drogen exchange can occur without necessarily involving a complete conversion of one tautomer into the other. This is, of course, consistent with the hypothesis of an intermediate anion, and on this basis the observed rate relations can be understood from Fig. 47-1. This indicates that only a small proportion of the anions formed from the thermodynamically unstable $\beta\gamma$-compound will pass forward over the high barrier into the thermodynamically stable $\alpha\beta$-product; most will return over the low barrier to the original $\beta\gamma$-isomer. The reverting anions will not contribute to the isomerisation rate; yet every anion formed leads to hydrogen exchange. Thus hydrogen exchange of the convertible isomer will be faster than its isomeric conversion. Furthermore, the isomeric conversion will be faster than hydrogen exchange of the conversion product. For, as can also be followed from Fig. 47-1, the complete forward process from the $\beta\gamma$-unsaturated factor to the $\alpha\beta$-product, that is, the isomerisation, has to surmount a smaller energy hill than has the partial reverse change from the $\alpha\beta$-unsaturated product to the ions, the process necessary for hydrogen exchange.

(47f) The Bimolecular Mechanism of Prototropy.—The bimolecular mechanism, B–S_E2', has been investigated by generally similar methods in the example of the aryl-flanked methyleneazomethine system, which is one of the less mobile of the known triad systems, but can be brought to equilibrium under catalysis by strong bases, such as ethoxide ions, in ethyl alcohol. Two methods have been used. In one, a chemically measured rate of isomerisation is compared with the rate of racemisation of an optically active tautomer. In the other, either of these rates is compared with the rate of hydrogen exchange between the tautomers and the medium.

The examined examples are as indicated in Table 47-7. They are all thermodynamically more or less balanced systems, yielding measurable proportions of both tautomers at equilibrium, as is shown in the table.

The relation between chemically followed isomerisation rates and racemisation rate was studied[88] in examples (a), (b), and (c). In each case, optically active (I), on isomerisation catalysed by ethoxide ions in ethyl alcohol, gave inactive (II): this was true even in case (a), in which (II) has a centre of asymmetry. There were therefore three rates which could be measured, namely, the chemically-followed rate of the reaction (I)→(II), the rate of the reverse reaction (II)→(I), and

[88] C. K. Ingold and C. L. Wilson, *J. Chem. Soc.*, **1933**, 1493; *idem*, *ibid.*, **1934**, 93; S. K. Hsü, C. K. Ingold, and C. L. Wilson, *ibid.*, **1935**, 1774.

TABLE 47-7.—EQUILIBRIA IN ETHYL ALCOHOL OF THE METHYLENEAZOMETHINES WHOSE BASE-CATALYSED ISOMERISATION, RACEMISATION, AND HYDROGEN-EXCHANGE RATES ARE COMPARED.

$$\text{(I)}\quad \begin{matrix}R\\R'\end{matrix}\!\!>\!CH\cdot N\!:\!C\!<\!\!\begin{matrix}R''\\R'''\end{matrix} \;\underset{}{\overset{OEt^-}{\rightleftharpoons}}\; \begin{matrix}R\\R'\end{matrix}\!\!>\!C\!:\!N\!-\!CH\!<\!\!\begin{matrix}R''\\R'''\end{matrix}\quad \text{(II)}$$

Example	R	R′	R″	R‴	*Equilib.*, (I):(II)
(a).........	C_6H_5	CH_3	C_6H_5	p-Cl·C_6H_4	50:50 at 85°
(b).........	C_6H_5	CH_3	C_6H_5	C_6H_5	68:32 at 85°
(c).........	p-Ph·C_6H_4	C_6H_5	C_6H_5	H	56:44 at 25°
(d).........	p-MeO·C_6H_4	H	C_6H_5	H	24:76 at 74°
	(1) $KO(CH_2)_2OH$ in $HO(CH_2)_2OH$; (2) $KOBu^t$ in $HOBu^t$				
(e).........	C_6H_5	CH_3	p-Cl·C_6H_4	pCl·C_6H_4	50:50, 75° (2)

the rate of loss of optical activity from (I). The decision required was whether optical activity is lost from (I) only as fast as it would be by conversion into inactive (II) and regeneration from (II), or whether it is lost faster. The bimolecular mechanism B–S_E2' provides no opportunity for faster racemisation: optical activity should be lost just as fast as can be calculated from chemically measured rates of isomerisation in both directions. The unimolecular mechanism B–S_E1' provides an intermediate anion in which optical activity would be lost, so that the full cycle of conversion into and regeneration from (II) can be short-circuited by conversion into and regeneration from the intermediate ions, thus producing faster racemisation. Experiment showed that in every case under catalysis by ethoxide ions in alcohol, the rate of racemisation accompanying isomerisation was just what it would be if no such short-circuiting occurred. This shows that there is no reversibly formed intermediate in which optical activity can be lost, and therefore that, either (i) there is no intermediate anion, or (ii) its formation is not detectably reversible, *i.e.*, that, when formed from I, it undergoes protonation in all cases only to give II, though this means protonation only at the benzhydryl position in cases (a) and (b), and only at the benzyl position in case (c). The investigators thought possibility (ii) to be so unlikely that they favoured the alternative (i) of a one-step isomerisation by Lowry's mechanism, B-S_E2'.

The relation between either the chemical isomerisation rates in both directions, or the corresponding racemisation rate, on the one hand, and the rates of hydrogen exchange between the total tautomeric system and the medium, on the other, has been examined in examples (c), (d) and (e) of Table 47-7. The unimolecular mechanism provides an intermediate anion, and so requires hydrogen exchange with the reacting system to be faster than any *directly* measurable isomerisation. The bimolecular mechanism requires initial equality between the rate of isomerisation of one tautomer and the rate of uptake by the total isomerising system of hydrogen from the solvent, in particular, of deuterium from a deuteroxylic solvent. Obviously, if the solvent can supply only deuterons and not any protons, then, for every original molecule once converted by the bimolecular mechanism, one deuteron is admitted to the system:[89]

$$\begin{array}{ccc} \bar{E}tO\ \ H \quad\quad D\text{—}OEt & & EtO\text{—}H \quad\quad D\ \ OEt^- \\ RR'C\text{—}N\text{=}CR''R''' & \rightarrow & RR'C\text{=}N\text{—}CR''R''' \end{array}$$

The first attempt[90] to diagnose the bimolecular mechanism using this principle was made by de Salas and Wilson with system (d) of Table 47-7. Chemically measured isomerisation rates were compared with the rate of uptake of deuterium by the total system from an incompletely deuterated hydroxylic solvent. The relative rates of transference of protons and deuterons from the solvent to the solute system being undetermined,[91] the results showed only that the initial rates of isomerisation and of hydrogen exchange were of the same order of magnitude. But Ossorio and Hughes[92] used complete deuteration in system (c) of Table 47-7. In this case the comparison of isomerisation rates with racemisation rate had been made already: and so Ossorio and Hughes compared the rate of loss of optical activity with the rate of uptake of deuterium, during the isomerisation of (I) under catalysis by ethoxide ions in the pure deuteroxylic solvent EtOD. They found that the initial rates of loss of optical activity and of uptake of deu-

[89] After this initial rate equality, the deuteration rate should run ahead of the isomerisation rate, as reaction proceeds. For, whilst at the beginning of the isomerisation of (I), practically all the formed (II) will have gone through the simple history (I)→(II), which allows only one deuterium atom to get into a molecule of (II), at all later times some (II) will be present which has gone through a more complicated history, such as (I)→(II)→(I)→(II), providing for the admission of more than one deuterium atom into one molecule of finally formed (II).

[90] E. de Salas and C. L. Wilson, *J. Chem. Soc.*, **1938**, 319.

[91] Protons and deuterons are transferred at different rates, whose ratio is in principle different for every transfer process, since it depends on hydrogen zero-point energy in the initial and transition states of the process. Without a knowledge of this ratio, a rate of hydrogen exchange cannot be determined by the isotopic marking of only a sample of the exchanging hydrogen.

[92] R. P. Ossorio and E. D. Hughes, *J. Chem. Soc.*, **1952**, 426.

terium were exactly equal.[93] It follows that the initial rates of isomerisation and of deuterium uptake were equal; and that therefore the single process I→II admits exactly one deuterium atom, as is required by the single-stage bimolecular mechanism, B-S_E2'.

Cram and Guthrie have proposed to reverse these conclusions on account of a study which they have made of example (e). As noted in Table 47-7, they employed other base-solvent systems, but their prototropic system was very similar to that of example (a). Their work was without kinetic support,[94] but they did obtain the rate pattern: H-exchange of II ≫ conversion II → I ≫ H-exchange of I; which shows that, in the conditions, II has a mechanism of exchange that does not entail conversion to I. Their interpretation is that the exchange of II goes through a carbanion, the same carbanion through which the unimolecular mechanism of isomerisation B-S_E1' takes II into I; and that this isomerisation is so much slower than exchange only because the carbanion is protonated almost wholly in the benzhydryl position, *i.e.*, with reversion to II, rather than conversion to I. The discrepancy must be pointed out between this finding and Ossorio and Hughes's results in example (c), to account for which an assumed intermediate carbanion would have to have the opposite property of protonating only in the benzyl position. It is to be hoped that this apparent contradiction can be resolved and that a pending kinetic reinvestigation will throw light on the matter.

(48) PSEUDO-BASICITY AND ANIONOTROPY

(48a) Pseudo-basicity.—Hantzsch was the first to recognise a form of tautomeric change in the reversible conversion between ionised quaternary ammonium hydroxides having double-bonded nitrogen, and the isomeric non-ionic carbinols. The latter he termed *pseudo-bases*. One of his original examples was that of 5-phenyl-10-methylacridinium hydroxide and its salts.[95] The salts with strong acids, such as hydrochloric acid, are typical quaternary ammonium salts. When an aqueous solution of such a salt, say, the chloride, is basified, for example, with silver oxide, the resulting solution has at first the properties of a solution of a quaternary ammonium hydroxide: it has a high electrical conductance, and is strongly alkaline. But with time, the con-

[93] After about 10% of isomerisation the deuteration rate ran markedly ahead of the racemisation rate, indicating the uptake of several deuterium atoms per molecule by to-and-fro isomerisation.

[94] D. J. Cram and R. D. Guthrie, *J. Am. Chem. Soc.*, 1965, **87**, 397; 1966, **88**, 5760. (Their argument was in terms of "one-point rate constants," though one point is not enough to show that anything is constant.)

[95] A. Hantzsch, *Ber.*, 1899, **32**, 575; A. Hantzsch and M. Kalb, *ibid.*, p. 3109.

ductance falls away, and the solution becomes more nearly neutral: the covalent carbinol, which is formed, may crystallise out:

Ph | Ph OH

$+ \bar{O}H \rightarrow$

+N | N

Me | Me

This slow production of a neutral carbinol from the cation and a hydroxide ion is reminiscent of the slow formation of normal phenylnitromethane from its anion and hydrogen ion. The pseudo-basic carbinol corresponds to the pseudo-acidic phenylnitromethane; and the ions that give the carbinol correspond to the ions of the nitro-compound. What is missing in the analogy is that there is no second covalent, but very easily ionising, form of base to correspond to the covalent *aci*-form of the nitro-compound: in pseudo-basicity the "isomeric change" is only between the electrovalent ion-pair and the covalent carbinol.

When the carbinol is treated with strong acids, the acridinium ion is regenerated with loss of hydroxide ion. Thus we have to think of the above change as reversible. With anions of high stability, such as perchlorate or chloride, the ion-pair is favoured. In the presence of a strongly nucleophilic anion, such as hydroxide, the covalent molecule is predominantly produced. The anion need not be hydroxide: the cyanide ion, for instance, is sufficiently nucleophilic to produce a covalent cyanide. Hantzsch called such compounds *pseudo-salts:*

Me—N (X, Ph) $\underset{X^- = OH^-,\ CN^-,\ \text{etc.}}{\overset{X^- = Cl^-,\ ClO_4^-,\ \text{etc.}}{\rightleftharpoons}}$ Me—$\overset{+}{N}$ —Ph + $\bar{X}$

Pseudo-base or pseudo-salt | Ammonium hydroxide or salt

Further features of pseudo-basic systems may be illustrated by another of Hantzsch's leading examples, namely, that of N-alkylquinolinium derivatives. The salts of this cation on basification yield alkaline solutions, which in course of time lose alkalinity with the production of pseudo-bases. The latter can be oxidised by ferricyanide to α-quinolones,[96] and are therefore regarded as 2-carbinols:

$\xrightarrow{OH^-}$ (H, C, OH) $\xrightarrow{Fe(CN)_6^{---}}$ C=O

+N | N | N

R | R | R

[96] H. Decker, *Ber.*, 1892, 25, 443; *J. prakt. Chem.*, 1893, 47, 28.

The greater thermodynamic stability of the 2-carbinols than of the 4-carbinols, which is indicated by this general result, can be understood on the basis that the former alone preserves the phenyl-to-vinyl conjugation. The same type of structure is preserved in ethers, such as those formulated below, which are very readily produced from the carbinol, probably through anion exchange, either by reaction with solvent alcohol or by self-reaction if no other alcohol is available:

H C OEt N Me   H H N O N Me Me

Pseudo-salt formation can be seen in the reactions of methylquinolinium salts with various sources of carbanions, for instance Grignard reagents,[97] or pseudo-acidic carbonyl or nitro-compounds,[98] as in the following examples:

N^+ Me — MeMgI ⟶ CHMe N Me; — $MeNO_2$ ⟶ $CH \cdot CH_2 \cdot NO_2$ N Me

Pseudo-salt formation with cyanide ion takes the exceptional course of producing, not a 2-cyanide, but a 4-cyanide, proved so to be by successive oxidation, demethylation, and hydrolysis to cinchonic acid.[99] One suspects that the isolated cyanide is really the prototropic tautomer of the 4-pseudo-salt: there seems to be nothing in the literature to prove the contrary. Having more conjugation, the tautomer would be thermodynamically more stable than either the 4-pseudo-salt itself, or the 2-pseudo-salt, or any accessible prototropic tautomer of the latter:

[97] M. Freund, *Ber.*, 1904, **37**, 4666; M. Freund and L. Richard, *Ber.*, 1909, **42**, 1101.

[98] A. Kaufmann, German Patent, 1912, No. 250154.

[99] A. Kaufmann and A. Albertini, *Ber.*, 1909, **42**, 3776; A. Kaufmann and R. Widmer, *Ber.*, 1911, **44**, 2058.

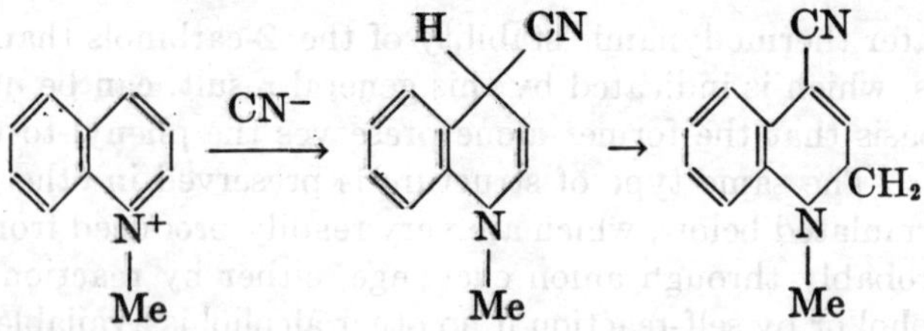

Free cyclic pseudo-bases formed by hydroxyl co-ordination in the 2-position contain a ring-chain prototropic system: the cyclic 2-carbinols are tautomeric with decyclised amino-carbonyl compounds:

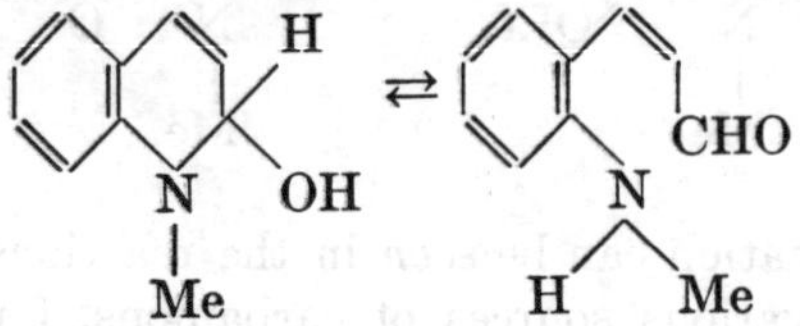

In fact, methylquinolinium salts react with hydroxylamine and with phenylhydrazine to give respectively an oxime and phenylhydrazone, which are themselves members of ring-chain prototropic systems, and are probably more stable in their cyclic hydroxylamino- and phenylhydrazino-forms, just as are the corresponding derivatives of mutarotating sugars (Section **47b**):[100]

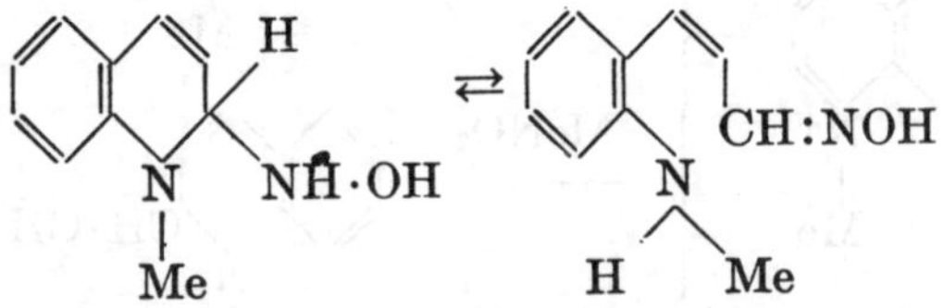

Whether these compounds are formed by anion exchange in the cyclic pseudo-base, or through carbonyl reactions of the open-chain amino-aldehyde, has not yet been determined.

As Hantzsch and Kalb pointed out,[101] alkylpyridinium ions seem to have a definitely smaller tendency than alkylquinolinium ions to pass into covalent pseudo-forms. When a solution of a methylpyridinium salt is basified, the alkalinity and electrical conductance persist; yet the existence of some pseudo-base in equilibrium with the pair of ions is indicated by the formation of an α-pyridone on oxidation with ferricyanide:

[100] A. Kaufmann and P. Strüber, *Ber.*, 1911, **44**, 680; H. Decker and A. Kaufmann, *J. prakt. Chem.*, 1911, **84**, 219.
[101] A. Hantzsch and M. Kalb, *Ber.*, 1899, **32**, 3109.

This difference from the quinoline analogues probably means that a greater loss of aromatic stability results from the partial saturation of a simple pyridine ring than from that of the pyridine part of the quinoline system, wherein the benzene ring is likely to gain stability from the destruction of aromatic character in the hetero-ring.

Some pseudo-basic systems possess another property, of which the α-pyridones, and likewise the γ-pyridones, provide illustrations. The general principle of the matter is that, when a quaternary ammonium ion contains some acidic centre, for instance, a phenolic or other acidic hydroxyl group, then the ammonium hydroxide will undergo a dehydration of the nature of an internal acid-base neutralisation, deprotonating the acidic centre, and forming what is called an *anhydro-base.* For example, when 2-hydroxypyridine, or α-pyridone, as it is usually named after its prototropic tautomer, is alkylated in the usual manner of a pyridine, the formed quaternary ammonium ion passes into its anhydro-base, the N-alkyl-α-pyridone:[102]

This might be represented by the betaine valency structure, as here, or by the carbonyl structure, as previously: the real structure is, of course, mesomeric between the two.

Hantzsch and Kalb discussed cotarnine,[103] an example of pseudobasicity in a hydroaromatic ammonium system. The salts of cotarnine with strong acids are definitely ionic, but the hydroxide, cotarnine itself, is a pseudo-base, and the cyanide is a covalent pseudo-salt. The cation reacts with almost any source of a reactive anion, for example, with alcohols, and mercaptans,[104] with pseudo-acidic carbonyl[105]

[102] H. v. Pechmann and O. Baltzner, *Ber.*, **1891**, **24**, **3144**.

[103] A. Hantzsch and M. Kalb, *loc. cit.*

[104] M. Freund and P. Bamberg, *Ber.*, **1902**, **35**, **1739**.

[105] C. Liebermann and A. Glawe, *Ber.*, **1904**, **37**, **2738**; F. Kropf, *ibid.*, p. **2744**

and nitro-compounds, with indene,[106] and with Grignard reagents,[107] forming covalent products of the standard pattern:

MeO, CH, $\overset{+}{\text{N}}$Me, O, CH_2, O, CH_2, CH_2 $+ \bar{X}$

$\bar{X} = \bar{Cl}$, etc. (←)

(→) $\bar{X} = \bar{OH}, \bar{CN}, \bar{OEt}, \bar{SEt}$, $RCO\cdot\bar{CH}_2$, $NO_2\cdot\bar{CH}_2$, $\bar{Alk}$.

MeO, CH—X, NMe, O, CH_2, O, CH_2, CH_2

Cotarnine, as a cyclic pseudo-basic 2-carbinol, is a member of a ring-chain prototropic system, the other tautomer being an amino-aldehyde:[108]

MeO, CH·OH, NMe, O, CH_2, O, CH_2, CH_2 ⇄ MeO, CHO, NHMe, CH_2, O, CH_2, O, CH_2

Actually, cotarnine reacts with hydroxylamine[109] and with aniline,[110] to form respectively an oxime and an anil, which are themselves ring-chain tautomers, and are probably most stable in their cyclic forms, as in other similar cases. The question of whether they are formed from the carbinol cotarnine by anion exchange, or through the aldehydic modification of cotarnine, has been discussed, but no certain conclusion has been reached.

A pseudo-basic 2-carbinol need not be cyclic: but what was, in the cyclic case, a ring-chain prototropic system, becomes, in the acyclic

[106] E. Hope and R. Robinson, *J. Chem. Soc.*, 1911, **99**, 2119; 1913, **103**, 361.
[107] M. Freund, *Ber.*, 1903, **36**, 4257.
[108] H. Decker, *Ber.*, 1900, **33**, 2273.
[109] W. Roser, *Ann.*, 1889, **254**, 334.
[110] M. Freund and F. Becker, *Ber.*, 1903, **36**, 1522.

case, a protolytic system: the carbinol, indeed, is the unstable adduct in a reversible addition, as of amines to aldehydes or ketones:

$$>\overset{+}{N}=\overset{|}{\underset{|}{C}} + \overset{-}{O}H \rightleftarrows >N-C-OH \rightleftarrows >NH + \overset{|}{\underset{|}{C}}=O$$

This is the basis of the *Mannich reaction*, in which ammonia or a primary or secondary amine, together with formaldehyde, will interact with nearly any anion which is sufficiently accessible and sufficiently nucleophilic to displace hydroxide ion from a pseudo-base. The usual sources of anions are pseudo-acidic carbonyl compounds, but pseudo-acidic nitro-compounds have been employed, and also alcohols, and, using the pseudo-alkoxides or ethers thus produced, Grignard reagents. Some examples are formulated:

$$PhCO \cdot CH_3 + CH_2O + HNMe_2 \rightarrow PhCO \cdot CH_2 \cdot CH_2 \cdot NMe_2$$

$$NO_2 \cdot CH_2Me + CH_2O + HN(CH_2)_5 \rightarrow NO_2 \cdot CHMe \cdot CH_2 \cdot N(CH_2)_5$$

$$n\text{-}BuOH + CH_2O + NHEt_2 \rightarrow n\text{-}BuO \cdot CH_2 \cdot NEt_2$$

$$CH_2{:}CH \cdot CH_2 \cdot MgCl + n\text{-}BuO \cdot CH_2 \cdot NEt_2 \rightarrow CH_2{:}CH \cdot CH_2 \cdot CH_2 \cdot NEt_2$$

The triphenylmethane dyes, such as malachite green and pararosaniline, were discussed as pseudo-basic systems by Hantzsch and Osswald.[111] These systems present certain formal differences from those mentioned already. The centre of co-ordination is further from the nitrogen atom: with the previous numbering (N = 1) the carbinols would be 6-carbinols. Also, it is not now the ammonium ions, but the covalent pseudo-forms, which are fully aromatic; the cations derive their stability (and their colour) from a form of mesomerism which makes them largely quinonoid. However, in most of their reactions these systems are similar to others. The dyes themselves are the electrovalent ammonium salts of strong acids, such as hydrochloric acid. When an alkali hydroxide is added to a solution of any of them, crystal violet, for example, the colour fades, but not instantaneously: the colour, the electrical conductance, and the alkalinity diminish together, and the colourless covalent carbinol, which is formed, may be precipitated. This is the pseudo-base. The addition to the dye of cyanide ion similarly produces a colourless covalent cyanide, that is, a pseudo-salt. Other sources of reactive anions, for example, Grignard reagents,[112] interact with the dye cation to form analogously constituted covalent products:

[111] A. Hantzsch and G. Osswald, *Ber.*, 1900, **33**, 278.

[112] M. Freund and H. Beck, *Ber.*, 1904, **37**, 4679.

$$\left(Me_2\overset{+}{N}{=}C_6H_4{=}\right)(Me_2NC_6H_4)_2C + X^- \underset{\bar{X} = \bar{O}H,\ \bar{C}N,\ \bar{A}lk,\ etc.}{\overset{X^- = Cl^-,\ etc.}{\rightleftarrows}} (Me_2NC_6H_4)_3C{-}X$$

(Crystal violet and its pseudo-forms: single valency structures are written. In the mesomeric state of the cation, the charge is shared by the three nitrogen atoms, and also to some extent by the three α-, the six meta-, and the single ω-carbon atoms.)

Turgeon and La Mer showed that the cation of crystal violet and hydroxide ion combine according to a second-order kinetic law, and with the negative salt effect appropriate for the combination of singly charged counter-ions to give a neutral adduct.[113]

A case of pseudo-basicity involving co-ordination on a second nitrogen atom, instead of on carbon, was recognised by Hantzsch[114] in the chemistry of the aromatic diazo-compounds. The diazonium salts of strong acids are the ammonium ionic forms of this system. The diazohydroxides, which must be covalent as formed from the diazonium and hydroxide ions, even though they are afterwards ionised as acids in an alkaline medium to form the diazotates, are the pseudo-bases of the system. The covalent diazocyanides and diazosulphonates are examples of pseudo-salts:

$$Ar{-}\overset{+}{N}{\equiv}N + \overset{-}{X} \underset{X^- = OH^-,\ CN^-,\ etc.}{\overset{X^- = Cl^-,\ etc.}{\rightleftarrows}} Ar{-}N{=}N{-}X$$

The presence of a triple bond in the ionic form, and therefore of a double bond in the pseudo-forms, leads to certain special consequences, which Hantzsch pointed out. One is that the pseudo-basic diazohydroxide is a member, not of a protolytic system, the adduct in a reversible addition, but of a prototropic system. Having regard to the moderate acidity of diazohydroxides, that is, the facile formation of

[113] J. C. Turgeon and V. K. La Mer, *J. Am. Chem. Soc.*, 1952, **74**, 5988.
[114] A. Hantzsch, *Ber.*, 1899, **32**, 3132.

diazotate ions, we may confidently assume that the prototropic interconversion will take place by the ionic mechanism B–S_E1':

$$Ar{-}N{=}N{-}OH \rightleftarrows [Ar{-}\dot{N}{-}N{-}O]^- + H^+ \rightleftarrows Ar{-}NH{-}N{=}O$$

The knowledge that protons separate very readily from nitrogen and from oxygen, and analogy with tautomerism in diazoamino-compounds, in amidines, and in amides, suggest that the diazohydroxide-nitrosamine system, like the other prototropic systems mentioned, would be very mobile, and that separate isomers would be extremely difficult if not impossible to prepare and to preserve.

The second important consequence of the unsaturation in the pseudo-forms is that they all should be capable of geometrical isomerism, similar in type to that shown by oximes and by azobenzene. That the known two series of diazotates, the two series of diazocyanides, and the two of diazosulphonates are indeed to be understood in this way, is a thesis which Hantzsch advanced originally, and defended to the end of his life; and it is one which, despite the many attacks made upon it, is today generally believed to be correct.[115]

Not only ammonium, but also oxonium pseudo-basic systems are well known. Xanthydrol forms an ionic xanthylium tribromide and ferrichloride.[116] However the lesser relative stability of the xanthylium than of the N-alkylacridinium ion is indicated by the fact that xanthydryl chloride and bromide have been isolated as covalent pseudo-salts.[117] The carbinol itself is, of course, an entirely covalent pseudo-base. However, it undergoes most of the usual anion-exchange reactions of pseudo-bases, for instance, with keto-enols, such as acetylacetone, and with pseudo-acids of a number of different kinds:[118]

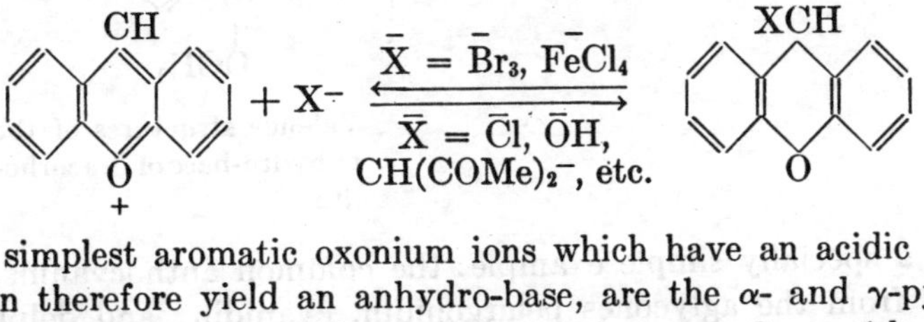

CH ... O^+ (xanthylium) $+ X^-$ $\underset{\bar{X} = \bar{C}l,\ \bar{O}H,\ CH(COMe)_2^-,\ \text{etc.}}{\overset{\bar{X} = \bar{B}r_3,\ FeCl_4}{\rightleftarrows}}$ XCH ... O (xanthene)

The simplest aromatic oxonium ions which have an acidic centre, and can therefore yield an anhydro-base, are the α- and γ-pyrones. They form salts with acids, and the cations are 2- or 4-hydroxypyrylium ions.[119] They are easily deprotonated by weak bases, for

115 R. J. W. LeFevre, R. Roper, and I. H. Reece, *J. Chem. Soc.*, **1959**, 4104.

116 A. Werner, *Ber.*, 1901, **34**, 3301; J. T. Hewitt, *ibid.*, p. 3820

117 M. Gomberg and L. H. Cone, *Ann.*, 1910, **376**, 188.

118 R. Fosse, *Bull. soc. chim.* (France), 1906, **35**, 1005.

119 J. N. Collie and T. Tickle, *J. Chem. Soc.*, 1899, **75**, 710; A. Werner, *Ber.*, 1901, **34**, 3300; A. Hantzsch, *Ber.*, 1919, **52**, 1535; F. Arndt, E. Scholtz and P. Nachtwey, *Ber.*, 1924, **57**, 1903.

example, by water, to give anhydro-bases, that is, the pyrones themselves, which, like most other anhydro-bases, can be represented by betaine or by carbonyl valency structures, and are actually mesomeric between the two. The general relationship may be illustrated thus:

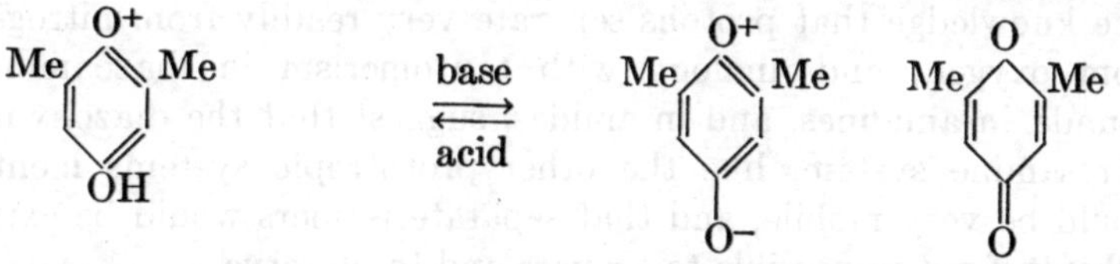

O+ Me Me OH base ⇄ acid O+ Me Me O− O Me Me O

Hydroxypyrylinium ion

Valency structures of a pyrone

The anthocyanins are constituted as polynuclear hydroxypyrylium ions, in particular, as hydroxyflavylium ions, and the derived anhydro-bases. The acidic centres in the cations are for the most part in other rings than that which contains the oxonium centre, so that the anhydro-bases have an inter-nuclear quinonoid character as illustrated below for dracorhodin:

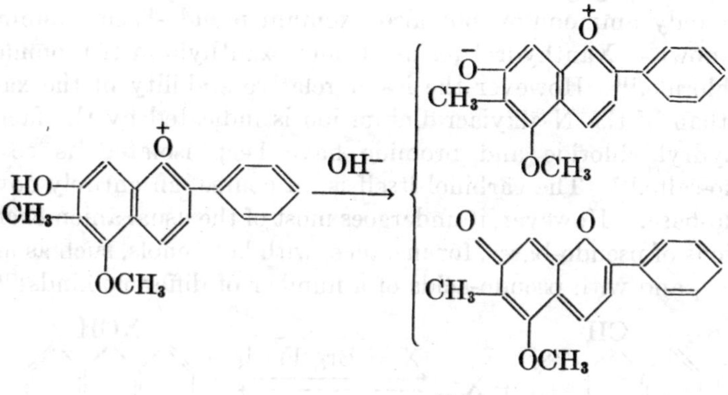

HO— CH_3— $\overset{+}{O}$ OCH_3 $\xrightarrow{OH^-}$ $\overset{-}{O}$— CH_3— $\overset{+}{O}$ OCH_3 ; O= CH_3— O OCH_3

Valency structures of the anhydro-base of dracorhodin

This is a specially simple example: the common anthocyanins, those derived from the aglycones pelargonidin, cyanidin, and delphinidin possess several acidic centres, with the consequence that the anhydro-base is not merely mesomeric, but also prototropic. For example, the anhydro-base of callestephin, that is, pelargonidin 3-glucoside, could exist in three tautomeric forms, differing in the distribution of the phenolic protons, each tautomer being mesomeric between betainoid and quinonoid valency structures as illustrated below. The mobility of the prototropic system is likely to be much too great to permit isolation and preservation of the separate tautomers:

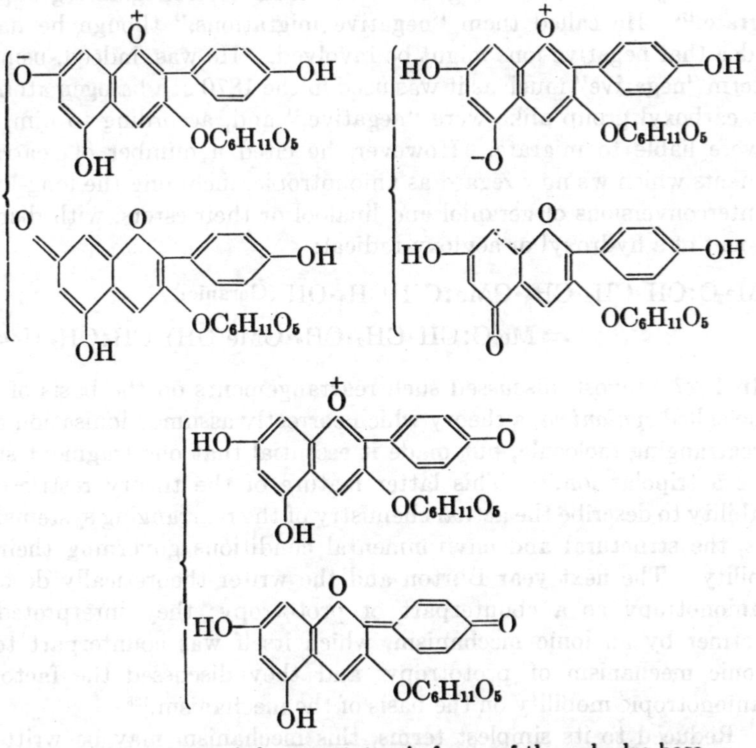

Valency structures of three prototropic forms of the anhydro-base of callestephin

Sulphonium pseudo-basic systems are known. Thioxanthydrol forms sulphonium salts with loss of its hydroxyl group, exactly as xanthydrol forms oxonium salts.[120] 2-Phenylbenzdithiylium salts on basification give a covalent carbinol:[121]

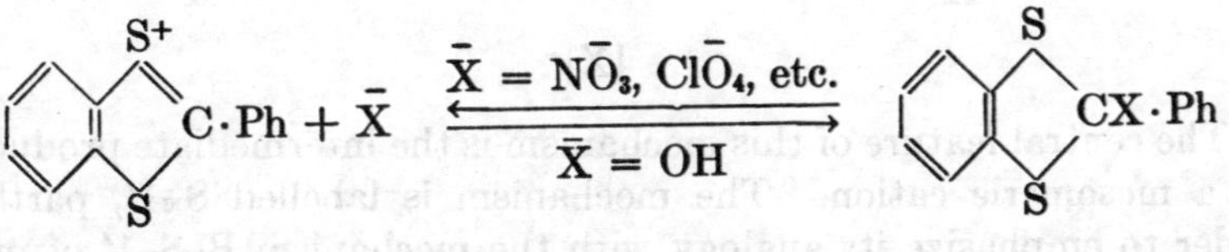

$\bar{X} = NO_3^-, ClO_4^-$, etc.; $\bar{X} = OH$

(48b) Anionotropy: Growth of the Concept: The Unimolecular

[120] A. Werner, *Ber.*, 1901, **34**, 3301; T. P. Hilditch and S. Smiles, *J. Chem. Soc.*, 1911, **99**, 160.

[121] W. R. H. Hurtley and S. Smiles, *J. Chem. Soc.*, **1926**, 1821

Mechanism:[122]—In 1922 Gillet directed attention to the formal similarity of some rearrangements in which electronegative groups migrate.[123] He called them "negative migrations," though he had no idea that negative ions might be involved. He was, indeed, using the term "negative" much as it was used in the 1870's: a halogen atom and a carboxyl group alike were "negative," and, according to him, both were liable to migrate. However, he cited a number of rearrangements which we now regard as anionotropic, including the long-known interconversions of geraniol and linalool or their esters, with displacement of a hydroxyl or acyloxy-radical:

$$Me_2C{:}CH{\cdot}CH_2{\cdot}CH_2{\cdot}CMe{:}CH{\cdot}CH_2{\cdot}OH \text{ (Geraniol)}$$

$$\rightleftarrows Me_2C{:}CH{\cdot}CH_2{\cdot}CH_2{\cdot}CMe(OH){\cdot}CH{:}CH_2 \text{ (Linalool)}$$

In 1927 Prévost discussed such rearrangements on the basis of what he called *synionism*, a theory which correctly assumed ionisation of the rearranging molecule, but made it essential that one fragment should be a tripolar ion.[124] This latter feature of the theory restricted its ability to describe the actual chemistry of the rearranging systems, that is, the structural and environmental conditions governing their mobility. The next year Burton and the writer theoretically described anionotropy as a counterpart of prototropy; they interpreted the former by an ionic mechanism, which itself was counterpart to the ionic mechanism of prototropy; and they discussed the factors of anionotropic mobility on the basis of the mechanism.[125]

Reduced to its simplest terms, this mechanism may be written as follows: it is formulated for the three-carbon system, since this is the only one yet studied in any detail:

$$\underset{X}{\overset{|}{C}}\text{—}C\text{=}C \rightleftarrows \begin{matrix}[C\text{—}C\text{—}C]^+\\ \\ [X]^-\end{matrix} \rightleftarrows C\text{=}C\text{—}\underset{X}{\overset{|}{C}} \qquad (S_N1')$$

The central feature of this mechanism is the intermediate production of a mesomeric cation. The mechanism is labelled S_N1', partly in order to emphasize its analogy with the mechanism $B\text{–}S_E1'$ of proto-

[122] An extensive review of the subject of anionotropy has been given by P. B. D. de la Mare in "Molecular Rearrangements," Editor P. de Mayo, Interscience, New York, 1963, Chap. 2.

[123] A. Gillet, *Bull. soc. chim.* (Belges), 1922, **31**, 366.

[124] C. Prévost, *Compt. rend.*, 1927, **185**, 132.

[125] H. Burton and C. K. Ingold, *J. Chem. Soc.*, **1928**, 904.

tropy, which involves a mesomeric anion; and there is another reason, which is as follows. Obviously, the mechanism would not be essentially different if, after a particular anion has separated, another anion, possibly one of a different kind, returned to the system. If the new anion returned to where the old one came from, the total process would be a unimolecular nucleophilic substitution, and we should label it S_N1. If the new anion returned to the other end of the mesomeric cation, it would seem natural to consider the resulting substitution with rearrangement as a derivative form of the non-rearranging substitution, and so to label it S_N1'. In either event, it would be illogical to exclude from the designation given the special case in which the anion returning to the system is identical in kind with that eliminated. In other words, the anion X^- in the above scheme is to be regarded as representing a general anion, whose identity may or may not be altered in different parts of the total process. With these generalisations in mind, we give the ionic mechanism of anionotropic rearrangement the label S_N1'.

The above mechanism was originally advanced on the basis of four arguments:[126] others were adduced later. First, for a fixed three-carbon system and a variable migrating group, mobility increases markedly with the stability of the latter as an anion. It was already known that geraniol and linalool can be interconverted in water only at temperatures near 200°, whereas geranyl acetate and linalyl acetate are interconverted at much lower temperatures in acetic anhydride. It was found that the nearly irreversible conversions of 1-phenylallyl to cinnamyl (3-phenylallyl) compounds,

$$\mathrm{Ph\cdot CH(X)\cdot CH{:}CH_2 \rightarrow Ph\cdot CH{:}CH\cdot CH_2(X)}$$

were difficult to realise with the alcohols (as distinct from their conjugate acids), easy to observe with the acetates, and so facile with the bromides that the less stable isomer could not be isolated: mobility followed the order (X=)Br>OAc>OH.

Secondly, for a variable three-carbon system and a fixed migrating group, namely, acetoxyl, mobility was markedly increased by structural modifications which could increase the supply of electrons to the centre from which the migrating group was required to separate. Thus starting from the 1-phenylallyl system formulated above (X=OAc), mobility was increased by a *p*-methyl, and much more by a *p*-chloro-substituent. It was greatly reduced if a phenyl group was replaced by a methyl group. Mobility accorded with the following se-

[126] H. Burton, and C. K. Ingold, *loc. cit.*; H. Burton, *J. Chem. Soc.*, **1928**, 1650; C. K. Ingold, *Ann. Repts. on Progress Chem.* (Chem. Soc. London), **1928**, **25**, 127.

quence of groups terminally attached to the three-carbon system:[127] $p\text{-ClC}_6\text{H}_4 \gg p\text{-MeC}_6\text{H}_4 > \text{C}_6\text{H}_5 \gg \text{Me} > \text{H}$.

Thirdly, the effects of solvents and catalysts could easily be understood on the basis of the ionic mechanism. In the absence of significant catalysis by solutes, the above-written conversion of 1-phenylallyl acetate (X = OAc) into cinnamyl acetate took place in a series of solvents at rates agreeing in order with the dielectric constants of the solvents: benzonitrile > acetic anhydride > chlorobenzene > *p*-xylene. The typical solute catalysis of anionotropy was a general catalysis by strong acids, as by H_2SO_4 or HBr, or by the solvated hydrogen ion; and its effect was more pronounced the more basic the mobile group, for example, large for alcohols and small for esters. The following example, due to J. W. Cook,[128] brings out the opposition of prototropy and anionotropy in relation to catalysis. The central structure written below is capable of two alternative isomerisations, one anionotropic and the other prototropic. For the alcohol of the series, its methyl ether, and its acetate (X = OH, OMe, OAc), the anionotropic conversions were realised: they were catalysed by strong acids. For the alcohol (X = OH), the prototropic conversion was observed: it occurred under catalysis by strong alkali:

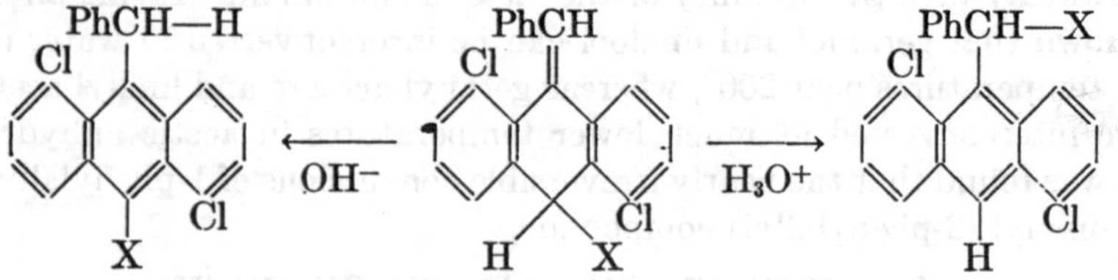

PhCH—H, Cl, Cl, X ⟵ (OH^-) — PhCH, Cl, Cl, H X — (H_3O^+) ⟶ PhCH—X, Cl, Cl, H

Fourthly, Burton showed that the isomerisation of 1-phenylallyl *p*-nitrobenzoate to cinnamyl *p*-nitrobenzoate, in solvents such as benzonitrile or acetic anhydride, could be largely diverted into a non-isomeric substitution with rearrangement by the introduction of tetramethylammonium acetate. The interpretation offered was as follows:

$$\text{PhCH(X)}\cdot\text{CH:CH}_2 \rightarrow [\text{Ph}\cdot\text{CH}\text{—}\text{CH}\text{—}\text{CH}_2]^+ + \begin{matrix}\bar{\text{X}} \\ \text{Y}^-\end{matrix} \longrightarrow \begin{cases}\text{PhCH:CH}\cdot\text{CH}_2\text{(X)} \\ \text{PhCH:CH}\cdot\text{CH}_2\text{(Y)}\end{cases}$$

$$\text{X} = \text{O}\cdot\text{CO}\cdot\text{C}_6\text{H}_4\cdot\text{NO}_2\text{-p};\ \text{Y} = \text{O}\cdot\text{CO}\cdot\text{CH}_3$$

[127] Other orders have since been obtained for acid-catalysed isomerisations of substituted allyl alcohols, but, of course, different alcohols yield their conjugate acids to different equilibrium extents, so that the mobility comparison is in this case not straightforward.

[128] J. W. Cook, *J. Chem. Soc.*, **1928**, 2798.

Burton subsequently confirmed by rate comparisons that the diverted reaction was not a step-wise rearrangement and substitution, and must therefore be simultaneous with the undiverted isomerisation.[129]

The conjugative mechanism of electron supply, by which ortho- or para-halogen in an aryl carbinyl compound promotes mobility in some of the above examples, is a reminder that the phenomena of pseudo-basicity and anionotropy merge into each other. Two anionotropic carbinols, thus activated by halogen, or by methoxyl, or by some other group (X) having the requisite unshared electrons, can be regarded as pseudo-bases of the same 'onium ion:

$$\left.\begin{array}{c}\overset{+}{X}{=}C_6H_4{=}C{-}C{=}C{-}\\ +\ OH^-\end{array}\right\} \begin{array}{l}\rightleftarrows X{-}C_6H_4{-}\underset{OH}{\underset{|}{C}}{-}C{=}C{-}\\ \rightleftarrows X{-}C_6H_4{-}C{=}C{-}\underset{OH}{\underset{|}{C}}{-}\end{array}$$

The further evidence supporting the S_N1' mechanism, which has been built up since 1928, refers to (1) reaction kinetics in conjunction with the product compositions, including the kinetics of reactions followed by the isotopic tracer method, and (2) to changes in optical activity accompanying rearrangement.

A number of the kinetic studies are directly confirmatory of mechanism. De la Mare and Vernon have shown[130] that the data by Braude, Jones, and Stern[131] for relative rates of the rearrangement

$$RC_6H_4{\cdot}CH(OH){\cdot}CH{:}CHMe \rightarrow RC_6H_4{\cdot}CH{:}CH{\cdot}CHMe(OH)$$

in acidified aqueous ethanol, *viz.*,

R	*p*-OMe	*p*-Me	*m*-Me	H	*p*-F	*p*-Cl	*m*-Cl
Rel. rate	105	9	1.2	1	0.8	0.22	0.17

correlate very closely with values for the kinetic effect of the same substituents in unimolecular nucleophilic substitutions in an aromatic side-chain. Vernon's data[132] for effects of substituents on the solvolysis rates of allyl chlorides in aqueous ethanol or in formic acid provide, as de la Mare and he point out[130] using the data in Table 48-1, a

[129] H. Burton, *J. Chem. Soc.*, **1934, 1268.**

[130] P. B. D. de la Mare and C. A. Vernon, "Studies in Chemical Structure and Mechanism," Editor J. H. Ridd, Methuen, London, 1966, Chap. 2.

[131] E. A. Braude, E. R. H. Jones, and E. S. Stern, *J. Chem. Soc.*, 1946, 396.

[132] C. A. Vernon, *J. Chem. Soc.*, 1954, 423.

Table 48-1.—Relative Rates of Solvolysis of Allyl Chlorides (de la Mare and Vernon).

	H	Cl	*t*-Bu	Me	Ph	$\alpha\alpha$-Me_2
α-............	1	—	—	5900	—	$\sim 8 \times 10^7$
β-............	1	—	—	0.5	—	$\gamma\gamma$-Me_2
trans-γ-........	1	3.1	2300	3600	$\sim 5\times 10^5$	$\sim 1.5 \times 10^7$

clear picture of the need for electron release towards the α- or γ-carbon atom.

A different type of kinetic investigation establishes the S_N1' character of the acid-catalysed rearrangement of 1-phenylallyl alcohol to cinnamyl (3-phenylallyl) alcohol. The rearrangement was conducted in oxygen-18 water by Bunton, Dahn, and Pocker,[133] and also by Goering and Dilgren.[134] The common result was that the oxygen in the formed cinnamyl alcohol came entirely or almost entirely from the ^{18}O water, whilst the oxygen of unconverted 1-phenylallyl alcohol became partly exchanged with the oxygen-18. The relative rates of oxygen exchange and rearrangement showed that 60% of the formed carbonium ions went back to the original alcohol:

$$CH_2{:}CH\cdot CHPh\cdot \overset{+}{O}H_2 \rightleftharpoons [CH_2\!\!-\!\!-CH\!\!-\!\!-CHPh]^{+} \rightarrow H_2\overset{+}{O}\cdot CH_2\cdot CH{:}CHPh$$

The basic evidence of mechanism provided by the study of changes of optical activity in anionotropic rearrangement was provided by Kenyon and his coworkers. They thus showed the generality of mechanism S_N1' by demonstrating in numerous cases its expected steric course of racemisation when an asymmetric three-carbon system was the seat of the change. It will be convenient to consider the evidence relating to non-isomeric and isomeric rearrangements in turn.

As to non-isomeric rearrangements, the basic observation is that optical activity, dependent on asymmetry which would be destroyed by ionisation, is actually lost in the rearrangement process. In a symmetrical example, such as the solvolytic substitution of 1, 3-dimethylallyl hydrogen phthalate in formic acid, or acetic acid, or methyl alcohol, it is impossible to prove by chemical methods that a rearrangement has occurred:

$$\underset{\displaystyle O\cdot CO\cdot C_6H_4\cdot CO_2H}{\overset{\displaystyle MeCH\cdot CH{:}CHMe}{|}} \rightarrow \underset{\displaystyle OR}{\overset{\displaystyle MeCH\cdot CH{:}CHMe}{|}} \equiv \underset{\displaystyle OR}{\overset{\displaystyle MeCH{:}CH\cdot CHMe}{|}}$$

[133] C. A. Bunton, H. Dahn, and Y. Pocker, *Chem. and Ind.*, **1958,** 1516.
[134] H. L. Goering and R. E. Dilgren, *J. Am. Chem. Soc.*, **1960,** 82, 5744.

But Kenyon and his collaborators showed,[135] not only that the solvolytic product was completely or very nearly completely racemised, but also that original ester, recovered from an incomplete reaction, was largely racemised, just as though most of it had once been ionised. It is significant that with the best ionising solvents, such as formic acid, the activity of the product was vanishing, while it was only with poorly ionising solvents, such as *n*-butyl alcohol, that racemisation was appreciably incomplete (greatest observed activity 9%). These small residual activities undoubtedly arise because the main reaction, S_N1, S_N1', is accompanied by a small amount of the side reaction, S_N2, that is, bimolecular substitution without rearrangement. The sign of the residual activity always corresponded to an inverted configuration at the original asymmetric centre. Furthermore, for the solvolyses of 1-*n*-propyl-3-methylallyl chloride, and of the corresponding hydrogen phthalate, in the same solvents, it was proved[136] that the residual activity found in some cases (maximum 2%) was definitely due to substitution without rearrangement, because it was lost on hydrogenation, a process which would destroy asymmetry in the unrearranged structure (by producing a second propyl group), but not in the rearranged structure.

As to isomeric rearrangements, the main group of examples[137] consists in the conversion of four 1-phenyl-3-methylallyl compounds, namely, the alcohol in acid solution (presumably the active entity is the conjugate acid of the alcohol), the acetate, the *p*-nitrobenzoate, and the hydrogen phthalate, into their 1-methyl-3-phenyl-isomerides. The general result was that, when the isomerisations were allowed to proceed in dilute solution in solvents such as aqueous acid for the alcohol, acetic acid for the acetate, chloroform for the *p*-nitrobenzoate, and carbon disulphide for the hydrogen phthalate (many other solvents were also employed), the products were inactive or nearly so, with one notable exception, the hydrogen phthalate, which showed retentions of activity up to 58%.

This last result may disclose the operation of another mechanism to which we shall come in Section **48d**.

(48c) The Bimolecular Mechanism of Anionotropy.—The idea of anionotropic change by a bimolecular mechanism, S_N2', which, on the one hand, is counterpart to the bimolecular mechanism $B\text{–}S_E2'$ of

[135] M. P. Balfe, H. W. Hills, J. Kenyon, H. Phillips, and B. C. Platt, *J. Chem. Soc.*, **1942**, 556.

[136] C. L. Arcus and J. Kenyon, *J. Chem. Soc.*, **1938**, 1912.

[137] J. Kenyon, S. M. Partridge, and H. Phillips, *J. Chem. Soc.*, **1937**, 207.

prototropy, and, on the other, is a derivative form of bimolecular nucleophilic substitution S_N2, was first suggested by Hughes.[138]

$$\underset{X}{C}-C{=}C \quad X^- \rightleftarrows X^- \quad C{=}C-\underset{X}{C} \qquad (S_N2')$$

As before, we have to think of X^- as a general anion, so that the two X's appearing in this equation may or may not be chemically identical.

Consideration of this mechanism is relevant to the evidence derived from the study of kinetics and product compositions. The earlier attempts to detect the bimolecular mechanism of rearrangement by this means led (*a*) to the production of new evidence for the unimolecular mechanism, and (*b*) to the conclusion that bimolecular rearrangement is relatively unimportant in the systems studied. The following illustration will suffice.

One carefully examined group of reactions[139] was the non-isomeric conversions of 1-methylallyl and of crotyl (3-methylallyl) chlorides (which, though interconvertible, are stable enough to be studied separately) into 1-methylallyl and crotyl ethyl ethers, by interaction with ethyl alcohol containing sodium ethoxide: the latter was introduced either in such small concentration as to give first-order kinetics, or in such large concentration as to secure second-order kinetics. It was found that either chloride, by first-order substitution, gave a similar mixture of ethers, as would be expected if, in accordance with the unimolecular mechanisms S_N1 and S_N1', the substitutions without and with rearrangement go through a common intermediate ion. But by second-order substitution, each chloride yielded only its own unrearranged ether. In short, mechanisms S_N1, S_N1', and S_N2 were observed, but not mechanism S_N2':

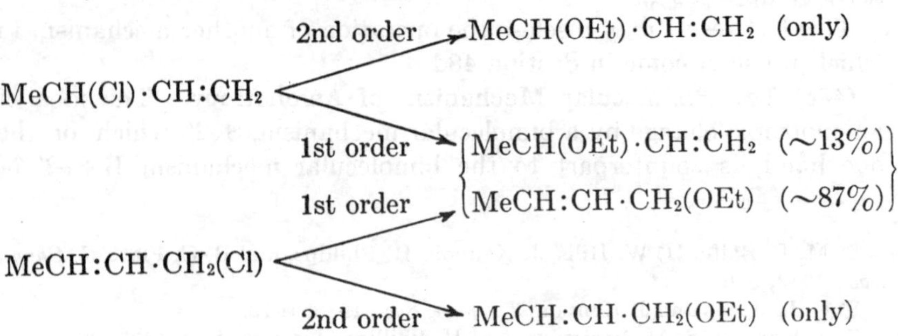

[138] E. D. Hughes, *Trans. Faraday Soc.*, 1938, **34**, 194.

[139] A. G. Catchpole and E. D. Hughes, *Trans. Faraday Soc.*, 1941, **37**, 629; *J. Chem. Soc.*, **1948**, 4.

Substitutions by the S_N2' mechanism have been claimed in which the entering substituent is derived from a pseudo-acid. Cinnamyl alcohol has been converted through its esters to 1-phenylallylacetone by treatment with ethyl acetoacetate and basic catalysts, and 1-phenylallyl alcohol has been similarly converted to cinnamylacetone.[140] 1-Methylallyl chloride has been converted by treatment with ethyl malonate and sodium ethoxide, partly into the normal substitution product, but partly also into the rearranged product, ethyl crotylmalonate.[141] 1-Ethylallyl choride has been shown to undergo similar reactions. However, as Dewar pointed out[142]—his argument has been contested, but not refuted—such experiments prove nothing, because a pseudo-acid has two reactive centres, and the product of an S_N2 O-allylation of the pseudo-acid, followed by a Claisen rearrangement (Section 49) would be the same as the product of an S_N2' C-allylation. Other similarly insubstantial claims have been made.

The reason for the difficulties which have attended the establishment of mechanism S_N2' is, not that it does not exist, but that, under conditions conducive to bimolecular substitution, it is usually masked by the much more rapid reaction S_N2. Such masking can be avoided by the following method.[143] The allyl compound, for example, 1-methylallyl bromide, is allowed to interact under conditions leading only to bimolecular substitution with a supplied anion, for example, radiobromide ion, identical but for an isotopic distinction with the anion that could be given by the allyl compound. This ensures that every individual molecular act of substitution by mechanism S_N2 will, for all ordinary chemical purposes, replace the original molecule by an identical one; so that the original substance never becomes used up by mechanism S_N2, but continues to be available indefinitely for the observation, at any necessary temperature, of isomerisation by mechanism S_N2'. The kinetics of the latter reaction can be controlled, and its rate determined by ordinary chemical means; and this S_N2' rate can be compared with the rate of the also kinetically controlled S_N2 exchange, as determined by radio-chemical means. This programme has been carried through by England and Hughes for the reactions

[140] F. M. Carroll, *J. Chem. Soc.*, **1940**, 266; C. L. Wilson, *Trans. Faraday Soc.*, 1941, **37**, 631.

[141] R. E. Kepner, S. Winstein, and W. G. Young, *J. Am. Chem. Soc.*, 1949, **71**, 115.

[142] M. J. S. Dewar, *Bull. soc. chim.* (France), 1951, **18**, p. C43.

[143] P. B. D. de la Mare, B. D. England, L. Fowden, E. D. Hughes, and C. K. Ingold, *J. chim. phys.*, 1948, **45**, 236; B. D. England and E. D. Hughes, *Nature*, 1951, **168**, 1002; B. D. England, *J. Chem. Soc.*, **1955**, 1615.

TABLE 48-2.—RATE CONSTANTS AND ARRHENIUS PARAMETERS OF BIMOLECULAR BROMINE EXCHANGE (S_N2) AND BIMOLECULAR ISOMERISATION (S_N2') OF ALLYL BROMIDES WITH LITHIUM BROMIDE IN ACETONE (ENGLAND AND HUGHES). k_2 and A_2 are in sec.$^{-1}$ mole^{-1} l., and E_A is in kcal. mole^{-1}.

Bromide	Reaction	$10^6\,k_2(25°)$	$\log_{10} A_2$	E_A
1-Methylallyl	S_N2	879	9.06	16.5
	S_N2'	14.9	9.40	19.4
Crotyl	S_N2	141000	9.93	14.7
	S_N2'	5	~9	~19

both of 1-methylallyl bromide and of crotyl bromide with lithium bromide in acetone. Their kinetic data are in Table 48-2.

It can be seen that both of the isomeric halides undergo both bimolecular reactions. But for 1-methylallyl bromide the S_N2 reaction goes 60 times faster than the S_N2' process, while for crotyl bromide the S_N2 exchange proceeds 28,000 times faster than the S_N2' isomerisation. It is easy to understand why the S_N2' mechanism is difficult to observe when a concomitant S_N2 substitution can mask it. It is also clear that the difference in the two rate-ratios S_N2/S_N2' arises mainly from the difference of S_N2 rates. Thus the considerable factor by which the S_N2' process is less unfavourable to observation for 1-methylallyl than for crotyl bromide can be attributed chiefly to a local effect of the 1-methyl substituent in repressing the local S_N2 reaction. A larger 1-substituent should do this better, and a large enough 1-substituent should knock out this S_N2 reaction altogether. A local polar effect might help, but such effects are somewhat weak in S_N2 substitutions. This general picture has been well verified by de la Mare and Vernon and their collaborators. Allylidene chloride (1-chloro-allyl chloride), on treatment with ethoxide ion in ethanol, underwent a second-order reaction to form about equal amounts of the S_N2 and S_N2' ethoxy-products, the former of which underwent, as should be expected, further conversion to an acetal:[144]

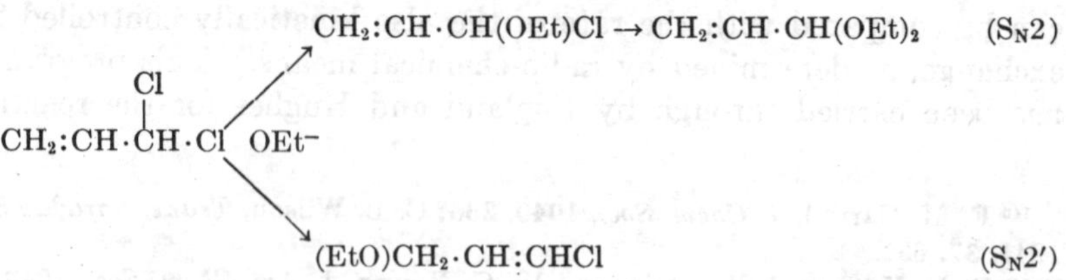

[144] P. B. D. de la Mare, E. D. Hughes, and C. A. Vernon, *Nature*, 1952, 169, 672; P. B. D. de la Mare and C. A. Vernon, *J. Chem. Soc.*, 1952, 3325.

.-*t*-Butylallyl chloride, on similar treatment, gave only the S_N2' ethoxy somer:[145]

$$CH_2{:}CH\cdot\underset{}{\overset{t\text{-Bu}}{\overset{|}{C}H}}\cdot Cl \xrightarrow{OEt^-} (EtO)CH_2\cdot CH{:}CH\cdot Bu^t \qquad (S_N2')$$

De la Mare and Vernon have given several further examples of the substantial or complete take-over of second-order substitution by the rearranging mechanism S_N2', when steps are taken to reduce by substitution the rate of the competing mechanism S_N2.[146]

(48d) The Internal Mechanism of Anionotropy.—One of the early suggestions concerning this mechanism arose out of the observations of Kenyon and his collaborators[137] on the changes of optical activity accompanying anionotropic rearrangement. As mentioned in Section **48b**, they noted one exception to the rule of essentially total racemisation in rearrangements of 1-phenyl-3-methylallyl esters. The exception applied to the acid-ester of phthallic acid, and the suggestion was made[147] that the free carboxyl group is involved in its isomerisation, acting as an internal acid catalyst in assisting the fission of the old CO bond, and also as a nucleophilic reagent in forming the new one:

```
R—CH——CH═CH—R'        R—CH═CH——CH—R'
  |                                   |
  O        H—O      →       O—H       O
  |          |              |         |
  CO—C6H4—CO                CO—C6H4—CO
```

This type of internal mechanism has been labelled S_Ni', because it is related to the substitution mechanism S_Ni—internal substitution leading to group replacement on a single carbon atom (Section **33h**)—just as mechanism S_N2' is related to S_N2, or S_N1' to S_N1.

Another line of development arose from the study of the reactions in which a substituted allyl alcohol is converted by hydrogen or phos-

[145] P. B. D. de la Mare, E. D. Hughes, P. C. Merriman, L. Pichat, and C. A. Vernon, *J. Chem. Soc.*, **1958**, 2513.

[146] P. B. D. de la Mare and C. A. Vernon, *J. Chem. Soc.*, **1952**, 3331, 3628; **1953**, 3555.

[147] E. D. Hughes, *Trans. Faraday Soc.*, 1941, **37**, 725; A. G. Catchpole, E. D. Hughes, and C. K. Ingold, *J. Chem. Soc.*, **1948**, 13. The suggestion applies essentially to rearrangements in solution. Kenyon and his coworkers have recorded several examples of retentions of optical activity during anionotropic rearrangements of undiluted substances, sometimes with adventitious catalysts (see, for example, R. S. Airs, M. P. Balfe, and J. Kenyon, *J. Chem. Soc.*, **1942**, 18), but the mechanisms involved in such conditions are far from obvious.

phorus halides or by thionyl chloride into either or both of the anionotropic halides. These reactions of 1- and 3-ethylallyl alcohol were studied by Meisenheimer and Link,[148] and of 1- and 3-methylallyl alcohol by Young and Lane.[149] With hydrogen and phosphorus halides the results can be understood, as Young and Lane recognised, on the basis of mechanisms S_N1 and S_N1', which proceed through a common carbonium ion, together with mechanism S_N2, which involves attack by halide ion on a hydrogen-bond complex or ester (Section **33j**). Just as with saturated alcohols, so with these allyl alcohols, the presence of pyridine during the reactions with phosphorus halides increases the prominence of bimolecular processes; and thus, mechanism S_N2' being unimportant, there is a facilitation of mechanism S_N2, and a reduction in the amount of rearrangement. However, with thionyl chloride, which brings mechanism S_Ni into prominence in the reactions of saturated alcohols (Section **33h**), Meisenheimer and Link obtained an *increase* in the amount of rearrangement; and this worked in both directions with the result that their primary alcohol gave mainly the secondary chloride, and their secondary alcohol mainly the primary chloride. In solvent ether the cross conversions are practically quantitative, as Young and his coworkers showed subsequently.[150] Evidently rearrangement was inherent in the mechanism of substitution, independently of the relative stabilities of the products. As Roberts, Winstein, and Young have noted,[151] this seems rather a clear indication of the rearrangement of a first-formed chlorosulphinic ester in accordance with mechanism S_Ni':

$$\begin{array}{l} \text{R—CH—CH═CH—R}' \\ \quad | \\ \quad \text{O—SO—Cl} \end{array} \rightarrow \text{SO}_2 + \begin{array}{l} \text{R—CH═CH—CH—R}' \\ \qquad\qquad\qquad | \\ \qquad\qquad\qquad \text{Cl} \end{array} \qquad (S_Ni')$$

Goering and his collaborators have claimed[152] that optical activity is preserved, as well as geometrical isomerism in the *cyclo*hexene series, when the conversion to chlorides by thionyl chloride in ether is applied to *cis*- and *trans*-5-methyl*cyclo*hex-2-en-1-ol:

[148] J. Meisenheimer and J. Link, *Ann.*, 1930, **479**, 211.

[149] W. G. Young and J. F. Lane, *J. Am. Chem. Soc.*, 1937, **59**, 2051; 1938, **60**, **847**.

[150] F. F. Caserio, C. E. Dennis, R. H. de Wolfe, and W. G. Young, *J. Am. Chem. Soc.*, 1955, **77**, 4182.

[151] J. D. Roberts, W. G. Young, and S. Winstein, *J. Am. Chem. Soc.*, 1942, **64**, **2157**.

[152] H. L. Goering, T. D. Newitt, and E. F. Silversmith, *J. Am. Chem. Soc.*, 1955, **77**, 4042.

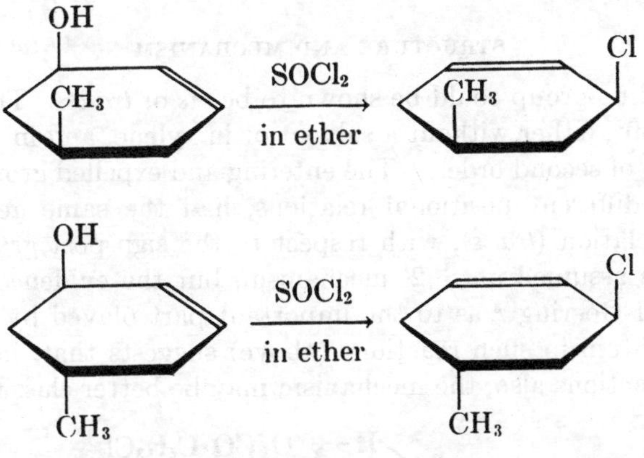

$$\text{(cis-5-methylcyclohex-2-enol)} \xrightarrow[\text{in ether}]{SOCl_2} \text{(chloride)}$$

$$\text{(trans-5-methylcyclohex-2-enol)} \xrightarrow[\text{in ether}]{SOCl_2} \text{(chloride)}$$

This is as expected for mechanism S_Ni', and demonstrates the essentially configuration-retaining stereochemistry of that mechanism:

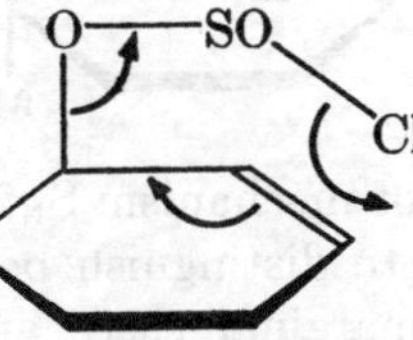

$$\text{O—SO—Cl (cyclic transition state)}$$

Another type of example of mechanism S_Ni' may be seen in the observation of Young, Webb, and Goering that 1-methylallyl chloride, on treatment with diethylamine in solvent benzene, gives crotyldiethylamine.[153] This reaction was originally discussed as an instance of mechanism S_N2', but the amino-hydrogen atom appears to be necessary to the mechanism, and hence the mechanism is better regarded as involving a cyclic transition state, and accordingly is better classified as of S_Ni' type:

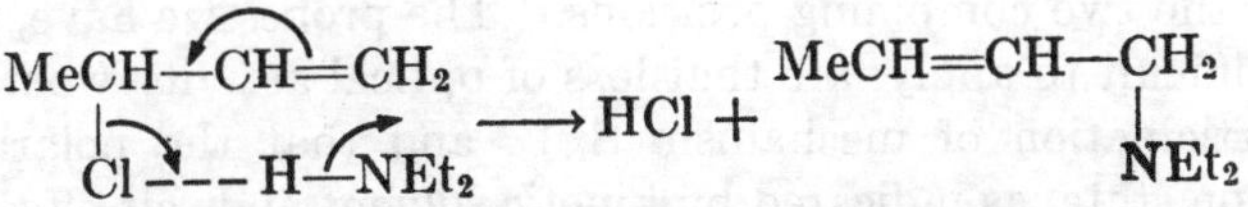

$$\begin{matrix} \text{MeCH—CH=CH}_2 \\ | \\ \text{Cl - - H—NEt}_2 \end{matrix} \longrightarrow \text{HCl} + \begin{matrix} \text{MeCH=CH—CH}_2 \\ | \\ \text{NEt}_2 \end{matrix}$$

Stork and White have demonstrated[154] the configuration-retaining stereochemistry of this reaction, using piperidine as the substituting agent and allyl-type *cyclo*hexenyl esters as the anionotropic system. A methyl or higher alkyl group (R) was present, to retard S_N2 substitution, and also to act as a stereochemical sign-post, with respect to which the expelled group (X = 2,6-dichlorobenzoate) and the enter-

[153] W. G. Young, I. D. Webb, and H. L. Goering, *J. Am. Chem. Soc.*, 1951, **73**, 1076.

[154] G. Stork and W. N. White, *J. Am. Chem. Soc.*, 1953, **75**, 4119; 1956, **78**, 4609.

ing piperidino-group could be shown to be *cis* or *trans*. The reactions went at 130°, either without a solvent or in xylene, and in xylene were kinetically of second order. The entering and expelled groups, though they had different positional relations, had the same geometrically isomeric relation (*trans*), with respect to the sign-post group. Stork and White assumed an S_N2' mechanism, but the evidence of Young, Webb, and Goering[153] as to the important part played by the amino-hydrogen atom in such reactions (above) suggests that, in Stork and White's reactions also, the mechanism may be better classified as S_Ni':

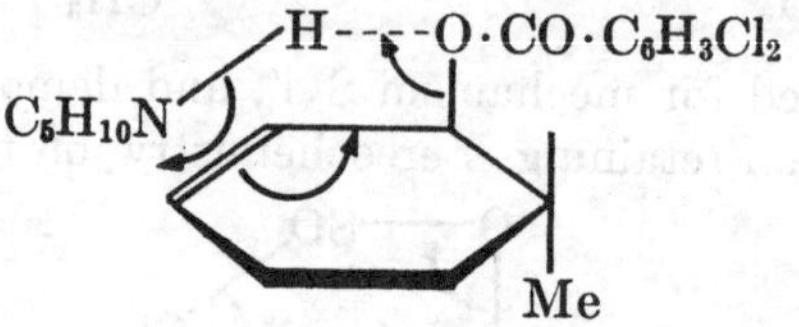

H---O·CO·$C_6H_3Cl_2$

$C_5H_{10}N$

Me

Though the diagnosis of mechanism S_N2' is usually fairly clear, it is sometimes very difficult to distinguish between mechanism S_N1' and mechanism S_Ni'. The marginal cases arise when a reaction which indubitably goes by mechanism S_N1' in dissociating solvents, is put into such low-dielectric solvents, that ions, if formed, recombine, largely or perhaps even totally without dissociating. They may then, after having been bound together only by fluctuating, ill-directed, but still strong electrostatic forces, recombine in part with rearrangement. Alternatively, the rearranged product might arise in mechanism S_Ni' by the formation, in the transition state, of a cycle of well-directed bonds having some covalent character, by which the mobile group bridges the two combining positions. The probes we have, which are often difficult to apply, are that loss of optical activity would point to the participation of mechanism S_N1', and that the polarity of the transition state, as indicated by kinetic solvent and salt effects, should be higher in this mechanism than in mechanism S_Ni'.

A case belonging to this nebulous region of mechanism was described in 1951 by Young, Winstein, and Goering.[155] The solvolysis of 1,1-dimethylallyl chloride in acetic acid (which has a dielectric constant of about 6), was accompanied by a considerable isomerisation to 3,3-dimethylallyl chloride; and this isomerisation did not involve the kinetic participation of external halide ions. The phenomenon was shown to depend on the acetic acid solvent in an essential way: it was not reproduced in anything like the same degree in solvent ethanol.

[155] W. G. Young, S. Winstein, and H. L. Goering, *J. Am. Chem. Soc.*, 1951, **73**, 1958.

Goering and his coworkers have followed up the matter with a study[156] of the solvolysis in acetic acid and in ethanol of *cis*- and *trans*-5-methyl*cyclo*hex-2-en-1-yl chlorides (the alcohols are formulated on p. 859). They gave mixtures of stable *cis*- and *trans*-products of the same composition; but optical activity was lost faster than *cis-trans*-specificity. A study[157] of the isomerisation in acetonitrile of *cis*- and *trans*-5-methyl*cyclo*hex-2-en-1-ol hydrogen phthalates (alcohols formulated on p. 859) again showed that optical activity was lost faster (very much faster in this case) than *cis-trans* specificity; and that added 3-nitrophthalate ion intervened in the reaction to give nitrophthalate esters. All this means that mechanism S_N1' is involved, and that, in terms of this mechanism, a larger degree of counter-ion separation is needed to allow the *cyclo*hexene ring to turn over relatively to the anion than is required to allow the anion to reach the other end of the three-carbon system on the same side of the *cyclo*hexene ring (so producing racemisation). But, of course, the question of whether, in order to achieve this last result, the ions have really to be formed, or whether the bridging of the three-carbon system can occur covalently before the ions are formed, remains unanswered. The answer may even be different for the chloride, and for the hydrogen phthalates, since in the latter the mobile group is much better adapted for bridging in the manner suggested by Hughes (p. 857).

(48e) Anionotropic Equilibria.—Such equilibria can, of course, be considered quite independently of the mechanism of rearrangement. The equilibria between cinnamyl and 1-phenylallyl isomers always contain undetectably little of the latter:

$$(100\%)\ \mathrm{Ph\cdot CH{:}CH\cdot CH_2X \rightleftarrows Ph\cdot CHX\cdot CH{:}CH_2}\ (0\%)$$

This would be expected on any reasonable estimate of the extra stability which the cinnamyl isomers derive from the phenyl-to-vinyl conjugation they contain. (Taking the free-energy difference as 6 kcal. /mole, the 1-phenylallyl/cinnamyl ratio at ordinary temperature would be $e^{-6000/600} = e^{-10} = 10^{-4.3} = 1/20{,}000$.) The equilibria between crotyl and 1-methylallyl chlorides, and between the corresponding bromides, are in a corresponding direction, but are so much less extreme that the proportions of the isomerides are easily measurable. The exact proportions depend on the halide, the solvent, and the temperature, but they lie in the neighbourhood indicated below:

[156] H. L. Goering, T. D. Newitt, and E. F. Silversmith, *J. Am. Chem. Soc.*, 1955, **77**, 5026.

[157] H. L. Goering, J. P. Blanchard, and E. F. Silversmith, *J. Am. Chem. Soc.*, 1954, **76**, 5409.

$$(75\text{–}85\%)\ CH_3{\cdot}CH{:}CH{\cdot}CH_2X \rightleftarrows CH_3{\cdot}CHX{\cdot}CH{:}CH_2\ (15\text{–}25\%)$$

Here, the main energetic distinction between the isomers will be one of methyl hyperconjugation, and it can at least be said that our scant knowledge of such energy factors is not inconsistent with the equilibrium data. (Allowing 1 kcal./mole for the free-energy difference, the equilibrium ratio would be 1/5.)

(49) VALENCY TAUTOMERISM

(49a) The Claisen Rearrangement.—This consists in rearrangements of O-allyl to ortho-allyl derivatives of phenols, and of O-allyl to C-allyl derivatives of keto-enols,[158] including rearrangements of vinyl allyl ethers to allyl-acetaldehydes:[159]

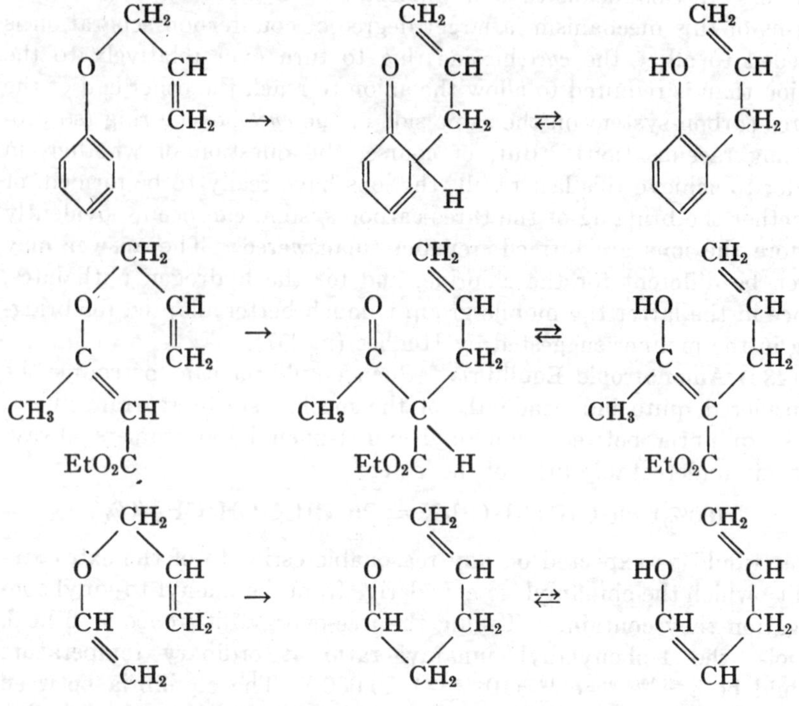

```
    CH2                    CH2                   CH2
  /    \                  //                    //
 O      CH          O     CH          HO      CH
 |      ||          ||    |           |       |
 |      CH2   →     ||    CH2    ⇄    |       CH2
 C6H5 (phenyl)     (cyclohexadienone,   (o-allylphenol)
                    H at ring C)

    CH2                    CH2                   CH2
  /    \                     \\                     \\
 O      CH           O        CH          HO        CH
 |      ||     →     ||       |     ⇄     |         |
 C      CH2          C        CH2         C         CH2
/ \\                / \      /           / \\      /
CH3 CH              CH3 C                CH3  C
    |                  / \                    |
  EtO2C            EtO2C  H                 EtO2C

    CH2                    CH2                   CH2
  /    \                     \\                     \\
 O      CH           O        CH          HO        CH
 |      ||     →     ||       |     ⇄     |         |
 CH     CH2          CH       CH2         CH        CH2
   \\                  \     /              \\     /
    CH2                 CH2                   CH
```

These rearrangements take place on heating the O-allyl compounds to temperatures near 200°, either alone, or in some inert solvent, such as

[158] L. Claisen, *Ber.*, 1912, **45**, 3157; *Ann.*, 1919, **418**, 69; L. Claisen and O. Eisleb, *Ann.*, 1913, **401**, 21; L. Claisen and E. Tietze, *Ber.*, 1925, **58**, 275.

[159] C. D. Hurd and M. A. Pollack, *J. Am. Chem. Soc.*, 1938, **60**, 1905; *J. Org. Chem.*, 1938, **3**, 550.

diphenyl ether or diethylaniline: no catalyst is necessary. In the rearrangements of phenolic ethers, the allyl group moves to an ortho-position, if one is free: in none of the simpler examples for which this is true has any accompanying para-isomerisation been detected.[160]

Allyl migrations of the types indicated, that is, from oxygen to ortho-carbon in a phenol, and from oxygen to carbon in a keto-enol, have been shown, by the use of substituted allyl groups, always to involve the represented 1, 3-reversal of bonding in the allyl group. Thus the O-cinnamyl and O-crotyl ethers of phenol give the ortho-1-phenylallyl and ortho-1-methylallyl substitution products of phenol.[161] The O-cinnamyl derivative of ethyl acetoacetate yields by rearrangement the C-1-phenylallyl derivative of the ester.[162]

As to these rearrangements, the following points have been established. First, they follow first-order kinetics, as has been verified for the conversion of allyl *p*-cresyl ether into *o*-allyl-*p*-methylphenol in solvent diphenyl ether.[163] Furthermore, the gaseous conversion of allyl vinyl ether to allylacetaldehyde is a homogeneous gas reaction of the first order, and the same has been shown for some homologous ethers.[164] This shows that each individual molecular act of rearrangement involves but one molecule. Secondly, when two of the rearrangements are carried out together, each behaves as if it were alone, and no crossed products are formed; thus a mixture of 2-naphthyl allyl ether and phenyl cinnamyl ether, on heating without a solvent, gave only 1-allyl-2-naphthol and ortho-1-phenylallylphenol.[165] It is clear from this that the molecules do not split each into two fragments. Thirdly, the 1,3-reversal of bonding of the allyl group works both ways, and not alone in the direction that might lead to a more stable product: not only does phenyl 3-ethylallyl ether give ortho-1-ethylallylphenol,[166] but also phenyl 1-ethylallyl ether gives ortho-3-ethylallylphenol.[167] This shows that the reversal of bonding in the allyl group is a necessity of the mechanism of rearrangement. Fourthly, optically active 1,3-dimethylallyl phenyl ether has yielded active ortho-1,3-

[160] W. M. Lauer and R. M. Leekly, *J. Am. Chem. Soc.*, 1939, **61**, 3042.

[161] L. Claisen and E. Tietze, *Ber.*, 1925, **58**, 275; 1926, **59**, 2344; C. D. Hurd and F. L. Cohen, *J. Am. Chem. Soc.*, 1931, **53**, 1917.

[162] W. M. Lauer and E. I. Kilburn, *J. Am. Chem. Soc.*, 1937, **59**, 2580.

[163] J. F. Kincaid and D. S. Tarbell, *J. Am. Chem. Soc.*, 1939, **61**, 3085.

[164] F. W. Schuler and G. W. Murphy, *J. Am. Chem. Soc.*, 1950, **72**, 3155; L. Stein and G. W. Murphy, *ibid.*, 1952, **74**, 1041; H. M. Frey and B. M. Pope, *J. Chem. Soc.*, **1966, B**, 209.

[165] C. D. Hurd and L. Schmerling, *J. Am. Chem. Soc.*, 1937, **59**, 107.

[166] C. D. Hurd and M. A. Pollak, *J. Org. Chem.*, 1937, **3**, 550.

[167] W. M. Lauer and W. F Filbert, *J. Am. Chem. Soc.*, 1936, **58**, 1388.

dimethylallylphenol.[168] This result proves that the ortho-bond begins to be formed before the ether-bond is fully broken.

These results make clear that the skeletal rearrangement, which may or may not be succeeded by a prototropic change, is a one-step, unimolecular reaction, proceeding through a cyclic six-atom transition state, in which three alternately situated bonds are concertedly migrating to the remaining three positions, as formulated on page 862.

The further question may be asked as to how polar this transition state is. Apparently it is not very polar. This is shown by many observations to the effect that strongly polar substituents in the aromatic ring make only very moderate differences to the rate of the Claisen rearrangements. Thus, Goering and Jacobson[169] measured the rates of rearrangements in diphenyl ether at 185° of a large number of monosubstituted phenylallyl ethers, containing substituents ranging from accelerating *p*-dimethylamino-, *p*-amino-, and *p*-methoxyl groups to retarding *p*-cyano- and *m*-nitro-groups; and the whole spread of the rates lay within a ratio of 16:1.

Efforts have been made to establish the stereochemistry of the Claisen rearrangement, and in particular to answer the question of whether, in the absence of special structural influences, the chair-like or boat-like conformation of the six-membered ring in the transition state is the more stable, and hence characterises the effective transition state for the rearrangement:

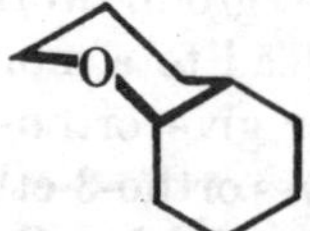

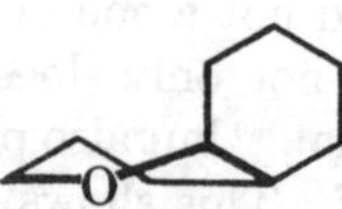

Schematic illustration of chair-like (left) and boat-like (right) conformations which might be adopted in the course of the Claisen rearrangement.

The evidence is not fully conclusive, but appears to favour the chair-like form.[170] This conclusion is indirectly supported by analogy with the Cope rearrangement (Section **49b**), for which the stereochemistry can be, and has been, determined more simply.

Claisen and Eisleb showed that, when an allyl aryl ether having substituents in both ortho-positions is heated alone or in solvents at temperatures such as 200° the allyl group migrates to the para-position.[158] It has been shown by the use of substituted allyl groups that, in con-

[168] E. R. Alexander and R. W. Kluiber, *J. Am. Chem. Soc.*, 1951, **73**, 4304.

[169] H. L. Goering and R. R. Jacobson, *J. Am. Chem. Soc.*, 1958, **80**, 3277.

[170] *Cf.*, *e.g.*, E. N. Marvell and J. L. Stephenson, *J. Org. Chem.*, 1960, **25**, 676; *idem* and J. Ong, *J. Am. Chem. Soc.*, 1965, **87**, 1267.

trast to the 1,3-reversal of bonding which occurs in ortho-migrations, no such reversal occurs in para-migration.[171] The para-migration has been shown to be a first-order reaction.[172] Optically active 1,3-dimethylallyl 2,6-dimethylphenyl ether has been shown to yield an optically active para-rearrangement product.[168]

Hurd and Pollak were the first to have the right idea about the mechanism of these para-migrations, namely, that the first step consists in an ortho-migration to a *cyclo*hexadiene, which, prototropic reversion to a phenol being excluded by the ortho-substitution, suffers further migration of the allyl group, by way of another cyclic transition state, to give the para-alkylated product, at first also in dienone form, which finally undergoes prototropic change to the phenol:[166]

$$\text{O}\cdot\text{CH}_2\cdot\text{CH}:\overset{*}{\text{C}}\text{H}_2 \text{ (2,6-R}_2\text{C}_6\text{H}_3\text{)} \longrightarrow \text{2,6-R}_2\text{-6-}(\overset{*}{\text{C}}\text{H}_2\cdot\text{CH}:\text{CH}_2)\text{-cyclohexa-2,4-dienone} \longrightarrow \text{2,6-R}_2\text{-4-H-4-}(\text{CH}_2\cdot\text{CH}:\overset{*}{\text{C}}\text{H}_2)\text{-cyclohexa-2,5-dienone}$$

$$\rightarrow \text{2,6-R}_2\text{-4-}(\text{CH}_2\cdot\text{CH}:\overset{*}{\text{C}}\text{H}_2)\text{C}_6\text{H}_2\text{OH}$$

One sees how this idea accommodates the absence of allyl reversal in the para-position by the assumption of reversal in each of the two cyclic steps.

This mechanism has been thoroughly established in several ways. Schmid, Haegele, and Schmid demonstrated that a single ortho-α ^{14}C-label in allyl 2,6-diallylphenyl ether became divided between the ortho-α and para-ω positions in its rearrangement product, 2,4,6-triallylphenol.[173] This proves the intervention of the triallyl*cyclo*hexadienone shown in brackets:

[171] O. Masson, H. Hornhardt and J. Diederichsen, *Ber.*, 1939, **72**, 100; O. Masson and J. Diederichsen, *ibid.*, 1523; J. P. Ryan and P. R. O'Connor, *J. Am. Chem. Soc.*, 1952, **74**, 5866; H. Conroy and R. A. Firestone, *ibid.*, 1953, **75**, 2530; S. J. Rhoads, R. Raulins, and R. D. Reynolds, *ibid.*, 2531.

[172] D. S. Tarbell and J. F. Kincaid, *J. Am. Chem. Soc.*, 1940, **62**, 728.

[173] K. Schmid, W. Haegele, and H. Schmid, *Experientia*, 1953, **9**, 414; *Helv. Chim. Acta*, 1954, **37**, 1080.

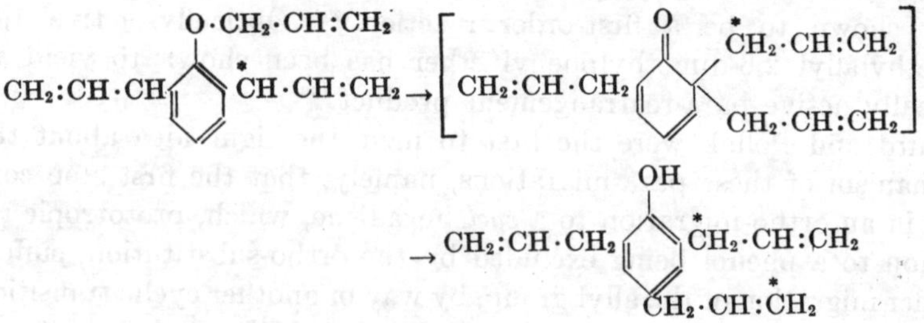

$$CH_2{:}CH\cdot CH\text{-}C_6H_2(O\cdot CH_2\cdot CH{:}CH_2)\text{-}\overset{*}{C}H\cdot CH{:}CH_2 \rightarrow \left[CH_2{:}CH\cdot CH_2\text{-}C_6H_3O(\overset{*}{C}H_2\cdot CH{:}CH_2)(CH_2\cdot CH{:}CH_2) \right]$$

$$\rightarrow CH_2{:}CH\cdot CH_2\text{-}C_6H_2(OH)(\overset{*}{C}H_2\cdot CH{:}CH_2)\text{-}CH_2\cdot CH{:}\overset{*}{C}H_2$$

Analogous demonstrations have also been given by the use of ordinary substituents as labels on the allyl groups.[174] In the para-rearrangement of allyl 2,6-dimethylphenyl ether, Conroy and Firestone were able to trap some of the intermediate *cyclo*hexadienone as its Diels-Alder adduct with maleic anhydride, and also to prove the constitution of the isolated adduct by synthesis.[175] Nothing could be more conclusive.

The general reversibility of the cyclic mechanism, as it operates in one or both steps of Claisen rearrangements, at least when such reversibility cannot be obscured by prototropic changes, was neatly proved by Kalberer, Schmid, and Schmid.[176] They showed that allyl 2,6-dimethyl-4-allylphenyl ether having a ^{14}C-label in the ω-position of the 4-allyl group, on heating at 168°, gave back a chemically identical ether, which, however, had the ^{14}C-label distributed between its original position and the ω-position of the O-allyl group.

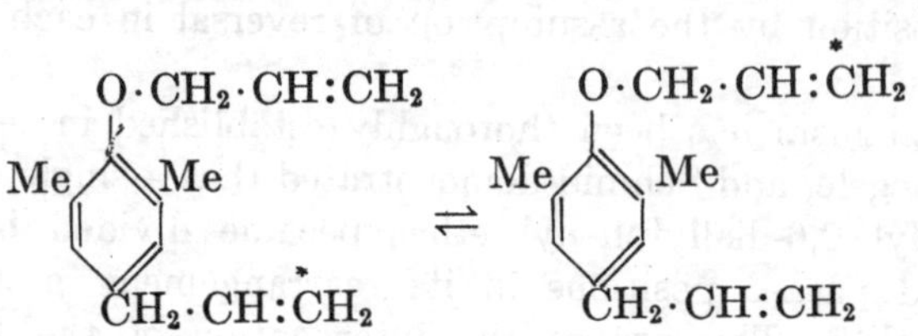

$$O\cdot CH_2\cdot CH{:}CH_2\text{-}C_6H_2(Me)_2\text{-}CH_2\cdot CH{:}\overset{*}{C}H_2 \rightleftharpoons O\cdot CH_2\cdot CH{:}\overset{*}{C}H_2\text{-}C_6H_2(Me)_2\text{-}CH_2\cdot CH{:}CH_2$$

We may take as the essential and defining characteristic of the Claisen rearrangement that it proceeds through a cyclic transition state consisting of one oxygen atom and five carbon atoms. As we have seen, examples of this process are to be found in both the aliphatic and the aromatic series. In Claisen's para-rearrangement, however, which is a definitely aromatic phenomenon, the Claisen rearrangement

174 E. N. Marvell and R. Teranishi, *J. Am. Chem. Soc.*, 1954, **76**, 6165; D. Y. Curtin and H. W. Johnson jr., *ibid.*, 1956, **78**, 2611.

175 H. Conroy and R. A. Firestone, *J. Am. Chem. Soc.*, 1953, **75**, 2550; 1956, **78**, 2290.

176 von F. Kalberer, K. Schmid, and H. Schmid, *Helv. Chim. Acta*, 1956, **39**, 555.

proper, as just defined, is succeeded by an allied, but different kind of rearrangement, namely, one which proceeds through a cyclic transition state of six carbon atoms. This is a rearrangement in its own right, and does not have to be studied only as a sequel to the Claisen rearrangement proper, and only in the aromatic series: it is the subject of the next Sub-section.

(49b) The Cope Rearrangement.—Rearrangement through a cyclic transition state of six carbon atoms was discovered as a simple process by Cope and Hardy in 1940. The main characteristics of this rearrangement were established by Cope and his coworkers within the next few years.[177]

The first examples were vinyl-allyl-substituted malonic esters, cyanoacetic esters, and malononitriles. The vinyl and allyl substituents often carried alkyl groups. These esters and nitriles, when heated alone or in solution at temperatures between 135° and 200°, underwent a rearrangement in which the allyl group became transferred from the malonic carbon atom to the β-carbon atom of its vinyl substitutent, so that an alkenylidene-malonic ester or nitrile resulted. As could be shown by reference to the alkyl groups often carried by the allyl substituents, these substituents underwent a 1,3-reversal of bonding in the rearrangement, as in the following illustration:

$$\begin{array}{l} CH_2{=}CMe{-}C(CO_2Et)_2 \\ \qquad\qquad\qquad | \\ MeCH{=}CH{-}CH_2 \end{array} \rightarrow \begin{array}{l} CH_2{-}CMe{=}C(CO_2Et)_2 \\ \quad | \\ MeCH{-}CH{=}CH_2 \end{array}$$

Kinetically, the rearrangements were first-order processes. When two different rearrangements of comparable rate were run in the same solution, they proceeded independently, each giving its own product, without any formation of cross-products.

First impressions were that the electronegative ("activating") groups CN and CO_2Et characteristically facilitated the rearrangement; but it soon emerged that their activating action was due, not so much to their electronegativity, as to their unsaturation, and capacity for conjugation with one of the ethylenic double bonds in the final product. For when these strongly polar groups were replaced by a single phenyl group, the rearrangements went about as easily, and still at temperatures not above 200°:

[177] A. C. Cope and E. M. Hardy, *J. Am. Chem. Soc.*, 1940, **62**, 441; A. C. Cope, K. E. Hoyle, and D. Heyl, *ibid.*, 1941, **63**, 1843; A. C. Cope, E. M. Hardy, and C. M. Horstmann, *ibid.*, p. 1852; D. E. Whyte and A. C. Cope, *ibid.*, 1943, **65**, 1999; H. Levy and A. C. Cope, *ibid.*, 1944, **66**, 1684; E. G. Forster, A. C. Cope, and F. Daniels, *ibid.*, 1947, **69**, 1893.

$$\begin{array}{ccc} CH_2{=}CH{-}CHPh & & CH_2{-}CH{=}CHPh \\ \qquad\quad | & \rightarrow & | \\ CH_2{=}CH{-}CH_2 & & CH_2{-}CH{=}CH_2 \end{array}$$

$$\begin{array}{ccc} CH_2{=}CH{-}CHPh & & CH_2{-}CH{=}CHPh \\ \qquad\quad | & \rightarrow & | \\ MeCH{=}CH{-}CH_2 & & MeCH{-}CH{=}CH_2 \end{array}$$

It seems obvious that the transition state of the Cope rearrangement, like that of the Claisen rearrangement, is not particularly polar. There can be no doubt that the phenyl group in these and similar examples, by its capacity for conjugation, reduces the energy of the product, relative to that of the factor, so creating favourable thermodynamics for the left-to-right reaction. It is also obvious, from qualitative observations of the rates, that it reduces the energy of the transition state, relative to that of the factors, so accelerating the left-to-right reaction.

When the phenyl group was replaced by a methyl group, those differences were observed which should be expected. The reaction still went; but it went more slowly, requiring temperatures approaching 300°. And now the reaction was appreciably incomplete, and could be shown to proceed to an equilibrium.

$$\begin{array}{ccc} CH_2{=}CH{-}CHMe & & CH_2{-}CH{=}CHMe \\ \qquad\quad | & \rightleftharpoons & | \\ CH_2{=}CH{-}CH_2 & & CH_2{-}CH{=}CH_2 \end{array}$$

The "parent" Cope rearrangement, to be obtained by leaving out the methyl substituent in this example, is symmetrical, and would proceed, probably still more slowly, to a 1:1-equilibrium mixture of chemically identical substances:

$$\begin{array}{ccc} CH_2{=}CH{-}CH_2 & & CH_2{-}CH{=}CH_2 \\ \qquad\quad | & \rightleftharpoons & | \\ CH_2{=}CH{-}CH_2 & & CH_2{-}CH{=}CH_2 \end{array}$$

It would be demonstrable by isotopic labelling, or perhaps by the nuclear-magnetic-resonance spectrum at a high enough temperature, using a principle explained in Section **49d**. As far as the writer knows, neither experiment has yet been done.

The stereochemistry of the Cope rearrangement, and in particular, the question of whether the cyclic transition state has a chair-like or boat-like conformation, has been determined by Doering and Roth.[178] Their example was 2,3-dimethyl-1,5-hexadiene, which, having two equivalent asymmetric carbon atoms, exists in racemic and *meso*-forms. They undergo the Cope rearrangement at 180° and 225°, respectively, giving equilibria in which the rearrangement products,

[178] W. von E. Doering and W. R. Roth, *Tetrahedron*, **1962, 18, 67.**

which consist of isomeric 2,6-octadienes, strongly predominate:

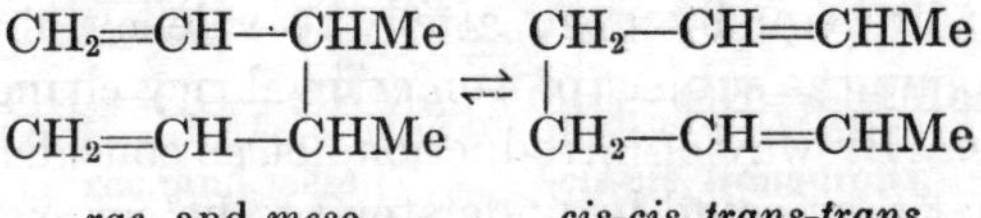

$$\begin{matrix} CH_2{=}CH{-}CHMe \\ | \\ CH_2{=}CH{-}CHMe \end{matrix} \rightleftharpoons \begin{matrix} CH_2{-}CH{=}CHMe \\ | \\ CH_2{-}CH{=}CHMe \end{matrix}$$

rac. and *meso* — *cis-cis, trans-trans,* and *cis-trans*

The test of transition-state conformation is this: if it is chair-like, the racemic factor should yield *cis-cis-* and *trans-trans*-products, whilst the *meso*-factor should give the *cis-trans*-product only, as can be seen from the accompanying diagrams; whereas, if the transition-state conformation were boat-like, then (as other diagrams can be drawn to show) the racemic factor would yield the *cis-trans*-product only, whilst the *meso*-factor would give the *cis-cis-* and *trans-trans*-products. In fact, the racemic factor gave 10% of the *cis-cis*-product and 90% of the *trans-trans*-product, whilst the *meso*-factor gave the *cis-trans*-product only. This is a clear verdict in favour of the chair-like transition state.[179]

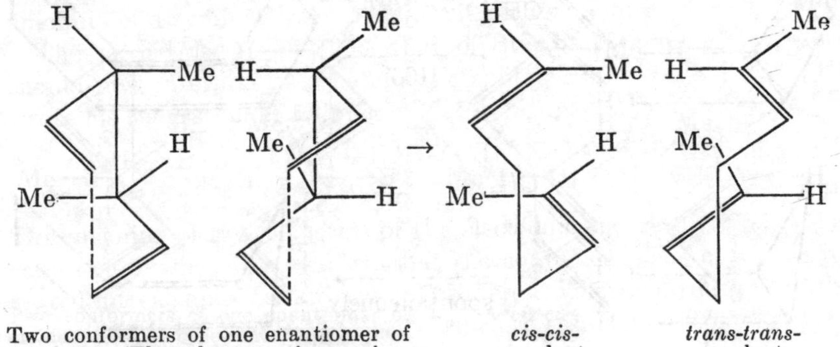

Two conformers of one enantiomer of *rac.*-factor (The other enantiomer gives identical inactive products.) → *cis-cis*-product; *trans-trans*-product

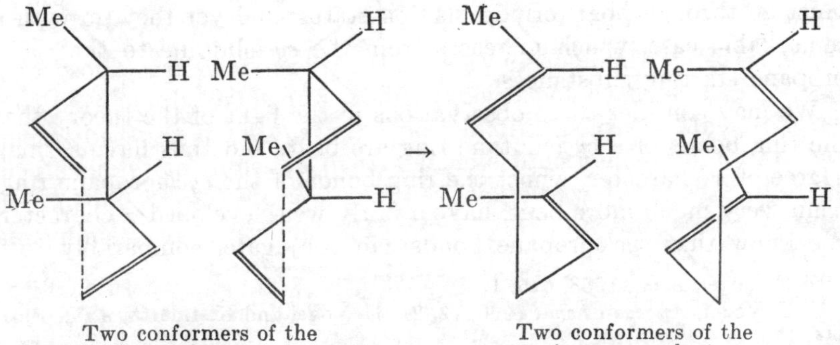

Two conformers of the *meso*-factor → Two conformers of the *cis-trans*-product

[179] For a theoretical discussion of its normally greater stability, see R. Hoffmann and R. B. Woodward, *J. Am. Chem. Soc.*, 1965, **87,** 4389

(49c) Ring-Chain Valency Tautomerism.—In the two preceding Sections we have been dealing with valency tautomerism in open-chain systems which are equally open after the valency change. In this Section we take up the subject of isomeric valency changes which open and close rings. By way of introduction, let us consider two examples so marginal that they could be understood to belong either to the preceding Section or to this one. Both are due to Vogel, and they are both Cope rearrangements in which side-chains of small aliphatic rings (which have vestigial similarity to double bonds) become included in larger rings. The *cis*-form of 1,2-divinyl*cyclo*butane passed readily at 100° into *cis*-*cyclo*-octa-1,5-diene. The *trans*-divinyl isomer underwent no reaction in these conditions, but at 240° broke down to two molecules of 1,3-butadiene.[180] Still more strikingly, the *cis*-form of 1,2-divinyl*cyclo*propane passed so readily into *cis*-*cyclo*hepta-1,4-diene that the former could not be isolated. The *trans*-form of the divinyl compound could be isolated, and only on heating at 200° did it pass into the same *cyclo*heptadiene.[181]

CH_2 CH_2 CH CH —100°→

CH_2 CH_2 CH CH —spontaneously→

These cyclising reactions of the *cis*-side-chains cannot avail themselves of the normally more stable chair-form transition state. They must go through boat-form transition states; and yet they go with a remarkable ease, which increases from the *cyclo*butane to the *cyclo*propane starting substances.

We may consider these observations in the light of the theory that the ring bonds of a *cyclo*butane ring are bent, and thus have a small degree of π character, whilst the ring bonds of the *cyclo*propane ring, being very much more bent, have a fairly well-developed π character. We know that *cyclo*propane bonds can conjugate, comparably to a

[180] E. Vogel, *Ann.*, 1958, **615**, 1.

[181] E. Vogel, *Angew. Chem.*, 1960, **72**, 21; E. Vogel and K. H. Ott, *Ann.*, 1961, **644**, 172.

double bond, with suitably situated double bonds. So it is more than a purely formal extrapolation to pass on to the case in which the place of the *cyclo*butane and *cyclo*propane rings in the foregoing examples is taken by a double bond, or even to the case in which the rings are omitted altogether, so that the vinyl double bonds are allowed to conjugate directly. So we reach unambiguous ring-chain processes, which Woodward and Hoffmann term *electrocyclic* transformations,[182] and define as comprising the formation of a single bond between the terminal atoms of a linear conjugated system, together with the retrogression of that process. We refer to these transformations as ring-chain processes, because they are always in principle and often in practice reversible, so that the question of whether we can observe them most conveniently as ring closures or ring fissions is a matter of thermodynamics, which makes no difference to mechanism, nor to any property dependent on mechanism, such as the stereochemical characteristics of the processes.

Woodward and Hoffmann dealt with the stereochemistry of these transformations by reference to the need to match the symmetries of the involved molecular orbitals, and, most importantly, that of the highest occupied conjugated π orbital, which in ring closure is dominantly involved in the formation of the new σ bond.[182] In explaining their theory,[183] we shall at first consider only thermal isomerisations, and therefore, by London's principle, the adiabatic interconversion of electronic ground states.

Let us consider the conversion of 1,3-butadiene to *cyclo*butene (though, in fact, this transformation goes practically wholly in the opposite direction). The four π electrons of butadiene occupy in pairs its two lowest moecular π orbitals. The lowest orbital of all has the plane of conjugation as its only nodal plane. It has the same symmetry as the π orbital of the double bond of the notionally formed *cyclo*-butene, and must be regarded as parent of that double bond in the cyclisation product. The upper of the two occupied π orbitals of butadiene has the same nodal plane, and also a second one, which lies in the plane of molecular symmetry at right angles to the plane of conjugation. The two nodal planes, the two-fold axes of symmetry to which they give rise, and the resultant phase-signs at the carbon atoms, will be clear from the diagram below. This orbital has to be

[182] R. B. Woodward and R. Hoffmann, *J. Am. Chem. Soc.*, 1965, **87**, 395.

[183] They mention that L. J. Oosterhoff is quoted by E. Havinga and J. L. M. A. Schlatmann (*Tetrahedron*, 1961, 16, 151) as suggesting that orbital symmetries may have an important influence on stereochemistry in ring-chain valency tautomerism.

the parent of the new σ bond of *cyclo*butene, and one can see that it must be terminally concentrated, and also twisted so that like phase-signs overlap between the terminal atoms of butadiene. The required sense of twisting (like at each terminal) is described by Woodward and Hoffmann as "conrotatory";

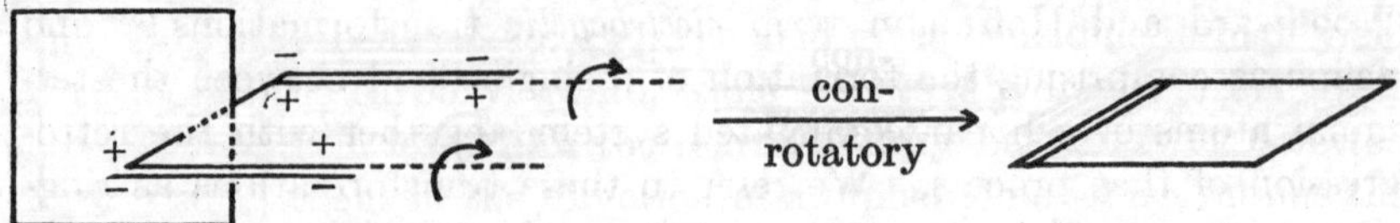

Its stereochemical consequence is that two pairs of groups, A, B and C, D, bound to the 1- and 4-carbon atoms of a butadiene, will be turned in a conrotatory manner when carried by ring closure into the *cyclo*butene. And naturally the same groups, when they start in the *cyclo*butene, will undergo conrotation as this ring opens to give the butadiene:

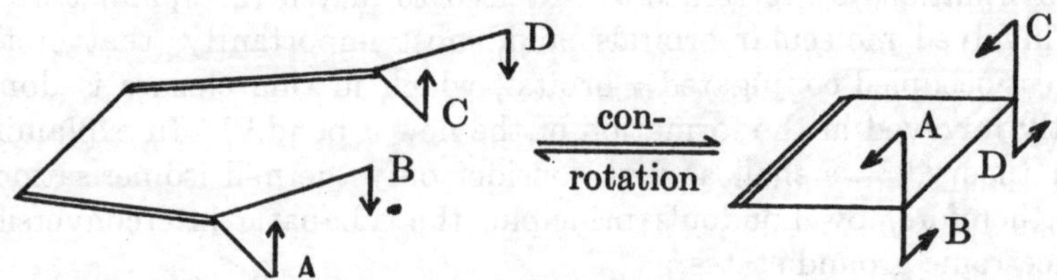

It is known that such transformations occur with a high degree of stereospecificity. As far as has been elucidated, they exhibit the stereochemical behaviour described. Thus methyl *cis-cyclo*butene-3,4-dicarboxylate ($A=C=CO_2Me$; $B=D=H$), on being heated at 120°, yields, out of the three methyl muconates, *cis-cis*, *trans-trans*, and *cis-trans*, which are all very well known, only the *cis-trans*-muconate.[184] Again, the *cis-* and *trans*-1,2,3,4-tetramethyl*cyclo*butenes, on being heated at 200°, yield, respectively, the *cis-trans-* and *cis-cis*-3,4-dimethylhexa-2,4-dienes.[185] All these changes are conrotatory.

Turning next to the conversion of *cis*-1,3,5-hexatriene to *cyclo*hexa-1,3-diene (normally this is the thermodynamically favoured direction of reaction), we note that the six π electrons of hexatriene will fill the lowest three molecular π orbitals. The lowest of them all has the plane of conjugation as its only nodal plane, whilst the second lowest has this nodal plane and also another in the plane of molecular sym-

[184] E. Vogel, *Ann.*, 1958, 615, 14.

[185] R. Criegee and K. Noll, *Ann.*, 1959, 627, 1.

metry perpendicular to the plane of conjugation. These two orbitals correspond, point for point in symmetry, to the two which compose the π electron system of the butadiene moiety contained in the formed *cyclo*hexadiene—this is explained above for butadiene itself—and hence these two hexatriene orbitals must be considered the parents of the π shell of the eventual butadiene residue. Thus the highest occupied hexatriene orbital, the third up in the energy sequence of π orbitals, must be taken as the parent of the σ bond which closes the *cyclo*hexadiene ring. This hexatriene orbital has the plane of conjugation as one nodal plane, and it has two other nodal surfaces which are perpendicular to the plane of conjugation, and which cut through the line of bonds, as shown:

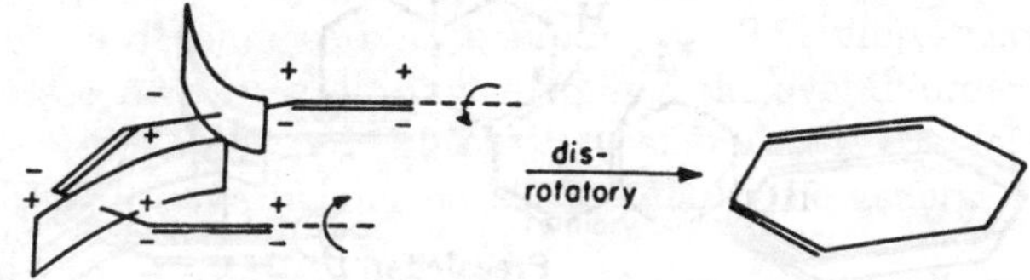

Thus the ring-closing orbital has a plane of symmetry, replacing the two-fold axis of the ring-closing orbital of butadiene, and so the phase relations between the different parts of the orbital are altered.

In order to produce the ring-closing σ bond, the π orbital of hexatriene must concentrate terminally, and must twist to make like phase-signs overlap between the terminal atoms. Woodward and Hoffmann call the required mode of twisting "disrotatory" (unlike senses at the terminals). It follows that two pairs of groups A, B and C, D bound to the 1- and 6-carbon atoms of a hexatriene will suffer a disrotatory twist when ring closure takes them into the corresponding *cyclo*hexadiene; and, of course, such a disrotatory twist must equally characterise the reverse reaction:

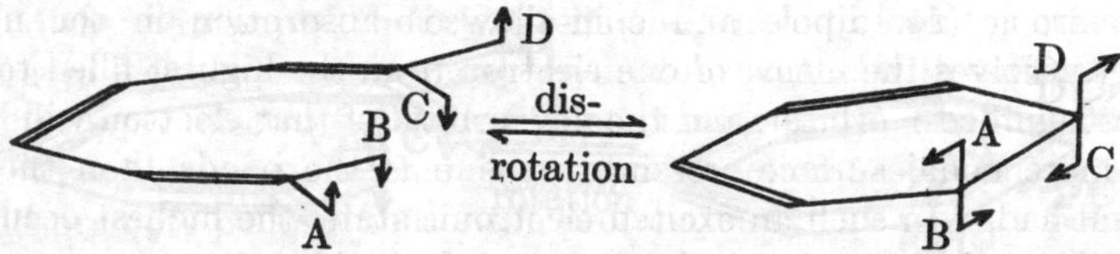

Ring closures of this kind have a high degree of stereospecificity, which in the known simple cases is of the kind predicted. Thus *trans-cis-trans*-1,6-dimethylhexa-1,3,5-triene (A = D = Me and B = C = H) gives *cis*-1,2-dimethyl*cyclo*hexa-3,5-diene, whilst *cis-cis-trans*-1,6-dimethylhexa-1,3,5-triene (B = D = Me, A = C = H) gives the *trans*-

dimethylcyclohexadiene.[186] These are clearly disrotatory stereo-changes. Other illustrations come from the vitamin-D field. Pre-calciferol (photochemically obtainable from ergosterol) is converted by being heated at 150–200° into a mixture of two stereoisomers of ergosterol: in one of them, pyrocalciferol, the 10-Me and 9-H are *cis*-α (both "down" in the formula below), and in the other, *iso*pyrocalciferol, the same side-groups are *cis*-β (both "up").[187] These groups started from the plane of conjugation of precalciferol, and therefore must have undergone disrotation:

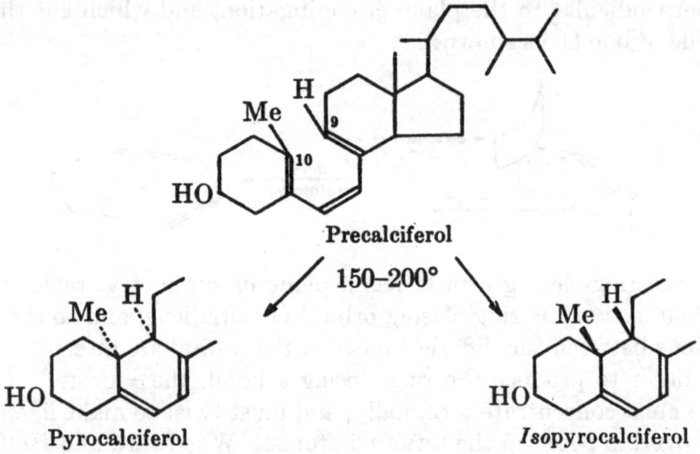

Precalciferol

150–200°

Pyrocalciferol

*Iso*pyrocalciferol

The third point of support for the theory, which Woodward and Hoffmann cited in their first paper on the subject, consists in the indications that the stereochemical rules for ring-chain valency isomerisations of the ground states of π electron systems become reversed in the corresponding photo-induced transformations. In a conjugated π electron system, without easily excited unshared electrons, the first strong (*i.e.* dipole and spin-allowed) absorption in the ultraviolet involves the lifting of one electron from the highest filled to the lowest unfilled π orbital: and the new orbital of that electron will have one more nodal surface crossing the line of the bonds than the old orbital had. In such an excited electronic state, the highest occupied orbital has a symmetry relation between the ends of the π system which is the opposite of that of the highest occupied orbital of the electronic ground state; and so, *if* such a symmetry relation still controls the stereochemistry in a non-adiabatic reversible ring closure through first

[186] E. Vogel and E. Marvell, personal communication quoted by Woodward and Hoffmann (ref. 182).

[187] E. Havinga and J. L. M. A. Schlatmann, *Tetrahedron*, 1961, 16, 146.

excited electronic states (this is not a foregone conclusion), then the stereochemical rules should be the opposite of those applying to the corresponding transformation through electronic ground states; that is, photochemically, a buta-1,3-diene should correlate in a disrotatory way with a *cyclo*butene, and a hexa-1,3,5-triene should correlate in a conrotatory fashion with a *cyclo*hexa-1,3-diene.

Some examples of the former correlation will be mentioned in the next Section. Woodward and Hoffmann have given several examples of the latter correlation.[182] One is that *trans-cis-trans*-1,6-dimethylhexa-1,3,5-triene on irradiation gives *trans*-1,2-dimethyl*cyclo*hex-3,5-diene.[183,188] A number of examples are known among the polyunsaturated steroids; for example, both ergosterol, in which 10-Me and 9-H are *trans* with β-Me and α-H (Me "up" and H "down"), and its stereoisomer, lumisterol, in which the same side-groups are also *trans* but now with α-Me ("down") and β-H ("up"), on irradiation (*e.g.*, by mercury 2537 *A* light) give precalciferol, the reaction of ergosterol being reversible.[189] All these stereo-changes are evidently conrotatory:

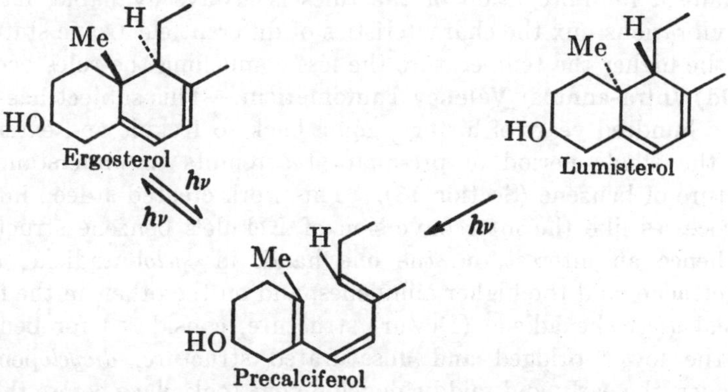

Me H HO **Ergosterol** $h\nu$ $h\nu$ Me H HO **Lumisterol** $h\nu$ Me H HO **Precalciferol**

Woodward and Hoffmann noted that the described control of stereochemistry by orbital symmetry may be over-ridden by other factors. Thus, although, as we have seen, *cis*-1,2,3,4-tetramethyl*cyclo*butene smoothly undergoes conrotatory ring-opening at 200°, the related dimethyl*dicyclo*heptene formulated below, being incapable of such a reaction for stereochemical reasons, undergoes disrotatory ring-opening, but only slowly at 400°.[190]

[188] G. J. Fonken, *Tetrahedron Letters*, 1962, 549.
[189] E. Havinga, R. J. de Kock, and M. P. Rappolatt, *Tetrahedron*, 1960, 11, 276.
[190] R. Criegee and H. Furrer, *Chem. Ber.*, 1964, 97, 2949.

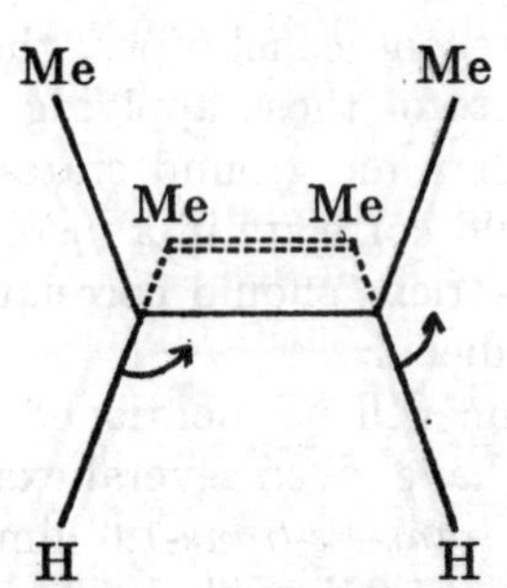

Conrotatory at 200° to
cis-trans-3,4-dimethylhexa-2,4-diene

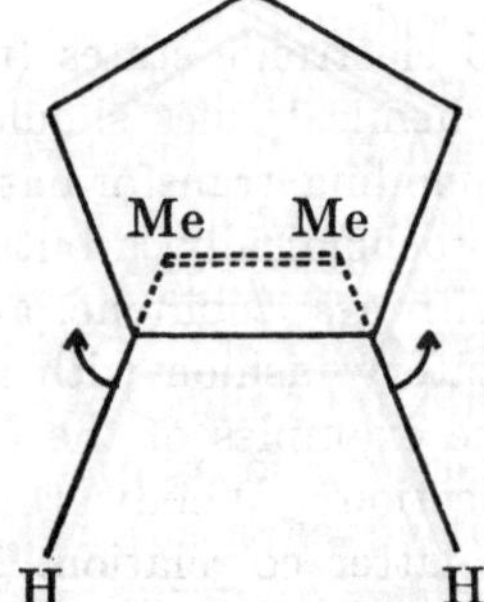

Disrotatory at 400° to
1,2-dimethyl*cyclo*hepta-2,7-diene

One can foresee that special electronic situations could of themselves lead to an abrogation of the stereochemical rules in their simple form, for instance, in some systems of cross-conjugation, in which out-of-plane nodes cross within the system, and so could give the "wrong" number of nodes between a pair of butadiene termini. One general mechanism for abrogation of the rules is always available, namely, that vibrations mix the characteristics of different electronic states, so that the higher the temperature the less compelling the rules become.

(49d) Intra-annular Valency Tautomerism.—This subject has more than a hundred years of history, going back to Kekulé and extending over the whole period of pre-quantal attempts to understand the structure of benzene (Section **13**). This work created a deep interest in processes like the interconversion of Kekulé's benzene structures, and hence an interest, on the one hand, in *cyclo*butadiene, *cyclo*-octatetraene, and the higher annulenes, and on the other, in the hypothetical *dicyclo*hexadiene (Dewar) structure, considered for benzene, and the lower bridged and unsaturated structure, *dicyclo*pentene. However, the early and middle development took place before the distinction had been made between mesomerism, that is, valency change at electronic rates and thus inseparably from the general electronic motion, and valency tautomerism, that is, valency change at the much lower rates of activated nuclear movements, and hence between isomers. And this may be one reason, and the need for more powerful experimental techniques was certainly another, why the earlier background, despite its extent, set the stage largely in a general way for later developments, and touched the details of those developments only at a few points.

As one such point: Farmer and the writer found in 1920 that a keto-enolic dicarboxylic acid,[191] which Perkin and Thorpe had synthesised as a *dicyclo*pentene derivative by closing the three-membered and four-membered component rings one at a time,[192] and which by decarboxylation gave a ketomonocarboxylic acid, subsequently synthesised by Toivonen by simple closure of a five-membered ring,[193] on oxidation gave either *trans*-caronic acid or $\alpha\alpha$-dimethylaconitic acid, according to the oxidising agent:

CO_2Et | $C-CH(CO_2Et)_2$ | Me_2C | $CH-CO_2Et$

Dieckmann and hydrolysis ↓

CO_2H | $C-C\cdot CO_2H$ | Me_2C | $CH-C\cdot OH$ ⇌ CO_2H | $C{=}C\cdot CO_2H$ | Me_2C | $CH{=}C\cdot OH$ → CO_2H | $C{=}CH$ | Me_2C | CH_2-CO

(formed by aldol and H_2O-loss from: CO_2H | CO CH_3 | Me_2C | CH_2-CO)

$K_3Fe(CN)_6$ ↓ $CH\cdot CO_2H$ | Me_2C | $CH\cdot CO_2H$

$KMnO_4$ ↓ $C(CO_2H):CH$ | Me_2C | CO_2H CO_2H

Separate dicyclic or monocyclic isomers were never isolated in this or in any of the similar systems studied, and the two types of synthesis and the two of degradation were taken to indicate an *intra-annular valency tautomerism* (the name is due to Thorpe), mobile enough to defeat the attempts then made to separate the postulated valency isomers.

The parent example of valency tautomerism in the *cyclo*pentadiene-*dicyclo*pentene system has been described more recently by van Tamelen and his associates.[194] On irradiation in ethanol, *cyclo*pentadiene underwent partial conversion to *dicyclo*pentene, which came over with the first runnings on distillation and was finally purified

[191] E. H. Farmer and C. K. Ingold, *J. Chem. Soc.*, 1920, **117**, 1302; *idem* and J. F. Thorpe, *ibid.*, 1922, **121**, 128.

[192] W. H. Perkin jr. and J. F. Thorpe, *J. Chem. Soc.*, 1901, **79**, 729.

[193] N. J. Toivonen, *Ann.*, 1919, **419**, 176.

[194] J. Braumann, L. E. Ellis, and E. E. van Tamelen, *J. Am. Chem. Soc.*, 1966, **88**, 846.

by vapour chromatography. Its nuclear-magnetic-resonance spectrum showed that it contained four kinds of hydrogen atoms, rather than the three kinds of *cyclo*pentadiene. Reduction by di-imine (from azodicarboxylic acid) gave the known hydrocarbon *dicyclo*pentane. In the dark, *dicyclo*pentene reverted to *cyclo*pentadiene, with some concurrent polymerisation, its half-life being about two hours at room temperature:

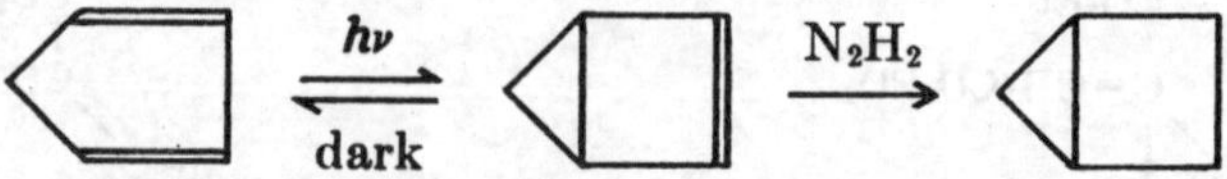
hν
dark
N₂H₂

The slowness of the dark reaction, despite an undoubtedly strong thermodynamic drive, is ascribed to the stereochemical necessity for a disrotatory bond change, contrary to orbital symmetry requirements in a ground-state conversion:

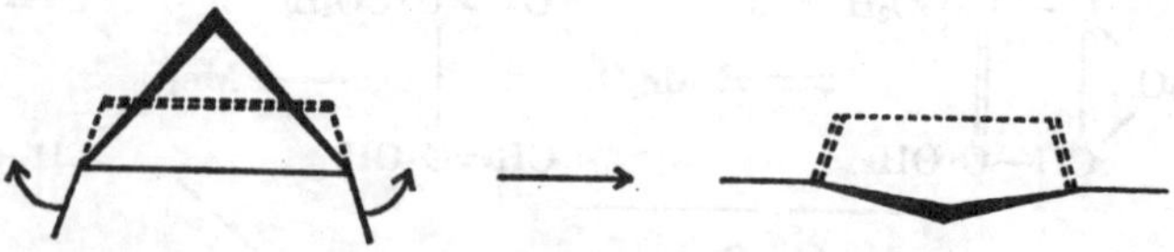

The next higher case of importance is that of the interconversion of benzene and *dicyclo*hexadiene, the isomer with the bond articulation of the Dewar structure of benzene, but, of course, with a very different geometry from that of benzene. The writer tried to make a derivative of *dicyclo*hexadiene in 1922, by the Dieckmann closing of one four-membered ring on another, but obtained only the benzene derivative (orcinol):[195]

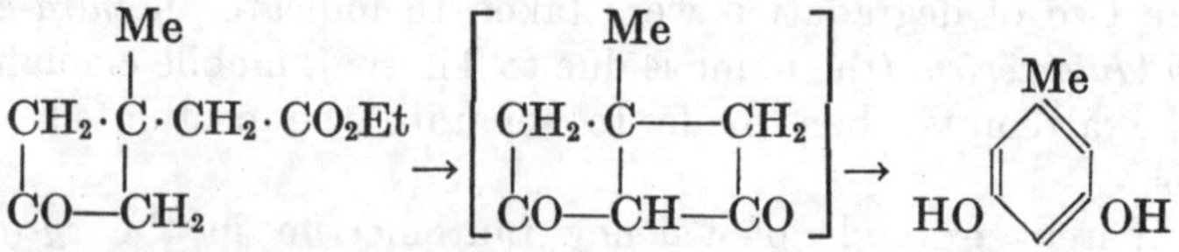
Me
CH₂·C·CH₂·CO₂Et
CO—CH₂
Me
CH₂·C—CH₂
CO—CH—CO
Me
HO
OH

More recently Cookson and his coworkers added methyl acetylenedicarboxylate to tetramethyl*cyclo*butadiene, but again obtained only the benzenoid product (methyl tetramethylphthalate):[196]

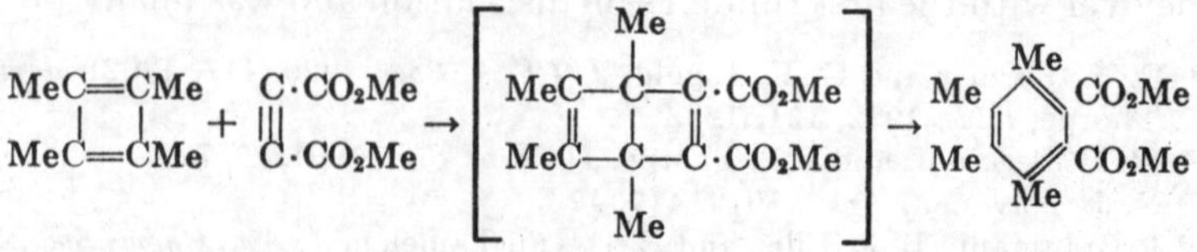
MeC═CMe
MeC═CMe
C·CO₂Me
C·CO₂Me
Me
MeC—C—C·CO₂Me
MeC—C—C·CO₂Me
Me
Me
Me
Me
Me
CO₂Me
CO₂Me

[195] C. K. Ingold, *J. Chem. Soc.*, 1922, 121, 1143.

[196] C. E. Berkhoff, R. C. Cookson, J. Hudee, and R. O. Williams, *Proc. Chem. Soc.*, 1961, 312.

Success in the isolation of the *dicyclo*hexadiene system belongs to the decade of the 1960's. Not the first preparation of that system, but the first rational step-wise synthesis, starting from a monoalicyclic compound, was accomplished by van Tamelen and Pappas[197] in 1963. The initial step consisted in the irradiation of *cis*-1,2-dihydrophthalic anhydride to give a *dicyclo*hexene anhydride, which was singly unsaturated and gave a proton-magnetic-resonance spectrum that corroborated the bridged structure:

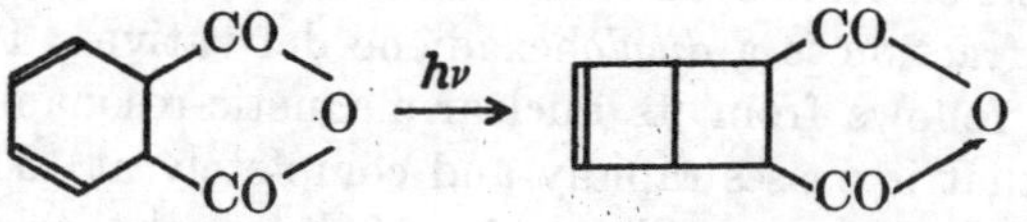

$$\text{(cyclohexadiene-}CO\text{-}O\text{-}CO) \xrightarrow{h\nu} \text{(bicyclic-}CO\text{-}O\text{-}CO)$$

This is an intra-annular valency change in its own right, being homologous in type with the photoconversion of *cyclo*pentadiene to *dicyclo*pentene. The place of the three-membered ring in that conversion is taken by a four-membered ring. As in the simpler system, the conversion would be allowed by the symmetry of a first excited π orbital.

Conversion of the bridged anhydride to *dicyclo*hexadiene was achieved by oxidative removal of the anhydride group by means of lead tetra-acetate in pyridine. On distillation, the *dicyclo*hexadiene came over with the first runnings, and gave a proton-magnetic-resonance spectrum confirmatory of the structure. It was reduced by di-imine to the known hydrocarbon *dicyclo*hexane. It underwent spontaneous conversion to benzene with a half-life of two days at room temperature, and this conversion could be run to completion in half an hour at 90°. Therefore the change must possess quite a large energy of activation, despite its expected large exothermicity:

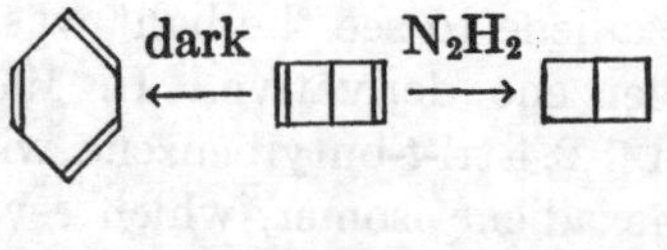

$$\text{(benzene)} \xleftarrow{\text{dark}} \text{(dicyclohexadiene)} \xrightarrow{N_2H_2} \text{(dicyclohexane)}$$

It has been shown by Pettit and his collaborators[198] that *cyclo*butadiene, which when free rapidly dimerises, may be presented for reaction as its stable tricarbonyliron complex, and with ceric ion liberated therefrom to trapping agents. They have shown also that this somewhat elusive hydrocarbon can be trapped thus by acetylene derivatives, including phenylacetylene, methyl propiolate, and methyl acetylenedicarboxylate, to give *dicyclo*hexadiene derivatives. These,

[197] E. E. von Tamelen and S. P. Pappas, *J. Am. Chem. Soc.*, 1963, **85**, 3297.

[198] L. Watts, J. D. Fitzpatrick, and R. Pettit, *J. Am. Chem. Soc.*, 1965, **87**, 3253; G. D. Burt and R. Pettit, *Chem. Comm.*, **1965**, 517.

though isolable, thermally revert more or less easily to benzene compounds:

$$(CO)_3Fe(C_4H_4) \xrightarrow{Ce^{4+}} [\square] \xrightarrow{RC:CR'} \text{(R, R'-dicyclohexadiene)} \rightarrow \text{(R, R'-benzene)}$$

A derivative of a second valency isomer of benzene was obtained by Viehe and his associates[199] in the course of their study of the spontaneous polymerisation of *t*-butylfluoroacetylene. Two-thirds of the product consists of trimers, and the rest of tetramers. About one-half of the trimer fraction is a *dicylo*hexadiene derivative. Its structure, shown below, follows from its nuclear-magnetic-resonance spectrum, and the fact that it passes rapidly and completely at 100° into 1,2,3-tri-*t*-butyltrifluorobenzene. The other half of the trimer fraction proved to be a derivative of *tricyclo*hexene, which Viehe has named "benzvalene." The spectral and chemical behaviour of this trimer gave good support for the proposed structure. This trimer is more stable than the other: but it aromatises rapidly at 220° to 1,2,4-tri-*t*-butyltrifluorobenzene:

3 t-Bu–C≡C–F → (dicyclohexadiene: t-Bu, t-Bu, Bu-t, F, F, F) —100°→ (benzene: t-Bu, t-Bu, Bu-t, F, F, F)

3 t-Bu–C≡C–F → (benzvalene: F, t-Bu, Bu-t, Bu-t, F, F) —220°→ (benzene: F, t-Bu, Bu-t, Bu-t, F, F)

The first *dicyclo*hexadiene to see the light was produced by photoisomerisation of a benzene derivative. In 1962 Pappas and van Tamelen[200] irradiated 1,2,4-tri-*t*-butylbenzene with 2537-*A* light and obtained the *dicyclo*hexadiene isomer, which reverted to the original benzene derivative in the dark at 200°. This work has been extended by Wilzbach and Kaplan,[201] who have shown that either 1,2,4- or 1,3,5-tri-*t*-butylbenzene, on irradiation by 2537-*A* light, gives a photostationary mixture of three valency isomers. One is a *dicyclo*hexadiene, which, as noted above, thermally reverts to 1,2,4-tri-*t*-butyl-

[199] H. G. Viehe, R. Merényi, J. F. M. Oth, J. R. Senders, and P. Valange, *Angew. Chem. internat. Edit.*, 1964, **3**, 755; H. G. Viehe, *ibid.*, 1965, **4**, 746.

[200] S. P. Pappas and E. E. van Tamelen, *J. Am. Chem. Soc.*, 1962, **84**, 3789.

[201] K. E. Wilzbach and L. Kaplan, *J. Am. Chem. Soc.*, 1965, **87**, 4004.

benzene. The second is the *tricyclo*hexene or benzvalene, which also thermally reverts to the 1,2,4-tri-*t*-butylbenzene. The third is a *tetracyclo*hexane, or "prismane," having the bond articulation of Ladenburg's prism structure of benzene. This isomer thermally reverts at 115° in the course of hours, by way of *dicyclo*hexadiene isomers, formed intermediately but in isolable amount, to a mixture of 1,2,4- and 1,3,5-tri-*t*-butylbenzene. The identified valency isomers are the following:

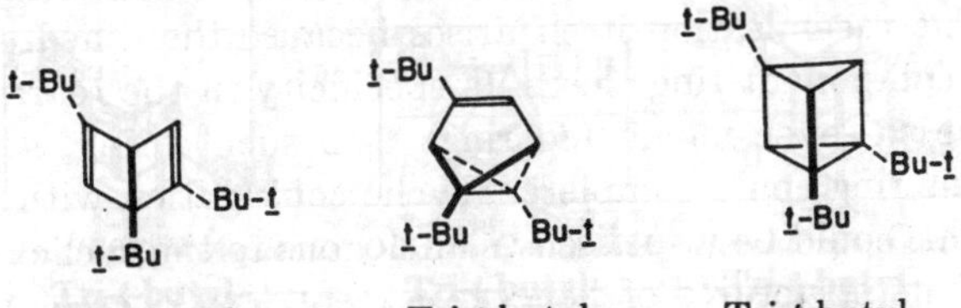

Tri-*t*-butyl-*dicyclo*hexadiene

Tri-*t*-butyl-benzvalene

Tri-*t*-butyl-prismane

When di- and tri-methylbenzenes are irradiated with ultraviolet light, the methyl groups change their relative positions: *o*-xylene gives a mixture of *m*- and *p*-xylene, and mesitylene gives pseudocumene.[202] In the latter case, it has been proved by isotopic labelling that the rearrangement is not one of methyl groups, but is one of the ring carbon atoms, which carry their methyl groups with them (the asterisks mark positions of ^{14}C isotopic labels):

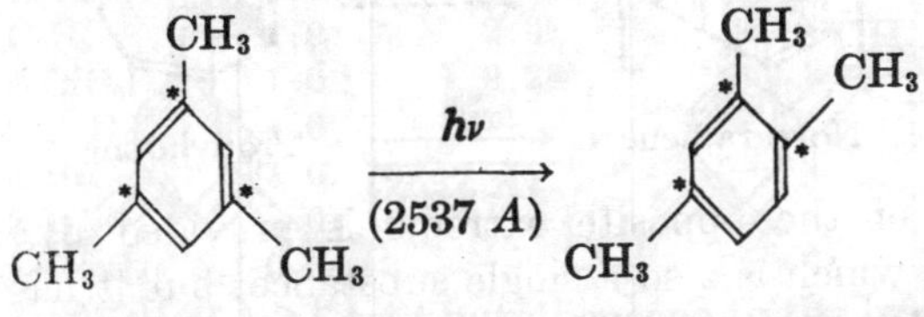

$$\xrightarrow[(2537\ A)]{h\nu}$$

The photoconversion of 1,3,5-tri-*t*-butylbenzene to the bridged valency isomers, and their thermal reversion to 1,2,4-tri-*t*-butylbenzene, provides a model for these isomerisations. They could proceed either by way of a benzvalene, or through a prismane, formed through one *dicyclo*hexadiene and reverting through a different one.

The *cyclo*propane ring has an appreciable capacity for conjugation with a double bond. We might therefore expect the double bond and *cyclo*propane ring contained in the six-membered ring of α-thujene to be capable of completing a cyclic conjugation. It could be visualised as similar to the cyclic conjugation of the *cyclo*pentadiene-*dicyclo*-

[202] K. E. Wilzbach and L. Kaplan, *J. Am. Chem. Soc.*, 1964, 86, 2307; *idem.*, W. G. Brown and S. S. Yan, *ibid.*, 1965, 87, 675.

pentene system, except that a *cyclo*propane ring takes the place of a double bond in the *cyclo*pentadiene isomer:

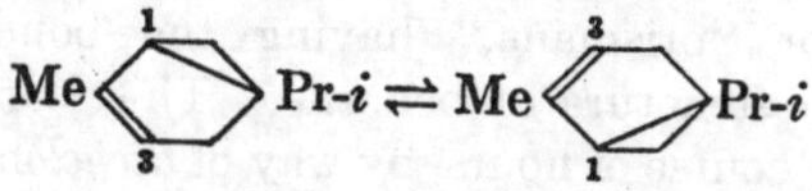

Me⟨1,3⟩Pr-*i* ⇌ Me⟨3,1⟩Pr-*i*

Doering and Lambert showed that this is the mechanism by which α-thujene racemises at 250°: they introduced a deuterium into position 3 and found it distributed between positions 1 and 3 after the racemisation.[203] The racemisation itself arises because the dihedral angle between the component rings loses its specificity in the rearrangement.

We come to seven-membered rings. In such a ring, a component *cyclo*propane ring could complete a cyclic conjugation with two double bonds. This could be visualised as analogous to the cyclic conjugation of the Kekulé structures of benzene, except that a *cyclo*propane ring takes the place of a double bond in one isomer. The form of tautomerism which we are thus led to contemplate is between *nor*caradiene and tropylidene. Actually the equilibrium in this particular case appears to be entirely on the side of tropylidene; for the one known substance, which can be synthesised either from benzene or *cyclo*heptadiene, is shown by its proton-magnetic-resonance spectrum to have only the tropylidene structure:[204]

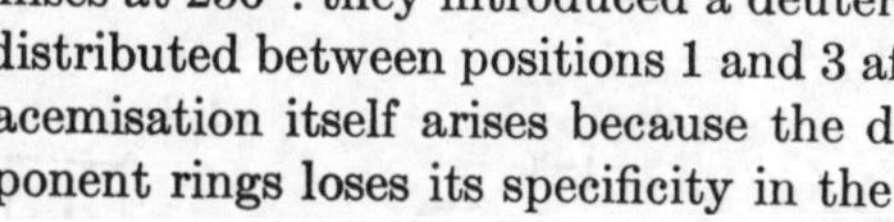

Norcaradiene Tropylidene

An example of the opposite extreme is provided by 7,7-dicyanonorcaradiene, which is also a single substance; but it has the bridged structure, and not the tropylidene structure.[205] We may suppose that quasi-conjugation of the *cyclo*propane ring with the cyano-groups has reversed the free-energy difference:

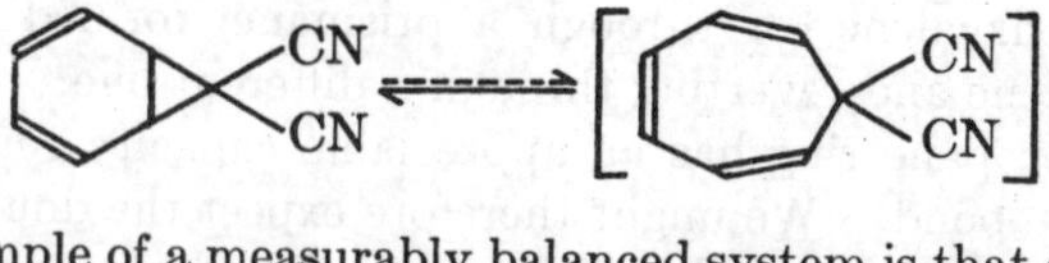

CN CN ⇌ CN CN

The first example of a measurably balanced system is that of Ciganek's 7-cyano-7-trifluoromethyl derivatives.[206] The interconversion is so

[203] W. von E. Doering and J. B. Lambert, *Tetrahedron*, 1963, **19**, 1989.

[204] F. A. L. Anet, *J. Am. Chem. Soc.*, 1964, **86**, 438; F. R. Jenson and L. A. Smith, *ibid.*, p. 956.

[205] E. Ciganek, *J. Am. Chem. Soc.*, 1965, **87**, 652.

[206] E. Ciganek, *J. Am. Chem. Soc.*, 1965, **87**, 1149.

rapid that the proton magnetic spectrum is diffuse at room temperature and incompletely resolved into the superposed spectra of the tautomers even at −80°. The equilibrium does become "frozen" at −112°, and the mixture of tautomers then contains the proportions shown below:

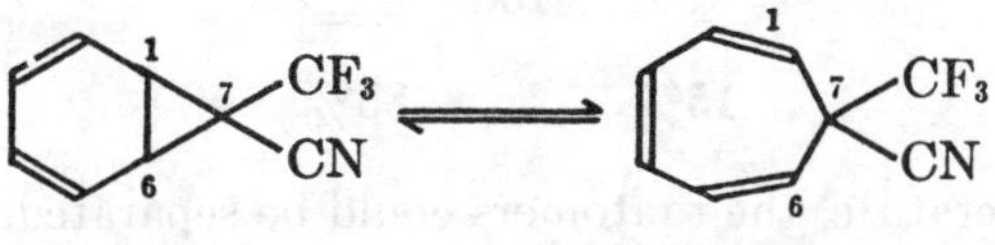

$$\text{(7-CF}_3\text{-7-CN norcaradiene)} \rightleftharpoons \text{(7-CF}_3\text{-7-CN cycloheptatriene)}$$

60% 40%

The identity of the bridged structure is confirmed by the presence of the norcarane derivative, as well as of the *cyclo*heptane derivative, and the *cyclo*hexylmethyl derivative, in the product of catalytic hydrogenation.

Vogel and his collaborators have found another balanced system in the equilibrium between benzene oxide and oxepin.[207] Günther has carried through a kinetic investigation of this interconversion,[208] by the nuclear-magnetic-resonance method. At 0° the equilibrium is as follows:

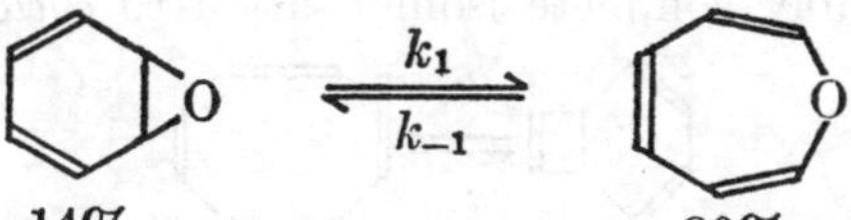

$$\text{(benzene oxide)} \underset{k_{-1}}{\overset{k_1}{\rightleftharpoons}} \text{(oxepin)}$$

14% 86%

The rate constants were $k_1 = 14.1 \times 10^6$ sec.$^{-1}$, and $k_{-1} = 2.29 \times 10^6$ sec.$^{-1}$. Thus the lives of the isomers are less than a microsecond.

The eight-membered ring admits various distributions of unsaturation. Let us refer first to a system which is simply homologous to the conversion of norcaradiene to tropylidene, in that the place of the *cyclo*propane ring is taken by a *cyclo*butane ring. As is not surprising, the higher homologous intra-annular tautomeric system differs from the lower one in two main aspects: first, the thermodynamic balance is much less uneven, and second, the mobility is much lower. The *cyclo*butane ring is less unsaturated than the *cyclo*propane ring. Our knowledge of the case is due to Cope and his collaborators,[209] who found that *cyclo*-octatriene, the first hydrogenation product of *cyclo*-

[207] E. Vogel, W. A. Böll, and H. Günther, *Tetrahedron Letters,* **1965,** 609.

[208] H. Günther, personal communication cited by G. Schroder, ref. 213.

[209] A. C. Cope, A. C. Haven, F. L. Ramp, and E. R. Trumbull, *J. Am. Chem. Soc.,* 1952, **74,** 4867.

octatetraene, came into equilibrium with its bridged isomer on brief heating at 80–100°:

100°

15% 85%

At room temperature, the tautomers could be separated. (The triene forms a complex with silver nitrate.) The structure of the bridged tautomer was shown by its reduction to the *dicyclo*-octane, and its oxidation to *cis-cyclo*butane-1,2-dicarboxylic acid.

Vogel and also Huisgen, and their respective collaborators, have shown that *cyclo*-octatetraene itself is involved in intra-annular valency tautomerism with much less stable *dicyclo*-octatriene. Vogel and his coworkers prepared *dicyclo*-octatriene by debrominating its synthetically obtained dibromide at a low temperature.[210] Its constitution was established by its reduction to the expected and already known *dicyclo*-octane, and by its proton-magnetic-resonance spectrum. At temperatures above −20°, *dicyclo*-octatriene underwent spontaneous and sensibly complete isomerisation to *cyclo*-octatetraene:

k_1

k_{-1}

At 0° the rate constant k_1 of this thermodynamically favoured process was 7.5×10^{-4} sec.$^{-1}$, a value which corresponds to a half-life of 15 minutes. The activation energy of the reaction was 18.7 kcal./mole. The equilibrium constant [*cyclo*-octatetraene]/[*dicyclo*-octatriene] is not well known, but it is believed to be near $10^{5.5}$ at 0°, or about 10^4 at 100°. Nevertheless, Huisgen and Mietzsch succeeded in measuring at 100° and other raised temperatures the rate constant k_{-1} of isomerisation of *cyclo*-octatetraene, that is, isomerisation in the thermodynamically unfavourable direction. This they did by a trapping technique.[211] They showed that dienophiles act on *cyclo*-octatetraene by adding to the *dicyclo*-octatriene formed from it. The adduct with maleic anhydride, for example, has the constitution

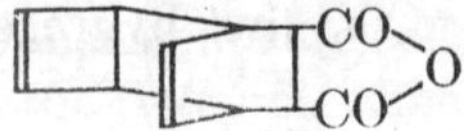

[210] E. Vogel, H. Kiefer, and W. R. Roth, *Angew. Chem. internat Edit.*, 1964, **3**, 442.

[211] R. Huisgen and F. Mietzsch, *Angew. Chem. internat. Edit.*, 1964, **3**, 83.

Maleic anhydride is not so reactive that it could trap off formed *dicyclo*-octatriene fast enough fully to forestall reversion to *cyclo*-octatetraene; but by going over to dienophiles, such as tetracyanoethylene and dicyanomaleimide, which we know to react with simple dienes some thousands of times faster than maleic anhydride does, such reversion could be fully forestalled. The measured rate of the addition then became independent of the concentration and nature of the dienophile, and equal to the rate of isomerisation, as given by the rate constant k_{-1}. At 100° in dioxan k_{-1} had the value 4.4×10^{-4} sec.$^{-1}$. In an analogous reaction with phenyl*cyclo*-octatetraene, instead of *cyclo*-octatetraene itself, the activation energy was determined as 27.2 kcal./mole. One sees that the activation energies for reaction in both directions are fairly high, in conformity with the considerable changes of geometry associated with this tautomeric system.

The eight-membered ring allows valency tautomerism to include the displacement of a component *cyclo*propane ring, without its reduction to a double bond. The change contemplated is the vinylogue of that in α-thujene: two double bonds are included in the cycle, instead of only one. The simplest example is that of homotropylidene, which Doering and Roth obtained in 1963 by the action of diazomethane and cuprous chloride on tropylidene.[212] Its proton-magnetic-resonance spectrum showed that fast tautomerism between equivalent tautomers was under observation:

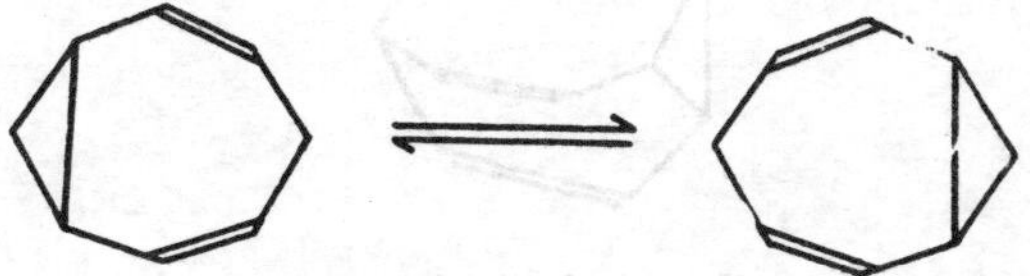

The spectroscopic principle applying to the fast interconversion of equivalent tautomers is this. In any spectrum, *e.g.*, infra-red, for which the uncertainty principle, $\Delta E\cdot\Delta t\sim h$, makes the time of observation very much shorter than the lifetime of a tautomer, the observed spectral frequencies will be those of a single tautomer, and will be independent of temperature. But in proton magnetic resonance, the energies are so low that times of observation are relatively long, running from milliseconds to seconds. If, at a certain temperature, the lifetime of a tautomer is comparable to the time of observation, then below a lower temperature the spectrum will be discrete and temperature-invariant, and will record the classes of protons contained in an individual tautomer; and above a higher temperature, the different

[212] W. von E. Doering and W. R. Roth, *Tetrahedron*, 1963, **19**, 715.

spectrum will again be discrete and temperature-invariant, but will record the classes of protons as they would be under the extra symmetry (a plane of symmetry) gained by averaging the structures, *i.e.*, "smearing out" the mobile bonds; and between these threshold temperatures, the spectrum will be diffuse and changing with temperature. In the case in point, different discrete spectra, related in the required way, were obtained at $-50°$ and $+180°$; and well in between these temperatures the spectrum was diffuse and temperature-dependent. Though the spectra were not analysed quantitatively, they showed qualitatively that the life of a tautomer at 0° must be of the order of a centisecond.

Doering and Roth suggested that homotropylidene should have two conformations, one chair-like and more stable, and the other boat-like, and although less stable, better suited for the valency change. The favourable conformation of an individual tautomer would therefore be present only in small concentration. Accordingly, it was predicted that the introduction of a 1,5-bridge, by preserving the boat-like conformation of the homotropylidene structure, would provide a more mobile tautomeric system. This prediction has been verified by Schröder and others in several examples,[213] for instance, with a —$CH_2 \cdot CH_2$— bridge, as in dihydrobullvalene, represented below:

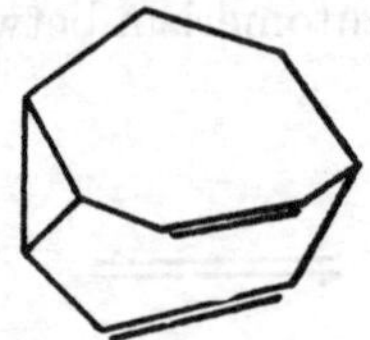

Dihydrobullvalene

The proton magnetic spectrum of this compound was quantitatively analysed, and rate-constants for interconversion of the tautomers were obtained. At 0° the first-order constant was 330,000 $sec.^{-1}$, corresponding to a tautomer life of three microseconds. On the other hand, the valency change is still dependent on nuclear movement which the structure resists, because the activation energy is 12.6 kcal./mole.

Doering and Roth made another prediction. This was that if the 1,5-bridge were made a —CH:CH-bridge, so to give the trigonally symmetrical structure represented below, which, while still hypothetical, they called "bullvalene," the number of equivalent tautomers would be raised to 1,209,600, inasmuch as all the ten carbon atoms

[213] G. Schröder, *Angew. Chem. internat. Edit.*, 1965, **4**, 752.

could be permuted by successive bond changes of homotropylidene type:

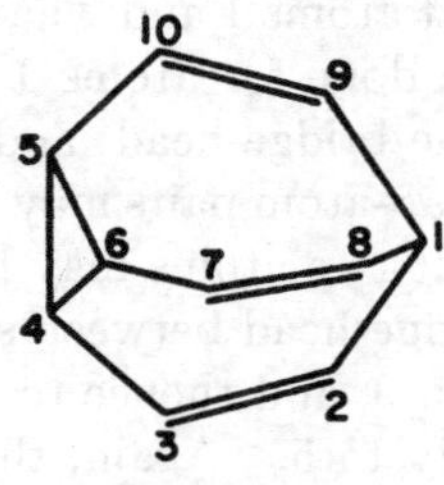

Bullvalene

This arises as follows. By one such change, the bridge-head 1 may be transferred to position 4, 5, or 6, and by a following one, back to 2, 8, or 9; and by yet another to 3, 7, or 10; and so any of the ten carbon atoms can become the bridge-head.

Then, two next-but-one carbon atoms can so change their binding in a succession of such processes that they themselves become interchanged. Thus, atoms 2 and 4 can, by means of two homotropylidene-type valency changes, shift their binding from 1 and 5,6, respectively, to 1,9 and 6, and then back to 9 and 6,7, respectively, without any other changes in bond articulation. Another pair of such valency changes will shift the binding of atoms 2 and 4 by another such rotatory step to 10 and 7,8; and yet another pair by yet another step to 5 and 8,1, respectively. And then one more valency change, the seventh, will carry the binding to 5,6 and 1, respectively, all without other bond changes. Atoms 2 and 4 have now changed places. By symmetry, atoms 9 and 5, and atoms 8 and 6, can be similarly interchanged, when atom 1 is still the bridge-head; and since any carbon atom may be made the bridge-head, all $\alpha\gamma$-atom pairs may be interchanged.

Next, by a succession of $\alpha\gamma$-exchanges, two adjacent atoms may be interchanged. Thus we can, by $\alpha\gamma$-exchange as described, carry carbon atom 2 to position 4, and then, after suitably adjusting the position of the bridge-head, to position 10, and after a further such adjustment, on to position 1; and this last exchange is also the first of three which will take carbon atom 1 back along the same route to position 10, then to 4, and then to 2. The bridge-head shifts that must be effected between the five sets of seven bond changes each that constitute the $\alpha\gamma$-exchanges, 2-4, 4-10, 10-1, 4-10, 2-4, are either $1\rightarrow9\rightarrow2\rightarrow3\rightarrow1$ or $1\rightarrow9\rightarrow5\rightarrow9\rightarrow1$; and the numbers of homotropylidene changes that are needed in order to effect these shifts of the bridge-head are either two, four, two, and four, or two, four, four, and two, in order. The total number of homotropylidene changes in the sequence is therefore forty-seven; and their result is to leave all atoms where they were, except that atoms 1 and 2 have become interchanged. Obviously the same can be done for atoms 1 and 8, and for atoms 1 and 9, atom 1 being still the bridge-head; and since any carbon atom may be the bridge-head, all $\alpha\beta$-atom pairs may be interchanged.

Furthermore, the next-but-two atoms may be interchanged. Thus, by suitably shifting the bridge-head between steps of $\alpha\gamma$-exchange, we can carry atom 5 to position 9, and thence to 2, so carrying atom 2 to position 9, and subsequently to 5. Again, the overall result of these sequences, which involve twenty-nine individual homotropylidene rearrangements, is to leave all atoms where they were, except that atoms 2 and 5 have become interchanged. As before, it follows that all $\alpha\delta$-atom pairs may be exchanged. No two atoms can be further apart than next-but-two.

So at the end of the day (less time for chess players) the conclusion reached is that any pair of carbon atoms chosen from the whole ten may be interchanged, that is, that the ten as a whole may be freely permuted. The number of equivalent isomers is thus factorial 10 divided by the symmetry number 3, that is, 1.2 million. The consequence for the proton magnetic spectrum is that, above the temperature needed to make tautomer life much shorter than the time of observation, all ten hydrogen atoms will act as if equivalent, and the spectrum will consist of one line. The low-temperature spectrum will show four kinds of hydrogen, but the main distinction will be between the four olefinic and the six *cyclo*alkanic hydrogen atoms.

A few months after the publication of these theoretical considerations, Schröder had obtained bullvalene by an unexpected and highly practical method, had established its structure, and had verified Doering and Roth's predictions.[214] An easily accessible dimer of *cyclo*octatetraene, thermally formed in major amount, was proved to be a 1,2-1,5 adduct, and thus to be, as shown below, a symmetrically 1,5-bridged homotropylidene. It displayed the appropriate tautomeric behaviour in the proton-magnetic-resonance spectrometer. Its mobility was very similar to that of dihydrobullvalene. On photolysis, it gave bullvalene and benzene in high yield:

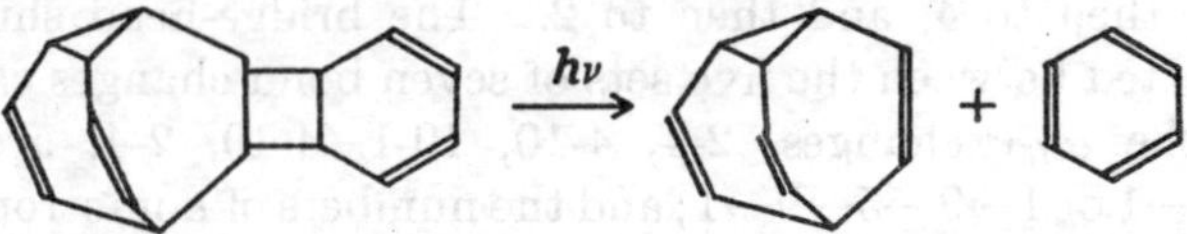

[214] G. Schröder, *Angew. Chem. internat. Edit.*, 1963, **2**, 481; *idem*, *Chem. Ber.*, 1964, **97**, 3130, 3140; R. Merenyi, J. F. M. Oth, and G. Schröder, *ibid.*, p. 3150.

The structure of bullvalene was confirmed chemically, first, by reduction of the double bonds with the aid of di-imine (from cupric-ion catalysed autoxidation of hydrazine), successively to the dihydro-, tetrahydro-, and hexahydro-derivatives, and secondly, by ozonolysis at the double bonds, followed by reduction to *cis*-1,2,3-tri(hydroxymethyl)*cyclo*propane. The proton-magnetic-resonance spectrum at 120° consisted of a single line. At −85°, the spectrum consisted of two pairs of partly merged lines, the pairs having intensities in the ratio 4:6. The weaker pair had unequal components, and the stronger pair apparently equal components. The former of these doublets is, of course, due to *cyclo*alkanic hydrogen, and its components should contribute to the intensity in the ratio 1:3. The latter doublet arises from the olefinic hydrogen, and its components should contribute equally to the intensity.

The mobility of the tautomeric system of bullvalene lies between that of homotropylidene and those of the examined 1,5-bridged homotropylidenes. The rate-constant for tautomer conversion in bullvalene at 0° has been determined[215] as 790 $sec.^{-1}$, corresponding to a tautomer lifetime of about a millisecond. The rate was thus 400 times smaller for bullvalene than for dihydrobullvalene. The activation energy of the valency change had the value 11.7 kcal./mole, that is, 0.9 kcal./mole lower than for dihydrobullvalene. Thus the main cause of the lower interconversion rate of bullvalene appears to lie in the entropy factor. This may be because the nuclear-magnetic-resonance spectrometer is measuring the rate of approach to effective equivalence between all the ten hydrogen atoms, and only certain sequences, that is, only a small fraction of all the possible sequences, of individual homotropylidene-type interconversions can produce this result.

[215] J. M. Gilles and J. F. M. Oth, unpublished work cited by G. Schröder in ref. 213.

CHAPTER XII

Aromatic Rearrangements

(50) AROMATIC ELECTROPHILIC REARRANGEMENTS

WE shall be concerned in this Chapter mainly with rearrangements of the following types,

$$\bigcirc\text{—NRX} \xrightarrow{\text{acid}} \overset{\text{X}}{\bigcirc}\text{—NRH} \quad \text{and} \quad \text{X}\bigcirc\text{—NRH}$$

where X = Cl, Br, I, N_2Ar, NO, Alk, OH, NO_2, NRAr, and

$$\bigcirc\text{—OX} \xrightarrow{\text{acid}} \overset{\text{X}}{\bigcirc}\text{—OH} \quad \text{and} \quad \text{X}\bigcirc\text{—OH}$$

where X = Alk. It is obvious that there is a considerable family of such rearrangements: the list given could be extended. It is obvious also that they are formally all very similar: a part of a side-chain replaces hydrogen in the aromatic ring, and is replaced by hydrogen in the side-chain: in the original side-chain there is only one atom between the migrating group and the ring, and it possesses unshared electrons: the migrating group enters ortho- and para-positions exclusively: and the reactions are all catalysed by acids.

However, when we examine the mechanism of these processes, we find that they are not all as similar as might be thought. There is a primary distinction of polar type. Of a number of the rearrangements it is true that the migrating group moves as an electrophilic fragment, separating from the side-chain without the electrons by which it was there bound, and uniting with aromatic carbon by means of electrons which the latter has to supply. We shall call these reactions *aromatic electrophilic rearrangements;* and the property signalised being treated as a primary classificatory character, they will be our concern in this Section.

Among the rearrangements listed above is represented another class, in which the group migrates as a nucleophilic fragment, taking with it the electrons with which it was bound in the side-chain, and using its own electrons for the purpose of establishing a bond with a carbon kernel in the aromatic ring. These reactions will be called *aromatic nucleophilic rearrangements,* and they will be discussed in Section **51.**

The rearrangements to which reference has been made are often (somewhat illogically) called "intermolecular" rearrangements, in order to distinguish them from the class next to be mentioned. These are the *aromatic intramolecular rearrangements*, which are to be discussed in Section **52**. They proceed through a cyclic transition state, in which one cannot be certain which way round the electrons move, or even whether they move heterolytically in pairs, or homolytically by uncoupling and recoupling of the pairs. Indeed, the uncertainty principle teaches that the denying of this knowledge to us is one of Nature's ways of making the cyclic transition state as stable as it is, and thus of enabling the intramolecular reaction to go as easily as it does. Accordingly, it is unphysical to try to classify intramolecular rearrangements as exclusively electrophilic or nucleophilic, or even as heterolytic or homolytic: if they are typically intramolecular they will have all these characters, though cases may arise in which one character seems to predominate.

With these introductory remarks, we may proceed to the main subject of this Section, aromatic electrophilic rearrangements.

(50a) Rearrangements of Halogenoamines (Orton).—A typical example is the conversion of N-chloroacetanilide into a mixture of *o*- and *p*-chloroacetanilide, in the presence of hydrochloric acid, and usually in hydroxylic solvents, such as acetic acid, or water, or aqueous acetic acid:[1]

$$C_6H_5\cdot NClAc \xrightarrow{HCl} (o\text{- and } p\text{-})Cl\cdot C_6H_4\cdot NHAc$$

Up to 1909, the side-chain-to-nucleus migrations of halogen, which this example illustrates, were regarded as true intramolecular rearrangements. But in that year a different view of the reaction was advanced by Orton and W. J. Jones.[2] This was that it commenced with a reversible acidolysis of the N-chloro-compound to give acetanilide and elemental chlorine, and that then the latter attacked the former in an ordinary process of aromatic C-chlorination:

$$C_6H_5\cdot NClAc + HCl \underset{(2)}{\overset{(1)}{\rightleftarrows}} C_6H_5\cdot NHAc + Cl_2$$

$$\xrightarrow{(3)} (o\text{-}, p\text{-})ClC_6H_4\cdot NHAc + HCl$$

[1] G. Bender, *Ber.*, 1886, **19**, 2272; F. D. Chattaway and K. J. P. Orton, *J. Chem. Soc.*, 1899, **75**, 1046; H. E. Armstrong, *ibid.*, 1900, **77**, 1047.

[2] K. J. P. Orton and W. J. Jones, *Proc. Chem. Soc.*, 1909, **25**, 196, 233, 305; *J. Chem. Soc.*, 1909, **95**, 1456; *Brit. Assoc. Advancement Sci., Rept.*, **1910**, 85; K. J. P. Orton, *ibid.*, **1911**, 94; **1912**, 116; **1913**, 136; **1914**, 105; **1915**, 82; K. J. P. Orton, and H. King, *J. Chem. Soc.*, 1911, **99**, 1185.

This interpretation, though it has often been attacked, holds good to-day; while there is naturally more that can be added.

In the early work of Orton and Jones, it was pointed out that the overall isomeric change is specifically catalysed by hydrochloric acid: there was but little general acid catalysis in the investigated conditions. Acetanilide was isolated from a solution in which N-chloroacetanilide was undergoing rearrangement. Elemental chlorine was aspirated from such a solution. And by going over from N-chloroacetanilide to a derivative with a deactivated ring, N-chloro-2,4-dichloroacetanilide, for example, it was found possible to use the chlorine liberated from it to chlorinate some other more reactive aromatic ring, for instance that of acetanilide itself, or that of anisole. It was subsequently shown[3] that the proportions in which ortho- and para-chloroacetanilide are formed are the same whether the starting materials are N-chloroacetanilide and hydrochloric acid or acetanilide and chlorine, provided that the solvent and temperature are the same.

Here a mildly subtle point arises. Let us rewrite the Orton mechanism, labelling the component reactions (1), (2), (3), as is done above, but adding, as reaction (4), the hypothetical intramolecular rearrangement:

$$\begin{array}{ccc} C_6H_5\cdot NClAc + HCl & \xrightarrow{(4)} & (o\text{-}, p\text{-})ClC_6H_4\cdot NHAc + HCl \\ (1)\downarrow\quad\uparrow(2) & \nearrow & \\ C_6H_5\cdot NHAc + Cl_2 & (3) & \end{array}$$

Then, *if* the equilibrium (1) – (2) were always established much more rapidly than the isomerisation is observed to proceed, we could not distinguish between routes (3) and (4) for the formation of the rearrangement products. For reaction (4) would have the same factors, products, and rate laws as reaction sequence (1+3), and reaction (3) would have the same factors, products, and rate laws, as reaction sequence (2+4). However, fortunately, reactions (1) and (2) are *not* always, or even usually, very fast in comparison with reaction (3). The equilibrium (1) – (2) depends much on the solvent: in water the stable system is PhNClAc+HCl, as is doubtless determined by the strong ionic solvation of HCl; but in acetic acid the stable system is $PhNHAc + Cl_2$. The rate of reactions of form (3) can be varied over a great range by introducing substituents into the aromatic ring.

In their original work, Orton and Jones showed that, in aqueous acetic acid containing less than 65% of the acid, the rate of isomerisation of N-chloroacetanilide is less than the rate of C-chlorination of

[3] K. J. P. Orton and A. E. Bradfield, *J. Chem. Soc.*, 1927, 986.

acetanilide by chlorine. This means that reaction (1) is at least partly rate-determining. An incursion of the intramolecular process (4) would make the total rate of isomerisation greater than the rate of the chlorination. Soper subsequently showed[4] that, in water as solvent, reaction (1) becomes wholly rate-determining, the rate of isomerisation of N-chloroacetanilide in the presence of hydrochloric acid being just equal to the rate of production of chlorine. Orton, Soper, and Williams[5] found several ring-substituted acetanilides, namely, *o*-, *m*-, and *p*-chloroacetanilide, *p*-bromoacetanilide, and aceto-*o*- and aceto-*p*-toluidide, for which the rates of reactions (2) and (3) were both measurable in the medium they were to use; and by employing a strongly aqueous medium, 40% acetic acid, they secured that the rate of reaction (1) would be negligibly small in comparison. Then, starting with the acetanilide and chlorine, they showed in each case that the ratio of the N- to the C-chlorinated product was independent of the time, thus satisfying Wegscheider's test for the simultaneity of two reactions of the same order. Reactions (2) and (3) were simultaneous, and (3) was not being mistaken for (2) followed by (4). This completes Orton's case for the intermolecular mechanism (1) – (2) – (3), as against the intramolecular mechanism (4), for the chloroamine rearrangement in hydroxylic solvents.

Confirmation has been furnished by Olson and his collaborators,[6] who have examined the isomerisation of N-chloroacetanilide in the presence of hydrochloric acid isotopically labelled with radiochlorine. They found that the final ring-bound chlorine had approximately the radioactivity it would possess if it had once been pooled with the inorganic chlorine in the medium.

As remarked already, hydrochloric acid is a specific reagent for the isomeric transformation of N-chloroacetanilide. However, other halogen acids bring about transformations, if not the isomeric one: hydrobromic acid produces *o*- and *p*-bromoacetanilide, and hydriodic acid gives *o*- and *p*-iodoacetanilide.[7] This can be understood on the basis of Orton's mechanism, since the intermediate halogens would in these cases be bromine monochloride and iodine monochloride, which are respectively brominating and iodinating agents.

Of the three reactions, (1), (2), and (3), involved in the Orton mech-

[4] F. G. Soper, *J. Phys. Chem.*, 1927, **31**, 1192.

[5] K. J. P. Orton, F. G. Soper, and Gwyn Williams, *J. Chem. Soc.*, **1928**, 998.

[6] A. R. Olson, C. W. Porter, F. A. Long, and R. S. Halford, *J. Am. Chem. Soc.*, **1936**, **58**, 2467; A. R. Olson, R. S. Halford, and J. C. Hornel, *ibid.*, 1937, 59, 1613; A. R. Olson and J. C. Hornel, *J. Org. Chem.*, 1938, 3, 76.

[7] A. E. Bradfield, K. J. P. Orton, and I. C. Roberts, *J. Chem. Soc.*, **1928**, **782**, M. Richardson and F. G. Soper, *ibid.*, **1929**, **1873**.

anism, reaction (3) needs little comment, aromatic C-chlorination having already been discussed in Section 24a. We know that molecular chlorine has a combination of thermodynamic stability and electrophilic reactivity that makes it a very effective chlorinating agent; so much so that, if we want to observe chlorination by specifically more reactive though less stable reagents, such as Cl^+ or $ClOH_2^+$, we have to take steps carefully to remove every trace of molecular chlorine. The effectiveness of chlorine for chlorination is, we may believe, one of the reasons for the importance of the Orton mechanism in chloroamine rearrangements.

However, reaction (1) deserves further comment. From the qualitative fact of the specificity of hydrochloric acid, it follows that, if this substance reacts as its ions, as seems probable in view of the highly aqueous conditions to which much of the evidence of mechanism applies, then the reaction needs both ions. This conclusion is supported by the kinetics: the reaction is of third order,[8] that is, first with respect to the chloroamine and second with respect to hydrochloric acid, or, if we prefer the ionic interpretation, first in chloroamine, first in hydrogen ion, and first in chloride ion:

$$\text{Rate} \propto [\text{chloroamine}][\text{HCl}]^2 \propto [\text{chloroamine}][\text{H}^+][\text{Cl}^-]$$

Actually Richardson and Soper have confirmed the ionic interpretation in the following way.[7] They examined the kinetics of the conversion of N-chloroacetanilide by means of hydrogen bromide into *o*- and *p*-bromoacetanilide, in various essentially aqueous media, under conditions in which reaction (1), leading to bromine monochloride, is rate-determining, while reaction (3), in which the aromatic ring is brominated with liberation of hydrochloric acid, is instantaneous:

$$C_6H_5\cdot NClAc + HBr \xrightarrow[\text{slow}]{} C_6H_5\cdot NHAc + BrCl$$

$$\xrightarrow[\text{fast}]{} BrC_6H_4\cdot NHAc + HCl$$

The rate obeyed the expression

$$\text{Rate} \propto [\text{chloroamine}][\text{H}^+][\text{Br}^-]$$

which cannot be put into an alternative molecular form, because two acids are supplying the proton, while one has the outstandingly reactive anion, namely, bromide ion.

[8] J. J. Blanksma, *Rec. trav. chim.*, 1903, **22**, 290; A. C. D. Rivett, *Z. physik. Chem.*, 1913, **82**, 201; H. S. Harned and H. Seltz, *J. Am. Chem. Soc.*, 1922, **44**, 1475; F. G. Soper and D. R. Pryde, *J. Chem. Soc.*, 1927, 2761; H. M. Dawson and H. Millet, *ibid.*, 1932, 1920.

On this evidence we can plausibly regard[9] reaction (1) as a bimolecular nucleophilic substitution by halide ion at the chlorine atom of a chloroammonium ion, a kind of S_N2 substitution in an 'onium salt, but at chlorine instead of at carbon:

$$\mathrm{Hal^- + Cl{-}\overset{+}{N}HAcAr \rightarrow Hal{-}Cl + NHAcAr}$$

This being accepted, it follows, by the principle of microscopic reversibility, that reaction (2) is a bimolecular nucleophilic substitution by the acylanilide molecule at one halogen atom in the halogen molecule.

Reaction (1) is, then, certainly not a hydrolysis, as it is sometimes loosely called. But Soper and Pryde showed[8] that it is accompanied in aqueous solutions by a comparatively unimportant side-reaction of the nature of hydrolysis: this gives hypochlorous acid, which, in the presence of hydrochloric acid, undergoes further conversion to chlorine. Their evidence was that the rate of acidolytic displacement of halogen from N-chloroacetanilide by aqueous acids other than the halogen acids increased with the acid strength and was identical for the strong acids, nitric, sulphuric, and perchloric acids: clearly this was a hydrogen ion reaction, the anions of the strong acids taking no part. However, if such a reaction were assumed for hydrochloric acid, it would account at most for a few units per cent of the observed rate of chlorine production. The mechanism of this relatively slow hydrolytic process is not known. It might, as before, be an S_N2-type substitution in the chloroammonium ion, but with water as the substituting agent:

$$\mathrm{H_2O + Cl{-}\overset{+}{N}HAcAr \rightarrow H_2\overset{+}{O}{-}Cl + NHAcAr}$$

Or, it might be an S_N1-type substitution:

$$\mathrm{Cl{-}\overset{+}{N}HAcAr \rightarrow \overset{+}{Cl} + NHAcAr}$$

$$\mathrm{H_2O + \overset{+}{Cl} \rightarrow H_2\overset{+}{O}{-}Cl}$$

Clearly it is still correct to speak of hydrochloric acid as a specific catalyst for the rearrangement, not only because the acidolysis with the aid of chloride ion is so much faster than that involving water, but also because, in the absence of any chloride ion, the product is hypochlorous acid, a poor chlorinating agent of itself, and one insufficiently

[9] Professor E. D. Hughes, personal communication.

converted in equilibrium into active cationic forms to produce a chlorinating agent of efficiency comparable to the chlorine which would be given by chloride ion.

In 1912 Orton wrote[2] of the chloroamine rearrangement: "Whether a true intramolecular change is possible under certain conditions has not yet been discovered, but it must not be supposed that the possibility is excluded." Orton was one of the earliest workers on reaction mechanism explicitly to repudiate the assumption, apparent in some more recent writings, that no reaction can have more than one mechanism. And the position with respect to the chloroamine rearrangement remains to this day almost as he expressed it.

For halogenoamine rearrangements in aprotic solvents, such as chlorobenzene, evidence for a one-stage intramolecular process, with general acid catalysis, has been claimed by Bell[10] in the examples N-chloroacetanilide, N-bromoacetanilide, N-bromobenzanilide, and N-iodoformanilide. It is contended that the concentration of halogen detected in the system would not account for the observed reaction rates. But according to Soper and his collaborators,[11] inadequate account is taken of the formation of acylhypohalites, HalOAc, which, as they have shown in this and in other connexions, are undoubtedly produced in such conditions, and are good halogenating agents. Dewar has discussed the position several times, at first supporting Bell's views,[12] and more latterly Soper's.[13] Thus the matter remains where Orton left it: intramolecular rearrangement is a possibility.

On the other hand, the proposition that mechanisms other than the Orton mechanism exist, even if we do not know exactly what they are, can be unequivocally supported. For example, the existence of some kind of homolytic mechanism is made clear by the known effect of light in promoting the transformation of N-chloroacetanilide.[14]

(50b) Rearrangements of Diazoamino-Compounds.—The standard

[10] R. P. Bell, *Proc. Roy. Soc.* (London), 1934, **A, 143, 377**; R. P. Bell and R. V. H. Levinge, *ibid.*, 1935, **A, 151,** 211; R. P. Bell, *J. Chem. Soc.*, **1936,** 1154; R. P. Bell and J. F. Brown, *ibid.*, p. 1520; R. P. Bell and P. V. Danckwerts, *ibid.*, **1939,** 1774.

[11] G. C. Israel, A. W. N. Tuck, and F. G. Soper, *J. Chem. Soc.*, **1945, 547.**

[12] M. J. S. Dewar, *Nature*, 1946, **156,** 784; *J. Chem. Soc.*, **1946,** 406; *Disc. Faraday Soc.*, 1947, **2,** 50; "Electronic Theory of Organic Chemistry," Clarendon Press, Oxford, 1949, p. 233; *Bull. soc. chim.* (France), **1951,** p. 71C.

[13] M. J. S. Dewar and J. M. W. Scott, *J. Chem. Soc.*, **1957,** 2676; "Theoretical Organic Chemistry: Kekulé Symposium," Butterworths, London, 1959, p. 195; "Molecular Rearrangements," Editor P. de Mayo, Interscience, New York, 1963, p. 295.

[14] J. J. Blanksma, *Rec. trav. chim.*, 1902, **21,** 366; J. H. Mathews and R. V. Williams, *J. Am. Chem. Soc.*, 1923, **45,** 2574.

illustration is the conversion of diazoaminobenzene into *p*-aminoazobenzene:

$$C_6H_5\cdot N{:}N\text{—}NH\cdot C_6H_5 \xrightarrow[\text{HCl + PhNH}_2]{\text{HCl or}} (p\text{-})NH_2\cdot C_6H_4\text{—}N{:}N\cdot C_6H_5$$

The reaction can be effected, for example, by treatment with alcoholic hydrochloric acid, or, better, by treatment with aniline together with aniline hydrochloride or some other salt of aniline.[15] In most examples of the change, the azo-group migrates to the para-position. Ortho-migration is less facile; but it does occur, if the para-position is blocked.

Although this reaction has not been investigated as fully and accurately as has the chloroamine rearrangement, it has had a much less controversial history: since 1885 no-one seems seriously to have doubted that the diazoamino-aminoazo-conversion is intermolecular. In that year, Friswell and Green[15] advanced the view that the acid-catalysed reaction went in stages, an acidolysis, which reverses the usual mode of formation of a diazoamino-compound, being succeeded by an ordinary process of aromatic diazo-coupling. Their mechanism is formulated below in a way which leaves open the question, to which we shall return, of whether (as in the Orton mechanism) the anion of the catalysing acid is directly utilised in the acidolysis, or is not so utilised. In other words, the question left open is whether the primary acidolysis product is the covalent diazo-pseudo-salt or the ionised diazonium salt:

$$C_6H_5\cdot N{:}N\text{—}NH\cdot C_6H_5 + HX \underset{(2)}{\overset{(1)}{\rightleftarrows}} \left\{\begin{matrix} C_6H_5\cdot N{:}N\cdot X \\ \updownarrow \\ C_6H_5\cdot N_2^+ + X^- \end{matrix}\right\} + NH_2\cdot C_6H_5$$

$$C_6H_5\cdot N_2^+ + NH_2\cdot C_6H_5 \xrightarrow{(3)} NH_2\cdot C_6H_4\text{—}N{:}N\cdot C_6H_5$$

The earliest observation of special significance in relation to the question of mechanism was that of Nietzski,[16] who demonstrated the transference of the diazo-group from a rearranging diazoamino-compound to a foreign aniline molecule: by treating *p*-diazoaminotoluene with the hydrochloride of aniline, or of *o*-toluidine, he obtained the transfer products,

[15] P. Griess and C. A. Martius, *Zeit. Chem.*, 1866, **2**, 132; A. Kekulé, *ibid.*, p. 688; O. N. Witt and E. G. B. Thomas, *J. Chem. Soc.*, 1883, **43**, 112; R. J. Friswell and A. G. Green, *ibid.*, 1885, **47**, 917.

[16] R. Nietzski, *Ber.*, 1877, **10**, 662.

$$CH_3\langle C_6H_4\rangle N{:}N\text{—}\langle C_6H_4\rangle NH_2 \quad \text{and} \quad CH_3\langle C_6H_4\rangle N{:}N\text{—}\langle C_6H_3(CH_3)\rangle NH_2$$

It was subsequently shown[17] that the foreign molecule receiving the transferred azo-group need not be an aromatic amine, but could be a phenol: from diazoaminobenzene and phenol, 4-benzeneazophenol and aniline were obtained:

$$C_6H_5\cdot N{:}N\text{—}NH\cdot C_6H_5 + \langle C_6H_5\rangle OH \rightarrow C_6H_5\cdot N{:}N\langle C_6H_4\rangle OH + NH_2\cdot C_6H_5$$

A modification of the Friswell-Green mechanism has been developed by Heinrich Goldschmidt,[18] particularly as an interpretation of the marked facilitating effect, on which all observers agree, of aniline and similar bases on the reactions catalysed by such bases in association with acids. In Goldschmidt's mechanism, the aromatic base is assumed to act in just the way in which we allowed that the anion of the catalysing acid might act in the Friswell-Green mechanism; but when aniline fulfils this function there is no uncertainty about whether a covalent or ionic azo-compound is going to be formed: the product is covalent, and is the final product, so that the second stage of the general Friswell-Green mechanism disappears:

$$H_2N\langle C_6H_5\rangle + N(=N\text{—}C_6H_5)\text{—}\overset{+}{N}H_2\cdot C_6H_5 \rightarrow H_2N\langle C_6H_4\rangle\text{—}N{=}N\text{—}C_6H_5 + NH_2\cdot C_6H_5 + H^+$$

The Goldschmidt mechanism can thus be regarded as a particular case of the Friswell-Green mechanism, the general acid catalyst, HX, having been specialised to the anilinium ion, $PhNH_3^+$: this, in essence, was Goldschmidt's final view. The theory implies that the Friswell-Green mechanism of the diazoamino-rearrangement is able to assume a form completely analogous to that of the Orton mechanism of the

[17] K. Hewmann and L. Oeconomides, *Ber.*, 1887, **20**, 372; B. Fischer and H. Wimmer, *ibid.*, p. 1579; H. V. Kidd, *J. Org. Chem.*, 1937, **2**, 198.

[18] H. Goldschmidt, *Ber.*, 1891, **24**, 2317; H. Goldschmidt and B. Bardack, *Ber.*, 1892, **25**, 1347; H. Goldschmidt and R. U. Reinders, *ibid.*, 1896, **29**, 1369, 1899; H. Goldschmidt and R. M. Salcher, *Z. physik. Chem.*, 1899, **29**, 89; H. Goldschmidt, S. Johnsen, and E. Overwien, *ibid.*, 1924, **110**, 251.

chloroamine rearrangement. Just as in stage (1) of the latter, the acidolysis of chlorine was assumed to involve an S_N2-like substitution by chloride ion at the chlorine atom of a chloroammonium ion, so in stage (1) of the diazoamino-rearrangement the acidolysis of the azo-group is represented as involving the S_N2-like substitution by a nucleophilic conjugate-base at the azo-group of an azo-ammonium ion.

The evidence on the matter is kinetic, and is due entirely to Goldschmidt and his coworkers.[18] They used mainly aniline, or some other such base, as their solvent. They observed the reaction to be of first order with respect to the diazoamino-compound, and to be subject to general acid catalysis. With the strong acids, hydrochloric acid, hydrobromic acid, and nitric acid, as catalysts, the reaction was approximately of first order with respect to the acid; but the three acids had not quite the same absolute kinetic effect, and careful examination of the matter showed that a part of the reaction was of second order with respect to acid. Then, when these strong acids were replaced by successively weaker acids, namely, 3,5-dinitrobenzoic acid, *o*-nitrobenzoic acid, *m*-nitrobenzoic acid, and *o*-bromobenzoic acid, the order with respect to the catalysing acid rose, so that with the weakest acid, at not too low concentration, the order was more nearly two than one. All this is consistent with the view that, for the formation of the transition state of the acidolysis, there is needed the diazoamino-compound, a proton, and a nucleophile; that when strong acids, having weakly nucleophilic anions, are used, the nucleophilic function is fulfilled mainly by the solvent aniline, though halide ions do intervene, in place of the aniline, to a small extent; but that when weak acids, having strongly nucleophilic anions, are employed, these anions intervene, in place of the aniline, to a much larger extent. This interpretation makes the kinetics and mechanism entirely analogous to those of the chloroamine rearrangement.

(50c) Rearrangements of Nitrosamines (Fischer-Hepp).—It was discovered by Otto Fischer and Hepp[19] that certain aromatic nitrosamines undergo rearrangement on treatment with acids, particularly hydrochloric and hydrobromic acids, to give ring-nitrosated isomerides, as in the following example:

$$C_6H_5\cdot NMe(NO) \xrightarrow{HCl} (p)NO\cdot C_6H_4\cdot NHMe$$

The main products are usually para-nitroso-compounds in the simpler examples of the benzene series, but N-nitroso-N-alkyl-2-naphthyl-

[19] O. Fischer and E. Hepp, *Ber.*, 1886, 19, 2291

amines give 1-nitroso-N-alkyl-2-naphthylamines.[20] The reaction is usually carried out with ethyl alcoholic hydrogen chloride or bromide as catalyst; but ethyl ether, acetic acid, and water, have been used as solvents, instead of alcohol.

Fischer and Hepp first believed their isomerisations to be intramolecular rearrangements. But in 1912 Fischer showed[21] that the halogenated by-products, which are usually formed, can be understood as arising from the action of free halogen, produced by oxidation of the catalysing halogen acid by nitrous acid liberated during the reaction. In 1913 Houben showed[22] that in certain examples in which the yield of rearrangement product was poor, a much improved yield could be secured by adding sodium nitrite to the reacting system. As to the mechanism of rearrangements, the evidential value of these observations is, of course, very slight; but, on such evidence, Houben set up the theory that the reaction is intermolecular, consisting of an acidolytic denitrosation, reversing the ordinary method of formation of the nitrosamine, followed by direct ring-nitrosation of the formed secondary amine by the simultaneously formed nitrosyl halide, or perhaps by some conversion product of the latter, such as nitrous acid:

$$C_6H_5\cdot NR\cdot NO + HX \underset{(2)}{\overset{(1)}{\rightleftarrows}} C_6H_5\cdot NHR + NOX$$

$$\xrightarrow{(3)} NO\cdot C_6H_4\cdot NHR + HX$$

Such further evidence as has since been secured has tended to confirm this theory. Neber and Rauscher found that hydrogen chloride and bromide are much more effective as catalysts than other strong acids, in agreement with general experience to the effect that nitrosyl chloride and bromide have a combination of stability and reactivity which makes them particularly useful nitrosating agents.[23] It has been found that on acidolysing an aromatic nitrosamine in the presence of urea, no C-nitroso-isomeride is produced, but only the secondary amine.[24] Various transfers of the nitroso-group to a foreign aromatic molecule have been reported. When N-nitroso-N-methylaniline is treated with ethyl alcoholic hydrogen chloride in the presence

[20] O. Fischer and E. Hepp, *Ber.*, 1887, **20**, 1247, 2471; G. T. Morgan and F. D. Evens, *J. Chem. Soc.*, 1919, **115**, 1142.

[21] O. Fischer, *Ber.*, 1912, **45**, 1098.

[22] J. Houben, *Ber.*, 1913, **46**, 3984.

[23] P. W. Neber and H. Rauscher, *Ann.*, 1942, **550**, 182.

[24] W. Macmillen and T. H. Reade, *J. Chem. Soc.*, **1929**, 585

of dimethylaniline, the products are methylaniline and *p*-nitrosodimethylaniline.[23] Corresponding products are formed when N-nitroso-N-methyl-2,4-dinitroaniline is treated with ethereal hydrogen chloride in the presence of dimethylaniline.[25] What is now needed in order to establish the mechanism firmly is a kinetic study of the rearrangement, and, as far as possible, of the separate reactions, (1), (2), and (3), just as in the example of the chloroamine rearrangement.

(50d) Rearrangements of Alkylanilines (Hofmann-Martius).—The rearrangements which the hydrochlorides and hydrobromides of NN-dialkylanilines and N-alkylanilines undergo by thermal decomposition, to give salts of ring-alkylated secondary or primary aniline derivatives, were discovered by Hofmann and Martius.[26]

$$C_6H_5 \cdot NR_2 \xrightarrow{HX} (o\text{- or } p\text{-})R \cdot C_6H_4 \cdot NHR$$

$$C_6H_5 \cdot NHR \xrightarrow{HX} (o\text{- or } p\text{-})R \cdot C_6H_4 \cdot NH_2$$

Our further knowledge of them is due mainly to Hickinbottom.

The required temperatures are usually high, around 250–300° when the alkyl groups are primary, though temperatures below 200° may suffice for the displacement of secondary and tertiary alkyl groups. The alkyl groups enter mainly into para-positions, if such are free; but ortho-migration will occur if the para-position is occupied; and a minor proportion of ortho-migration may accompany para-migration. Thus N-methylaniline, when rearranged by heating its hydrobromide, gives salts of *p*-toluidine and a little *o*-toluidine. Polyalkylation may occur, not only in the successive conversions of a tertiary amine, through secondary amines, to primary amines, but also in conversions starting from secondary amines. In the latter case there must be alkyl transfer; for whereas, before the change, every molecule of base contained one alkyl group, after the change some molecules contain none, and some two or more. Thus N-*n*-butylaniline, rearranged through its hydrochloride, yields *p*-*n*-butylaniline as the principal basic product, while as by-products aniline and N-*p*-di-*n*-butylaniline are found, together with smaller amounts of more highly butylated anilines.[27] Hickinbottom has shown that alkyl halides, and, for ethyl and higher alkyl groups, olefins, are produced in the course of re-

[25] J. Glazer, E. D. Hughes, C. K. Ingold, A. T. James, G. T. Jones, and E. Roberts, *J. Chem. Soc.*, **1950**, 2657.

[26] A. W. Hofmann and C. A. Martius, *Ber.*, 1871, **4**, 742; A. W. Hofmann, *Ber.*, 1872, **5**, 704, 720; 1874, **7**, 526.

[27] J. Reilly and W. J. Hickinbottom, *J. Chem. Soc.*, 1920, **117**, 103

arrangement: they can be drawn off, and identified, naturally with a diminished yield in the actual rearrangement.[28] He has also shown that alkyl groups isomerise during rearrangement in just the way to be expected if they should pass through a carbonium ionic form. Thus, when N-*iso*butylaniline is rearranged as its hydrobromide, *iso*butyl bromide and *iso*butylene can be drawn off, but the rearrangement product is *p*-*t*-butylaniline.[29] And when N-*iso*amylaniline is similarly rearranged, the products are *iso*amyl bromide, trimethylethylene, and *p*-*t*-amylaniline.[30] It is to be noted that the alkyl group in the alkyl bromide is not rearranged, but that the olefin, and the alkyl group in the C-alkyl aniline, are rearranged. Hickinbottom has shown that the easily ionising alkyl halide, triphenylmethyl chloride, can be used to introduce the triphenylmethyl group into the para-position of dimethylaniline.[30] Finally, he has shown that the various olefins encountered in the study of the rearrangement can be condensed with aniline in the presence of its hydrobromide, under conditions fairly similar to those of the rearrangements, to give the actual products of the rearrangements, *iso*butylene, for example, yielding *p*-*t*-butylaniline.[30]

The Hofmann-Martius rearrangement has long been regarded as intramolecular, and this view still has its adherents. Dewar supported it,[12] adding that the reactions exemplify his "π-bond" theory of rearrangements.[31] But his arguments were inconclusive.

The opposite view, that the reaction is intermolecular, was first suggested by Michael.[32] He thought of the alkyl halides as the active intermediates, and this idea has received support since.[33] Hickinbottom has suggested[30] that the alkyl group is split off from the anilinium ion as a carbonium ion, which may then undergo various independent reactions, combining with halide ion to give the alkyl halide, losing a proton to yield an olefin, and attacking the benzene ring to give the rearrangement product. The carbonium ion would react in its internally rearranged form, if it is one of those which usually do so. This theory explains all the facts except one, namely, that when an alkyl group undergoes internal rearrangement during migration, it may appear in its unrearranged form in the isolated alkyl halide, though it is represented entirely by its rearranged form in the olefin

[28] W. J. Hickinbottom and S. E. A. Ryder, *J. Chem. Soc.*, **1931**, 1281.

[29] W. J. Hickinbottom and G. H. Preston, *J. Chem. Soc.*, **1930**, 1566.

[30] W. J. Hickinbottom, *J. Chem. Soc.*, **1932**, 2396; **1934**, 1700; **1935**, 1279; **1937**, 404.

[31] The support is much qualified in the later statements.

[32] A. Michael, *Ber.*, 1881, **14**, 2105; *J. Am. Chem. Soc.*, 1920, **42**, 787.

[33] E. Beckmann and E. Correns. *Ber.*, 1922, **55**, 852.

and in the *p*-alkylaniline. Hughes suggested[9] a mechanism which is a combination of those of Michael and Hickinbottom, and which takes account of our general knowledge of nucleophilic substitution and elimination. Recalling that the halide ion is strongly nucleophilic towards carbon, but not towards hydrogen, it is assumed that the decomposition of the anilinium salt, in the high concentrations used, proceeds by the S_N2 mechanism:

$$Ph\overset{+}{N}H_2R + \overset{-}{Hal} \rightarrow PhNH_2 + RHal$$

This makes the first step of the rearrangement analogous to that of the Orton rearrangement, and probably also to those of the diazoamino-rearrangement and the Fischer-Hepp rearrangement. It is to be noted that, if R is the kind of alkyl group which is ultimately to suffer an internal rearrangement, as of *iso*butyl to *t*-butyl, it would not yet be rearranged in the alkyl halide. Next, noting that an anilinium salt at a high temperature is to be regarded as a highly polar medium, it is suggested that the alkyl halide attacks the aniline by an S_N1 process, that, is by way of an intermediate carbonium ion, which is also the source of the olefin, formed, according to this theory, in a reversible side-reaction:

$$RHal \rightleftarrows R^+ + Hal^-$$
$$R^+ + PhNH_2 \rightleftarrows \text{Olefin} + PhNH_3^+$$
$$R^+ + PhNH_2 \rightarrow R \cdot C_6H_4 \cdot NH_2 + H^+$$
$$H^+ + PhNH_2 \rightleftarrows PhNH_3^+$$

(50e) Rearrangements of Alkyl Aryl Ethers.—When alkyl aryl ethers are treated with strong acids, such as sulphuric acid, or with Friedel-Crafts catalysts, such as aluminium chloride, in general, with strong electrophiles, dealkylation is the usual result; but in a number of cases this reaction is partly or wholly replaced by a rearrangement, in which the alkyl group enters an ortho- or para-position of the aromatic ring:

$$C_6H_5 \cdot OR \xrightarrow[\text{acid}]{\text{strong}} (o\text{- or } p\text{-})R \cdot C_6H_4 \cdot OH$$

With tertiary alkyl groups the reaction is fairly facile under the conditions indicated; but secondary alkyl groups migrate less easily; and the simplest primary alkyl groups do so with difficulty, or not at all, even in the presence of the more powerful catalysts. Hartmann and Gattermann found that, while anisole and phenetole are totally dealkylated by aluminium chloride, *iso*butyl phenyl ether is only partly dealkylated, the aromatic product containing, besides phenol, a butylphenol, which was subsequently recognised to be *p-t*-butylphenol.[34,35]

A number of circumstances suggest that the catalysed phenolic ether rearrangement is more or less similar in mechanism to the Hofmann-Martius reaction, and in particular that it involves the formation of an alkyl carbonium ion. First, there is the indication of general experience that those alkyl groups migrate more easily from which the derived carbonium ions are more stable. Secondly, not only are alkyl chlorides formed side by side with rearrangement products when aluminium chloride is employed as catalyst, but also olefins have been obtained as by-products in the example of the rearrangement of 2-butyl phenyl ether under catalysis by sulphuric acid in acetic acid.[36] Thirdly, alkyl transfer reactions have been observed. Thus, when *iso*propyl phenyl ether is rearranged under catalysis by aluminium chloride, the phenolic product contains, not only *iso*propyl phenol, but also phenol and a di*iso*propylphenol.[35,37] When the same rearrangement is conducted in the presence of diphenyl ether, some *p-iso*-propylphenyl phenyl ether is formed; and when excess of benzene is present, some *iso*propylbenzene is obtained.[35] Fourthly, those alkyl groups which, in carbonium-ion reactions, normally undergo rearrangement, appear in rearranged form in these migrations. Thus, while 2-butyl phenyl ether, on treatment with aluminium chloride, yields *p*-2-butylphenol, both *iso*butyl phenyl ether and *t*-butyl phenyl ether yield the common rearrangement product, *p-t*-butylphenol.[35] In view of all this it seems certain that, in these acid-catalysed rearrangements, the O-alkyl group leaves its oxygen atom as a carbonium ion, or at least becomes a carbonium ion in some stage of its migration.

The alkyl groups of tertiary alkyl phenyl ethers will migrate to the ring under the action of heat alone, usually at about 200–250°. Thus, *t*-butyl phenyl ether may be thermally rearranged to *p-t*-butylphenol,[35] and *neo*pentyldimethylcarbinyl phenyl ether to *p-neo*-pentyldimethylcarbinylphenol,

$$(CH_3)_3C\cdot CH_2\cdot C(CH_3)_2\cdot C_6H_4\cdot OH$$

In the last case,[38] it was shown that, when diphenyl ether was present,

[34] C. Hartmann and L. Gattermann, *Ber.*, 1892, **25**, 253; Beilstein's "Handbuch der Organischen Chemie," 4th Edn., **6**, 143.

[35] R. A. Smith, *J. Am. Chem. Soc.*, 1933, **55**, 3718; 1934, **56**, 717.

[36] M. M. Sprung and E. S. Wallis, *J. Am. Chem. Soc.*, 1934, **56**, 1715.

[37] F. J. Sowa, H. D. Hinton, and J. A. Nieuwland, *J. Am. Chem. Soc.*, 1933, **55**, 3402; R. A. Smith, *ibid.*, 1934, **56**, 717.

[38] S. Natelson, *J. Am. Chem. Soc.*, 1934, **56**, 1583.

no transfer of the alkyl group to the diphenyl ether molecule took place, contrary to what would presumably have happened in a catalysed rearrangement: apparently pyrolytic rearrangement goes by a different mechanism. It has been found[39] that optically active 1-phenylethyl phenyl ether and the 2,6-xylyl ether, heated at 200°, respectively give incompletely racemised ortho-1-phenylethyl-phenol and para-1-phenylethyl-2,6-xylol, among other products; and from this the conclusion has been drawn that the pyrolytic rearrangements are partly intramolecular. But the details are far from clear.

(51) AROMATIC NUCLEOPHILIC REARRANGEMENTS

(51a) Rearrangements of Hydroxylamines.—When phenylhydroxylamine is treated with dilute aqueous sulphuric acid, *p*-aminophenol is the chief product, as was first observed by Bamberger:[40]

$$C_6H_5\cdot NH\cdot OH \xrightarrow{\text{acid}} (p\text{-})OH\cdot C_6H_4\cdot NH_2$$

The subsequent investigation of this, and of a number of closely related reactions is due chiefly to Bamberger.[41]

The question of the mechanism of these processes has evoked contrary opinions. Bamberger[42] regarded them as proceeding in an "intermolecular" manner, through a univalent nitrogen nitrene Ar-N. His reasons will be mentioned later; and his conclusion, as we shall then see, comes fairly close to what we believe today. The question of polar classification did not arise when Bamberger propounded this theory in 1921. Much more recently, in 1949, Dewar[12] classified the rearrangements, firstly, as intramolecular and, secondly, as electrophilic, with the corollary that they illustrate his "π-bond" theory. His reasons were that the transference of hydroxyl from an arylhydroxylamine to a foreign amine or phenol has not been achieved, and that the production of hydrogen peroxide during rearrangement in aqueous solution has not been observed. However, the conclusions do not follow from the evidence;[43] and they are at variance with what we believe today.

Our present view, first expressed in 1950 by Yukawa,[44] is, indeed, quite the opposite, namely, that the reactions are "intermolecular," and nucleophilic (and have nothing to do with the π-bond theory).

[39] H. Hart and H. S. Eleuterio, *J. Am. Chem. Soc.*, 1954, **76**, 519.

[40] E. Bamberger, *Ber.*, 1894, **27**, 1347, 1548.

[41] E. Bamberger, *locc. cit.*, and many subsequent papers, including three summarising articles: *Ann.*, 1921, **424**, 233, 297; 1925, **441**, 207.

[42] E. Bamberger, *Ann.*, 1921, **424**, 233.

[43] They have been abandoned in the later statements.

[44] Y. Yukawa, *J. Chem. Soc.* (Japan), 1950, **71**, 603.

With the customary ellipsis of allowing single valency structures to stand for mesomeric molecules, this view may be formulated for a para-rearrangement as follows:

$$\text{H}-\text{C}_6\text{H}_4-\text{NH}\cdot\overset{+}{\text{O}}\text{H}_2 \rightarrow \text{H}-\overset{+}{\text{C}_6\text{H}_4}=\text{NH} \xrightarrow{\text{Y:}} \overset{+}{\text{Y}}(\text{H})\text{C}_6\text{H}_4=\text{NH}$$

$$\rightarrow \overset{+}{\text{Y}}-\text{C}_6\text{H}_4-\text{NH}_2$$

In the strictly isomeric change, the nucleophilic reagent, Y:, would be a water molecule; but taking into account closely related non-isomeric substitutions with rearrangement, Y: would be any sufficiently accessible and reactive nucleophilic molecule or anion. In conformity with the acid catalysis of the reactions, they are formulated as starting from the ionic conjugate acid of the arylhydroxylamine, which is here written in the form in which it would undergo the indicated heterolysis, rather than in its probably more stable form with the extra proton carried by nitrogen. The heterolysis product, represented by the second formula, is mesomeric, having its carbonium ionic charge, not only as indicated at the para-position, but also in the ortho-positions; so that, by the use of a different valency structure for the carbonium ion, the formation, in the general case, of ortho- as well as of para-products can be accommodated. The transition from the third to the fourth formula represents an ordinary prototropic change, here written without reference to mechanism. When Y: contains a hydroxyl group, a proton can, of course, be lost from the last product formulated.

The first two steps as written above express a heterolysis to give a mesomeric carbonium ion, which subsequently takes up a nucleophilic reagent in a position other than that of the heterolysis: this is a familiar form of change, a unimolecular nucleophilic substitution with rearrangement, S_N1'. It is conceivable that, in some circumstances, the same two steps would become telescoped into a single step, so that the change would be a bimolecular nucleophilic substitution with rearrangement, S_N2'. The mechanism in this form would be expressed thus:

$$\text{H}-\text{C}_6\text{H}_4-\text{NH}\cdot\overset{+}{\text{O}}\text{H}_2 \xrightarrow{\text{Y:}} \overset{+}{\text{Y}}(\text{H})\text{C}_6\text{H}_4=\text{NH} \rightarrow \overset{+}{\text{Y}}-\text{C}_6\text{H}_4-\text{NH}_2$$

Both mechanisms are well-known routes of anionotropic change (Sections **40b** and **c**), within which major category of organic reactions the arylhydroxylamine rearrangement furnishes an aromatic example. Actually, a decision between these two forms of the nucleophilic mechanism can at present only tentatively be made—in favour of the S_N1' form as the more usual: really crucial distinguishing tests have not yet been applied.

The present evidence for this mechanism derives from a study of the products and kinetics of the reaction. The significant work on products was done many years ago, chiefly by Bamberger.[41] It has more recently been confirmed and extended by Yukawa.[44] When phenylhydroxylamine was rearranged by means of dilute aqueous sulphuric acid, *p*-aminophenol was the main product. However, when ethyl alcohol was used to dilute the acid, *o*- and *p*-phenetidines, and with methyl alcohol, anisidines were formed; and when the acid employed was hydrochloric acid, *o*- and *p*-chloroanilines were produced. When phenol was added, the product was observed to contain $(p)OH \cdot C_6H_4 \cdot C_6H_4 \cdot NH_2(p)$ and some $C_6H_5 \cdot NH \cdot C_6H_4 \cdot OH(p)$, and when aniline was introduced, it contained some $C_6H_5 \cdot NH \cdot C_6H_4 \cdot NH_2(p)$. Formed *p*-aminophenol was in some cases accompanied by the ether, $(p)NH_2 \cdot C_6H_4 \cdot O \cdot C_6H_4 \cdot NH_2(p)$. The fact that so many fragments can appear in place of OH in the arylhydroxylamine-aminophenol conversion, strongly suggests that the latter is not an intramolecular rearrangement. Furthermore, since all the fragments come from obvious nucleophiles,

$$Y: = H_2O,\ EtOH,\ MeOH,\ Cl^-,\ PhOH,\ PhNH_2,\ NH_2 \cdot C_6H_4OH(p)$$

one is led to assume an active electrophilic intermediate.

Bamberger made an extensive comparison between the products obtained from arylhydroxylamines and those produced by nitrogen loss from the corresponding aryl azides in similar conditions. He found the two sets of products to be essentially (and strikingly) identical, and was accordingly led to assume a common univalent-nitrogen intermediate, Ar-N. Now if we supply this nitrene with the extra proton shown by the kinetics to be involved, it becomes $Ar\text{-}\overset{+}{N}H$, which is only another valency structure for the mesomeric carbonium ion already assumed as the active electrophilic intermediate.

By rearranging *p*-tolylhydroxylamine in aqueous acid at low temperatures, Bamberger demonstrated the formation of the methyl iminoquinol and quinol,

$$\underset{HO}{\overset{CH_3}{>}}C_6H_4{=}NH \quad \text{and} \quad \underset{HO}{\overset{CH_3}{>}}C_6H_4{=}O$$

along with products derived from them. This is where the sequence of reactions representing the nucleophilic mechanism would have to stop, when the final prototropic change is blocked by methyl substitution.

It should be mentioned that Bamberger usually found aniline and azoxybenzene among the products obtained from phenylhydroxylamine. However, these substances probably arose from an irrelevant oxidation-reduction of phenylhydroxylamine.

This is one of the points established by a kinetic examination of the reaction.[45] The redox conversion is a chain-reaction, easily started by short exposures to atmospheric oxygen, but avoidable by arranging that the phenylhydroxylamine has never been exposed to oxygen. The acid-catalysed rearrangements of phenylhydroxylamine are completely separate, and are not dependent on oxygen or other oxidants.

The kinetic study also shows that rearrangement depends on the conjugate acid of phenylhydroxylamine. At low acidities, the rate is proportional to the acidity; but it ceases to increase proportionally to the acid when enough acid has been added to ionise nearly the whole of the base.

Obviously the matter needs further study: yet it seems a reasonable presumption that the general character of the arylhydroxylamine rearrangement has been correctly outlined.

(52) AROMATIC INTRAMOLECULAR REARRANGEMENTS

(52a) Rearrangements of Nitroamines.—It was found by Bamberger that phenylnitroamine, phenylmethylnitroamine, and similar arylnitroamines undergo rearrangement on treatment with aqueous strong acids, or with hydrogen chloride in organic solvents, to yield mainly *o*-nitroaniline or its derivatives, sometimes with a small amount of *p*-nitroaniline or its derivatives:[46]

$$C_6H_5\cdot NH\cdot NO_2 \xrightarrow{\text{acids}} o\text{-}NO_2\cdot C_6H_4\cdot NH_2$$

Having found in a parallel series of researches that treatment of primary and secondary amines with neutral or not strongly acid nitrating agents, such as dinitrogen pentoxide, will often lead to N-nitration, he made the suggestion[47] that the aromatic C-nitration of these amines by strongly acidic nitrating agents consists of an N-nitration followed

[45] H. E. Heller, E. D. Hughes, and C. K. Ingold, *Nature*, 1951, **168**, 909.

[46] E. Bamberger and K. Landsteiner, *Ber.*, 1893, **26**, 485; E. Bamberger, *Ber.*, 1894, **27**, 359; 1897, **30**, 1248.

[47] E. Bamberger, *Ber.*, 1894 **27**, 584; 1895, **28**, 399.

by an acid-catalysed intramolecular rearrangement of the N-nitro-compound to the C-nitro compound.

Now this hypothesis of "indirect nitration," as it has been called, was obviously not necessitated by the facts. It would have been equally possible, on the same facts, to set up the alternative hypothesis that, in analogy with the chloroamine rearrangement or the diazo-amino-aminoazo-rearrangement, for example, the nitroamine rearrangement is not intramolecular, but is one of the so-called "intermolecular rearrangements," that is, a composite process, consisting of an acidolysis of the N-nitro-group to give a nitrating agent, followed by participation of the latter in an ordinary aromatic nitration. In terms of the scheme written below, instead of assuming "indirect nitration," that is, that reaction (3) is really (2+4), Bamberger might have assumed "intermolecular rearrangement," that is, that (4) is really (1+3):

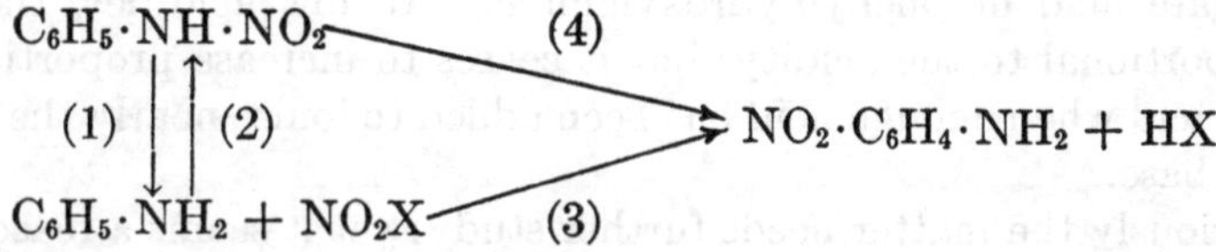

A third alternative hypothesis is equally open, namely, that both the preceding assumptions are incorrect, and that reactions (3) and (4) both exist as independent processes, reactions (1) and (2) taking no part in the process.

Orton attempted to test the second alternative hypothesis, namely, that the isomerisation of the nitroamine might be an "intermolecular rearrangement," *i.e.*, the hypothesis that reaction (4) is really(1+3). An answer in this sense would have corresponded with that which he had established for the chloroamine rearrangements (Section **50a**). However, he and his collaborators quickly found that the nitroamine rearrangement was very different.[48] They noted that it was subject to catalysis by any strong acid. Their main conclusion was that, although in special cases nitroamines in acid solution could be observed to nitrate a foreign aromatic compound, thus proving that a nitrating agent is present in these conditions, "no nitrating agent invariably and normally appears in the system in which a nitroamine is undergoing isomeric change."

Hughes and Jones have further examined[49] the matter in two ex-

[48] K. J. P. Orton and A. E. Smith, *J. Chem. Soc.*, 1905, **87,** 389; K. J. P. Orton and C. Pearson, *ibid.*, 1908, **93,** 725; K. J. P. Orton, *Brit. Assoc. Advancement Sci., Rept.*, **1912,** 116; *Chem. News*, 1912, **106,** 236; A. E. Bradfield and K. J. P. Orton, *J. Chem. Soc.*, **1929,** 915.

[49] E. D. Hughes and G. T. Jones, *J. Chem. Soc.*, **1950,** 2678.

amples, which, illustrating complementary kinetic situations, further elucidate Orton's statement. Their first example was that of *p*-nitrophenyl-N-methylnitroamine, which underwent rearrangement to 2, 4-dinitro-N-methylaniline,

$$(4\text{-})NO_2\cdot C_6H_4\cdot NMe\cdot NO_2 \rightarrow (2,4\text{-})(NO_2)_2C_6H_3\cdot NHMe$$

in the presence of a variety of acids, ranging in strength from formic acid to sulphuric acid, and in a number of solvents, including water, ethyl alcohol, acetic acid, and ethyl ether. However, they found that under no conditions could any denitration of the nitroamine be detected, either by the formation of *p*-nitro-N-methylaniline in the presence of an easily nitrated foreign substance, or by the actual nitration of the added substance. The second example was that of 2, 4-dinitrophenyl-N-methylnitroamine, which suffered rearrangement to 2, 4, 6-trinitro-N-methylaniline,

$$(2,4\text{-})(NO_2)_2C_6H_3\cdot NMe\cdot NO_2 \rightarrow (2,4,6\text{-})(NO_2)_3C_6H_2\cdot NHMe$$

either in 80% aqueous sulphuric acid or in pure sulphuric acid. They found that the nitroamine readily underwent denitration in these conditions, as shown both by the isolation of the denitration product, 2,4-dinitro-N-methylaniline, in the presence of added easily nitratable substances, such as *p*-xylene, phenol, or dimethylaniline, and also by the isolation of nitration products of such added materials. However, they found that neither the produced nitrating agent, nor nitric acid added in equivalent amount, was able to nitrate the denitration product, 2,4-dinitro-N-methylaniline, to the rearrangement product, 2,4,6-trinitro-N-methylaniline, under the conditions in which the rearrangement itself readily took place. Thus, in terms of a scheme of the type of that given above, Hughes and Jones's first case established that reaction (4) could not be replaced by (1+3), because (1) was too slow, while their second case proved that it could not when (1) was fast enough, because (3) was too slow.

Holleman, Hartogs, and van der Linden attempted to test the hypothesis of "indirect nitration," by measuring the proportions of *o*-, *m*-, and *p*-nitro-products, as obtained by the nitration of aniline, and by the action of acids on phenylnitroamine.[50] They obtained the results given in the upper part of Table 52-1, and concluded that the C-nitration of aniline does not always proceed by way of an initial N-nitration. The caution apparent in this statement reflects the circumstance that the conditions of nitration and rearrangement were not identical, and that the proportions of isomers formed by nitration are sensitive to the conditions. However, Hughes and G. T. Jones

[50] A. F. Holleman, J. C. Hartogs, and T. van der Linden, *Ber.*, 1911, **44**, 704.

TABLE 52-1.—PROPORTIONS OF NITRO-COMPOUNDS FORMED BY NITRATION OF ANILINE AND BY REARRANGEMENT OF PHENYLNITROAMINE.

Process	Conditions	o-%	m-%	p-%
Holleman, Hartogs, and Linden (1911)				
Nitration	$PhNH_3NO_3$, 95% aq.H_2SO_4, −20°	4	39	56
Nitration	$PhNH_3NO_3$, 80% aq.HNO_3	5	32	62
Nitration	$PhNH_3NO_3$, Ac_2O	82	3	15
Rearrangement	$PhNH\cdot NO_2$, 74%, aq.H_2SO_4, −20°	95	1.5	3.5
Hughes and Jones (1950)				
Nitration	$PhNH_3NO_3$, 85% aq.H_2SO_4, 10°	6	34	59
Rearrangement	$PhNH\cdot NO_2$, 85% aq.H_2SO_4, 10°	93	0	7

have conducted similar experiments in which the same conditions were used for nitration and for rearrangement.[49] Their results, given in the lower part of Table 52-1, leave no doubt that reactions (3) and (4) are essentially independent processes.

It follows that, of the three hypotheses originally open, we have to choose the third: reactions (3) and (4) are independent processes.

At this stage of the investigation, the main question was why the nitroamine rearrangement in particular should have an easy intramolecular route, which is denied to all the rearrangements discussed in the two preceding Sections. It was supposed that the reason might be the same as the reason why the nitroamine rearrangement gave such an outstandingly high proportion of ortho-product, namely, that, just as in the Claisen rearrangement, the migrating group contains an unsaturated three-atom system,[51] which could bridge to an ortho-position. The small amount of para-product might arise through some intermolecular nitration process, or by a second step of intramolecular bridging. Brownstein, Bunton, and Hughes rearranged N-nitroaniline in aqueous sulphuric acid containing ^{15}N-nitric acid. No uptake of ^{15}N occurred, either into ortho- *or into the para*-rearrangement product. The conclusion was drawn that both isomers arose by intramolecular routes; and in explanation they formulated a theory, based on a proposal made by Hughes a few years earlier,[52] of successive bridging by nitrito-groups.[53]

[51] The migrating group in the diazoamino-rearrangement has such a system, but its third atom is an α-benzenoid atom which might be unable to function.

[52] E. D. Hughes, recorded in the first edition of this book, 1953, p. 628.

[53] S. Brownstein, C. A. Bunton, and E. D. Hughes, *Chem. and Ind.*, **1956**, 981: *J. Chem. Soc.*, **1958**, 4354.

$$H_2\overset{+}{N}-N^{+}(O^-)=O \rightleftharpoons H_2\overset{+}{N}-O-N=O \rightleftharpoons H_2\overset{+}{N}=C_6H_5(H)(O-N=O) \rightleftharpoons H_2\overset{+}{N}=C_6H_5(H)(O-N=O)$$

$+H^+$ ⇅ $-H^+$ $C_6H_5\cdot NH\cdot NO_2$; $-H^+$ ↓ $o\text{-}NO_2\cdot C_6H_4\cdot NH_2$; $-H^+$ ↓ $p\text{-}NO_2\cdot C_6H_4\cdot NH_2$

The first step in this scheme describes specific hydrogen-ion catalysis. It is an open question whether the N-nitrito-intermediate should be retained or short-circuited as it could be. In the final C-nitrito-to-C-nitro reconversions, with aromatising deprotonations, the order of the steps is left as another open question.

Banthorpe and Hughes and their coworkers have established several further points relating to the rearrangement of N-nitroaniline, N-nitro-1-naphthylamine, and N-nitro-N-methyl-1-naphthylamine.[54] All give mainly ortho- or 2-nitro-rearrangement products along with minor amounts of the para- or 4-nitro-products. These workers proved that the catalysis is of the specific hydrogen-ion, rather than of the general acid, type in all cases. They applied both of the standard tests for making this distinction. First, they found that the rate followed Hammett's h_0 rather than $[H^+]$. The slopes of the plots of log k versus $-H_0$ were about 1.3, but the excess slope could be a salt effect, because, in a similar study of catalysis in the benzidine rearrangement (Section **50b**), such an apparent excess of slope disappeared when the Hammett function was determined in the salt conditions of the rate measurements. Secondly, it was found that the rate was increased in a deutero-acid medium. This indicated that a proton was being taken up in pre-equilibrium, and a deuteron more extensively so, because D_3O^+ is a stronger acid in D_2O than H_3O^+ is in H_2O. The same demonstration has been given in the same two ways by White and his associates for the rearrangement of N-nitro-N-methylaniline.[55]

A second group of findings by Banthorpe and Hughes, though in agreement with previous observations by Orton[48] and by Hughes and Jones,[49] contradicted a common assumption, probably based on the

[54] D. V. Banthorpe, E. D. Hughes, and D. L. H. Williams, *J. Chem. Soc.*, 1964, 5349; D. V. Banthorpe, J. A. Thomas, and D. L. H. Williams, *ibid.*, 1965, 6135; D. V. Banthorpe and J. A. Thomas, *ibid.*, p. 7149.

[55] W. N. White, J. K. Klink, D. Lazdins, C. Hathaway, J. T. Golden, and H. S. White, *J. Am. Chem. Soc.*, 1961, 83, 2024.

behaviour of the N-nitro-derivatives of polynitroanilines such as picramide, that if the N-nitro-group of N-nitroaniline or a simple derivative were heterolysed by acid, it would appear as nitric acid. On the contrary, it appears as nitrous acid, and products, such as diazonium ions, that are obviously formed from nitrous acid; and these substances arise along with phenols, and such coloured oxidation products and tars as would arise from an *o*- or *p*-aminophenol in the presence of nitrous acid. Now the rearrangement in high yield of N-nitroaniline requires somewhat high acidities (*e.g.*, 75% aqueous sulphuric acid). At much lower acidities, losses of rearrangement yields of up to 40% can arise through the side-chain breakdown described. At very high acidities side-chain breakdown becomes prominent again, now in a drastic fashion in which oxides of nitrogen are visibly evolved. The Hughes mechanism allows an easy loss of nitrite ion from a rearranging N-nitroaniline at various intermediate stages of its rearrangement.[56]

A third section of the work consisted in the testing of the intramolecular nature of these rearrangements by the ^{15}N method over wide ranges of acidity, including acidities at which concurrent side-chain breakdown is considerable. The ^{15}N was introduced into the rearrangment medium both as nitrite and as nitrate; but in no case could any uptake of that isotope into any rearrangement product be detected.

A fourth group of results by these investigators related to the effects of substrate deuteration in those aromatic positions to which the nitro-group would migrate. Deuteration of N-nitroaniline in the 2,4,6-positions, and of N-nitro-1-naphthylamine in the 2,4-positions, had no effect on rates of rearrangement. It was concluded that the final proton losses, and the ortho-para nitrito-interchange in competition with them, are all fast processes subsequent to the rate-controlling step of the Hughes mechanism. In the reaction of N-nitro-1-naphthyl-

[56] Dewar (ref. 12) has raised, as a *complaint* against the mechanism, that it allows easy nitrite loss. He may have been unaware of the evidence that the labile nitro-group, when it separates, does so as nitrite ion, to leave the tars and other products that he says he would predict from the Hughes mechanism, and does *not* (except in polynitro-examples) leave as nitronium ion, convertible to nitrate ion. He has also objected to the postulated nitrite-to-nitro isomerisations on the ground that they are unrealised among alkyl nitrites. But in spite of that, such conversions should be possible, because the nitrite ion can certainly combine with the carbonium ion to form either a nitro-compound or a nitrite, and in retrogression of this process a sufficient polarisation of a nitrito-group in the direction of nitrite-ion formation should allow isomerisation to the thermodynamically more stable nitro-form.

amine, 2,4-deuteration substantially increased side-chain breakdown. This was taken to mean that eliminated nitrite ion comes largely from the C-nitrites of the Hughes mechanism; wherefore such elimination is in competition with the aromatising proton losses, and gains an advantage when the proton losses suffer the handicap of becoming deuteron losses. In the reaction of N-nitroaniline, either ortho- or para-deuteration diverts rearrangement to the other position, the effect of para-deuteration being the larger. This dissymmetry could be understood on the basis that, in the benzene series, para-quinonoid bond arrangements are more stable than ortho-quinonoid (Section 22d), and, on aromatisation, must need more activation energy, entailing a greater loss of zero-point energy, and a greater primary isotopic retardation.

All this implies that the rate-controlling step in the Hughes mechanism lies somewhere between the first conjugate acid of the nitroamine and the first C-nitrite.

There is one other recurrent observation on which some suggestion should be offered, and that is that side-chain breakdown, *i.e.*, the failure of its lost nitro-group to arrive in the aromatic ring, is minimised at an acidity optimum. As to this, Banthorpe, Hughes, and Williams have proposed that the added proton must be retained in the system long enough to retard nitrite-ion loss from the C-nitrites, but that the aromatising ortho- and para-proton losses must not be impeded by too high an acidity.

Other theories of the nitroamine rearrangement have been propounded. White and his associates suggested homolysis of the conjugate acid of the nitroamine to an aromatic radical-cation acid and a nitrogen dioxide molecule, which are held together by the solvent prior to their recombination.[55] These investigators found that side-chain breakdown was increased by added substances, such as iodine, that could be thought to destroy radicals. Nitrite might be sensitive to the same additives, but the nitrate, which should be formed in equivalence from nitrogen dioxide, should survive. It has not been found to do so. Banthorpe and his collaborators have searched for radical intermediates in several examples, both by looking for electron spin resonance signals, and by seeking kinetic effects on radical chain polymerisations. These attempts have been uniformly unsuccessful.

Dewar had applied his π-bond theory to this as to most other intramolecular rearrangements.[12] In this particular application the nitro-group migrates as a π-complexed nitronium ion. Its uncoupling from the system should therefore produce nitrate, and not nitrite, contrary to the observations. It is also not clear why the π-complex of a nitronium ion with an aniline molecule should behave so very differently (Table 52-1) according to whether it is produced directly from these entities or from protonated N-nitroaniline, the medium being the same.

The nitroamine rearrangement can occur otherwise than under acid catalysis. Banthorpe and Thomas have recorded some information about the rearrangement of N-nitro-N-methyl-1-naphthylamine in neutral media at 100°, and also about the photochemically promoted rearrangement of the same substance at 20°. The mechanisms in operation under these conditions are not yet understood.[57]

(52b) The Benzidine Rearrangement.—Hydrazobenzene was discovered, and its conversion to benzidine under the influence of acids was first observed, by Hofmann[58] in 1863. Benzidine was known already, Fittig[59] having identified it as a diaminobiphenyl. The positions of its amino-groups were established later by Schultz.[60] Schmidt and Schultz[61] noted the formation, along with benzidine, of a minor proportion of a second diaminobiphenyl, so-called diphenyline; and with Strasser[62] they determined the positions of its amino-groups. The further investigation of these and related rearrangements is due chiefly to Jacobson,[63] who established the formation, not indeed from hydrazobenzene, but from many other benzenoid hydrazo-compounds, of two other types of isomerisation products. These were both amino-diphenylamines, and are usually called ortho- and para-semidines.

Under the name "benzidine rearrangement," it is customary to summarise the whole family of rearrangements, in which aromatic hydrazo-compounds, on treatment with acids, yield either diaminobiphenyls or aminodiphenylamines, by ortho- or para-coupling of the two arylamine residues of which the hydrazo-compound can be considered composed. The possible products are 2,2′-, 2,4′-, and 4,4′-diaminobiphenyls, respectively known as ortho-benzidines, diphenylines, and benzidines, and 2- and 4-aminodiphenylamines, known as ortho-semidines and para-semidines. Not all these need arise in any one example, but the types can all be found among known examples, and hence their relation may be represented by the omnibus scheme below, in which A and B stand for substituents in general:

[57] D. V. Banthorpe and J. A. Thomas, *J. Chem. Soc.*, **1965**, **7158**.

[58] A. W. Hofmann, *Proc. Roy. Soc.* (London), 1863. **12**, **576**.

[59] R. Fittig, *Ann.*, 1862, **124**, **282**.

[60] G. Schultz, *Ann.*, 1874, **174**, **227**.

[61] H. Schmidt and G. Schultz, *Ber.*, 1878, **11**, **1754**.

[62] H. Schmidt and G. Schultz, *Ann.*, 1881, **207**, **320**; *idem* and H. Strasser, *ibid.*, p. 348.

[63] P. Jacobson, many papers from 1892 to 1922, including the summarising paper. *Ann.*, 1922, **428**, **76**.

ortho-Semidine: NH_2 on ring A ortho to ·NH·, linked to ring B (A·NH·B)

para-Semidine: A·NH·BNH_2

A NH·NH B → ortho-Benzidine (NH_2 NH_2, A—B); Diphenyline (NH_2 on A, A—BNH_2); Benzidine (NH_2A—BNH_2)

Alongside of these isomerisations, reactions of disproportionation may occur: some of the hydrazo-compound becomes reduced to aniline bases (the "fission amines"), and some becomes oxidised to the azo-compound:

$$\text{A}\,NH\cdot NH\,\text{B} \rightarrow \begin{cases} \text{A}\,NH_2 + NH_2\,\text{B} \\ \text{A}\,N = N\,\text{B} \end{cases}$$

The acids used to effect these changes are often dilute aqueous or aqueous-alcoholic solutions of strong acids, such as hydrochloric or sulphuric acids. Hydrogen chloride in an organic solvent is sometimes employed. With such strong acids the rearrangements are usually rapid. Some of them can be effected by weak acids, such as acetic acid. A method, which has been considerably employed on account of its convenience, for investigating the products formed by the rearrangements of hydrazo-compounds, side-steps the actual preparation of the hydrazo-compounds, and proceeds by reducing the related, usually easily prepared azo-compounds with an acid reducing agent: the hydrazo-compound is produced, and is at once rearranged, though a certain amount of reductive fission into primary amines often comes into competition with the processes of rearrangement.

When hydrazobenzene itself is rearranged, the formed mixture of isomers contains about 70% of benzidine and 30% of diphenyline, along with other isomers in chromatographic traces. Few ortho-benzidines have been obtained in substantial amount in the benzene series, though ortho-semidines, diphenylines, and parasemidines are not infrequently encountered. In the naphthalene series, on the contrary, products of ortho-benzidine type appear, but no isomer of diphenyline type has ever been established as an important product.

Substituents play a large part in determining the course followed by the rearrangement of a hydrazobenzene. They would play a larger part, but for the circumstance that these rearrangements are very "strong" processes, often able to cause the ejection of a substituent which stands in their way. The groups SO_3H and CO_2H are thus ejected more easily than most groups, Cl and OAc rather less easily, OR less easily still, and NRAc, NR_2, and Alk, not at all. For example, hydrazobenzene-4-carboxylic acid gives benzidine in high yield with loss of the carboxyl group, while 4-acetoxyhydrazobenzene gives benzidine only in low yield, the rearrangement being largely diverted by the substituent in the direction of a diphenyline which retains the substituent. There is evidence here that both polarities occur in the benzene rings involved in rearrangement. For the groups SO_3H and CO_2H appear as H_2SO_4 and H_2CO_3, having left their bond electrons behind them on being ejected. The groups Cl and OAc, on the other hand, appear as HCl and HOAc, and must have carried their bond electrons away with them on their expulsion.

Two firm-standing para-substituents in a hydrazobenzene block all the commonly observed rearrangements, except that leading to an ortho-semidine. One firm-standing para-substituent blocks the formation of a benzidine: and whether the main rearrangement product will be a diphenyline or an ortho-semidine depends on the nature of the para-substituent. Para-semidines are usually minor products. Substituents in ortho- or meta-positions in the hydrazobenzene considerably affect the orientation of rearrangement. A large body of qualitative and semiquantitative data on the composition of products of rearrangements of hydrazobenzenes was recorded by Jacobson.[63] In spite of the need for reserve in drawing conclusions from data, obtained as these were, before multiplicity of mechanism in benzidine rearrangements was appreciated, one does gain from them the impression that the property of substituents most important for their orienting action is the property of polarity, as in most other heterolytic aromatic reactions.

The question of the *mechanism of the benzidine rearrangement* has been a challenge since the beginning of this century. The immediate difficulty was to understand how the hydrazobenzene molecule could turn itself inside out without coming to pieces. The earliest theories, both of 1903, assumed that in fact it fell into pieces, which subsequently rejoined.

Tichwinsky[64] assumed what we should now understand as a preliminary homolysis of the N—N bond of the hydrazine. He wrote his mechanism as follows:

[64] M. Tichwinsky, *J. Russ. Phys. Chem. Soc.*, 1903, 35, 667.

$$\begin{matrix} C_6H_5\cdot NH \\ | \\ C_6H_5\cdot NH \end{matrix} + 2HCl \rightarrow 2(\cdot C_6H_4\cdot NH_2\cdot HCl) \rightarrow \begin{matrix} C_6H_4\cdot NH_2\cdot HCl \\ | \\ C_6H_4\cdot NH_2\cdot HCl \end{matrix}$$

The precise mode of incursion of the acid is an adjustable detail in this theory: what is essential is the assumed dissociation into radicals, whose radical centres are transferred to ortho- and para-positions. Jacobson[63] advanced two arguments against theories of this type. First, he cited the work of Wieland[65] on the tetra-arylhydrazines, which freely dissociate in solution to radicals in measurable equilibrium proportions, but do not undergo the benzidine rearrangement in these conditions:

$$(C_6H_5)_2N\cdot N(C_6H_5)_2 \rightleftharpoons 2(C_6H_5)_2N\cdot$$

Secondly, Jacobson pointed out that he had studied the products of rearrangement of many unsymmetrically substituted hydrazo-compounds AB, and had obtained only unsymmetrical benzidines AB, never a symmetrical benzidine AA or BB. This finding has since been confirmed[66,67] with systems designed for the easy detection of small amounts of a symmetrical benzidine, if such were formed.

The second theory of 1903, that of Stieglitz,[68] assumed what we should now interpret as a heterolytic splitting of the NN-bond. He wrote his suggestion as follows:

$$C_6H_5\cdot NH\cdot NH\cdot C_6H_5 + HX \rightarrow C_6H_5\cdot N< + XH_3N\cdot C_6H_5$$
$$H_2N\cdot C_6H_5 + >C_6H_4{:}NH \rightarrow H_2N\cdot C_6H_4\cdot C_6H_4\cdot NH_2$$

The meaning of this, in terms of the electronic theory of valency, becomes clear when it is realised that the conjugate acids of the represented nitrene and carbene, are only different valency structures of the heterolysis fragment $(C_6H_5{:}NH)^+$, which is assumed to combine with the other heterolysis fragment $C_6H_5\cdot NH_2$:

$$C_6H_5\cdot NH\cdot NH\cdot C_6H_5 \xrightarrow{H^+} (C_6H_5{:}NH)^+ + NH_2\cdot C_6H_5 \rightarrow \text{Benzidine etc.}$$

Jacobson's arguments against the theory of homolytic dissociation are not particularly damaging to this theory, not even his second argument; because, if an unsymmetrical hydrazobenzene AB heterolysed in its preferred direction, it would give functionally complementary fragments, A^+ and B^-, say; and they would have to reunite to give the unsymmetrical benzidine AB. But in 1933 Kidd and the writer

[65] H. Wieland, *Ann.*, 1912, 392, 127; *Ber.*, 1915, **48**, 1095.
[66] G. W. Wheland and T. R. Schwartz, *J. Chem. Phys.*, 1949, **17**, 425.
[67] G. J. Bloink and K. H. Pausacker, *J. Chem. Soc.*, **1950**, 950.
[68] J. Stieglitz, *Am. Chem. J.*, 1903, **29**, 62–63, footnote.

carried out the test of rearranging two closely similar, symmetrical hydrazobenzenes, AA and BB, in the same solution. The product was a mixture of the symmetrical benzidines AA and BB, and contained none of the unsymmetrical benzidine AB, which should have been formed if the hydrazo-compounds had undergone any form of dissociation, homolytic or heterolytic. So, since 1933 it has been generally agreed that the hydrazobenzene molecule does not come to pieces in the course of the benzidine rearrangement. And thus the result of the first 30 years of research since the earliest theories of the rearrangement were promulgated was simply to close the way of escape, provided by those theories, from the difficulty of understanding the stereochemical convolution which rearrangement involves.

The demonstration of 1933 was simply that, when 2,2′-dimethoxy- and 2,2′-diethoxy-hydrazobenzene,

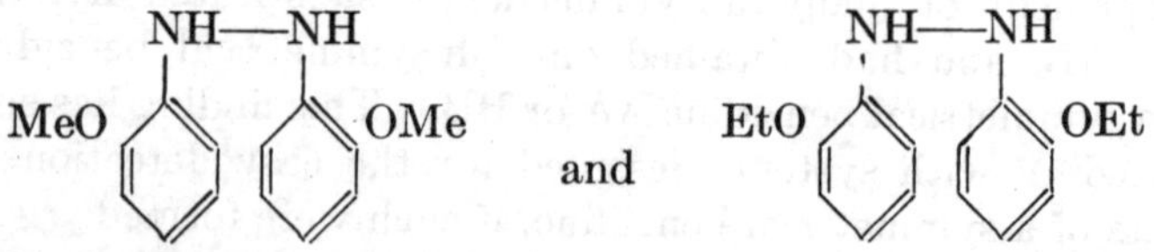

NH—NH (MeO, OMe) and NH—NH (EtO, OEt)

were rearranged with acid in the same solution, the product was a binary mixture of 3,3′-dimethoxy- and 3,3′-diethoxy-benzidine,

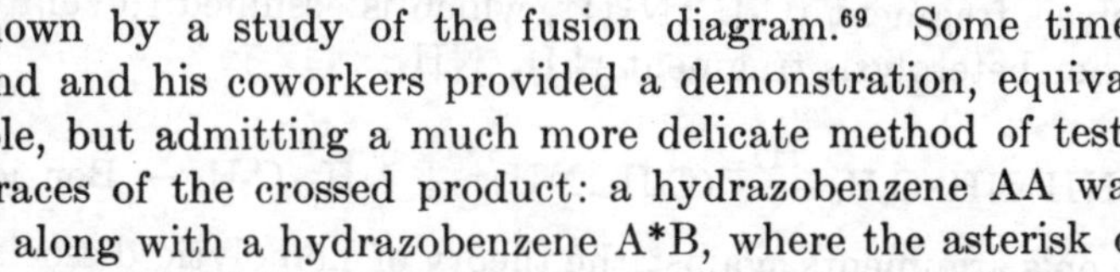

NH_2 NH_2 (MeO, OMe) and NH_2 NH_2 (EtO, OEt)

The absence of the crossed product, 3-methoxy-3′-ethoxybenzidine, was shown by a study of the fusion diagram.[69] Some time later, Wheland and his coworkers provided a demonstration, equivalent in principle, but admitting a much more delicate method of testing for even traces of the crossed product: a hydrazobenzene AA was rearranged along with a hydrazobenzene A*B, where the asterisk denotes a label of radioactivity; and the recovered benzidine AA was checked for radioactivity. The initial substances were 2,2′-dimethylhydrazobenzene and 2-^{14}C-methylhydrazobenzene. The recovered 3,3′-dimethylbenzidine was not radioactive.[70] Still later, after multiplicity of mechanism in benzidine rearrangements had been recognised, and after the rearrangements of hydrazonaphthalenes had assumed an in-

[69] C. K. Ingold and H. V. Kidd, *J. Chem. Soc.*, **1933**, 984.

[70] D. H. Smith, J. R. Schwartz, and G. W. Wheland, *J. Am. Chem. Soc.*, 1952, **74**, 2282.

creased importance in the developing study of the mechanism of the benzidine rearrangement, Banthorpe extended the demonstrations into this field. He rearranged pairs of the three isomeric hydrazonaphthalenes, the 1,1′-, 1,2′-, and 2,2′-isomers, in the same solution, and, once again, obtained no crossed products. For the detection of minor products, he used paper chromatography, which shows trace products in the tenths percent range.[71] It would be a misdirection of effort to strive after a greater delicacy of detection, since it would be almost impossible to prove that a very small trace product, if such were formed, arose from the main reaction and not from some minor independent reaction.

For some time after 1933, the main contributions to the problem of the benzidine rearrangement were theoretical. It was necessary to understand how a drastic stereochemical convolution could occur in an intramolecular reaction. Three ways of meeting this challenge were proposed.

One was the polar-transition-state theory,[72] incepted by Hughes and the writer in 1941, and modified since, notably by the incorporation of a suggestion by Hammick and Mason[73] in 1946. This theory assumes only intermediates having only ordinary benzenoid or quinonoid bonding. But it assumes, between such, transition states having certain bonds of a strongly polar character. This strong electrostatic content will confer on the bonds considerably greater lengths, and very much lower bending force-constants, than those possessed by ordinary bonds. These characteristics can be shown to permit energetically cheap shape-changes drastic enough to meet the stereochemical requirements. The transient polar bonds resemble those of unimolecular solvolysis (Section **32d**).

Another theory, proposed by Dewar in 1946, is the "π-complex" theory.[12] It has been modified in detail, but its distinguishing feature is that rearrangement is supposed to go through a protonated π-complex. This complex is a definite intermediate: it is not a transition state. In it, the original N—N bond is replaced by a delocalised covalency, called a "π-bond," between the aromatic rings. The π-bond holds the rings in parallel planes, with the possibility of relative rotation. Products follow when the π-bond is replaced by a localised interatomic bond.

[71] D. V. Banthorpe, *J. Chem. Soc.*, **1962,** 2413.

[72] E. D. Hughes and C. K. Ingold, *J. Chem. Soc.*, **1941,** 608; **1950,** 1638; C. K. Ingold, *Chem. Soc. Special Pubs.*, 1962, **16,** 118.

[73] D. Ll. Hammick and S. F. Mason, *J. Chem. Soc.*, **1946,** 638; D. Ll. Hammick and D. C. Munro, *ibid.*, **1950,** 2049.

The remaining theory, which has been discussed on a number of occasions since 1950, but was first seriously advocated by Večera and his coworkers in 1960, is the "caged-dissociation" theory.[74] It assumes homolytic splitting of the protonated hydrazo-molecule into protonated radicals, which are structurally independent, but are restrained from kinetic independence by a solvent "cage." The most evident objection to this theory is the difficulty of understanding the absence of attack on the walls of the cage, indeed, on those of a variety of cages; for many benzidine rearrangements have been conducted in many solvents, no single characteristic fragment of any of which has ever appeared in combination in a rearrangement product. A further objection is that sensitive methods for the detection of radical intermediates have failed to detect any.[75] Dewar has criticised the theory on the ground that it is inconsistent with the products of rearrangements.[12] The theory runs into further difficulties in connexion with the kinetics of rearrangements, as we shall see.[76] It is no longer exclusively supported by Večera.[74]

The *kinetics* of the acid rearrangement of hydrazobenzene were first examined in 1904 by van Loon,[77] who found a kinetic order of two in acid:

$$-(d[\mathrm{Hz}]/dt)/[\mathrm{Hz}] = k_1 = k_3[\mathrm{H}^+]^2$$

This finding remained largely forgotten until it was made again in 1950 by Hammond and Shine.[78] A number of investigators at once took up the work of generalising this result; and within a few years it was generalised over a number of substituted hydrazobenzenes in a number of solvents. In the course of this work, Carlin and Odioso encountered the anomaly that the rearrangement of 2,2′-dimethylhydrazobenzene (*o*-hydrazotoluene) in "95%" aqueous ethanol showed an order in acid, not of 2, but of 1.6, in their conditions.[79] The search now became one for the limits of validity of the Loon-Hammond-Shine kinetics. But this problem proved less easy: indeed, it needed the guidance of theory to solve it. In the meantime, for nearly a decade, Carlin and Odioso's example of an order in acid of less than two remained unique.

[74] M. Večera, L. Synek, and J. Sterba, *Coll. Czech. Chem. Comm.*, 1960, **25**, 1992. Cf. *ibid.*, 1966, **31**, 3486.

[75] D. V. Banthorpe, R. Bramley, and J. A. Thomas, *J. Chem. Soc.*, **1964**, 2900.

[76] For a review of these theories in relation to the data on rates and products known in 1963, see D. V. Banthorpe, E. D. Hughes, and C. K. Ingold, *J. Chem. Soc.*, **1964**, 2864.

[77] J. P. van Loon, *Rec. trav. chim.*, 1904, **23**, 62.

[78] G. S. Hammond and H. J. Shine, *J. Am. Chem. Soc.*, 1950, **72**, 220.

[79] R. B. Carlin and R. C. Odioso, *J. Am. Chem. Soc.*, 1954, **76**, 100.

It was nevertheless considerably discussed. Blackadder and Hinshelwood saw in it an indication that the benzidine rearrangement had in principle a second mechanism, which was kinetically of first order in acid.[80] This mechanism rarely contributed to the observed kinetics of rearrangement; but in Carlin and Odioso's example, it did, for some unexplained reason, contribute substantially to an overall rate given by the equation,

$$-(d[\mathrm{Hz}]/dt)/[\mathrm{Hz}] = k_1 = k_2[\mathrm{H}^+] + k_3[\mathrm{H}^+]^2$$

Dewar discussed the case from the viewpoint of the π-complex theory.[12] He thus saw in it, not two mechanisms, but one mechanism, *viz.*, the π-complex mechanism, of two potentially rate-controlling steps. One proton was needed to form his π-complex, and another was needed to decompose it into products. Therefore, according as the first or second step was rate-controlling, the overall order would be first or second in acid; and if both steps shared rate-control, then the apparent kinetic order would be intermediate, the general rate equation being

$$\frac{1}{-(d[\mathrm{Hz}]/dt)/[\mathrm{Hz}]} = \frac{1}{k_1} = \frac{1}{k_a[\mathrm{H}^+]} + \frac{1}{k_b[\mathrm{H}^+]^2}$$

This equation of summed reciprocal rates has consequences quite different from those of the Blackadder-Hinshelwood equation of summed rates, as we note below. Why rate-control should, peculiarly in the Carlin-Odioso example, be shared comparably between the steps, was not explained.

Banthorpe, Hughes, and the writer took the Blackadder-Hinshelwood approach, but started by asking why the Carlin-Odioso example had remained unique, persistent attempts over eight years to find a second example of an order in acid of less than two having failed. The tentative answer was that the polar-transition-state theory had not guided these attempts, though it tells one where to look for other low orders in acid, namely, among hydrazobenzenes with substituents which supply electrons to their phenylamine rings, and weaken an aniline base by impairing charge solvation (Section **57e**).[81] Either factor would promote polarisation of the protonated N—N bond, a polarisation that would be transferred to other bonds in the course of rearrangement as pictured in the polar-transition-state theory. Either

[80] D. A. Blackadder and Sir C. Hinshelwood, *J. Chem. Soc.*, **1957**, 2898.

[81] The reason for the latter effect (cf. Chapter XIV) is that the ortho-substituent reduces external neutralisation of the cationic charge by electrostriction of the dipolar solvent, so increasing the internal electron-affinity of the charge.

factor, if strong enough, could sufficiently so act without help from the other. But the two factors collaborate in the *o*-methyl substituent, and hence any other substituent in which *both* effects are stronger could be predicted to reduce kinetic order more efficaciously. The following series of orders of efficacy of aryl groups in hydrazoarenes were thus predicted:

$$\alpha\text{-naphthyl} > \beta\text{-naphthyl} > o\text{-tolyl} > \text{phenyl}$$
$$o\text{-anisyl} > o\text{-tolyl} > \text{phenyl}$$

The first of these series was established in 1962, and by its use, the one-proton mechanism of the benzidine rearrangement was completely isolated.[82] The rearrangement of 1,1′-hydrazonaphthalene was found to be accurately of first order in acid over the investigated 10^4-fold range of hydrogen-ion concentration. 1,2′-Hydrazonaphthalene and 2,2′-hydrazonaphthalene were in much the same case, though for the latter, the order in acid rose to near 1.2 at the highest of the investigated acidities. But for N-1-naphthyl-N′-phenylhydrazine and for N-2-naphthyl-N′-phenylhydrazine, the kinetics were characteristically transitional, the order in acid rising from near one at the lower end to near two at the upper end of the investigated range of acidities. Carlin and Odioso's 2,2′-dimethylhydrazobenzene was shown to be essentially similar: a rise in the order in acid from about 1.3 to near 2.0 with rising acidity was followed experimentally. Carlin and Odioso's figure of 1.6 was a result of the particular narrow range of acidities which they used.

These results are in Table 52-2. Some data due to Bunton,[83] to Carlin,[79,84] and to Shine,[85] and their respective collaborators, as well as a number of results obtained by Banthorpe and his coworkers[86] since 1962 are included in the table.

In the last group of results one finds confirmation of the second of the predicted series, that is, of the superiority of the *o*-anisyl group over the *o*-tolyl group in promoting the one-proton mechanism. One *o*-anisyl group acts like two *o*-tolyl groups in producing transitional

[82] D. V. Banthorpe, E. D. Hughes, and C. K. Ingold, *J. Chem. Soc.*, **1962,** 2386, 2418; D. V. Banthorpe and E. D. Hughes, *ibid.*, p. 2402; D. V. Banthorpe, *ibid.*, pp. 2407, 2429; *idem*, C. K. Ingold, J. Roy, and S. M. Somerville, *ibid.*, p. 2436; D. V. Banthorpe, E. D. Hughes, C. K. Ingold, and J. Roy, *ibid.*, p. 3294.

[83] C. A. Bunton, C. K. Ingold, and M. M. Mhala, *J. Chem. Soc.*, **1959,** 1906.

[84] R. B. Carlin, R. G. Nelb, and R. C. Odioso, *J. Am. Chem. Soc.*, 1951, **73,** 1002; R. B. Carlin and R. C. Odioso, *ibid.*, 1954, **76,** 2345; R. B. Carlin and G. S. Wich, *ibid.*, 1958, **80,** 4023.

[85] H. J. Shine and J. T. Chamness, *J. Org. Chem.*, 1967, **52,** 901; H. J. Shine and J. P. Stanley, *ibid.*, p. 905.

[86] D. V. Banthorpe, A. Cooper, and C. K. Ingold, *Nature*, 1967, **216,** 232.

kinetics. Two *o*-anisyl groups give the one-proton mechanism exclusive dominance.

In the same series of results, we see the two factors of polarisation acting independently. A single *p*-anisyl group and a single *p*-acetaminophenyl group give pure one-proton kinetics, obviously because the substituents in these aryl groups sufficiently strongly release electrons from the *p*-position which theory shows, as we shall see, to be the most effective position for electron release. Two *o*-bromophenyl groups lead to transitional kinetics, and two *o*-iodophenyl groups to pure one-proton kinetics, evidently because the substituents, increasingly in this order, impair charge solvation (reduce base strength) in the position which, as we shall later see, is most inhibitory to the retention of a second added proton in the transition state. In each type of case in which one factor is essentially responsible for the reduced kinetic order, the other factor is either equivocal or weakly contrary.

Some further data, not easily included in Table 52-2, are the follow-

TABLE 52-2.—KINETIC ORDERS IN HYDROGEN ION OF HYDRAZOARENE CONVERSIONS.

R·NH·NH·R′		"%" Aq.-org. solvent		Range of $[H]^+$	Order in H^+	Ref.
R	R′					
C_6H_5	C_6H_5	60	dioxan	0.05—1.0	2	82
		95	EtOH	0.05—0.10		84
1-$C_{10}H_7$	1-$C_{10}H_7$	60	dioxan	0.000,003—0.03	1	82
1-$C_{10}H_7$	2-$C_{10}H_7$	60	dioxan	0.003—0.04	1	82
2-$C_{10}H_7$	2-$C_{10}H_7$	60, 70	dioxan	0.001—0.2	1.0–1.2	82
1-$C_{10}H_7$	C_6H_5	60	dioxan	0.001—0.3	1.0–1.9	82
2-$C_{10}H_7$	C_6H_5	60, 70	dioxan	0.01—0.3	1.2–1.9	82
2-MeC_6H_4	2-MeC_6H_4	60	dioxan	0.02—0.5	1.4–2.0	82
		95	EtOH	0.03—0.1	1.6	79
3-MeC_6H_4	3-MeC_6H_4	95	EtOH	0.05—0.1	2	84
4-MeC_6H_4	4-MeC_6H_4	60	dioxan	0.005—0.07	2	83
		95	EtOH	0.007—0.03		84
4-*t*-BuC_6H_4	4-*t*-BuC_6H_4	95	EtOH	0.01—0.05	2	85
2-$MeOC_6H_4$	2-$MeOC_6H_4$	60	dioxan	0.000,1—0.05	1	86
2-$MeOC_6H_4$	C_6H_5	60	dioxan	0.002—0.3	1.1–2.0	86
4-$MeOC_6H_4$	C_6H_5	60	dioxan	0.000,007—0.005	1	86
4-$NHAcC_6H_4$	C_6H_5	60	dioxan	0.007—0.1	1	86
2-FC_6H_4	2-FC_6H_4	60	dioxan	0.1—0.8	2	86
2-ClC_6H_4	2-ClC_6H_4	60	dioxan	0.8—2.8	2	86
4-ClC_6H_4	4-ClC_6H_4	60	dioxan	0.1—1.0	2	86
4-ClC_6H_4	C_6H_5	60	dioxan	0.07—1.0	2	86
2-BrC_6H_4	2-BrC_6H_4	60	dioxan	0.2—2.0	1.2–1.9	86
4-BrC_6H_4	4-BrC_6H_4	60	dioxan	0.1—0.5	2	86
2-IC_6H_4	2-IC_6H_4	60	dioxan	0.7—1.6	1	86
4-IC_6H_4	4-IC_6H_4	60	dioxan	0.05—0.5	2	86
2-PhC_6H_4	2-PhC_6H_4	60	dioxan	0.9—1.6	2	86
4-PhC_6H_4	4-PhC_6H_4	95	EtOH	0.01—0.5	2	85
4-PhC_6H_4	C_6H_5	60	dioxan	0.004—0.6	2	86
4-$NO_2C_6H_4$	C_6H_5	60	dioxan	2.0—4.0	2	86

ing. Transitional kinetics in the acidity range 0.0003–0.06N in "25%" aqueous methanol have been reported for the rearrangement of N-methylhydrazobenzene.[87] Kinetics of first order in acid described the overall reaction of 4,4′-divinylhydrazobenzene under catalysis by hydrochloric acid in "95%" aqueous ethanol; the product, however, was a polymer.[88] Kinetics of inverse-first order in acid described the rearrangement of 3,3′-diaminohydrazobenzene by acid in "95%" aqueous ethanol.[89] If we assume the amine to be stored in doubly protonated form, this implies a one-proton mechanism of rearrangement.

The kinetic findings as a whole have consequences for mechanism.[76] The well-established result that, in transitional kinetics, the order in acid rises as acidity rises is obviously to be expected from the Blackadder-Hinshelwood equation, with which, in fact, all examined cases of transitional kinetics agree quantitatively. The same result is just as obviously inconsistent with the equation which Dewar derived from the π-complex theory. It requires that the order in acid should fall as the acidity rises. Moreover, a π-complex with a naphthalene residue should be more stable than with a benzene residue, and should be more difficultly converted to products by the action of a proton. Thus the kinetic order in acid should not fall, but should, if anything, rise, from hydrazobenzene to a hydrazonaphthalene. The caged-dissociation theory is also in difficulties, in that it relies on the second-added proton to create the electrical symmetry, combined with the N—N-bond weakening, that are necessary for homolysis. An easy concurrence of one-proton and two-proton mechanisms would be incredible on this theory. The polar-transition-state theory is not in the same case, because this mechanism starts with a heterolytic loosening of the N—N bond. It therefore regards the first-added proton as the more important activator of rearrangement. The second-added proton is less important, because it acts only through the difference of its contrary effects in destroying dissymmetry and creating bond weakening. The concurrence of one-proton and two-proton mechanisms is therefore comprehensible on this theory.

All catalytic protons, even the second when there are two, are added in pre-equilibria. That is, all acid catalysis is of the specific hydrogen-ion type. Proton addition in the transition state of rearrangement, that is, general acid catalysis of the rearrangement, does not occur, not even in respect of the second-added proton, in the conditions of any of the listed kinetic investigations. The first proofs of this were given

[87] W. N. White and R. Preisman, *Chem. and Ind.*, **1961,** 1752.
[88] H. J. Shine and J. T. Chamness, *J. Org. Chem.*, 1963, **28,** 1222.
[89] G. S. Hammond and J. S. Clovis, *Tetrahedron Letters*, **1962,** 945.

in 1957 by Bunton, Mhala, and the writer,[83] whose demonstrations have been much extended by Banthorpe.[82]

Two independent methods of demonstration were applied with mutually supporting results. First, it was shown that the rates of benzidine rearrangements follow Hammett's thermodynamic measure of acidity. Thus, under two-proton catalysis, rates follow the square of the equilibrium acidity function h_0, as is appropriate for proton-transfer equilibria, rather than the square of the concentration function $[H^+]$, as would be more appropriate for a purely kinetic form of proton intervention. Even the mixed function $h_0[H^+]$ was found to be quite inapplicable. The second type of demonstration consisted in showing that when catalysis by H^+ in solvent H_2O is replaced by catalysis by D^+ in solvent D_2O, the reactions go faster. If the proton uptake were to occur in the transition state, then, when it became a deuteron uptake, a kinetic primary-isotope effect should cause the reaction to go more slowly. However, the isotope effect works oppositely in pre-equilibrium: a deuteron is transferred from D_3O^+ in D_2O more extensively than a proton is from H_3O^+ in H_2O. The observed factors by which benzidine rearrangements were accelerated when they were changed from a protium solvent to a deuterium solvent were about 2 per catalytic proton. Typical factors of acceleration were 2.3 for the one-proton rearrangement of 1,1′-hydrazonaphthalene, and $4.8 = (2.2)^2$ for the two-proton rearrangement of hydrazobenzene.

The short summary of all this is that we know when the catalytic protons impinge on the reaction co-ordinate for rearrangement. They impinge at the beginning.[90] The opening sequence of events in the mechanism is the uptake of a first proton, followed in many cases by that of a second proton, to form, in pre-equilibrium, the first or second conjugate acid of the hydrazo-compound.

We turn now to the losses of protons from the rearranging system. We shall find that these events belong to the last stages of the mechanism. Two aromatic protons have to be lost in order to establish any one biaryl bond. We can learn something of these processes by putting deuterium atoms in those aromatic positions which the eventual biaryl bond will connect. The following two sets of results illustrate the situation.

Hydrazobenzene rearranged in aqueous-organic solvents with quad-

[90] Nevertheless, general acid catalysis in respect of the second-added proton was maintained by Dewar (ref. 12) up to 1963, but more in relation to his theory than on experimental grounds. A revised π-complex theory has since been proposed which is so fluid as to be without distinctive predictions (M. J. S. Dewar and A. P. Marchand, *Ann. Rev. Phys. Chem.*, 1965, 16, 338).

ratic dependence on hydrogen ions, to give 73–76% of the 4,4′-linked biaryl, benzidine, and 27–24% of the 2,4′-linked biaryl, diphenyline. The exact figures depend on the solvent, but are independent of the acidity. It was found[91] that when all four ortho-positions in the substrate were furnished with deuterium atoms, both the overall rate, and the product proportions remained the same. Likewise, when the two para-positions in the substrate were provided with deuterium atoms, both the rate, and the product proportions, remained unchanged.

The second series of results, which related to 1,1′-hydrazo-naphthalene, were only partly parallel. This substrate rearranges in aqueous organic solvents with linear dependence on hydrogen ion, to give three products, whose proportions vary a little with the solvent but are independent of the acidity. For "60%" aqueous dioxan as solvent, the products consisted of 64% of the 4,4′-linked biaryl, naphthidine, 18% of the 2,2′-linked biaryl diamine, called dinaphthyline, and 18% of the corresponding 2,2′-linked biaryl imine, which is, of course, a dibenzocarbazole.[92] It was found [93] that, when the 4- and 4′-positions in the substrate were supplied with deuterium atoms, both the overall rate and the product proportions remained the same. But further, when the 2- and 2′-positions in the substrate were provided with deuterium atoms, then the overall rate remained unchanged, but the products suffered a partial change, as follows. The proportions of 4,4′-linked naphthidine, and of total 2,2′-linked products, remained the same; but the internal ratio of the two 2,2′-linked products, the diamine and related imine, was changed by a factor of 5 (the figure would be higher if fully corrected) in favour of the imine. This is clearly a primary isotope effect discriminating against the loss of an aromatic deuterium atom when in competitition with loss of ammonia:

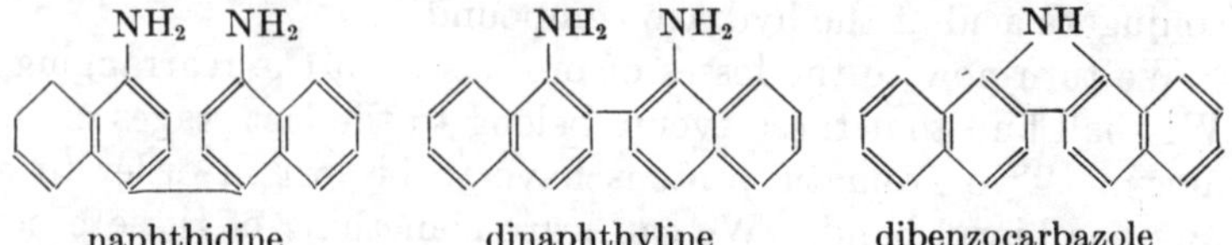

	naphthidine	dinaphthyline	dibenzocarbazole
Parent	64%	18%	18%
4,4′-D_2	63%	18%	19%
2,2′-D_2	64%	6%	30%

These results give a picture of the closing series of events in the mechanism of benzidine rearrangements. The two aromatic protons

[91] D. V. Banthorpe and E. D. Hughes, *J. Chem. Soc.*, **1962,** 3308.

[92] It has been shown that the imine is an independent product of the rearrangement, and is not produced from already formed diamine. This can be deaminated, but not in the conditions of this rearrangement (ref. 82).

[93] D. V. Banthorpe, E. D. Hughes, C. K. Ingold, and R. Humberlin, *J. Chem. Soc.*, **1962,** 3299.

uents are in either meta- or ortho-positions. This suggests that, in the transition state of the two-proton mechanism, a cationic charge is concentrated on a para-carbon atom, which, as a near-carbonium ion,

TABLE 52-3.—RATE-CONSTANTS, k_3 FOR THE TWO-PROTON MECHANISM, AND k_2 FOR THE ONE-PROTON MECHANISM OF HYDRAZO-ARENE CONVERSIONS. (μ = formal ionic strength)

R·NH·NH·R′		μ	10^3k_3 with k_3 in sec.$^{-1}$, mole^{-2} l.^{2}			Ref.
			$k_3 = k_1/[H^+]^2$	$k_3 = k_1/h_0^2$		
R	R′		0°	0°	25°	
In "60%" Aqueous Dioxan Containing Perchloric Acid						
C_6H_5	C_6H_5	0.1	1.6	—	—	82
C_6H_5	C_6H_5	1.0	30[b]	1,580	30,000[a]	83
1-$C_{10}H_7$	C_6H_5	0.1	130	—	—	82
2-$C_{10}H_7$	C_6H_5	0.1	5.0	—	—	82
2-MeC_6H_4	2-MeC_6H_4	0.1	8.5	—	—	82
2-MeC_6H_4	2-MeC_6H_4	0.5	53[b]	8,400	—	82
4-MeC_6H_4	4-MeC_6H_4	0.05	1,400	—	—	83
2-$MeOC_6H_4$	C_6H_5	0.4	1,350	—	—	86
2-FC_6H_4	2-FC_6H_4	1.0	—	—	47	86
2-ClC_6H_4	2-ClC_6H_4	1.0	0.002[b]	0.034	—	86
4-ClC_6H_4	C_6H_5	0.1	0.066	—	—	86
4-ClC_6H_4	C_6H_5	1.0	2.9[b]	150	—	86
4-ClC_6H_4	4-ClC_6H_4	1.0	0.24[b]	12.8	—	86
2-BrC_6H_4	2-BrC_6H_4	1.0	—	—	0.60	86
4-BrC_6H_4	4-BrC_6H_4	1.0	—	—	102	86
2-IC_6H_4	2-IC_6H_4	2.0	—	—	<0.01[c]	86
4-IC_6H_4	4-IC_6H_4	0.5	—	—	230	86
2-PhC_6H_4	2-PhC_6H_4	>1	—	4.8	—	86
4-PhC_6H_4	C_6H_5	1.0	140[b]	12,000	—	86
4-$NO_2C_6H_4$	C_6H_5	>2	—	0.0041	—	86
In "95%" Aqueous Ethanol Containing Hydrochloric Acid						
C_6H_5	C_6H_5	0.1	2.4	—	—	84
2-MeC_6H_4	2-MeC_6H_4	0.05	7.5	—	—	79
3-MeC_6H_4	3-MeC_6H_4	0.05	15	—	—	84
4-MeC_6H_4	4-MeC_6H_4	0.05	1,240	—	—	84
4-*t*-BuC_6H_4	4-*t*-BuC_6H_4	0.05	1,200	—	—	85
4-PhC_6H_4	4-PhC_6H_4	0.05	380	—	—	85

[a] Extrapolated for temperature.
[b] At low acidities.
[c] HCl replacing $HClO_4$.

TABLE 52-3.—(*continued*)

			10^2k_2 with k_2 in sec.$^{-1}$ mole^{-1} l.			
			$k_2 = k_1/[H^+]$	$k_2 = k_1/h_0$		
			0°	0°	25°	
In "60%" Aqueous Dioxan Containing Perchloric Acid						
C_6H_5	C_6H_5	0.05	<0.002	—	—	83
1-$C_{10}H_7$	1-$C_{10}H_7$	0.05	180[d]	—	—	82
1-$C_{10}H_7$	2-$C_{10}H_7$	0.05	100	—	—	82
2-$C_{10}H_7$	2-$C_{10}H_7$	0.06	46	—	—	82
1-$C_{10}H_7$	C_6H_5	0.1	2.0	—	—	82
2-$C_{10}H_7$	C_6H_5	0.1	0.050	—	—	82
2-MeC_6H_4	2-MeC_6H_4	0.1	0.021	—	—	82
2-MeC_6H_4	2-MeC_6H_4	0.5	0.14[b]	—	—	82
4-$NHAcC_6H_4$	C_6H_5	0.1	46	—	—	86
2-$MeOC_6H_4$	C_6H_5	0.4	1.0[b]	—	—	86
2-$MeOC_6H_4$	2-$MeOC_6H_4$	0.1	170[d]	—	—	86
4-$MeOC_6H_4$	C_6H_5	0.1	480[d]	—	—	86
2-BrC_6H_4	2-BrC_6H_4	1.0	—	—	0.008	86
2-IC_6H_4	2-IC_6H_4	2.0	—	0.00015[c]	0.0054[c]	86
In "95%" Aqueous Ethanol Containing Hydrochloric Acid						
2-MeC_6H_4	2-MeC_6H_4	0.05	—	0.025	—	79

[d] Buffers used at some acidities.

is much more stable when tertiary than when secondary. The same kind of rate difference is shown by para- and ortho-halogeno-substituents, which, in spite of their inductive electronegativity, exert electropositive conjugative effects.

When the one-proton mechanism becomes prominent or dominating on account essentially of strong electron release by substituents, the change of kinetic form is associated with high absolute rates, as in the presence of benzo-, *p*-acetamino-, and *o*- or *p*-methoxy-substituents. When the dominant factor producing such a change of kinetic form is reduced basicity, then the change is associated with low absolute rates, as in the presence of *o*-bromo- and *o*-iodo-substituents. The *o*-methyl substituent is marginal, bridging these two classes.

In reading Table 52-3, one must allow for the kinetic effects of ionic strength, and the fact that some rate-constants are defined in terms of [H+] and some in terms of h_0. The table is arranged accordingly.

The *products* of benzidine rearrangements show some curious and much-discussed patterns. The most celebrated is Jacobson's puzzle of the contrast in biaryl orientation between hydrazobenzenes and hydrazonaphthalenes, both having free 2- and 4-positions in both aryl residues. Different biaryl-diamine isomers are missing from the two series. In the benzene series, the 4,4′-linked biaryl, benzidine, is the main product, and the 2,4′-biaryl-linked isomer, diphenyline, is an important minor product; and these products are normally unaccompanied by any 2,2′-linked ortho-benzidine, or, indeed, anything else at all above the level of traces. In the naphthalene series, three comparably important products are formed, the 4,4′-linked biaryl, naphthidine, the 2,2′-biaryl-linked diamine called dinaphthyline, and the corresponding 2,2′-biaryl-linked imine, *i.e.*, the carbazole (formulae p. 928); and these products are unaccompanied by any 2,4′-linked biaryl-diamine, or, indeed, by anything else at all above the level of traces. The above descriptions apply typically to hydrazobenzene and 1,1′-hydrazonaphthalene. The mixed-type naphthyl-phenylhydrazines act as if they belonged to the naphthalene series rather than to the benzene series. Thus N-1-naphthyl-N′-phenylhydrazine gives a set of products just like those of 1,1′-hydrazonaphthalene. 2,2′-Hydrazonaphthalene gives only the 1,1′-biaryl-linked diamine and its imine. N-2-naphthyl-N′-phenylhydrazine behaves completely similarly. None of these findings, not even those for hydrazobenzene, can be understood by assigning relative reactivities to the 2- and 4-positions of the individual rings. They show that orientation must depend on the inter-relation of the rings, that is, on the whole molecular system.

The only known cases in the benzene series in which ortho-benzidine formation rises to several units percent are among the 3,5,3′,5′-tetrahalo- and tetra-alkyl-hydrazobenzenes.[94] The reason for this is not understood.

Among the few cases for which transitional kinetics can conveniently be observed, product composition depends on mechanism. Thus, among the naphthyl hydrazines, when the kinetic order in acid is lifted from one to two by an increase in acidity, the proportion of 4,4′-linked biaryl is mildly increased, and the proportion in which the total ortho-linked product appears as imine is reduced sharply to zero. The latter result is easy to understand. For, as we have noted already, ammonia loss in the course of rearrangement requires that one nitrogen atom (the nucleophile) should be in free-basic form, whilst the other

[94] R. B. Carlin and W. O. Forshay jr., *J. Am. Chem. Soc.*, 1950, 72, 793; R. B. Carlin and S. A. Hessinger, *ibid.*, 1955, **77**, 2272.

one (that eliminated) should be in ammonium ionic form. Therefore, one is the right number of added protons for imine formation: two is one too many.

Turning next to examples in the benzene series in which one 4-position is substituted, the first point to note is that the substituents CO_2H and SO_3H are eliminated from the 4-position, just as hydrogen would be; and so the 4,4′-linked benzidine is still the main product. The eliminated substituents leave their bonding electrons behind: one may suppose that these electrons are needed to allow a quinonoid intermediate to recover benzenoid character.

A single firm-standing 4-substituent cuts out benzidine formation. The 2,4′-linked diphenyline would then be the main rearrangement product were it not replaced in part or totally by the 2,N′-linked ortho-semidine. The replacement is partial if the 4-substituent is electron-attracting (*e.g.*, halogens), but total if it is freely electron-releasing (*e.g.*, OR). In the latter case, the ortho-semidine becomes the main rearrangement product. In both cases, however, another isomer, the N,4′-linked para-semidine, constitutes a minor, but far from negligible, product.[95] Finally, in both types of case, substantial amounts of the disproportionation products, that is, of the fission amines and the azo-compound, usually appear.

The substituent being in position-4, it will be obvious that the diphenyline must be 2,4′-linked, and the para-semidine N,4′-linked. The ortho-semidine, which might have been either 2,N′- or N,2′-linked, has in all known cases the 2,N′-linked structure. In the known cases, the general polarity of the substituent R, in particular its base-strengthening or base-weakening properties, makes no difference to this result:

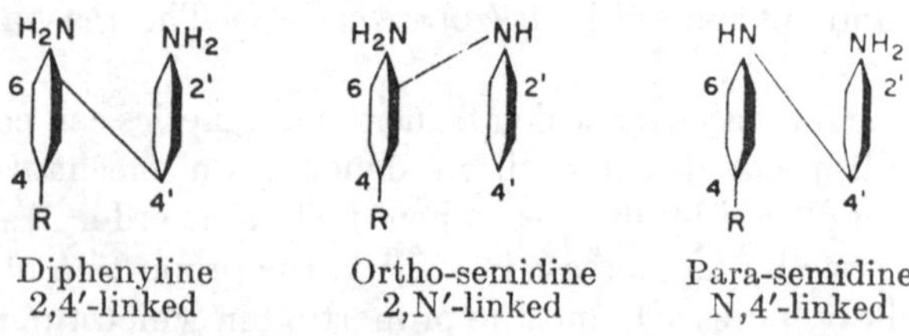

Diphenyline 2,4′-linked — Ortho-semidine 2,N′-linked — Para-semidine N,4′-linked

(The numbering above is as for the parent hydrazobenzenes.)

[95] The suggestion was made by Hammick and Munro (ref. 73) that para-semidines are not formed in benzidine rearrangements in the absence of heavy-metal ions. This generalisation was subsequently questioned by Večera and his coworkers, (ref. 96) and by Shine and Stanley (ref. 85). Banthorpe and Cooper have confirmed (ref. 86) that para-semidines are normal, though usually minor, products of one-proton and two-proton rearrangements of those hydrazobenzenes which carry a single firm-standing para-substituent.

Two firm-standing substituents occupying 4- and 4′-positions in the hydrazobenzene cut out all rearrangement products except the ortho-semidine. Disproportionation is now comparable with, and may exceed, rearrangement.

In the presence of either one or two substituents in 2- or 2′-positions, rearrangement yields the 4,4′-linked benzidine nearly exclusively. Disproportionation occurs, if at all, only in small amount.

The fact that an accelerating substituent capable of strong electromeric electron release, for example, methoxyl, when in position-4 directs the accelerated rearrangement to produce substitution in its own ring in position-2, and when in position-2 so directs it as to produce substitution in position-4, gives a superficial appearance of selective electromeric meta-activation, a phenomenon forbidden in the general theory of electrophilic aromatic substitution (Section **21c**). However, that would be an incorrect reading of the facts, inasmuch as it treats the two aromatic moieties as independent reactants, which they are not: orientation is an affair of the whole molecule. In particular, the electron-releasing substituent is helping to put electrons into the other aromatic ring, not into its own ring.

For rearrangements proceeding in any one kinetic form, the product composition is independent of the acidity. This was first shown by Carlin and his coworkers for the formation of benzidine and diphenyline from hydrazobenzene, and for the formation of ortho-semidine and disproportionation products from 4,4′-dimethylhydrazobenzene.[84] It has been further demonstrated over a larger number of examples by Banthorpe and Cooper for all the types of product formed from substituted hydrazobenzenes.[86]

Most of this pattern of product compositions was qualitatively uncovered by Jacobson early in the present century.[63] He examined about eighty benzidine rearrangements. Nothing was then known of duality of mechanism or of the need to define conditions on that account. Separations were incomplete, wherefore Jacobson attempted no more than to distinguish between major, minor, and trace products, which he symbolised as +++, ++, and +, respectively. Today, we understand the need to define conditions. By a combination of spectroscopy and chromatography, we can make analyses more quantitatively than he could. Some of Jacobson's examples have been re-examined with the use of these advantages, and some of his findings have thus been made more precise, with results which are given in Table 52-4. Some rearrangements not previously examined by him are included in the table.

---

[96] M. Večera, J. Gasparič, and J. Petránek, *Coll. Czech. Chem. Comm.*, 1957, **22**, 1603.

TABLE 52-4.—PRODUCTS OF HYDRAZOARENE CONVERSIONS. (The figures are percentages. Jacobson's signs are used where the data do not warrant a figure.)

Hydrazobenzenes

Substituents in phenyl groups		Medium[a]	Order in H⁺	4,4′-Linked	2,4′-Linked	2,N′-Linked	N,4′-Linked	Disprop.	Ref.
—	—	D	2	76	24	—	—	—	91
		E	2	73	27	—	—	—	
2-Me	2-Me	D	1, 2	100	—	—	—	—	82
		E	1, 2	100	—	—	—	—	79
3-Me	3-Me	E	2	100	—	—	—	—	84
4-Me	4-Me	E	2	—	—	40	—	60	84
4-*t*-Bu	4-*t*-Bu	E	2	—	—	49	—	50	85
2-MeO	2-MeO	D	1	95	—	—	—	5	85
2-MeO	—	D	1, 2	~100	—	—	—	+	85
4-MeO	—	D	1	—	—	55	24	20	85
4-NHAc	—	D	1	—	+[bd]	+++[b]	++[d]	70	85
2-F	2-F	D	2	86	—	—	—	14	86
2-Cl	2-Cl	D	2	94	—	—	—	6	86
4-Cl	4-Cl	D	2	—	—	22	—	75	86
4-Cl	—	D	2	—	~19	30	20	31	86
2-Br	2-Br	D	1, 2	95	—	—	—	5	86
4-Br	4-Br	D	2	—	—	~30	—	~70	86
2-I	2-I	D	1	100	—	—	—	—	86
4-I	4-I	D	2	—	—	—	—	100	86
2-Ph	2-Ph	D	2	90	—	—	—	10	86
4-Ph	4-Ph	E	2	—	—	25	—	75	85
4-Ph	—	D	2	—	+++	+++[c]	—	38	86
4-NO_4	—	D	2	—	+++	+++[c]	~20	~40	86

Hydrazonaphthalenes and N-Naphthyl-N′-phenylhydrazines

Aryl groups		Medium[a]	Order in H⁺	4,4′-Linked	2,4′-Linked	ortho-Linked		Disprop.	Ref.
						Diamine	Imine		
1-Naph	1-Naph	D	1	64	—	18	18	—	82
1-Naph	2-Naph	D	1	—	1(?)	55	44	—	82
2-Naph	2-Naph	D	1	—	—	94	6	—	82
1-Naph	Ph	D	1	45	—	43	11	—	82
2-Naph	Ph	D	1	—	—	99	0.5	—	82

[a] D = "60%" aqueous dioxan containing perchloric acid. E = "95%" aqueous ethanol containing hydrochloric acid.

[b] Identity was not confirmed by comparison with a synthetic isomer.

[c] Whether 2,N′- or N,2′-linked was not determined.

[d] Noticeable only at acidities well above the kinetic range.

We must now consider how the most successful of the theories we have of the benzidine rearrangement, the polar-transition-state theory, deals with this orientational pattern.[72,76] Let us start with Jacobson's conundrum.

In the two-proton mechanism of rearrangement of hydrazobenzene, it is assumed that, after protonation, the N—N bond heterolytically becomes highly electrostatic and hence long and flexible, in the approach to the transition state. One of the loosely bound aromatic moieties then carries nearly two units of positive charge, and the other a nearly zero nett charge. It is important to note that the two charges in the quasi-cationic moiety are essentially localised: one is the ammonium-ionic charge; and this electrostatically reinforces quantal direction of the other,[97] which is the electron-deficiency charge, to the para-position. One sees how important solvation of the ammonium ionic charge is for the stability of the doubly protonated transition state: the proton which produces the charge on nitrogen in the quasi-cation would be lost if solvation in that region were seriously impaired. The quasi-molecular moiety of the transition state will have widely distributed fractional dipolar charges, as in the aniline molecule. It follows from the distribution of charges shown below that, as the system passes over the transition state, the only positions in which largely electrostatic bonds can be incepted, to become covalencies as they shorten, are the 4,4′- and 2,4′-positions: there can be little or no 2,2′-bonding. In the transition state some longitudinal displacement of the converging rings should occur, as is allowed by their flexible interconnexion, because the localised electron-deficiency charge will draw to itself the centroid of the negative charges in the other ring:

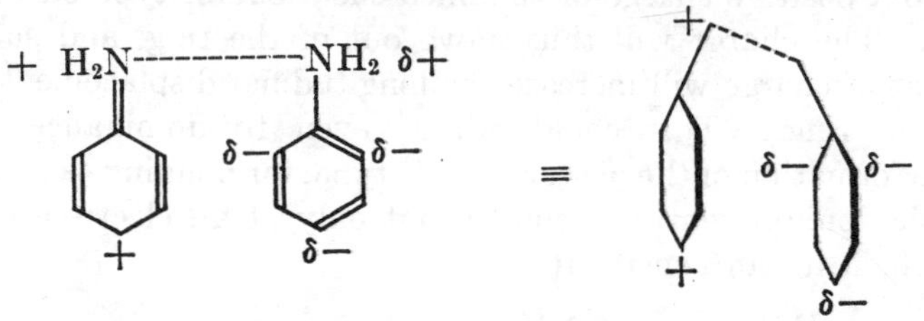

$+\ H_2N$----------$NH_2\ \delta+$

The contrasting situation arises in the one-proton rearrangement of 1,1′-hydrazonaphthalene. This system, on approaching its transition state, will have a quasi-cationic moiety containing only the electron-deficiency charge, which will be comparably distributed between the 2- and 4-positions.[98] The complementing quasi-molecular moiety will have its negative partial charges similarly distributed. Therefore the rings will converge without longitudinal displacement, and such congruence will restrict bond inception to 4,4′- and 2,2′-positions: there can be little or no 2,4′-bonding:

[97] The reference is to the quantal reason why, in uncondensed benzenoid rings, para-quinonoid bond arrangements are more stable than ortho-quinonoid (cf. Section **22g**).

[98] This is again a quantal matter: in a benzene ring that is within a naphthalene nucleus, α- and β-quinonoid bond arrangements are about equally stable.

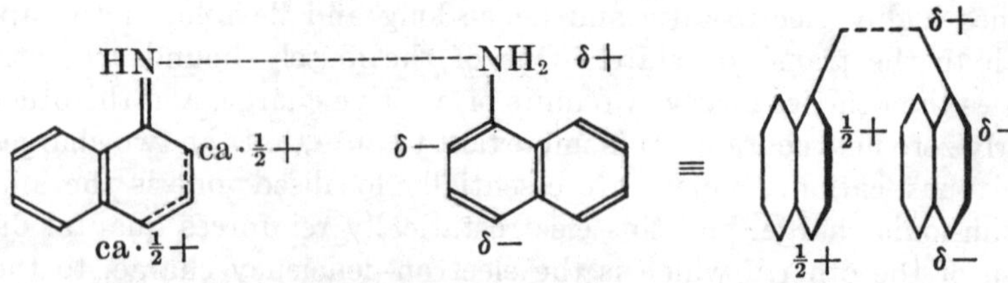

An essentially similar discussion would apply to the rearrangement of N-1-naphthyl-N′-phenyl hydrazine.

We return to the benzene series in order to discuss effects of substituents more generally. In the reaction of any unsymmetrically substituted hydrazobenzene one has the preliminary problem of the direction of N—N polarisation. For the time being, let us suppose that the N—N bond electrons move away from a substituent that can supply electrons ($+E$ effect) towards an electron-deficient centre. On this assumption, a single such para-substituent will determine that its ring becomes the quasi-cationic moiety in the transition state. This will be true whether the transition state is that of the two-proton mechanism or of the one-proton mechanism. In either transition state, the electron-deficiency positive charge will be considerably converted to a positive charge of the filled-shell 'onium type on the substituent. The charge will thus move out of the ring, and such displacement of charge will increase the longitudinal displacement of the converging rings. This could admit, even to dominance, ortho-semidine formation of the observed 2,N′-type; for bonding can develop, not at the 'onium centre of course, but only at an electron-deficient centre which it can constitute:

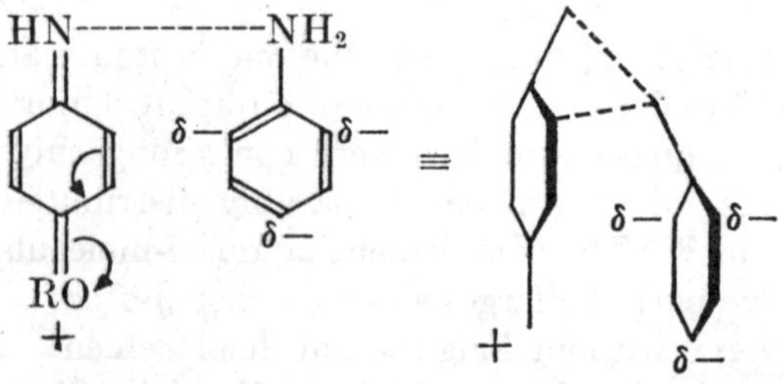

Para-semidines are not the most important rearrangement products but may be minor products from 4-monosubstituted hydrazobenzenes, under both one-proton and two-proton catalysis[86] (see Table 52-4). They are so far unknown among the products from the homogeneous acid-catalysed rearrangements of hydrazonaphthalenes. This suggests that a causal factor in their appearance may be the relatively high stability of para-quinonoid bond arrangements in the uncondensed benzene ring.[97] For that reason alone a strong concentration on the 4-position of any existing electron-deficiency, and of the positive charge associated with it, is to be expected. This in turn suggests that para-semidines may be formed when the basic N—N polarisation takes the bond electrons towards the 4-substituted ring. With a 4-nitro-substituent under two-proton catalysis, this is a favoured direction of polarisation; and with a 4-chloro-substituent, it is inductively favoured. With a 4-methoxy-substituent, it would not be favoured, unless the single catalytic proton effective in that case were to add to the substituted and more basic aniline residue first, as it is likely in some degree to do. And even disfavoured polarisations must be considered seriously, because one has always to reckon with the countervailing effects of stability and reactivity: the more difficult polarisation will be, relatively to its extent, the more activating for rearrangement. So we can picture that an approach to the transition state might take some such form as the following:

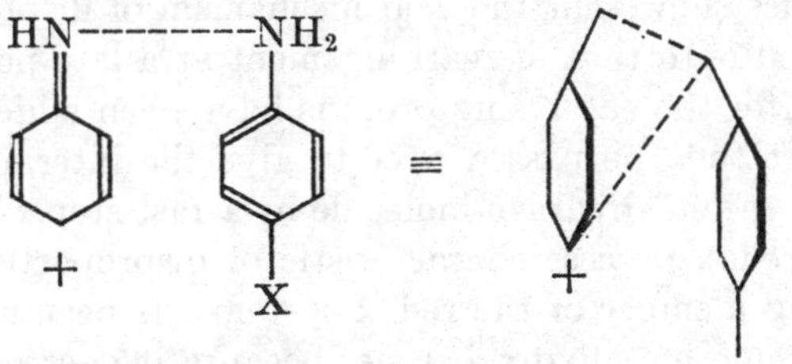

HN--------NH₂ … + … X ≡ … +

The N-p broken-line bond in the above "perspective" diagram might, for example, have a length of about 3 *A*. An isolated pair of unit-charges of this separation has an energy of 111 kcal./mole, so that a polar bond of, say, one-quarter or less of this maximum electrovalent strength could be quite strong enough, even allowing for a little bending energy, to stop dissociation during rearrangement.

It is implied in the diversity of some of the diagrams here drawn for transition states leading to various rearrangement products that what we often shortly call "the" transition state of rearrangement might in reference to one product be represented by a simple energy col, but may when several products are collectively considered be better represented by a family of cols, all within a few times kT of one another. A knowledge of the temperature dependence of the isomer ratios in rearranged products would help to define (or delimit) this picture.

The *disproportionation* of hydrazoarenes to azo-compounds and fission amines has base-catalysed, uncatalysed, and acid-catalysed mechanisms. We know very little about the first two. Through the last, disproportionation accompanies many acid-catalysed rearrangements, as will be clear from Table 52-4. The acid mechanisms of rearrangement and disproportionation are closely related.

Like the rearrangements, the accompanying disproportionations are kinetically of first order in hydrazo-compound. This is notable; for whereas the stoicheiometry of rearrangement involves only one hydrazo-molecule, that of disproportionation involves two. The kinetics show that only one of the two can be concerned in the rate-controlling step of disproportionation. The second must enter into a subsequent fast step. There must, then, be an intermediate compound characteristic of disproportionation.

Like rearrangements, disproportionations may be either of second order or first order in hydrogen ions. In fact, the kinetic dichotomy of rearrangement applies identically to disproportionation, the latter process taking its whole kinetic form from the rearrangement which it is accompanying.[86]

These kinetics show that the acid mechanism of disproportionation must be grafted onto that of rearrangement at a late point in the reaction path, after the catalysing protons have been added. A transition state must then be passed over to give the intermediate, which will involve a second hydrazo-molecule in a fast step. This step will comprise the redox process characteristic of disproportionation.

The reducing member of the redox system has been shown to be a complete molecule of a hydrazoarene, because it goes into the corresponding azoarene without any intermixing of aryl residues.[86] The oxidising member of the system must be derived from another molecule of hydrazoarene, but, in case a mixture of hydrazoarenes is employed, not necessarily and exclusively one of the particular species which supplied the reducing agent (and so became an azo-compound).[85,86] The precise identity of the oxidising member of the redox system is not finally established; but, according to a current investigation by D. V. Banthorpe and Mrs. J. G. Winter, it is definitely not one of the quinonoid intermediates postulated for rearrangement, and therefore may arise from NN-fission without the concurrent closure of a quinonoid bond. One of these fission products would be an aromatic amine, and the other would be a doubly or singly charged cation,

$$H_2\overset{+}{N}=\langle\ \ \rangle^{+} \quad \text{or} \quad HN=\langle\ \ \rangle^{+}$$

according to mechanism. The cation would be the oxidising reactant in the redox process; and, in accepting two electrons from the reducing hydrozoarene, it would produce the second of the two molecules of aromatic amine that have to be formed.

There exists a *no-proton mechanism* of benzidine rearrangements. It proceeds without acid in protic and aprotic solvents, such as ethanol, acetone, and benzene, at temperatures in the range 80–130°. This was discovered by Krolik and Lukashevich,[99] and was first studied on quantitative lines by Shine[100] in 1956. He observed kinetics of first order in hydrazo-compounds, and higher rates in alcoholic than in aprotic solvents. His work on products was extended by Lukashevich and Krolik,[101] and that on kinetics and products by Banthorpe and Hughes.[102] The last-named workers carried out rearrangements of mixtures that should have given crossed products had a dissociative mechanism been in operation. They obtained no crossed products, and concluded that the non-catalytic mechanism, like the two acid-catalysed mechanisms, is intramolecular.

The general situation concerning kinetics is that the reactions are of first order with respect to hydrazo-compounds in alcoholic solvents, and in polar aprotic solvents, such as acetonitrile and acetone. More complicated, still unelucidated, kinetics prevail in benzene. Electron-releasing substituents increase rearrangement rate. An increase in the polarity of the solvent increases rearrangement rate.

All investigations of the products of non-catalytic rearrangements have brought out the striking similarity of these products to those of acid-catalysed rearrangements, and particularly to products of reactions by the one-proton mechanism. Thus hydrazobenzene gives 4,4′- and 2,4′- but no 2,2′-biaryl-linked diamines, whereas 1-naphthylhydrazines give 4,4′- and 2,2′-linked diamines, and 2,2′-linked imines, but no 2,4′-linked diamines. The major and secondary products from the five hydrazines of the naphthalene series listed at the foot of Table 52-4 are qualitatively identical, having nothing extra and nothing missing, with those obtained under one-proton catalysis. In general,

[99] L. G. Krolik and V. O. Lukashevich, *Doklady Akad. Nauk S.S.S.R.*, 1949, **65**, 37.

[100] H. J. Shine, *J. Am. Chem. Soc.*, 1956, **78**, 4807; H. J. Shine and J. C. Trisler, *ibid.*, 1960, **82**, 4054; H. J. Shine, F.-T. Huang, and R. L. Snell, *J. Org. Chem.*, 1961, **26**, 380.

[101] V. O. Lukashevich and L. G. Krolik, *Doklady Akad. Nauk S.S.S.R.*, 1962, **147**, 1090.

[102] D. V. Banthorpe and E. D. Hughes, *J. Chem. Soc.*, **1964**, 2849, 2860; D. V. Banthorpe, *ibid.*, p. 2854.

the mild quantitative differences which are observed are not significant, because in both mechanisms the proportions of products are solvent-dependent. Some particular differences, which seem significant, are mentioned below.

This correspondence of products has been a main cause for the belief[76] that the mechanism of the non-catalytic rearrangements belongs to the same family of heterolytic mechanisms of which the acid-catalysed rearrangements have afforded two examples. By extension from the two-proton and one-proton mechanisms, this new mechanism is a "no-proton" mechanism, to which essentially the same polar-transition-state theory is taken to apply. The relationship between the three envisaged mechanisms may be expressed in terms of the approximate distributions of charge among the two aromatic moieties composing the three transition states:

(2+)(±)	(+)(±)	(+)(−)
Two-proton	One-proton	No-proton

It is expected that the no-proton mechanism will differ from the one-proton more widely than the latter will from the two-proton, because, as we have seen, the first-added proton is regarded as a more important activator for rearrangement than the second-added proton. This is borne out by experience. For, unlike the two-proton and one-proton mechanisms, which can be observed to run concurrently, the one-proton and no-proton mechanisms have rates which are so different, and hence temperatures of observation which are so different, that to observe them running concurrently and thus to show transitional kinetics is quite impossible.

A few further observations on the non-catalytic rearrangement may be mentioned. One is that its rate is reduced by factors up to 6 by putting deuterium into those positions from which it must be eliminated to form a biaryl bond.[102] As we have noticed already, no such rate reductions could thus be induced in either catalytic form of rearrangement. This kinetic isotope effect means that, in the non-catalytic reaction, the first proton loss has been pushed back on the reaction co-ordinate to the region of the transition states: proton transfer co-operates with biaryl bond formation. One can see a reason for this. The aromatic moiety, which in the transition state provides the electrons required to form the biaryl bond, will be the more negative of the two. For a no-proton mechanism uniquely, that moiety is quasi-anionic. The electrons which it supplies will be recouped from its C—H bond, and can be released therefrom co-operatively by the easy shift of the proton to the main anionic centre of the moiety, the adjacent nitrogen atom. No such facility is offered in other mechanisms.

Among rearrangements of hydrazo-compounds of the naphthalene series, a general difference in the proportions of products given by the no-proton and one-proton mechanisms has been noted.[76] The no-proton reaction gives smaller percentages of 4,4′-linked products and larger of 2,2′-linked. This could be ascribed to the tighter binding in the quasi-counter-ionic transition state of the no-proton mechanism.

One other observation may be mentioned, and it is that the formation of imines (that is, of carbazoles) is suppressed by added strong bases.[101] If a rearrangement in ethanol is conducted in the presence of ethoxide ions, what would have appeared as imine in the absence of the added base is recovered as extra ortho-diamine. One can see a reason for that too. As noted already, imine formation depends on an optimal degree of nitrogen protonation: two extra protons are too many; and no extra would be too few. The non-catalytic mechanism starts with no extra nitrogen protons. But immediately after passage through the transition state, one arrives, which is in fact the first aromatic proton to be lost. Normally, its arrival would allow imine formation to compete as usual with the loss of the second aromatic proton. This will be so, unless the medium immediately deprotonates the system. If the medium is basic enough, it will do that.

CHAPTER XIII

Additions and Their Retrogression

(53) ELECTROPHILIC ADDITIONS TO OLEFINIC COMPOUNDS[1]

WE are to deal with addition reactions, and shall be concerned in this Section with the addition of electrophiles to simple and conjugated unsaturated systems, typically olefins and polyolefins. For brevity, we call such reactions *electrophilic additions*, symbolised Ad_E. It is convenient to sub-divide electrophilic addenda into two classes, namely, the acid electrophiles, which are all strong acids, adding as such in the parts H-X, and the non-acid electrophiles, such as halogens, which add in the parts X-Y. Also it will be found convenient to consider additions to simple and conjugated unsaturated systems separately.

(53a) Additions of Strong Acids, Notably of Hydrogen Halides and of Hydroxonium Ion, to Mono-olefinic Compounds.—Orientation in olefinic additions began to receive attention at least as long ago as did orientation in aromatic substitutions. By 1870 a few relevant facts had been established: it was known, for example, that propylene and hydrogen iodide gave *iso*propyl iodide.[2] In that year Markownikoff advanced his *rule of orientation* for the *addition of hydrogen halides* to olefins: it was that the addition would be so oriented that the halogen combines with the less hydrogenated of the ethenoid carbon atoms.[3] It is noteworthy that Markownikoff gave his rule in this form only for additions to hydrocarbons. The addition to vinyl bromide of hydrogen chloride and of hydrogen bromide, to give ethylidene halides, was established about this time;[4] but Markownikoff preferred to classify such cases separately.

The subsequent study of the additions of hydrogen halides to olefinic compounds has been much confused by the circumstance that one of the commonly employed addenda, hydrogen bromide, can not only add to a double bond in a "normal" manner, that is, with an orientation agreeing with the Markownikoff rule and resembling that shown by the additions of hydrogen chloride and hydrogen iodide: it can also add in a second, so-called "abnormal" manner, which usually leads to an oppositely oriented hydrobromide. For a long time the condi-

[1] This subject is now enriched by a comprehensive and compendious monograph: P. B. D. de la Mare and R. Bolton, "Electrophilic Additions to Unsaturated Systems," Monograph 4, Editor C. Eaborn, Elsevier, London, 1966.

[2] E. Erlenmeyer, *Ann.*, 1866, **139**, 228; A. Butlerow, *ibid.*, 1868, **145**, 271.

[3] W. Markownikoff, *Ann.*, 1870, **153**, 256.

[4] E. Reboul, *Ann.*, 1870, **155**, 29.

tions controlling the incursion of this abnormal reaction remained obscure: they were finally tracked down by Kharasch and Mayo in 1933. These investigators showed that the *abnormal addition of hydrogen bromide* is dependent on peroxides, which are nearly always present in olefinic substances that have at any time been exposed to air. The interpretation which was developed in order to account for this action,[5] is that the peroxides oxidise the hydrogen bromide with liberation of bromine atoms, which start a homolytic chain reaction of addition of the hydrogen bromide (Section 55a). Hydrogen chloride and hydrogen iodide do not usually participate in similar homolytic chain reactions, not even when peroxides are deliberately introduced.[6] The assumed reason is that chlorine atoms are not formed easily enough, while easily formed iodine atoms are not reactive enough. Having discovered what caused the abnormal addition of hydrogen bromide, Kharasch and his coworkers knew how to exclude this reaction. In principle, it was necessary to operate in the dark, having removed air and peroxides; and in practice it was useful to work in the presence of antioxidants. Thus it became possible for the first time to make accurate studies of orientation in the normal addition reactions of hydrogen bromide.

Propylene and hydrogen iodide yield *iso*propyl iodide exclusively.[7] The additions of hydrogen iodide to 1-*n*-butylene (but-1-ene) and to *neo*pentylethylene proceed similarly.[7] Abnormal addition being suppressed, propylene and hydrogen bromide yield *iso*propyl bromide.[8] With the same precautions, the additions of hydrogen bromide to 1-*n*-butylene[9] and to *iso*butylene[9] proceed similarly. These results hold whether no solvent, or a solvent, is used. In all cases the Markownikoff rule is followed, the halogen combining non-terminally with a terminally unsaturated olefin:

$$\text{Alk}\cdot\text{CH:CH}_2 \xrightarrow{\text{HX}} \text{Alk}\cdot\text{CHX}\cdot\text{CH}_3$$

[5] M. S. Kharasch and F. R. Mayo, *J. Am. Chem. Soc.*, 1933, **55**, 2468; and a number of subsequent papers by M. S. Kharasch and others. The subject has been reviewed by F. R. Mayo and C. Walling, *Chem. Revs.*, 1940, **27**, 351; C. Walling, "Free Radicals in Solution," Wiley, New York, 1957, Chap. 7.

[6] Peroxide effects on the addition of hydrogen chloride to certain olefins have, however, been reported (J. H. Raley, F. F. Rust, and W. E. Vaughan, *J. Am. Chem. Soc.*, 1948, **70**, 2767; G. G. Ecke, N. C. Cook, and F. C. Whitmore, *ibid.*, 1950, **72**, 1511).

[7] M. S. Kharasch and C. Hannum, *J. Am. Chem. Soc.*, 1934, **56**, 1782.

[8] M. S. Kharasch, M. C. McNab, and F. R. Mayo, *J. Am. Chem. Soc.*, 1933, **55**, 2531.

[9] M. S. Kharasch and J. A. Hinckley, *J. Am. Chem. Soc.*, 1934, **56**, 1212.

Allyl bromide displays the same orientation in its additions. The formation of 1,2-dihalides has been established for the addition of hydrogen iodide,[10] and also for that of hydrogen bromide when precautions are taken to suppress the abnormal reaction, which leads to the 1,3-dihalide.[11] Here again, orientation remains the same whether no solvent, an aprotic solvent, or a hydroxylic solvent is employed:

$$BrCH_2 \cdot CH:CH_2 \xrightarrow{HX} BrCH_2 \cdot CHX \cdot CH_3$$

The union of hydrogen bromide with vinyl bromide to give ethylidene bromide has been proved to be the normal form of this addition:[12] the peroxide-promoted reaction leads to ethylene bromide. The addition of hydrogen iodide to vinyl chloride, and the normal addition of hydrogen bromide to vinyl chloride, have also been shown to produce ethylidene dihalides:[13]

$$Hal \cdot CH:CH_2 \xrightarrow{HX} Hal \cdot CHX \cdot CH_3$$

It was shown in the 1870's by Linnemann, and in part by Wisliscenus, that the addition of hydrogen chloride, hydrogen bromide, and hydrogen iodide to acrylic acid gives in each case the terminally halogenated propionic acid:[14]

$$HO_2C \cdot CH:CH_2 \xrightarrow{HX} HO_2C \cdot CH_2 \cdot CH_2X$$

This type of orientation seems to have been felt by Thiele to be sufficiently remarkable to merit special discussion, and in his first paper on conjugation, published in 1898, he suggested[15] that it arose in consequence of a 1,4-addition of HX to the conjugated system O:C·C:C, such addition placing X where it is finally found because the additive affinity of H is for oxygen, though a subsequent shift of hydrogen is necessary for restoration of the carboxyl group.

Such an interpretation could not, of course, be applied to the addition of hydrogen iodide to neurine, which, as Schmidt had already shown,[16] yields a terminally iodinated ammonium ion:

[10] M. S. Kharasch and C. Hannum, *J. Am. Chem. Soc.*, 1934, **56**, 1782.

[11] M. S. Kharasch and F. R. Mayo, *J. Am. Chem. Soc.*, 1933, **55**, 2461.

[12] M. S. Kharasch, M. C. McNab, and F. R. Mayo, *J. Am. Chem. Soc.*, 1933, **55**, 2521.

[13] M. S. Kharasch and C. Hannum, *J. Am. Chem. Soc.*, 1934, **56**, 712.

[14] E. Linnemann, *Ann.*, 1872, **163**, 96; J. Wisliscenus, *ibid.*, 1873, **166**, 1.

[15] J. Thiele, *Ann.*, 1898, **306**, 87.

[16] E. Schmidt, *Ann.*, 1892, **267**, 300

$$Me_3\overset{+}{N}\cdot CH{:}CH_2 \xrightarrow{HI} Me_3\overset{+}{N}\cdot CH_2\cdot CH_2I$$

It has been established by Henne and Kay that trifluoromethylethylene adds hydrogen chloride and hydrogen bromide in the manner of neurine, rather than in that of propylene:[17]

$$CF_3\cdot CH{:}CH_2 \xrightarrow{HX} CF_3\cdot CH_2\cdot CH_2X$$

The electronic interpretation of the Markownikoff rule was first given in an acceptable form by Lucas and Jameson in 1924. They assumed[18] that an electropositive alkyl group would bias the polarisation of an adjacent double bond, so that the carbon atom more remote from the alkyl group would the more easily acquire π electrons for use in uniting with the protonic part of the electrophilic addendum. By an obvious extension, this theory can be made to cover the other orientational effects illustrated:

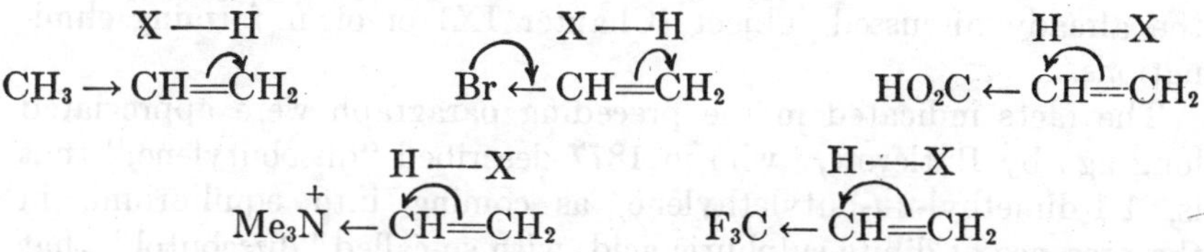

$$\overset{X\text{—}H}{CH_3 \rightarrow CH{=}CH_2} \qquad \overset{X\text{—}H}{Br \leftarrow CH{=}CH_2} \qquad \overset{H\text{—}X}{HO_2C \leftarrow CH{=}CH_2}$$

$$\overset{H\text{—}X}{Me_3\overset{+}{N} \leftarrow CH{=}CH_2} \qquad \overset{H\text{—}X}{F_3C \leftarrow CH{=}CH_2}$$

The difference between this explanation and Thiele's for the $\alpha\beta$-unsaturated acid is unimportant in view of the difficulty of tracing the detailed movements of the keto-enolic proton; while the explanation here applied to the halogenoethylene reaction can be regarded as an extension of Thiele's basic idea that conjugation may determine the direction of addition to the olefinic unit in a conjugated system. This is as in electrophilic aromatic substitution, in which the electronegativity (−I) of halogens reduces the rate of substitution, but leaves the predominating ortho-para-orientation as determined by their electropositive polarisability effect (+E), provided that they are conjugated with the aromatic system. Just as ω-nitrostyrene is in the same case (−I+E) with bromobenzene as regards aromatic substitution, so p-nitrostyrene is in the same case with vinyl bromide (−I+E) as regards addition to the ethylenic bond. Eliel and his collaborators have shown[19] that the introduction of a p-nitro-group into styrene greatly reduces the rate of hydrogen bromide addition, but leaves the orienta-

[17] A. L. Henne and S. Kaye, *J. Am Chem. Soc.*, 1950, **72**, 3369.

[18] H. J. Lucas and A. Y. Jameson, *J. Am. Chem. Soc.*, 1924, **46**, 2475

[19] E. L. Eliel, A. H. Goldkamp, L. E. Carosins, and M. Eberhardt, *J. Org. Chem.*, 1961, **26**, 5188.

tion of addition as in styrene;

$$p\text{-}NO_2\text{—}C_6H_4\text{—}CH\text{=}CH_2 \xrightarrow{HBr} NO_2\cdot C_6H_4\cdot CHBr\cdot CH_3$$

Strong acids other than halogen acids will add to the olefinic double bond. The most important examples are the *addition of the hydroxonium ion*, and of the sulphuric acid molecule, to form respectively the ionic conjugate acid, and the hydrogen sulphate, of an alcohol, the product actually isolated in the presence of water being in either case the alcohol. The orientation of these additions is the same as for halogen acids. Thus Markownikoff's rule would apply in the form that the hydroxyl group of the alcohol is bound to the less hydrogenated of the originally unsaturated carbon atoms. The acidic hydration of olefins to alcohols is often measurably reversible. And thus we are led to realise the close connexion between this subject of addition and the already discussed subject (Chapter IX) of olefin-forming eliminations.

The facts indicated in the preceding paragraph were appreciated long ago by Butlerow,[20] who in 1877 described "di*iso*butylene," that is, 1,1-dimethyl-2-*t*-butylethylene, as coming into equilibrium, in the presence of dilute sulphuric acid, with so-called "di*iso*butol," that is, dimethyl*neo*pentylcarbinol, or with the hydrogen sulphate of the latter:

$$(CH_3)_2C\!:\!CH\cdot C(CH_3)_3 \underset{H_2SO_4}{\overset{\text{dilute}}{\rightleftharpoons}} (CH_3)_2C(OH)\cdot CH_2\cdot C(CH_3)_3$$

More recently the equilibrium between *iso*butylene and *t*-butyl alcohol in excess of $0.2N$ aqueous nitric acid has been quantitatively studied by Eberz and Lucas.[21] At ordinary temperatures this equilibrium lies well over towards the alcohol:

$$(CH_3)_2C\!:\!CH_2 \underset{HNO_3}{\overset{\text{dilute}}{\rightleftharpoons}} (CH_3)_2C(OH)\cdot CH_3$$

Considerable effort has been devoted to study of the *kinetics* of additions of hydrogen halides and hydroxonium ion to olefins. The kinetics of the addition of hydrogen chloride to *iso*butylene,[22] and of hydrogen bromide to propylene,[23] in solvent heptane, have been examined by Mayo and his coworkers. They observed in each case a

[20] A. Butlerow, *Ann.*, 1877, **189**, 76.
[21] W. F. Eberz and H. J. Lucas, *J. Am. Chem. Soc.*, 1934, **56**, 1230.
[22] F. R. Mayo and J. J. Katz, *J. Am. Chem. Soc.*, 1947, **69**, 1339.
[23] F. R. Mayo and M. G. Savoy, *J. Am. Chem. Soc.* 1947, **69**, 1348.

reaction of first order in the olefin, and of a somewhat indefinite order, averaging about three, in the hydrogen halide. Such a result might have been expected for the following reason (Section **31a**). In any definitely heterolytic reaction, the transition state is always highly polar. If the solvent is non-polar, then the most polar available solute molecules will cluster round the transition state. If the most polar solute happens to be a reactant, we shall observe an enhanced, and possibly somewhat indefinite, order in that reactant (as is here illustrated). If the most polar solute is a product of the reaction, we shall observe autocatalysis, possibly with a high and rather indefinite order in the catalyst (as was illustrated in Section **23e**).

Less complex kinetics are observed when polar solvents are employed, as in the experiments of Lucas and his coworkers on the rate of acid-catalysed hydration of *iso*butylene[24] and of trimethylethylene[25] in solvent water. They established that the reaction is of first order with respect alike to olefin and to acid, and made it highly probable that the main, if not the only, effective acid in the aqueous conditions used is the hydroxonium ion:

$$\text{Rate} \propto [\text{olefin}][H_3O^+]$$

These kinetics alone do not tell us whether the proton of the strong acid, namely, the hydroxonium ion, adds ahead of its conjugate base, the water molecule, the whole addition involving two steps, or whether the proton and the conjugate base simultaneously "clap" on to the olefinic double bond. However, since the addition is reversible, we cannot consider it separately from elimination: the principle of microscopic reversibility teaches that the easiest way over any potential barrier from a factor to a product is the easiest way back from the product to the factor. Now there is a considerable weight of evidence[26] that the substitutions and eliminations undergone by the ionic conjugate acids of secondary and tertiary alcohols are normally two-stage unimolecular processes, S_N1 and E1. It is therefore indicated that the additions which reverse these eliminations are also two-stage processes:

$$R\cdot CH\!=\!CH_2 + H\cdot OH_2^+ \rightarrow R\cdot\overset{+}{C}H\text{—}CH_3 + OH_2$$

$$R\cdot\overset{+}{C}H\text{—}CH_3 + OH_2 \rightarrow R\cdot CH(\overset{+}{O}H_2)\cdot CH_3$$

Whitmore and Johnston have provided a special piece of evidence[27]

[24] H. J. Lucas and W. F. Eberz, *J. Am. Chem. Soc.*, 1934, **56**, 460.
[25] H. J. Lucas and Yun-Pu Liu, *J. Am. Chem. Soc.*, 1934, **56**, 2138.
[26] See particularly Sections **28d** and **29e**.
[27] F. C. Whitmore and F. Johnston, *J. Am. Chem. Soc.*, 1933, 55, 5020.

to the effect that the same conclusion applies to hydrogen halide additions. They showed that, while the addition of hydrogen chloride to *iso*propylethylene in the absence of a solvent yields *iso*amyl chloride accompanied by much *t*-amyl chloride, the latter is not produced by way of the former, which remains completely stable under the experimental conditions. Therefore the rearrangement leading to *t*-amyl chloride can take place only in some intermediate product of addition, and this can scarcely be anything else than the carbonium ion, which the step-wise mechanism provides:

$$\mathrm{Me_2CH\cdot CH{=}CH_2 + HCl}$$

$$\rightarrow \mathrm{Me_2CH\cdot \overset{+}{C}H\cdot CH_3 + Cl^- \rightarrow Me_2CH\cdot CHCl\cdot CH_3}$$

$$\downarrow$$

$$\mathrm{Me_2\overset{+}{C}\cdot CH_2\cdot CH_3 + Cl^- \rightarrow Me_2CCl\cdot CH_2\cdot CH_3}$$

The addition of hydrogen iodide to *t*-butylethylene also gives[28] both the unrearranged iodide $\mathrm{Me_3C\cdot CHI\cdot Me}$ and the rearranged iodide $\mathrm{Me_2CI\cdot CHMe_2}$. Hughes and Peeling, after conducting the addition at −80° in the absence of a solvent, found 50% of each isomer.[29]

A point of mechanism which one always tries to settle for any reaction that depends on proton uptake is that of whether the proton transfer is completed in a pre-equilibrium, before the system rises to its transition state (specific hydrogen-ion catalysis), or whether the proton transfer is the slow process going on in the transition state (general-acid catalysis). A problem was created, which it took nearly a decade to solve, when, in 1952, Taft observed[30] that the rates of acidic hydration of olefins followed Hammett's h_0 more closely than $[H^+]$. Hammett's h_0 scale is constructed as a measure of acidity for equilibrium proton transfers to nitrogen bases. The conclusion drawn (practically automatically at that date) from Taft's observation was that rates of olefin hydration depend on equilibrium proton transfers (specific hydrogen-ion catalysis). The first difficulty then was to make a reasonable suggestion as to what could be the slow process which was going on in the transition state. The suggestions made—perhaps the only ones that could be made—were not reasonable. More seriously, all attempts to check the inferred pre-equilibria by other approaches

[28] G. G. Ecke, N. C. Cook, and F. C. Whitmore, *J. Am. Chem. Soc.*, **1950, 72,** 1511.

[29] E. D. Hughes and Marion G. Peeling, results personally communicated.

[30] R. W. Taft, *J. Am. Chem. Soc.*, 1952, **74,** 5372; R. W. Taft, E. L. Purlee, P. Riesz, and C. A. de Fazio, *ibid.*, 1955, **77,** 1584; R. H. Boyd, R. W. Taft, A. P Wolf, and D. R. Christman, *ibid.*, 1960, **82,** 4729.

failed to confirm them. Taft, as well as others, tried several independent approaches.

One was to examine the kinetic effect of solvent deuterium. Reactions dependent on pre-equilibrium proton uptake normally go two to three times faster in deuterium water than in ordinary water, essentially because D_3O^+ is a considerably stronger acid in D_2O than H_3O^+ is in H_2O. Rate-controlling proton-transfers go more slowly when they become deuteron transfers in deuterium water. It was found that acid hydrations of olefins go more slowly in deuterium water.[31,33,34]

Taft applied tests for interconversion ahead of hydration of two olefins which should give the same carbonium ion, and do give the same alcohol:

$$(CH_3)_2C{=}CH{-}CH_3 \underset{(-1)}{\overset{(1)}{\rightleftharpoons}} (CH_3)_2\overset{+}{C}{-}CH_2{-}CH_3 \underset{(-1)}{\overset{(1)}{\rightleftharpoons}} CH_2{=}C(CH_3){-}CH_2{-}CH_3$$

$$(CH_3)_2\overset{+}{C}{-}CH_2{-}CH_3 \xrightarrow{(2)} (CH_3)_2C(OH){-}CH_2{-}CH_3$$

It the proton transfers are pre-equilibrium processes, the transition fsate must be in the reaction labelled (2), and nearly all the formed carbonium ion will revert to olefin, only a small proportion mounting the energy hill to the transition state, so to give the alcohol. Therefore the olefins should undergo interconversion much faster than hydration; but experiment showed that there was no interconversion of olefins at 50% of hydration.[32] An equivalent test is to run either of the hydrations in deuterium water. If protonation is a pre-equilibrium process, deuterium should get incorporated into the olefin much faster than the olefin undergoes hydration. Experiment showed that no deuterium got incorporated into the olefin.[31] The only possible con-

[31] J. S. Coe and V. Gold, *J. Chem. Soc.*, **1960,** 4571; V. Gold and M. A. Kessick, *Proc. Chem. Soc.*, **1964,** 295.

[32] J. B. Levy, R. W. Taft, and L. P. Hammett, *J. Am. Chem. Soc.*, 1953, **75,** 1253.

[33] E. L. Purlee and R. W. Taft, *J. Am. Chem. Soc.*, 1956, **78,** 5807.

[34] W. M. Schubert, Bo Lamm, and J. R. Keefe, *J. Am. Chem. Soc.*, 1964, **86,** 4727.

clusion is that reactions (-1) do not occur, *i.e.*, that the transition states have been passed over by the time the carbonium ion is produced, *i.e.*, that the proton transfers are rate-controlling.

This implies general-acid catalysis. If the transition state composition includes, besides the olefin, the complete acid H_3O^+, which is transferring a proton to the olefin, then other transition states containing other complete acids HA should be possible. (In specific hydrogen-ion catalysis, the transition state contains the substrate and the proton from the acid, so that all acids lead to the same transition state.) The usual difficulty in detecting a multiplicity of transition states is that rate terms dependent on molecular acids are often inconveniently low. Although the discovery came after the original difficulty of the Hammett-type kinetics had been cleared up, we may note here that Schubert and his coworkers were able, by the use of the very reactive olefin, *p*-methoxy-α-methylstyrene, and of formate buffers, to establish hydration catalysed by the formic acid molecules.[34] This is clear evidence that olefin hydration is in principle general-acid catalysed.

Concurrently with this problem concerning the manner and timing of proton transfers in acid-catalysed olefin hydration, a similar problem arose in regard to acid-catalysed aromatic hydrogen-exchanges, as already described in Section **24c**. Rates appeared to follow h_0 rather than $[H^+]$, though it had been known since the discovery of this reaction (but many ignored this) that it was general-acid catalysed. In 1961 Bunnett cleared up both these problems.[35] He showed that acidity scales applying to equilibria in aqueous acid depend largely on the changes in the activity of solvent water, and hence on the amount of bound, including solvation, water that is released or acquired by the solutes as a result of the proton transfer. A given release of bound water is more favourable to reaction at higher acidities when the free solvent water is less plentiful. The h_0 scale was constructed to represent equilibrium proton transfers from the strongly hydrophilic water molecule to more mildly hydrophilic organic nitrogen bases. In these processes some bound water is released, and that is a main reason why the h_0 scale rises with increasing steepness above $[H^+]$ with rising acidity. The h_0 scale does represent fairly well equilibrium proton transfers to similarly mildly hydrophilic organic nitrogen and organic oxygen bases. But so much more bound water is released when a proton is transferred from water to a hydrophobic carbon base, that the h_0 function does not take care of that case at all. A much more steeply rising function than h_0 would be required to represent equi-

[35] J. F. Bunnett, *J. Am. Chem. Soc.*, 1961, **83**, 4056 (4 papers).

libria in such proton transfers to carbon. It is, Bunnett concludes, to be considered as coincidental that Hammett's h_0 does approximately describe the pseudo-equilibrium of the partial proton transfer, and the associated partial water release, in the formation of the transition state of a proton transfer to carbon.

If we write out the Bunnett mechanism,

$$R_2C{=}CR_2 + H_3O^+ \underset{\text{slow}}{\rightleftharpoons} R_2CH{-}CR_2^+ + H_2O$$

$$R_2CH{-}CR_2^+ + H_2O \rightleftharpoons R_2CH{-}CR_2{\cdot}OH_2^+$$

$$R_2CH{-}CR_2{\cdot}OH_2^+ + H_2O \rightleftharpoons R_2CH{-}CR_2{\cdot}OH + H_3O^+$$

and read the result backwards, we obtain the mechanism for olefin elimination from the conjugate acid of an alcohol. Even though it goes through a carbonium ion, it is not mechanism E1, because a water molecule, as well as the carbonium ion, is involved in the transition state. It is a bimolecular mechanism based on pre-equilibrium formation of a carbonium ion, and therefore we label it $E_2(C^+)$. It is the counterpart for elimination of a substitution mechanism, $S_N2(C^+)$, that is fairly well known (Section **29c**). It may be written as follows, its distinguishing feature being that the last step (marked "slow") is rate-controlling:

$$\left.\begin{aligned} R_2CH{\cdot}CR_2{\cdot}OH + H_3O^+ &\rightleftharpoons R_2CH{\cdot}CR_2{\cdot}OH_2^+ \\ &\rightleftharpoons R_2CH{\cdot}CR_2^+ + H_2O \\ &\underset{\text{slow}}{\rightleftharpoons} R_2C{:}CR_2 \end{aligned}\right\} \quad [E2(C^+)]$$

Turning to the *stereochemistry* of the additions of hydrogen halides and hydroxonium ion to cyclic olefinic compounds, we may note first some observations[36] to the effect that cyclic $\alpha\beta$-olefinic acids, such as *cyclo*hexene-1-carboxylic acid, add hydrogen chloride in a *trans*-fashion:

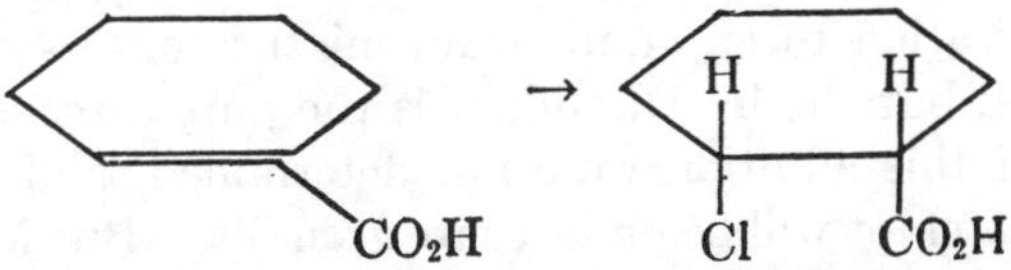

CO_2H → H, H, Cl, CO_2H

The difficulty of interpretation in such cases is to know whether we are dealing with a reaction localised in the olefinic bond, or whether, as Thiele would have said (cf. the next Section), the initial uptake of

[36] W. R. Vaughan, R. L. Cravan, R. Q. Little, and A. C. Schoenthaler, *J. Am. Chem. Soc.*, 1955, **77**, 1594.

hydrogen is at carboxyl oxygen, though it subsequently undergoes prototropic migration to the α-carbon atom, at which it is found.

This difficulty does not occur in additions to olefinic hydrocarbons. As to these, two types of result have been obtained. The first may be represented by Collins and Hammond's demonstration that the addition of water to 1,2-dimethyl*cyclo*hexene in aqueous nitric acid gives nearly equal amounts of the diastereoisomeric alcohols formed by *cis*- and *trans*-addition.[37] There can be no question here of isomerisation of the adducts after their formation. To this reaction we can surely apply the already described kinetic findings concerning olefin hydration, which show that the rate-controlling step is a proton transfer, the immediate product thus formed being a carbonium ion:

The stereochemistry therefore corresponds to that expected for the reversal of an E1 elimination, in which the intermediate carbonium ion has time to settle to its equilibrium configuration, so that dissymmetric shielding is not important.

The second type of stereochemistry may be illustrated by a result by the same workers for the addition of hydrogen chloride in pentane to 1,2-dimethyl*cyclo*pentane.[38] This reaction gave the *trans*-1,2-hydrochloride. When formed, it does at suitable temperatures undergo partial isomerisation to an equilibrium mixture of *cis*- and *trans*-1,2-hydrochlorides; but the initial adduct is the pure *trans*-isomer. Now the kinetics of this addition were not determined, and so any interpretation we attempt will be on insecure grounds. But Mayo's kinetic investigation of additions of hydrogen bromide in somewhat similar conditions suggests that the order in hydrogen chloride is likely to be at least two. This, if confirmed, would suggest a concerted process, the stereochemistry of which would be that of an E2 elimination in reverse. Where the chlorine enters, one has a local S_N2 substitution

[37] C. H. Collins and G. S. Hammond, *J. Org. Chem.*, 1960, **25,** 911.
[38] G. S. Hammond and C. H. Collins, *J. Am. Chem. Soc.*, 1960, **82,** 5323.

with inversion, and where the hydrogen enters, a local S_E2 substitution with retention of configuration: the result is *trans*-addition:

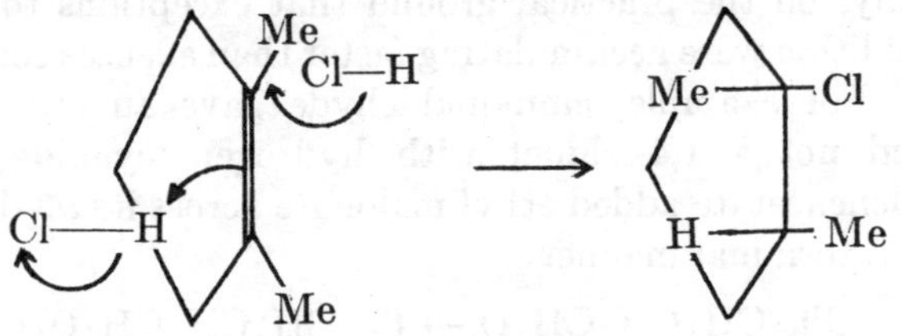

Similar *trans*-additions have been reported[39] for additions of hydrogen bromide in pentane or acetic acid to 1,2-dimethyl*cyclo*hexene and other *cyclo*hexenes. Although the stereochemistry of a reaction is a property of its mechanism and not of its stoicheiometry, no kinetic investigations are associated with these stereochemical determinations.

(53b) Additions of Strong Acids, in Particular of Hydrogen Halides, to Conjugated Polyolefinic Compounds.—This is the first of several Sections, in which we shall be dealing with one branch or another of the general subject of additions to conjugated unsaturated systems; and hence it will be convenient here to introduce the whole matter with a note on the development of the study of such additions.

The most eventful period in the study of the additive reactions of conjugated unsaturated systems began with the group of papers[40] published by Thiele in 1898, in the first of which he presented his theory of the residual affinity possessed by double-bonded carbon, and of its internal satisfaction along a chain of conjugated double bonds, except at the ends of the chain, where, accordingly, additions should occur. Originally Thiele meant his theory, not only to explain how terminal addition could occur, but also to carry the consequence that terminal addition would occur when the necessary molecular system was provided. He went to some pains to show that various exceptions to this rule, cases of 1,2-addition despite the structural possibility of 1,4-addition, could be explained as 1,4-additions succeeded by tautomeric changes, as in the following representation of the reduction of benzil to benzoin:

$$\mathrm{Ph\cdot CO\cdot CO\cdot Ph \rightarrow Ph\cdot C(OH){:}C(OH)\cdot Ph \rightarrow Ph\cdot CO\cdot CH(OH)\cdot Ph}$$

During the next decade, Thiele's theory was strongly attacked,

[39] G. S. Hammond and T. D. Nevitt, *J. Am. Chem. Soc.*, 1954, **76**, 4121; R. C. Faheg and R. A. Smith, *ibid.*, **86**, 5035.

[40] J. Thiele, *Ann.*, 1898, **306**, 87, *et seq.* (12 papers); 1899, **308**, **333**; 1900, **314**, 298; 1901, **319**, 129.

notably by Michael[41] and by Hinrichsen,[42] first, on the theoretical ground that it attached too little weight to specific affinities between atoms of the addendum and of the unsaturated molecule, affinities which might be understood as disclosing electrochemical influences; and secondly, on the practical ground that exceptions to the rule of terminal addition were accumulating faster than excuses could be found for them. For example, cinnamaldehyde gave an ordinary cyanohydrin, and not a 1,4-adduct with hydrogen cyanide; and ethyl cinnamylideneacetate added ethyl malonate across its $\alpha\beta$-double bond, and not in a terminal manner:

$$\mathrm{Ph\cdot CH{:}CH\cdot CH{:}O \rightarrow Ph\cdot CH{:}CH\cdot \underset{\displaystyle CN}{\underset{|}{CH}}\cdot OH}$$

$$\mathrm{Ph\cdot CH{:}CH\cdot CH{:}CH\cdot CO_2Et \rightarrow Ph\cdot CH{:}CH\cdot \underset{\displaystyle CH(CO_2Et)_2}{\underset{|}{CH}}\cdot CH_2\cdot CO_2Et}$$

Obviously it was necessary at least to concede that an unsymmetrically constituted and highly polar addendum, or an unsymmetrical and polar unsaturated system, or both in conjunction, could produce unsymmetrical modes of addition, the specific, possibly electrochemical, affinities causing variation from the terminal form of addition to which Thiele's distribution of affinity should lead. But in 1909 it was made clear that even this concession would not meet the situation: Straus showed[43] that the symmetrical molecule, bromine, adds to the symmetrical diolefin, 1,4-diphenylbutadiene, in an unsymmetrical manner, forming exclusively the 1,2-dibromide:

$$\mathrm{Ph\cdot CH{:}CH\cdot CH{:}CH\cdot Ph \rightarrow Ph\cdot CHBr\cdot CHBr\cdot CH{:}CH\cdot Ph}$$

So it became recognised that Thiele's theory, though it could still provide a mechanism for terminal addition when observed, could neither require such addition, nor explain its frequent non-occurrence. In short, one had no theory of orientation, nor even any orientation rules, for addition to conjugated unsaturated systems, comparable in range and definition to the rules which had by that time been developed for substitution in aromatic systems. And there the position remained until 1928, when Burton and the writer noted, in their first paper on anionotropic change,[44] that the addition of an electrophile to a conjugated polyene can produce anionotropic tautomers; and that if

[41] A. Michael, *J. prakt. Chem.*, 1899, **60**, 467.

[42] F. W. Hinrichsen, *Ann.*, 1904, **336**, 168.

[43] F. Straus, *Ber.*, 1909, **42**, 2866.

[44] H. Burton and C. K. Ingold, *J. Chem. Soc.*, **1928**, 910.

addition follows the simplest possible two-stage mechanism, the second stage of addition, which is a union of two ions, is identical with the second stage of the usual S_N1' mechanism of anionotropic isomerisation, as illustrated in the following example:

$$CH_2{:}CH\cdot CH{:}CH_2 + HBr \rightarrow [CH_3\cdot CH \frown CH \frown CH_2]^+ + Br^-$$
$$\rightleftarrows CH_3\cdot CHBr\cdot CH{:}CH_2 \text{ and } CH_3\cdot CH{:}CH\cdot CH_2Br$$

They discussed the problem of orientation in additions to conjugated systems from this point of view. This discussion was subsequently restated[45] in an improved form, which will be followed in the present text.

In this Section we shall be concerned only with the additions Ad_E of acid electrophiles to conjugated polyolefins. We will outline the theory of orientation for these additions. Then we will notice a number of experimental observations relating to the additions of hydrogen halides.

The theoretical problem has two parts corresponding to the two stages of addition. The first is concerned with the position of uptake of the adding proton by the conjugated system. This is assumed to be determined by a straightforward application of the electrochemical principles of orientation in additions to unsaturated systems, as set forth for simple mono-olefinic systems in the preceding Section. The addendum is an electrophile: where it first attacks, it demands electrons. Therefore each vinyl group of butadiene, for example, will act electropositively towards the other, contributing a $+E$ effect, through which electrons will be made most available to the adding proton at the ends of the conjugated system. If the two ends of such a system are rendered non-equivalent by alkyl or aryl substitution, then that end at which the substituent itself can contribute a hyperconjugative or conjugative $+E$ effect will be preferred as the point of initiation of addition. Thus in 2-methylbuta-1,3-diene we must expect electrophilic addition to be initiated in the 1-position, in 1-phenylbuta-1,3-diene in the 4-position, and so on:

$$\overset{(1)}{CH_2}{=}\overset{CH_3}{\overset{\downarrow}{C}}{-}CH{=}CH_2 \qquad Ph{-}CH{=}CH{-}CH{=}\overset{(4)}{CH_2}$$

The experimental evidence supporting this part of the theory is, briefly, that no normal adduct which disagrees with it has ever been isolated. Thus, butadiene has three possible monohydrochlorides,

[45] P. B. D. de la Mare, E. D. Hughes, and C. K. Ingold, *J. Chem. Soc.*, 1948, 17.

which we can distinguish as the 1-hydro-2-chloride, the 1-hydro-4-chloride, and the 2-hydro-1-chloride. The first two are indeed formed, but the third is not. 2-Methylbutadiene (isoprene) has six possible hydrochlorides, only two of which could arise following proton uptake in the 1-position. These two are in fact found, but no others. 1-Phenylbutadiene likewise has six possible hydrochlorides, only two of which would arise from addition initiated in the 4-position. The one hydrochloride which in fact is formed is one of these two. We shall be referring to these examples again later.

The second orientational problem is concerned with the alternatives left open by the first: they relate to the position in which the conjugate base of the adding acid is taken up. In the example of hydrogen halide additions, the ions of the products, which are anionotropic halides, are assumed to have been formed, and it has to be considered how the ions will unite. At first their union will be kinetically controlled: that isomeride which is formed more quickly will appear in greater amount. But if the halides can re-ionise freely, their proportions will become thermodynamically controlled: the more stable will be present in greater amount.

In simple cases it is usually possible to foretell which of two anionotropic isomerides is the more stable by comparing the structures with respect to the known factors of stability, such as conjugation and hyperconjugation. Thus, of the two hydrohalides of butadiene which could arise following terminal proton uptake, the 1-hydro-4-halide, $CH_3 \cdot CH:CH \cdot CH_2X$, should be somewhat more stable than the 1-hydro-2-halide, $CH_3 \cdot CHX \cdot CH:CH_2$, because of the methyl-hyperconjugation in the former structure. Of the two hydrohalides of 2-methylbutadiene which could arise following proton uptake in the 1-position, the 1-hydro-4-halide $(CH_3)_2C:CH \cdot CH_2X$ should be considerably more stable than the 1-hydro-2-halide $(CH_3)_2CX \cdot CH:CH_2$, because of a double methyl-hyperconjugation in the former. Of the two hydrohalides of 1-phenylbutadiene which could arise after proton uptake in the 4-position, the 4-hydro-3-halide, $Ph \cdot CH:CH \cdot CHX \cdot CH_3$, is much more stable than $Ph \cdot CHX \cdot CH:CH \cdot CH_3$, the 4-hydro-1-halide, because only the former structure retains the phenyl-to-vinyl conjugation. Such deductions would conclude a qualitative discussion of the orientational problem, if one were sure that the system, and the conditions, were such that the anionotropic system will attain equilibrium.

When the anionotropic system does not move into equilibrium, so that orientation in the second stage of addition is kinetically controlled, our basis for predicting the structure of the main product is less secure.

However, it seems reasonable to expect that the rule, illustrated for prototropic systems in Section **47d**, namely, that an unstable ionic form of a tautomeric system passes more quickly into the less stable, than into the more stable, covalent form, will hold also for anionotropic systems. This would mean that the less stable tautomer, decided as illustrated in the preceding paragraph, would appear as the predominating addition product.

Whether the final stage of orientation will be kinetically or thermodynamically controlled depends on the capacity, and opportunities, of the anionotropic products for ionisation: $+E$ substituents in the order phenyl > methyl, easily liberated anions, in particular, bromide > chloride, and polar solvents, are among the factors which should promote thermodynamic control.

With these considerations in mind, let us notice some of the observations. The addition of hydrogen chloride to buta-1,3-diene, both in the absence of a solvent, and in acetic acid, has been investigated by Kharasch and his coworkers.[46] As already indicated, they found the 1-hydro-4-chloride, and the 1-hydro-2-chloride, but no 2-hydro-1-chloride. The proportion of 1-hydro-4-chloride was 20–25%, and was independent of temperature between $-80°$ and $+25°$; and the separated chlorides underwent no measurable conversion under the conditions of their formation. However, prolonged treatment with hydrogen chloride at the upper end of the temperature range caused conversion, finally, into an equilibrium mixture containing 75% of the 1-hydro-4-chloride. We see here initial kinetic control, giving mainly the less stable 1-hydro-2-chloride, followed, after a sufficient time at a high enough temperature, by the thermodynamically controlled production in major amount of the more stable 1-hydro-4-chloride.

The addition of hydrogen bromide to buta-1,3-diene leads to a more mobile anionotropic system. The same investigators obtained a kinetically controlled mixture of products only at low temperatures such as $-80°$, and (since the abnormal addition of hydrogen bromide had to be guarded against) with careful exclusion of oxidant catalysts. This mixture contained 20% of the 1-hydro-4-bromide. At higher temperatures larger proportions of this compound were produced, and the separated isomers could be observed to suffer interconversions, leading towards the equilibrium mixture, which has been shown[47] to contain about 80% of the 1-hydro-4-bromide.

[46] M. S. Kharasch, J. Kritchevsky, and F. R. Mayo, *J. Org. Chem.*, 1938, **2**, 489.

[47] S. Winstein and W. G. Young, *J. Am. Chem. Soc.*, 1936, **58**, 104. B. D. England and E. D. Hughes, results personally communicated.

The addition of hydrogen chloride to 2-methylbutadiene (isoprene) also shows a phase of kinetic control, as has been proved by Ultrée.[48] The earlier literature of the reaction is confused: some authors have reported the formation of the 1-hydro-4-chloride only, and one author of the 1-hydro-2-chloride only, while one group of authors reported the production of both substances. Ultrée showed that, with a deficit of hydrogen chloride at a low temperature, the 1-hydro-2-chloride is predominantly produced, but that this undergoes a facile isomerisation under catalysis by hydrogen chloride to give the 1-hydro-4-chloride, which, therefore, is the product isolated when excess of hydrogen chloride is used in the process of addition. Thus there is initial kinetic control to give the less stable, and ultimate thermodynamic control to give the more stable, of the two adducts allowed by proton uptake in position-1, under orientation by the 2-methyl substituent. As theoretically expected, the relative thermodynamic stability of the 1,4-adduct is greater for isoprene than for butadiene, with the result that, in equilibrium, the proportion of 1,2-adduct is inappreciably low.

The addition of hydrogen bromide to isoprene, to 2,3-dimethylbuta-1,3-diene, and to 1,4-dimethylbuta-1,3-diene, has been investigated.[49] But in none of the recorded results can any phase of kinetic control be recognised: the chief product is always that which is expected to be the more stable, out of those allowed by the rule giving the position of proton uptake. Thus 2-methylbutadiene (isoprene) gives the 1-hydro-4-bromide only; 2,3-dimethylbutadiene gives the 1-hydro-4-bromide only; while 1,4-dimethylbutadiene yields mainly the 1-hydro-2-bromide, $CH_3 \cdot CH_2 \cdot CHBr \cdot CH{:}CH \cdot CH_3$, with a minor proportion of the 1-hydro-4-bromide, $CH_3 \cdot CH_2 \cdot CH{:}CH \cdot CHBr \cdot CH_3$. In this last case, we should expect the 1-hydro-2-bromide to be the somewhat more stable of the two isomers, because the methyl group should be more effective in hyperconjugation than the ethyl group.

The addition of hydrogen chloride to 1-methylbutadiene (piperylene) is stated to give only the 4-hydro-3-chloride or 4-hydro-1-chloride:[50] these are two names for the same compound, *viz.*, $CH_3CHCl \cdot CH{:}CH \cdot CH_3$. The one clear conclusion is that the proton addition occurs where expected, namely, in the 4-position.

The addition of hydrogen chloride to 1-phenylbutadiene has been

[48] A. J. Ultrée, *J. Chem. Soc.*, **1948,** 530. This paper gives a review of the earlier literature of the reaction.

[49] L. Claisen, *J. prakt. Chem.*, 1922, **105,** 65; E. H. Farmer and F. C. B. Marshall, *J. Chem. Soc.*, **1931,** 129.

[50] A. L. Henne, H. Chanan, and A. Turk, *J. Am. Chem. Soc.*, 1941, **63,** 3474; A. N. Pudovik and N. B. Shavipova, *Zh. Obshch. Khim.*, 1955, **25,** 589.

examined,[51] as also has the addition of hydrogen bromide.[52] Again no phase of kinetic control can be seen in the results. In each case, the exclusive product is the 4-hydro-3-halide, $Ph \cdot CH{:}CH \cdot CHX \cdot CH_3$. This is the more stable of the two halides which could arise following proton uptake in the 4-position.

The termination of a butadiene by an electron-absorbing substituent, such as carboxyl in sorbic acid, cuts out anionotropy in formed hydrochlorides.[53] Therefore these adducts have structures determined by mechanism, and not by thermodynamics. The proton adds where Thiele would have supposed, namely, in the electronegative substituent, for instance at oxygen in a carboxyl group, though it subsequently undergoes prototropic migration to the α-position, in which it is found. The chloride ion enters where maximal electron deficiency can be developed, namely, at the other end of the conjugated system, the δ-position. So we obtain α-hydro-δ-chloride adducts to sorbic acid and like systems:[53]

$$CH_3 \cdot CH{:}CH \cdot CH{:}CH \cdot CO_2H \rightarrow CH_3 \cdot CHCl \cdot CH{:}CH \cdot CH_2 \cdot CO_2H$$

The *kinetics* of acid-catalysed 1,4-hydration have been definitively investigated in the example of the conversion of furan to succindialdehyde, presumably by ring-chain and keto-enol prototropy through 1,4-dihydroxybutadiene:

$$\text{CH}\overset{\text{CH—CH}}{=\quad\quad=}\text{CH}\ (\text{ring O}) \xrightarrow{\text{slow}} \overset{\text{H}}{\text{CH}}\text{—CH=CH—}\overset{+}{\text{CH}}\ (\text{ring O}) \rightarrow \overset{\text{H}}{\text{CH}}\text{—CH=CH—CH}\cdot\text{OH}\ (\text{ring O})$$

$$\rightarrow \overset{\text{H}}{\text{HO}\cdot\text{CH}}\text{—CH=CH—CH{:}O} \rightarrow \text{HO}\cdot\text{CH=CH—CH=CH}\cdot\text{OH} \rightarrow \text{CHO—CH}_2\text{—CH}_2\text{—CHO}$$

Stamhaus, Drenth, and Van den Berg have shown[54] that the rate of this reaction follows h_0 rather than $[H^+]$, and is reduced in deuterium water ($k_H/k_D = 1.7$), just as in the acid hydration of simple olefins (Section **52a**). The conclusion is the same, namely, that the reaction depends on rate-controlling proton uptake at an unsaturated carbon

[51] I. E. Muskat and K. A. Huggins, *J. Am. Chem. Soc.*, 1934, **56**, 1239.
[52] C. N. Riiber, *Ber.*, 1911, **44**, 2974.
[53] C. K. Ingold, G. J. Pritchard, and H. G. Smith, *J. Chem. Soc.*, **1934**, 79.
[54] E. J. Stamhaus, W. Drenth, and H. Van den Berg, *Rec. trav. chim.*, 1964, **83**, 107.

atom. No kinetic investigation of the 1,4-addition of hydrogen halides has yet been recorded.

The *stereochemistry* of acidic 1,4-hydration has not yet been studied, but that of 1,4-addition of a hydrogen halide has. The stereochemistry must, of course, depend on mechanism, and in particular on whether the reaction occurs in steps, or is concerted. Corresponding to the already discussed, concerted, termolecular *trans*-1,2-addition of hydrogen chloride, one can envisage a concerted, termolecular, *cis*-1,4-addition:

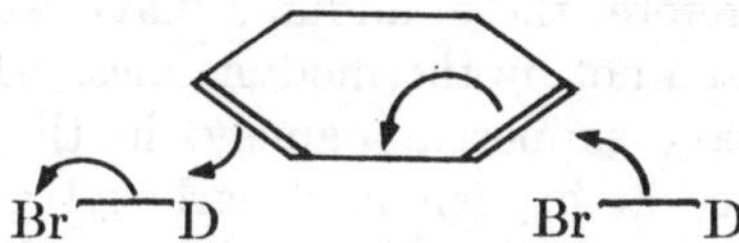

It has been shown[55] that the primary product of addition of deuterium bromide to *cyclo*hexa-1,4-diene in pentane consists of 80% of the *cis*-1,4-hydrobromide plus 20% of the *trans*-1,2-hydrobromide. Kinetic control of the mechanism in operation is not available.

(53c) Additions of Non-acid Electrophiles, in Particular of Halogens, to Mono-olefinic Compounds.—The halogens, apart from fluorine, form a leading group of non-acidic electrophilic addenda, which include a number of other substances, such as nitrosyl chloride and acetyl nitrate. (The reactions of fluorine seem to be entirely homolytic.) The addition of chlorine and bromine to olefinic substances may be promoted photochemically or by chemically produced radicals, and it then occurs in homolytic chain reactions. We shall here be concerned, however, with "dark" reactions in the absence of radical initiation. As is shown by their obvious need for a polar environment, these reactions are heterolytic. We know that the so-called gaseous additions of chlorine and bromine to ethylene are actually surface reactions, which moreover need a polar surface.[56] It has been established that the addition of bromine and iodine to olefinic compounds in non-polar solvents is markedly sensitive to polar surfaces,[57] and to adventitious polar solutes, such as hydrogen halides[58] and water.[59] Simpler situa-

[55] G. S. Hammond and J. Warkentin, *J. Am. Chem. Soc.*, 1961, **83**, 2554.

[56] T. D. Stewart and K. R. Edlund, *J. Am. Chem. Soc.*, 1923, **45**, 1014; T. D. Stewart and R. D. Fowler, *ibid.*, 1926, **48**, 1187; R. G. W. Norrish, *J. Chem. Soc.*, 1923, **123**, 3006; R. G. W. Norrish and G. G. Jones, *ibid.*, **1926**, 55.

[57] P. W. Robertson, N. T. Clare, K. J. McNaught, and G. W. Paul, *J. Chem. Soc.*, **1937**, 335.

[58] J. J. Sudborough and J. Thomas, *J. Chem. Soc.*, 1910, **97**, 715, 2450; M. D. Williams and T. C. James, *ibid.*, **1928**, 343; N. W. Hanson and T. C. James, *ibid.*, p. 1955; N. W. Hanson and D. M. Williams, *ibid.*, **1930**, 1059; D. M. Wil-

tions arise when we allow the heterolytic process what it clearly needs, namely, a polar solvent, such as water, or methyl alcohol, or acetic acid: it is in such circumstances that some knowledge of the heterolytic mechanism is most easily obtained.

When acting as heterolytic addenda, the halogens behave as electrophilic reagents, except, as will be mentioned later, towards certain quite special, unsaturated systems. This conclusion is consistent with the general classification of halogens as electrophilic reagents (Chapter V). It has been specifically supported for halogen additions to simple ethylene derivatives by a demonstration[60] that electron-releasing substituents in the olefin, substituents such as Ph and Me, accelerate addition, while electron-withdrawing substituents, such as Br, CO_2H, and NMe_3^+, retard addition. This thesis has since been much more fully documented by P. W. Robertson and his collaborators, who since 1937 studied the kinetics, and measured rate-constants in comparative conditions, for a large number of additions of halogens to olefinic substances.[61] We shall refer to this work again later.

In polar solvents, halogen additions to olefins can be proved to follow a two-stage mechanism, which involves a carbonium ionic intermediate, and is entirely similar to that already illustrated with reference to the additions of strong acids to olefins:

$$CH_2{:}CH_2 + Br_2 \rightarrow \overset{+}{C}H_2\cdot CH_2Br + \bar{B}r$$

$$\overset{+}{C}H_2\cdot CH_2Br + \bar{B}r \rightarrow CH_2Br\cdot CH_2Br$$

Though the first and rate-controlling step requires elaboration in certain circumstances, this outline has been established by means of demonstrations to the effect that the second stage can be diverted by any sufficiently ample source of active foreign anions. Such anions might be provided as an added salt, as in the experiments of Francis[62] on the reaction between bromine and ethylene in aqueous solutions of sodium chloride, iodide, or nitrate, to give the products indicated below:

---

liams, *ibid.*, **1932**, 2911; S. V. Anantakrishnan and R. Venkataraman, *ibid.*, **1939**, 224.

[59] H. S. Davis, *J. Am. Chem. Soc.*, 1928, **50**, 2769.

[60] C. K. Ingold and E. H. Ingold, *J. Chem. Soc.*, **1931**, 2354; S. V. Anatakrishnan and C. K. Ingold, *ibid.*, **1935**, 984, 1396.

[61] P. W. Robertson and his coworkers published about twenty papers, mainly in the *J. Chem. Soc.* A collection of their rate-constants is given on pp. 84–85 (and the original references on pp. 108–109) of de la Mare and Bolton's monograph (ref. 1).

[62] A. W. Francis, *J. Am. Chem. Soc.*, 1925, **47**, 2340.

$$Br_2 + CH_2{:}CH_2 \begin{cases} \xrightarrow{\text{aq. NaCl}} CH_2Cl\cdot CH_2Br \\ \xrightarrow{\text{aq. NaI}} CH_2I\cdot CH_2Br \\ \xrightarrow{\text{aq. NaNO}_3} CH_2(NO_3)\cdot CH_2Br \end{cases}$$

Again, the diverting anion may be taken from a hydroxylic solvent molecule, a hydroxide ion from solvent water, methoxide ion from methyl alcohol, or acetate from acetic acid, as when chlorine water or bromine water is used in order to add the elements of hypohalous acid,[63] or when a methyl alcoholic[64] or an acetic acid[65] solution of the halogen is employed in order to add the elements of methyl or acetyl hypohalite to an olefinic double bond as in the following examples:

$$Br_2 + CH_2{:}CH_2 \xrightarrow{H_2O} H^+ + CH_2(OH)\cdot CH_2Br$$

$$Br_2 + CHPh{:}CHPh \xrightarrow{MeOH} H^+ + CHPh(OMe)\cdot CHPhBr$$

$$Cl_2 + CH_2{:}CH_2 \xrightarrow{MeCO_2H} H^+ + CH_2(OAc)\cdot CH_2Cl$$

It is necessary to show that such reactions are indeed diverted additions, and are not the ordinary additions of a modified addendum, namely, of a molecular hypohalite formed by solvolysis of the halogen:

$$Hal_2 + ROH \rightleftarrows ROHal + H^+ + Hal^-$$

Now in all these solvolytic halogenations of olefin compounds, a certain amount of dihalide accompanies the oxy-halogen addition products; and an examination of the proportions, and rates of formation, of the different products enables this matter to be tested. In the aqueous halogenations, it has been found that the proportion of halogenohydrin in the product is independent of the acidity, as it obviously

[63] E. Biilmann, *Rec. trav. chim.*, 1917, **36**, 313; M. Gomberg, *J. Am. Chem. Soc.*, 1919, **41**, 1414; J. Read and M. M. Williams, *J. Chem. Soc.*, 1920, **117**, 359; J. Read and R. G. Hook, *ibid.*, p. 1214; J. Read and A. C. P. Andrews, *ibid.*, **1921**, 1774; J. Read and E. Hurst, *ibid.*, **1922**, 989, 2550; J. Read and W. G. Reid, *ibid.*, **1928**, 745; E. M. Terry and L. Eichelberger, *J. Am. Chem. Soc.*, 1925, **47**, 1067.

[64] J. B. Conant and E. L. Jackson, *J. Am. Chem. Soc.*, 1924, **46**, 1727; E. L. Jackson, *ibid.*, 1926, **48**, 3166; K. Meinel, *Ann.*, 1934, **510**, 129; P. D. Bartlett and D. S. Tarbell, *J. Am. Chem. Soc.*, 1936, **58**, 466; 1937, **59**, 407.

[65] H. J. Backer and J. Strating, *Rec. trav. chim.*, 1934, **53**, 525; W. Bockemüller and F. W. Hoffmann, *Ann.*, 1935, **519**, 165.

should not be, if the formation of halogenohydrin depended on molecular hypohalous acid, produced in the reversible reaction written above.[62,63] The proportion of halogenohydrin is, however, depressed (as we should in any case expect) by the addition of halide ions.[63] In the example of the methyl alcoholic bromination of stilbene, Bartlett and Tarbell showed[64] that the rate of formation of the methoxy-bromide was independent of the acidity; and furthermore that the proportional yield of methoxy-bromide was independent of the acidity, but was depressed by added bromide ion in a way which could be quantitatively understood on the assumption that bromide ion was competing with methyl alcohol for the carbonium ionic intermediate. The same investigators[64] made the reality of such intermediates very evident when they produced β-lactones from the reactions of sodium dimethylmaleate and of sodium dimethylfumarate with chlorine water and with bromine water, although it was impossible to obtain these lactones from the fully formed halogenohydrins, consistently with the general experience that β-lactones cannot be prepared by the dehydration of β-hydroxy-acids, not even when other modes of dehydration are precluded:

$$\bar{O}_2C\cdot CMe{:}CMe\cdot C\bar{O}_2 \xrightarrow[H_2O]{Hal_2} \begin{matrix} Me \\ \bar{O}_2C \end{matrix}\!\!>\overset{+}{C}-\underset{Me}{\overset{C\bar{O}_2}{C}}\cdot Hal \rightarrow \begin{matrix} Me \\ \bar{O}_2C \end{matrix}\!\!>\underset{}{C}-\underset{Me}{C}\cdot Hal \;\; (\text{with } O-CO \text{ bridging the two carbons})$$

These early conclusions have been confirmed in all subsequent work. As an instance, one may cite Bell and Pring's kinetic and product studies[66] of the action of aqueous bromine on various olefinic substances, both without added nucleophiles, and with added bromide and chloride ions. Their results clearly confirm that there is in general no connexion between rates and products. Rates are determined by substrate constitution, as would be expected for the rate-controlling attack of an electrophilic reagent. Products depend on the competition of the available nucleophiles in fast succeeding reactions, that cannot affect the rate. The one exception found was ethyl fumarate, on which the attack by the bromine molecule, on the one hand, and that by the water or bromide ion, on the other, appear to be concerted and jointly rate-controlling. This seems not unreasonable: the affinity of the fumarate structure for the nucleophiles suffices to bring them into reaction, without the need to wait for the prior formation of a carbonium ion.

[66] R. P. Bell and M. Pring, *J. Chem. Soc.*, 1966, B, 1119.

The *kinetics of halogen addition* take their simplest form in the case of the addition of *chlorine* to olefins in *solvents not less polar than acetic acid.* These reactions are of second order, as has been established by P. W. Robertson and his coworkers[61] for a wide range of olefinic compounds mainly in solvent acetic acid:

$$\text{Rate} \propto [\text{olefin}][\text{Hal}_2]$$

The kinetics indicate that the entity which attacks the olefin is the halogen molecule. The addition of water and of ionised salts increases reaction rate, consistently with the picture of a heterolytic process, having a polar transition state. The effects of constitutional changes in the olefin on rate of addition, as illustrated in Table 53-1, confirm the view that the halogen is acting as an electrophilic reagent towards the olefin.

TABLE 53-1.—RELATIVE RATES OF CHLORINE ADDITION TO OLEFINS, $R\cdot C_6H_4\cdot CH{:}CH\cdot R'$, IN ACETIC ACID.

R′ =	COPh	CO_2H	CHO	CN	NO_2	SO_2Cl
R = *p*-Me	800	103	—	—	—	—
H	61	4.9	1.8	0.022	0.020	0.001
p-Cl	23	2.5	—	—	—	—
p-NO_2	—	0.001	—	—	—	—

The addition of *bromine* to olefins in *water, methanol, formic acid, and aqueous lower alcohols and acids*[67,68] follows the same second-order kinetic law provided that the concentration of bromine is low (*e.g.*, *M*/1000).[61] As we shall see below, more complex kinetic forms of bromination can arise in other conditions; and they have been interpreted by Robertson and others through the assumption of a pre-equilibrium molecular association of olefin and bromine to give a complex, which various catalysts break up in various rate-controlling ways. In the absence of such a catalyst, the same pre-equilibrium must occur. But now the rate-controlling step can hardly be other than the ionisation of the complex (having regard to the many demonstrations that the last-combining anion plays no part in the rate control of addition):

$$A + Br_2 \rightleftharpoons A, Br_2 \qquad A, Br_2 \rightarrow ABr^+ + Br^-$$

[67] A. Berthoud and M. Mosset, *J. chim. phys.*, 1936, **33**, 272; P. D. Bartlett and D. S. Tarbell, *J. Am. Chem. Soc.*, 1936, **58**, 466; J. R. Atkinson and R. P. Bell, *J. Chem. Soc.*, **1963**, 3260.

[68] J. E. Dubois and F. Garnier, *Spectrochim. Acta*, 1967, **23**, A, 2279; *Chem. Comm.*, **1968**, 241. Cf. R. H. Boyd, R. W. Taft, A. P. Wolf, and D. R. Christman, *J. Am. Chem. Soc.*, 1960, **82**, 4729.

This view has been directly supported by Dubois,[68] who has adduced spectroscopic evidence of the pre-equilibrium and evidence based on the large kinetic solvent effect of rate-control by ionisation. Thus, the first step of the original two-step mechanism of bromine addition in highly polar solvents becomes elaborated into two steps. They may be illustrated as below, though the precise nature of the pre-equilibrium complex remains speculative:

$$R_2C{=}CR_2 + Br_2 \rightleftharpoons R_2C{-}\overset{+}{C}R_2 \text{ (complexed with } {}^{-}Br{-}Br)$$

$$R_2C{-}\overset{+}{C}R_2 \,(\cdots {}^{-}Br{-}Br) \xrightarrow{\text{slow}} R_2C{-}\overset{+}{C}R_2 \,(\text{bridged by } Br) + Br^-$$

Unlike additions of chlorine and bromine, additions of *iodine* commonly have perceptible reversibility. However, the forward reaction has been shown to follow the same second-order kinetics *in water*.[67]

In *solvent acetic acid*, but not in more polar solvents, the addition of *bromine*, in a certain range of concentrations (around $M/40$), proceeds[61] according to a third-order law:

$$\text{Rate} \propto [\text{olefin}][\text{Hal}_2]^2$$

Dilution, or an increase of temperature, or the addition of water to the solvent tends to break down the order from three towards two. The effects of constitutional changes in the olefin on the rate of this third-order bromine addition are strikingly similar to their effects on the rate of second-order chlorine addition in acetic acid: indeed the two rates bear to each other a nearly constant ratio. This suggests that the extra unit of order in the bromine reaction signalises some not very fundamental change in the mechanism of addition, though certainly another molecule of halogen has to be accommodated in the transition state of the rate-determining stage of the reaction.

In solution *in acetic acid*, the addition of *iodine* follows the same third-order form.[61] So also does the addition of *bromine chloride*, of *iodine chloride*, and of *iodine bromide*, the relative rates of addition, in this kinetic form, by the different halogens being as follows:[61]

Halogen	I_2	IBr	Br_2	ICl	BrCl
Rate	1	3000	10000	100000	4000000

The rate sequence $ICl > IBr > I_2$ is expected to be a general order of iodinating power, as $BrCl > Br_2$ is of brominating power, in accordance with the principle that X−Y will be a better electrophilic "X-ating" agent the more strongly Y attracts electrons. Thus the above rate relations suggest that addition starts with an electrophilic introduction of the more electropositive halogen.

As far as has been disclosed, these additions of halogens higher than chlorine, whether by second-order or third-order processes, show constitutional effects similar to those found in the additions of chlorine: electron-releasing substituents accelerate, and electron-attracting substituents retard. They also show similar positive salt effects, with the one difference that halide ions may exert a specific catalytic effect, as is mentioned below.

The circumstance that the third-order reaction is not given by chlorine, but requires a halogen containing at least one bromine or iodine atom, suggests that the reaction mechanism in the third-order process makes use of those higher co-ordination numbers which are reached more easily by heavier atoms. The usually accepted interpretation[69] is that the halogen molecule adds reversibly by an octet-expansion of one of its atoms, thereby forming a small stationary concentration of an adduct, which fails, of itself, to eject its second halogen atom as an anion, and only does so when another halogen molecule arrives to complete the addition (A = olefin):

$$A + X_2 \rightleftarrows A, X_2 \qquad A, X_2 + X_2 \rightarrow \text{products}$$

We may illustratively elaborate this formal scheme, as follows:

$$R_2C{=}CR_2 + Br_2 \rightleftharpoons R_2C{-}\overset{+}{C}R_2 \ (\text{with } {}^{-}Br{-}Br \text{ bridging})$$

$$R_2C{-}\overset{+}{C}R_2 \ (\text{with } {}^{-}Br{-}Br \text{ bridging}) + Br_2 \xrightarrow{\text{slow}} \underset{Br}{R_2C}{-}\underset{Br}{CR_2} + Br_2$$

The second step of this scheme may in fact consist of two steps.

For some olefinic substances, notably vinyl and allyl halides, the addition of ***bromine in acetic acid*** is ***catalysed by bromide ions and by chloride ions.*** This catalytic process,[70] discovered by Nozaki and Ogg, and further investigated by Swedlund and Robertson, has the following kinetic form:

[69] E. P. White and P. W. Robertson, *J. Chem. Soc.*, **1939**, 1509; Gwyn Williams, *Trans. Faraday Soc.*, 1941, **37**, 749.

[70] K. Nozaki and R. A. Ogg jr., *J. Am. Chem. Soc.*, 1942, **64**, 637, 704, 709; R. W. Swedlund and P. W. Robertson, *J. Chem. Soc.*, **1945**, 131; **1947**, 630.

$$\text{Rate} \propto [\text{olefin}][Br_2][\text{Hal}^-]$$

Over the range of compounds for which this catalysis is prominent, the catalysed rate varies with structure in a manner quite similar to that of the uncatalysed third-order rate of addition, as is illustrated by the following relative rates of bromine addition in acetic acid at 25°. Here, the olefin and the bromine are at concentration $M/80$, and the lithium bromide or chloride, when introduced, is at concentration $M/20$:

	$CH_2{:}CH{\cdot}CH_2Cl$	$CH_2{:}CH{\cdot}CH_2CN$	$CH_2{:}CHBr$
Br_2	1.6	0.23	0.001
Br_2+LiBr	4	1.2	0.005
Br_2+LiCl	10	2.4	0.007

The figures show that each reaction suffers the same drop in rate by a factor of 10^3 from the allyl to the vinyl halide. It would therefore appear that the catalysed reactions are still electrophilic processes, and therefore probably do not depend on pre-formed perhalide ions, $ClBr_2^-$ and Br_3^-, which are expected to behave in a nucleophilic manner. Accordingly it is supposed that these catalysed reactions are simply variants of the uncatalysed third-order process: they arise when a halide ion springs more quickly than does a halogen molecule to the task of completing the second stage of addition:

$$A + Br_2 \rightleftarrows A, Br_2 \qquad A, Br_2 + \text{Hal}^- \rightarrow \text{products}$$

We may illustrate the formal scheme, as follows:

$$R_2C{-}CR_2 + Br_2 \rightleftharpoons R_2C{-}\overset{+}{C}R_2 \text{ (with } {}^-Br{-}Br \text{ bridging)}$$

$$R_2C{-}\overset{+}{C}R_2 \text{ (with } {}^-Br{-}Br\text{)} + X^- \xrightarrow{\text{slow}} \underset{Br\quad X}{R_2C{-}CR_2} + Br^-$$

The second step of this scheme may consist of two steps.

Halogens are typically electrophilic reagents; yet it could be foreseen that, if an olefinic bond could be sufficiently polarised by an electron-demanding group, a *nucleophilic addition of halogen* Ad_N might be realised. Evidence of such a form of addition is most strikingly given by the additions of *chlorine* and *bromine* to *αβ-unsaturated aldehydes and ketones in acetic acid in the presence of a strong acid.*[71] In the absence of a strong acid, addition is slow; but it is powerfully catalysed by strong acids; and the catalysis is suppressed by water. The rate of catalysed addition varies with structure quite differently from that of any of the ordinary electrophilic additions, for example, the second-order addition of chlorine, as is illustrated by the following list of relative rates for bromine addition, as catalysed by sulphuric acid, and for uncatalysed chlorine addition, all reactants, including the sulphuric acid, being at concentrations $M/80$ in acetic acid:

	PhCH=HC·COPh	PhCH=HC·CO_2Et	PhCH=HC·CHO	MeCH=HC·CHO	PhCH=HC·NO_2
$Br_2+H_2SO_4$	32	<0.02	27	>1000	0.005
Cl_2	61	10	1.8	0.41	0.020

The figures indicate that basicity, as well as polarisation of the double bond, in the original unsaturated molecule, is necessary for high catalytic sensitivity. The interpretation offered is that the rate-determining step is a nucleophilic attack by the halogen molecule on the carbonium ion formed by the addition of a proton to the basic group in the original molecule, as illustrated by the following formulae:

$$\begin{matrix} RCH{:}CH{\cdot}CR'{:}O \\ + H^+ \end{matrix} \rightleftharpoons R\overset{+}{C}H{\cdot}CH{:}CR'{\cdot}OH \xrightarrow{Br_2} \begin{matrix} RCH{\cdot}CH{:}CH{\cdot}OH \\ {}^{+}| \\ Br{\cdot}Br \end{matrix} \rightarrow \text{products}$$

As acid catalysts for these halogen additions, hydrogen bromide and hydrogen chloride are much more efficient, relatively to other acids, than would be expected from the known order of acid strengths in acetic acid, namely,

$$HClO_4 > HBr > H_2SO_4 > HCl > HNO_3$$

Thus the relative rates of addition of bromine to cinnamaldehyde in acetic acid, with the reactants at concentration $M/80$, and the acid catalyst at concentration $M/320$, are as follows:

$HClO_4$	HBr	H_2SO_4	HCl	HNO_3
7.3	300	3.4	24	0.8

It is suggested that catalysis by the halogen acids arises, not only through the already described protonation of the cinnamaldehyde, but also on account of the formation of the complex anions, Br_3^-, $ClBr_2^-$,

[71] P. B. D. de la Mare and P. W. Robertson, *J. Chem. Soc.*, **1945**, 888; H. P. Rothbaum, I. Ting, and P. W. Robertson, *ibid.*, **1948**, 980.

$BrCl_2^-$, and Cl_3^-. These act as nucleophilic reagents for the purpose of introducing halogen into the carbonium ion, for which task they should be better suited than neutral halogen molecules.

Leaving these matters of kinetics and catalysis, let us now turn to the *products of uncatalysed halogen additions*, and first of all to the problem of the *orientation* of addition without reference to possible stereochemical specificity.

Unsymmetrical halogens are oriented in additions so that the more electropositive atom, for example, the iodine atom of iodine monochloride, is found mainly where the hydrogen atom would be in a normal addition of a hydrogen halide,[72] as is illustrated by the following examples:

$$CH_3\cdot CH{:}CH_2 \rightarrow CH_3\cdot CHCl\cdot CH_2I$$

$$C_6H_5\cdot CH{:}CH_2 \rightarrow C_6H_5\cdot CHCl\cdot CH_2I$$

$$CH_2{:}CH\cdot SO_3H \rightarrow CH_2Cl\cdot CHI\cdot SO_3H$$

$$CH_3\cdot CH{:}CH\cdot CO_2H \rightarrow CH_3\cdot CHCl\cdot CHI\cdot CO_2H$$

These orientations are not quantitative, but are sufficiently dominant to make it clear that, whatever detailed mechanism the reactions may adopt, the iodine is introduced as an electrophilic fragment I^+, and the chlorine as a nucleophilic fragment Cl^-.

According to the two-step mechanism of the formation of halogenohydrins by the action of halogens in water on olefinic substances, the halogen atom and the hydroxyl group might be expected to go respectively where the hydrogen and the halogen atoms go in the electrophilic additions of hydrogen halides. To some extent, this happens. Thus *iso*butylene, which gives nothing but *t*-butyl chloride on addition of hydrogen chloride, gives nothing but chloro-*t*-butyl alcohol on addition of the elements of hypochlorous acid by reaction with chlorine and water. But as the electropositivity of the groups at one end of the ethylenic bond becomes progressively reduced, the orientations of the two electrophilic additions diverge, until, at a certain stage, they become qualitatively opposite. This is illustrated by some data collected from various sources by de la Mare and Bolton[1,73] and reproduced in Table 53-2. Throughout the series illustrated, the orientation of hydrogen-halide addition remains that of terminal hydrogen uptake, but the orientation of the hypochlorous acid addition starts the series with complete terminal chlorine uptake and ends it with nearly complete non-terminal chlorine uptake.

[72] C. K. Ingold and H. G. Smith, *J. Chem. Soc.*, **1931**, 2742.

[73] With the warning (ref. 1, p. 87) that some of the older values may be inexact. This applies mainly to the HX additions.

TABLE 53-2.—PERCENTAGE TERMINAL UPTAKE OF HYDROGEN BY OLEFINS IN THE ELECTROPHILIC ADDITION OF HYDROGEN HALIDES, AND PERCENTAGE TERMINAL UPTAKE OF CHLORINE IN ADDITIONS OF HYPOCHLOROUS ACID BY REACTION OF OLEFINS WITH CHLORINE AND WATER.

$\frac{R}{R'}>$ in $\frac{R}{R'}>C:CH_2$	CH_3, CH_3	CH_3, H	$HOCH_2$, H	$ClCH_2$, H	Cl_2CH, H
Terminal H from HX	100	100	100	100	100
Terminal Cl of HOCl	100	91	73	30	2

Obviously one cannot explain this by an assumption about the different powers of the electrophilic reagents to *discriminate* between favoured and disfavoured directions of polarisation of the olefins. One must start from some fundamental difference between adding hydrogen and adding chlorine; and the effective difference is probably that the latter alone possesses unshared electrons. The halogen, when added, is the halogen of a β-halogeno-carbonium ion, and therefore must possess configuration-holding properties, as described in Section **33g**. According to the picture there presented, the β-chloro-carbonium ion, as formed, will have in its structure a long, loose, largely electrostatic bond. And this will give the chlorine atom a helpful start, which similarly situated hydrogen would not enjoy, towards the β-to-α shift which would allow reversal of orientation of the addition. A variant of this idea will be considered below; but let us keep it in this form for the moment, assuming, with de la Mare and Pritchard,[74] that (A) is the first-formed carbonium ion, and that although, within its lifetime, it can undergo some conversion to isomer (B), the latter is thermodynamically less stable:

$$\text{(A)}\quad R-\overset{+}{C}H-CH_2(\cdots Cl) \rightleftharpoons R-CH(Cl)-\overset{+}{C}H_2 \quad\text{(B)}$$

The small proportion of (B) at equilibrium (supposing that equilibrium should ever be attained) will not prevent a disproportionately large fraction of the addition from taking place by way of (B); for (B), as a primary carbonium ion, will be trapped by the solvent, or by any anion, at a much greater specific rate than will its secondary carbonium isomer (A).

[74] P. B. D. de la Mare and J. G. Pritchard, *J. Chem. Soc.*, **1954,** 3910, 3990.

This description is well confirmed by a critical study[75] by de la Mare, Naylor, and Llyn Williams of hypochlorous-acid additions to allyl halides, including an example of particular importance, allyl chloride containing the isotopic label ^{36}Cl. In all cases, they obtained three products: first, a 1,3-dihalopropan-2-ol, with no central halogen, corresponding therefore to the carbonium ion (A); secondly, 1,2-dihalopropan-3-ol, in which the central halogen has come from the addendum, so that it corresponds to the carbonium ion (B); and thirdly, another 1,2-dihalopropan-3-ol, in which the terminal halogen from the olefinic substrate has migrated to occupy the central position. This shows the reality of the process of halogen migration. Furthermore, the proportions of the products show that the main path of the reaction at no stage goes through a symmetrically bonded intermediate. In the case in which the substrate is allyl chloride with ^{36}Cl, and the addendum contains ordinary, unlabelled Cl, it is possible to *write* various intermediate structures in which the ^{36}Cl and the Cl are completely equivalent (apart from the isotopic label), the one on one terminal carbon and the other on the other. But the product compositions show that the newly added Cl atom is better situated for moving over to the central carbon atom than is the originally present ^{36}Cl atom. Thus, we cannot assume that the first product of chlorine addition is an open carbonium ion, for that would be symmetrical; and if it developed a largely electrostatic bond subsequently, it would do so equally in two directions, to give 50% of the carbonium ion which we call (A), and 50% of an isotopic modification, which we will call (A′):

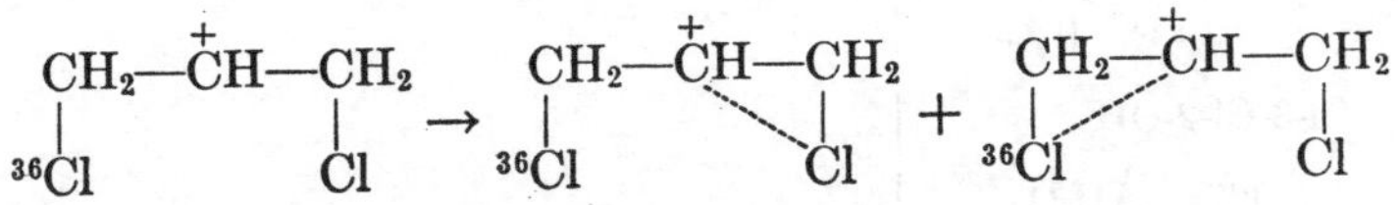

$$\underset{^{36}Cl}{CH_2}-\overset{+}{C}H-\underset{Cl}{CH_2} \rightarrow \underset{^{36}Cl}{CH_2}-\overset{+}{C}H\cdots\underset{Cl}{CH_2} \ (A) \quad + \quad \underset{^{36}Cl}{CH_2}\cdots\overset{+}{C}H-\underset{Cl}{CH_2} \ (A')$$

And then the proportions of Cl migration and of ^{36}Cl migration to the central carbon atom would be equal, which they are certainly not. Again, we cannot assume that carbonium ion (A), if first formed, establishes effective symmetry through an equilibrium of rapid bond changes,

$$A \rightleftharpoons A'$$

Nor can we assume that it passes into a symmetrical electrostatically bonded intermediate,

[75] P. B. D. de la Mare, P. G. Naylor, and D. L. H. Williams, *J. Chem. Soc.*, **1962**, 443; **1963**, 3429; C. A. Clarke and D. L. H. Williams, *ibid.*, **1966**, **B**, 1126.

$$\overset{+}{\text{CH}}\text{—}$$

$CH_2—\overset{+}{C}H—CH_2$ (bridged: ^{36}Cl and Cl)

which could then establish equilibrium relationships with (A) and (A′). The products show that the symmetry to which all these ideas lead is not present. All this is consistent with de la Mare and Pritchard's original picture, that the first-formed carbonium ion is dissymmetric (A), and that it has its desymmetrising electrostatic bond built into it *as it is formed.*

The proportions of products found by de la Mare, Naylor, and Llyn Williams for hypochlorous-acid addition to allyl ^{36}Cl-chloride in solvent water are set out below. There is 70% of end-to-middle chlorine migration. In the short lifetime of the first-formed carbonium ion (A), there is time for only 6% of it, instead of the equilibrium proportion of 50%, to undergo the bond change needed to produce the isomeric carbonium ion (A′). During this time, 94% of (A) becomes either trapped by the solvent, or isomerised to (B), which is even more quickly trapped by the solvent, probably so quickly that it cannot appreciably revert to (A):

Factors → (A) $CH_2—\overset{+}{C}H—CH_2$ (^{36}Cl, Cl) —66%→ (B) $CH_2—CH—\overset{+}{C}H_2$ (^{36}Cl, Cl) —H_2O→ 1-^{36}Cl-2-Cl-3-OH (66%)

(A) —28%, H_2O→ 1-^{36}Cl-3-Cl-2-OH (30%)

(A) —6%→ (A′) $CH_2—\overset{+}{C}H—CH_2$ (^{36}Cl, Cl) —2%, H_2O→ 1-^{36}Cl-3-Cl-2-OH

(A′) —4%→ (B′) $\overset{+}{C}H_2—CH—CH_2$ (^{36}Cl, Cl) —H_2O→ 1-Cl-2-^{36}Cl-3-OH (4%)

With higher halogens than chlorine, we would expect an increased capacity for liaison with the carbonium ionic centre, and hence an increased proportion of halogen migration, and an increased exchange of such liaison between the halogen of the substrate and the halogen of the added hypohalous acid. Clarke and Llyn Williams[75] have studied the aqueous addition to allyl bromide of the elements of hypobromous acid, through the agency of bromine in water acidified with perchloric acid. As an isotopic label, they employed ^{82}Br, placed alternatively in the allyl bromide and in the bromine, with identical results. They found 79% of bromine migration, and 30% of the bond change which permutes the functions of the two halogen atoms. The break-down is as follows:

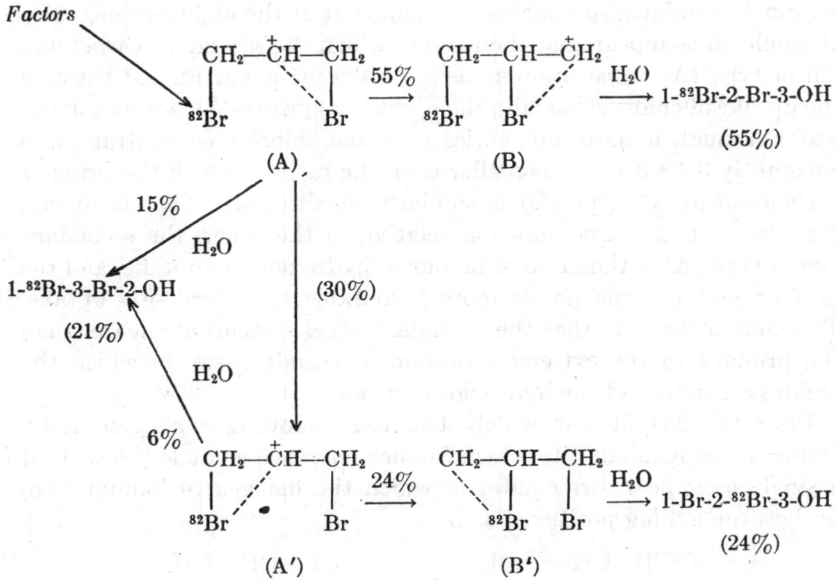

When hypochlorous acid is added to allyl bromide or allyl iodide the tendency of the electrostatic bond to pass over in the sense (A)→→(A′) is expected to be still more increased. De la Mare and Llyn Williams have examined these reactions.[75] We have now no longer the principle of the chemical identity of isotopes to allow us to calculate the whole break-down of what occurs, but we can calculate upper and lower limits. The shift (A)→(A′) of the electrostatic bond from chlorine to bromine goes to the extent of 28–60%, and from chlorine to iodine to the extent of 48–79%, before all carbonium ions are trapped by the solvent. Evidently, the rate of trapping is too great to allow the establishment of equilibria between the various carbonium ions.

De la Mare and Galandauer have examined[76] the compositions of the products of the reactions of addition of hypobromous acid and of bromine chloride to propylene, reactions which occur together when that hydrocarbon is treated with a solution of bromine in aqueous hydrochloric acid. As the concentration of hydrochloric acid is

[76] P. B. D. de la Mare and S. Galandauer, *J. Chem. Soc.*, 1958, 36.

raised from $1N$ to $3N$, the proportion in which bromochloropropane is formed rises from 30% to 59%. That is to say, the ratio, (total BrCl addition)/(total BrOH addition), rises from 0.43 to 1.44. The rise by a factor of 3.35 is about what one might expect. But the proportion in which the formed bromochloropropane has terminal bromine remains constant at 54%, over the three-fold range of chloride concentration; and the proportion in which the formed bromohydrin has terminal bromine also remains constant, but at the higher value, 79%. It would thus appear that the ratio in which the secondary carbonium ion of type (A) (with bromine as the halogen) is partitioned between the uptake of chloride ion, and the uptake of hydroxide ion from solvent water, though it naturally varies with the chloride concentration, is constantly 3.1 ± 0.1 times smaller than the ratio in which the primary carbonium ion of type (B) is similarly partitioned. That is to say, considering each carbonium ion relative to the other, the secondary one of type (A) is the more in favour of hydroxide-ion uptake, and the primary one of type (B) is more favourable to chloride-ion uptake. This may mean only that the secondary alkyl systems are nearer than the primary to the extreme situation in pseudo-bases, in which the halides are ionic and the hydroxides are not.

Prior to 1954, it was widely believed, following a suggestion by Roberts and Kimball,[81] to which further reference is made below, that a single cationic intermediate, in which the halogen in 'onium form bridges the adding positions, as in

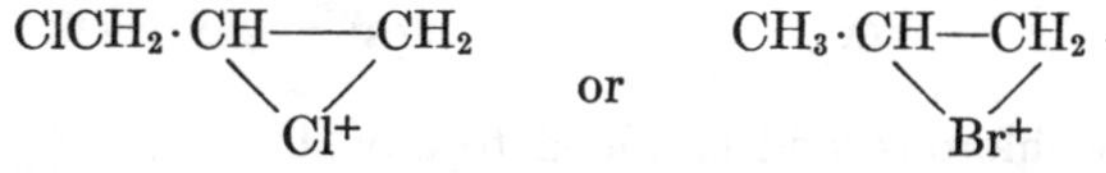

$$\underset{\diagdown\ Cl^+\ \diagup}{ClCH_2\cdot CH\text{——}CH_2} \quad \text{or} \quad \underset{\diagdown\ Br^+\ \diagup}{CH_3\cdot CH\text{—}CH_2}$$

would suffice for the interpretation of halogen additions. In advancing their theory of the two carbonium ions (A) and (B), de la Mare and Pritchard pointed out that the behaviour which one would have to ascribe to the Roberts-Kimball ions is out of analogy with the known behaviour of epoxides,[77] such as

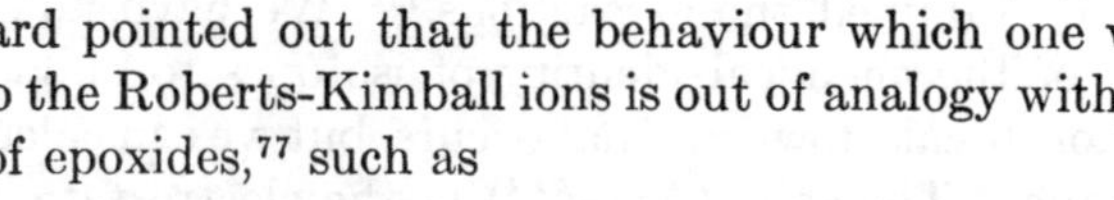

$$\underset{\diagdown\ O\ \diagup}{ClCH_2\cdot CH\text{—}CH_2} \quad \text{or} \quad \underset{\diagdown\ O\ \diagup}{CH_3\cdot CH\text{—}CH_2}$$

Ring-opening by nucleophilic attack occurs, predominantly or exclusively in epichlorohydrin and in propylene oxide, at the primary carbon atom, as expected for S_N2-type substitution.

We could consider modifying the Roberts-Kimball ions by making

[77] They are summarised in the first edition of this book (p. 341, *et seq.*), but the subject is one of those dropped in attempting to limit the size of the present edition.

them *synartetic*, so that some charge is borne by the carbon atoms, as in

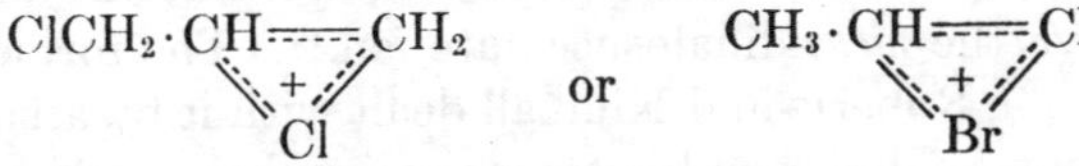

$$\mathrm{ClCH_2\cdot CH{=\!=\!=}CH_2}\ \text{(bridged by } \overset{+}{\mathrm{Cl}}\text{)} \qquad \text{or} \qquad \mathrm{CH_3\cdot CH{=\!=\!=}CH_2}\ \text{(bridged by } \overset{+}{\mathrm{Br}}\text{)}$$

We can then say, if we choose, that most of the charge carried by carbon is on the secondary carbon atom, although such charge as is carried by the primary carbon atom has a disproportionately large effect in producing reactivity. We can, indeed, make reasonable assumptions which reproduce all the results of the de la Mare-Pritchard interpretation. The only trouble with this theory is in the matter of principle, particularly urged by H. C. Brown,[78] that one should not accept an ion as synartetic, unless the evidence imperatively so characterises it. His point is sound. Overclaiming has been so rife and has caused such controversy that one avoids risking it.

The *stereochemistry* of the electrophilic additions of, or initiated by, halogens is dominated by a general, though not universal, prevalence of *trans*-additions. The addition of chlorine and bromine in hydroxylic solvents to maleic acid gives more than 80% of *rac.*-dihalosuccinic acid, and to fumaric acid more than 80% of the *meso*-isomer.[79] The addition of chlorine in the absence of solvent to *cis*- and *trans*-2-butene gives, nearly exclusively, *rac.*- and *meso*-2,3-dichlorobutanes, respectively.[80] These are all *trans*-additions. Such additions were interpreted by Roberts and Kimball[81] on the basis that configuration is held by the first-added halogen atom in an intermediate cation, which, as already mentioned, they regarded as a halogenium ion:

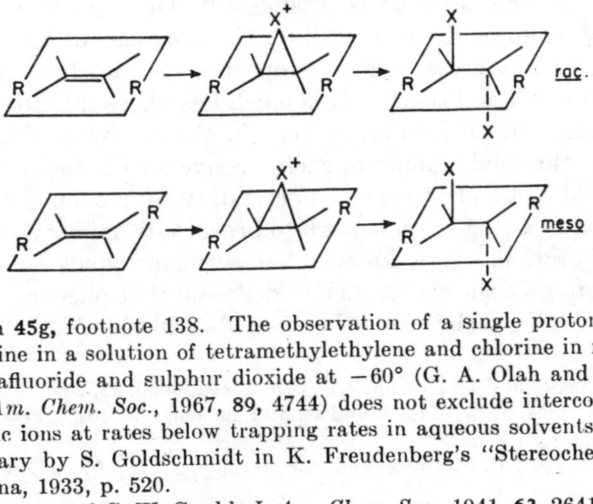

[78] Section **45g**, footnote 138. The observation of a single proton-magnetic-resonance line in a solution of tetramethylethylene and chlorine in mixed antimony pentafluoride and sulphur dioxide at −60° (G. A. Olah and J. M. Bollinger, *J. Am. Chem. Soc.*, 1967, **89**, 4744) does not exclude interconversion of disymmetric ions at rates below trapping rates in aqueous solvents.

[79] Summary by S. Goldschmidt in K. Freudenberg's "Stereochemie," Deuticke, Vienna, 1933, p. 520.

[80] H. J. Lucas and C. W. Gould, *J. Am. Chem. Soc.*, 1941, **63**, 2641.

[81] I. Roberts and G. E. Kimball, *J. Am. Chem. Soc.*, 1937, **59**, 947.

The maleate ion and the fumarate ion *both* add chlorine and bromine in water to give the *meso*-dihalosuccinate ion.[79] The former reaction is a *cis*-addition. Roberts and Kimball dealt with it by assuming that the configuration-holding bond becomes uncoupled, so that the structure can suffer internal rotation under the forces between the *cis*-carboxylate ion groups.[81] This is probably not the complete explanation, because Bell and Pring observed *cis*-addition of bromine in water to ethyl maleate.[66] Competition for the configuration-holding function between the first-added halogen and a carboxylate-ion or carbonyl group might play some part. These configuration-holding bonds cannot always be strong, or the additions would be more nearly sterospecific than they are.

A limited area of prevalent *cis*-additions of molecular halogens, or at least of chlorine, is that in which the carbonium ionic centre that could be formed by an initial attack of the halogen is conjugated with the continuing unsaturation of the polysaturated system. Possibly other conditions, for instance, concerning the kinetic form of the addition, and the ion-dissociating power of the solvent, have also to be satisfied; but we do not yet know enough to say what all the requirements are. Another troublesome point is that the olefin itself may undergo isomeric change during addition, for instance, by reversal of the first step of addition. Thus the addition of chlorine to *cis*-stilbene in ethylene dichloride is non-stereospecific, but gives a large proportion of *meso*-dichlorodibenzyl, the product of *cis*-addition.[82] But it is known that, during the addition of bromine, which is also not stereospecific, some *trans*-stilbene is produced.[83] On the other hand, the addition of chlorine to *trans*-stilbene in ethylene dichloride is not stereospecific, but gives a large proportion of *rac.*-dichlorodibenzyl, the product of *cis*-addition.[82] It is much less likely that *trans*-stilbene undergoes conversion into *cis*-stilbene in the course of this reaction, because the thermodynamics of such a conversion is against it.

We get rid of this last type of uncertainty by including the adding double bond in a ring small enough to prevent its having anything but a *cis*-configuration. It is known that acenaphthylene adds chlorine in benzene to give the *cis*-7,8-dichloride,[84] and that phenanthrene adds chlorine in acetic acid to give the *cis*-9,10-dichloride:[85]

[82] R. E. Buckles and D. F. Knaak, *J. Org. Chem.*, 1960, **25**, 20.

[83] R. E. Buckles, J. M. Badar, and R. J. Thurmeier, *J. Org. Chem.*, 1962, **27**, 4523.

[84] S. J. Cristol, F. R. Stermitz, and P. S. Ramey, *J. Am. Chem. Soc.*, 1956, **78**, 4939.

[85] P. B. D. de la Mare, N. V. Klassen, and R. Koenigsberger, *J. Chem. Soc.*, **1961**, 5285; P. B. D. de la Mare and R. Koenisberger, *ibid.*, **1964**, 5327.

$$\text{Acenaphthylene} \xrightarrow[C_6H_6]{Cl_2} \text{dichloride (Cl, Cl)} \qquad \text{Phenanthrene} \xrightarrow[\text{HOAc}]{Cl_2} \text{9,10-dichloride (Cl, Cl)}$$

In both these cases, as also in the example of *trans*-stilbene[82] (which is planar, as its *cis*-isomer is not—Sections **9b** and **11c**), any carbonium ionic charge, developed in a first step of chlorine addition, would be widely distributed in the aromatic systems. This would be expected to weaken, perhaps to destruction, any configuration-holding bond that might have been developed between the added halogen and the adjacent carbonium ionic centre.

The addition of chlorine to phenanthrene in acetic acid has been investigated by de la Mare and his collaborators in sufficient detail to provide an approximate idea of what is occurring.[85] The reaction was kinetically of second order, first in phenanthrene and first in chlorine. Experiments with radical inhibitors disclosed no sign of homolytic processes. The products contained 34% of the main substitution product, 9-chlorophenanthrene, 42% of the main addition product, the 9,10-dichloride, which consists wholly or almost wholly of the *cis*-isomer, and 14% of a 9-chloro-10-acetoxy-addition product, which was predominantly the *trans*-adduct, though the presence of some *cis*-isomer was established. On conducting the chlorination in the presence of added lithium chloride, the ratio of addition to substitution was not increased.

Let us assume that aromatic conjugation renders negligible the usual one-sided configuration-holding in a first-formed monochloro-cation. Such a cation must either add an anion to give a product of addition, or lose a proton to give the product of substitution. As the amount of addition was not increased at the expense of substitution by supplying chloride ion in added lithium chloride, it is inferred that free chloride ion cannot enter the structure, and that the second chlorine atom in the dichloride comes out of the adding chlorine molecule. This chlorine atom receives an electron from the other, but is never further away from the first-entering chlorine atom than is appropriate for counter-ions in an ion-pair. We know that ion-pairs tend to be somewhat tight in acetic acid, because of its low dielectric constant (about 6) (Section **32g**). One can then understand why the formed dichloride is a *cis*-adduct. The chloroacetoxy-adduct is in a different case, inasmuch as the two parts of its addendum must come from different places. Here the picture is that the ion-paired chloride ion, as long as it remains uncombined, is shielding its own side of the carbonium ion from reaction with the acetic acid solvent. However, the solvent can react freely on the other side. There is thus a competition between reaction of the carbonium ion with ion-paired chloride ion on one side, and its reaction with solvent acetic acid predominantly on the other side; and so one observes the concurrent formation of a *cis*-dichloride and a chloride-acetate which is mainly of *trans*-form.[86]

(53d) Additions of Non-acid Electrophiles, in Particular of Halogens, to Conjugated Polyolefinic Compounds.—The addition of halogens to conjugated polyenes was discussed in the already cited papers by Burton, de la Mare, Hughes, and the writer, particularly with reference to the orientation of addition, and its relation to equilibrium in, and the mobility of, anionotropic systems.

The theory of orientation in these conjugative Ad_E additions follows the same general lines as that of orientation in the addition of hydrogen halides to polyenes (Section **52b**). It is assumed that the first halogen atom to become combined to carbon enters as an electrophilic fragment, and is therefore taken up in the position in which the proton would be, in an addition of a hydrogen halide, that is, always at an end of the conjugated system, and, if the ends are different, at that end at which the strongest $+E$ effect can be developed. The experimental support for this rule is, as before, that no addition product which disagrees with it has been obtained.

As to the position assumed by the second halogen atom, there are obviously two possibilities in additions to a conjugated diene, three in additions to a triene, and so on; and the alternative products are anionotropic isomers. If the anionotropic system is not mobile under the conditions of the addition, the proportions of these isomers will be kinetically controlled: the chief product will be that which is formed faster in the final stage of addition. If the system is mobile under the experimental conditions, the proportions of the isomers will be thermodynamically controlled: the predominating product will be the more stable product.

The question of the relative stability of the alternative products can usually be decided by comparing their structures with respect to the recognised factors of stability, particularly conjugation and hyperconjugation. In this connexion, it is necessary to take account both of alkyl and of halogen hyperconjugation, as illustrated in the formulae

$$H_3C—C=C \quad \text{and} \quad C=C—C—Br$$

[86] This is the investigators' theory, except for the inessential detail that instead of regarding the interhalogen bond in the intermediate as ionic, they take it as a covalency requiring the expansion of a valency octet.

Halogen hyperconjugation could be neglected in the foregoing discussion (Section **52b**) of hydrogen halide additions, because it was always a balanced factor in the systems compared; however in the products of halogen additions, such balancing no longer obtains. Thus, of the two dibromides of butadiene,

$$BrCH_2\cdot CH{:}CH\cdot CH_2Br \quad \text{and} \quad BrCH_2\cdot CHBr\cdot CH{:}CH_2$$

the 1,4-dibromide is expected to be slightly the more stable, for the reason that it has two halogen-hyperconjugated systems, whereas the 1,2-isomer has only one system of this kind. In the example of 2-methylbutadiene (isoprene), either of the dibromides,

$$BrCH_2\cdot \overset{\overset{CH_3}{|}}{C}{:}CH\cdot CH_2Br \quad \text{and} \quad BrCH_2\cdot \overset{\overset{CH_3}{|}}{C}Br\cdot CH{:}CH_2$$

would be a structurally possible product, following uptake of the first bromine atom in the 1-position. Of these, the 1,4-dibromide will again be the more stable, but by a larger margin than before, because it has two halogen-hyperconjugated systems and one methyl-hyperconjugated system, whereas the 1,2-dibromide has only one halogen-hyperconjugated system. The dominating influence of ordinary conjugation enters in the example of hexa-1,3,5-triene. Three dibromides could conceivably arise, following a terminal initiation of reaction, namely, the 1,6-, 1,4-, and 1,2-dibromides,

$$\overset{\overset{Br}{|}}{C}H_2\cdot CH{:}CH\cdot CH{:}CH\cdot \overset{\overset{Br}{|}}{C}H_2, \quad \overset{\overset{Br}{|}}{C}H_2\cdot CH{:}CH\cdot \overset{\overset{Br}{|}}{C}H\cdot CH{:}CH_2$$

$$\overset{\overset{Br}{|}}{C}H_2\cdot \overset{\overset{Br}{|}}{C}H\cdot CH{:}CH\cdot CH{:}CH_2$$

But of these, only the 1,6- and 1,2-compounds preserve a butadienoid conjugation. They are therefore much more stable than the 1, isomeride. Similarly, much the more stable dibromide of 1-phen; butadiene, out of those which could arise following an initial attack the 4-position, is the 3,4-dibromide, which alone preserves the styre type of conjugation. And of the two possible dibromides of 1 diphenylbutadiene, the 1,2-dibromide will, for the same reason, much more stable than its 1,4-isomer.

We have to expect some additions in which a phase of kinetic contro of orientation can be seen to arise, before the products have had an adequate opportunity to come into equilibrium. The general rule is then expected to apply, that the thermodynamically less stable isomer will be formed in excess.

The kinetic control of orientation should be observed more easily among the additions of butadiene, or of its 1- or 1,4-alkyl derivatives, the halogen adducts of which are primary or secondary alkyl halides, than among the 2- or 2,3-alkyl derivatives of butadiene, whose less stable adducts are the easily ionising, and therefore easily isomerising, tertiary halides. One could scarcely expect to observe kinetic control in additions to 1- or 1,4-phenylated butadienes, wherein the phenyl substituent strongly promotes ionisation of halogen. Kinetic control should be more prevalent in the additions of chlorine, than in those of bromine. And it should be more easily observed in poorly ionising, than in the best ionising solvents.

Coming now to the observations, the addition of chlorine to buta-1,3-diene has been investigated by Muskat and Northrop,[87] whose work has been confirmed and extended by Pudovik.[88] The mixtures produced by addition contained about 40% of 1,4-dichloride and 60% of the 1,2-isomer. The dichlorides underwent no interconversion under the conditions of their formation; but on heating at 200°, or on treatment with zinc chloride at much lower temperatures, they became converted into an equilibrium mixture, which contained about 70% of the 1,4-dichloride and 30% of the 1,2-isomer. The proportions of the additively formed isomerides are evidently kinetically determined, and, as expected, the 1,4-dichloride is the principal product in equilibrium.

The addition of bromine to butadiene was first studied by Griner, who obtained the liquid 1,2 dibromide, and observed its further conversion to the crystalline 1,4-isomer.[89] Thiele later reported that in similar conditions he obtained the 1,4-dibromide directly.[90] Subsequently he agreed, as is noted in a paper by Strauss, that the 1,2-dibromide is also formed directly.[91] Farmer, Lawrence, and Thorpe re-examined the matter,[92] as Hatch, Gardner, and Gilbert did subsequently.[93] It was found that, in conditions which exclude isomerisation of the dibromide, they are formed in similar amounts, the exact proportions depending on the solvent. When conversion to equilibrium is allowed to occur, or is deliberately effected, the final mixture contains 80% of the 1,4-isomer. These results illustrate the sensitivity to solvent influences of the kinetically controlled product-ratio, the

[87] I. E. Muskat and H. E. Northrop, *J. Am. Chem. Soc.*, 1930, **52**, 4043.

[88] A. N. Pudovik, *J. Gen. Chem.* (U.S.S.R.), 1949, **19**, 1179.

[89] G. Griner, *Compt. rend.*, 1893, **116**, 723; **117**, 553.

[90] J. Thiele, *Ann.*, 1899, **308**, 333.

[91] F. Straus, *Ber.*, 1909, **42**, 2872.

[92] E. H. Farmer, C. D. Lawrence, and J. F. Thorpe, *J. Chem. Soc.*, 1928, 729.

[93] L. F. Hatch, P. D. Gardner, and R. E. Gilbert, *J. Am. Chem. Soc.*, 1959, **81**, 5943.

greater mobility of the bromides than of corresponding chlorides, the initial production of an excessive proportion of the thermodynamically less stable product, and the final production of excess of that isomer which would be expected to be the more stable.

The addition of iodine to butadiene gives the 1,4-adduct.[94] The involved anionotropic system is expected to be very labile, and the obtained product was probably the equilibrium product. The addition of iodine monochloride to butadiene in water gave a mixture of 80% of $ClCH_2 \cdot CH:CH \cdot CH_2I$ and 20% of $CH_2:CH \cdot CHCl \cdot CH_2I$, a mixture which was probably also the equilibrium product.[95]

The addition of bromine to terminally alkylated butadienes has been studied in the examples of 1,4-dimethylbutadiene,[96] *cyclo*pentadiene,[97] and *cyclo*hexa-1,3-diene.[97] In the last two examples, mixtures of 1,2- and 1,4-dibromides were obtained, which were much out of equilibrium. In all these cases the equilibrium products consisted predominantly of the 1,4-dibromides.

The addition of chlorine[98] and of bromine[99] to isoprene, and of bromine to 2,3-dimethylbutadiene,[96,100] has been examined. In each case, the main first addition product was the 1,4-dihalide. In the addition of chlorine to 2-methylbutadiene (isoprene), the 1,4-dichloride was accompanied by a smaller amount of the 1,2-dichloride and a still smaller of the 3,4-dichloride. The bromides would almost certainly have been equilibrium products. The chlorides might not have been.

A study of the addition of bromine to hexa-1,3,5-triene led to the isolation of 1,6- and 1,2-dibromides only.[101] These are expected to be much the most stable of the conceivable dibromides.

The addition of chlorine[102] and bromine [103] to 1-phenylbutadiene has been found to yield 3,4-dihalides exclusively. The addition of bro-

[94] A. A. Petrov, *Doklady Akad. Nauk S.S.S.R.*, 1950, **72**, 515.

[95] C. K. Ingold and H. G. Smith, *J. Chem. Soc.*, **1931**, 2752.

[96] P. Duden and R. Lemme, *Ber.*, 1902, **35**, 1335; E. H. Farmer, C. D. Lawrence, and W. D. Scott, *J. Chem. Soc.*, **1930**, 510.

[97] J. Thiele, *Ann.*, 1900, **314**, 296; E. H. Farmer and W. D. Scott, *J. Chem. Soc.*, 1929, 172.

[98] W. J. Jones and H. G. Williams, *J. Chem. Soc.*, **1934**, 829; A. J. Ultrée, *Rec. trav. chim.*, 1949, **68**, 125; E. G. E. Hawkins and M. D. Philpot, *J. Chem. Soc.*, **1962**, 3204.

[99] H. Staudinger, O. Muntwyler, and O. Kupfer, *Helv. Chim. Acta*, 1922, **5**, 756.

[100] I. Kondakow, *J. prakt. Chem.*, 1900, **62**, 166; A. D. Macallum and G. S. Whitby, *Trans. Roy. Soc. Can.*, 1928, **22**, 33.

[101] E. H. Farmer, B. D. Laroia, T. M. Switz, and J. F. Thorpe, *J. Chem. Soc.*, **1927**, 2937.

[102] I. E. Muskat and K. A. Huggins, *J. Am. Chem. Soc.*, 1929, **51**, 2496.

[103] F. Strauss, *Ber.*, 1909, **42**, 2866.

mine to 1,4-diphenylbutadiene has been found to give only the 1,2-dibromide.[103] All these dihalides are undoubtedly equilibrium products.

The chlorination of butadiene in solvent methyl alcohol has been shown to yield a mixture containing 70% of 1-chloro-2-methoxybut-3-ene and 30% of 1-chloro-4-methoxybut-2-ene. Preponderating quantities of 1,2-isomer are likewise obtained in solvent ethyl alcohol or in *n*-butyl alcohol, and also in bromination and iodination in the alcoholic solvents.[104] The alkoxy-group being immobile, the proportions of the products in all these reactions may be assumed to be kinetically determined. Similarly, Arbuzov and Zoroastrova found[105] that the main product of chlorination of butadiene in acetic acid containing sodium acetate was 1-chloro-2-acetoxybut-3-ene, whilst the secondary product was 1-chloro-4-acetoxybut-2-ene. Kadesch has shown[106] that the main product of addition of hypochlorous acid to butadiene in water is 1-chloro-2-hydroxybut-3-ene. The formation of these products is evidently kinetically controlled.

Muskat and Grimsby showed that the main product of addition of hypochlorous acid and of hypobromous acid to 1-phenylbutadiene in water is the phenyl-4-halo-3-hydroxybut-1-ene.[107] Among the probable adducts, this is thermodynamically much the most stable, though its formation (probably in less than the thermodynamic proportion) is doubtless controlled kinetically.[108]

Two questions of *stereochemistry* concerning 1,4-additions of halogens have been considered. The first relates to the carbon skeleton and applies only to additions to open-chain (or large-ring) dienes. It is the question of whether the singly-olefinic product will be *cis* or *trans*. As Mislow and Hellman showed,[109] the addition of chlorine to butadiene in carbon tetrachloride produces a 1,4-dichloride which is a dichloro-derivative of *trans*-but-2-ene. The chlorine atoms are so far apart in this structure that they must have come from different chlorine molecules. It follows that either the reaction is termolecular, or it

[104] A. A. Petrov, *J. Gen. Chem.* (U.S.S.R.), 1949, 19, 1046.

[105] B. A. Arbuzov and V. M. Zoroastrova, *Compt. rend. acad. sci., U.S.S.R.*, 1946, 53, 41.

[106] K. G. Kadesch, *J. Am. Chem. Soc.*, 1946, 68, 44.

[107] I. E. Muskat and L. B. Grimsby, *J. Am. Chem. Soc.*, 1930, 52, 1574.

[108] O. Grummitt and R. V. Vance, *J. Am. Chem. Soc.*, 1950, 72, 2669, confirmed Muskat and Grimsby's finding for hypochlorous acid addition, and added the conclusion that a minor amount of another isomer, 1-phenyl-1-hydroxy-2-chlorobut-3-ene, is formed. However, this conclusion was based, not on direct measurement, but on a further reaction with alkali, that might have pursued a more complicated course than was supposed.

[109] K. Mislow and H. M. Hellman, *J. Am. Chem. Soc.*, 1951, 73, 244.

goes in two steps. A kinetic study that could be correlated with this stereochemical result is not available.

The other question is that of whether the two adding halogen atoms enter on the same side of the plane of conjugation (*cis*-addition) or on opposite sides (*trans*-addition). Young and his collaborators have made a careful study of the addition of chlorine to *cyclo*pentadiene in light petroleum and in chloroform.[110] The main products were of 1,4-addition, and their main component was one of *cis*-1,4-addition, though it was accompanied by the *trans*-1,4-isomer. It was also accompanied by some 1,2-dichloride, and this was the *trans*-1,2-isomer. The principal stereoisomers obtained in 1,4- and 1,2-addition, the *cis*-1,4- and *trans*-1,2-, are required by the termolecular mechanism, and can be accommodated by the two-step mechanism. The fact that 1,4-addition is not stereospecific points to the presence of the two-step mechanism, but again the check of kinetics is not available.

The chlorination of naphthalene, like that of phenanthrene (Section **53c**), involves concurrent substitution and addition. The main substitution product is 1-chloronaphthalene. The addition products are said to include dichlorides, but these substances are not well characterised. The well-characterised products of addition are 1,2,3,4-tetrachlorides. Six stereoisomers are possible, five of them have been described, and the configurations of four of them have been determined.[111,112] The particular stereoisomers which arise by addition depend on the conditions, in particular, on whether the conditions are conducive to heterolytic or homolytic addition. The heterolytic reaction in acetic acid in the dark has been studied by de la Mare and Michael Johnson and their coworkers.[112] Two-thirds of the reaction leads to substitution and one-third to addition, and of the total products of addition, two-thirds are tetrachlorides, and one-third consists of acetoxypolychlorides, mainly an acetoxytrichloride. Of the tetrachlorides, two-thirds consists of the α-isomer, that is, the (1,2/3,4)- or *cis-trans-cis*-tetrachloride, and one-third of the δ-isomer, shown to be the (1,2,4/3)- or *cis-trans-trans*-tetrachloride. The dominant acetoxytrichloride was shown to be the 4-acetoxy-(1,2,4/3)-1,2,3-trichloride. These structures are formulated below. When the chlorination was conducted in the presence of lithium chloride, the

[110] W. G. Young, H. K. Hall, and S. Winstein, *J. Am. Chem. Soc.*, 1956, **84**, 109.

[111] M. A. Lasheen, *Acta Cryst.*, 1952, **5**, 593.

[112] P. B. D. de la Mare, R. Koenigsberger, J. S. Lomas, V. Sanchez del Olmo, and A. Sexton, *Rec. trav. chim.*, 1965, **84**, 109; P. B. D. de la Mare, M. D. Johnson, J. S. Lomas, and V. Sanchez del Olmo, *Chem. Comm.*, 1965, 483; *J. Chem. Soc.*, **1966**, 827.

proportion of the α-tetrachloride was reduced and that of the δ-isomer increased: it was even possible then to make the latter isomer the preponderating one.

The interpretation offered is that the α-tetrachloride is formed by a duplication of the process operating in the addition of chlorine to phenanthrene. The first chlorine molecule starts adding at 1 (end of a butadiene system), and, because conjugation withdraws the formed carbonium ionic charge so largely from 2, the first-added chlorine atom does not form an electrostatic bond there, and the second chlorine does not dissociate, but does combine there, in the *cis*-position. The second chlorine molecule starts adding at 3 (end of a styrene system), and similarly ends at 4. But because the first-formed carbonium ionic charge is withdrawn less extensively from 4, some dissociation of chloride ion does occur; and therefore the δ-tetrachloride is formed by *trans*-uptake of chloride in a substantial proportion, which can be increased by added chloride ion; and the acetoxytrichloride is formed by a similar *trans*-uptake of an acetate ion from the acetic acid solvent.

(53e) Acid-Initiated Polymerisation of Olefinic Compounds by Self-Addition.—It has been known since the last century[113] that some olefinic substances could be converted to materials of high molecular weight by very small amounts of strong proton acids, and also by Friedel-Crafts catalysts. These substances are all acids in the nomenclature of G. N. Lewis; that is, they are all strong electrophiles. The olefinic substances that can be thus polymerised most readily include alkyl vinyl ethers, *iso*butylene, styrene, α-methylstyrene, butadiene, and, generally, those alkenes in which the substituents would render electrons freely available at the other end of the double bond. Obviously, the nature of these processes could not be understood before Staudinger had made clear in 1920 the general character of polymerisation as a chain process.[114] The specific nature of this particular form of polymerisation could not be appreciated for some time after that, *viz.*, until the general theory of heterolytic reactions

[113] For example, in 1839, Deville polymerised "spirits of turpentine" to "colophony" with sulphuric acid (*Ann. chim.*, 1839, **75**, 37).

[114] H. Staudinger, *Ber.*, 1920, **53**, 1073.

in organic chemistry, which began its rapid move forward in 1926, had made some progress.

By about 1940 it was becoming clear that, should the electron-rich carbon atom here actually combine with the electrophilic catalyst, the carbon atom at the substituted end of the double bond would become a carbonium ion. That is to say, it would itself become a strong electrophile, possibly capable of combining with the electron-rich carbon atom of a second olefinic molecule, and so effecting the first growth-step in what might become a continuing polymerisation. This process, as catalysed by proton acids, may be illustrated as follows:

$$H_2SO_4 + CH_2{:}CMe_2 \rightarrow CH_3\cdot CMe_2^+\}HSO_4^-$$
$$\rightarrow CH_3\cdot CMe_2\cdot CH_2\cdot CMe_2^+\}HSO_4^-$$
$$\rightarrow CH_3\cdot CMe_2\cdot CH_2\cdot CMe_2\cdot CH_2\cdot CMe_2^+\}HSO_4^- \rightarrow \ldots$$

The expression for polymerisation catalysed by Friedel-Crafts reagents used to be written in the similarly simple way illustrated below, although, as we shall see, this expression has had to be modified.

$$BF_3 + CH_2{:}CMe_2 \rightarrow \overset{-}{B}F_3\cdot CH_2\cdot \overset{+}{C}Me_2 \rightarrow \overset{-}{B}F_3\cdot CH_2\cdot CMe_2\cdot CH_2\cdot \overset{+}{C}Me_2$$
$$\rightarrow \overset{-}{B}F_3\cdot CH_2\cdot CMe_2\cdot CH_2\cdot CMe_2\cdot CH_2\cdot \overset{+}{C}Me_2 \rightarrow \ldots$$

The proton acid catalysts include most very strong inorganic acids, such as $HClO_4$ and H_2SO_4, down to much less strong ones, such as H_3PO_4, and also the stronger organic acids down at least to dichloroacetic acid. One needs larger quantities of the weaker of these acids, and they will even then work only with the most easily polymerising olefins. All the stronger Friedel-Crafts catalysts are effective: BF_3, $AlCl_3$, $AlBr_3$, $TiCl_4$, $TiBr_4$, $SbCl_5$, $FeCl_3$, $SnCl_4$, and so on.

The polymerisations are usually very fast. Thus the polymerisation of *iso*butylene under catalysis by BF_3 or $AlCl_3$ at $-100°$ goes instantly, that is, as fast as the reagents can be mixed, to a degree of polymerisation (average number of monomer units in the polymer) of the order of a million. It was discovered by Evans and Polanyi[115] in 1946–47 that such Friedel-Crafts-catalysed polymerisations do not go at all, except in the presence of a "co-catalyst," which is frequently a proton acid, and in the commonest case is, or arises from, adventitious water. Thus, nothing happens when *iso*butylene and boron trifluoride are mixed, if the materials and containers are thoroughly dried. This

[115] A. G. Evans, D. Holden, P. Plesch, M. Polanyi, H. A. Skinner, and M. A. Weinberger, *Nature*, 1946, **157**, 102; A. G. Evans, G. W. Meadows, and M. Polanyi, *ibid.*, 1946, **158**, 94; A. G. Evans and M. Polanyi, *J. Chem. Soc.*, **1947**, 252; A. G. Evans and G. W. Meadows, *Trans. Faraday Soc.*, 1950, **46**, 327.

finding has been contested, but there is no doubt that it is correct. Evans and Polanyi ascribed the catalysis to the extremely strong proton acids that the catalyst and co-catalyst will together produce, and reformulated the Friedel-Crafts polymerisations, as in the following illustration:

$$H_2O + BF_3 + CH_2{:}CMe_2 \rightarrow CH_3{\cdot}CMe_2^+\}BF_3OH^-$$
$$\rightarrow CH_3{\cdot}CMe_2{\cdot}CH_2{\cdot}CMe_2^+\}BF_3OH^-$$
$$\rightarrow CH_3{\cdot}CMe_2{\cdot}CH_2{\cdot}CMe_2{\cdot}CH_2{\cdot}CMe_2^+\}BF_3OH^- \rightarrow \ldots$$

The possibility of a third type of catalysis follows from these explanations. Each step of propagation depends on a carbonium-ion electrophile, and so one should be able to organise a similar step of initiation, that is, to use a pre-formed carbonium ion as catalyst. This was done first by Eley and Richards,[116] who used triphenylmethyl chloride in solvent *m*-cresol, in which it forms the triphenylmethylium ion, in order to polymerise vinyl 2-ethylhexyl ether. It has been done since with a variety of carbonium ions, including the *t*-butylium, acetylium, and benzoylium ions, introduced as perchlorate,[117] and the acetylium ion introduced as tetrafluoroborate.[118] A typical formulation is the following:

$$Ph_3\overset{+}{C} + CH_2{:}CHOR \rightarrow Ph_3C{\cdot}CH_2{\cdot}CHOR^+$$
$$\rightarrow Ph_3C{\cdot}CH_2{\cdot}CH(OR){\cdot}CH_2{\cdot}CHOR^+$$
$$\rightarrow Ph_3C{\cdot}CH_2{\cdot}CH(OR){\cdot}CH_2{\cdot}CH(OR){\cdot}CH_2{\cdot}CHOR^+ \rightarrow \ldots$$

An alkyl chloride will act as a co-catalyst to a Friedel-Crafts catalyst, presumably on account of pre-conversions, such as

$$RCl + AlCl_3 \rightarrow R^+\{AlCl_4^-$$

to carbonium ions. Colclough and Dainton showed this for the polymerisation of styrene by stannic chloride co-catalysed by various rigorously dried alkyl chlorides.[119] *t*-Butyl chloride as co-catalyst gave the highest rate, *iso*propyl chloride a considerably lower one, and ethyl chloride lower still. Again, Kennedy and Thomas showed that *iso*butylene is polymerised at low temperatures by aluminium chloride dissolved in ethyl chloride, and even in methyl chloride, again with rigorous exclusion of water; and that the use of ^{14}C-methyl chloride as solvent and co-catalyst led to a polymer containing ^{14}C-radioactivity.[120]

[116] D. D. Eley and A. W. Richards, *Trans. Faraday Soc.*, 1949, **45**, 425.
[117] W. R. Longworth and P. H. Plesch, *Proc. Chem. Soc.*, **1958**, 117.
[118] G. A. Olah, H. W. Quinn, and S. J. Kuhn, *J. Am. Chem. Soc.*, 1960, **82**, 426.
[119] R. O. Colclough and F. S. Dainton, *Trans. Faraday Soc.*, 1958, **54**, 886.
[120] J. P. Kennedy and R. M. Thomas, *J. Polymer Sci.*, 1960, **45**, 227, 229; **46**, 233, 481.

Confirmation that propagation proceeds through a series of carbonium ionic intermediates is evident in Kennedy and Thomas's examination of the proton-magnetic-resonance spectrum of the polymer of *iso*propylethylene.[121] They found that the repeating unit of the structure was not 1,2-linked with one secondary and two tertiary carbon atoms:

$$CH_2{:}CH{\cdot}CH(CH_3)_2 \rightarrow CH_2{\cdot}\overset{+}{C}H{\cdot}CH(CH_3)_2 \rightarrow CH_2{\cdot}CH{\cdot}CH(CH_3)_2 \text{ (bearing } CH_2{\cdot}\overset{+}{C}H{\cdot}CH(CH_3)_2)$$

It was 1,3-linked with two secondary and no tertiary carbon atoms. This means that each new secondary carbonium ionic group, formed as shown above by a newly added monomer molecule, before growth continues, suffers the hydride shift that might be expected in such a carbonium ion, to give a tertiary carbonium ion, through which, in the same two steps of monomer addition and hydride shift, growth does continue:

$$CH_2{\cdot}\overset{+}{C}H{\cdot}CH(CH_3)_2 \rightarrow CH_2{\cdot}CH_2{-}\overset{+}{C}(CH_3)_2 \rightarrow CH_2{\cdot}CH_2{\cdot}C(CH_3)_2 \text{ (bearing } CH_2{\cdot}CH_2{\cdot}\overset{+}{C}(CH_3)_2)$$

Polymer growth ends by proton loss to give a double bond at what was the growing end of the polymer chain. This was established for necessarily fairly low polymers of *iso*butylene by Dainton and Sutherland's examination of their infra-red specta.[122] They found, not only the end-group $(CH_3)_3C$—, but also the end group $\cdot CH_2{\cdot}C(CH_3){:}CH_2$.

If we are dealing with polymerisation initiated by an acidic catalyst or catalyst-co-catalyst complex in the absence of a basic solvent, the most obvious base for reception of the eliminated proton is the counter-anion, which the growing polymer derived from the catalysing acid, and thereafter carried in the ion-pair at its growing point. To distinguish it from another possibility, this is called "chain termination." The other possibility is that the proton is received by a monomer molecule, so to start the growth of a new polymer molecule. This is described as "chain transfer." It is characteristic of both modes of growth-ending that the catalysing acid, apart from its proton, never gets incorporated into the polymer molecule, and therefore that one molecule of catalyst can make many molecules of polymer. This is the observation.[122,123] It is also characteristic that the acidic proton does

[121] J. P. Kennedy and R. M. Thomas, *Makromol. Chem.*, 1962, **53**, 28.
[122] F. S. Dainton and G. B. B. M. Sutherland, *J. Polymer Sci.*, 1949, **4**, 37.
[123] R. O. Colclough, *J. Polymer Sci.*, 1952, **8**, 467.

get incorporated into the polymer. It has been shown that fairly low polymers of *iso*butylene, obtained with the aid of the BF_3—D_2O complex, contain deuterium.[122]

High polymers are formed in acid-initiated polymerisation, because growth-stopping processes are rare events in the life of a growing polymer, relative to growth extension processes. The former are rare; but not for the reason for which they are in radical polymerisations, in which two intermediate radicals, present in very low concentration, have to be brought together. Chain termination is internal to the growing ion-pair, and is slow, because its activation energy is greater than that of the growth process. The ratio of the rates of growth-continuing and growth-stopping processes, which is equal to the degree of polymerisation, will therefore fall with rise of temperature. This is, indeed, one of the striking characteristics of acid-initiated polymerisations. Thus the degree of polymerisation of *iso*butylene with a boron trifluoride catalyst fell from 5,000,000 to 50,000 when the temperature was raised from $-100°$ to $0°$.[124] By plotting the logarithm of the degree of polymerisation against the reciprocal of the absolute temperature, it can be computed that the activation energy of growth-stopping exceeds that of growth-continuation by 4.6 kcal./mole.[125] Of course, such a plot presumes a single stopping process: if the stopping by chain transfer of continued chain extension were comparable with its stopping by the termination of polymerisation, we should not expect to obtain a good Arrhenius plot from the degree of polymerisation. More detailed kinetic studies in a variety of cases show that activation energies of chain propagation are generally low.[126]

If the rate R_i of initiation by an acid HA of polymerisation of a monomer M is given by

$$R_i = k_i[\mathrm{HA}][\mathrm{M}]$$

and the rate of chain growth in the ion-pair $\mathrm{HM}_r^+\}\mathrm{A}^-$ is given by

$$R_p = k_p[\mathrm{HM}_r^+\}\mathrm{A}^-][\mathrm{M}]$$

the rate of chain termination by

$$R_t = k_t[\mathrm{HM}_r^+\}\mathrm{A}^-]$$

and the rate of chain transfer by

[124] R. M. Thomas, W. J. Sparks, P. K. Frolich, M. Otto, and M. Mueller-Conradi, *J. Am. Chem. Soc.*, 1940, **62,** 276.

[125] P. J. Flory, "Principles of Polymer Chemistry," Cornell Univ. Press, Ithaca, New York, 1953, p. 218.

[126] P. H. Plesch, *J. Chem. Soc.*, 1950, 543.

$$R_{tr} = k_{tr}[\mathrm{HM}_r{}^+\}\mathrm{A}^-][\mathrm{M}]$$

then, assuming that $k_i \ll k_p$, a stationary-state treatment gives the results that the rate R of polymerisation is

$$R = \frac{k_i k_p}{k_t}[\mathrm{HA}][\mathrm{M}]^2$$

and the degree of polymerisation $\overline{DP}$ is

$$\overline{DP} = \frac{k_p[\mathrm{M}]}{k_t + k_{tr}[\mathrm{M}]}$$

One sees that according as the main way of ending the continued growth of a chain is by termination or transfer, the degree of polymerisation is proportional to or independent of the concentration of monomer.

One of the first illustrations of these equations, which represent the simplest stationary-state conditions, was given in 1949 by Pepper on the polymerisation of styrene under catalysis by stannic chloride. In this case chain transfer was the more important means of arresting continued chain growth.[127] Pepper has shown in various examples that, when the dielectric constant of the solvent is increased, both the rate of polymerisation and the degree of polymerisation are increased. This should be expected, because initiation involves charge separation, and termination involves charge destruction. Other examples of the kinetics formulated above, notably the polymerisation of vinyl 2-ethylhexyl ether by stannic chloride catalyst, were described by Eley and Richards in the same period.[127]

As Pepper pointed out in 1954,[128] many variations in these kinetic phenomena, variations which must represent changes in, or complications added to, the simple kinetic conditions assumed above, are apparent in particular cases. Hayes and Pepper have elucidated one group of such variations.[128] It relates to the polymerisation of styrene catalysed by strong but stable molecular acids, such as sulphuric acid and perchloric acid. Initiated by sulphuric acid, this polymerisation in its early stages is very fast; but it dies away rapidly, and ceases before all the monomer is consumed, to give a well-defined "yield" of polymer, related to the initial acid concentration. When the initiation

[127] D. C. Pepper, *Trans. Faraday Soc.*, 1949, **45**, 397, 404; D. D. Eley and A. W. Richards, *Trans. Faraday Soc.*, 1949, **45**, 436.

[128] D. C. Pepper, *Quart. Revs. Chem. Soc.*, 1954, **8**, 88; M. J. Hayes and D. C. Pepper, *Proc. Chem. Soc.*, **1958**, 228; *Proc. Roy. Soc.* (London), 1961, **A, 263**, 63; D. C. Pepper, "Friedel-Crafts and Related Reactions," Editor G. A. Olah, Interscience, New York, 1964, Vol. 2, Chap. 30.

is by perchloric acid, the phenomenon of the limited yield is not shown; instead the rate of monomer consumption is of simple first-order form throughout the whole conversion. Both results can be explained by the same assumption, namely, that the stationary-state condition is now reversed, *i.e.*, that the specific rate of propagation, instead of being much greater, is now much smaller than the specific rate of initiation, $k_i \gg k_p$. In these conditions, there is formed immediately a concentration of growing carbonium ionic centres equal to the initial concentration, $[HA]_0$, of the catalysing acid, and the rate R, the fractional yield Y of polymer, and the degree of polymerisation $\overline{\overline{DP}}$, are given by the expressions

$$R = k_p[\mathrm{HA}]_0[\mathrm{M}] \exp(-k_t \cdot t)$$

$$\ln \frac{1}{1-Y} = \frac{k_p}{k_t[\mathrm{HA}]_0}$$

$$\frac{1}{\overline{\overline{DP}}} = \frac{k_{tr}}{k_p} + \frac{k_t}{k_p} \cdot \frac{\ln[\mathrm{M}]_0 - \ln[\mathrm{M}]}{[\mathrm{M}]_0 - [\mathrm{M}]}$$

The difference between the two acids reflects their difference of acidity, or, in other words, the different basicities of their anions. In initiation by sulphuric acid, k_t is large, and hence the die-away factor, exp $(-k_t \cdot t)$, in the rate equation is powerfully retarding, whilst the fractional yield Y falls much below unity. In initiation by perchloric acid, k_t is small, presumably because the perchlorate ion has but little proton affinity; wherefore the die-away factor is unity, and the rate equation is of first order, whilst the fractional yield is unity, and the degree of polymerisation is limited by chain-transfer only.

(54) NUCLEOPHILIC ADDITIONS TO CARBONYL AND OLEFINIC COMPOUNDS

Nucleophilic addenda are taken up typically by the carbonyl group, and by olefinic bonds so polarised by conjugation with carbonyl, or with other groups of $-M$ type, such as cyano- or nitro-groups, as to give the addenda access to an ethenoid carbon kernel:

$$\mathrm{X} \curvearrowright \mathrm{C{=}O} \qquad \mathrm{X} \curvearrowright \mathrm{C{=}C{-}C{=}O}$$

Such additions are for brevity called *nucleophilic additions*, symbolised $\mathrm{Ad_N}$. Grignard reactions, in which X is a carbanion R^- derived from the Grignard reagent RMgHal, are nucleophilic additions:

$$\mathrm{R^-} + \mathrm{C{=}O} \rightarrow \mathrm{R{-}C{-}O^-} \xrightarrow{\mathrm{H_2O}} \mathrm{R{-}C{-}OH}$$

A most important class of nucleophilic addenda are certain weak acids, such as hydrogen cyanide or ammonium ion, including pseudo-acids, such as acetone or ethyl malonate. They add in the parts H—X across the carbonyl group to give CX—OH, or across a double bond conjugated with carbonyl to give CX—CH—C=O; but it is the conjugate base of HX, and not the proton, which now leads the attack, and gives to the addendum its nucleophilic character. These additions, whether to a simple carbonyl group, or to a conjugated system involving carbonyl, are in general easily reversible. Therefore we cannot separate the study of these additions from that of eliminations which produce carbonyl or conjugated olefin-carbonyl systems: the two matters must be considered together. A most important non-acidic nucleophilic addendum is hydrogen, as provided by metals dissolving in hydroxylic media, by reducing metallic cations in such media, by complex anions able to liberate hydride ion, and in a few other ways, but *not* by molecular hydrogen with surface catalysis, In ordinary conditions nucleophilic hydrogen addition is not appreciably reversible. Very strong bases, such as amide ions or alkylide ions, will often add, not only to olefinic bonds which are conjugated with strongly electronegative unsaturated groups such as carbonyl, cyano-, or nitro-groups, but also, less easily, to olefinic bonds which are not so conjugated. A frequent result is then addition-polymerisation.

(54a) Reversible Additions of Bases or Weak Acids to Simple Carbonyl Compounds.—In 1903 Lapworth[129] described the marked effect of basic catalysts on the *formation of cyanohydrins* from carbonyl compounds and hydrocyanic acid. He examined, among other cases, the reaction of "camphor-quinone" (1,2-diketocamphane), using the discharge of colour which accompanied its conversion to its cyanohydrin, in order to follow the reaction. He concluded that the rate-determining step in cyanohydrin formation is the uptake of cyanide ion by the carbonyl group to give the anion of the cyanohydrin. He knew that cyanohydrin formation is reversible, and wrote the mechanism accordingly, thus illustrating nucleophilic addition Ad_N:

$$CN^- + R_2CO \underset{\text{slow}}{\overset{\text{slow}}{\rightleftharpoons}} R_2C\begin{matrix} \diagup CN \\ \diagdown O^- \end{matrix}$$

$$R_2C(CN)\cdot O^- + H^+ \underset{\text{fast}}{\overset{\text{fast}}{\rightleftharpoons}} R_2C(CN)\cdot OH$$

The implied kinetic equation:

[129] A. Lapworth, *J. Chem. Soc.*, 1903, **83**, 995; 1904, **85**, 1206.

$$\text{Rate} \propto [\text{carbonyl}][\text{CN}^-]$$

was not quantitatively verified owing to the great sensitivity of the rate to small, not accurately known, amounts of cyanide ion; though a demonstration of kinetic form was given later[130] for the addition of hydrogen cyanide to conjugated olefinic ketones, as we shall note below. But before this, a significant kinetic investigation was conducted on the benzoin reaction, which in principle includes both cyanohydrin formation and the aldol reaction.

The *benzoin reaction* consists in the union of two molecules of benzaldehyde to give benzoin under the specific catalytic influence of cyanide ions. In his paper of 1903, Lapworth discussed this reaction, suggesting that the first step was the production of benzaldehyde cyanohydrin, which then acted as an aldol adduct towards a second molecule of benzaldehyde, and thus gave the unstable cyanohydrin of benzoin, which at once broke down into benzoin and hydrogen cyanide. In 1904 Bredig and Stern examined the kinetics of the process,[131] and established the rate law

$$\text{Rate} \propto [\text{benzaldehyde}]^2[\text{CN}^-]$$

They showed that non-ionised cyanides such as mercuric cyanide had no effect on the rate, and that hydroxide ions, as such, had no effect. Lapworth's mechanism, adapted to this kinetic law, would run as follows:[132]

$$\bar{\text{C}}\text{N} + \text{Ph}\cdot\text{CH}:\text{O} \rightleftarrows \text{Ph}\cdot\text{CH(CN)}\cdot\text{O}^-$$

$$\text{Ph}\cdot\text{CH(CN)}\cdot\text{O}^- \rightleftarrows \text{Ph}\cdot\bar{\text{C}}\text{(CN)}\cdot\text{OH}$$

$$\text{Ph}\cdot\bar{\text{C}}\text{(CN)}\cdot\text{OH} + \text{Ph}\cdot\text{CH}:\text{O} \rightleftarrows \text{Ph}\cdot\text{CH}(\text{O}^-)\cdot\text{CPh}(\text{OH})(\text{CN})$$

$$\text{Ph}\cdot\text{CH}(\text{O}^-)\cdot\text{CPh}(\text{OH})(\text{CN}) \rightleftarrows \text{Ph}\cdot\text{CH}(\text{OH})\cdot\text{CPh}:\text{O} + \text{CN}^-$$

The first equation represents the slow step of cyanohydrin formation.

[130] W. J. Jones, *J. Chem. Soc.*, 1914, **105**, 1547, 1560.

[131] G. Bredig and E. Stern, *Z. Elektrochem.*, 1904, **10**, 582; E. Stern, *Z. physik. Chem.*, 1905, **50**, 513.

[132] R. W. L. Clarke and A. Lapworth, *J Chem. Soc.*, 1907, **91**, 694.

Its product, after a prototropic change, is correctly constituted to participate in what is often the slow step of an aldol addition, as represented in the third equation. The kinetics require that either the third or the fourth step be the slowest of the sequence; but, knowing how rapidly cyanohydrin equilibria are set up in the presence of as much cyanide ion as is usually here employed, we cannot doubt that the slowest step is actually the third.

Although the rates of formation of simple cyanohydrins are difficult to study, valuable results have been obtained by quantitative measurements on *cyanohydrin equilibria.* Lapworth and Manske[133] examined equilibria of the form

$$R \cdot C_6H_4 \cdot CHO + HCN \rightleftarrows R \cdot C_6H_4 \cdot CH(OH) \cdot CN$$

for which they determined equilibrium constants, and thence the free-energy changes, in 96% ethyl alcohol at 20°, with various substituents R in ortho-, meta- and para-positions. The effects of ortho-substituents are complicated by specific local interactions, but those of meta- and para-substituents can be given a fairly simple interpretation. The effects of para-substituents are generally somewhat large, and are clearly dominated by the unsaturation of R: subject to modification from minor influences, these free-energy values measure the extra stability that the aldehyde, but not its cyanohydrin, can gain by through-conjugation between an unsaturated R and the unsaturated group CHO. The recognisable minor influence is polarity, permanently electron-attracting groups R tending to de-stabilise the aldehyde relatively to the cyanohydrin, presumably because the group $\cdot$CHO is itself more strongly electron-attracting than the group $\cdot$CH(OH)$\cdot$CN. The observed effects of meta-substituents are generally smaller: they cannot display any effect of through-conjugation; and therefore they leave in isolation the effect of polarity just mentioned. The following free-energy changes for para-substituted systems will in part illustrate these points:

p-Substituent........	NMe_2	OH	OMe	CH_3	Cl	H
$-\Delta G$(kcal./mole).....	0.55	1.5	2.0	2.7	3.1	3.1

A low figure means that the aldehyde has been made relatively stable. We see that all the groups which can conjugate (or hyperconjugate) through the benzene ring with the aldehyde group make the aldehyde more stable, excepting chlorine, for which one may presume that the weak conjugative effect is just annulled by the electronegativity effect. The effect of polarity can be seen in the free-energy changes

[133] A. Lapworth and R. H. F. Manske, *J. Chem. Soc.*, **1928**, 2533.

for meta-substituted systems:

m-Substituent........	CH_3	H	OH	OMe	NO_2	Cl
$-\Delta G$(kcal./mole)......	3.0	3.1	3.1	3.2	3.4	3.5

As mentioned in Section **7i,** Baker and Hemming employed this reaction in order to establish the principle of hyperconjugation as a permanent mode of electron displacement.[134] Using *p*-alkyl-substituents, they obtained the following free-energy differences in 96% ethyl alcohol:

p-Substituent...........		H	Me	Et	*i*-Pr	*t*-Bu
$-\Delta G$(kcal./mole)	35°....	2.90	2.39	2.48	2.51	2.57
	20°....	3.15	2.75	2.80	2.81	2.85

One sees that the alkyl groups stabilise the aldehyde relatively to its cyanohydrin, in the order Me > Et > *i*-Pr > *t*-Bu.

Baker and Hopkins have employed cyanohydrin equilibria in order to measure the relative extents to which the halogens exert their $+M$-effect when bound to the benzene ring. Such mesomeric conjugation should stabilise the aldehyde relatively to the cyanohydrin. For para- and meta-halogeno-benzaldehydes, they determined[135] the following free-energy changes in cyanohydrin formation in constant-boiling ethyl alcohol at 20°:

Substituent............		H	F	Cl	Br	I
$-\Delta G$(kcal./mole)	para...	3.16	2.95	3.24	3.34	3.36
	meta..	3.16	3.59	3.63	3.66	3.62

The meta-halogen substituents here show the already-mentioned electronegativity effect ($-I$), which de-stabilises the aldehyde relatively to the cyanohydrin. The para-halogen substituents can be seen always relatively to de-stabilise the aldehyde less than when the halogen is acting from the meta-position; and one halogen, para-fluorine, relatively stabilises the aldehyde. Evidently the mesomeric effect ($+M$) of halogen acts, as it should, in the direction of producing a relative stabilisation of the aldehyde; and this effect is greatest in fluorine and least in iodine. In short, the mesomeric effects stand in the order F > Cl > Br > I, as stated in Section **7e.** We shall note in Chapter XIII that this order is confirmed by data on acid strengths.

Baker, Barrett, and Tweed have used the same reaction in order

[134] J. W. Baker and M. L. Hemming, *J. Chem. Soc.*, **1942,** 191.
[135] J. W. Baker and H. B. Hopkins, *J. Chem. Soc.*, **1949,** 1089.

to confirm that the $+M$ effect of neutral groups $\cdot$**XR**, containing elements X of the Mendeléjeff group VI, follows the sequence OR>SR>SeR, as given in Section **7e**. For cyanohydrin formation from substituted benzaldehydes in ethanol, they have measured the following free-energy changes,[136] which show that the *p*-substituents relatively stabilise the aldehyde according to the sequence stated:

Substituents		H	OMe	SMe	SeMe
$-\Delta G$(kcal./mole), 20°	*p*-	3.16	0.81	0.90	1.94
	m-	3.16	3.18	3.20	3.22

As we shall see in the next chapter, this order also is confirmed by measurements of acid strengths.

By the principle of microscopic reversibility, the retrograde cyanohydrin reaction, which is a carbonyl-forming elimination, proceeds through the conjugate base of the cyanohydrin, by a rate-determining unimolecular loss of cyanide ion. This is what, in Section **38a**, was labelled the E1cB mechanism of elimination, a mechanism not at all well known in application to olefin-forming eliminations, though it is one of the normal mechanisms of carbonyl-forming eliminations.

All that is known of the *aldol addition reaction* is consistent with the assumption that it is analogous to cyanohydrin formation, and that it often follows the general anion-addition mechanism of Lapworth. The reversibility of the process has long been known in the example of the conversion of acetone into its ketol, diacetone-alcohol:[137] it was recognised as a general property after the demonstration of a number of equilibria involving simple aldols, such as *iso*butyraldol:[138]

$$(CH_3)_2C{:}O + CH_3\cdot CO\cdot CH_3 \rightleftarrows (CH_3)_2C(OH)\cdot CH_2\cdot CO\cdot CH_3$$

$$(CH_3)_2CH\cdot CH{:}O + (CH_3)_2CH\cdot CHO \rightleftarrows (CH_3)_2CH\cdot CH(OH)\cdot C(CH_3)_2\cdot CHO$$

The additions were shown to be exothermic, and therefore to be thermodynamically favoured by low temperatures. The difficulty in formally establishing such equilibria in all cases, is that many aldols and ketols are easily dehydrated to $\alpha\beta$-unsaturated carbonyl compounds, as in the conversion of acetaldol to crotonaldehyde, or of diacetone-alcohol to mesityl oxide; and that many aldols and ketols react further with their factors to give higher aldols or ketols, or dehydration products

136 J. W. Baker, S. F. C. Barrett, and W. T. Tweed, *J. Chem. Soc.*, **1954**, 3831.
137 K. Koelichen, *Z. physik. Chem.*, **1900, 33,** 129.
138 E. Hilda Ingold (Usherwood), *J. Chem. Soc.*, 1923, **123,** 1717; 1924, **125,** 435.

of the latter, as in the conversion of acetaldol to the dimeric "octaldol," and of diacetone-alcohol to phorone.

The aldol reaction is catalysed in a number of different ways, but typically by bases. The aqueous alkaline addition of acetaldehyde to formaldehyde,

$$CH_2{:}O + CH_3\cdot CHO \rightarrow CH_2(OH)\cdot CH_2\cdot CHO$$

can be approximately isolated from subsequent processes, and Bell and McTigue have shown[139] that the forward reaction follows the second-order rate law:

$$\text{Rate} \propto [\text{acetaldehyde}][OH^-]$$

The concentration of formaldehyde is absent from the rate equation. It follows that the only aldehyde consumed in the slow step is acetaldehyde, and that the formaldehyde is converted in a subsequent fast step. This is consistent with the generalised Lapworth mechanism, under the kinetic condition that the second forward step, that of addition, is fast compared to the reversal of the initial step of ionisation:

$$CH_3\cdot CHO + OH^- \rightleftharpoons \bar{C}H_2\cdot CHO + H_2O$$

$$CH_2{:}O + \bar{C}H_2\cdot CHO \rightleftharpoons CH_2\begin{cases} O^- \\ CH_2\cdot CHO \end{cases}$$

$$CH_2\begin{cases} O^- \\ CH_2\cdot CHO \end{cases} + H_2O \rightleftharpoons CH_2(OH)\cdot CH_2\cdot CHO + OH^-$$

Different relations between the rates of the stages apply to the alkaline aqueous ketolisation of acetone, for which we may set down the corresponding mechanism:

$$CH_3\cdot CO\cdot CH_3 + OH^- \rightleftarrows CH_3\cdot CO\cdot CH_2^- + H_2O$$

$$(CH_3)_2C{:}O + \bar{C}H_2\cdot CO\cdot CH_3 \rightleftarrows (CH_3)_2C\begin{cases} O^- \\ CH_2\cdot CO\cdot CH_3 \end{cases}$$

$$(CH_3)_2C\begin{cases} O^- \\ CH_2\cdot CO\cdot CH_3 \end{cases} + H_2O \rightleftarrows (CH_3)_2C(OH)\cdot CH_2\cdot CO\cdot CH_3 + OH^-$$

[139] R. P. Bell and P. T. McTigue, *J. Chem. Soc.*, 1960, 2983.

The kinetics of this reaction have been investigated in the backward direction, because the equilibrium renders this approach the more convenient.[137,140] The rate-law is as follows:

$$\text{Rate} \propto [\text{ketol}][\text{OH}^-]$$

This rate of deketolisation of diacetone-alcohol is unaffected by acetone. It is inferred that the anion $CH_3 \cdot CO \cdot CH_2^-$ reacts with a water molecule faster than with acetone, since the latter process would retard deketolisation. Hence, the rate-determining step in deketolisation is either the first (lowest of the above three lines of formulae) or the second; and it surely cannot be the first, which is only a proton transfer between oxygen atoms. Then, from the rate of deketolisation and the equilibrium constant, one can calculate the rate of ketolisation of acetone. This is only about one-thousandth of the rate of iodination, or of the identical rate of deuteration (Section **47e**), reactions which should measure the rate of the first step of ketolisation.[141] Thus, the second step of ketolisation is slower than either the first or the reversal of the first. So we can see that the second step is rate-determining for both ketolisation and deketolisation. It follows that, if the kinetics of ketolisation were directly investigated, the following third-order rate-law would be found:

$$\text{Rate} \propto [\text{acetone}]^2[\text{OH}^-]$$

The aqueous alkaline aldolisation of acetaldehyde bridges these two limiting kinetic situations. The reaction was first investigated by Bell,[142] who established the second-order kinetic equation. Bonhoeffer and Walters showed that when the reaction is run in deuterium water, deuterium is not taken up.[141] Both results can be understood on the basis that the second forward step is fast enough to forestall reversal of the first step (which would admit deuterium), so leaving the first forward step in control of the rate. However, Broche and Gibert showed[143] that this was not the general situation; which is that the kinetics are transitional between the second- and third-order equations as limits, the "order in acetaldehyde," an approximate concept now, tending downwards as the concentration of acetaldehyde is raised. Moreover, although deuterium is not taken up from deuterium water if the concentration of acetaldehyde is fairly high, it is taken up more strongly as the concentration is reduced. A reduction in the concentration of acetaldehyde will slow down the second forward step of the

140 V. K. LaMer and M. L. Miller, *J. Am. Chem. Soc.*, 1935, 57, 2674.

141 K. F. Bonhoeffer and W. D. Walters, *Z. physik. Chem.*, 1938, A, 181, 141; A, 182, 265.

142 R. P. Bell, *J. Chem. Soc.*, 1937, 1637; *Trans. Faraday Soc.*, 1941, 37, 716.

143 A. Broche and R. Gibert, *Bull. soc. chim.* (France), 1955, 131.

mechanism relative to the first step, or to the reversal of the first step, and so rate control will move over from the first step towards the second. By the use of buffers, Bell and McTigue were able to carry this transfer of rate control almost all the way,[139] and thus to observe a close approximation to the limiting third-order equation:

$$\text{Rate} \propto [\text{acetaldehyde}]^2[\text{OH}^-]$$

The aldol addition of ethyl malonate to formaldehyde in water,

$$CH_2{:}O + CH_2(CO_2Et)_2 \rightarrow CH_2(OH)\cdot CH(CO_2Et)_2$$

has been found[144] to follow a kinetic equation similar to that deduced for the ketolisation of acetone. The reaction tends to go beyond the first stage, but by studying initial rates in phosphate buffers, the following law has been established

$$\text{Rate} \propto [\text{aldehyde}][\text{ester}][\text{OH}^-]$$

This means that the anion of ethyl malonate is formed quickly, but adds slowly.

The condensation of benzaldehyde with acetophenone in ethyl alcohol under catalysis by ethoxide ions has also been studied kinetically.[145] The isolated product is benzilidene-acetone, and it is assumed that the ketol is formed intermediately:

$$Ph\cdot CH{:}O + CH_3\cdot CO\cdot Ph \rightarrow Ph\cdot CH(OH)\cdot CH_2\cdot CO\cdot Ph \rightarrow Ph\cdot CH{:}CH\cdot CO\cdot Ph$$

The rate-law is as follows:

$$\text{Rate} \propto [\text{aldehyde}][\text{ketone}][\text{OEt}^-]$$

This means that the anion of acetophenone is formed quickly, and that either its addition, or (improbably) the final dehydration, is slow.

These studies have been much extended by Patai and others. Patai, Israeli, and Zabicky showed[146] that, if the weakly acidic adduct is acidic enough, it will function in a hydroxylic solvent, such as water or ethanol, without an added basic catalyst: the solvent will be basic enough. Malononitrile will thus add without a basic catalyst to benzaldehyde or to substituted benzaldehydes. Of course, the reaction is reversible: catalysis is irrelevant to thermodynamics, and thus the formed aldol will come to pieces in the solvent, without an added catalyst. The kinetics of the forward reaction are of second order:

[144] K. N. Welch, *J. Chem. Soc.*, **1931, 653.**

[145] E. Coombs and D. P. Evans, *J. Chem. Soc.*, **1944, 1295.**

[146] S. Patai, Y. Israeli, and J. Zabicky, *Chem. and Ind.*, **1957**, 1671; S. Patai and Y. Israeli, *J. Chem. Soc.*, **1960,** 2020, 2025; S. Patai and J. Zabicky, *ibid.*, p. 2030; *idem* and Y. Israeli, *ibid.*, p. 2038.

$$\text{Rate} \propto [\text{malononitrile}][\text{aldehyde}]$$

This corresponds, except for the absence of a catalytic factor, to third-order kinetics in the presence of a basic catalyst: its meaning is that the ionisation of the malononitrile is rapid, the slow step being the attack of the anion on the aldehyde. Ethyl cyanoacetate is less acidic than malononitrile, but will also function without an added catalyst, and more or less according to the same form of kinetics. But now there are signs of transitional kinetics, the apparent order in ethyl cyanoacetate tending to fall with increasing concentration of the ester. On increasing its concentration, the rate of the step of addition begins to catch up with the rate of the preliminary ionisation, and so control of the rate begins to shift from the second step towards the first step of the mechanism. Cyanoacetamide is less acidic still, and its addition discloses thorough-going transitional kinetics. Ethyl malonate is even less acidic and in practice needs a basic catalyst.

The same workers have shown that the aldol dehydrations, which succeed the additions in these reactions, are also freely reversible. Such dehydrations are in general base-catalysed, and are also powerfully acid-catalysed; and so, in the cases considered, dehydration is effected with the aid of a solvent that can function as either an acid or a base.

By the principle of microscopic reversibility, the base-catalysed retrograde aldol reaction, a carbonyl-forming elimination, proceeds by unimolecular anion-loss from the pre-formed conjugate base of the aldol. This is the mechanism of elimination which we labelled E1cB in Chapter IX.

The aldol reaction is catalysed by acids. It has been made clear that the Lapworth mechanism, as adapted for acid catalysis, applies, that is, that the first step is the conversion of the carbonyl compound into its conjugate acid, which is in part an oxonium ion and in part a carbonium ion, and in the latter capacity is so strongly electrophilic that it can act as a substituting agent on the enol of the carbonyl compound:

$$Me_2CO + H^+ \rightleftarrows Me_2\overset{+}{C}(OH)$$

$$Me_2\overset{+}{C}(OH) + CH_2{=\!=}CMe{-}OH \rightleftarrows Me_2C(OH)\ CH_2{\cdot}CMe{:}O + H^+$$

These acid-catalysed reactions often proceed further, the aldol or ketol undergoing a dehydration, which in the example of acetone, leads to mesityl oxide, or by further ketolisation and dehydration, to phorone.

Noyce and his coworkers studied the kinetics of the acid-catalysed reactions between acetone or methyl ethyl ketone and benzaldehyde, and *p*-methoxy- and *p*-nitro-benzaldehyde.[147] Their results are consistent with this mechanism, provided that the step of addition is rate-controlling. In this group of examples, the aldol additions are succeeded by dehydration of the ketols to benzylidene-ketones, the whole sequence of reactions being reversible.

The same investigators have made an analysis of the effects of substituents on the kinetics, and on the thermodynamics, of some of the component processes. As to the reversible reaction between the benzaldehyde and a ketone, on the one hand, and the ketol adduct, on the other, the indication is that substituents have a thermodynamic effect similar to that which they exert on the equilibria between benzaldehydes and their cyanohydrins. In either case, a *p*-methoxy-substituent holds back the addition; as we can understand, because the methoxy-group will conjugate through the benzene ring with the aldehyde group, thereby stabilising the aldehyde in a way that the cyanohydrin or ketol cannot be stabilised, because in them the unsaturation of the original aldehyde function has been destroyed by addition.

When this effect on equilibrium was separated into rate effects on the opposing reactions, it was found that the *p*-methoxy-substituent mildly accelerates the addition but accelerates its reversal very much more strongly. This indicates that the *p*-methoxy-group conjugates with the partial carbonium-ionic centre of the transition state of the addition step of the mechanism somewhat more strongly than it conjugates with the aldehyde group in the initial state. Thus the substituent will stabilise the initial state: it will more strongly stabilise the transition state; and it will not stabilise the final state of the acid-catalysed aldol-addition process.

The kinetics of the reversible dehydration of the ketols to benzylidene ketones were studied only in the direction of dehydration. Again, the methoxy-substituent had a mildly accelerating effect. As will be explained, this is to be expected even though we do not know the mechanism of the acid-catalysed dehydration.

There are two possible mechanisms. One is as follows. We noted in Section **53a** that the acid hydration of simple olefins is general-acid catalysed; and, by applying the principle of microscopic reversibility, we deduced that the acid dehydration of similarly simple alcohols had a carbonium-ion mechanism, which was not the well-studied mechanism E1, but was the less familiar mechanism $E2(C^+)$. If this were

[147] D. S. Noyce and L. R. Snyder, *J. Am. Chem. Soc.*, 1958, **80**, 4033, 4324; 1959, **81**, 620; D. C. Joyce and W. I. Reed, *ibid.*, 1958, **80**, 5539; 1959, **81**, 624; D. C. Noyce and W. A. Pryor, *ibid.*, p.618.

true for the acid dehydration of a ketol, it would be expressed as follows:

$$\left.\begin{array}{l} \mathrm{ArCH(OH)\cdot CH_2\cdot CO\cdot CH_3} \overset{+\mathrm{H}^+}{\rightleftharpoons} \mathrm{ArCH(\overset{+}{O}H_2)\cdot CH_2\cdot CO\cdot CH_3} \\ \rightleftharpoons \mathrm{Ar\overset{+}{C}H\cdot CH_2\cdot CO\cdot CH_3} \underset{\text{slow}}{\overset{-\mathrm{H}^+}{\rightleftharpoons}} \mathrm{ArCH{:}CH\cdot CO\cdot CH_3} \end{array}\right\} [\mathrm{E2(C^+)}]$$

Here the transition state is in the third step; and the transition state must be in part a carbonium ion, such that the *p*-methoxyl group can conjugate with its electron-deficient centre. Since no such conjugation is possible in the initial state of the dehydration, the methoxy substituent must exert an accelerating effect. How large the effect will be must depend on the unknown extent to which the positive charge on the transition state is represented by an electron deficiency at the benzyl carbon atom.

However, one cannot confidently expect to be able to carry over to ketols the conclusions reached for the acid dehydration of simple alcohols. Mechanism E2(C+) rests on the difficulty of extracting a proton from alkanic hydrogen, a difficulty which makes the proton transfer the slowest step in the process. In the acid dehydration of ketols, the corresponding step is the extraction of a proton from prototropic (keto-enolic) hydrogen. This must be very much easier, and might be fast enough to allow an earlier step of the mechanism to be rate-controlling. The mechanism could then be E1, in which the same intermediates are involved, but the second step is rate-controlling:

$$\left.\begin{array}{l} \mathrm{ArCH(OH)\cdot CH_2\cdot CO\cdot CH_3} \overset{+\mathrm{H}^+}{\rightleftharpoons} \mathrm{ArCH(\overset{+}{O}H_2)\cdot CH_2\cdot CO\cdot CH_3} \\ \overset{\text{slow}}{\rightleftharpoons} \mathrm{Ar\overset{+}{C}H\cdot CH_2\cdot CO\cdot CH_3} \overset{-\mathrm{H}^+}{\rightleftharpoons} \mathrm{ArCH{:}CH\cdot CO\cdot CH_3} \end{array}\right\} (\mathrm{E1})$$

The transition state is now a different one, but it is still in part a carbonium ion, and therefore the *p*-methoxy-substituent should accelerate the dehydration, though, once again, the amount of such acceleration depends on the unknown proportion in which the cationic charge has been accepted by the benzyl carbon atom.

Mechanism E1 requires specific hydrogen-ion catalysis of the hydration of an $\alpha\beta$-unsaturated ketone. Mechanism E2(C+) requires general-acid catalysis in hydration. Hence a determination of the type of acid catalysis operative in this reaction would be decisive for the choice between the two mechanisms of elimination.

There appears to be a correspondence between the orientation of aldol addition to an unsymmetrical ketone, and the orientation of halogenation of the ketone. This should be so, insofar as aldol products are kinetically, rather than thermodynamically, controlled; for both reactions are electrophilic processes, occurring through the anion in basic catalysis, and through the enol in acid catalysis. In Section **47d** we saw that methyl ethyl ketone was halogenated faster in the methyl group in alkaline media (Hofmann-like control of the orientation of ionisation) and in the methylene group in acid media (Saytzeff-like control). It has been known since 1902 that methyl ethyl ketone condenses with benzaldehyde to give $PhCH{:}CH\cdot CO\cdot CH_2\cdot CH_3$ in alkaline solution, and to give $CH_3\cdot CO\cdot C({:}CHPh)\cdot CH_3$ in acid solution.[148]

The amines, apart from tertiary amines, constitute a third type of catalyst for the aldol reaction, and for the reactions which so often succeed it. The behaviour of these catalysts has been quantitatively investigated in the example of the dektolisation of diacetone-alcohol.[149] Tertiary amines as such do not catalyse the reaction: any apparent catalysis is due to hydroxide ions contained in the solutions of tertiary amines. But ammonia, and primary and secondary amines, are catalysts in their own right, each contributing a rate of the form,

$$\text{Rate} \propto [\text{ketol}][\text{amine}]$$

It has been suggested that they condense at the carbonyl group to form an immonium ion, which accomplishes the rate-determining step of reaction more quickly than would the carbonyl compound:

$$(CH_3)_2C\begin{cases} O^- \\ CH_2\cdot C({:}\overset{+}{N}R_2)\cdot CH_3 \end{cases} \rightleftarrows (CH_3)_2C{:}O + \bar{C}H_2\cdot C({:}\overset{+}{N}R_2)\cdot CH_3$$

The aldol reaction, essentially the addition of a keto-enol or other pseudo-acid, H—CXYZ, to the group C=O of an aldehyde or ketone, together with the dehydrations and further reactions that frequently succeed it, is the basis of a very important group of synthetic methods. Historically, the aldol reaction was discovered in 1872 by Wurtz.[150] The use of alkali for the purpose of effecting aldol addition, and the condensations based on it, was introduced by Schmidt,[151] and was developed particularly by Claisen.[152] Thus conducted, the reaction

[148] C. Harries and G. H Müller, *Ber.*, 1902, **35,** 966.

[149] J. G. Miller and M. Kilpatrick, *J. Am. Chem. Soc.*, 1931, **53,** 3217; F. H. Westheimer and H. Cohn, *ibid.*, 1938, **60,** 90.

[150] A. Wurtz, *Jahresber.*, **1872,** 449.

[151] J. G. Schmidt, *Ber.*, 1880, **13,** 2342.

[152] L. Claisen, *Ber.*, 1881, **14,** 2468.

is sometimes, though somewhat ambiguously, termed the *Claisen reaction.* Claisen also developed the use of acid catalysts for the aldol reaction and succeeding processes.[153] The use of ammonia was introduced by Japp and Streatfield;[154] but a much more complete investigation on the use of ammonia and primary and secondary amines was carried out by Knoevenagel,[155] after whom the reaction, conducted by such means, is usually known as the *Knoevenagel reaction.*

Yet another form of the aldol reaction, which it is convenient to consider separately, partly because of its history, and partly because of the distinctive nature of the experimental conditions, is the *Perkin reaction.* It was introduced by W. H. Perkin sr.[156] in 1875 for the preparation, typically, of cinnamic acid, the process being to heat benzaldehyde with acetic anhydride and sodium acetate at 180°. Attempts were made by Perkin, and by Fittig, to find out something about the mechanism of this reaction, particularly whether it was the anhydride or the sodium salt which underwent the condensation. Perkin thought the former,[156] and Fittig the latter.[157] The method which both investigators tried was to use the sodium salt of one acid in conjunction with the anhydride of another, and to see which cinnamic acid analogue appeared. It transpired that this depended on the temperature, and the main result of work along these lines was the discovery,[156,158] which has more recently been confirmed,[159] of a facile interchange between anhydride and salt:

$$\text{anhydride of A} + \text{salt of B} \rightleftarrows \text{salt of A} + \text{anhydride of B}$$

Thus it became obvious that the original problem could not easily be solved this way. However, it was made clear that when benzaldehyde is condensed with propionic anhydride and sodium propionate, or with butyric anhydride and sodium butyrate, it is the α-carbon atom of the fatty-acid structure which interacts with the aldehyde molecule.

Fittig made a strong case for the view that the first phase of the reaction is an aldol-like addition. From benzaldehyde, succinic anhydride, and sodium succinate, at 100°, he obtained the γ-lactone of the hydroxy-acid adduct.[160] From benzaldehyde, *iso*butyric anhydride, and sodium *iso*butyrate, also at 100°, he secured the hydroxy-

153 L. Claisen, *Ann.*, 1883, **218,** 172.

154 F. R. Japp and F. W. Streatfield, *J. Chem. Soc.*, 1883, **43,** 27.

155 E. Knoevenagel, *Ann.*, 1894, **281,** 25; *Ber.*, 1904, **37,** 4461; and many other papers to which references are given in the second of those cited.

156 W. H. Perkin sr., *Chem. News*, 1875, **32,** 258; *J. Chem. Soc.*, 1877, **31,** 388; 1886, **47,** 317.

157 R. Fittig, *Ber.*, 1881, **14,** 1824; *Ann.*, 1885, **227,** 48.

158 R. Fittig and F. L. Slocum, *Ann.*, 1885, **227,** 53.

159 C. R. Hauser and D. S. Breslow, *J. Am. Chem. Soc.*, 1939, **61,** 786.

160 R. Fittig and H. W. Jayne, *Ann.*, 1882, **216,** 97.

acid adduct itself.[161] The latter result has since been confirmed.[162]

$$\mathrm{Ph\cdot CHO + CH_2(CO_2H)\cdot \underset{\displaystyle CO_2H}{\underset{|}{CH_2}} \rightarrow Ph\cdot CH\cdot CH(CO_2H)\cdot CH_2}$$
$$\mathrm{O\text{———————}CO}$$

$$\mathrm{Ph\cdot CHO + CHMe_2\cdot CO_2H \rightarrow Ph\cdot CH(OH)\cdot CMe_2\cdot CO_2H}$$

The question of the respective roles of the anhydride and the salt remained unsolved until 1928. In that year Kalnin demonstrated[163] that, while the anhydride is essential to the reaction, the sodium salt of the carboxylic acid can be replaced by a variety of other bases, for instance, by sodium carbonate, phosphate, or sulphite, or by triethylamine, pyridine, or quinoline. Thus, as we should expect from general electrochemical principles, the anhydride is the pseudo-acidic addendum, and the salt is the basic catalyst. Presumably a proton from the anhydride becomes transferred to the anion of the salt, while the anion of the anhydride engages in addition to the carbonyl group of the aldehyde.

Turning to additions of H—N to C═O, we have to consider the *reversible formation of azomethines, oximes, arylhydrazones, and semicarbazones.* All these reactions follow the general pattern of aldol condensations: addition to give a carbinolamine, or an N-hydroxy- or N-amino-substituted derivative of it, is succeeded by a dehydration of the simple or substituted carbinolamine to the double-bonded condensation product. This sequence of reactions, like that of the aldol condensation, is completely reversible.

The *formation of azomethines* shows some general differences from the other reactions. With simpler aliphatic aldehydes or ketones and primary amines, the condensation may often proceed beyond the first-formed azomethine, inasmuch as the additive properties of the groups >C:NR and >C:O are similar. Generally speaking, the simplest factors can thus give the relatively most complicated products, as is illustrated *par excellence* in the reactions between formaldehyde and ammonia.

Insofar as azomethine formation does not proceed beyond a single-stage condensation, the equilibrium in aqueous solution lies well over on the side of the factors; but it can be shifted towards the product by removing water. The carbinolamines are not formed at all completely before they start undergoing either dehydration or return to the factors, unless they are formed, as, for example, acetaldehyde-ammonia can so easily be, under conditions in which they crystallise.

[161] R. Fittig and H. W. Jayne, *Ann.*, 1882, **216**, 115; R. Fittig and P. Ott, *Ann.*, 1885, **227**, 61.

[162] D. S. Breslow and C. R. Hauser, *J. Am. Chem. Soc.*, 1939, **61**, 793.

[163] P. Kalnin, *Helv. Chim. Acta*, 1928, **11**, 977.

Unlike aldol condensations, azomethine condensations, and their reversal by hydrolysis, are not characteristically base-catalysed. For the amines are bases in their own right, and do not have to be deprotonated in order to add to a carbonyl group. This is not to say that the azomethine condensations and hydrolyses cannot be base-catalysed: some can be at very high pH, as in the example of the formation of benzylidene-aniline.[164] For although the amines are bases, the amide ions formed from them by deprotonation are much stronger bases. However, from moderately basic pH's to the neutral point, the addition reactions, and indeed the whole sequence through to the azomethines, and, of course, the retrograde processes, are uncatalysed.

On the acid side of the neutral point, the sequence of reactions is acid-catalysed; but, as Jencks has shown, the acid catalysis belongs to the dehydration step.[165] This is natural enough, because a carbinol-amine is a pseudo-base, and hence is very sensitive to acids (Section **48a**).

As the concentration of acid is raised, the rate of the condensation may pass through a maximum, at some point, which seems to be related to the basicity of the adding amine. At high acidities, the acid may so accelerate dehydration that rate control is passed back to the step of addition; and then, this gets retarded because the excess of acid will put the primary amine out of action as a nucleophile.

Except for quantitative differences, the phenomena described apply not only to reversible azomethine formation, but also oxime, semicarbazone, and probably arylhydrazone formation, and we may therefore formulate the mechanisms common to all these reactions in a single set of formulae, by writing the nucleophile as NH_2X, where X may be H, Alk, Ar, OH, NHAr, or $NH \cdot CO \cdot NH_2$:

Base-catalysed addition:

$$NH_2X + OH^- \overset{1}{\rightleftharpoons} NHX^- + H_2O$$

$$RR'C{:}O + NHX^- \overset{2}{\rightleftharpoons} RR'C\begin{matrix} \diagup O^- \\ \diagdown NHX \end{matrix}$$

$$RR'C\begin{matrix} \diagup O^- \\ \diagdown NHX \end{matrix} + H_2O \overset{3}{\rightleftharpoons} RR'C\begin{matrix} \diagup OH \\ \diagdown NHX \end{matrix} + OH^-$$

[164] B. Kesterning, L. Holleck, and G. A. Melkonian, *Z. Elektrochem.*, 1956, **60**, 130.

[165] E. H. Cordes and W. P. Jencks, *J. Am. Chem. Soc.*, 1962, **84**, 832; 1963, **85**, 2843.

Uncatalysed addition:

$$\mathrm{RR'C{:}O + NH_2X \overset{4}{\rightleftharpoons} RR'C\begin{matrix}\diagup O^- \\ \diagdown NH_2X^+\end{matrix} \overset{5}{\rightleftharpoons} RR'C\begin{matrix}\diagup OH \\ \diagdown NHX\end{matrix}}$$

Uncatalysed dehydration:

$$\mathrm{RR'C\begin{matrix}\diagup OH \\ \diagdown NHX\end{matrix} \overset{6}{\rightleftharpoons} RR'C{:}\overset{+}{N}HX + \overset{-}{O}H \overset{7}{\rightleftharpoons} RR'C{:}NX + H_2O}$$

Acid-catalysed dehydration:

$$\mathrm{RR'C\begin{matrix}\diagup OH \\ \diagdown NHX\end{matrix} + H_3O^+ \overset{8}{\rightleftharpoons} RR'C\begin{matrix}\diagup OH_2^+ \\ \diagdown NHX\end{matrix} + H_2O}$$

$$\mathrm{RR'C\begin{matrix}\diagup OH_2^+ \\ \diagdown NHX\end{matrix} \overset{9}{\rightleftharpoons} RR'C{:}\overset{+}{N}HX + H_2O \overset{10}{\rightleftharpoons} RR'C{:}NX + H_3O^+}$$

When the addition is base-catalysed, the rate equation for the condensation is:

$$\text{Rate} \propto [\text{carbonyl cpd.}][\text{amine}][\mathrm{OH^-}]$$

When the addition and the dehydration are both uncatalysed, the rate equation is:

$$\text{Rate} \propto [\text{carbonyl cpd.}][\text{amine}]$$

no matter whether the addition (step 4) or the dehydration (step 6) is rate-controlling. When the dehydration is acid-catalysed, the rate equation may be either of the following:

$$\text{Rate} \propto [\text{carbonyl cpd.}][\text{amine}][\mathrm{HA}]$$

$$\text{Rate} \propto [\text{carbonyl cpd.}][\text{amine}][\mathrm{HA}]/[\mathrm{A^-}]$$

according to whether the catalysis is of the general-acid type (step 8 rate-controlling), or of the specific hydrogen-ion type (step 9 rate-controlling).

Both forms of acid catalysis have been demonstrated for the hydrolysis of various azomethines, in various solvents, and at various degrees of acidity, usually obtained with the aid of buffers.[166,167] Presumably both apply to the corresponding azomethine-forming condensation, though this has not been directly and formally proved. If, in the condensations, rate-control, at a particular acidity, is in the acid-catalysed dehydration, then an increase in the acidity will accelerate the step of dehydration, and may make it faster than the step of addition, when rate-control will pass back to the step of addition. The rate will now cease to increase with the acidity; and, if an excess of acid is putting the adding amine out of action as a free base to an appreciable degree, the rate may decrease with further increase in acidity. These effects are well known.[165]

The step of rate-control in azomethine formation or hydrolysis can often be located by the effects of substituents on rate. Thus in azomethine formation from derivatives of benzaldehyde, a *p*-methoxy-substituent in the benzaldehyde will reduce the rate at which the aldehyde group will add the amine (reaction 4), but will increase the rate at which the carbinolamine will undergo dehydration (reaction 6, or reactions 7 and 8). Many other substituents will show a like contrast in their effects on the two main steps in the overall process. Suppose that rate-control, *i.e.*, the transition state, is in the step of reversible addition (step A):

$$\text{Aldehyde} + \text{Amine} \underset{\text{A}}{\rightleftharpoons} \text{Carbinolamine} \underset{\text{B}}{\rightleftharpoons} \text{Azomethine}$$

Then, if we are considering the left-to-right reaction, *i.e.*, the formation of an azomethine, the only substituent effect that will count will be that on step A; and therefore observed substituent effects should be fairly large, and as predicted for step A. If, however, we are concerned with the right-to-left reaction, *i.e.*, the hydrolysis of an azomethine, then the effect of substituents on what is now the pre-equilibrium step B may increase the stationary concentration of carbinolamine when it is going to decrease its rate of fission in step A, or decrease the stationary concentration when it is going to increase the rate of fission. The nett effect of substituents on the hydrolysis is then a difference of opposites and is likely to be small and irregular. Starting again, let us suppose that rate-control, *i.e.*, the transition state, is in the step of reversible dehydration of the carbinolamine (step B). Then by a similar argument, substituent effects on azomethine formation should be small and complicated, and those on azomethine hydrolysis should be large and regular, as predicted for the right-to-left step B.

[166] R. L. Reeves, *J. Am. Chem. Soc.*, 1962, **84**, 3332.

[167] A. V. Willis and R. E. Robertson, *Can. J. Chem.*, 1953, **31**, 361; O. Bloch-Chaudé, *Compt. rend.*, 1954, **239**, 804.

Some of these expected effects can be illustrated. The uncatalysed condensation of benzaldehyde with aniline in benzene obeyed the second-order rate law, and the rate-constants for the condensations of substituted benzaldehydes disclosed just the kinetic substituent effects which are expected for the formation of azomethine when the step of addition (step 4) is rate-controlling.[168] The hydrolysis of benzylidene-aniline and its substitution products in nearly neutral conditions, or in weakly acid buffers, showed only small and complicated substituent effects.[167] Both results point to rate-control in step 4. The condensation of substituted benzaldehydes with 2-butylamine in methanol with acetate buffers showed small and confused substituent effects, indicating rate-control in step 6.[169] Conditions have been found for the hydrolysis of benzylidene-aniline by dilute acid in aqueous methanol, without buffers, in which the kinetic control is being shared between steps 4 and 6, and is moving from step 6 towards step 4 with rising acidity.[170]

The reaction of *formation of oximes, arylhydrazones, and semicarbazones* shows two general differences from the formation of azomethines. One is that the formation of oximes and hydrazones, including semicarbazones, shows little tendency to run beyond the first condensation product to a further stage of addition. Subsequent reactions are usually of other types. Thus an aldoxime may be dehydrated to a nitrile, and an arylhydrazone may tautomerise to the azo-compound. The other general difference is that, even in highly aqueous media, the equilibria in carbonyl reactions with hydroxylamine and hydrazines, including semi-carbazide, lie much more towards the oxime or hydrazone or semi-carbazone, than the equilibria in azomethine formation lie towards the azomethine. (Because of its relatively small extent, the simplest way to demonstrate reversibility in the formation of an oxime or hydrazone is to trap the hydroxylamine or hydrazine formed from these derivatives by hydrolysis, with excess of another carbonyl compound.) We may connect both these differences from azomethine formation with the circumstance that, when we condense hydroxylamine or a hydrazine with a carbonyl compound, we provide the introduced group with a new internal conjugated system, $\ddot{O}-N=C$ or $\ddot{N}-N=C$, from which it will derive thermodynamic stability. We do not do that when we condense an amine to make an azomethine.

[168] E. F. Pratt and M. J. Kamlet, *J. Org. Chem.*, 1961, **26**, 4029.

[169] G. M. Santerre, C. J. Hamstote, and T. I. Crowell, *J. Am. Chem. Soc.*, 1958, **80**, 1254.

[170] A. V. Willi, *Helv. Chim. Acta*, 1956, **39**, 1193.

The *formation of oximes* has a special distinction from the formation of hydrazones in the prominence of its *base catalysis*. This came out in the first definitive investigation of mechanism in the whole group of these carbon-nitrogen condensations, that of Barrett and Lapworth in 1908 on the formation of oximes.[171] These workers observed both basic and acid catalysis. For the former, they assumed the mechanism written above (p. 1009). We may connect the peculiar importance of base catalysis in oxime formation with the circumstance that the anion of hydroxylamine is "anticonjugated" (p. 552, note) in that its high concentration of unshared electrons drives two into an antibonding molecular orbital where they will make the anion an abnormally powerful nucleophile (Section **28c**). A hydroxylamine anion cannot avoid this situation by twisting, as a hydrazine anion could, and doubtless does (Section **28c**). A small equilibrium concentration of the hydroxylamine anion will thus have a disproportionately large effect in reactions with a highly polarisable electrophilic centre.

The *acid catalysis* of the *formation of oximes*,[171,174] *arylhydrazones*,[172] and *semicarbazones*[173,174,175] follows a common pattern. At low acidities, where the acid catalysis is linear, a rapid disappearance of the carbonyl compound is followed by a slow appearance of the oxime or hydrazone compound. This means that an N-substituted carbinolamine is rapidly formed, and that it is the slow dehydration of this addition product that is acid-catalysed. With increasing acidity, linearity fails, and the rates pass through maxima, and then decline. With the speeding up of the dehydration, the control of rate is being passed back to the step of addition, where, as the acidity is further increased, rate becomes depressed by protonation of the nucleophilic addendum. In the case of semicarbazone formation from substituted benzaldehydes, Anderson and Jencks showed[175] that the kinetic effects of substituents at acidities on the two sides of the rate maximum are different: on the more acid side, these effects are appropriate for rate-control by the step of addition; and on the less acid side they are consistent with rate-control in the step of pseudo-base dehydration.

Turning to the H—O additions of the carbonyl group, we have to refer to the *formation of carbonyl hydrates and alcoholates*. The best

[171] E. Barrett and A. Lapworth, *J. Chem. Soc.*, 1908, **93**, 85; A. Ölander, *Z. physik. Chem.*, 1927, **129**, 1.

[172] S. Bodforss, *Z. physik. Chem.*, 1924, **109**, 223.

[173] J. B. Conant and P. D. Bartlett, *J. Am. Chem. Soc.*, 1932, **54**, 2881; F. H. Westheimer, *ibid.*, 1934, **56**, 1962; F. P. Price jr. and L. P. Hammett, *ibid.*, 1941, **63**, 2387.

[174] W. P. Jencks, *J Am. Chem. Soc.*, 1959, **81**, 475.

[175] F. M. Anderson and W. P. Jencks, *J. Am. Chem. Soc.*, 1960, **82**, 1773.

investigated example is the hydration of acetaldehyde,

$$CH_3{\cdot}CH{:}O + H_2O \rightleftarrows CH_3{\cdot}CH(OH)_2$$

which has been studied by Bell and his coworkers.[176] They have followed the kinetics in both directions, taking advantage of the circumstance that the reaction goes largely towards the hydrate in solvent water, but largely towards the aldehyde in 92% aqueous acetone. In each direction the reaction shows general basic and general acid catalysis. It would thus appear that we have to contemplate two groups of mechanisms. Fundamental for basic mechanisms is the reversible addition of a hydroxide ion to a neutral aldehyde molecule:

$$CH_3{\cdot}CH{:}O + OH^- \rightleftarrows CH_3{\cdot}CH\begin{cases} O^- \\ OH \end{cases}$$

But this scheme has to be generalised in order to allow for general basic catalysis, and, as usual, there are several ways in which this can be done. Since hydroxide ion comes from the solvent, a plausible way in this case is to assume that the general basic catalyst B^- acts on solvent water to generate a hydroxide ion synchronously with the addition of the latter in a termolecular reaction:

$$^-B \curvearrowright H{-}OH \curvearrowright \overset{|}{\underset{|}{C}}{=}O \rightleftarrows B{-}H + HO{-}\overset{|}{\underset{|}{C}}{-}O^-$$

Equally fundamental for acid mechanisms is the reversible addition of the conjugate acid of the aldehyde to a neutral water molecule:

$$CH_3{\cdot}\overset{+}{C}H{\cdot}OH + OH_2 \rightleftarrows CH_3{\cdot}CH\begin{cases} OH \\ OH_2^+ \end{cases}$$

This mechanism also has to be generalised in order that it shall express general acid catalysis. Again there are several possibilities: but the assumption, analogous to that described for basic catalysis, would be that the general acid HA generates the cation of the aldehyde as this cation binds a molecule of solvent water in a synchronous termolecular process:

$$A{-}H \curvearrowleft O{=}\overset{|}{\underset{|}{C}} \curvearrowleft OH_2 \rightarrow \bar{A} + H{-}O{-}C{-}\overset{+}{O}H_2$$

[176] R. P. Bell and W. C. E. Higginson, *Proc. Roy. Soc.* (London), 1949, **A, 197,** 141; R. P. Bell and B. de B. Darwent, *Trans. Faraday Soc.*, 1950, **46,** 34.

Termolecular reactions involving one solvent molecule are not improbable. If we should split this reaction into a bimolecular rate-controlling proton transfer succeeded by a fast water uptake, it would conform in reverse to the general mechanism given on p. 1010 for acid-catalysed (including general-acid catalysed) dehydration.

(54b) Reversible Additions of Bases or Weak Acids to Conjugated Olefinic Carbonyl Compounds.—The simplest conjugative Ad_N additions of nucleophilic acid addenda might be typified by the *addition of hydrogen cyanide to αβ-unsaturated* ketones, esters, or nitriles. Lapworth examined a number of these reactions in 1903 and subsequently, for example, the additions of hydrogen cyanide to mesityl oxide, phorone, 1-cyanostilbene, and carvone.[177]

$$\mathrm{Me_2C{:}CH{\cdot}COMe \rightarrow Me_2C(CN){\cdot}CH_2{\cdot}COMe}$$

$$\mathrm{(Me_2C{:}CH)_2CO \rightarrow \{Me_2C(CN){\cdot}CH_2\}_2CO}$$

$$\mathrm{PhCH{:}CPh{\cdot}CN \rightarrow PhCH(CN){\cdot}CHPh{\cdot}CN}$$

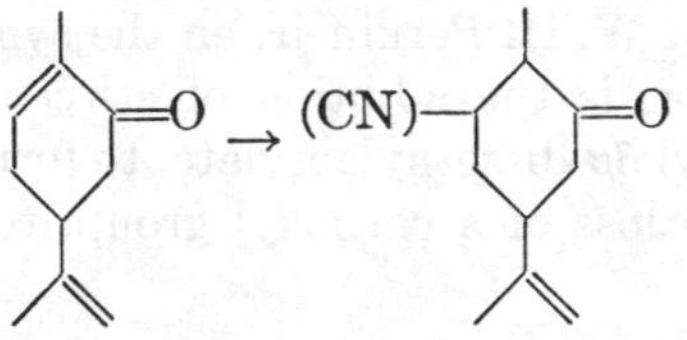

=O → (CN)— =O

The direction of these additions is always the same, the cyano-group going to the β-position. Most of them seem to go substantially to completion: no study of equilibria has hitherto been reported. As to rate, it was shown by Lapworth, in each of the examples he examined, that while the addition would scarcely go when hydrogen cyanide and the unsaturated substance were brought together, it went very easily when potassium cyanide was introduced. W. J. Jones[178] later made a kinetic study in the example of the addition of hydrogen cyanide to sodium α-cyanocinnamate. He was able to establish that the rate was proportional to the concentration of free cyanide ions:

$$\text{Rate} \propto [\mathrm{PhCH{:}C(CN){\cdot}CO_2^-}][\mathrm{CN^-}]$$

Thus he confirmed Lapworth's view that the rate-controlling step was the addition of cyanide to the β-end of the αβ-double bond:

$$\bar{\mathrm{C}}\mathrm{N} + \mathrm{Ph{\cdot}CH{=}C}\genfrac{}{}{0pt}{}{\diagup \mathrm{CN}}{\diagdown \mathrm{CO_2^-}} \rightarrow \mathrm{Ph{\cdot}}\underset{\mathrm{CN}}{\underset{|}{\mathrm{CH}}}\mathrm{{-}\bar{C}}\genfrac{}{}{0pt}{}{\diagup \mathrm{CN}}{\diagdown \mathrm{CO_2^-}}$$

[177] A. Lapworth, *J. Chem. Soc.*, 1903, **83**, 995; 1904, **85**, 1214; 1906, **89**, 945.
[178] W. J. Jones, *J. Chem. Soc.*, 1914, **105**, 1547.

The *Michael reaction*, essentially the base-catalysed addition of a pseudo-acidic ketone, ester, nitrile, or nitro-compound, to the $\alpha\beta$-double bond of a conjugated unsaturated ketone, ester, or nitrile, stands in the same relation to the above-mentioned additions of hydrogen cyanide to an $\alpha\beta$-double bond, as does the aldol addition reaction to ordinary cyanohydrin formation. Michael's original example,[179] discovered in 1887, was the addition of ethyl malonate to ethyl cinnamate, under the influence of sodium ethoxide in ethyl alcohol, to give an addition product, which could be hydrolysed, and decarboxylated, to β-phenylglutaric acid:

$$\mathrm{Ph\cdot CH{:}CH\cdot CO_2Et + CH_2(CO_2Et)_2 \rightarrow Ph\cdot CH}\Big\langle\begin{matrix}\mathrm{CH_2\cdot CO_2Et}\\ \mathrm{CH\cdot(CO_2Et)_2}\end{matrix}$$

Another example, one which found distinguished employment in the course of the work of W. H. Perkin jr. on the synthesis of degradation products of camphor, is the addition of ethyl malonate or of ethyl cyanoacetate to ethyl $\beta\beta$-dimethylacrylate, to form an ester, which can be hydrolysed, with loss of a carboxyl group, to $\beta\beta$-dimethylglutaric acid:

$$\mathrm{Me_2C{:}CH\cdot CO_2Et + CH_2(CN)\cdot CO_2Et \rightarrow Me_2C}\Big\langle\begin{matrix}\mathrm{CH_2\cdot CO_2Et}\\ \mathrm{CH(CN)\cdot CO_2Et}\end{matrix}$$

The direction of these additions is always as illustrated, the anionic part of the pseudo-acidic addendum going to the β-end of the $\alpha\beta$-double bond.

There are three standard ways of carrying out a Michael reaction. Michael's original method employed one molecular proportion of sodium ethoxide. Then there is the so-called "catalytic" method, in which one uses a much smaller amount of sodium ethoxide. And then there is Knoevenagel's method,[180] in which the catalyst is, not sodium ethoxide, but some secondary amine, such as piperidine. Reaction by the second and third of these methods is slower than by the first method.

The reversibility of the Michael reaction was first noticed by Vorländer;[181] it was studied further by Powell, Perren, and the writer.[182]

179 A. Michael, *J. prakt. Chem.*, 1887, **35**, 251.

180 E. Knoevenagel and S. Mottek, *Ber.*, 1904, **37**, 4460.

181 D. Vorländer, *Ber.*, 1900, **33**, 3185.

182 C. K. Ingold and W. J. Powell, *J. Chem. Soc.*, 1921, **119**, 1976; C. K. Ingold and E. A. Perren, *ibid.*, 1922, **121**, 1414.

Most Michael additions are exothermic, and so a larger yield of addition product results at lower temperatures, provided that one can wait the extra time that the reaction then requires. In his original experiments with ethyl cinnamate and ethyl malonate, Michael records a high yield of addition product obtained by reaction at room temperature, and a poor yield obtained by reaction at the boiling point of the alcoholic solution. Equilibrium also depends on the experimental method, in a way that can be understood if one assumes, as seems probable, that the adding pseudo-acid is a stronger acid than the pseudo-acidic adduct, or, in other words, that the former has the more stable anion. In a reaction conducted in the presence of one equivalent of sodium ethoxide, the equilibrium which determines the eventual composition of the bulk of the material is not between the three esters, in examples such as those formulated above, but between the unsaturated ester and the anions of the other two esters; and so, the stability difference just mentioned between the anions is thermodynamically inhibitory to addition. Suppose now that we change the method, employing only "catalytic" amounts of sodium ethoxide, or alternatively, using the Knoevenagel method; then the composition-determining equilibrium will really be between the three esters, and the thermodynamically inhibitory factor will have been removed; and therefore, provided that equilibrium is attained, we shall get a better yield of addition product.

As to the effect of structure on equilibrium, certain relations are fairly well established. Alkyl groups, and still more aryl groups, in either the α- or the β-position of the unsaturated ester are thermodynamically inhibitory towards addition. Presumably this is because they hyperconjugate or conjugate with the double bond, thereby tending towards its preservation. A primary steric effect may contribute to the result.[182] Preparative yields of Michael addenda with ethyl malonate or ethyl cyanoacetate may be obtained, when one conjugated phenyl group is, or two hyperconjugated methyl groups are, present in the unsaturated ester, as illustrated for cinnamic and $\beta\beta$-dimethylacrylic esters; but not when two such phenyl groups, or three methyl groups, are present. Cyanoacetic esters give generally higher equilibrium yields of addition products than do malonic esters: why this is so, is not known definitely.

The kinetics have been studied of a number of Michael additions to acrylonitrile. In these reactions the addition is thermodynamically strongly favoured. The addition of a pseudo-acid to acrylonitrile is often called the "cyanoethylation" of the pseudo-acid. We may note as an example the addition of acetylacetone to acrylonitrile in water containing potassium hydroxide.[183] The addition obeys the equation written below, which is quite similar to that found by W. J. Jones for the addition of hydrogen cyanide to the α-cyanocinnamate ion:

$$\text{Rate} \propto [\text{CH}_2{:}\text{CH}\cdot\text{CN}][(\text{CH}_3\cdot\text{CO})_2\text{CH}^-]$$

The second factor in this expression represents the concentration of acetylacetonate ion, as calculated from the basicity of the solution and the known acidity constant of acetylacetone. This kinetic form confirms the theory of the mechanism of Michael additions.

Ammonia, and primary and secondary amines, can be added to the ethenoid double bond of the $\alpha\beta$-unsaturated ketones and esters. The nitrogen atom of the amine always takes the β-position. Thus ammonia, methylamine, and dimethylamine add to mesityl oxide to give diacetonamine and its methylation products,[184] and aniline and phenylhydrazine add to methyl benzylidenemalonate to give analogously constituted addition compounds:[185]

$$(\text{CH}_3)_2\underset{\displaystyle\text{NRR}'}{\underset{|}{\text{C}}}\text{—CH}_2\cdot\text{CO}\cdot\text{CH}_3 \qquad \text{Ph}\cdot\underset{\displaystyle\text{NHPh}}{\underset{|}{\text{CH}}}\text{—CH}(\text{CO}_2\text{Me})_2$$

Ogata and his collaborators found[183] that the addition of ethanolamine to acrylonitrile (the "cyanoethylation" of ethanolamine) in water at pH 7.5–9.4 takes place through the nitrogen atom of the ethanolamine, which adds to the β-position of the acrylonitrile, to give finally $\text{HO}\cdot\text{CH}_2\cdot\text{CH}_2\cdot\text{NH}\cdot\text{CH}_2\cdot\text{CH}_2\cdot\text{CN}$. They found that this reaction obeys the rate equation,

$$\text{Rate} \propto [\text{CH}_2{:}\text{CH}_2\cdot\text{CN}][\text{NH}_2\cdot\text{CH}_2\cdot\text{CH}_2\cdot\text{OH}]$$

It is clear from this result that all additions of amines to $\alpha\beta$-unsaturated ketones, esters, or nitriles, in no more than moderately basic media, take place through the free base, rather than its anion, as the nucleophile.

The unsaturated ketones, esters, and nitriles also add alcohols in the presence of their alkoxide ions. The alkoxy-group enters the β-position. Thus, methyl benzylidenemalonate adds methanol in methanolic sodium methoxide.[186] The adduct has the structure, $\text{PhCH(OMe)}\cdot\text{CH(CO}_2\text{Me)}_2$.

The kinetics of the addition to acrylonitrile of a number of the

[183] Y. Ogata, M. Okanu, Y. Furuya, and L. Tabushi, *J. Am. Chem. Soc.*, 1956, 78, 5426.

[184] A. Hochstetter and M. Cohn, *Monatsh.*, 1903, 24, 773.

[185] R. Blank, *Ber.*, 1885, 28, 145.

[186] C. Liebermann, *Ber.*, 1893, 26, 1876.

simpler aliphatic alcohols ("cyanoethylation" of the alcohols), in the alcohols as solvent, and in the presence of an alkali-metal alkoxide as catalyst, has shown[187] that the rate obeys the equation,

$$\text{Rate} \propto [\text{CH}_2\text{:CH}_2\cdot\text{CN}][\text{OR}^-]$$

In all these cases the adding nucleophile is evidently the alkoxide ion, rather than the alcohol molecule.

We may add a note applying to all these basic mechanisms of Michael and related additions, for which we presume, and in many cases can prove, reversibility. This is that the principle of microscopic reversibility requires that the retrograde process must occur by way of a preliminary loss of a proton from the decomposing molecule to give its anionic conjugate base, followed by the unimolecular loss of an anion from the conjugate base. This is the elimination mechanism, which was labelled E1cB in Chapter IX but could not be well illustrated there. Here, however, we see it operating generally, to form an olefinic double bond, but, of course, one on which special properties are conferred by its conjugation with a carbonyl or cyano- or nitro-group (cf. Section **38a**, footnote 12).

An acid-catalysed mechanism is known for the addition of alcohols, and of water, to the $\alpha\beta$-double bond conjugated to carbonyl or carboxyl. Alcohols have been added preparatively to mesityl oxide by the use of a small amount of sulphuric acid as catalyst, the products being ethers of diacetone alcohol.[188] The addition of water under catalysis by acids to the $\alpha\beta$-double bond of acrolein and of acrylic acid and their homologues, to give hydracrolein or hydracrylic acid or their homologues, has been investigated by Lucas and his coworkers.[189] These additions are markedly reversible:

$$\text{CH}_2\text{:CH}\cdot\text{CH:O} + \text{H}_2\text{O} \overset{\text{H}^+}{\rightleftharpoons} \text{CH}_2(\text{OH})\cdot\text{CH}_2\cdot\text{CH:O}$$

$$\text{CH}_2\text{:CH}\cdot\text{CO}_2\text{H} + \text{H}_2\text{O} \overset{\text{H}^+}{\rightleftharpoons} \text{CH}_2(\text{OH})\cdot\text{CH}_2\cdot\text{CO}_2\text{H}$$

Water being the solvent, the rate in each direction was found to be proportional to the concentration of the strong acid, which was usually perchloric or nitric acid in concentrations of the order of 0.1 M to 1 M:

[187] B. A. Fett and A. Zilkha, *J. Org. Chem.*, 1963, **28**, 406.

[188] A. Hoffman, *J. Am. Chem. Soc.*, 1927, **49**, 552.

[189] S. Winstein and H. J. Lucas, *J. Am. Chem. Soc.*, 1937, **59**, 1461; D. Pressman and H. J. Lucas, *ibid.*, 1939, **61**, 2271; 1940, **62**, 2069; D. Pressman, L. Brewer, and H. J. Lucas, *ibid.*, 1942, **64**, 1117, 1122; D. Pressman and H J. Lucas, *ibid.*, p. 1953; H. J. Lucas, W. T. Stewart, and D. Pressman, *ibid.*, 1944, **66**, 1818.

$$\text{Forward rate} \propto [\alpha\beta\text{-unsat. comp.}][H^+]$$

$$\text{Backward rate} \propto [\beta\text{-hydroxy-comp.}][H^+]$$

Though formulated here as hydrogen-ion catalysed, they might in fact be general-acid catalysed. In any case, they would start with the uptake of a proton on carbonyl oxygen, so to create a carbonium ionic centre at which a water molecule could be taken up:

$$\overset{+}{H} + CH_2{:}CH{\cdot}CH{:}O \rightleftarrows \overset{+}{C}H_2{\cdot}CH{:}CH{\cdot}OH$$

$$\rightleftarrows \underset{{}^{+}OH_2}{CH_2}{\cdot}CH{:}CH{\cdot}OH \rightleftarrows \underset{OH}{CH_2}{\cdot}CH_2{\cdot}CH{:}O + H^+$$

In base-catalysed Michael and related additions to conjugated polyolefinic ketones, esters, or nitriles, such as sorbic, cinnamylidene-acetic, or cinnamylidene-malonic ester, a problem of orientation arises. Either the β- or the δ-position, in conjugated compounds such as those mentioned, is in principle positively polarisable, and is therefore a potential place of attachment of the nucleophilic addendum or the anionic portion of the weakly acidic or pseudo-acidic addendum:

X⁻ β-attack

R—C=C—C=C—C=O

X⁻ δ-attack

The reactions under consideration being strongly reversible, the question to be discussed is that of which position will actually receive, *and will succeed in holding*, the anionic portion of the addendum.

If the anionic portion enters the β-position, the protonic part of the addendum will necessarily enter the α-position, supposing the enolic form of the addition product to be thermodynamically unstable:

$$—C{=}C—\underset{}{\overset{X}{C}}—\overset{H}{C}—C{=}O$$

However, in case the anionic fragment becomes bound at the δ-carbon atom, there are two positions which the proton might enter, namely, the α- and γ-positions, again assuming the enol to be unstable:

$$—\overset{X}{C}—C{=}C—\overset{H}{C}—C{=}O \quad \text{and} \quad —\overset{X}{C}—\overset{H}{C}—C{=}C—C{=}O$$

The question of which of these forms will in fact appear is one of the kinetic and thermodynamic control of the formation of prototropic tautomers in the pentad keto-enol system, so thoroughly studied by Kon and Linstead. The principles of this matter were discussed in Section **47d,** where it was noted that kinetic control would send the proton into the α-position, while its thermodynamically most stable position depended on the substituents present. We shall therefore concern ourselves now mainly with the previous question of where the anionic part of the addendum becomes first bound, and where it finally settles down.[190]

If the orientation of uptake of the anion or other nucleophile to a conjugated polyene chain containing a carbonyl or similar end-group were kinetically controlled, the nucleophile would attach itself exclusively to the other end of the conjugated system. The reason, as we have seen before (Section **53b**), is that, in a freely conducting linear system, polarity is necessarily developed at the ends. In order to test this prediction, it would be necessary to run an addition of the type described only to conversions which are small relative to the equilibrium conversions. But as far as the writer knows, a study of products formed in such conditions has not yet been undertaken.

However, in ordinary preparative work, Michael additions are almost always run to equilibrium; and thus, in seeking an interpretation of existing observations, it is necessary to consider the orientation of addition as thermodynamically controlled, that is, as depending on the relative free energies of the end-products. In the case of certain additions, for example, of a malonic ester to a β-vinylacrylic ester, $CH_2{:}CH{\cdot}CH{:}CH{\cdot}CO_2R$, we have to think of the relative stabilities of structures of the following types:

$$
\begin{array}{ccccc}
[\beta\text{-adduct}]^- & \rightleftarrows & \text{Factors} & \rightleftarrows & [\delta\text{-adduct}]^- \\
\downarrow H^+ & & & & \downarrow H^+ \\
CH_2{:}CH{\cdot}\underset{\substack{|\\ CH(CO_2R)_2}}{CH}{\cdot}CH_2{\cdot}CO_2R & & \underset{\substack{|\\ CH(CO_2R)_2}}{CH_2}{\cdot}CH{:}CH{\cdot}CH_2{\cdot}CO_2R & \rightleftarrows & \underset{\substack{|\\ CH(CO_2R)_2}}{CH_2}{\cdot}CH_2{\cdot}CH{:}CH{\cdot}CO_2R
\end{array}
$$

Some approximately quantitative observations are available[191] concerning the proportions in which the β- and δ-adducts are present in the equilibrium product of Michael additions of malonic and cyanoacetic esters to β-vinylacrylic ester, and to various methylated homologues of the latter, namely, to the δ-methyl derivatives, that is, sorbic esters, and to α-, β-, and γ-methyl-sorbic esters. The data are summarised in Table 54-1.

[190] J. Bloom and C. K. Ingold, *J. Chem. Soc.*, **1931,** 2765; P. B. D. de la Mare. E. D. Hughes, and C. K. Ingold, *ibid.*, **1948,** 17.

[191] E. H. Farmer and T. N. Mehta, *J. Chem. Soc.*, **1931,** 1904; J. Bloom and C. K. Ingold, *ibid*, p. 2765.

TABLE 54-1.—EFFECT OF METHYL SUBSTITUTION IN β-VINYLACRYLIC ESTERS ON THE PERCENTAGE OF β-ADDUCT IN MICHAEL ADDITIONS.

$$\text{VAE (=vinylacrylic ester):— } \overset{\delta}{C}{=}\overset{\gamma}{C}{-}\overset{\beta}{C}{=}\overset{\alpha}{C}{-}CO_2R$$

VAE	Parent	δ-Me	αδ-DiMe	βδ-DiMe	γδ-DiMe
VAE+malonate[1]	0	9	—	—	—
VAE+cyanoacetate[2]	—	10	0	0	72

[1] Methyl esters used. [2] Ethyl esters used.

The exclusive δ-addition to the parent vinylacrylic ester may be interpreted on the basis that one of the prototropic tautomers of the δ-adduct is stabilised by conjugation between the olefinic bond and the terminal carboxyl group, while the β-adduct has no such compensating factor of stability. However, the δ-methyl substituent present in the sorbic esters, by its hyperconjugation with the γδ-olefinic bond of the β-adduct, confers on the latter a partly compensating stability, with the result that an appreciable proportion is present in the equilibrium product. What is thus done by a δ-methyl substituent, is undone again when an α- or a β-methyl substituent is additionally present to confer extra stability on the more stable form of the δ-adduct, by hyperconjugation with its αβ-olefinic bond. On the other hand, a γ-methyl substituent, in addition to the δ-methyl substituent, further stabilises the β-adduct by hyperconjugation, making this product actually more stable than any form of the δ-adduct.

The effect of a δ-phenyl substituent in a vinylacrylic ester on the course of Michael and similar addition processes is quite well defined: it determines the practically exclusive production of the β-adduct in equilibrium. Thus the addition of hydrogen cyanide through the agency of potassium cyanide to ethyl cinnamylidenemalonate,[192] the addition of ethyl malonate in the presence of sodium ethoxide to ethyl cinnamylideneacetate,[193] and the addition of ethyl alcohol to methyl cinnamylidenemalonate through the action of ethoxide ions in alcohol,[194] lead to the addition products formulated below:

$$Ph{\cdot}CH{:}CH{\cdot}\underset{\displaystyle CN}{\underset{|}{CH}}{\cdot}CH(CO_2Et)_2 \qquad Ph{\cdot}CH{:}CH{\cdot}\underset{\displaystyle CH(CO_2Et)_2}{\underset{|}{CH}}{\cdot}CH_2{\cdot}CO_2Et$$

$$Ph{\cdot}CH{:}CH{\cdot}\underset{\displaystyle OEt}{\underset{|}{CH}}{\cdot}CH(CO_2Me)_2$$

[192] J. Thiele and J. Meisenheimer, *Ann.*, 1899, **306**, 247.
[193] D. Vorländer and P. Groebel, *Ann.*, 1906, **345**, 206.
[194] F. W. Hinrichsen and W. Trepel, *Ann.*, 1904, **336**, 196.

This uniform result is doubtless determined by the dominating energy effect of the phenyl-to-vinyl conjugation, which only the β-adducts preserve.

The addition of methyl malonate to the hexatriene ester, methyl sorbylideneacetate, $CH_3 \cdot CH{:}CH \cdot CH{:}CH \cdot CH{:}CH \cdot CO_2Me$, yields, according to Farmer and Martin, the β-adduct and the ζ-adduct, the former preponderating, but no detected amount of δ-adduct.[195] The absence of this last can be understood, because its formation would break up a butadienoid conjugation, which either of the other two adducts can preserve.

(54c) Addition of Metal-Alkyls to Carbonyl and Conjugated Olefinic Carbonyl Compounds.—These additions lead to 1,2-adducts to carcarbonyl groups and to 1,2- and 1,4-adducts to conjugated olefinic carbonyl systems (M = metal):

$$>C{=}O + RM \rightarrow >C(R){-}O(M)$$

$$>C{=}C{-}C{=}O + RM \rightarrow >C{=}C{-}C(R){-}O(M) \quad \text{and} \quad >C(R){-}C{=}C{-}O(M)$$

There can be no doubt that they are nucleophilic additions: the organo-metal reagent delivers its alkyl group *as a carbanion*—whether preformed or not is another question—to an electrophilic centre in the unsaturated substrate, that is, either to the carbonyl carbon atom or the β-carbon atom of the conjugated olefin-carbonyl group.

In the hydrocarbon and ether solvents usually employed for these additions, any pre-formation of a carbanion would be as a member of an ion-pair in equilibrium with the original organo-metal molecule:

$$RM \rightleftharpoons R^{-}\}M^{+}$$

The ion-pair will be much the more specifically active for nucleophilic addition. But in case the equilibrium lies far to the left, the difference of concentration may outweigh that of specific reactivity sufficiently to allow nucleophilic addition to occur through the molecule.

The outstandingly important metal-alkyl reagent for carbonyl compounds is the Grignard reagent. Lithium alkyls are also important. Alkyls of metals of Groups I and II heavier than lithium and magnesium have practical value for special purposes.

To remark first on the field in general, let us note some points of

[195] E. H. Farmer and S. R. W. Martin, *J. Chem. Soc.*, 1933, 960.

comparison between alkali-metal alkyls and Grignard reagents. For a given alkyl group, the order of reactivity is believed to be

$$M = MgX < Li < Na < K$$

This series is not based on systematic measurements made under uniform conditions, but is compiled from unrelated, usually qualitative comparisons. For instance, the fact that *t*-butyl-lithium will not add to hexamethylacetone, whereas *t*-butyl-sodium adds preparatively to give (after protolysis of the adduct) tri-*t*-butylcarbinol, leads to the deduction, Li<Na. The series has, however, the support of theory, because it must represent the degree to which, with a given alkyl group in a given solvent, the equilibrium, molecule$\rightleftharpoons$ion-pair, lies towards the side of the more specifically reactive ion-pair. The same series probably also represents the order of ease of separation of the counter-ions of an ion-pair in an environment in which there is any possibility of their coming apart.

It is obvious that, for a given metal and a given solvent, the position of the equilibrium, molecule$\rightleftharpoons$ion-pair, will depend on the hydrocarbon group R in RM. If, for a particular metal and solvent, when R is a phenyl or small alkyl group, the equilibrium lies well over to the side of the molecule, then, when R = 9-fluorenyl or triphenylmethyl, which both have very much more stable anions than unsubstituted aryl or alkyl groups do, the equilibrium should be relatively displaced towards the ion-pair side. The large size and wide dispersal of charge, which help to make these anions stable, will also help to make their ion-pairing weak, wherefore in such cases we can even contemplate additions dependent on separated ions.

The physical study of the molecule$\rightleftharpoons$ion-pair equilibrium of metal-alkyls has not yet made much progress, and therefore these statements of general principle lack specific confirmation. But we can try them in tentative explanation of a main feature of difference, which many investigators have emphasized, between alkali-metal-alkyls and Grignard reagents. This has reference to the extent to which each type of reagent gives 1,2- and 1,4-adducts, when both are possible, as in additions to conjugated olefinic carbonyl compounds. The two types of reagent usually do different things in this respect, but the difference is not always the same way round.[196] A collection of recorded results is given in Table 54-2.

Grignard reagents with unsubstituted phenyl or alkyl groups give mainly 1,4-adducts with $\alpha\beta$-unsaturated ketones. At one time, this

[196] T. Eicher, "Chemistry of the Carbonyl Group," Editor S. Patai, Interscience Publishers, Chap. 13, p. 621.

TABLE 54-2.—1,2-ADDITION AND 1,4-ADDITION OF GRIGNARD REAGENTS AND OF ORGANO-LITHIUM AND ORGANO-SODIUM COMPONENTS TO $\alpha\beta$-UNSATURATED KETONES.

Addendum	$\alpha\beta$-Unsaturated ketone	Solvent	Mode addn.	Yield*	Ref.	Assignment reacting species†
Phenyl-MgBr	Chalcone‡	Et_2O	1,4	94	197	molecule
i-Propyl-MgBr	*cyclo*Hex-2-en-1-one	Et_2O	1,4	65	198, 199	molecule
	Pent-3-en-2-one	Et_2O	1,4	66	199	molecule
	Hex-3-en-2-one	Et_2O	1,4	57	199	molecule
9-Fluorenyl-MgBr	Mesityl oxide	Xylene	1,2	30	200	ion-pair
Trityl-MgCl	Cinnamaldehyde	C_6H_6	1,2	?	202	ion-pair
Phenyl-Li	Chalcone	Et_2O	1,2 1,4	69 13	197	mainly ion-pair
Phenyl-Na	Chalcone	Et_2O	1,2 1,4	60 14	197	mainly ion-pair
9-Fluorenyl-Li	Mesityl oxide	Ligroin	1,4	32	200	sepd. ions
	Benzalacetone	Ligroin	1,4	17	200	sepd. ions
	Chalcone	Ligroin	1,4	?	200	sepd. ions
9-Fluorenyl-Na	Chalcone	EtOH	1,4	27	201	sepd. ions
Trityl-Na	Cinnamaldehyde	?	1,4	?	196	sepd. ions

* Preparative yields of the products specified, *i.e.*, lower limits to the amounts formed. Where a second product is not mentioned, its presence could not be detected.

† Tentative: see text.

‡ Chalcone = ω-benzylidene-acetophenone. (The old, short name is too convenient to drop for the sake of "official" nomenclature.)

was explained on the basis that the Grignard reagent spanned the 1- and 4-atoms of the conjugated system in a transition state involving a six-membered ring. This would require that conjugated double bonds, originally of the ketone, are *cis*-related in the transition state, and would exclude 1,4-addition to *cyclo*hex-2-en-1-one, in which the double bonds are necessarily *trans*-related. In fact, 1,4-addition in that case is just about as easy as in the open-chain analogues, pent-3-en-2-one and hex-3-en-2-one, in which the double bonds could come into *cis*-relation if they were required to do so. The suggestion in Table 54-2 is that these Grignard reagents go as molecules to where most of the

[197] E. P. Kohler, *Am. Chem. J.*, 1907, **38**, 511; H. Gilman and R. H. Kirby, *J. Am. Chem. Soc.*, 1941, **63**, 2046; W. I. Sullivan, F. W. Swanner, W. J. Humphlett, and C. R. Hauser, *J. Org. Chem.*, 1961, **26**, 2306.

[198] F. C. Whitmore and G. W. Pedlar, *J. Am. Chem. Soc.*, 1941, **63**, 758.

[199] E. R. Alexander and G. R. Coroar, *J. Am. Chem. Soc.*, 1951, **73**, 2721.

[200] H. S. Tucker and M. Whalley, *J. Chem. Soc.*, **1949**, 50.

[201] R. S. Taylor and R. Connor, *J. Org. Chem.*, 1941, **6**, 696.

[202] J. Schmidlin and H. H. Hodgson, *Ber.*, 1908, **41**, 430.

positive charge in the ketone will develop, the β-position, and there deliver their carbanions, so liberating the $MgBr^+$ cation subsequently to co-ordinate with the oxygen atom of the carbonyl group. The fluorenyl and trityl Grignard compounds may, on the other hand, combine as ion-pairs, through their pre-formed cations, with the only oxygen atom there is in the systems investigated, that of the carbonyl group, when the ion-pairing forces will constrain the carbanion to combine at carbonyl carbon.

Turning to the alkali-metal-alkyl series, the suggestion in Table 54-2 is that phenyl-lithium and phenyl-sodium act in ion-pair form, and thus co-ordinate through their cations with the oxygen atom of the substrate. We have to suppose that any partial positive charges on the substrate are insufficient easily to pull the paired ions apart, and that therefore the nucleophilic attack is largely constrained to the location of the carbonyl carbon atom. For the fluorenyl- and trityl-lithium and sodium addenda, it is suggested that the attack is either by the ion-pair or by the dissociated ions, according to the solvent, but that, in hydrocarbon solvents, the ions of the ion-pairs get separated by the charges on the substrate, so that in all cases the nucleophilic addition is by a separated anion; and it will occur where the positive charge on the substrate is strongest, the 4-position. It is difficult to go beyond such tentative interpretations, until some definitive electrochemical work is done on the materials involved.

There is more to be said of *Grignard additions to carbonyl compounds.* As explained in Section **26e**, it is at length clear that simple aliphatic and aromatic Grignard compounds are essentially tetrahedral monomeric co-ordination structures, of the type $[Mg^{II}RX(OEt_2)_2]^0$, in efficiently co-ordinating ether solvents. The chlorides have a marked tendency to dimerise, probably by halogen bridging, but in the bromides and iodides this tendency is relatively weak. All Grignard halides are participants in a somewhat mobile equilibrium (called the Schlenk equilibrium),[203] which may be formulated,

$$2RMgX \rightleftharpoons R_2Mg + MgX_2$$

Here, then, is a problem: Grignard addition might go either through RMgX, or through R_2Mg, even when the latter is only a minor component of the equilibrium. For the dialkyl of any Group II metal will split off a carbanion more easily than will the monoalkyl-halide of the metal (Section **26**).

There is another apparent problem in a complication that may be

[203] W. Schlenk and W. Schlenk jr., *Ber.*, 1929, **62**, 920.

more apparent than real. It has been shown spectrally[204] that substituted benzophenones and methylmagnesium bromide in ethyl ether are partly associated into a complex, and that, as the normal Grignard addition takes place, the uncomplexed ketones and the complex disappear together, at a rate which is of first order when the Grignard compound is in great excess. Obviously, the ketone is partly replacing one ether molecule, in an instantaneously established co-ordination pre-equilibrium. This will make no essential difference to the Grignard addition. The observed rate-constant will be a weighted mean of the rate-constant of addition of the ether-co-ordinated reagent, and of the ether-ketone-co-ordinated reagent; but the two rates are probably closely similar to each other, and hence to their weighted mean. The first-order rate-constants were found to rise with the concentration of Grignard reagent, present in excess, linearly up to 0.1 M, and after that less steeply. This implies second-order kinetics overall in dilute solution. The tendency of the kinetic order to fall in more concentrated solution probably reflects the tendency of the Grignard bromides to dimerise appreciably at higher concentrations.

Kinetic results on Grignard additions have been reported in several investigations, which have been considered by the investigators concerned as mutually discrepant; but this is not necessarily so. Anteunis showed[205] that the reactions of methylmagnesium bromide and iodide with benzophenone in ether-benzene, and with pinacolone in ether, have overall third-order kinetics:

$$\text{Rate} \propto [\text{ketone}][\text{stoich. RMgX}]^2$$

But when, in the work with methylmagnesium bromide and pinacolone in ether, an excess of magnesium bromide was added initially, the kinetics became overall of second order:

$$\text{Rate} \propto [\text{ketone}][\text{ stoich. RMgX}]$$

Bikales and Becker examined the addition of methylmagnesium bromide to benzophenone in tetrahydrofuran,[206] and obtained results fitting the same second-order kinetic equation, though only now over the earlier portion of the reaction. Later, the reaction rate dropped

[204] S. G. Smith, *Tetrahedron Letters*, **1963**, 409; S. G. Smith and G. Su, *J. Am. Chem. Soc.*, 1964, **86**, 2750. Kinetics characteristic of addition of methyl magnesium bromide in excess to acetone in ethyl ether by way of a pre-equilibrium Grignard-acetone complex have been demonstrated by E. C. Ashby, R. B. Duke, and H. M. Neumann, *ibid.*, 1967, **89**, 1904.

[205] M. Anteunis, *J. Org. Chem.*, 1961, **26**, 4214; 1962, **27**, 596.

[206] N. M. Bikales and E. I. Becker, *Can. J. Chem.*, 1963, **41**, 1329.

sharply. In these equations [stoich. RMgX] means the stoicheiometric concentration of the Grignard reagent, as calculated without taking the Schlenk equilibrium into account.

The Schlenk equilibrium embraces three kinetic cases, between which transitional situations are possible. The cases are as follows. Case (a): The Grignard reagent is stored mainly as the alkylmagnesium halide, but reacts through the minor equilibrium concentration of the dialkylmagnesium. Case (b): The Grignard reagent is stored almost wholly as alkylmagnesium halide, and it reacts in this form. Case (c): The Grignard reagent is stored mainly as the dialkylmagnesium, and it reacts in that form. There is, of course, no case in which the dialkylmagnesium is the storage form but the alkylmagnesium halide is the reaction form, because of the greater specific reactivity of the dialkylmagnesium. In cases (a) and (c) the addition reaction is

$$R_2'C{=}O + R_2Mg \rightarrow R_2'CR{-}OMgR$$

whilst in case (b) it is

$$R_2'C{=}O + RMgX \rightarrow R_2'CR{-}OMgX$$

If case (a) obtains, and if the concentration of the magnesium halide of the Schlenk equilibrium is buffered for any reason, for instance, because the solution is saturated with that salt, as Anteunis's ether-benzene solvent would be saturated with magnesium bromide, or because, after an initial period, the concentration of magnesium bromide has so grown that its proportional variation is relatively slow, then $[R_2Mg] \propto [RMgX]^2 \approx [\text{stoich. } RMgX]^2$, and one observed the third-order kinetics, which Anteunis did in fact observe.

Suppose, however, that, in an ether solvent, in which magnesium bromide is easily soluble, one adds enough magnesium bromide so to suppress the dimethylmagnesium that case (b) obtains. Then the storage and reaction forms of the Grignard reagent will be identical, and one will observe the second-order kinetics, which Anteunis did in fact observe in such conditions.

Again, suppose that one works in tetrahydrofuran, in which magnesium bromide is so sparingly soluble that the Schlenk equilibrium becomes drawn over to the side of the dialkylmagnesium. One then establishes case (c), in which, once again, the storage and reaction forms of the Grignard reagent will be identical, so that second-order kinetics will be observed, as, in fact, Bikales and Becker did observe them in that solvent. But now there will be a difference, in that one alkyl group in every two will be held up in the residue —OMgR of the adduct, until a slower reaction of addition to another ketone molecule liberates it therefrom. Bikales and Becker found that their second-order law failed at around 40% of reaction of the ketone, and that then the reaction began to go much more slowly, so that at 60% of reaction of the ketone it was going at only about 1% of its original specific rate. This small residual rate would be that of the addition of $RMgOCRR_2'$, as a Grignard reagent, to $R_2'C{:}O$.[196]

(54d) Heterolytic Addition of Hydrogen to Carbonyl and Conjugated Olefinic Carbonyl Compounds.—Any compound capable of transferring a hydride ion, H^-, to positively polarised carbon, as of a carbonyl group, acts as a nucleophilic reducing agent. One thinks at once of *metal hydrides*, such as lithium aluminium hydride, and of *metal alkyls having β-hydrogen*, such as Grignard reagents having that feature, which usually waste some of the experimenter's hard-won ketone by reducing it:

$$M\text{—}H \; \overset{|}{\underset{|}{C}}\text{=}O \rightarrow M^+ + H\overset{|}{\underset{|}{C}}\text{—}O^-$$

$$M\text{—}CR_2\text{—}CR_2\text{—}H \; \overset{|}{\underset{|}{C}}\text{=}O \rightarrow M^+ + CR_2{:}CR_2 + H\overset{|}{\underset{|}{C}}\text{—}O^-$$

Alkaline solutions of aldehydes constitute a wide class of reducing agents. They will reduce a carbonyl group, in particular, that of the aldehyde itself:

$$RCHO + OH^- \rightleftharpoons R\text{—}\overset{OH}{\underset{O^-}{C}}\text{—}H \; \overset{R}{\underset{H}{C}}\text{=}O \rightarrow R\text{—}\overset{OH}{\underset{O}{C}} + H\overset{R}{\underset{H}{C}}\text{—}O^-$$

This is the *Cannizzaro reaction*:

$$2R\cdot CHO \xrightarrow{OH^-} R\cdot CH_2\cdot OH + R\cdot CO_2^-$$

It was discovered in 1853 by Cannizzaro[207] in the example of benzaldehyde. It is shown by most aldehydes that do not undergo the aldol reaction, or suffer other interfering conversions under the influence of alkali: typical examples are formaldehyde, pivalaldehyde (trimethylacetaldehyde), benzaldehyde and substituted benzaldehydes, and furfuraldehyde.

[207] S. Cannizzaro, *Ann.*, 1853, **88**, 129.

The problem of mechanism presents its simplest aspect in the reaction as ordinarily conducted without surface catalysts, in homogeneous solution in hydroxylic solvents. The solvents include notably water, supposing the aldehyde to be soluble, methyl alcohol, and aqueous dioxan. In such conditions, the kinetics of the Cannizzaro reaction of benzaldehyde and some of its substitution products, of furfuraldehyde, and of formaldehyde have been examined. It would appear that there are two rate laws, which can be observed separately, in one case or another, at suitable alkali concentrations. One is the third-order law,

$$\text{Rate} \propto [\text{aldehyde}]^2[\text{OH}^-]$$

the other the fourth-order law,

$$\text{Rate} \propto [\text{aldehyde}]^2[\text{OH}^-]^2$$

The reaction of benzaldehyde in methyl alcohol, and in aqueous methyl alcohol or dioxan, follows the third-order law at the usual alkali concentrations.[208] The reaction of furfuraldehyde in water or in aqueous methyl alcohol follows the fourth-order law,[209] but in aqueous dioxan exhibits mixed-order kinetics, which can be brought close to a limiting third-order form.[210] The reaction of formaldehyde would appear to have a limiting fourth-order form,[211] and also lower reaction orders down to third.[212] The internal Cannizzaro reaction, in which phenylglyoxal is converted by means of aqueous methyl alcoholic alkali into mandelic acid, has a rate proportional to the product [phenylglyoxal][OH^-], a kinetic law which corresponds to the third-order law for the ordinary intermolecular Cannizzaro reaction.[213] In some of these kinetic studies it has been shown that the reactions measured are not affected either by peroxides or by antioxidants.

The effect of substituents on the rate of the Cannizzaro reaction of benzaldehyde seems qualitatively straightforward: electropositive groups of $+I$ or $+M$ type retard reaction, while electronegative of $-I$ or $-M$ type accelerate it, as the following reaction-rate series[208,214]

[208] E. L. Molt, *Rec. trav. chim.*, 1937, **56**, 233; A. Eitel and G. Lock, *Monatsh.*, 1939, **72**, 392; E. Tommila, *Ann. Acad. Sci. Fennicae*, 1942, **A**, **59**, No. 8.

[209] K. H. Geib, *Z. physik. Chem.*, 1934, **A**, **169**, 41.

[210] A. Eitel, *Monatsh.*, 1942, **74**, 136.

[211] H. v. Euler and T. Lövgren, *Z. anorg. Chem.*, 1925, **127**, 123.

[212] I. I. Paul, *J. Gen. Chem.* (U.S.S.R.), 1941, **11**, 1121; V. Pajunen, *Ann. Acad. Sci. Fennicae*, 1950, **A**, **2**, No. 87; R. J. L. Martin, *Austral. J. Chem.*, 1954, **7**, 335.

[213] E. R. Alexander, *J. Am. Chem. Soc.*, 1947, **69**, 289.

[214] A. Weissberger and R. Hasse, *J. Chem. Soc.*, **1934**, 535.

illustrates:

$$p\text{-Me}_2\text{N} < p\text{-MeO} < p\text{-Alk} < \text{H} < p\text{-Cl} < m\text{-Cl} < m\text{-NO}_2$$

It was shown by Fredenhagen and Bonhoeffer[215] that, when the Cannizzaro reaction of formaldehyde, and that of benzaldehyde, are conducted in deuterium water, no carbon-bound deuterium appears in the products. The same was true of the internal Cannizzaro reaction, which glyoxal undergoes when it is converted in alkaline aqueous solution into glycollic acid. These experiments showed that the hydrogen is transferred from one aldehyde molecule to the other, or from one aldehydic group to the other, directly, and not by a sequence of exchanges involving the medium.

On the basis of such of these facts as were known in 1940, Hammett[216] suggested the mechanism, which is today generally believed to be a correct representation of the uncatalysed homogeneous reaction in aqueous solvents. It is assumed that the aldehyde, by interaction with hydroxide ions, can produce two reducing anions, the first more easily than the second. The first is an anion of moderate hydride-ion-donating power, formed by simple addition of a hydroxide ion; and the second, which has the same capacity more strongly developed, is formed from the first by the transfer of its proton to another hydroxide ion. The reducing function of these hypothetical intermediates may be represented as follows:

```
      O⁻                  O⁻
      |                   |
  R—C—H               R—C—H
      |                   |
      OH                  O⁻
```

The ions are assumed to arise in rapidly established equilibria between the aldehyde molecule and the hydroxide ions: the concentrations of the singly and doubly charged ions are therefore proportional to [aldehyde][OH^-] and [aldehyde][OH^-]^2, respectively. It is supposed that neither of these anions is capable of splitting off a hydride ion in a unimolecular way, but that either will transfer a hydride ion in bimolecular fashion to a suitable acceptor, in particular to a carbonyl carbon atom of another aldehyde molecule. The observed rate-laws follow:

[215] H. Fredenhagen and K. F. Bonhoeffer, *Z. physik. Chem.*, 1938, A, 181, 379.

[216] L. P. Hammett, "Physical Organic Chemistry," McGraw-Hill, New York, 1940, p. 350.

$$\text{R}\cdot\overset{\displaystyle\text{O}^-}{\underset{\displaystyle\text{OH}}{\text{C}}}\text{—H} + \text{R}\cdot\text{CH}{=}\text{O} \xrightarrow[\text{order}]{\text{3rd}} \text{R}\cdot\text{C}\begin{matrix}{=}\text{O}\\ \text{—OH}\end{matrix} + \text{R}\cdot\overset{\displaystyle\text{H}}{\text{C}}\text{H—O}^-$$

$$\text{R}\cdot\overset{\displaystyle\text{O}^-}{\underset{\displaystyle\text{O}^-}{\text{C}}}\text{—H} + \text{R}\cdot\text{CH}{=}\text{O} \xrightarrow[\text{order}]{\text{4th}} \text{R}\cdot\text{C}\begin{matrix}{=}\text{O}\\ \text{—O}^-\end{matrix} + \text{R}\cdot\overset{\displaystyle\text{H}}{\text{C}}\text{H—O}^-$$

The intramolecular Cannizzaro reaction, as of phenylglyoxal to mandelic acid under the influence of alkali, is, according to this mechanism, nothing other than a saturated nucleophilic rearrangement, of the type of many of those discussed in Chapter X, notably the benzil-benzilic acid rearrangement, in which the shifting group is phenyl, instead of hydrogen as here:

$$\text{O}{=}\underset{\displaystyle\text{Ph}}{\text{C}}\text{—}\overset{\displaystyle\text{H}}{\underset{\displaystyle\text{OH}}{\text{C}}}\text{—O}^- \rightarrow \bar{\text{O}}\text{—}\overset{\displaystyle\text{H}}{\underset{\displaystyle\text{Ph}}{\text{C}}}\text{—}\underset{\displaystyle\text{OH}}{\text{C}}{=}\text{O}$$

Reduction by *metals dissolving in protic media* superficially seems a very different kind of process from the hydride-ion transferring reactions just considered: but the difference may be more apparent than real. We have an immediate hint that dissolving-metal reductions, like the hydride-transfer reactions, are nucleophilic additions, in the types of substrate which are most easily reduced by dissolving metals—carbonyl and conjugated olefinic carbonyl compounds, and analogous cyano- and nitro-compounds.

The idea that hydrogen generated at the surface of a dissolving metal is a distinct, chemically active form of hydrogen is of early origin. The specialisation of that view which regards "nascent" hydrogen as atomic hydrogen was that most widely considered in the first three decades of the present century. One did not know then the tests for homolytic processes, nor, for much of the time, the way to recognise and classify heterolytic processes by the nature of the substrates on which reagents most easily act (Chapter V). In 1929, Burton and the writer developed the view that the "nascent" hydrogen of dissolving metals consists, not of atoms, but of electrons and protons supplied from different sources.[217]

[217] H. Burton and C. K. Ingold, *J. Chem. Soc.*, **1929**, 2022.

A metal was represented by the model of an electron gas enclosed in potential walls. It was assumed that the electrons can escape through any sufficient breach in these walls, which is created by the adsorption of an electrophilic cation or molecule. They may so escape to an adsorbed hydrogen ion, which thereby yields atomic and finally molecular hydrogen. Or they may escape to a hydrogen ion, through an adsorbed, unsaturated, and therefore electrically conducting organic molecule, which thereby becomes reduced. This molecule must be electrophilic: typically it needs a $-E$ group, such as a carbonyl, carboxyl, cyano-, nitroso-, or nitro-group, in order that it will be able to create the positively polarised, electrophilic centre required for an adsorption that will provide a way of escape for the conduction electrons of the metal. The needed level of electrophilic reactivity will depend much on the work-function of the metal. For a metal such as sodium, dissolving in alcohol, even an aryl group at the end of an unsaturated system, as in styrene, or stilbene, is sufficiently polarisable to allow effective adsorption of the olefinic unit; for we know that these and similar unsaturated aromatic hydrocarbons can be reduced by dissolving sodium.[218] For a metal such as magnesium, an aryl group does not suffice, but the carbonyl group is adequately electrophilic, as is shown by the reduction of acetone by magnesium alone to the magnesium salt of pinacol.[219] For metals such as amalgamated zinc or tin, even the carbonyl group does not possess a sufficient electron-affinity, except with the assistance of a strong acid: it is a plausible hypothesis that the conjugate acid of the carbonyl compound is then the actual electron acceptor, as in the example of the reduction of an aldehyde or ketone by Clemmensen's method.[220]

Whether the first proton enters the reducible system before, during, or after the transfer of electrons from the metal, its presence will normally be required to hold the transferred electrons during desorption. This may take place after the reception of only one electron, as in pinacol formation. It occurs more usually when two electrons have been taken up, octets have been completed, and a negative charge has been acquired by the organic system. The components, $H^+ + 2e$, of a hydride ion, H^-, have now been added in this surface reaction, which is evidently to be classified as heterolytic, and, more particularly, as a nucleophilic addition, Ad_N. After desorption, the reduction may be assumed to be completed homogeneously by the uptake of a second proton H^+ from the medium:

[218] A. Klages, *Ber.*, 1902, **35**, 2642; A. Klages and R. Keil, *Ber.*, 1903, **36**, 1632.
[219] F. Couturier and L. Meunier, *Compt. rend.*, 1905, **140**, 721.
[220] E. Clemmensen, *Ber.*, 1913, **46**, 1837; 1914, **47**, 51, 681.

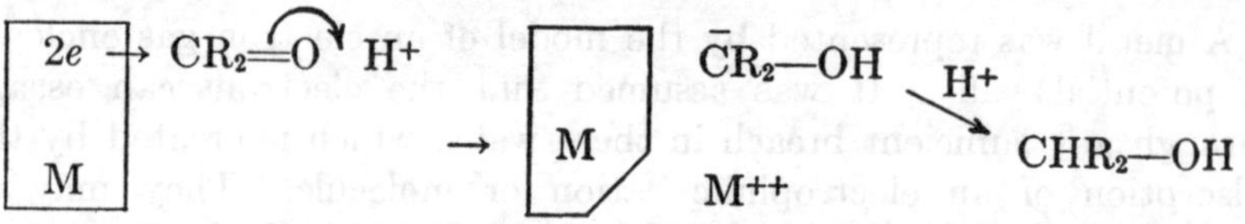

$$\boxed{2e \rightarrow CR_2{=}O\ \ H^+ \quad M} \rightarrow \boxed{M}\ \ \bar{C}R_2{-}OH \ \ M^{++} \xrightarrow{H^+} CHR_2{-}OH$$

The main application which was made of this picture of the reduction process was to the orientation of such reductions of conjugated unsaturated systems. Reduction by dissolving metals was regarded as a nucleophilic addition: the initial uptake of H^- corresponded to that of CN^- or $CH(CO_2Et)_2^-$ in cyanohydrin formation or the Michael reaction, while the final uptake of H^+ was of the same nature as the final step in the other nucleophilic additions. However there was one great difference between the reductions and the other additions: for once the hydride ion enters the reducible system, it remains there. Furthermore, neither it, nor the finally added proton, can usually be re-ionised, or re-transferred, as a proton, under the conditions of the reduction: whether we think of, say, the reduction of muconic acid by sodium amalgam in water, or the reduction of 1,4-diphenylbuta-1,3-diene by sodium amalgam in alcohol, the conditions are scarcely ever basic enough, nor is the temperature high enough, to produce prototropic equilibrium in the reduction product. Therefore orientation in the reduction of conjugated systems by dissolving metals is normally controlled kinetically and not thermodynamically, quite unlike the cyanohydrin reaction, or the Michael reaction.[221]

The significance of this cannot be better illustrated than by recounting some of the early history of the study of the reduction of conjugated unsaturated systems. The matter began in the course of Baeyer's investigation of the structure of the benzene ring (Section **13a**). He was led to examine the reduction of the terephthalic acid. He showed[222] that the primary reduction product given by sodium amalgam was the 2,5-diene acid having the two added hydrogen atoms adjacent to the carboxyl groups. This was not the thermodynamically most stable dihydro-compound, because on treatment with alkali it underwent an isomerisation, which could be followed through two stages:

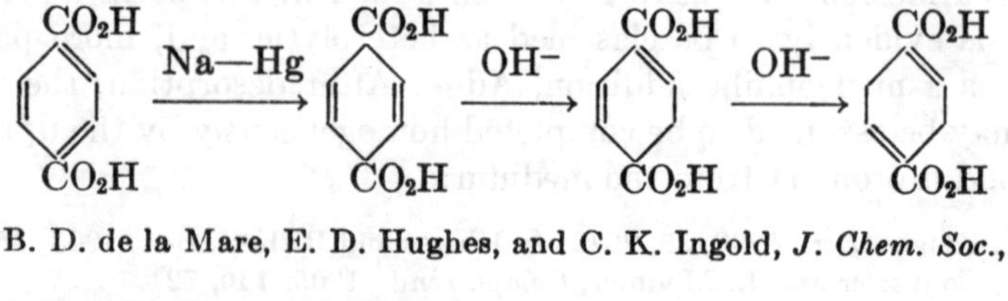

$$C_6H_4(CO_2H)_2 \xrightarrow{Na-Hg} \text{(2,5-diene)} \xrightarrow{OH^-} \text{(isomer)} \xrightarrow{OH^-} \text{(isomer)}$$

[221] P. B. D. de la Mare, E. D. Hughes, and C. K. Ingold, *J. Chem. Soc.*, **1948**, 17.

[222] A. v. Baeyer, *Ann.*, 1889, **251**, 257.

Baeyer and Rupe then examined muconic acid,[223] the simplest butadiene derivative having terminal carboxyl groups. On reduction by sodium amalgam, it gave the $\beta\gamma$-unsaturated dihydro-compound, again with added hydrogen atoms adjacent to the carboxyl groups. And this was not the stable dihydro-derivative, because it could be converted by means of alkali into the $\alpha\beta$-unsaturated isomer:

$$CO_2H\cdot CH{:}CH\cdot CH{:}CH\cdot CO_2H \xrightarrow[\text{Hg}]{\text{Na-}} CO_2H\cdot CH_2\cdot CH{:}CH\cdot CH_2\cdot CO_2H$$

$$\xrightarrow{OH^-} CO_2H\cdot CH{:}CH\cdot CH_2\cdot CH_2\cdot CO_2H$$

Shortly afterwards it was shown that cinnamylideneacetic acid,[224] and also cinnamylidenemalonic acid,[225] on reduction by sodium amalgam in nearly neutral solution, gave $\beta\gamma$-unsaturated dihydro-acids, with the added hydrogen adjacent to the carboxyl and phenyl groups. These products were thermodynamically unstable, and were converted by alkali into their $\alpha\beta$-unsaturated isomers:

$$Ph\cdot CH{:}CH\cdot CH{:}CH\cdot CO_2H \xrightarrow[\text{Hg}]{\text{Na-}} Ph\cdot CH_2\cdot CH{:}CH\cdot CH_2\cdot CO_2H$$

$$\xrightarrow{OH^-} Ph\cdot CH_2\cdot CH_2\cdot CH{:}CH\cdot CO_2H$$

$$Ph\cdot CH{:}CH\cdot CH{:}C(CO_2H)_2 \xrightarrow[\text{Hg}]{\text{Na-}} Ph\cdot CH_2\cdot CH{:}CH\cdot CH(CO_2H)_2$$

$$\xrightarrow{OH^-} Ph\cdot CH_2\cdot CH_2\cdot CH{:}C(CO_2H)_2$$

It was known[226] that naphthalene on reduction by means of sodium in boiling ethyl alcohol gives a 1,4-dihydro-derivative. Strauss showed[227] that 1,4-diphenylbutadiene, on reduction by sodium amalgam in alcohol, gives the 2,3-unsaturated dihydro-compound, with added hydrogen atoms adjacent to the phenyl groups:

$$PhCH{:}CH\cdot CH{:}CH\cdot Ph \rightarrow Ph\cdot CH_2\cdot CH{:}CH\cdot CH_2\cdot Ph$$

Although this product was not isomerised, one may feel sure that it is

[223] A. v. Baeyer and H. Rupe, *Ann.*, 1890, **256**, 1.

[224] R. Fittig and T. Hoffmann, *Ann.*, 1894, **283**, 308.

[225] J. Thiele and J. Meisenheimer, *Ann.*, 1899, **306**, 225; C. N. Riiber, *Ber.*, 1904, **37**, 3120.

[226] E. Bamberger and W. Lodter, *Ann.*, 1895, **288**, 74.

[227] F. Strauss, *Ann.*, 1905, **342**, 190.

TABLE 54-3.—EFFECT OF METHYL SUBSTITUTION IN β-VINYLACRYLIC ACID OR ITS ANION ON THE PERCENTAGE OF αβ-DIHYDRO-DERIVATIVE FORMED IN AQUEOUS REDUCTION BY SODIUM AMALGAM.

VAA (=vinylacrylic acid):— $\overset{\delta}{C}=\overset{\gamma}{C}-\overset{\beta}{C}=\overset{\alpha}{C}-CO_2H$

VAA	Parent	δ-Me	αδ-DiMe	βδδ-TriMe
Alkaline medium	0	40	28	38
Acidic medium	18	55	—	—

thermodynamically unstable, and could be completely converted by strong bases at high temperatures into its 1,2-double-bonded isomer. Finally, Kuhn and Winterstein showed[228] that 1,6-diphenylhexatriene, 1,8-diphenyloctatetraene, and 1,10-diphenylpentadecaene gave, by reduction with sodium amalgam in alcohol, their 1,6-, 1,8-, and 1,10-dihydro-derivatives respectively: in each case hydrogen entered the positions adjoining the phenyl groups.

All these examples illustrate a kinetically controlled orientation of reduction. The polyene chain will, for reasons given already in relation to other addition processes, develop positive polarisation, and will therefore become adsorbed by the dissolving metal, at one end or the other; and it will be at the δ-end in an example such as cinnamylideneacetic acid. The first proton to be taken up by the polyene chain will, then, add at the other end; and the second proton will add at the first end, after its release by desorption. These proton co-ordinations can occur more quickly where stated than elsewhere. For, as has been discussed in relation to prototropy, and to certain other conjugative additions, the transition states for co-ordination (and heterolysis) at carbon adjoining a strongly electron-absorbing group are stabilised by electronic resonance with the latter, thus allowing faster reaction there than in other positions.

The effect of methyl groups on orientation in amalgam reductions is not even qualitatively similar to that of phenyl groups. This may be illustrated by some measurements[217] summarised in Table 54-3. They relate to the proportions of αβ- and αδ-dihydro-derivatives produced by the reduction of β-vinylacrylic acid, $CH_2{:}CH\cdot CH{:}CH\cdot CO_2H$, and some of its methylated homologues, by means of sodium amalgam, either in aqueous sodium carbonate solution, or in aqueous acetic acid. The first hydrogen atom adds to the α-position in every case, and the second hydrogen atom to either the β- or the δ-position. One sees that, on passing from vinylacrylic acid to sorbic acid, the δ-methyl group present in the latter, far from favouring αδ-addition as

[228] R. Kuhn and A. Winterstein, *Helv. Chim. Acta*, 1928, **11**, 123.

would a δ-phenyl group, actually displaces the point of combination of the second hydrogen atom from the δ-position over to the β-position: a β-methyl substituent, additionally introduced, partly displaces it back again; while an extra δ-methyl group reverses this effect.

From the viewpoint of theory, we have to consider, in its kinetic aspect, the reactivity of a desorbed anion of a type which could react either as though its charge were in the δ-position and its double bond in the βγ-position, or as though it had the other possible distribution of charge and double bond:

$$\overset{\delta-}{C_\delta}\text{—}C_\gamma\text{—}\overset{\delta-}{C_\beta}\text{—}CH_2\text{—}X$$

As to this, we should expect a qualitative difference between the effect of a phenyl and of a methyl group, situated, for example, in the δ-position. For the hyperconjugation of methyl is unidirectional, and this group cannot do by hyperconjugation what phenyl can do by conjugation, namely, stabilise a *negative* charge on an adjoining atom, and therefore stabilise the transition states of reactions which create or destroy such a charge. All that a δ-methyl group can do is to hyperconjugate with the double bond, thereby tending to localise it in the γδ-position, and the negative charge in the β-position. That is the explanation given of why a δ-methyl group, unlike a δ-phenyl group, favours the addition of the second hydrogen atom in the β-position. The application to a β-methyl group is similar. As to the general difference that alkaline reduction gives more αδ-addition than does acid reduction, the suggestion is that the electrostatic effect of the carboxylate-ion group present in the alkaline medium, relatively to that of the carboxyl group in the acid medium, tends to set the negative charge on carbon in the desorbed mesomeric carbanion in the more remote of the two possible positions.

(54e) Base-Initiated Polymerisation of Olefinic Compounds by Self-Addition.[229]—The polymerisation of olefinic compounds by strong bases has been recorded in scattered observations since the turn of the century.[230] Thus, von Pechmann polymerised ethyl crotonate by means of sodium ethoxide, Bruylants allyl cyanide by the agency of sodium ethoxide, and by that of a Grignard reagent, and Schmidt and Reitz nitro-olefins by the use of aqueous sodium hydroxide.[231] Of

[229] M. Szwarc and J. Smid, "Progress in Reaction Kinetics," Vol. 2, Pergamon Press, London, 1964, p. 219.

[230] D. C. Pepper, *Quart. Revs. Chem. Soc.*, 1954, **8**, 114.

[231] H. v. Pechmann, *Ber.*, 1900, **33**, 3329; P. Bruylants, *Bull. Soc. chim. Belges*, 1923, **32**, 317; E. Schmidt and G. Rutz, *Ber.*, 1928, **61**, 2142.

course, one could not know what was happening in such reactions, until after Staudinger's elucidation of the chain character of polymerisation generally in 1920.[114] Nor could the chemical nature of the initiation and propagation of chain growth be appreciated, until the general theory of the heterolytic reactions of organic chemistry, which began its rapid development in 1926, had made some progress. In fact, it was not until the late 1940's that it became understood that the function of the strong base was to add as a nucleophile to a monomer molecule, so to give a carbanion, which then became the nucleophile that would add to a second monomer molecule, and so on.

The polymerisation of olefins by means of alkali metals has been known since 1910.[232] The important work of Harries on the polymerisation of butadiene and of isoprene with sodium[233] became for a time the basis of the large-scale production of synthetic rubber in Germany. About that time Schlenk described the polymerisation of styrene and of 1-phenylbutadiene with finely divided sodium suspended in ether.[234]

The nature of these alkali-metal-initiated polymerisations, and their essential identity in mechanism of chain growth with base-initiated, in particular, organo-metal-initiated, polymerisations, were largely elucidated by Ziegler in the years around 1930.[235] There was a preconception at the time, which Schlenk supported, that, alkali-metals being odd-electron atoms, the polymerisations which they initiated were radical-propagated processes. Ziegler adduced evidence for the view that the starting molecule from which polymer growth proceeded contained two atoms of the alkali metal. It was therefore an even-electron molecule. Ziegler's interpretation was on the following lines:

$$2Na + CH_2{:}CH \cdot CH{:}CH_2 \rightarrow NaCH_2 \cdot CH{:}CH \cdot CH_2Na$$

$$2Na + CH_2{:}CHPh \rightarrow NaCH_2{:}CH(Ph)Na$$

The molecules with two atoms of sodium had two growing points; and growth by addition of successive monomer molecules took place at both. It was supposed that a metal-carbon bond became split as addition took place to a monomer molecule, to form a new metal-carbon bond at the end of the growing chain. All this is nearly as we would describe it today. One point of difference is that the disodio-compounds are today considered to be formed by dimerisation of first-

[232] F. E. Matthews and E. H. Strange, British Patent, 1910, No. 24,790.

[233] C. Harries, *Ann.*, 1911, **383**, 213.

[234] W. Schlenk, J. Appenrodt, A. Michael, and A. Thal, *Ber.*, 1914, **47**, 473.

[235] W. Ziegler, many papers since 1928, summarised in *Chem. Zeitg.*, 1938, **62**, 125.

formed radical-anions, and therefore to contain twice as much carbon and hydrogen as is represented above, *e.g.*,

$$CH_2{=}CH{-}CH{=}CH_2 + N\dot{a} \rightarrow \dot{C}H_2{\cdot}CH{=}CH{-}CH_2^-\}Na^+$$

$$2\,\dot{C}H_2{\cdot}CH{=}CH{-}CH_2^-\}Na^+ \rightarrow Na^+\{^-CH_2{-}CH{=}CH{-}CH_2{-}CH_2{-}CH{=}CH{-}CH_2^-\}Na^+$$

The other difference is that we would take the sodio-compounds to add, like any metal-alkyl, through their carbanions, the sodium counter-ion following the outward-moving negative charge as polymerisation continues, *e.g.*,

$$R^-\}Na^+ \xrightarrow{CH_2:CHPh} R{-}CH_2{-}CHPh^-\}Na^+ \xrightarrow{CH_2:CHPh}$$

$$R{-}CH_2{-}CHPh{-}CH_2{-}CHPh^-\}Na^+ \xrightarrow{CH_2:CHPh}$$

$$R{-}CH_2{-}CHPh{-}CH_2{-}CHPh{-}CH_2{-}CHPh^-\}Na^+ \xrightarrow{CH_2:CHPh} \text{etc.}$$

Ziegler's point remains that metal initiation is simply a duplicated form of metal-alkyl initiation.

That all this is a specialisation of initiation by bases, in particular, of strongly nucleophilic anions, whether of carbon, nitrogen, or oxygen, was set down clearly for the first time[236] by Beaman in 1948. He had investigated the polymerisation of methacrylonitrile by initiation with Grignard reagents, with triphenylmethyl-sodium in ether, and with sodium in liquid ammonia. Sanderson and Hauser followed with a demonstration of the polymerisation of styrene by means of sodamide in liquid ammonia.[237] They explained it similarly, as initiated by addition of the highly basic amide ion, and showed that the reaction with sodamide failed in very much less ionising solvents than liquid ammonia.

In 1950 the experiments on copolymerisation were done, concurrently in two laboratories, which very simply exposed the distinction between acid-initiated, base-initiated, and radical-initiated addition-polymerisations of olefinic compounds. Walling, Mayo, and their coworkers,[238] and also Landler,[239] polymerised, for example, a 1:1-molar mixture of

236 R. G. Beaman, *J. Am. Chem. Soc.*, 1948, **70**, 3115.

237 J. J. Sanderson and C. R. Hauser, *J. Am. Chem. Soc.*, 1949, **71**, 1595.

238 C. Walling, E. R. Briggs, W. Cummings, and F. R. Mayo, *J. Am. Chem. Soc.*, 1950, **72**, 48.

239 Y. Landler, *Compt. rend.*, 1950, **280**, 539.

TABLE 54-4.—POLYMERISATION OF 1:1-MIXTURE OF STYRENE AND METHYL METHACRYLATE.

Catalyst	Solvent	Temp.	% Styrene in copolymer
BF_3-Et_2O	None	30°	>99
$SnCl_4$	None	30°	>99
$SnBr_4$	Nitrobenzene	25°	*99*
K	Metal suspended in benzene	30°	< 1
Na	(Metal suspended in benzene)	30°	< 1
Na	Liquid NH_3	−50°	*2*
Bz_2O_2	None	60°	51
Bz_2O_2	None	?	*54*

NOTE. Roman figures are from reference 140, and the italic figures from reference 141.

styrene and methyl methacrylate. The point of this choice of monomers is that one of them is an olefinic hydrocarbon, typically susceptible to electrophilic reagents, whilst the other is an $\alpha\beta$-unsaturated ester, characteristically vulnerable to nucleophilic reagents. When the monomer mixture was treated with boron trifluoride, or stannic chloride, or stannic bromide (a co-catalyst is not mentioned, but no steps were taken to exclude it), the product was almost pure polystyrene. Evidently the reactive end of the growing polymer was an electrophile, presumably a carbonium ion, which picked out the styrene molecules, but neglected nearly all the methyl methacrylate molecules. When the mixture of monomers was treated with sodium or potassium, the polymer obtained was essentially pure methyl polymethacrylate. The growing end was now a nucleophile, presumably a carbanion, with a strong affinity for the β-carbon atom of methyl methacrylate, but relatively little affinity for styrene. When the monomer mixture was treated with benzoyl peroxide, an approximately equimolar copolymer was produced. In this case, the growing end must have been a radical, very ready to accept either type of monomer molecule. The data are in Table 54-4.

Abkin and Medvedev first studied, in 1936–1940, the kinetics of a base-initiated addition polymerisation, in the example of the polymerisation of butadiene, in the gas phase or in hydrocarbon solvents, on initiation with metallic sodium.[240] The reaction was heterogeneous with respect, at least, to initiation, but from its qualitative kinetic features some support was adduced for the Ziegler mechanism.

[240] A. Abkin and S. Medvedev, *Trans. Faraday Soc.*, 1936, **21**, 286; *J. Phys. Chem. U.S.S.R.*, 1939, **13**, 705; *idem* and O. Manontova, *Acta Physicochim. U.S.S.R.*, 1940, **12**, 269.

A kinetic study with supplementary observations that collectively amount to a complete proof of mechanism of a base-promoted polymerisation was put on record by Higginson and Wooding in 1952.[241] They examined the polymerisation of styrene, as initiated by potassamide in liquid ammonia. (Note the choice of styrene: a monomer such as methyl methacrylate would have polymerised much too rapidly to have admitted kinetic study in the conditions.) The rate equation was

$$\text{Rate} \propto [\text{KNH}_2]^{1/2}[\text{styrene}]^2$$

and the mean degree of polymerisation was given by

$$\overline{DP} \propto [\text{styrene}]$$

It was shown further that every polymer molecule contained an amino-group, but that potassamide was not consumed. Conductance studies on potassamide confirmed that this is a weak electrolyte in liquid ammonia, and gave the free energy and an approximate value for the heat of its ionic dissociation. Temperature coefficients were also determined for the polymerisation.

These data determine the mechanism. It is standard to the extent that it consists of initiation, propagation, and termination steps. The one-half power in the rate equation shows that initiation is by the dissociated amide ion, not by the potassamide molecule or its ion-pair. The second power in the rate equation shows that the propagation step is bimolecular. The first power in the equation for the degree of polymerisation ($\overline{DP} = k_p/k_t$) shows that termination is a first-order process, that is, that it is of first order in the terminating polymer, and that the only other material that could be involved in termination is the solvent. That the solvent is involved is shown by the stoicheiometry: termination is a proton transfer from the solvent to the growing polymer anion:

$$\text{NH}_2^- + \text{CH}_2\text{:CHPh} \xrightarrow{k_i} \text{NH}_2\cdot\text{CH}_2\cdot\text{CHPh}^-$$

$$\text{NH}_2\cdot\text{CH}_2[\text{CH}_2\cdot\text{CHPh}]_r\text{CHPh}^- + \text{CH}_2\text{:CHPh} \xrightarrow{k_p} \text{NH}_2\text{–CH}_2[\text{CH}_2\text{–CHPh}]_{r+1}\text{CHPh}^-$$

$$\text{NH}_2\cdot\text{CH}_2[\text{CH}_2\cdot\text{CHPh}]_n\text{CHPh}^- + \text{NH}_3 \xrightarrow{k_t} \text{NH}_2\cdot\text{CH}_2[\text{CH}_2\cdot\text{CHPh}]_n\text{CH}_2\text{Ph} + \text{NH}_2^-$$

241 W. C. E. Higginson and N. S. Wooding, *J. Chem. Soc.*, **1952,** 760, 1178.

The temperature-coefficient studies gave 13±4 kcal./mole for the activation energy of initiation E_i, and 4±1 kcal./mole for the difference $E_t - E_p$ between the activation energies of termination and propagation. One sees that, in base-initiated polymerisation, just as in acid-initiated polymerisation, termination is slow enough to allow a high polymer to be formed, because the activation energy of the terminating process is high, not as in radical-carried polymerisations, when termination is by radical colligation, a reaction of very low activation energy, which is nevertheless slow because the radicals are of such low concentration.

A similar kinetic investigation[241] of the polymerisation of styrene under initiation by potassium in liquid ammonia pointed to the mechanism described above as the more modern elaboration of Ziegler's mechanism.

Sodium naphthalene is an odd-electron substance, which has been much used in place of sodium or potassium in later work on the addition-polymerisation of olefins by base initiation. This substance contains the radical-anion, $C_{10}H_8^-$, the extra electron being in an antibonding orbital. Two of these anions initiate polymerisation, just as two sodium atoms do by producing a di-carbanion from two olefin molecules. The di-carbanion then polymerises at both ends. This has been succinctly proved by Szwarc and his collaborators[242] in the example of the polymerisation of α-methylstyrene by sodium naphthalene in tetrahydrofuran. They showed that the degree of polymerisation is equal to 2×[monomer]/[initiator], the factor 2 representing the number of growing points in a single growing polymer molecule.

The kinetic course of addition polymerisation in the absence of any chain-terminating or chain-transfer step was discussed in 1943 by Flory,[243] and later by Bauer and Magat,[244] who illustrated the matter with certain acid-initiated polymerisations. But the best examples of terminationless addition polymerisation are in the field of base-initiated polymerisations. For, in these, chain-transfer steps are frequently impossible, and it is easy to arrange that nothing is present which, by transferring a proton, could terminate the chain.

This situation was demonstrated by Ziegler and Bähr as early as 1928.[245] They showed that the polymerisation of butadiene, initiated

[242] R. Waack, A. Rembaum, J. D. Coombes, and M. Szwarc, *J. Am. Chem. Soc.*, 1957, **79**, 2026; H. Brody, M. Ladacki, R. Milkovich, and M. Szwarc, *J. Polymer Sci.*, 1957, **25**, 221.

[243] P. J. Flory, *J. Am. Chem. Soc.*, 1943, **65**, 372.

[244] E. Bauer and M. Magat, *J. chim. phys.*, 1950, **47**, 841.

[245] K. Ziegler and K. Bähr, *Ber.*, 1928, **61**, 253.

with sodium, proceeded until the monomer was consumed; and that then, on the addition of fresh monomer, the polymerisation continued, so to produce a polymer of increased molecular weight. Nearly 30 years later, this phenomenon was rediscovered by Szwarc and his collaborators,[246] who used it for the preparation of block polymers, and of polymers with chosen end-groups, as well as for thermodynamic and kinetic studies, as indicated below. They referred to polymers having carbanionic ends capable of continuing polymerisation if supplied with monomer by the convenient name of "living" polymers, and to their reactive ends by the name of "living" ends. They showed that the red colour seen in base-initiated polymerised styrene is the colour of the living ends, that is, benzylide ions in ion-pairs, such as $—CHPh^{-}\}Na^{+}$. They showed that styrene, base-polymerised until polymerisation ended on near-exhaustion of the styrene, could be further polymerised with more styrene to give a higher polymer, or, alternatively, further polymerised with isoprene to give a styrene-isoprene block-polymer.

If the propagation steps of a base-initiated addition polymerisation, which are in principle reversible, are in practice appreciably so, the collective effect of such reversibility may limit the size to which the polymer can grow, and the degree of completeness with which the monomer can be exhausted, by the polymerisation in the absence of termination or chain-transfer. A determination of the equilibrium, between monomer and polymer of determined degree of polymerisation, allows the equilibrium constant of a propagation step to be deduced, and, from the temperature coefficient of that constant, the entropy and enthalpy of the step of propagation.[247] For high degrees of polymerisation, as of styrene, butadiene, or isoprene, the values are independent of molecular weight, but they vary for the first few steps in the formation of a low polymer, as of α-methylstyrene.[248]

It will be remembered that, in the work of Higginson and Wooding, the kinetics of the amide-ion-initiated polymerisation of styrene in liquid ammonia allowed the difference between the activation energies of termination and propagation to be determined. In the absence of

[246] M. Szwarc, *Nature*, 1956, **178,** 1168; M. Szwarc, M. Levy, and R. Milkovich, *J. Am. Chem. Soc.*, 1956, **78,** 2656.

[247] H. Brody, M. Ladack, R. Milkovich, and M. Szwarc, *J. Polymer Sci.*, 1957, **25,** 221; H. W. McCormick, *ibid.*, 448; D. J. Worsfold and S. Bywater, *ibid.*, **26,** 299; *idem, ibid.*, 1962, **58,** 571; R. Waack, A. Rembaum, J. D. Coombes, and M. Szwarc, *J. Am. Chem. Soc.*, 1957, **79,** 2026; A. Vraneken, J. Smid, and M. Szwarc, *ibid.*, 1961, **83,** 2772; *Trans. Faraday Soc.*, 1962, **58,** 2036.

[248] D. J. Worsfold and S. Bywater, *Can. J. Chem.*, 1958, **36,** 1141; G. Allen, G. Gee, and C. Stretch, *J. Polymer Sci.*, 1960, **48,** 189; C. Geacinov, J. Smid, and M. Szwarc, *J. Am. Chem. Soc.*, 1962, **84,** 2508.

termination, a study of kinetics will allow the rate and activation parameters of the propagation itself to be deduced. Initial conditions can be set up in which the number of living ends in a pre-formed polymer is determined by the amount of initiator supplied, and may be analytically (*e.g.*, spectrophotometrically) checked. The concentration of living ends will then remain constant in the polymerisation which ensues when more monomer is added. For styrene or α-methylstyrene in dioxan or in tetrahydrofuran, these polymerisations are of first order in monomer; and the first-order rate-constants are nearly proportional to the concentration of living ends. Proportionality would mean that propagation proceeds through the living end in ion-pair form, —$CPh^-\}Na^+$. However, in the example of the polymerisation of styrene in tetrahydrofuran the second-order rate-constant of the equation, Rate $\propto$ [living ends][monomer], rises appreciably with dilution, and this might mean that, even in ether solvents, a proportion of the reaction proceeds through a minute amount of highly active dissociated carbanion.

(55) HOMOLYTIC ADDITION TO OLEFINIC COMPOUNDS[249]

It was noted in Section **18h** that homolytic additions comprise two main classes. In the first, *mono-addition*, an addendum XY adds to a carbon-carbon double bond, X adding as a pre-formed radical to give the adduct-radical XC—C·, which then extracts Y from the molecule XY, to give the addition product XC—CY. In the second class of additions, *polyadditions*, the same first-formed adduct-radical, instead of decomposing a molecule XY, adds to another olefin molecule, to form a higher adduct-radical, XC—C—C—C·, and from this, by a succession of similar additions, a polymer-radical is formed, before an end-group Y is acquired to give the final polymer. We shall describe these two types of addition largely separately, but they merge in *tele-additions*, the name applied when the originally formed adduct-radical XC—C· takes up only a few olefin molecules, before it acquires the end-group Y in the telemer (low polymer), $X(C—C)_nY$ (n small).

(55a) Mono-additions of Hydrogen Bromide and Sulphides, Halogens, Polyhaloalkanes, and Aldehydes to Olefinic Compounds.—In the early 1930's, the additions of hydrogen halides to olefins were generally understood to follow the Markownikoff rule (Section **53a**). Nevertheless, reports relating to additions of *hydrogen bromide* had appeared, which were inconsistent with this rule, and in some cases

[249] C. Walling, "Free Radicals in Solution," Wiley, New York, 1957, Chaps. 3–7; J. I. G. Cadogan and M. J. Perkins, in "Chemistry of Alkenes," Editor S. Patai, Interscience Publishers, London, 1964, Chap. 9.

seemed inconsistent with one another. In 1933, Kharasch and Mayo, whose concern was to clear up such discrepancies in the literature, made an examination, *inter alia*, of the addition of hydrogen bromide to allyl bromide.[250] They observed that this reaction could take different directions in different conditions. In the dark, and in the absence of oxygen or peroxides, or of anything else of the class, unrecognised then, which we now know as radical initiators, addition took place in the course of some days at room temperature to give the Markownikoff product, propylene dibromide:

$$CH_2{:}CH\cdot CH_2Br + HBr\ (\text{dark, no initiator}) \xrightarrow{\text{slow}} CH_3\cdot CHBr\cdot CH_2Br$$

Under illumination, or in the presence of small amounts of oxygen and/or peroxides, addition took place in a matter of minutes, but in the opposite direction, to give trimethylene dibromide:

$$CH_2{:}CH\cdot CH_2Br + HBr\ (\text{light or initiation}) \xrightarrow{\text{fast}} CH_2Br\cdot CH_2\cdot CH_2Br$$

Four years later, the interpretation of such findings was given concurrently by Hey and Waters in a review which did much to incorporate and rationalise the then new subject of homolytic reactions,[251] and by Kharasch, Engelmann, and Mayo in the development of their own work.[252] The reaction in the absence of light or initiators was an ordinary electrophilic addition, incepted by the proton of the hydrogen bromide molecule. The reaction in the presence of light or initiators was incepted by bromine atoms, and attained its high rate because its mechanism involved long kinetic chains:

$$\left.\begin{aligned} HBr + h\nu &\rightarrow H + \dot{B}r \\ HBr + O_2 &\rightarrow \dot{O}_2H + \dot{B}r \end{aligned}\right\}\ \text{initiation}$$

$$\left.\begin{aligned} \dot{B}r + CH_2{:}CH\cdot CH_2Br &\rightarrow BrCH_2\cdot \dot{C}H\cdot CH_2Br \\ BrCH_2\cdot \dot{C}H\cdot CH_2Br + HBr &\rightarrow BrCH_2\cdot CH_2\cdot CH_2Br + \dot{B}r \end{aligned}\right\}\ \text{chain propagation}$$

As other examples accumulated, it became clear that bromine atoms always add terminally, when that is possible. And the presumed reason was, and is, that the formed electron-deficient radical-centre will tend to set itself where it can best be stabilised by conjugation or hyperconjugation, and therefore at a secondary, rather than at a primary, carbon atom. The reason why the homolytic addition of hy-

[250] M. S. Kharasch and F. R. Mayo, *J. Am. Chem. Soc.*, 1933, **55,** 2468.

[251] D. H. Hey and W. A. Waters, *Chem. Revs.*, 1937, **21,** 169.

[252] M. S. Kharasch, H. Engelmann, and F. R. Mayo, *J. Org. Chem.*, 1957, **2,** 288.

drogen bromide takes the anti-Markownikoff direction is thus analogous to the reason why the electrophilic addition obeys the Markownikoff rule, namely, that the electron-deficient carbonium-ionic centre, on which that mechanism depends, is again more stable at secondary than at primary carbon: $Br^{\cdot}$, like H^+, is electrophilic.

If we examine the steps of chain propagation written above, taking account of the bond energies in Table 18-3 of Section **18g**, we see that both chain steps are exothermic. Thus, the propagation process is expected to be rapid, as indeed it is. It leads to long kinetic chains. If we similarly consider the energetics of the same reactions with other hydrogen halides, one sees immediately that the reaction with *hydrogen fluoride* should be unable to proceed, because the hydrogen fluoride bond is too strong. Homolytic additions of hydrogen fluoride have not been observed.

For like reasons, the homolytic addition of *hydrogen chloride* must needs be a difficult reaction. The first chain step would be strongly exothermic, but the second chain step would be endothermic by about 10 kcal./mole. Thus the radical-adduct will be produced; but it is difficult for it rapidly to decompose hydrogen chloride; and an easier reaction is open to it. For it can add to a new olefin molecule, thereby taking the first step in a succession of steps that will lead to a polymer. If, at any one of the successive steps of chain growth, the polymer-radical, instead of taking up yet one more olefin molecule, did decompose a hydrogen chloride molecule, the formation of that polymer molecule would be terminated:

$$\dot{Cl} + CH_2{:}CHR \rightarrow ClCH_2\cdot\dot{C}HR$$

$$ClCH_2\cdot\dot{C}HR + CH_2{:}CHR \rightarrow ClCH_2\cdot CHR\cdot CH_2\cdot\dot{C}HR$$

$$\cdots$$

$$ClCH_2\text{—}[CHR\cdot CH_2]_n\text{—}\dot{C}HR + HCl \rightarrow ClCH_2\text{—}[CHR\cdot CH_2]_n\text{—}CH_2R + \dot{Cl}$$

There is overlap here between the subject of the present Section and that of Section **55b**; but we may add the remark that the degree of polymerisation will be determined by the ratio of the rates with which the radical reacts with olefin monomer and with hydrogen chloride, a ratio of absolute rates that can be influenced by adjustment of the relative concentration of the competing reactants. Some low polymers (telemers) have been produced in additions of hydrogen chloride to ethylene under high pressure of ethylene,[253] a fact which shows that the

[253] T. A. Ford, W. E. Hanford, J. Harmon, and R. D. Lipscomb, *J. Am. Chem. Soc.*, 1952, **74**, 4323.

specific rates (rate-constants) of the competing reactants are not extremely different.

The homolytic addition of *hydrogen iodide* is a difficult reaction for a different reason. The iodine atom is easily produced; but its addition to an olefin in the first chain step is endothermic. Hence the easiest reaction open to the radical-adduct, if formed, is to split off the iodine atom again, rather than to decompose hydrogen iodide, or to add to another olefin molecule. In fact, the homolytic addition of hydrogen iodide has not been observed.

Hydrogen sulphide and the *thiols* can not only add, like water and alcohols, as electrophiles to olefins in acid conditions, and as nucleophiles to conjugated olefinic carbonyl compounds in basic conditions, but also can add as radicals in a third set of conditions to most types of olefinic compounds. These conditions do not require the presence of strong acids or strong bases, but, as Ashworth and Burkhardt showed in 1928, do depend on the presence of light or air or both.[254] In 1934, Burkhardt recognised these additions as radical processes.[255] In 1938, Kharasch, Read, and Mayo applied to these reactions the chain-reaction scheme, which had been established a year earlier for additions of hydrogen bromide:[256]

$$\left.\begin{array}{l} \dot{R}S + CH_2{:}CXY \rightarrow RS\cdot CH_2\cdot \dot{C}XY \\ RS\cdot CH_2\cdot \dot{C}XY + HSR \rightarrow RS\cdot CH_2\cdot CHXY + R\dot{S} \end{array}\right\} \text{chain}$$

Initiation by means of organic peroxides, first used by Jones and Reid in 1938, has been commonly employed since that time.[257]

The reactions of hydrogen sulphide are similar to those of thiols, except that the former reactions may run to two steps of addition, as when hydrogen sulphide and vinyl chloride give "mustard gas," $ClCH_2\cdot CH_2\cdot S\cdot CH_2\cdot CH_2\cdot Cl$.

As can be seen in Table 18-3 (Section **18f**), the energies of bonds H—SH and H—Br are closely similar. We may assume that this will be generally true for the H—S bonds of thiols and the bond of hydrogen bromide. Likewise, the energies of the bonds C—SH and C—Br are closely similar. Thus both the steps of propagation in the radical-chain addition of hydrogen sulphide and of thiols to olefinic substances will be exothermic, and an essential condition for rapid propagation will be fulfilled. Therefore, we may expect hydrogen sulphide and the

[254] F. Ashworth and G. N. Burkhardt, *J. Chem. Soc.*, **1928**, 1791.

[255] G. N. Burkhardt, *Trans. Faraday Soc.*, 1934, **30**, 18.

[256] M. S. Kharasch, A. T. Read, and F. R. Mayo, *Chem. and Ind.*, 1938, **57**, 752.

[257] S. O. Jones and E. E. Reid, *J. Am. Chem. Soc.*, 1938, **60**, 2452.

thiols to do much as hydrogen bromide does in the matter of homolytic addition.

By arguments on lines already illustrated with respect to homolytic additions of hydrogen halides, one can understand why homolytic additions by O—H bond fission of water and alcohols have not been realised, and why similar additions of hydrogen selenide and of selenols, as well as of hydrogen telluride and of tellurols, have not hitherto been described.

Although the homolytic addition of thiols is broadly similar to that of hydrogen bromide, one can see vestigial resemblances in the homolytic behaviour of thiols to that of both hydrogen chloride and hydrogen iodide. Such a resemblance to hydrogen chloride is apparent in the fact that, although telemer formation is not a normal accompaniment of homolytic thiol additions to simple olefins, it has been realised in additions to ethylene by the use of high pressures of ethylene.[258] A vestigial analogy with hydrogen iodide may perhaps be seen in the circumstance that reversibility in the radical-addition chain step, reversibility which is strong enough to prevent the homolytic addition of hydrogen iodide, may in thiol additions suffice to cause the long-known effect of hydrogen sulphide in promoting *cis-trans* isomerisation in slowly adding olefinic substances, such as maleic acid.[259]

Qualitative observations make clear that, as homolytic addenda, both hydrogen bromide, and hydrogen sulphide along with the thiols, are predominantly electrophilic. Radicals to which correspond stable anions, but unstable electron-deficient cations, are expected to be predominantly electrophilic. The matter has been quantitatively illustrated for the homolytic addition of thioglycollic acid to simple and substituted styrenes:[260]

$$RC_6H_4\cdot CH{:}CH_2 + HS\cdot CH_2\cdot CO_2H \rightarrow RC_6H_4\cdot CH_2\cdot CH_2\cdot S\cdot CH_2\cdot CO_2H$$

Measurements of relative consumption, when pairs of these styrenes compete for the thiol, gave the following relative rates of addition at 60° of the thienyl radical to the substituted styrenes:

Substituent	*p*-MeO	*p*-Me	H	*p*-Br	*p*-F
Rel. rate	100	2.3	0	0.90	0.50

The ease with which a thiol may have its hydrogen atom abstracted by the adduct-radical can be assessed by setting the hydrogen abstraction, which completes an addition, in competition with addition to

[258] J. Harmon, U. S. Patent, 1945, No. 2,390,099.

[259] Z. H. Skraup, *Wien Akad. Sitzungber.*, 1891, **100**, 124.

[260] C. Walling, D. Seymour, and K. B. Wolfstirn, *J. Am. Chem. Soc.*, 1948, **70**, 2559.

another molecule of the olefin, a reaction which constitutes a step in the formation of a telemer. In the addition of thiols to styrene, and to butadiene, telemer formation is appreciable, and from the extent of it "transfer constants" can be computed. They are ratios of the rates of completion of addition to the rates of continuation of telemer formation. When the olefin remains the same, and only the thiol is varied, these transfer constants are, in effect, relative rates of abstraction of the hydrogen atom from the thiols. A number of such transfer constants have been measured,[261] and have been collected together by Walling.[262] For unsubstituted aryl and alkyl thiols, the values fall into three groups, as shown in Table 55-1.

TABLE 55-1.—TRANSFER CONSTANTS FOR TELEMERISATION WITH ADDITION OF THIOLS TO STYRENE AND TO BUTADIENE.*

R in RSH	Temp.	Const.	R in RSH	Temp.	Const.
Phenyl	60°	very high	*n*-Dodecyl	60°	20
n-Butyl	60°	22	*α*-Naphthylmethyl	50°	18
n-Amyl	60°	18	*t*-Butyl	60°	3.6
n-Octyl	50°	19, *16*	*t*-Octyl†	50°	4.5, *3.7*

* Constants in roman figures refer to reactions of styrene, and in italics to those of butadiene.

† 1,1,3,3-Tetramethylbutyl.

The three sets into which these values fall give for the relative rates of abstraction of H from RSH the order (R=)

$$\text{aryl} > \text{primary alkyl} > \text{tertiary alkyl}$$

The first item in this series may represent stabilisation of the radical RS· by conjugation, the second its stabilisation by hyperconjugation, and the third the absence of either of these forms of stabilisation, with a possible superposed steric effect.

Photochemical initiation is usually employed in order to effect the homolytic additions of *halogens* to olefins. The reactions are best studied in the gas phase or in non-polar solvents, because of the great ease of electrophilic additions in polar solvents. Telemer formation does not accompany these mono-additions.

The kinetics of the light-initiated addition of chlorine and of bromine to ethylene and to mono- and poly-chloroethylenes, mainly in the gas

[261] W. V. Smith, *J. Am. Chem. Soc.*, 1946, **68**, 2059, 2064; C. Walling, *ibid.*, 1948, **70**, 2561; R. A. Gregg, D. M. Alderman, and F. R. Mayo, *ibid.*, p. 3740; E. J. Mechan, I. M. Kohltoff, and P. R. Sinha, *J. Polymer Sci.*, 1955, **16**, 471; R. M. Pierson, A. J. Costanza, and A. H. Weinstein, *ibid.*, **17**, 221.

[262] C. Walling, ref. 249, p. 319.

phase but to some extent in solution, have been investigated by Schumacher and others.[263,265] For the addition of *chlorine* to ethylene, the rate equation is

$$\text{Rate} \propto I^{1/2}[Cl_2][C_2H_4]^{1/2}$$

where I is the intensity of the absorbed light. This means that, of the chain propagation steps,

$$\left.\begin{aligned} Cl^{\cdot} + C_2H_4 &\rightleftharpoons ClCH_2{\cdot}CH_2^{\cdot} \\ ClCH_2{\cdot}CH_2^{\cdot} + Cl_2 &\rightarrow ClCH_2{\cdot}CH_2Cl + Cl^{\cdot} \end{aligned}\right\} \text{chain}$$

the first is a pre-equilibrium, its reversal being faster than the second step, even though both forward steps are exothermic. Termination is by interaction of a chlorine atom and a chloroalkyl radical. The kinetic chain length runs to some millions of cycles. In the corresponding additions to vinyl chloride, to *cis*- and *trans*-di, to tri-, and to tetrachloroethylene, the olefin factor drops out from the rate equation:

$$\text{Rate} \propto I^{1/2}[Cl_2]$$

This shows, *inter alia*, that the reversal of the first chain step is now slower than the second chain step, *e.g.*,

$$\left.\begin{aligned} Cl + CH_2{:}CHCl &\rightarrow ClCH_2{\cdot}\dot{C}HCl \\ ClCH_2{\cdot}\dot{C}HCl + Cl_2 &\rightarrow ClCH_2{\cdot}CHCl_2 + \dot{C}l \end{aligned}\right\} \text{chain}$$

The accepted explanation is that the conjugative effect ($+M$) of the original chlorine substituent stabilises the electron-deficient radical centre in the radical-adduct more than it stabilises the original olefin, with the result that, not only is the first forward chain step more exothermic than in the reaction of ethylene, but also its free-energy increment is negative, despite the loss of translation entropy. Thus, rather than destroy itself, the radical-adduct must wait for a chlorine molecule to destroy it. The kinetic equation also shows that chain termination involves two chloroalkyl radicals, which presumably either colligate or disproportionate. The kinetic chains are still very long.

[263] J. A. Leernakers and R. G. Dickenson, *J. Am. Chem. Soc.*, 1932, **54,** 4648; R. G. Dickenson and J. L. Carrico, *ibid.*, 1934, **56,** 1473; 1935, **57,** 1343; J. Willard and F. Daniels, *ibid.*, p. 2240; K. L. Müller and H. J. Schumacher, *Z. Elektrochem.*, 1937, **43,** 807; *Z. physik. Chem.*, 1937, **B, 35,** 285, 455; 1939, **B, 42,** 327; C. Schott and J. H. Schumacher, *ibid.*, 1941, **B, 49,** 107; H. Schmitz, H. J. Schumacher, and A. Jäger, *ibid.*, 1942, **B, 51,** 281; H. Schmitz and H. J. Schumacher, *ibid.*, 1942, **B, 52,** 72.

The corresponding gas reactions of *bromine* with ethylene and the mono- and poly-chloroethylenes involve chain steps which are still both exothermic, but much less strongly so. Evidence for reversibility in the first chain step is now general. In the reaction between bromine and tetrachloroethylene, the overall addition, though it goes forward in the liquid phase at room temperature, is strongly reversed at temperatures as low as 100° in the vapour phase. However, the additions generally go forward through fairly long kinetic chains, of the order of tens of thousands of cycles. Added oxygen reduces the chain length.[265] The oxygen molecules are evidently competitive with the bromine atoms in providing a termination process by attacking the radical-adduct.

The homolytic addition of *iodine* to simple olefins would be endothermic in the first chain step; and, in fact, the overall addition is thermodynamically disfavoured at room temperature. However, the photo-initiated addition of iodine to ethylene, propylene, and the four isomeric butylenes has been realised[264] at −55°.

The function of reversibility in the formation of the radical-adduct from bromine atoms and olefins in providing a mechanism for *cis-trans* isomerisation of the olefin has been checked by Ketelaar and his collaborators. By a combined study of kinetics and product compositions in the action of bromine on *cis*-dichloroethylene in the liquid phase, they were able to show that bromine addition to the olefin, and the *cis*→*trans* isomerisation of the latter, go through the same intermediate.[265] A further check has been achieved by Steinmetz and Noyes, who, by the use of radioactive bromine for promoting the *cis*→*trans* isomerisation of *cis*-dibromoethylene in carbon tetrachloride at 40–60°, could show kinetically that the bromine exchange, which accompanies isomerisation of the olefin, goes through the same intermediate as the isomerisation.[266] The same methods, applied by Schomaker, Dickenson, and Noyes, to the *cis-trans* isomerisation of dichloro-, dibromo-, and di-iodo-ethylene in decalin, induced by iodine atoms, have shown that these isomerisations also proceed by reversible formation of a radical-adduct from the iodine atom and the olefin.[267]

Because of the great strength of the hydrogen-fluorine bond, the

[264] G. S. Forbes and A. F. Nelson, *J. Am. Chem. Soc.*, 1937, **59**, 693.

[265] J. A. A. Ketelaar, P. F. VanVerden, G. H. J. Broers, and H. R. Gersmann, *J. Phys. Colloid Chem.*, 1951, **55**, 987.

[266] H. Steinmetz and R. M. Noyes, *J. Am. Chem. Soc.*, 1952, **74**, 4141.

[267] R. E. Wood and R. G. Dickenson, *J. Am. Chem. Soc.*, 1939, **61**, 3259; R. M. Noyes and R. G. Dickenson, *ibid.*, 1943, **65**, 1427; *idem* and V. Schomaker, *ibid.*, 1945, **67**, 1319; R. G. Dickenson, R. F. Wallis and R. E. Wood, *ibid.*, 1949, **71**, 1238.

reactions of any organic compound containing hydrogen with elemental fluorine are dominated by the more or less indiscriminate abstraction of the hydrogen. Thus olefins form simple addition products with *fluorine* only when the olefins are perhalogenated. And then, as Miller and Koch have shown,[268] one has not, as in other homolytic additions of halogen, first to produce halogen atoms. The bond of molecular fluorine is so weak, and the carbon-fluorine bond is so strong, that the fluorine molecule itself will add to produce its own fluorine atom along with the fluorinated adduct-radical. The fluorine atom will then, on contact, add to the next-neighbouring olefin molecule to give another fluorinated adduct-radical. Thus, the adduct-radicals tend to be produced locally in pairs; and so, besides participating in the usual type of chain propagation, they combine with each other to form dimers:

$$CX_2{:}CX_2 + F_2 \rightarrow FCX_2{\cdot}CX_2^{\cdot} + F^{\cdot} \qquad \text{initiation}$$

$$\left.\begin{array}{r} CX_2{:}CX_2 + F^{\cdot} \rightarrow FCX_2{\cdot}CX_2^{\cdot} \\ FCX_2{\cdot}CX_2^{\cdot} + F_2 \rightarrow FCX_2{\cdot}CX_2F + F^{\cdot} \end{array}\right\} \qquad \begin{array}{l}\text{chain}\\ \text{propagation}\end{array}$$

$$FCX_2{\cdot}CX_2^{\cdot} + F^{\cdot} \rightarrow FCX_2{\cdot}CX_2F \qquad \text{normal termination}$$

$$2\,FCX_2{\cdot}CX_2^{\cdot} \rightarrow FCX_2{\cdot}CX_2{\cdot}CX_2{\cdot}CX_2F \qquad \text{dimer termination}$$

Dimer formation is the most characteristic feature of fluorine additions. Miller and Koch went far to prove their theory of the formation of local pairs of adduct-radicals by showing, for example, that, when a mixture of two olefins of very different reactivity, such as more reactive CFCl:CFCl and less reactive $CF_3{\cdot}CCl{:}CCl{\cdot}CF_3$, were treated with fluorine, the more reactive olefin monopolised the initiation step, and therefore gave much dimer along with the normal fluorine-addition product, whilst the less reactive olefin, presumably operating only in the steps of chain propagation, gave the normal addition product only. The other by-products formed when the olefin, for example, CFCl:CFCl, contains chlorine were easily understood. Any reversibility of adduct-radical formation would involve loss of the higher halogen, a chlorine atom rather than a fluorine atom:

$$\dot{F} + CFCl{:}CFCl \rightarrow CF_2Cl{\cdot}\dot{C}FCl \rightarrow CF_2{:}CFCl + \dot{C}l$$

The result is a substitution of fluorine for chlorine. The liberated chlorine atom will combine with the adduct-radical:

$$\dot{C}l + CF_2Cl{\cdot}\dot{C}FCl \rightarrow CF_2Cl{\cdot}CFCl_2$$

[268] W. T. Miller jr. and S. D. Koch jr., *J. Am. Chem. Soc.*, 1957, **79,** 3084.

The result of that is an apparent addition of chlorine fluoride. These were the other side reactions.

The *polyhaloalkanes* are an important group of substances capable of homolytic addition to olefins. As we have noticed, a halogen substituent stabilises an adjacent carbon radical. The radical to be derived by loss of an atom from a polyhaloalkane must be stable enough to be easily formed, and yet reactive enough to break the π component of an olefinic double bond. Either two or three halogen atoms bound to the same carbon atom will allow the carbon radical to be formed with the aid of the usual radical initiators, if the atom to be removed is iodine or bromine; but three halogens will be required if the atom to be removed is chlorine or hydrogen. The radical containing either two or three halogen atoms bound to the same carbon atom will usually open an olefinic double bond to form the adduct-radical.

The possibility of realising the homolytic addition of carbon tetrachloride was foreshadowed in observations that the presence of that substance during the polymerisation of styrene lowered the molecular weight of the polymer. The first record of such an addition was by Kharasch, Jensen, and Urry in 1945. They observed that carbon tetrachloride, and likewise chloroform, in the presence of radical initiators, added to 1-octene to give the products here formulated:[269]

$$CCl_4 + CH_2{:}CH\cdot C_6H_{13} \rightarrow Cl_3C\cdot CH_2\cdot CHCl\cdot C_6H_{13}$$
$$H\cdot CCl_3 + CH_2{:}CH\cdot C_6H_{13} \rightarrow Cl_3C\cdot CH_2\cdot CH_2\cdot C_6H_{13}$$

In both cases the first-adding radical is $Cl_3C^{\cdot}$, which takes the terminal position, so to produce a secondary alkyl radical, with which addition is completed in the second chain step.

Such additions of carbon tetrachloride have since been carried out with many kinds of acyclic, cyclic, polycyclic, and heterocyclic mono-olefins or poly-olefins. The usual initiators are acetyl or benzoyl peroxide at 60–100°. In some instances telemer formation accompanies simple addition.

Another tetrahalomethane which has been extensively investigated is trichlorobromomethane. It adds in the parts CCl_3 and Br. This tetrahalide is much more reactive than the tetrachloride, and, if a chemical initiator is used, only a small quantity is required. The energy of detachment of the bromine atom is sufficiently low that photo-initiation with light of wavelength long enough for transmission through Pyrex vessels may be used. Additions with carbon tetrabromide are in much the same case. Trifluoroiodomethane has also been employed. The general pattern of these additions is like that for carbon tetrachloride:

[269] M. S. Kharasch, E. V. Jensen, and W. H. Urry, *Science*, 1945, **102**, 128.

$$BrCCl_3 + CH_2{:}CH \cdot C_6H_{13} \rightarrow Cl_3C \cdot CH_2 \cdot CHBr \cdot C_6H_{13}$$
$$BrCBr_3 + CH_2{:}CH \cdot C_6H_{13} \rightarrow Br_3C \cdot CH_2 \cdot CHBr \cdot C_6H_{13}$$
$$I \cdot CF_3 + CH_2{:}CH \cdot CH_3 \rightarrow F_3C \cdot CH_2 \cdot CHI \cdot CH_3$$

Haloforms containing bromine or iodine do not act like chloroform, but split off a bromine or iodine atom in preference to the hydrogen atom. Peroxide initiation has usually been employed in additions of haloforms:

$$Br \cdot CHCl_2 + CH_2{:}CH \cdot CH_3 \rightarrow Cl_2CH \cdot CH_2 \cdot CHBr \cdot CH_3$$
$$Br \cdot CHBr_2 + CH_2{:}CH \cdot C_6H_{13} \rightarrow Br_2CH \cdot CH_2 \cdot CHBr \cdot C_6H_{13}$$
$$I \cdot CHI_2 + CH_2{:}CH \cdot CH_2 \cdot OBz \rightarrow I_2CH \cdot CH_2 \cdot CHI \cdot CH_2OBz$$

The perhalo-derivatives of some higher alkanes have been added to olefins, usually with the help of peroxide initiation; *e.g.*,

$$Br \cdot CFCl \cdot CF_2Br + CH_2{:}CH \cdot CH_3 \rightarrow BrF_2C \cdot CFCl \cdot CH_2 \cdot CHBr \cdot CH_3$$

The general mechanism of all these additions is as illustrated below for the addition of trichlorobromomethane:

$$Cl_3C \cdot Br \rightarrow Cl_3\dot{C} + \dot{B}r \qquad \text{initiation}$$

$$\left.\begin{aligned} Cl_3\dot{C} + CH_2{:}CHR &\rightarrow Cl_3C \cdot CH_2 \cdot \dot{C}HR \\ Cl_3C \cdot CH_2 \cdot CHR + Cl_3C \cdot Br &\rightarrow Cl_3C \cdot CH_2 \cdot CHBr \cdot Br + Cl_3\dot{C} \end{aligned}\right\} \qquad \text{chain steps}$$

$$\left.\begin{aligned} Cl_3\dot{C} + \dot{B}r &\rightarrow Cl_3C \cdot Br \\ Cl_3C \cdot CH_2 \cdot \dot{C}HR + \dot{B}r &\rightarrow Cl_3C \cdot CH_2 \cdot CHR \cdot Br \end{aligned}\right\} \qquad \text{termination}$$

Other termination processes may occur.[270]

The fact that the radicals $CX_3^{\cdot}$ and $CHX_2^{\cdot}$ add terminally already shows that they are predominantly electrophilic, that is, that they add to place the formed carbon radical centre at secondary carbon, where its electron déficiency has more opportunity of being stabilised by conjugation or hyperconjugation than it would have at primary carbon. This indication of the orientation of addition is confirmed by the relative rates of addition found by Kharasch and his coworkers by a competition method.[271] They put two olefins $CH_2{:}CRR'$ in admixture into competition for uptake of the radical $Cl_3C^{\cdot}$ in the reaction

$$Cl_3\dot{C} + CH_2{:}CRR' \rightarrow Cl_3C \cdot CH_2 \cdot \dot{C}RR'$$

Their figures have some dependence on the conditions, but lead to the rate order (R, R′ =)

[270] J. M. Tedder and J. W. Walton, *Trans. Faraday Soc.*, 1964, **60**, 1769.

[271] M. S. Kharasch and M. Sage, *J. Org. Chem.*, 1949, **14**, 537; M. S. Kharasch, E. Simon, and W. Nudenberg, *ibid.*, 1953, **18**, 328.

Ph, Me > Ph, H > C_6H_{13}, H > $PhCH_2$, H > CH_2Cl, H > CH_2CN, H

The favourable effect of electropositive conjugation ($+M$), and the unfavourable effect of inductive electronegativity ($-I$), on rate of addition are obvious. Pearson and Szwarc studied similar additions of the $F_3C^{\cdot}$ radical, which they generated by photolysis of hexafluoroazomethane:[272]

$$F_3C + CH_2{:}CRR' \rightarrow F_3C{\cdot}CH_2{\cdot}\dot{C}RR'$$

The reactions were run in the gas phase between 65° and 180°. With the slowest of the reactions examined as standard, the relative rates and activation-energy differences were as follows:

R,R′	Ph, Me	Ph, H	Me_2	Me, H	H_2	Cl, H	F,H
Rel. rate (65°) . . .	92	58	39	13	11	5	1
$-\Delta E$ (kcal./mole)	2.8	2.4	2.5	1.7	1.3	0.8	0

It was made clear by Huang, from studies on the orientation of the addition of the $Cl_3C{\cdot}$ radical in examples such as

$$CH_3{\cdot}\overset{\downarrow}{C}H{:}CH{\cdot}CO_2Et \quad \text{and} \quad Ph{\cdot}CH{:}\overset{\downarrow}{C}H{\cdot}CO_2Et$$

that the substituents in these examples stabilise an adjacent radical centre in the efficiency order,

$$Ph > CO_2Et > Me$$

It followed that even electronegative conjugation ($-M$) is of value in stabilising carbon radicals. Presumably the conjugation of CO_2Et is with the unshared electron of the radical. And so these perhalomethyl radicals, though predominantly electrophilic, have also a certain nucleophilic character.[273]

We conclude this Section with some remarks on oxygen compounds, particularly *aldehydes*, as homolytic addenda. In a mixture of a simple aldehyde and a simple olefin, the aldehydic C—H bond is usually the weakest in the system. Accordingly peroxide initiation will produce an acyl radical, $RCO^{\cdot}$, which will add to the olefin. The aldehydic C—H bond will usually be weak enough to allow the formed adduct-radical to extract a hydrogen atom, so completing a monoaddition of the aldehyde by the mechanism written below:

$$\left.\begin{array}{r} R'CO^{\cdot} + CH_2{:}CHR \rightarrow R'CO{\cdot}CH_2{\cdot}CHR^{\cdot} \\ R'CO{\cdot}CH_2{\cdot}CHR^{\cdot} + R'CHO \rightarrow R'CO{\cdot}CH_2{\cdot}CH_2R + R'CO^{\cdot} \end{array}\right\} \text{chain}$$

[272] J. M. Pearson and M. Szwarc, *Trans. Faraday Soc.*, 1964, **60**, 553.
[273] R. L. Huang, *J. Chem. Soc.*, **1956**, 1749.

Telemer formation is often an important competing process, to minimise which one may have to organise a countervailing concentration difference—as by gradual addition of the olefin with rapid stirring to excess of the aldehyde containing enough of the initiator to secure fairly rapid reaction.

The mono-addition of aldehydes was described in 1949 for additions to simple olefins by Kharasch, Urry, and Kuderna; and it was described in 1952 for additions to $\alpha\beta$-unsaturated esters and ketones by Patrick.[274] The following examples are typical:

$$n\text{-}C_4H_9\cdot CHO + CH_2{:}CH\cdot C_6H_{13} \rightarrow C_4H_9\cdot CO\cdot CH_2\cdot CH_2\cdot C_6H_{13}$$

$$CH_3\cdot CHO + cis\text{-}EtO_2C\cdot CH{:}CH\cdot CO_2Et \rightarrow \begin{matrix} CH_3\cdot CO \diagdown \\ CH\cdot CH_2\cdot CO_2Et \\ EtO_2C \diagup \end{matrix}$$

$$n\text{-}C_4H_9\cdot CHO + (CH_3)_2C{:}CH\cdot CO\cdot CH_3 \begin{matrix} \nearrow (CH_3)_2C(C_4H_9\cdot CO)\cdot CH_2\cdot CO\cdot CH_3 \quad (90\%) \\ \searrow (CH_3)_2CH\cdot CH(CO\cdot C_4H_9)\cdot CO\cdot CH_3 \quad (10\%) \end{matrix}$$

The generally higher yields of mono-addition products that have been obtained with $\alpha\beta$-unsaturated esters and ketones, such as ethyl maleate and mesityl oxide, than with simple olefins, such as 1-octene, led to an impression that the acyl radical is particularly strongly nucleophilic. The explanation may be that; but no direct comparison of the matter between acyl radicals and other radicals is known to the writer. Certainly the third of the examples cited above indicates that an acetyl substituent is somewhat better than two methyl substituents in stabilising an adjacent radical centre in the adduct-radical. This is the type of argument used by Huang,[273] who, by orientational studies on the addition of n-butaldehyde to various unsaturated ketones, acids, and esters, thus established the following order of efficiency in stabilising an adjacent carbon radical:

$$MeCO > CO_2Et > CO_2H > Me$$

It is again made clear that electronegative conjugation ($-M$) has an important stabilising action on a carbon radical.

The widespread autoxidisability of oxygen compounds suggests that their α-CH bonds are weak. The capacity of aldehydes for homolytic addition by splitting of their α-CH bonds has been shown to be shared

[274] M. S. Kharasch, W. H. Urry, and B. M. Kuderna, *J. Org. Chem.*, 1949, **14**, 248; T. M. Patrick jr., *ibid.*, 1952, **17**, 1009, 1269.

by *alcohols*.[275] Thus ethyl alcohol and ethylene, on peroxide initiation, give 2-butanol. Telemer formation is again an important competing process: in the example mentioned, 2-hexanol, 2-octanol, and 2-decanol are also produced. Higher primary alcohols, and also secondary alcohols, act similarly. Terminally unsaturated olefins up to 1-dodecane have been employed.

(55b) Polyaddition: Radical-Initiated Polymerisation of Olefinic Compounds by Self-Addition.—Polymerisations of unsaturated compounds in conditions in which these reactions must have been initiated and propagated by radicals have been observed and even recognised as polymerisations, since the preceding century.[276] But the chemical nature of the process, as a linear series of additions of olefin molecules to give an essentially saturated long-chain polymer molecule, was first made clear by Staudinger in 1920:[114]

$$n\mathrm{CH_2{:}CHR} \rightarrow (\mathrm{—CH_2{\cdot}CHR—})_n$$

In 1935 Staudinger and Steinhofer showed in the example of polystyrene that the linkings of the monomer units were all of the head-to-tail type; for by degradation at 300°, they obtained, besides styrene, the products

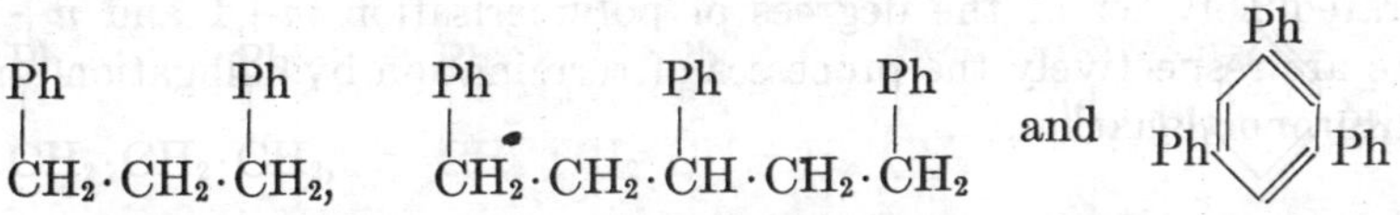

$$\underset{\mathrm{Ph}}{\mathrm{CH_2}}\cdot\mathrm{CH_2}\cdot\underset{\mathrm{Ph}}{\mathrm{CH_2}},\quad \underset{\mathrm{Ph}}{\mathrm{CH_2}}\cdot\mathrm{CH_2}\cdot\underset{\mathrm{Ph}}{\mathrm{CH}}\cdot\mathrm{CH_2}\cdot\underset{\mathrm{Ph}}{\mathrm{CH_2}}\quad \text{and}\quad \text{1,3,5-triphenylbenzene (Ph, Ph, Ph)}$$

and they failed to obtain any product having phenyl groups on adjacent carbon atoms.[277]

The olefins most readily polymerised by radical initiation are of the type CH_2CHR or $CH_2{:}CRR'$, where R or R′ or both will be capable of conjugating, electropositively or electronegatively or in both ways, with a radical centre produced on the carbon atom bearing R or R′. Examples of polymerising monomers with $+M$-type substituents are vinyl chloride, vinyl acetate, vinylidene fluoride, and vinylidene chloride. Examples with $-M$-type substituents are acrylonitrile, α-methacrylonitrile, methyl acrylate, and methyl α-methacrylate. Examples with $\pm M$-type groups are styrene, butadiene, isoprene, and neoprene.

[275] W. H. Urry, F. W. Stacey, E. S. Huyser, and O. O. Joveland, *J. Am. Chem. Soc.*, 1954, **76**, 450.

[276] For example, E. Simon, *Ann.*, 1839, **31**, 265. The description of such reactions as polymerisations seems first to have been made by M. Berthelot, *Bull. soc. chim.* (France), 1866, [ii], **6**, 294.

[277] H. Staudinger and A. Steinhofer, *Ann.*, 1935, **517**, 35.

The polymerisation may be initiated, in some cases by adventitious radicals, or radicals created by adventitious oxygen or light. Polymerisation may be initiated in all cases by radicals produced deliberately in any of the ways described in Section **18f**, for instance, by redox systems such as Fenton's reagent, by thermal homolysis of peroxides, by photolysis of halogens or aliphatic azo-compounds, or by high-energy irradiation of practically any organic material.

The addition of an initiating radical X˙ to an olefinic molecule (often called "the monomer" in this connexion) converts it to a monomeric carbon radical XC—C˙, so completing the initiation step of polymerisation. This carbon radical then adds to a second monomer in what becomes the first step of kinetic chain propagation, and the first step of structural chain growth, to give a dimeric carbon radical XC—C—C—C˙. After n such successive additions of the last-formed adduct-radical to a new monomer molecule, there is formed an adduct-radical having a degree of polymerisation $n+1$. Eventually two such radicals, of degrees of polymerisation $m+1$ and $n+1$, mutually annihilate their radical centres, either by colligation to give a final polymer of degree of polymerisation $m+n+2$, or by the transference of a hydrogen atom from one to the other to give an unsaturated and a saturated polymer of the degrees of polymerisation $m+1$ and $n+1$. There are respectively the processes of termination by colligation and by disproportionation:

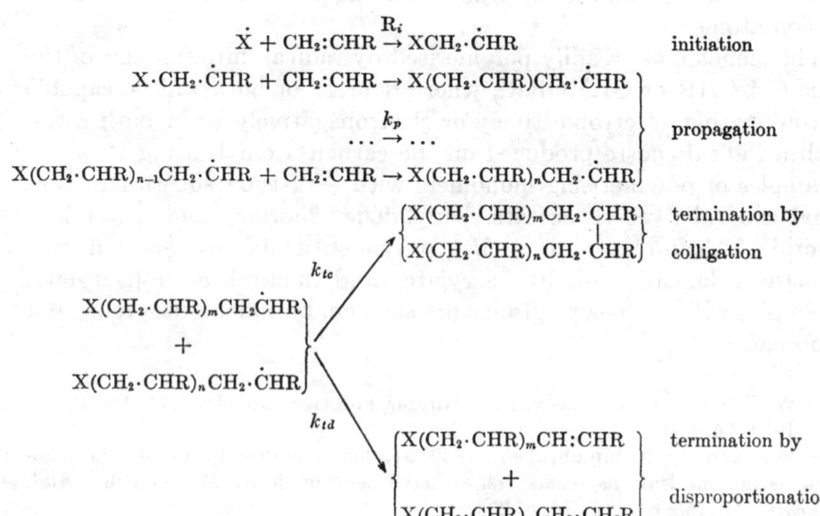

It is usually difficult to determine to what extent chain termination is by colligation and by disproportionation, even though colligation doubles the molecular weight of the eventual polymer. Kinetically, it makes no difference, and the rate of the sum of the two processes can be represented by a single second-order rate-constant for termination:

$$k_t = k_{tc} + k_{td}$$

There is another way of stopping structural chain growth, but now without stopping the kinetic chain. A polymeric adduct radical may transfer a hydrogen atom to a monomer molecule, so converting it to a radical from which a new polymer chain can grow:

$$X(CH_2\cdot CHR)_nCH_2\cdot \dot{C}HR + CH:CHR$$
$$\rightarrow X(CH_2\cdot CHR)_nCH:CHR + CH_3\cdot \dot{C}HR$$

Kinetically the original chain propagation just goes on as if the hydrogen transfer had never happened; but structural chain growth stops, and then starts from the beginning again. This is called "chain transfer." Whereas degrees of polymerisation are normally bound up with the kinetics, as we shall see below, so that in order to change a degree of polymerisation one has to change the rate, chain transfer results in a reduced degree of polymerisation without a change of rate.

It is common practice for the purpose of regulating the molecular weight of a polymer, without going outside convenient rates of polymerisation, to add to the polymerising system what is called a "chain transfer agent." This is a substance, YZ, usually a simple one, such as carbon tetrachloride, from which the polymerising adduct-radical can take an atom Y, so to produce a new initiating radical:

$$X(CH_2\cdot CHR)_nCH_2\cdot \dot{C}HR + YZ \rightarrow X(CH_2\cdot CHR)_nCH_2\cdot CHYR + \dot{Z}$$

$$\dot{Z} + CH_2:CHR \rightarrow ZCH_2\cdot \dot{C}HR$$

$$\cdots$$

Again, the kinetic chain, originally initiated with the radical $\dot{X}$, simply continues; but the chemical consequence of the intervention by YZ is to stop the old structural chain, and start a new one, with the result that the molecular weight of the eventual polymer becomes reduced.

In calculating the rate equation which follows from the mechanism given above for radical-carried addition-polymerisation, the assumption is made that the rate-constants of all steps of propagation are the same. This will be true, except at most for the first three or four steps. With the simplified assumption mentioned, the rate equation is of the standard form for chain reactions given in Section **37d**, *viz.*,

$$R_p = k_p[\mathrm{M}]\left(\frac{R_i}{2k_t}\right)^{1/2}$$

where R_p is the rate of polymerisation, R_i is the rate of initiation, k_p is the second-order rate-constant of a step of propagation, and k_t the second-order constant of total termination. Any chain transfer does not enter into the rate expression.

The kinetic chain length ν is given by

$$\nu = \frac{R_p}{R_i} = \frac{R_p}{R_t} = \frac{k_p^2}{2k_t}\cdot\frac{[\mathrm{M}]^2}{R_p} = \frac{k_p}{\sqrt{2k_t}}\cdot\frac{[\mathrm{M}]}{R_i^{1/2}}$$

For a given monomer concentration, the kinetic chain length is inversely proportional to the rate of polymerisation, or inversely to the square-root of the rate of initiation. For a given rate of initiation, it is proportional to the monomer concentration. In the absence of chain transfer, the average degree of polymerisation,

$$\overline{DP} = 2\nu \quad \text{or} \quad \nu$$

according as termination is by colligation or disproportionation. In the presence of chain transfer, the degree of polymerisation will be less, to an extent depending on the rate-constants of the chain-transfer processes, and the concentration of added chain-transfer agent if any.

Measurements of polymerisation rate, at known rates of initiation, give k_p^2/k_t. The individual rate-constants, k_p and k_t, have been determined by Bartlett and Melville's "sector method" of intermittent photo-initiation, and by other methods likewise based on relaxation of the steady-state condition on suddenly starting or stopping the initiation process (cf. Section **37d**). The sort of results obtained may be illustrated from Kwart, Broadbent, and Bartlett's study of the polymerisation at 25° of vinyl acetate initiated by photolysed di-*t*-butyl peroxide.[278] In the conditions used, the constants were $k_p = 1.0 \times 10^3$ sec.$^{-1}$ mole^{-1} l., and $k_t = 3.0 \times 10^7$ sec.$^{-1}$ mole^{-1} l. The concentration of polymerising radicals was about 0.5×10^{-8} mole/l. The half-life of a step of polymerisation was of the order of 10^{-4} sec., the average time of growth of a polymer was a very few seconds, and the degree of polymerisation was of the order of ten thousand. Some illustrative rate-constants for propagation and termination, taken from a critically selected compilation by Walling,[279] are given in Table 55-2.

The effect of substituents in a polymerising olefin on its rate of

[278] H. Kwart, H. S. Broadbent, and P. D. Bartlett, *J. Am. Chem. Soc.*, 1950, **72,** 1060.

[279] C. Walling, ref. 249, p. 95.

TABLE 55-2.—SECOND-ORDER RATE-CONSTANTS (IN SEC.$^{-1}$ MOLE^{-1} L.) FOR PROPAGATION AND TERMINATION IN ADDITION-POLYMERISATIONS AT 30°.

	k_p	$10^{-7}k_t$
Vinyl chloride	6800	1200
Vinyl acetate	990	2.0
Methyl acrylate	720	0.22
Methyl α-methacrylate	350	1.5
Styrene	49	0.24
Butadiene	25	

polymerisation is a complicated matter because of the prevalence of compensating effects, which Mayo and Walling have done much to disentangle.[280] A substituent that will stabilise the double bond of an olefinic monomer, let us say by conjugating with it, will thus stabilise much more strongly the adduct-radical into which an adding radical will convert the olefin; and therefore it will accelerate that conversion of the olefin into the adduct-radical. But the same conjugation with the radical centre on the adduct-radical will make the adduct-radical add more slowly to another molecule of the original olefin, or to a molecule of any other olefin. The same substituent therefore affects the reactivity of the two participants in the propagation steps of a homopolymerisation in opposite ways; but the effect on the unsaturation of the radical will be greater than that on the unsaturation of the olefin. Thus the effect of a substituent on the rate of a homopolymerisation is likely to be smaller than its effect on the rate of reaction of the radical with a standard olefin, but to be in the direction of the latter effect, and not in the direction of the effect of the substituent on the rate of reaction of the olefin with a standard radical. The field for making the required analyses of substituent effects is that of copolymerisation. In this process, each adduct-radical has a choice of monomers to which to add, and each monomer has a choice of types of radical to accept. It is because of the compensating effects described that copolymerisation occurs as freely as it does between monomers of widely different reactivities.

By a study of copolymer compositions, Mayo and Walling have deduced[280] that the effects of groups R on the rate of reaction of olefins $CH_2{:}CHR$ with a common adding radical stand in the order,

$$(R=)\ OMe < OAc < CH_3 < Cl < CO_2Me < CN$$
$$< CO\cdot CH_3 < CH_2{:}CH < Ph$$

[280] F. R. Mayo and C. Walling, *Chem. Revs.*, 1950, **46**, 191.

The relative rates that might be quoted to represent this series differ with the common adding radical; but some ranges of values, based on copolymerisation data involving 20 radicals and more than 30 olefins, have been given by Walling as follows:[281]

OMe	OAc, CH_3	Cl	CO_2Me	CN, COMe	$CH{:}CH_2$, C_6H_5
1	1.5–5	3–20	20–60	30–60	50–100

It is more difficult to obtain values representing the effects of substituents on the rates of addition of different adduct-radicals to a common olefin, because product composition and rates of propagation of polymerisation have to be combined; but the data available suggest that a series expressing the inequalities would be something like the reverse of that written above. Again, relative rate values differ with the common olefin; but some rather rough ranges can be given as follows:

OAc, Cl	CO_2Me	C_6H_5	$CH_2{:}CH$
100–2000	30–200	1	0.5–0.7

The spread of values from end to end of this series, besides being reversed, is larger than before, as we should expect from the explanation in the preceding paragraph. But on comparing the two series, one sees that, as regards homopolymerisation, there is a large degree of compensation. We may illustrate this by comparing the polymerisation of vinyl acetate with that of styrene. As an olefin, vinyl acetate reacts with a radical about 50 times more slowly than styrene does; but the adduct-radical of vinyl acetate reacts with an olefin about 1000 times faster than the adduct-radical of styrene does. The nett result is that the propagation rate for the polymerisation of vinyl acetate is about 20 times that for the polymerisation of styrene.

The addition polymerisation of olefins can be inhibited by added substances. It is presumed that the general mechanism of inhibition involves combination of the polymerising adduct-radical with the inhibitor to form either a non-radical or an unreactive radical, one which at least cannot participate in the continued propagation of polymerisation as easily as can the adduct-radical which it replaces. Triaryl or diphenylpicrylhydrazyl radicals will inhibit: in such cases combination of the adduct-radical with the radical inhibitor will produce a non-radical. Molecular oxygen is a notable inhibitor. This must form a peroxy-radical, which, though it will add to some olefins, styrene for instance, may not add to the particular olefinic substance that happens to be available.

Many molecules which are not radicals and are not in triplet states

[281] C. Walling, ref. 249, p. 121.

may be, and commonly are, used as inhibitors. They are well-conjugated, easily reducible electrophiles of the aromatic series, notably quinones and nitro-compounds. There are two ways in which they might act on the polymerising adduct-radical and so put it out of action as a carrier of the kinetic chain. One is by disproportionation: they could take a hydrogen atom out of the adduct-radical. Quinone would then become quinhydrone, and perhaps eventually hydroquinone, whilst the curtailed polymer would contain an unsaturated end-group. The other way is by simply adding the whole radical to give an addition radical in which mesomerism so spreads out the radical centre that it is incapable of adding to another olefin, even though it might be able to colligate with another radical.

A general point in favour of an explanation of this type is the common experience that the homopolymerisations which are most easily inhibited are those, such as the polymerisation of vinyl acetate, in which the adduct-radical is especially reactive, but the monomer is not.

The possible explanations based on disproportionation and addition are not mutually exclusive, but most positive indications show that addition is an effective mechanism. Among benzoquinones, chloranil is a somewhat poor inhibitor; but it copolymerises with styrene to give a polymer of the structure:[282]

$$\left[-\mathrm{O\cdot CH_2\cdot CHPh\cdot O}\langle \mathrm{C_6Cl_4} \rangle \mathrm{O}- \right]_n$$

Benzoquinone could terminate growing polymer chains by undergoing a similar O-alkylation. Chloranil could not undergo C-alkylation, but benzoquinone could do so; and there is evidence from polymer compositions that, when the polymerisation of allyl acetate is retarded by benzoquinone, both O- and C-alkylation of the inhibitor occur.[283] In a nitrobenzene inhibitor, addition of the carbon radical would be expected to occur ortho- and para- to the nitro-group, and it has been suggested that the addition can also occur in the nitro-group.[283,284] Studies of the stoicheiometry of inhibition show that either less than one, or more than one, molecule of inhibitor per molecule of polymer, according to the case, and according to the conditions, may be incorporated in the inhibited polymer. Of course, there is more than

[282] J. W. Breitenbach and A. J. Renner, *Can. J. Research*, 1950, **28**, **B**, 509.

[283] P. D. Bartlett, G. S. Hammond, and H. Kwart, *Disc. Faraday Soc.*, 1947, **2**, 342.

[284] P. D. Bartlett and H. Kwart, *J. Am. Chem. Soc.*, 1950, **72**, 1051.

one possible interpretation of any of these findings: multiple attack, disproportionation, and copolymerisation must all be kept in view.

(56) CYCLIC ADDITIONS TO OLEFINIC COMPOUNDS[285]

(56a) Additions of Carbenes to Give Three-Membered Rings.[286]— We noticed in Section **44** one of the two main methods of producing carbenes, *viz.*, by 1,1-elimination from substituted alkanes. The other main method is by the pyrolysis or photolysis of diazoalkanes or ketenes:

$$RR'C{:}N{:}N \rightarrow RR'C + N_2, \qquad RR'C{:}C{:}O \rightarrow RR'C + CO$$

The history of the cyclic additions of carbenes takes us back to the studies of Buchner and Curtius on the additions of diazoalkanes to aromatic compounds and olefins. From olefins, pyrazolines were obtained, which, on pyrolysis, lose nitrogen to form *cyclo*propanes. The work began with benzene and similar compounds in 1885. It yielded no intermediate pyrazolines.[287] It did yield what were taken to be norcaradienes, and were in fact their more stable valency-tautomers, tropylidenes. Eventually Buchner and Hediger reached the conclusion that the nitrogen loss occurred, not after, but before the addition, and that the effective addendum, for molecules such as benzene and naphthalene, was the carbene.[288]

The simplest carbene, methylene, was obtained by Herzberg and Shoosmith by flash photolysis of diazomethane. They were able to record its electronic absorption spectrum.[289] It has, indeed, two distinct spectra, that is, two different states long-lived enough to have their absorption spectra recorded. One of these spectra was in the vacuum ultraviolet (near 1415 *A*); and analysis of the bands showed that it was of a linear triplet state. The other spectrum was in the far red (bands at 6531, 7315, and 8190 *A*); and this proved to be the spectrum of a bent singlet state. When the inert gas pressure was increased, the far-ultraviolet band system gained intensity at the expense of the far-red system. Evidently gas collisions were overcoming spin conservation, and were converting a less stable singlet state to a more stable triplet state. The singlet state has an unshared electron-

[285] R. Huisgen, R. Grashey, and J. Sauer, "The Chemistry of Alkenes," Editor S. Patai, Interscience Publishers, London, 1964, p. 739.

[286] W. Kirmse, "Carbene Chemistry," Academic Press, New York, 1964.

[287] E. Buchner and T. Curtius, *Ber.*, 1885, **18**, 2377; E. Buchner, *Ber.*, 1897, **30**, 362; W. Barren and E. Buchner, *Ber.*, 1900, **33**, 684; 1901, **34**, 982.

[288] E. Buchner and S. Hediger, *Ber.*, 1903, **36**, 3502.

[289] G. Herzberg and J. Shoosmith, *Nature*, 1959, **183**, 1801; G. Herzberg, *Proc. Roy. Soc.*, 1961, **A**, **262**, 291; *idem* and J. W. C. Jones, *ibid.*, 1966, **A**, **295**, 107.

pair, as well as an unoccupied *p* orbital, whilst the triplet state has two singly occupied *p* orbitals:

C̈ (with H and H) — Singlet

H—C—H (with one dot above and one below C) — Triplet

In the singlet state, the CH length is 1.11 *A* and the bond angle 102.4°.

Though the triplet state is the more stable, the singlet state is the first to be formed from a singlet precursor, such as the ground state of diazomethane or keten, or an excited state of either reached by an allowed transition. Moreover, the singlet state, when formed, may often react in that condition, because the singlet-to-triplet conversion is a slow process, requiring many molecular collisions for its accomplishment.

There have been many earlier but less substantial claims for the production of methylene. In 1938 Pearson, Purcell, and Saigh photolysed diazomethane to a gas which removed deposited mirrors of selenium and tellurium.[290]

The two main general reactions of methylene are the so-called "insertion" reaction, in which C—H is converted to $C—CH_3$, and cyclic addition to an olefinic double bond, to give a *cyclo*propane ring. Meerwein and his coworkers observed the insertion reaction in 1942, when they noticed that, on photolysis of diazomethane in diethyl ether, some of the latter becomes converted to ethyl *n*-propyl ether and ethyl *iso*propyl ether.[291] Primary, secondary, and tertiary alkanic C—H bonds, as well as olefinic C—H bonds, are attacked with comparable ease. With an olefinic substrate, the most important reaction may be that of addition to the double bond. Thus, *cyclo*hexene takes up methylene from photolysed diazomethane to give all possible methyl*cyclo*hexenes together with norcarane:[292]

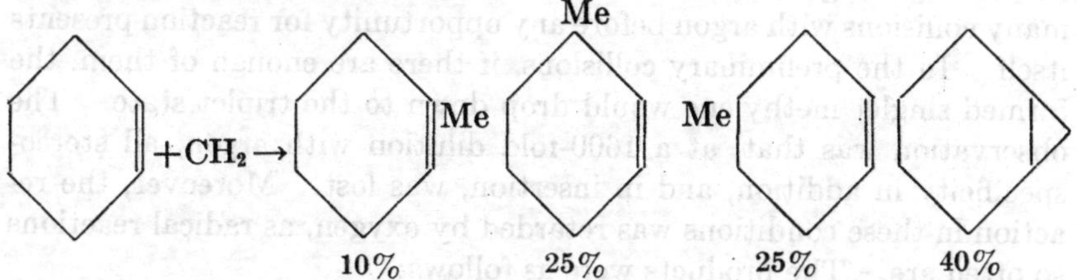

[290] T. G. Pearson, R. H. Purcell, and G. S. Saigh, *J. Chem. Soc.*, **1938**, 409.

[291] H. Meerwein, H. Rathjen, and H. Werner, *Ber.*, 1942, **75**, 1610.

[292] W. von E. Doering, R. G. Buttery, R. H. Laughlin, and N. Chaudhuri, *J. Am. Chem. Soc.*, 1956, **78**, 3224.

Something can be learned of the mechanism of these additions from their stereochemistry. If the conditions are so organised that first-formed methylene has the opportunity to react as soon as it is formed, the additions are stereospecific. It has been shown by Frey that, when diazomethane is photolysed in solution in *trans*-2-butene at −78°, the products are exclusively *trans*, and when the solvent is *cis*-2-butene, the products are exclusively *cis*:[293]

Me H / C:C / H Me $\xrightarrow{CH_2}$ Me H / C:C / Me Me (9%); Et H / C:C / H Me (40%); Me H / cyclopropane / H Me (51%)

Me Me / C:C / H H $\xrightarrow{CH_2}$ Me Me / C:C / Me H; Et Me / C:C / H H; Me Me / cyclopropane / H H

The proportions of the products from *trans*-2-butene were measured, and were as noted above. From this it is concluded that the addendum is singlet methylene, which adds, or inserts, in one step, without producing transiently any intermediate which could permit conformational change:

:CH₂ → C═C   :CH₂ → H—C≤

The contrasting conditions have been illustrated in the pyrolysis of diazomethane in the gas phase in the presence of *cis*-2-butene highly diluted with argon.[294] The first-formed methylene will now undergo many collisions with argon before any opportunity for reaction presents itself. In the preliminary collisions, if there are enough of them, the formed singlet methylene would drop down to the triplet state. The observation was that, at a 1600-fold dilution with argon, all stereospecificity in addition, and in insertion, was lost. Moreover, the reaction in these conditions was retarded by oxygen, as radical reactions so often are. The products were as follows:

[293] P. S. Skell and R. C. Woodworth, *J. Am. Chem. Soc.*, 1956, **78**, 4496; W. von E. Doering and P. La Flamme, *ibid.*, p. 5447; H. M. Frey, *ibid.*, 1958, **80**, 5005.

[294] H. M. Frey, *J. Am. Chem. Soc.*, 1960, **82**, 5947.

$$\begin{matrix}Me & & Me\\ & C{:}C & \\ H & & H\end{matrix} \xrightarrow[\text{in Ar}]{CH_2} \left\{\begin{matrix} \begin{matrix}Me & & Me\\ & C{:}C & \\ Me & & H\end{matrix} \quad 4\% & \begin{matrix}Et & & Me\\ & C{:}C & \\ H & & H\end{matrix} \quad 16\% & \text{Me, Me / H, H cyclopropane} \quad 27\% \\ CH_2{:}CH\cdot C(Me)(Et)(H){-}Me \quad 10\% & \begin{matrix}Et & & H\\ & C{:}C & \\ H & & Me\end{matrix} \quad 16\% & \text{H, Me / H, Me cyclopropane} \quad 27\% \end{matrix}\right.$$

The non-stereospecific addition to the double bond is interpreted on the basis that triplet methylene adds in two steps through an intermediate di-radical in which the conformational change occurs:

$$\dot{\underset{\cdot}{C}}H_2 + C{=}C \rightarrow CH_2{-}C{-}\dot{C} \rightarrow \text{ring}$$

The position with respect to insertion is less clear. There has been an impression that triplet methylene, as such, does not insert. But it may do, though less readily than singlet methylene does. If we assume that it inserts by hydrogen abstraction, after the model of the $H+H_2$ reaction, with concurrent colligation within the mesomeric di-radical thus formed, the geometrical *and positional* changes of the double bond, during insertion, are accounted for:

$$\dot{\underset{\cdot}{C}}H_2 + H{-}CH_2{-}C{=}C \rightarrow \dot{C}H_3 \ldots \left\{\begin{matrix}\dot{C}H_2{-}C{=}C\\ CH_2{=}C{-}\dot{C}\end{matrix}\right\} \rightarrow \text{products}$$

Alkyl and dialkyl carbenes spontaneously undergo rearrangements equivalent to intramolecular insertion reactions. Carbene insertion into β-CH leads to an olefin, and with a γ-CH to a *cyclo*propane derivative,[295] *e.g.*,

$$(CH_3)_2CH\cdot\ddot{C}H \rightarrow (CH_3)_2C{=}CH_2 \quad \text{and} \quad CH_3{-}CH{<}(CH_2)_2 \; (\text{CH}_3\text{-cyclopropane})$$

Diphenylcarbene, which is readily formed by pyrolysis or photolysis of diphenyldiazomethane, does not add in a stereospecific way to

[295] L. Friedman and H. Schechter, *J. Am. Chem. Soc.*, 1959, 81, 5512.

cis- and *trans*-2-butene.[296] The mixtures obtained from these isomers are not of identical composition, but must have been formed by a mechanism admitting some conformational change. Skell and his coworkers suggest that the ease of formation of the triplet state of diphenylcarbene is such that the reactions normally observed are reactions of that form. The observed additions are retarded by oxygen, as is consistent with this idea.

Carbalkoxycarbenes, which may be thermally or photolytically produced from alkyl diazoacetates, engage in cyclic additions to olefinic double bonds in much the same way as does methylene itself. Because of the substituent, more stereoisomers may be produced than from methylene: thus, addition of the ethyl diazoacetate to styrene gives ethyl *cis*- and *trans*-1-phenyl*cyclo*propane-2-carboxylate.[297] But when methyl diazoacetate was photolysed in solution in *cis*- or *trans*-2-butene, only those *cyclo*propane isomers were produced, two in the first case, and one in the second, which preserved the configuration, *cis* or *trans*, of methyl groups of the olefinic precursor.[298] The addition is still stereospecific, and it is concluded that the carbene is formed and reacts in the singlet state.

Dichlorocarbene and dibromocarbene, CCl_2 and CBr_2, are usually produced by Hine's method of 1,1-elimination from haloforms (Section **44**). Doering and Hoffmann showed that these carbenes would readily undergo cyclic addition to olefins if the competition of solvolysis to formates was excluded by the use of aprotic conditions.[299] Thus, when chloroform or bromoform was added to a suspension of potassium *t*-butoxide in *cyclo*hexene, good yields of 7,7-dichloro- or 7,7-dibromo-norcarane were obtained:

$$\text{(cyclohexene)} + CX_2 \rightarrow \text{(norcarane)}X_2$$

These reactions have been generalised over a wide range of olefins. Insertion reactions are not prominent, unless a particularly weak CH bond is present to participate, such as the benzylic CH of cumene,[300]

[296] R. M. Etter, H. S. Skovronek, and P. S. Skell, *J. Am. Chem. Soc.*, 1959, **81**, 1008; G. L. Closs and L. L. Closs, *Angew. Chem.*, 1962, **74**, 431.

[297] A. Burger and W. L. Yost, *J. Am. Chem. Soc.*, 1948, **70**, 2198; D. G. Markees, *ibid.*, p. 3329; H. L. de Waal and G. W. Perold, *Chem. Ber.*, 1952, **85**, 574.

[298] W. von E. Doering and T. Mole, *Tetrahedron*, 1960, **10**, 65.

[299] W. von E. Doering and A. K. Hoffmann, *J. Am. Chem. Soc.*, 1954, **76**, 6162.

[300] E. K. Fields, *J. Am. Chem. Soc.*, 1962, **84**, 1744.

or the α-CH_2 of an allyl ether[301] or allyl thio-ether.[302] It has been shown that dibromocarbene produced in solution in *cis*-2-butene, or in *trans*-2-butene, adds to these olefins in the completely stereospecific way characteristic of the addition of methylene in like conditions.[303] Evidently the dibromocarbene is produced and reacts in singlet form. Westcott and Skell have produced dichlorocarbene by pyrolysis of carbon tetrachloride, and of chloroform, at 1500°, and have collected the products on a liquid-nitrogen-cooled surface.[304] They established the presence of dichlorocarbenes by admitting ethylene, and obtaining 1,1-dichloro*cyclo*propene. They showed the dichlorocarbene to be in singlet form by demonstrating its addition to *cis*- and *trans*-2-butene with the complete stereospecificity characteristic of the singlet state of the carbene.

The relative rates of additions of dibromocarbene to different olefins have been determined by competition experiments with the following results:[303,305]

$Me_2C{:}CMe_2$	$Me_2C{:}CHMe$	$Me_2C{:}CH_2$	Butadiene	Styrene	*cyclo*Hexene	1-Hexene
3.5	3.2	(1)	0.5	0.4	0.4	0.07

In part, this series suggests that dibromocarbene is a mild electrophile, that is, that its reaction is facilitated by electropositive substituents in the substrate. But the low position of butadiene and styrene in such a series is most unusual. Huisgen, Grashey, and Sauer have discussed this,[285] pointing out that dibromocarbene has no nett charge and may have no field in the direction of the olefinic substrate, wherefore, although it can take advantage of a permanently present, electropositive, inductive effect (+I), it cannot excite an electromeric effect (+E) from the vinyl and phenyl substituents in butadiene and styrene.

The *Reimer-Tiemann* reaction,[306] by which phenols are converted by chloroform and alkali to ortho- and para-hydroxybenzaldehydes, almost certainly proceeds by way of first-formed dichlorocarbene, as illustrated below for the formation of salicylaldehyde:

$$\text{C}_6\text{H}_5\text{O}^- \xrightarrow[\text{slow}]{\text{CCl}_2} \text{(cyclohexadienone with CCl}_2^-\text{, H)} \longrightarrow o\text{-}^-\text{O}\text{C}_6\text{H}_4\text{CHCl}_2 \longrightarrow o\text{-HOC}_6\text{H}_4\text{CHO}$$

[301] J. C. Anderson and C. B. Reese, *Chem. and Ind.*, **1963**, 575.
[302] W. E. Pearson and E. Konces, *J. Am. Chem. Soc.*, 1961, **83**, 4034.
[303] P. S. Skell and A. Y. Garner, *J. Am. Chem. Soc.*, 1956, **78**, 3049, 5430.
[304] L. D. Westcott and P. S. Skell, *J. Am. Chem. Soc.*, 1965, **87**, 1721.
[305] W. von E. Doering and W. A. Henderson jr., *J. Am. Chem. Soc.*, 1958, **80**, 5274.
[306] K. Reimer, *Ber.*, 1876, **9**, 423; *idem* and F. Tiemann, *ibid.*, 824, 1285.

The last of the steps shown is simply a collective representation of the succession of steps involved in the hydrolysis of a benzal chloride (Section **28b**). Hine and van der Veen showed[307] that phenoxide ion reacts with chloroform only very slowly, and that the Reimer-Tiemann reaction requires the additional presence of hydroxide ions. The kinetics are consistent with the slow step shown above. In the experimental conditions, the *o-/p*-ratio was 1.9; but it was found to be sensitive to ion-pairing.

The *Hofmann* conversion of a primary amine by means of chloroform and alkali to an *iso*nitrile[308] also proceeds almost certainly through a preliminary addition of dichlorocarbene:

$$RNH_2 \xrightarrow{CCl_2} R\overset{+}{N}H_2\cdot\overset{-}{C}Cl_2 \rightarrow RNH\cdot CHCl_2 \begin{cases} \nearrow RN{:}C \\ \searrow RNH\cdot CHO \end{cases}$$

Nef believed this.[309] We have as yet no kinetic confirmation; but it has been shown[310] that the formamide by-product is formed simultaneously with, and not subsequently to, the *iso*nitrile.

As already noted in Section **45d**, the main importance of acylcarbenes is that they are the electron-deficient intermediates of the *Wolff rearrangement.* They may be formed by pyrolysis or photolysis of an α-diazoketone. Their rearrangement product is a ketene:

$$\underset{\substack{|\\ R}}{O{=}C}{-}CHN_2 \rightarrow \underset{\substack{|\\ R}}{O{=}C}{-}CH \rightarrow O{=}C{=}\underset{\substack{|\\ R}}{CH}$$

A special carbene is the source of the band system ("4050 group"), first observed in cometary spectra. It was produced later in laboratory discharges and flames. Its source has been identified by Douglas and others as the linear molecule C_3, that is, as carbon dicarbene, C:C:C.[311] Skell and his coworkers have shown that carbon vapour produced in a carbon arc consists to the extent of about 60% of C_3. The next most important constituent is C_2, the source of the blue "Swan bands," that anyone can see with a pocket spectroscope. Car-

[307] J. Hine and J. M. van der Veen, *J. Am. Chem. Soc.*, 1959, **81**, 6447.
[308] A. W. Hofmann, *Ann.*, 1887, **144**, 114; 1888, **146**, 107.
[309] J. U. Nef, *Ann.*, 1897, **298**, 202.
[310] P. A. S. Smith and N. W. Kalenda, *J. Org. Chem.*, 1958, **23**, 1599.
[311] A. Monnis and B. Rosen, *Nature*, 1949, **164**, 714; A. E. Douglas, *Astrophys. J.*, 1951; **114**, 406; K. Clusius and A. E. Douglas, *Can. J. Phys.*, 1954, **32**, 319; D. A. Ramsey, *Ann. New York Acad. Sci.*, 1957, **67**, 485.

bon atoms are also present, as well as some carbon molecules higher than C_3.[312]

The carbon dicarbene C_3 can be collected, and kept for days, in a matrix of neopentane on a surface at $-196°$. If an olefin is admitted, and the temperature is allowed to rise, cyclic addition occurs at one or both ends of the dicarbene.[312] In general several products are formed, but the addition to *iso*butylene goes particularly easily to give only one product, identified as the carbon bis*cyclo*propylidene:

$$C{=}C{=}C + 2\ \overset{CMe_2}{\underset{CH_2}{\|}} \rightarrow \begin{matrix} Me_2C & & & & CMe_2 \\ | & \diagdown & & \diagup & | \\ | & & C{=}C{=}C & & | \\ | & \diagup & & \diagdown & | \\ H_2C & & & & CH_2 \end{matrix}$$

(56b) Additions of Olefins to Give Four-Membered Rings.—Staudinger, who discovered the ketens, observed many examples of their capacity for cyclic dimerisation.[313] In general, the olefinic double bond of one keten molecule may add either to the carbonyl or to the olefinic double bond of another one. Keten itself dimerises in the first of these ways to give β-methylene-β-propiolactone. Dialkylketens dimerise in the second way to give *cyclo*butane-1,3-diones. Monoalkylketens usually dimerise in both ways, but the formed diketo-dimer monoenolises substantially completely, to give a moderately acidic enol, as already illustrated in Section 7e. Examples of these reactions are formulated below:

$$\begin{matrix} H_2C{=}C{=}O \\ + \\ H_2C{=}C{=}O \end{matrix} \rightarrow \begin{matrix} H_2C{-}CO \\ | \quad\ | \\ H_2C{=}C{-}O \end{matrix}$$

$$\begin{matrix} Me_2C{=}C{=}O \\ + \\ O{=}C{=}CMe_2 \end{matrix} \rightarrow \begin{matrix} Me_2C{-}CO \\ | \quad\ | \\ OC{-}CMe_2 \end{matrix}$$

$$2MeHC{=}C{=}O \rightarrow \begin{matrix} MeHC{-}CO \\ | \quad\ | \\ MeHC{=}C{-}O \end{matrix} \text{ and } \begin{matrix} MeHC{-}CO \\ | \quad\ | \\ OC{-}CHMe \end{matrix} \rightleftharpoons \begin{matrix} MeC{=}C{\cdot}OH \\ | \quad\ | \\ OC{-}CHMe \end{matrix}$$

A second group of compounds have become celebrated for their tendency to cyclic dimerisation. They are the perfluoro-olefins, as such, or with some partial replacement of fluorine by chlorine. The parent of the series, tetrafluoroethylene, smoothly dimerises at 200°

[312] P. S. Skell, L. D. Westcott jr., J. P. Goldstein, and R. R. Engel, *J. Am. Chem. Soc.*, 1965, **87**, 2829.

[313] H. Staudinger, many papers since 1908, summarised in his book "Die Ketene," F. Enke, Stuttgart, 1912. For a more recent review, see E. Enk and H. Spes, *Angew. Chem.*, 1961, **73**, 334.

to octafluoro*cyclo*butane.[314] Chlorotrifluoroethylene dimerises head-to-head, but the 1,2-dichlorohexafluoro*cyclo*butane appears in *cis*- and *trans*-forms.[315] 1,1-Dichloro-2,2-difluoroethylene gives only the head-to-head dimer 1,1,2,2,-tetrachlorotetrafluoro*cyclo*butane.[316] Hexafluoropropylene dimerises in both directions.[317]

$$2F_2C{:}CF_2 \rightarrow \begin{array}{c} F_2C-CF_2 \\ | \quad\;\; | \\ F_2C-CF_2 \end{array} \qquad 2Cl_2C{:}CF_2 \rightarrow \begin{array}{c} Cl_2C-CF_2 \\ | \quad\;\; | \\ Cl_2C-CF_2 \end{array}$$

$$2ClFC{:}CF_2 \rightarrow \begin{array}{c} ClFC-CF_2 \\ | \quad\;\; | \\ ClFC-CF_2 \end{array} \quad (\textit{cis and trans})$$

$$2F_3C\cdot CF{:}CF_2 \rightarrow \begin{array}{c} F_3C\cdot HC-CF_2 \\ | \quad\;\; | \\ F_3C\cdot HC-CF_2 \end{array} \quad \text{and} \quad \begin{array}{c} F_3C\cdot HC-CF_2 \\ | \quad\;\; | \\ F_2C-CH\cdot CF_3 \end{array}$$

Tetrafluoroethylene will add to propylene.[318] It will add at a lower temperature to butadiene, but only by cyclic 1,2-addition to give a *cyclo*butane derivative:[318]

$$\begin{array}{c} F_2C{:}CF_2 \\ + \\ H_2C{:}CHMe \end{array} \xrightarrow{225^\circ} \begin{array}{c} F_2C-CF_2 \\ | \quad\;\; | \\ H_2C-CHMe \end{array} \qquad \begin{array}{c} F_2C{:}CF_2 \\ + \\ H_2C{:}CH\cdot CH{:}CH_2 \end{array} \xrightarrow{125^\circ} \begin{array}{c} F_2C-CF_2 \\ | \quad\;\; | \\ H_2C-CH\cdot CH{:}CH_2 \end{array}$$

To *cyclo*pentadiene, however, tetrafluoroethylene adds largely in the same 1,2-manner, but also in part by cyclic 1,4-addition in the Diels-Alder manner.[318] Hexafluorobutadiene dimerises in two steps as follows:[319]

$$2F_2C{:}CF\cdot CF{:}CF_2 \xrightarrow{160^\circ} \begin{array}{c} F_2C-CF\cdot CF{:}CF_2 \\ | \quad\;\; | \\ F_2C-CF\cdot CF{:}CF_2 \end{array} \xrightarrow{200^\circ} \begin{array}{c} F_2C-CF-CF-CF_2 \\ | \quad\;\; | \quad\;\; | \quad\;\; | \\ F_2C-CF-CF-CF_2 \end{array}$$

It is not understood why ketens and polyfluoroethylenes in particular should have the property of engaging in cyclic 1,2-addition de-

[314] B. Atkinson and A. B. Trenwith, *J. Chem. Soc.*, **1953**, 2082.

[315] J. R. Lacher, G. W. Thompkin, and J. D. Park, *J. Am. Chem. Soc.*, 1952, **74**, 1693.

[316] A. L. Henne and R. P. Ruh, *J. Am. Chem. Soc.*, 1947, **69**, 279.

[317] M. Hauptschein, A. H. Fainberg, and M. Brand, *J. Am. Chem. Soc.*, 1958, **80**, 842.

[318] D. D. Coffman, P. L. Barrick, R. D. Cramer, M. S. Raasch, *J. Am. Chem. Soc.*, 1949, **71**, 490.

[319] M. Prober and W. T. Miller, *J. Am. Chem. Soc.*, 1949, **71**, 598.

veloped to the marked degree that has been illustrated. One may ask what common constitutional feature these two series share. By collecting cases of such additions that lie outside both series, one can see a possible regularity. Consider the following examples:[320,321,322]

$$2CH_2{:}C(SMe)(CN) \xrightarrow{20^\circ} \text{cyclobutane with MeS, CN (C-1) and MeS, CN (C-3)}$$

$$EtO{\cdot}CH{:}CH_2 + (NC)_2C{:}C(CN)_2 \xrightarrow{0^\circ} \text{cyclobutane with EtO; CN, CN; CN, CN}$$

$$t\text{-BuS}{\cdot}CH{:}CH_2 + (F_3C)(NC)C{:}C(CF_3)(CN) \xrightarrow{\text{room temp.}} \text{cyclobutane with } t\text{-BuS; } CF_3, CN; CF_3, CN \text{ and cyclobutane with } t\text{-BuS; } CN, CF_3; CN, CF_3$$

In these examples of very easy cyclic addition, two kinds of substituent are present. The first are strongly electron-attracting substituents, which may or may not be conjugated with the olefinic double bond (CN and CF_3). The second are strongly electron-releasing substituents, which definitely act by conjugation with the olefinic double bond (MeO and MeS). The two kinds of groups may both be present in each of the adding molecules, or one kind may be in one of them, and the other kind in the other. In the notation we sometimes use for signalising such distinctions, the total effect of the substituents would be summarised in the symbol $-I+K$. Now the carbonyl oxygen of a keten is a $-I+K$ substituent: it inductively attracts electrons, but conjugatively releases them (Sections **7e** and **8f**).

320 K. D. Grundermann and R. Thomas, *Chem. Ber.*, 1956, **89**, 1263; K. D. Grundermann and R. Huchting, *ibid.*, 1959, **92**, 415.

321 S. K. Williams, D. W. Wiley, and B. C. McKusick, *J. Am. Chem. Soc.*, 1962, **84**, 2210, 2216.

322 S. Proskow, H. E. Simmons, and T. L. Cavins, *J. Am. Chem. Soc.*, 1963, **85**, 2341.

The fluorine substituent in a fluoro-olefin is also a $-I+K$ substituent: it not only inductively attracts electrons more strongly than any other halogen, but also conjugatively releases electrons more strongly than any other halogen (Sections **7c** and **7e**). What seems to emerge is that the two kinds of polar effects co-operate to promote the transfer of electrons between the atoms of each pair that must unite when two double bonds undergo cyclic addition.

The two stereoisomers which constitute the total product in the third of the three examples given above show that each of the participating double bonds undergoes *cis*-addition to the other. When the place of the *cis*-dicyano-olefin in this reaction is taken by the *trans*-isomer, another pair of *cyclo*butane isomers is exclusively produced, which are again those required for *cis-cis*-addition.[322] This indicates that these 1,2-1,2 cyclic additions may go in a single step, and it at least shows that they do not go through any intermediate open-chain structure of sufficient life to admit conformational change.[323]

It should be emphaized that the effect of suitable substituents in promoting cyclic additions is a facilitating effect and not an absolute necessity for reaction. We have already noticed some spontaneous dimerisations and other rapid cyclic additions of highly strained, polyunsaturated, ring hydrocarbons. Thus *cyclo*butadiene dimerises very rapidly to *tricyclo*-octadiene, and adds acetylene derivatives to give *dicyclo*hexadienes (Section **49d**):

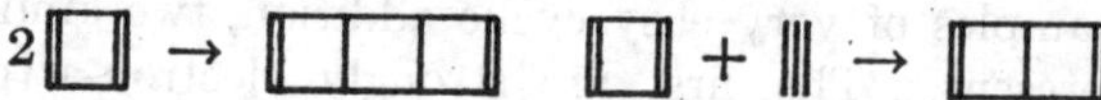

It is a general difficulty of classifying such reactions of *cyclo*butadiene to know whether they are really 1,2-1,2 cyclic additions or are 1,2-1,4 cyclic additions of Diels-Alder type. But this does not apply to the very rapid dimerisation of benzyne to diphenylene (Section **28d**):

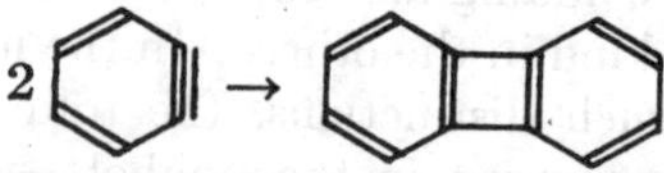

Many olefinic compounds, which cannot be thermally dimerised, do undergo photochemical cyclic dimerisation. Acenaphthylene is an example of a hydrocarbon which acts in this way on irradiation in benzene solution.[324] It gives both the possible stereoisomers:

[323] The opposite conclusion has been reached in consequence of stereochemical changes accompanying some cyclic 1,2-additions of 1,1-difluoro-2,2-dichloroethylenes to dienes (L. K. Montgomery, K. Schueller, and P. D. Bartlett, *J. Am Chem. Soc.*, 1964, **86**, 622, 628).

[324] E. J. Bowen and J. D. F. Marsh, *J. Chem. Soc.*, **1947**, 109.

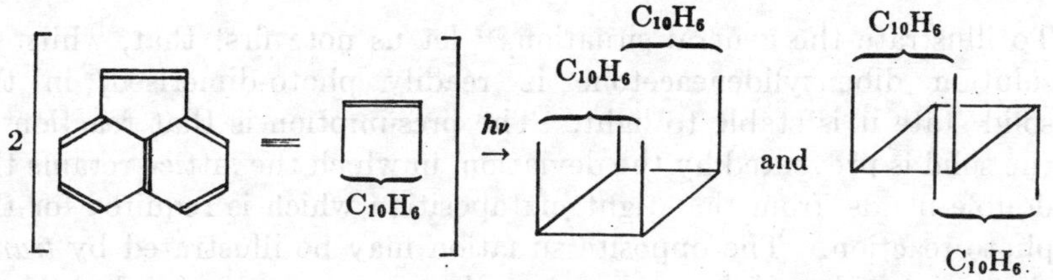

$$2\left[\ \text{(acenaphthylene)} \equiv \underbrace{\boxed{}}_{C_{10}H_6}\ \right] \xrightarrow{h\nu} \text{(cyclobutane dimer, } C_{10}H_6 \text{ bridges)} \text{ and } \text{(cyclobutane dimer, } C_{10}H_6 \text{ bridges)}$$

The majority of known examples, however, are among the conjugated unsaturated carbonyl, carboxyl, and cyano-compounds, including quinones. Thus chalcone, on irradiation in chloroform, undergoes a so-called "head-to-head" dimerisation:

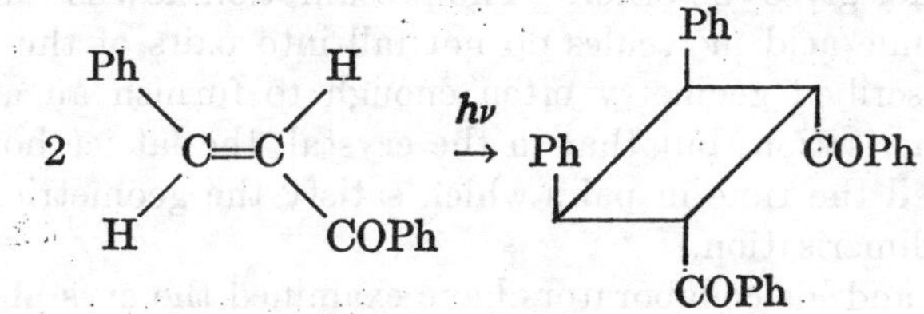

$$2\ \text{Ph(H)C=C(H)COPh} \xrightarrow{h\nu} \text{cyclobutane with Ph, Ph, COPh, COPh}$$

Dibenzylideneacetone, PhCH:CH·CO·CH:CHPh, behaves similarly.[325] Many photo-dimerisations are of this head-to-head type, but some are head-to-tail. A simple conjugated ketone, which photodimerises simultaneously in both directions, is *cyclo*pentenone.[326] It gives only one stereoisomer (*trans*) in each direction of addition.

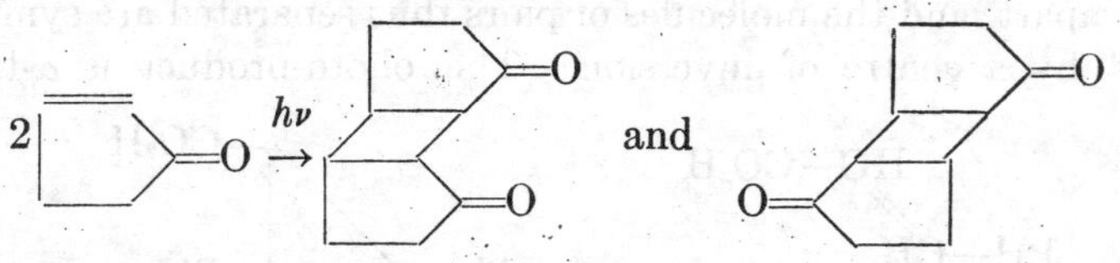

$$2\ \text{(cyclopentenone)} \xrightarrow{h\nu} \text{(head-to-head dimer)} \text{ and } \text{(head-to-tail dimer)}$$

Though we have no definite knowledge of the mechanisms involved in these reactions, it is certain that the precise geometrical presentation of the reactant molecules to each other at the moment when the electrons must make the traverse is highly critical. What shows this is that the fixed molecular geometry of the crystalline state can either destroy or create the capacity for photo-dimerisation, and, in the latter case, can direct it towards particular products. Schmidt and his collaborators have made an extensive study of these phenomena.

[325] H. Stobbe and K. Bremer, *J. prak. Chem.*, 1929, [2], **123**, 1; G. W. Reektenwald, J. N. Pitts, and R. L. Letsinger, *J. Am. Chem. Soc.*, 1953, **75**, 3028.
[326] P. E. Eaton, *J. Am. Chem. Soc.*, 1962, **84**, 2344, 2454.

To illustrate the general situation,[327] let us note first that, whilst in solution dibenzylideneacetone is readily photo-dimerised, in the solid state it is stable to light. The presumption is that reaction in the solid is prevented by the deviation, in which the lattice retains the double bonds, from that tight juxtaposition which is required for the photo-reaction. The opposite situation may be illustrated by *trans*-cinnamic acid, which, as has long been known, cannot be photo-dimerised in solution, but in the solid state readily gives both head-to-tail and head-to-head dimers, the truxillic and truxinic acids. Which of them one gets, depends on the kind of crystal irradiated; for *trans*-cinnamic acid is dimorphic, and one form of crystal gives one dimer, and the other gives the other. The presumption now is that, in solution, cinnamic acid molecules do not fall into pairs of the necessary, closely prescribed geometry often enough to furnish an appreciable rate of dimerisation; but that in the crystal, the lattice holds all the molecules all the time in pairs which satisfy the geometrical requirements for dimerisation.

Schmidt and his collaborators have examined the crystal structures and photo-products, not only of *trans*-cinnamic acid, but also of a large number of substituted *trans*-cinnamic acids.[328] Most of them are polymorphic. Collectively they show any or all of three types of crystal packing, called α, β, and γ. α-Packing may be illustrated by the more stable crystal modification of unsubstituted *trans*-cinnamic acid. In this crystal nearest-neighbour double bonds are centred 3.56 *A* apart, and the molecules of pairs thus separated are symmetry-related by a centre of inversion. The photo-product is α-truxillic acid:

HC—CO_2H
PH—CH
HC—Ph
HO_2C—CH

→

—CO_2H
Ph— —Ph
HO_2C—

α-Packing (schematic) α-Truxillic acid

β-Packing is represented in the less stable of the two crystal forms of *trans*-cinnamic acid, and it characterises the more stable, or the sole, crystal form of several of the substituted acids. The shortest double-bond distances are nearly as short as before, but the molecules of pairs

[327] M. D. Cohen and G. M. J. Schmidt, *J. Chem. Soc.*, **1964**, **1996**.

[328] M. D. Cohen, G. M. J. Schmidt, and F. I. Sonntag, *J. Chem. Soc.*, **1964**, 2000; G. M. J. Schmidt, *ibid.*, p. 2014.

so separated are now related by a translation. The photo-products are now truxinic acids:

HC—CO_2H
Ph—CH
HC—CO_2H
Ph—CH
→
—CO_2H
Ph—
—CO_2H
Ph—

β-Packing (schematic) β-Truxinic acid

In all cases of α- and β-packing of *trans*-cinnamic acids, the shortest double-bond distances lie in the range 3.6–4.1 *A*; and these crystals all give photo-dimers, with either a centre of symmetry or a plane of symmetry, according as the packing was α or β. In the third kind of packing, γ-packing, of which quite a number of examples were found, the shortest distances are greater, 4.7–5.1 *A*. These crystals do not give photo-dimers.

Similar, but less fully developed studies[329] of some substituted *cis*-cinnamic acids, and of a quinone, support the view that the double-bond separation required for cyclic photo-dimerisation is within the range 4.0 ± 0.4 *A*, and that, if this condition is fulfilled, photo-dimers will be formed which preserve the collective symmetry of the pair of combining monomers.

(56c) Additions of 1,3-Dipoles to Give Five-Membered Rings.—Some of these additions to olefins have a considerable history, but the additions were seen to comprise a group, the scope of which was much extended only in more recent times by Huisgen and his collaborators.[330] A 1,3-cyclic addendum must have a formal dipole, and it may, and usually does, have other unsaturation. With only nitrogen and oxygen as hetero-atoms, some dozens of types of 1,3-addenda are conceivable. Some of these types are represented in easily isolable compounds, but some types are less stable. However, compounds of these types can often be formed in the presence of, and intercepted by, an olefinic reactant, before they polymerise or decompose in some other way.

The *diazoalkanes* are the longest known of this group of addenda. The central atom of its three-atom unsaturated system has a pseudo-basic structure and hence will share its positive charge with either terminal atom, leaving the other to support the balancing negative

[329] J. Bregman, K. Osaki, G. M. J. Schmidt, and F. I. Sonntag, *J. Chem. Soc.*, **1964,** 3021; D. Rabinovich and G. M. J. Schmidt, *ibid.*, p. 2030.

[330] R. Huisgen, *Proc. Chem. Soc.*, **1961,** 357.

charge. The terminal atoms will thus be oppositely charged, and can be so charged in either of two ways as follows:

$$\overset{+}{\overbrace{R_2C{=}N}}{=}\bar{N} \qquad R_2\bar{C}{-}\overset{+}{\overbrace{N{\equiv}N}}$$

This is a common feature of unsaturated 1,3-addenda.

The addition of diazoalkanes to unsaturated esters to give pyrazoline derivatives, which are easily pyrolysed with loss of nitrogen to give *cyclo*propane derivatives, was first demonstrated by Buchner.[331] The addition of methyl diazoacetate to methyl maleate and to methyl fumarate gave the same Δ²-pyrazoline. The first products of addition must have been Δ¹-pyrazolines, but a prototropic change had supervened, with the result that all signs of a stereospecificity that would have differentiated the products from the maleic ester from those from the fumaric ester had been lost:

MeO₂C·CH:N:N + MeO₂C·CH:CH·CO₂Me → [MeO₂C·CH—N=N—CH·CO₂Me, ring closed by MeO₂C·CH—CH·CO₂Me] → [MeO₂C·CH—NH—N=C·CO₂Me, ring closed by MeO₂C·CH—C·CO₂Me]

The stereochemical course of addition was established by Auwers, who added diazomethane to methyl dimethylmaleate and dimethyl fumarate.[332] He obtained isomeric Δ¹-pyrazolines in which the original *cis*- or *trans*-relation between the carboxyl groups was preserved. This shows that the dipole adds in a *cis*-manner, as is consistent with the idea of addition in a single step:

CH_2N_2 + (Me)(MeO₂C)C=C(Me)(CO₂Me) → H₂C–N=N ring; Me, Me; MeO₂C, CO₂Me

CH_2N_2 + (MeO₂C)(Me)C=C(Me)(CO₂Me) → H₂C–N=N ring; CO₂Me, Me; Me, CO₂Me

[331] E. Buchner, *Ber.*, 1888, **21,** 2637; E. Buchner, M. Fritsch, A. Papendieck, and H. Witter, *Ann.*, 1893, **273,** 214.

[332] K. von Auwers and E. Cauer, *Ann.*, 1929, **470,** 284; K. von Auwers and F. Konig, *Ann.*, 1932, **496,** 27, 252.

Huisgen, Grashey, and Sauer[285] have advanced a strong argument against the alternative of a two-step mechanism. The analogy for such a mechanism would be the hydrolytic and other reactions of diazoalkanes, which are believed to be initiated by proton uptake at the carbon atom. If a dizaoalkane acted in a similarly nucleophilic way towards one carbon atom in the first step of a two-step cyclic addition to an olefinic bond, the intermediate product would be an aliphatic diazonium ion, which would surely never hold the nitrogen needed for the eventual production of a pyrazoline. For we know that aliphatic diazonium ions are very unstable, so much so that it has been doubted whether some of those produced from primary amines and nitrous acid have any free life at all, before they lose nitrogen to yield carbonium ions (Section **45b**).

Although the additions almost certainly go in one step, their rates suggest that diazoalkane addenda on the whole act in a predominantly nucleophilic way. The data by Huisgen and his coworkers given in Table 56-1 show that addition is accelerated by the introduction of electron-attracting substituents into the alkene.[333] But there are disturbances: the relation between the rates for ethyl acrylate and acrylonitrile is unusual; and it seems to be generally true that when ester groups are moved from *trans*- to *cis*-positions, rates are decreased, sometimes markedly so. The interpretation of these complications is not completely clear.

TABLE 56-1.—RATE-CONSTANTS (k_2 IN SEC.$^{-1}$ MOLE^{-1} L.) OF ADDITION OF DIPHENYLDIAZOMETHANE TO ALKENES IN FORMDIMETHYLAMIDE AT 40° (HUISGEN).

Alkene	10^5k_2	*trans*-Alkene	10^5k_2	*cis*-Alkene	10^5k_2
$Ph_2C:CH_2$	0.27	Et cinnamate	1.25	Maleic anhyd.	5830
$PhCH:CH_2$	1.40	Et crotonate	2.46	Et crotonate	0.95
$N\vdots C\cdot CH:CH_2$	484	Me_2 mesaconate	135	Me_2 citraconate	1.65
$EtO_2C\cdot CH:CH_2$	707	Me_2 fumarate	2450	Me_2 maleate	68.5

However, the predominatingly nucleophilic behaviour of diazoalkanes in additions to alkenes is confirmed by the orientation of addition to $\alpha\beta$-unsaturated esters, nitriles, and nitro-compounds. Auwers and Ungermach found as illustrated below, that ethyl diazoacetate and ethyl tiglate add to give a Δ^1-pyrazoline; and that diazomethane and cinnamonitrile yield a Δ^2-pyrazoline, the first-formed adduct having here suffered a prototropic change:[334]

[333] R. Huisgen, H. Stangl, H. J. Sturm, H. Wagenhofer, *Angew. Chem.*, 1961, **73**, 170; R. Huisgen, H. J. Sturm, and H. Wagenhofer, *Z. Naturforsch.*, 1962, **17b**, 202.

[334] K. von Auwers and O. Ungermach, *Ber.*, 1933, **66**, 1198.

$$EtO_2C\cdot CH{:}N{:}N + MeCH{:}CMe\cdot CO_2Et \rightarrow$$ (pyrazoline: EtO_2CH, N, N, MeH, $MeCO_2Et$)

$$CH_2{:}N{:}N + PhCH{:}CH\cdot CN \rightarrow$$ (pyrazoline: NH, N, H_2, PhH, CN)

Parham and Hasek observed that diazomethane and 1-nitropropene gave an isolable Δ^1-adduct, which readily lost nitrous acid to yield 4-methylpyrazole:[335]

$$CH_2{:}N{:}N + MeCH{:}CH\cdot NO_2 \rightarrow$$ (pyrazoline: N, N, H_2, MeH, HNO_2) $\rightarrow$ (pyrazole: NH, N, H, Me, H)

One sees that the positively polarised β-carbon atom of the conjugated ester, nitrile, or nitro-compound always receives the carbon atom of the diazoalkane system, as though that carbon atom were predominantly negatively charged, and the effective reaction formula of the diazoalkane were the right-hand one of the two mesomeric formulae on p. 1078.

The predominantly nucleophilic behaviour of diazoalkanes is again confirmed by the kinetic effect of introducing electron-absorbing groups into the diazoalkane. They must reduce the availability of the electrons of the diazoalkane, and they do reduce its rate of addition. This is illustrated by some rate-constants by Huisgen and Jung,[336] given in Table 56-2, for the reactions of various diazoalkanes with a common heterocyclic alkene:

(bicyclic alkene with $EtO_2C\cdot N$, $EtO_2C\cdot N$) $+ RR'CN_2 \rightarrow$ (adduct with $EtO_2C\cdot N$, $EtO_2C\cdot N$, N, N, R, R′)

[335] W. R. Parham and W. E. Hasek, *J. Am. Chem. Soc.*, 1954, **76**, 799.

[336] R. Huisgen and D. Jung, unpublished experiments cited by R. Huisgen, R. Grashey, and J. Sauer, ref. 285, p. 833.

TABLE 56-2.—RATE-CONSTANTS (k_2 IN SEC.$^{-1}$ MOLE^{-1} L.) OF ADDITIONS OF DIAZOALKANES TO ETHYL 5,6-DIAZONORBORNENE-5,6-DICARBOXYLATE IN FORMDIMETHYLAMIDE AT 60° (HUISGEN AND JUNG).

Diazoalkane	10^5k_2	Diazoalkane	10^5k_2
H_2CN_2	9700	$PhCO \cdot CHN_2$	1.8
Ph_2CN_2	102	$p\text{-}NO_2C_6H_4CO \cdot CHN_2$	0.85
$EtO_2C \cdot CHN_2$	9.3	$PhCO \cdot CN_2 \cdot COMe$	<0.1

The *additions of azides* to olefinic compounds follow the general pattern of the addition of diazoalkanes. The azides may be thought of as reacting in an approximation to one of the structures

$$R\overset{+}{N}{\equiv}N{=}\bar{N} \quad \text{and} \quad R\bar{N}{-}\overset{+}{N}{\equiv}N$$

The addition products are triazolines, which are easily pyrolysed with loss of nitrogen. The pyrolysis products are aziridines and azomethines, as may be illustrated by some additions of phenyl azide:[337,338,339]

PnN=N=N + cyclopentene → PhN(1)–N(2)=N(3) fused triazoline → (100°) PhN=C (cyclopentylidene)

PhN=N=N + PhCH=CH₂ → PhN–N=N, 5 PhH, 4 H₂ (triazoline) → (100°) PhN aziridine (PhH, H₂) and PhN=C(Ph)–CH₃

PhN=N=N + CH₂=CH·CO₂Me → PhN–N=N, 5 H₂, 4 HCO₂Me (triazoline) → (85°) PhN aziridine (H₂, HCO₂Me)

[337] K. Alder and G. Stein, *Ann.*, 1933, **501**, 1; 1935, **515**, 165, 185; K. Alder, H. K. Rieger, and H. Weiss, *Chem. Ber.*, 1955, **88**, 144.

[338] L. Wolff and G. K. Grau, *Ann.*, 1912, **394**, 68.

The addition products from acyl azides, such as benzazide, may lose nitrogen at a rate comparable to that of their formation. The isolable products from benzazide and norbornene are a benzoyl aziridine and an oxazoline:[339]

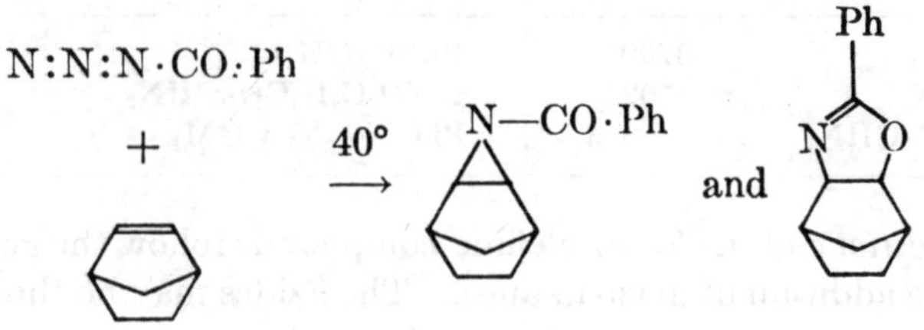

N:N:N·CO·Ph + norbornene $\xrightarrow{40°}$ N—CO·Ph (aziridine) and (oxazoline, N, O, Ph)

Phenyl azide adds to norbornene on the *exo*-side. It adds similarly to fenchene, and does not add to apobornene.[337,340]

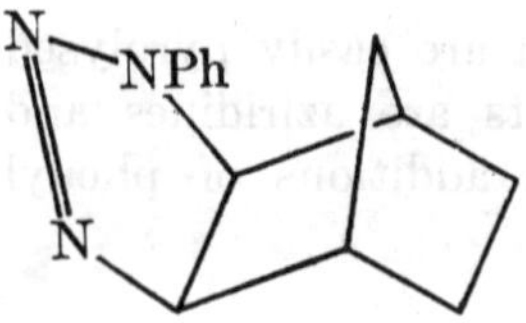

From norbornene 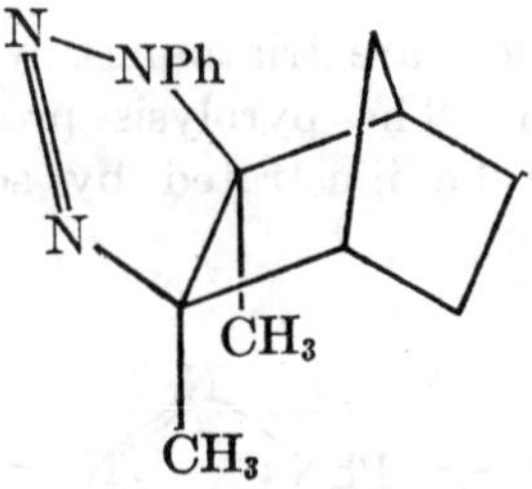 From fenchene 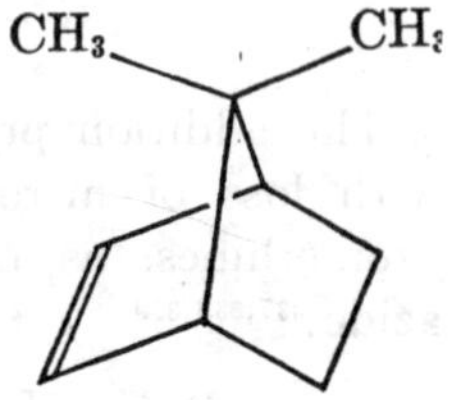 Apobornene

The double bond of norbornene is outstandingly reactive in this as in most other additions, a circumstance usually ascribed to Baeyer strain (the short bridge contracts lateral ring angles). But the absence of *endo*-addition, even though *exo*-addition may displace the methyl group of fenchene to *endo*-positions, and even when in apobornene *exo*-addition is (as we presume) sterically precluded, is not understood. Of course, *cis*-addition is a necessity in these examples. Whether *cis*-specificity would be maintained in additions that would allow conformational change in an intermediate of a two-step process of addition has not yet been determined.

The direction of addition of an azide to an unsymmetrically substituted alkene is illustrated above by the addition of phenyl azide to styrene and to ethyl acrylate. The directions are opposite: the phenyl

---

[339] R. Huisgen, G. Szeimies, G. Müller and L. Mobius, unpublished observations cited by R. Huisgen, R. Grashey, and J. Sauer, pp. 838–843 of ref. 285.

[340] K. Alder and G. Stein, *Ann.*, 1931, **485**, 211, 223; O. Diels and H. König, *Ber.*, 1938, **71**, 1179.

TABLE 56-3.—RATE-CONSTANTS (k_2 IN SEC.$^{-1}$ MOLE^{-1} L.) OF ADDITIONS OF PHENYL AZIDE TO ALKENES IN CARBON TETRACHLORIDE AT 25° (HUISGEN).

Alkene	10^7k_2	*trans*-Alkene	10^7k_2	*cis*-Alkene	10^7k_2
1-Heptene	0.24			*cyclo*Pentene	1.86
Styrene	0.40	Et crotonate	0.27	Norbornene	188
Et acrylate	9.85	Et_2 fumarate	8.36	Me_2 maleate	0.34

substituent of styrene appears in the 5-position, but the ester group of ethyl acrylate is found in the 4-position. The results combine to show that, of the two mesomeric formulae given on p. 1081 for an azide, that which has the negative charge on α-nitrogen is the more important as a reaction formula for cyclic addition. This is in analogy with the additions of diazoalkanes, which add to conjugated unsaturated carbonyl as though the diazoalkanes when reacting had predominantly negative carbon.

Huisgen and his coworkers have determined the rates of addition of phenyl azide to a number of alkenes,[339] and some of their results are in Table 56-3. The figures again give a picture of marked sensitivity to the stereochemistry of the alkene substrate, and of polar activation, weaker than in the additions of diazoalkanes, by an electronegative substituent.

We take, as our third example of polar 1,3-additions, the additions of *nitrile oxides*. The overall unsaturation is the same as in the two previous examples, but its distribution is different, as will be clear from the mesomeric formulae

$$\overset{+}{\overbrace{\text{RC}\equiv\text{N}}}-\bar{\text{O}} \quad \text{and} \quad \text{R}\bar{\text{C}}=\overset{+}{\overbrace{\text{N}=\text{O}}}$$

Benzonitrile oxide was first isolated by Wieland,[341] who obtained it by what is now the standard method. It consists in treating the corresponding hydroxamic acid chloride with a tertiary amine which removes the elements of hydrogen chloride. The nitrile oxide is not very easy to isolate, because it readily dimerises to 4,5-diphenylfurazan oxide:

$$\text{PhC}(=\text{NOH})\text{Cl} \xrightarrow{R_3N} \text{PhC}\equiv\overset{+}{\text{N}}-\bar{\text{O}} \rightarrow \text{PhC}(=\text{N}-\text{O}-)\,\text{PhC}=\overset{+}{\text{N}}-\bar{\text{O}} \ \ (\text{furazan oxide ring})$$

[341] H. Wieland, *Ber.*, 1907, **40**, 1667.

The study of the additions of nitrile oxides to alkenes would be much restricted by the tendency of the former to dimerise, were it not possible to produce the nitrile oxide by slow addition of the tertiary amine to the hydroxamic acid chloride *in situ*, that is, in low concentration, to be intercepted by the alkene already present in high concentration. The comprehensive exploration of the cyclic additions of nitrile oxides is due mainly to Quilico and his associates, who have used isolated nitrile oxides, and also, more largely, nitrile oxides produced *in situ*.[342] A few of their examples are formulated below; the products are isoxazolines:

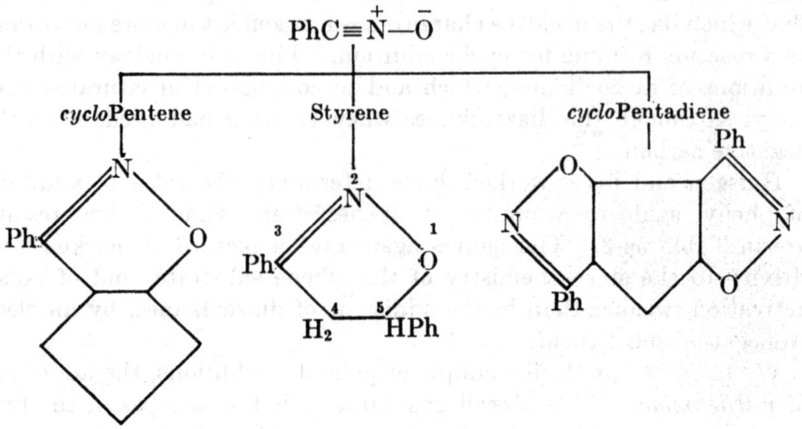

$$PhC\equiv\overset{+}{N}-\overset{-}{O}$$

*cyclo*Pentene — Styrene — *cyclo*Pentadiene

It has been shown[343] that the additions of benzonitrile oxide to methyl maleate and to methyl fumarate are completely stereospecific. This is the strongest single argument in favour of the theory of addition in a single step.

It has been found[344] that acetonitrile oxide adds to ethylenes having only one substituent, in such a way as to place that substituent in the 5-position of the isoxazole:

[342] A. Quilico and R. Fusco, *Gazz. chim. ital.*, 1937, **67**, 589; A. Quilicò and G. Speroni, *ibid.*, 1946, **76**, 148; G. Stagno d'Alcontres and P. Grunanger, *ibid.*, 1950, **80**, 741, 831; G. Stagno d'Alcontres and G. Fenech, *ibid.*, 1952, **82**, 175; A. Quilico, P. Grunanger, and R. Mezzini, *ibid.*, p. 349; G. Stagno d'Alcontres, *ibid.*, p. 627; P. Grunanger, *ibid.*, 1954, **84**, 359; *idem* and M. R. Langella, *ibid.*, 1961, **91**, 1112; *idem*, N. Barbulescu, and A. Quilico, *Tetrahedron Letters*, **1961**, 89.

[343] A. Quilico, G. Stagno d'Alcontres, and P. Grunanger, *Gazz. chim. ital.*, 1950, **80**, 479; A. Quilico and P. Grunanger, *ibid.*, 1952, **82**, 140; 1955, **85**, 1449.

[344] T. Mukaiyama and T. Hoshino, *J. Am. Chem. Soc.*, 1960, **82**, 5339; G. B. Bachman and L. E. Strom, *J. Org. Chem.*, 1953, **28**, 1150.

$$CH_3\cdot C\equiv \overset{+}{N}-\overset{-}{O} + CH_2{=}CHX \rightarrow \text{(isoxazoline ring: Me–C}{=}N\text{–O–C}^5HX\text{–C}^4H_2\text{)} \qquad X = \begin{cases} C_6H_5 \\ CN \\ OC_4H_9\text{-}n \end{cases}$$

There are reasons of analogy (see below) for thinking that this independence of polarity would not hold for ethylenes substituted at both ends; but the controlling observations have not yet been recorded.

Huisgen and his collaborators have employed a competition method to measure the relative rates of uptake of benzonitrile oxide by a series of alkenes.[345] Some of their figures are in Table 56-4. They present a pattern, generally similar to that shown for the azide reaction in Table 56-3, namely, one of great kinetic sensitivity to the stereochemistry of the olefinic substrate, and mild accelerating effects by conjugated ester groups, and also, in this case, a conjugated ether group.

TABLE 56-4.—RELATIVE RATE OF ADDITION OF BENZONITRILE OXIDE TO OLEFINS IN ETHER AT 20° (HUISGEN)

Alkene	Rel. rate	*trans*-Alkenes	Rel. rate	*cis*-Alkenes	Rel. rate
1-Hexene	2.6			*cyclo*Hexene	0.055
Styrene	9.3	*trans*-Stilbene	0.24	*cyclo*Pentene	1.04
Et acrylate	66	Et crotonate	≡ 1.00	Norbornene	97
Vinyl *n*-Bu ether	15	Me_2 fumarate	94	Me_2 maleate	1.61

As representative of the class of 1,3-dipolar adducts with a lower overall unsaturation than that of the class from which the previous examples come, we may consider the cyclic *additions of nitrones* (azomethine oxides; also called N-ethers of oximes). The system is like that in the nitrile oxides, except for the extra substituents accompanying the reduced unsaturation. We may represent it by the mesomeric formulae:

$$RR'C{=}\overset{+}{N}R''-\overset{-}{O} \quad \text{and} \quad RR'\overset{-}{C}-\overset{+}{N}R''{=}O$$

This system adds to alkene to produce isoxazolidines, as in the example:[346]

[345] R. Huisgen, W. Mack, K. Bast, and E. Kudera, unpublished experiments cited by R. Huisgen, R. Grashey, and J. Sauer, ref. 285, p. 826.

[346] R. Grashey, R. Huisgen, and H. Leitermann, *Tetrahedron Letters*, 1960, No. 12, 9; H. Hauck, Thesis, Munich, 1963.

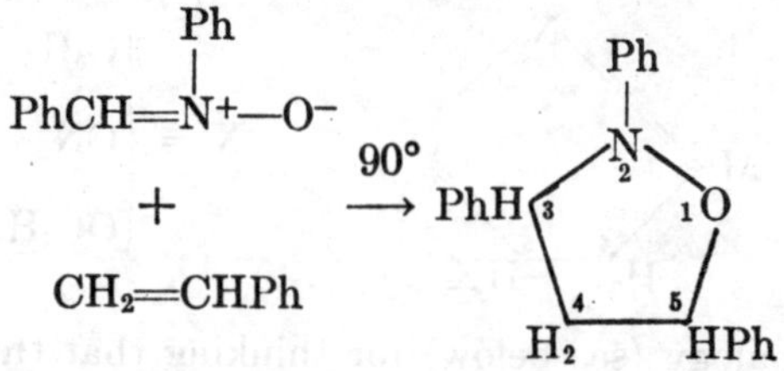

$$\underset{\substack{+\\ CH_2{=}CHPh}}{PhCH{=}\overset{\overset{\large Ph}{|}}{N^+}{-}O^-} \xrightarrow{90^\circ} \text{PhH}\!\!\underset{H_2\;\;\;\;\;HPh}{\overset{\overset{Ph}{|}}{\text{(isoxazolidine, N}_2\text{, O}_1\text{, C}_3\text{, C}_4\text{, C}_5)}} \quad (\textit{cis}\text{ and }\textit{trans})$$

The required nitrones are usually prepared from aldehydes and N-alkyl- or N-aryl-hydroxylamines, and it is sometimes more convenient, not to isolate them, but to make them in this way in the presence of excess of the alkene to which they will add. Thus *n*-butaldehyde and N-phenylhydroxylamine, condensed together in styrene, yield 2,5-diphenyl-3-*n*-propylisoxazolidine.[344]

The cyclic nitrones are conveniently reactive,[347] on the whole more reactive than open-chain nitrones, probably because the cyclic nitrones are necessarily *cis*, whereas open-chain nitrones are usually *trans*. Grashey has shown that 3,4-dihydro*iso*quinoline oxide adds to methyl maleate and to methyl fumarate quite stereospecifically, thereby providing a strong argument that the additions go in one step:[348]

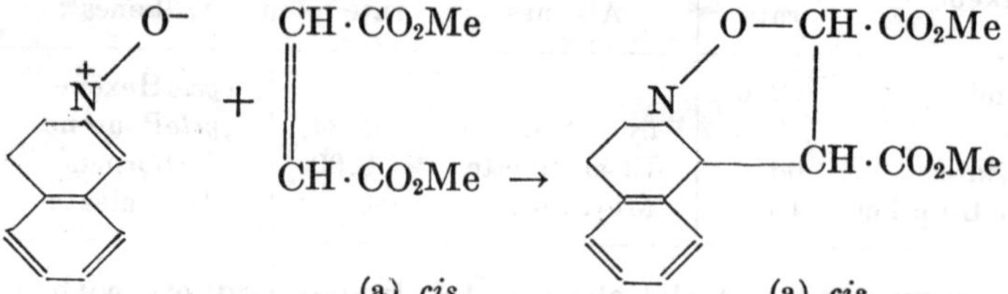

$$\text{3,4-dihydroisoquinoline N-oxide } (\overset{+}{N}{-}O^-) + \begin{matrix} CH\cdot CO_2Me \\ \| \\ CH\cdot CO_2Me \end{matrix} \rightarrow \text{adduct: } N{-}O{-}CH\cdot CO_2Me,\; {-}CH\cdot CO_2Me$$

(a) *cis*
(b) *trans*

(a) *cis*
(b) *trans*

A study has been made of the effect of substituents in the alkene on the direction of addition.[346] When the double bond of the alkene is terminal, as in $CH_2{:}CHPh$, $CH_2{:}CH\cdot CO_2Et$, and $CH_2{:}CMe\cdot CO_2Me$, the substituents are found in the 5-position of the isoxazolidine. But when both ends of the ethylene bear substituents, as in $CH_3\cdot CH{:}CH\cdot CO_2Et$ and $(CH_3)_2C{:}CH\cdot CO_2Et$, then the ester group appears in the 4-position, which is the position in which polar influences, acting alone, should place it, if a nitrone acts, like the addenda previously considered, as a nucleophile.

A large number of rate-constants for the addition of C-phenyl-N-

[347] C. W. Brown, K. Marsden, M. A. T. Rogers, C. M. B. Tyler, and R. Wright, *Proc. Chem. Soc.*, **1962,** 254.

[348] R. Grashey, unpublished experiments cited by R. Huisgen, R. Grashey, and J. Sauer, ref. 285, p. 863.

TABLE 56-5.—RATE-CONSTANTS (k_2 IN SEC.$^{-1}$ MOLE^{-1} L.) OF ADDITIONS OF C-PHENYL-N-METHYLNITRONE TO ALKENES IN TOLUENE (SEIDL).

Alkene	10^5k_2 120°	Alkene	10^5k_2 85°	10^5k_2 120°
1-Heptene	2.64	Me acrylate	44.0	—
*cyclo*Pentene	0.82	Me crotonate	3.96	36.4
Norbornene	4.90	Me_2 fumarate	72.5	—
p-MeO-styrene	8.7	Me_2 maleate	24.7	—
Styrene	11.7	Me_2 mesaconate	25.8	—
p-NO_2-styrene	51	Me_2 citraconate	3.17	13.4

methylnitrone to various alkenes have been measured by Seidl.[349] A selection of his values is in Table 56-5. They show a much weaker dependence of the rate on the stereochemistry of the accepting alkene than characterises the addition of nitrile oxides. Possibly the less unsaturated system is the more flexibly accommodating. It may be mainly on this account that kinetic polar effects come out more clearly in the additions of nitrones than in additions of nitrile oxides. The polar effect certainly characterises the nitrone as being predominantly a nucleophile.

Besides the four types of 1,3-dipoles exemplified above, quite a number of similar systems, such as nitrile imines, azomethine imines, and nitrile ylides, have been studied by Huisgen and his coworkers,[285] with respect to their cyclic additions.

(56d) 1,4-Addition of Dienes to Give Six-Membered Rings.[350]— This is the Diels-Alder reaction, celebrated for its great generality and synthetic value. By *diene* in this connexion is meant conjugated diene capable of adding through its 1- and 4-positions to an alkene, which in this context is termed the dienophile. An acetylenic group can take the place of the ethylenic group in the dienophile. The product in the case of an ethylenic dienophile is a *cyclo*hexene, and in that of an acetylenic dienophile is a *cyclo*hexa-1,4-diene. The active unsaturated portion of the dienophile, or that of the diene, or those in both, may be involved in rings: the adduct is then polycyclic. Some aromatic systems can furnish the buta-1,3-diene unit out of their more complex unsaturation: the furan ring and the central ring of anthracene can do so, as is illustrated below. Some aromatic systems can furnish

[349] R. Seidl, Thesis, Munich, 1963. Cited by R. Huisgen, R. Grashey, and J. Sauer, ref. 285, p. 865.

[350] A. Wassermann, "Diels-Alder Reaction," Elsevier Publishing Co., Amsterdam, 1965.

one double bond of the buta-1,3-diene unit: this will be illustrated later. Some aromatic systems can even furnish the dienophile double bond: an example in which 2-naphthol does so is formulated below. Some representative illustrations of diene addition are expressed in the following equations:

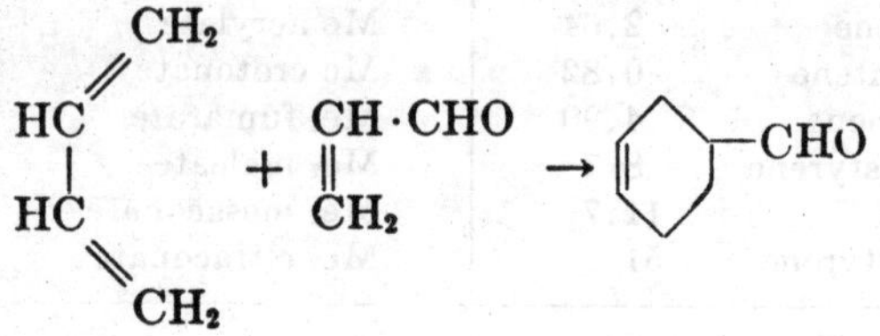

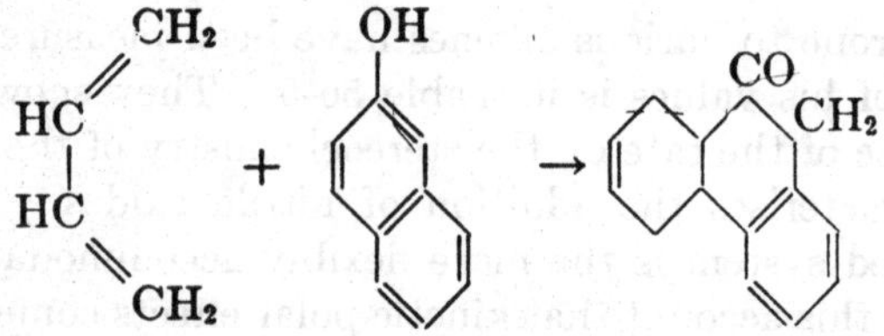

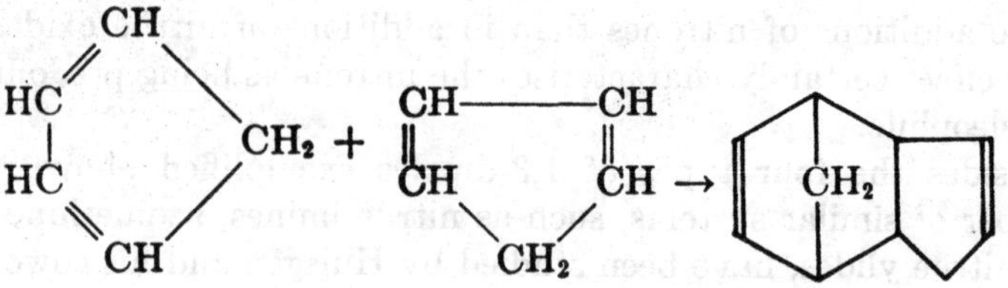

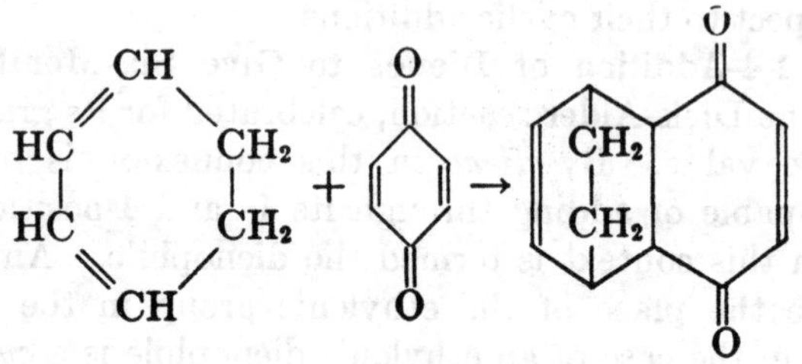

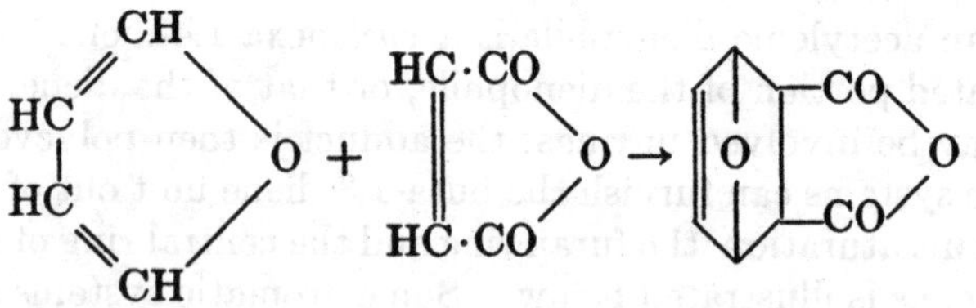

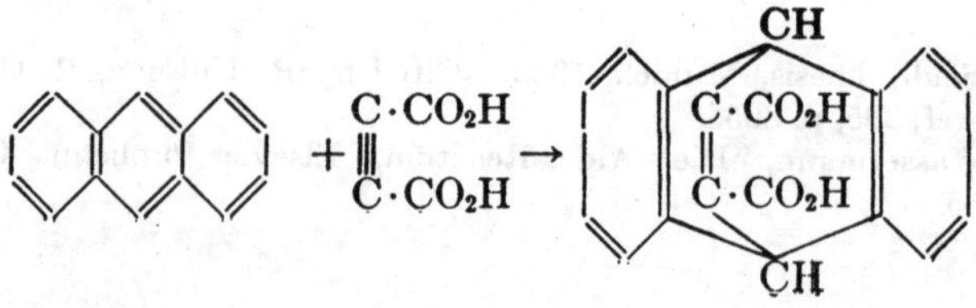

As to the history of the reaction, isolated examples of diene addition appear in the literature of the last century. Zincke discovered, and later correctly formulated, the dimerisation of tetrachloro*cyclo*pentadienone.[351] In the present century, Euler and Josephson recognised the nature of the addition products of isoprene to *p*-benzoquinone.[352] However, these observations remained uncorrelated, until Diels and Alder demonstrated the versatility of the reaction in 1928 and subsequently.[353]

Diene addition is stereochemically specific in several ways.[354] First, the addition is necessarily *cis*- with respect to the diene, as the cyclic structure of the product shows; that is, the diene must react in a synperiplanar conformation round its central, formally single, bond. Next, the addition is also *cis*- with respect to the unsaturation of the dienophile. This is shown by the observation that when, before addition, two groups are *cis*- or *trans*- with respect to the ethylenic bond of a dienophile, then these groups, after addition, preserve the same description, *cis*- or *trans*-, with respect to the formed alicyclic ring. Thus, adducts of maleic anhydride are anhydrides of cyclic *cis*-1,2-dicarboxylic acids, and adducts of fumaryl chloride are chlorides of cyclic *trans*-1,2-dicarboxylic acids. And next, the configuration of substituents in the diene is likewise retained in the adduct.[355] Thus, the addition of maleic anhydride to *trans-trans*-1,4-diphenylbutadiene yields a *cyclo*hexene derivative in which the phenyl groups are *cis* with respect to each other:

Ph Ph H H + CO·O·CO H H → Ph CO·O·CO Ph H H H H ≡ Ph Ph CO·O·CO

These rules of Alder and Stein prescribe a *cis* addition of reactants which otherwise carry their own stereochemistry into the adduct. No

[351] T. Zincke and H. Günther, *Ann.*, 1892, **272**, 243; T. Zincke, F. Bergmann, B. Francke, and W. Prenntzell, *ibid.*, 1897, **296**, 135; T. Zincke and K. H. Meyer, *Ann.*, 1909, **367**, 1; T. Zincke and W. Pfaffendorf, *ibid.*, 1912, **394**, 3.

[352] H. v. Euler and K. O. Josephson, *Ber.*, 1920, **53**, 822.

[353] O. Diels and K. Alder, *Ann.*, 1928, **460**, 98; and many later papers.

[354] K. Alder and G. Stein, *Angew. Chem.*, 1934, **47**, 837; 1937, **50**, 510.

[355] K. Alder and M. Schumacher, *Ann.*, 1951, **571**, 87.

exception to them has been found. There remains the question of whether the groups originally belonging to the dienophile might in the adduct be directed either towards the double bond surviving in what was originally the diene, that is, towards the *endo*-position in the usual terminology, or away from the surviving double bond, that is, to the *exo*-position. Here the rule is that any carbonyl, carboxyl, or other unsaturated groups, originally in the dieneophile, will be oriented, usually exclusively, to the *endo*-position in the adduct. This is illustrated schematically below for the addition of maleic anhydride to *cyclo*pentadiene, which gives exclusively the *endo*-adduct:

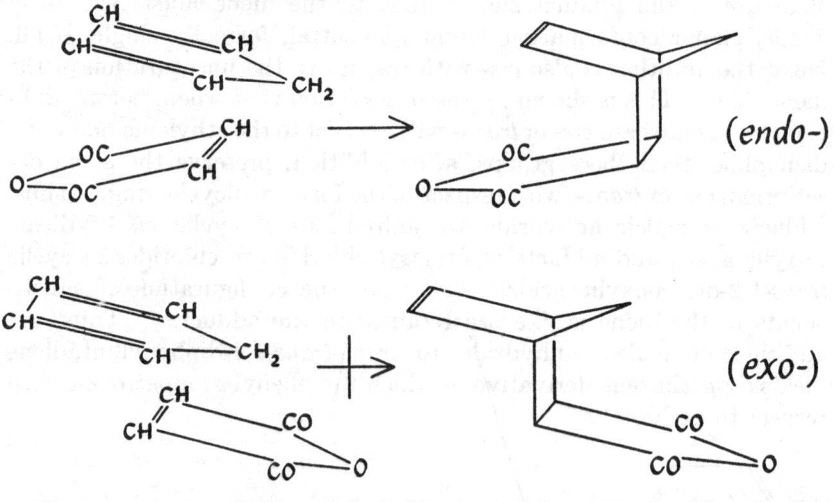

(*endo*-)

(*exo*-)

The same *endo*-addition rule is illustrated for an open diene in the previously formulated example of the addition of maleic anhydride to *trans-trans*-1,4-diphenylbutadiene. For, as will be seen, the phenyl groups are not only *cis* in relation to each other, but also *cis* in relation to the anhydride group, which, therefore, must have been directed towards the surviving ethylenic bond during the act of addition.

The scope of the *endo*-addition rule is, however, limited. The first limitation is the reasonable one that the rule is intended to prescribe the kinetically controlled products, that is, the products formed in a single act of addition, without reversal. But the Diels-Alder reaction is reversible, and the equilibrium to which it will run after a long enough time at a high enough temperature, the thermodynamically determined addition product, may not be identical with the first-formed product.

However, with all allowances made for this, the rule of *endo*-addition of first-formed adducts has such notable exceptions that it is still called a "rule" only for historical reasons.[356] In 1948, Woodward and Baer discovered that furan formed an *exo*-adduct with maleic anhydride in ether. This somewhat fast and easily reversed addition has been reinvestigated several times since with the object of determining the product which is formed first, before the retrograde reaction sets in; and the result obtained by Anet is that the first-formed product consists of 33% of the *endo*-adduct and 67% of the *exo*-isomer. The contrasting case in Woodward and Baer's original investigation was that of the addition of maleic acid to furan in water. In this case they obtained the *endo*-adduct. The more recent finding by Anet is that 75% of the kinetically controlled product is indeed the *endo*-adduct, which is accompanied by 25% of the *exo*-isomer. If isolation is delayed, for instance, by a week at room temperature, the product may contain approximately equivalent amounts of the two isomers. Presumably the proportion of *exo*-isomer at equilibrium is substantially more than 25%.

Alder and his coworkers found another group of exceptions to the *endo*-rule in the additions of open-chain $\alpha\beta$-unsaturated mononitriles and monocarboxylic esters to *cyclo*pentadiene.[357] Thus, the addition to this diene of acrylonitrile at 100° gave, apparently as first product, about equal amounts of the *endo*- and *exo*-adducts. Berson and his collaborators have examined a number of such additions quantitatively:[357] some of their results are given in Table 56-6. They show that the isomer ratio in the kinetically controlled product depends primarily on the dienophile, and to a not unimportant extent on the solvent, and also to some extent on the temperature. The rule of *endo*-addition has here but little importance. The addition of methyl acrylate obeys the rule in all solvents; that of methyl α-methacrylate disobeys it in all solvents, whilst that of methyl *trans*-crotonate exhibits borderline behaviour. In all cases a change to a more polar solvent increases the proportion of *endo*-isomer in the kinetically controlled product. This shows that the transition state of formation of the *endo*-adduct is more polar than that for the formation of the *exo*-isomer. Temperature acts usually as if enthalpy contributed more than entropy to the difference in the free energies of activation of formation of the isomers; that is, a rise of temperature usually increases the proportion of whichever isomer is formed in the smaller proportion.

[356] R. B. Woodward and M. Baer, *J. Am. Chem. Soc.*, 1948, **70**, 1161; H. Kwart and I. Burchuk, *ibid.*, 1952, **74**, 3094; J. A. Berson and R. Swidler, *ibid.*, 1953, **75**, 1721; P. A. L. Anet, *Tetrahedron Letters*, **1962**, 1219.

[357] K. Alder, K. Heinbach, and R. Reube, *Chem. Ber.*, 1958, **91**, 1516; J. A. Berson, Z. Hamlet, and W. A. Mueller, *J. Am. Chem. Soc.*, 1962, **84**, 297.

The differences in $\Delta H^{\neq}$ and $T\Delta S^{\neq}$ for the formation of the two isomers were, in fact, determined from the temperature coefficients, and were quite small, almost all of them less than 1 kcal./mole.

TABLE 56-6.—PERCENTAGES OF *endo* AND *exo*-ISOMERS IN KINETICALLY CONTROLLED PRODUCTS OF ADDITION OF DIENOPHILE TO *cyclo*-PENTADIENE (BERSON *et al.*)

(Contractions: N = *endo*, X = *exo*, $C_{10}H_{18}$ = decalin.)

Solvent	CH_2:CH·CO_2Me			CH_2:CMe·CO_2Me			*trans*-MeCH:CH·CO_2Me		
	Temp.	% N	% X	Temp.	% N	% X	Temp.	% N	% X
$C_{10}H_{18}$	−35°	80.3	19.7	56°	33.0	77.0	3°	52.6	47.4
	170	74.5	25.5	139	38.2	61.8	66	51.3	48.7
$MeNO_2$	3	84.6	15.4	3	30.5	69.5	3	62.0	38.0
	66	81.4	18.6	66	34.4	65.5	66	57.2	42.8
MeOH	0	89.8	18.2	0	41.5	58.5	3	66.4	33.6
	56	84.9	15.5	56	40.7	59.3	66	65.0	35.0

The *endo*-rule was originally developed for dienophiles having unsaturated substituents, which they carried into the adduct. It was described as a rule of "maximal accumulation of unsaturation" in the adduct. The various explanations of the rule which have been offered assume attractive non-bonding or secondary-bonding interactions between the unsaturated substituents (such as the anhydride group of maleic anhydride) thus carried into the adduct, and the double bond of the diene residue surviving in the adduct. Explanations have been suggested which postulate non-bonding interactions that would include electrokinetic attraction between single and double bonds in the transition state of formation of the *endo*-adduct. It is certainly not necessary to have unsaturation surviving from both partners to an addition in order to secure a predominating *endo*-orientation of that process. For *cyclo*pentene, a dienophile which contributes no surviving unsaturation, has been observed[358] to undergo strongly predominating *endo*-addition to *cyclo*pentadiene near 200°; and as this is the lower end of the range of temperature over which the addition is fast enough to be observed, there can be little doubt that the observations at such temperatures were of kinetically controlled products.

Our knowledge of the kinetics of diene addition, and of its retrogres-

[358] S. J. Cristol, W. K. Seifert, and S. B. Solonay, *J. Am. Chem. Soc.*, 1960, **82**, 2351.

sion, is due mainly to Wassermann, some of whose results[359] are collected in Table 56-7. First, as to the thermodynamic situation, diene addition is reversible and is exothermic, so that an increase of temperature shifts the equilibrium in the favour of the diene and dienophile. For the three reactions measured, $-\Delta H$ is about 17–18 kcal./mole.

TABLE 56-7.—ARRHENIUS PARAMETERS FOR DIENE ADDITION AND ITS RETROGRESSION (WASSERMANN).

Reaction	Solvent	Addition			Division		
		$\log_{10} A_2$	E_2	Temp. range	$\log_{10} A_1$	E_1	Temp. range
	EtOH	7.0	12.7	2– 30°	—	—	—
*cyclo*Pentadiene	AcOH	7.5	11.0	18– 30°	—	—	—
+benzoquinone	C_6H_6	6.5	11.6	8– 50°	12.6	29	55– 79°
	CS_2	4.0	8.5	3– 39°	—	—	—
	C_6H_6	6.1	16.4	12– 35°	—	—	—
*cyclo*Pentadiene	CS_2	5.7	17.7	0– 22°	—	—	—
+*cyclo*pentadiene	Paraffin	7.1	17.4	0– 17°	13.0	34.2	135–175°
	(Gas)	6.1	16.7	80–150°	13.1	35	27–111°
*cyclo*Pentadiene	C_6H_6	6.1	13.7	6– 77°	—	—	—
+acrolein	(Gas)	6.2	15.2	108–120°	12.3	33.6	102–242°
Isoprene +acrolein	(Gas)	6.0	18.7	218–333°	—	—	—
Butadiene +acrolein	(Gas)	6.2	19.7	155–333°	—	—	—
Butadiene +crotonaldehyde	(Gas)	6.0	22.0	242–299°	—	—	—

Kinetically, the reaction is almost unique in the facility with which its rate can be studied for both directions, and both in the homogeneous gas-phase and in solution in either non-polar or polar solvents. As some of the entries in Table 56-7 indicate, diene addition can be observed as a homogeneous gas-reaction of the second order:

$$\text{Rate addition} = k_2[\text{diene}][\text{dienophile}]$$

The same rate equation applies in solution. Division of a diene-adduct may be observed as a homogeneous gas-reaction of the first order:

[359] Those quoted are taken from a summarising article by A. Wassermann, *Trans. Faraday Soc.*, 1938, **34**, 128.

$$\text{Rate division} = k_1[\text{adduct}]$$

The same equation applies in solution. The parameters by which the temperature dependence of k_2 and k_1 can be expressed in the forms

$$k_2 = A_2 e^{-E_2/RT} \quad \text{and} \quad k_1 = A_1 e^{-E_1/RT}$$

are in the table, A_2 being in sec.$^{-1}$ mole^{-1} l., A_1 in sec.$^{-1}$, and E_2 and E_1 in kcal./mole.

As the table shows, most of the diene additions, including gas-phase reactions and the reactions in solution, have Arrhenius energies of activation lying in the range 10–20 kcal./mole. The Arrhenius frequency factors for the gas reactions, and for the reactions in solution, are of an order about 10^5 times smaller than the collision rate for a gas reaction: they are small enough to show that a highly special orientation of diene and dienophile is required for conversion into the transition state of reaction. The adduct divisions have Arrhenius energies of activation in the region 30–35 kcal./mole. The Arrhenius frequency factors, whether for the gas reactions, or for the reactions in solution, are of a normal order of magnitude for first-order gas-reactions. Clearly the adduct molecule has *not* to be brought to any unaccustomed configuration, before it can be energised to form the transition state. These relations indicate that the transition state has a geometrical form generally resembling that of the adduct.

The rates and Arrhenius parameters, both for diene addition, and for division of diene-adducts, are about the same in the gas phase and in solution in non-polar solvents. This shows that the transition state has a degree of polarity which is not so much different from that of the factors, or from that of the product, that induced dipole forces can cause a marked difference of solvation. Yet the rates of addition do differ somewhat in non-polar and polar solvents, and the Arrhenius parameters differ rather more markedly. There is, then, some change of polarity on passing from the reactants to the transition state, though not nearly as great a change as is common in purely heterolytic processes.

As to mechanism, the first question is that of the geometrical form of the transition state. Several suggestions have been made, but only one has survived. One of the abandoned ideas was that the reaction went in two steps through an intermediate open-chain diradical. Of course, the firm stereochemistry of a *cis* union between addenda each of which carried its own stereochemistry into the adduct, as well as the absence of any effect of radical scavengers on the reaction, are on the whole against any such two-step sequence as a general mechanism. The accepted idea is the one which Wassermann deduced from his kinetic data, namely, of one-step addition through a transition state of geometrical form resembling that of the adduct.[360] This implies that the new bonds between the diene and dienophile begin to be formed by overlap of molecular π orbitals in the direction which would involve endwise rather than lateral overlap of the relevant atomic *p*-orbitals. This will be obvious from the diagrams on p. 1090. The firm stereochemical rules follow from this mechanism. Attempts have been made to deduce from it the more dubious rule of *endo*-addition; but it has to be admitted that the interplay of factors which control *endo*- or *exo*-addition is not yet fully understood.

It has been qualitatively clear since the early 1940's that electron-absorbing substituents in the dienophile, and electron-releasing substituents in the diene, commonly accelerate diene additions. This was illustrated in the first edition of this book, and in 1955 was stated by Alder as a rule.[361] This rule certainly covered the data available up to that time. Rate-constants by which its validity can be controlled have since been provided by Sauer and his collaborators.[362] Some of their values are in Table 56-8.

TABLE 56-8.—RATE-CONSTANTS (k_2 IN SEC.$^{-1}$ MOLE^{-1} L.) OF DIENE ADDITIONS IN DIOXAN (SAUER).

Ethylene	*cyclo*Pentadiene 10^5k_2 (20°)	Butadiene	Maleic anhyd. 10^5k_2 (30°)
Cyano-	1.04	2-Chloro-	0.69
1,2-Dicyano-(*trans*)	81	(Parent)	6.83
1,2-Dicyano-(*cis*)	91	2-Methyl-	15.4
1,1-Dicyano-	45,000	1-Methyl-	22.7
Tricyano-	483,000	2,3-Dimethyl-	33.6
Tetracyano-	~43,000,000	1-Methoxy-	84.1

Additions to Hexachlorocyclopentadiene at 130°

Styrene	10^5k_2	Cyclic 'ene	10^5k_2
p-Methoxy	158	*cyclo*Pentene	5.9
(Parent)	79.3	Maleic anhydride	2.9
p-Nitro-	53.8		

[360] A. Wassermann, *J. Chem. Soc.*, **1942, 612**.

[361] K. Alder, *Experientia*, 1955, Suppl. II, 86.

[362] J. Sauer, H. Wiest, and A. Mielert, *Z. Naturforsch.*, 1962, **17b**, 203; *idem* and D. Lang, *Angew Chem.*, 1962, **74**, 352, 353· cf. ref. 285.

In the upper part of the Table, which deals with additions of cyano-substituted ethylenes, to *cyclo*pentadiene, and of maleic anhydride to variously substituted butadienes, we see the rule well illustrated: as we put more electron-absorbing cyano-groups into the dienophile, the rates increase strongly, and as we take chlorine out of the diene, or put electron-releasing methyl and methoxyl groups into the diene, the rates increase significantly. However, in the lower part of the table, wherein the values relate to the additions of some styrenes, and of two five-membered ring olefins, to hexachloro*cyclo*pentadiene, the rule is consistently disobeyed: the taking of an electron-releasing methoxyl group out of the dienophile, or the putting of an electron-absorbing nitro- or anhydride group into it, decreases the rate of its addition to the diene.

This situation may possibly be thought of in the following way. If we consider, first, the addition of ethylene to butadiene, we would expect that, as the system mounts to its transition state, the electrons which increasingly bridge the addenda during this activation will come mainly from the more nucleophilic of them, that is from the butadiene. We are, of course, not asking the question, which is an impossible one in such a reaction, as to whether the bond changes are homocyclic or heterocyclic. Nor are we failing to recognise that, when the transition state has been passed by, and the product has been fully formed, each reactant will have contributed just two electrons to the two bonds by which they are added together. But if the preferred direction of build-up of the bridging electron density during activation is as suggested, *viz.*, from the diene towards the dienophile, then that build-up should be facilitated if we put electron-absorbing substituents into the dienophile and electron-releasing substituents into the diene. But now suppose that the butadiene is already so heavily substituted with electronegative groups that it is no longer more nucleophilic than the dienophile. There will remain the other possibility, namely, that the bridging electron density is built up during activation, *i.e.*, from the initial to the transition state, mainly from the side of the dienophile. In that case, the reaction should be accelerated by electron-releasing substituents in the dienophile, and retarded by electron-absorbing substituents in that reactant.

Wassermann and his coworkers have made a considerable study of the catalysis of diene additions. The reaction is not highly sensitive to catalysts. Yet it is susceptible to a general acid catalysis,[363] which applies even to the dimerisation of *cyclo*pentadiene, where we have two

[363] A. Wassermann, *J. Chem. Soc.*, **1942**, 618; W. Rubin, H. Steiner, and A. Wassermann, *ibid.*, **1949**, 3046.

hydrocarbon reactants. The catalysed part of the rate is normally that of a third-order process:

$$\text{Rate} \propto [\text{acid}][\text{diene}][\text{dienophile}]$$

But in the case of the dimerisation of *cyclo*pentadiene, both this order, and an order one unit lower, have been realised:

$$\text{Rate} \propto [\text{acid}][\textit{cyclo}\text{pentadiene}]^2$$

$$\text{Rate} \propto [\text{acid}][\textit{cyclo}\text{pentadiene}]$$

This shows that the attack of the catalyst is on *one* of the two adding molecules: for such a process can be made rate-determining. As to the nature of the attack, the indications are as follows. First, catalytic activity increases with the strength of the acid, for example according to the sequence,

$$CH_3 \cdot CO_2H < CH_2Cl \cdot CO_2H < CHCl_2 \cdot CO_2H < CCl_3 \cdot CO_2H < HCl$$

Phenols are also moderately good catalysts in spite of their generally much lower acidity. Secondly, catalysis has been observed in the gas phase. Thirdly any solvent used must be non-basic for good catalysis: it could be carbon tetrachloride, but not dioxan. Fourthly, weakly basic neutral solutes and salts of the catalysing acid, retard catalysis. It is concluded that the catalysis depends on the entry of the acid proton into one reactant, to make an ion-pair in catalysis by carboxylic acids and by hydrochloric acid, or to make a hydrogen-bond complex in catalysis by phenols. The protonated reactant then takes up the second reactant, before the catalysing acid is finally split off again. There is some evidence that the attack of the protonated reactant on the second reactant takes place at one point first, so creating a further difference of mechanism from that of the uncatalysed addition.

CHAPTER XIV

Acids and Bases

PROTON transfers between electronegative atoms, such as nitrogen, oxygen, sulphur, and the halogens, occur so rapidly in solution that they can be kinetically examined only in special cases by special methods. However, they can be, and have been, extensively studied with respect to the equilibria attained. Acid-base proton transfers constitute, indeed, the most extensive organic-chemical field in which sufficient good measurements of equilibrium constants are available to allow a comprehensive study of constitutional effects on equilibria. This will be the subject of the present chapter, in which, therefore, the point of view will be wholly thermodynamic, instead of, as in most other chapters on reactions, predominantly kinetic.

(57) ACID-BASE EQUILIBRIA

(57a) Measurement of Acid-Base Equilibria.—In accordance with Brönsted's proposal, the equation,

$$HX \rightleftarrows H^+ + X^-$$

is allowed to define *acids* HX and *bases* X^-, which, thus related, are said to be *conjugate* to each other, independently of the absolute charges on the two species, the present minus sign being indicative only of the charge-relation between the acid and the base.

Water is the most important of the solvents in which acid-base equilibria have been studied. Water is defined as a base by the specialised equation,

$$H_3O^+ \rightleftarrows H^+ + H_2O$$

By combination of these two equations, one obtains an equation to which the mass-law can be conveniently applied:

$$HX + H_2O \rightleftarrows H_3O^+ + X^-$$

The acid HX transfers its proton to the base H_2O, to give the acid H_3O^+ and the base X^-. The process in principle is reversible, and the concentrations of all the species can in general be determined. The ***acidity constant of the acid*** HX in water, sometimes called alternatively the ***hydrolysis constant of the cation*** HX, in case HX is a cation, is just the equilibrium constant of this reaction, as defined for the special case in which water is the solvent:

$$K_a = \frac{\{H_3O^+\}\{X^-\}}{\{HX\}} \approx \frac{[H_3O^+][X^-]}{[HX]}$$

Here the braces { } denote activities: their values can easily be supplied when the concentrations [ ] are so low that activity coefficients depend on charge alone, being unity for neutral species, and having the standard Debye-Milner values for ions. The usual units of K_a are moles/litre. Values of K_a are often given in the form of negative logarithms, pK_a:

$$pK_a = -\log_{10} K_a$$

Water is defined as an acid by the specialised equation,

$$H_2O \rightleftarrows H^+ + OH^-$$

By combining this equation with the general equation of Brönsted, another equilibrium can be formulated to which the mass-law can be applied:

$$H_2O + X^- \rightleftarrows HX + OH^-$$

Here the acid H_2O transfers its proton to the base X^-, to give the acid HX and the base OH^-. The transfer is reversible, and the concentrations of the species can be found. This equation is useful for the purpose of making statements about the base X^-, which, we remember, may be in any state of electrical charge. The *basicity constant of the base* X^- in water, sometimes called alternatively the *hydrolysis constant of the anion* X^-, in case X^- is an anion, is simply the equilibrium constant of this reaction, as defined for the case in which water is the solvent:

$$K_b = \frac{\{HX\}\{OH^-\}}{\{X^-\}} \approx \frac{[HX][OH^-]}{[X^-]}$$

The usual units of K_b are moles/litre.

By combining the two specialised equations already given, an equation is obtained which represents water as both an acid and a base:

$$H_2O + H_2O \rightleftarrows H_3O^+ + OH^-$$

It is also an equation to which the mass-law can be applied. The *autoprotolysis constant* of water is the equilibrium constant of this reaction, as defined for the case in which water is the solvent:

$$K_{auto} = \{H_3O^+\}\{OH^-\} \approx [H_3O^+][OH^-]$$

The usual units of K_{auto} are (moles/litre)^2.

The three equilibrium constants already mentioned are connected by the relation,

$$K_a \cdot K_b = K_{auto}$$

It is a common practice, when K_{auto} is known with sufficient accuracy for the purpose, to express the basicity constants of bases in terms of the acidity constants of their conjugate acids, that is, to convert K_b into terms of K_a for the acid-base system.

The acidity constant of an acid is said to measure the *strength of the acid.* An acid is said to be *strong* or *weak* according as its acidity constant is high or low. The term "strength," as applied to an acid, is often made quantitatively synonymous with its acidity constant. The basicity constant of a base is said to measure the *strength of the base.* A base is said to be *strong* or *weak* according as its basicity constant is high or low. The term "strength," as applied to a base, is often quantitatively identified with its basicity constant. However, on account of the relation between K_a, K_b, and K_{auto}, the classifications of acids and bases as strong and weak are not independent: strong and weak acids necessarily have, respectively, weak and strong conjugate bases. Bases are often classified with reference to the strengths of their conjugate acids.

For the determination of the strength K_a of an acid, it is necessary to measure the concentration or activity of at least one of the three solute species involved in the expression for K_a: the concentrations of the other solute species can then be obtained from the stoicheiometry of mass and charge. The measurement of electrical conductance, as developed by Kohlrausch for electrolytic solutions, was applied by Ostwald to this purpose; and, with numerous subsequently introduced refinements of technique, this method has been much used in recent years for accurate determinations of K_a. Alternatively, the activity of H_3O^+ may be directly determined by measurement of the electromotive force of a cell which includes the electrolyte and a hydrogen electrode. Again, the concentration of any uniquely coloured species can be determined photometrically. Other methods of measurement, most of them less direct than those mentioned, are available.

If an acid HX is strong, and if, as is inevitable for nearly all electrically neutral acids, the concentration of HX is left to be determined from the stoicheiometry, it may in fact be impossible to determine it as a minute difference, and therefore impossible to obtain a K_a value for the acid. This difficulty arises with electrically neutral acids having K_a values of the order of 100 moles/litre or more. Thus two acids might have very different strengths, represented, say, by K_a values of 100 and 10,000 moles/litre: yet our measurements would tell us only that they are indistinguishably strong.

Comparisons among electrically neutral acids which are indistinguishably strong in water may be made in a solvent so much less basic than water that proton transfer from the acid to the solvent is appreciably incomplete, and a measurable equilibrium is thus attained. Perchloric acid, although of immeasurably great strength in water, is a weak acid, with a determinable acidity constant, in the much less basic solvent, sulphuric acid.[1] Again, neutral bases which in water are so weak that their conjugate acids are immeasurably strong, in other words, bases which will scarcely accept a proton from the water, may accept a proton to a measurable equilibrium extent from a more strongly acidic solvent. Thus nitrobenzene, although inappreciably basic in water, is an only moderately weak base, with a measurable basicity constant, in solvent sulphuric acid.[2]

Similarly, the equilibria in proton transfer from acids which are too weak, or to bases which are too strong, to permit a determination of acidity or basicity constants in water, may be amenable to measurement in a more basic or less acidic solvent, such as liquid ammonia.

A solvent which, like water, can either gain a proton or lose one, is called an *amphiprotic solvent*. Denoting such a solvent by LH, the equations defining K_a, K_b, and K_{auto} are those already given, except for the generalisation of replacing H_3O^+, H_2O, and OH^- by HLH^+, LH, and L^-, respectively. The autoprotolysis constants of a number of amphiprotic solvents are given in Table 57-1.

TABLE 57-1.—AUTOPROTOLYSIS CONSTANTS OF SOLVENTS.

Solvent	Temp.	pK_{auto}
Ammonia	−33°	22
Ethyl alcohol	+25°	19.[illegible]
Methyl alcohol	25°	16.7
Water	25°	14.0
Water	100°	12.3
Formic acid	25°	6.2
Sulphuric acid	10°	3.24

All but the last of these values are from L. P. Hammett's "Physical Organic Chemistry," McGraw-Hill, New York, 1940, p. 250. The value for sulphuric acid is as determined by R. J. Gillespie, *J. Chem. Soc.*, **1950**, 2516.

[1] R. J. Gillespie, *J. Chem. Soc.*, **1950**, 2537.

[2] A. Hantzsch, *Z. physik. Chem.*, 1907, **61**, 257; **62**, 626; 1908, **65**, 41; H. P. Treffers and L. P. Hammett, *J. Am. Chem. Soc.*, 1937, **59**, 1708; R. J. Gillespie, *J. Chem. Soc.*, **1950**, 2542.

The question has been discussed as to whether acids and bases always stand in the same order with respect to their strengths in different solvents. Obviously they need not: if one acid or base is replaced by another having a modification of structure which is local to the site of the proton transfer, the modification may have a specific effect on the concerned solvent molecule. This could apply, for instance, to the introduction of ortho-substituents into a benzoic acid. On the other hand, if the change of structure is not close to the site of proton transfer, acids and bases, provided that they are well separated with respect to strengths, are expected to preserve their order of strengths with a change of solvent. As far as is known, this is true.[3]

Equilibrium constants, such as acidity constants, depend on temperature; and from their temperature coefficients the two thermodynamic factors of equilibrium, the heat change and the entropy change, may be separately evaluated. The great majority of known acidity constants refer to the solvent water, and to the temperature 25°. Thus it is not at present possible to make the thermodynamic analysis indicated, except in a few cases, too few to allow the institution of a general comparison of constitutional effects on that basis. And so we shall make our comparisons with acidity constants directly, that is, with the free-energy differences. Theoretically, we have to expect that structural changes close to the site of proton transfer will influence both the enthalpy and the entropy changes, while structural changes at a distance will exert any large effect chiefly on the heat change The reason is that the entropy change depends mainly on the configurational latitude allowed, before and after reaction, to the units of the solvation shell, and that solvation is a local matter, depending on short-range forces.

We can go further in justifying a neglect of thermodynamic analysis, even to the limited extent to which it could be made. For there seems to be no doubt that the heat change at an experimental temperature is not so useful for structural comparisons as is the free-energy change, or its equivalent, the equilibrium constant. Evans and Polanyi[4] have offered a statistical thermodynamic argument leading to the conclusion that, under modifications of structure, the free-energy change follows more closely than does the heat change at a finite temperature, the heat change at zero temperature. This conclusion is certainly supported by the peculiar results obtained in even the most

[3] G. N. Burkhardt, *Chemistry & Industry*, 1933, **52**, 330; J. F. J. Dippy, *J. Chem. Soc.*, **1941**, 550.

[4] M. G. Evans and M. Polanyi, *Trans. Faraday Soc.*, 1936, **32**, 1333.

thorough attempts hitherto made, for example, that of Everett and Wynne-Jones,[5] to use the heat change at experimental temperatures. The difficulty in attempting to compute the heat change at zero temperature, from the observed variation in the heat change at finite temperatures, is that this variation, that is, the heat-capacity change, is large (mainly because water bound in ionic solvates has, like ice, a much lower heat capacity than liquid water); and the heat-capacity change cannot, of course, be assumed constant over the long extrapolation to zero temperature. Thus, the best practical procedure appears to be to use equilibrium constants in structural comparisons, but to remember that small differences may have no simple significance.

(57b) Long-Range Polar Effects: The Field Effect.—The existence of the field effect of a polar group on an acid-base centre, that is, of an electrostatic effect of the group acting on the centre, independently of inductive or conjugative relay through intervening bonds, was foreseen by Bjerrum, and was established by him with respect to the effect of a pole.[6] His argument was as follows. The two stages of ionisation of a dibasic acid, such as adipic acid, can be compared on the basis that the acid member of the acid-base system in the second stage is the same as that in the first, save for the unit of negative charge by which the charge of a combined proton can be imagined to have been cancelled:

$$HO_2C\cdot(CH_2)_4\cdot CO_2H \rightleftarrows HO_2C\cdot(CH_2)_4\cdot CO_2^- + H^+$$
$$^-O_2C\cdot(CH_2)_4\cdot CO_2H \rightleftarrows {}^-O_2C\cdot(CH_2)_4\cdot CO_2^- + H^+$$

If this extra negative charge had no effect on acid-base equilibrium, the ratio, K_{a1}/K_{a2}, of the acidity constants for the two stages would be 4, because the first acid has two positions permitting proton loss, and its conjugate base one position allowing proton gain, whereas the second acid has one position for proton loss, and its conjugate base two for proton gain. Bjerrum assumed that the electrostatic effect of the extra charge would add to the work of removal of the separating proton, and thus would relatively reduce K_{a2}, and so increase the ratio K_{a1}/K_{a2} above the value 4. All such ratios for symmetrical dicarboxylic acids are in fact greater than 4. By means of a simple electrostatic calculation of the work term, which was then counted as the relevant increment of free energy, Bjerrum derived the formula,

$$\ln (K_{a1}/4K_{a2}) = Ne^2/RTDr$$

[5] D. H. Everett and W. F. K. Wynne-Jones, *Trans. Faraday Soc.*, 1939, **35**, 1380.

[6] N. Bjerrum, *Z. physik. Chem.*, 1923, **106**, 219.

where D is the effective dielectric constant, and r is the distance between the acidic hydrogen atoms. Bjerrum took D as equal to the dielectric constant of the solvent, that is, 80, when acidity constants are measured in water at 25°. For a number of symmetrical dibasic acids, Bjerrum thus computed values of r which were of the right order of magnitude. For adipic acid the Bjerrum form of calculation gives $r=8A$, a quite reasonable value.

Gane and the writer studied the quantitative behaviour of the Bjerrum theory for a range of symmetrical dibasic acids, including all the homologous normal-chain acids up to azelaic acid, and a number of β-alkylated glutaric acids, and of alkylated malonic acids.[7] The longer normal-chain acids, from glutaric acid upwards, gave plausible values of r; but the shorter acids, and all the alkylated acids, gave values which were distinctly too small. This result suggests that, for the latter groups of acids, D was being given too great a value. The result might arise in part from a simultaneous operation of the inductive effect: no doubt it does in the malonic acids, and perhaps in succinic acid; but it is difficult to believe that the inductive effect would make a notable difference to acids with as many single bonds between the carboxyl groups as are present in the glutaric acids. A considerable, but still insufficient, improvement in the values was secured by allowing for electrical saturation, that is, the phenomenon that, under such strong forces as occur near an ionic centre, the molecular mechanism of dielectric polarisation begins to fail, so that the medium is physically incapable of increasing its induction in proportion to the field, and therefore the ratio of the two, which is the dielectric constant, falls.[8] However, there is another important cause of the quantitative failure, which was made clear in a different group of investigations, as we shall note below. It is that much of the space which Bjerrum's calculation assumes to be occupied by the solvent, is actually occupied by part of the molecule, the effective dielectric constant of which, especially as it is not free to rotate with respect to the field, must be much nearer 2 than 80.

Eucken[9] carried through a Bjerrum-type calculation to cover the field effect of a dipole. The principle may be illustrated by considering how the field effect of the chlorine substituent in chloroacetic acid can raise the acidity constant of this acid above that of acetic acid. The extra work term now arises from the carbon-chlorine dipole, of

[7] R. Gane and C. K. Ingold, *J. Chem. Soc.*, **1928**, 1594, 2267; **1929**, 1691.

[8] R. Gane and C. K. Ingold, *J. Chem. Soc.*, **1931**, 2153; C. K. Ingold, *ibid.* p. 2170; C. K. Ingold and H. G. G. Mohrhenn, *ibid.*, **1935**, 1482.

[9] A. Eucken, *Angew Chem.*, 1932, 45, 203.

moment μ, and inclination θ to the direction of the dissociable proton. Under this effect only, the ratio of the acidity constants should be given by equation:

$$\ln (K_a^{\text{chloroacetic}}/K_a^{\text{acetic}}) = Ne\mu \cos \theta/RTDr^2$$

If D is put equal to 80 in this equation, r takes the absurdly small value 0.6 A. However, Smallwood suggested that a value of D not much above 1 is appropriate in such a case, essentially for the reason that the space most relevant to the electrostatic calculation is largely occupied by part of the acid molecule.[10] Of course, it makes a great difference whether we take D as, say, 1, or 2, or 4; and by making D low enough one can formally take care of whatever the inductive effect of G. N. Lewis may be doing.

This dichotomy of D values is well illustrated by some figures given by Wheland,[11] here reproduced in Table 57-2. When a molecule is long and thin, most of the space relevant to the electrostatic calculation is indeed filled with solvent, and so a value of D somewhat near the upper limit of 80 is appropriate. But when a molecule is either short or thick, then the space most relevant to the calculation is filled mainly by the molecule itself, and thus a D value somewhat near the lower limit of 1 is preferable.

The best attempt yet made to provide a model which allows some of the space to be occupied by the molecule and some by the solvent, and yet permits the electrostatic work term to be computed in a closed form, is that of Kirkwood and Westheimer.[12] They consider the polar group and dissociating centre to be rigidly embedded in an ellipsoidal molecule of uniform dielectric constant 2, which is surrounded by an infinite medium of dielectric constant 80. Of course, the precise ellipsoidal shape, the location of the polar and dissociating centres within the ellipsoid, and the dielectric constant of 2, are arbitrarily adjustable features in this theory; but it does enable both long-and-thin molecules, and either short or thick molecules, to be treated on a common basis. Its numerical success in the examples already discussed is illustrated in Table 57-2.

All such calculations of field effects are of dubious quantitative significance, but there is a qualitative way to establish the existence of a

[10] H. M. Smallwood, *J. Am. Chem. Soc.*, 1932, **54**, 3048.

[11] G. W. Wheland, "Advanced Organic Chemistry," Wiley, New York, 1949, Chap. 11.

[12] J. G. Kirkwood, *J. Chem. Phys.*, 1934, **2**, 351; J. G. Kirkwood and F. H. Westheimer, *ibid.*, 1938, **6**, 506, 513; F. H. Westheimer and M. W. Shookhoff, *J. Am. Chem. Soc.*, 1939, **61**, 555; C. Tanford and J. G. Kirkwood, *ibid.*, 1957, **79**, 5333.

TABLE 57-2.—LENGTHS OF MOLECULES COMPUTED ASSUMING FULL CONTROL OF ACID STRENGTHS BY THE FIELD EFFECTS OF POLAR SUBSTITUENTS.[1]

Acid	Computed Lengths			Model Lengths	
	$D=80$ (Bjerrum)	$D=1$ (Smallwood)	D's 2 and 80 (K. and W.)	Maximum[2]	Average[3]
Adipic	8.1	635	7.8	9.0	5.6
Chloroacetic	0.6	5.1	3.0	3.4	3.0

[1] G. W. Wheland, *loc. cit.*
[2] Maximum with unstrained bonds.
[3] Average for rotation around unstrained bonds, but weighted for electrostatic interaction of end-groups.

field effect. This is to set it up in competition with a partly conjugative mechanism of internal polar transmission, to whose qualitatively known consequences a field effect is opposed, and if strong enough might qualitatively overturn. Two test points could be provided at which the internal polar effect would have magnitudes in one order, whilst a field effect would have magnitudes in the opposite order. Such experiments have been carried out by J. D. Roberts and his coworkers. We know that an internally transmitted polar effect, on traversing the benzene ring, appears more strongly at the more distant para-position than at the nearer meta-position. The field effect should appear with magnitudes in the opposite order in these two positions. The strength of an internally transmitted effect, and, more particularly, the difference in its strengths at para- and meta-positions may be great in the aromatic carbon atoms themselves. But such effects, including the relevant difference, can be weakened by providing the two positions with identical side-chains, and, with the increase of internal path-lengths thus furnished, testing for polar effects in the side-chains. This gives an improved opportunity to the field effect, provided that it is still strong at distances of the order of those involved, to show its distinctive differential action, as between meta- and para-positions, in a dominating way. And the best kind of field effect for producing such a result will be the strong effect of long range, which emanates from a free pole.

In the examples investigated,[13] the group $\cdot NMe_3^+$ was made the influencing pole in every case, while the meta- and para-side-chains, in which polar effects were tested by measurements on acidity constants, were $\cdot NH_3^+$ in one comparison and $\cdot CO_2H$ in another:

[13] J. D. Roberts, R. A. Clement, and J. J. Drysdale, *J. Am. Chem. Soc.*, 1951, 73, 2181. The authors offer a different explanation from that in the text.

$$(m\text{- or }p\text{-})\mathrm{Me_3\overset{+}{N}\cdot C_6H_4\cdot \overset{+}{N}H_3 \rightleftarrows Me_3\overset{+}{N}\cdot C_6H_4NH_2 + \overset{+}{H}}$$

$$(m\text{- or }p\text{-})\mathrm{Me_3\overset{+}{N}\cdot C_6H_4\cdot CO_2H \rightleftarrows Me_3\overset{+}{N}\cdot C_6H_4\cdot C\overset{-}{O_2} + \overset{+}{H}}$$

The results are in Table 57-3. In each case the trimethylammonium pole increases acidity, but does so more strongly from the meta- than

TABLE 57-3.—ILLUSTRATING DOMINATING FIELD EFFECTS OF A POSITIVE POLE ON ACID-BASE EQUILIBRIA IN META- AND PARA-AROMATIC SIDE-CHAINS.

Acid	pK_a		
	Parent	m-Me_3N^+	p-Me_3N^+
Anilinium ions in water at 25°	4.57	2.26	2.51
Benzoic acids in 50% EtOH at 25°	5.71	4.22	4.42

from the para-positions, as one might have hoped from the structure of the systems.

The first quantitative study of a pure field effect has been achieved by Beetlestone and Irvine.[14] They measured spectrophotometrically the ionisation equilibria of the acidic water ligand of the octahedrally coordinated iron in the (ferric) haems of methaemoglobins; and they made an associated theoretical development, starting from the dielectric theory of Kirkwood and Westheimer. Haemoglobins are known, which differ only in the identity of just one peptide unit in a particular position of a particular polypeptide sequence. Thus, the three human haemoglobins, known as *A* (the normal one), *S* (the abnormal one of sickle cell disease), and *C* (another abnormal one), differ only in the sixth peptide unit from the carboxyl end of the β-polypeptide chain. In *A* this unit is of glutamic acid,

$$\mathrm{HO_2C\cdot CH(NH_2)\cdot CH_2\cdot CH_2\cdot CO_2H}$$

in *S* it is of valine,

$$\mathrm{(CH_3)_2CH\cdot CH(NH_2)\cdot CO_2H}$$

and in *C* it is of lysine,

$$\mathrm{HO_2C\cdot CH(NH_2)\cdot (CH_2)_3\cdot NH_2}$$

In the region of pH 8, relevant to the measurements of methaemoglobin acidity, the free acid and basic centres in the peptide units of glutamic acid and lysine will be ionised, with the result that the ionic

[14] J. G. Beetlestone and D. H. Irvine, *Proc. Roy. Soc.*, 1964, A, **277**, 401, 414; *J. Chem. Soc.*, **1964**, 5086, 5090; **1965**, 3271; and subsequent papers.

charges carried by these units will be -1, 0, and $+1$, respectively. The ionic charges are 28.5 *A* from the iron atom of the haem structure, so that, by substituting *S* for *A* and *C* for *S*, one introduces two successive units of positive charge 30 *A* away from the ionising OH centre. At such distances, all types of intramolecular force which fade faster with distance than coulombic forces are completely negligible; and so one is left with a pure field effect. It is one of the rare cases in physical organic chemistry in which a high molecular weight aids quantitative study. For only a large molecule of rigid structure could provide such a large and accurately known intramolecular distance. Another simplification arises in that the globular protein approximates well in shape to an ellipsoid of the principal diameters 64, 55 and 50 *A*. Hence the dielectric constant which is effective between the known locations of the variable charge and the seat of acid-base dissociation can be closely calculated.

Beetlestone and Irvine developed formulae for calculating the effect of a coulombic field on the changes of free energy, entropy, and enthalpy in the methaemoglobin ionisation. Furthermore, they developed and illustrated a theoretically supported test for the situation in which the influence of the structural change on the acid-base equilibrium is wholly coulombic, coming as from a point, with a potential varying as the inverse first power of the distance, and no effective contribution from any type of interaction with a faster-fading force-law. When the structural change is of this type, the changes in ΔG, ΔH, and $T\Delta S$, should all be proportional, so that a plot relating any two of the quantities ΔG, ΔH, and $T\Delta S$, *e.g.*, one of ΔH against $T\Delta S$, for haemoglobins whose differences satisfy the pure-field condition should be linear (Cf. Chapter XVI).

The three human haemoglobins *A*, *S*, and *C*, whose structural differences are 30 *A* from the ionising centre, do in fact give such a linear plot. From the behaviour of some other abnormal human haemoglobins of known structure, some, like *S* and *C*, having their specific differences at points remote from the haem, and others having such differences close to the haem, it was concluded that modifications of electric charge made more than 10 *A* from any iron atom would satisfy the test for a pure field effect, whereas a modification made within that distance from an iron atom would in general not do so.

A number of animal haemoglobins, of unknown detailed structure, were examined. They all gave different thermodynamic parameters of ionisation. But when $T\Delta S$ was plotted against ΔE, all gave points lying, with those of the human haemoglobins *A*, *S*, and *C*, on the same straight line, as shown in Fig. 57-1. It was therefore suggested that

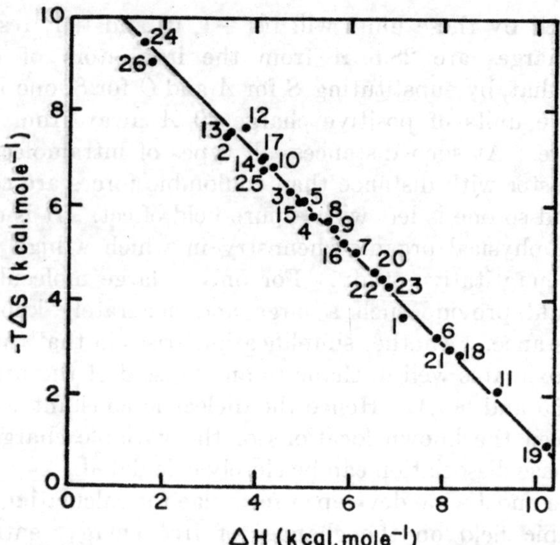

FIG. 57-1.—Plot of $T\Delta S$ against ΔE for methaemoglobin ionisations of the following vertebrate haemoglobins, in water at 20° and at ionic strength 0.05 mole l.$^{-1}$:

1. Mouse	10. Cat	19. Shrew
2. Rat	11. Pigeon	20. Duck
3. Baboon	12. Horse	21. Turkey
4. Patas monkey	13. Human *A*	22. Chicken
5. Mona monkey	14. Human *S*	23. Guinea fowl
6. Pig	15. Human *C*	24. Cow
7. Dog	16. Guinea pig	25. Mangabey monkey
8. Hyena	17. Lizard	26. Rabbit
9. Tantalus monkey	18. Bat	

(Reproduced with permission from Beetlestone and Irvine, *J. Chem. Soc.*, **1965**, 3273.)

within 10 *A* of each iron atom the structure of any normally functioning haemoglobin is characteristic, and that structural variations within this region would lead to important modifications in properties, perhaps in the vital property of oxygen binding.

(57c) Polar Effects Not Dependent on Conjugation: The Inductive Effect.—Ostwald's extensive measurements of the strengths of carboxylic acids showed that the strengths were markedly affected by substituents, in a way that appeared to be connected with the electropolar quality and unsaturation of the latter, and with their proximity to the carboxyl group. In 1899 Henrich[15] discussed the importance

[15] F. Henrich, *Ber.*, 1899, 32, 668.

of unsaturation in relation to the strengths of acids. In 1902 Vorländer[16] emphasized the connexion of carboxylic-acid strengths with the electropolar quality of substituents, as it was then recognised and assigned to substituents by reference to their behaviour in a wider range of chemical reactions. About the same time Wegscheider[17] attempted a quantitative analysis of the effects of substituents on acid strength: he calculated factors to express the influence, exerted by various substituents introduced at various positions along a saturated chain, on the acidity constants of carboxylic acids. In 1909 Flürscheim[18] included polar influences with other factors in a discussion of the strengths of aromatic acids and bases. Coming to the period of development of the electronic theory, Lewis in 1923 discussed[19] the transmission of polar influences by induction. In 1933 the writer discussed them[20] with reference to mesomerism. In the later 1930's and early 1940's more comprehensive discussions, all of which have the merit of treating the different aspects of the matter in combination, were presented by Waters,[21] by Watson,[22] by Dippy,[23] and by Branch and Calvin.[24] These later discussions still constitute the frame of any treatment which could be given today of internally transmitted polar effects on acid strengths.

TABLE 57-4.—THERMODYNAMICALLY CORRECTED ACIDITY CONSTANTS OF PARAFFINIC ACIDS IN WATER AT 25°.

Acid	10^5K_a	Acid	10^5K_a
Formic	17.72	*n*-Heptoic	1.28
Acetic	1.75	*n*-Octoic	1.27
Propionic	1.33	*n*-Nonoic	1.11
n-Butyric	1.50		
n-Valeric	1.44	*iso*Butyric	1.38
n-Hexoic	1.39	Pivalic	0.93

[16] D. Vorländer, *Ann.*, 1902, **320,** 99.

[17] R. Wegscheider, *Monatsh.*, 1902, **23,** 287.

[18] B. Flürscheim, *J. Chem. Soc.*, 1909, **95,** 722; 1910, **97,** 91.

[19] G. N. Lewis, "Valence and the Structure of Atoms and Molecules," Chemical Catalog Co., New York, 1923, Chap. 12.

[20] C. K. Ingold, *J. Chem. Soc.*, **1933,** 1120.

[21] W. A. Waters, "Physical Aspects of Organic Chemistry," Routledge, London, 1st Edn., 1935, Chap. 9.

[22] H. B. Watson, "Modern Theories of Organic Chemistry," Oxford Univ. Press, 1st Edn., 1937, Chap. 2.

[23] J. F. J. Dippy, *Chem. Revs.*, 1939, **25,** 151.

[24] G. E. K. Branch and M. Calvin, "The Theory of Organic Chemistry," Prentice-Hall, New York, 1941, Chap. 6.

The acidity constants of the paraffinic acids are in Table 57-4. The major distinctions can be summarised in the acidity series,

formic > acetic > higher acids

or in the statement that methyl substitution in formic or acetic acid leads to weaker acids.

This is in agreement with the recognised electropositivity of methyl and other alkyl groups ($+I$) in carboxylic acids, that is, the greater ease with which, compared to hydrogen, they yield electrons towards an electron-attracting centre (Section **7c**). The run of the figures for the first three homologues accords with the understood weakening of the inductive effect on relay through an intervening single bond; although it has to be remembered that hyperconjugation is expected appreciably to augment the first interval, and slightly to reduce the second. There could scarcely be a distinguishable field effect in such molecules as these, which have no intrinsically polar substituent apart from the dissociating centre itself. The minor differences between the higher homologues have never yet been explained in a satisfactory way: like most structurally produced differences of that order of smallness in thermodynamic or kinetic constants, their origin is undoubtedly complicated, and the analytical problem which it presents is beyond the present limits of our knowledge.

The introduction of ethylenic unsaturation causes a moderate increase in the strength of a carboxylic acid. The effect is reduced by an intercalation of single bonds between the unsaturated centre and the carboxyl group. These points are illustrated in the uppermost section of Table 57-5. The introduction of benzenoid unsaturation also produces an increase of acid strength, and it is the same order of magnitude as that caused by the olefinic bond. This effect of aromatic unsaturation is likewise diminished by the intercalation of single bonds. These points are exemplified in the second portion of the table. The introduction of acetylenic unsaturation leads to an altogether larger increase in acid strength, as is illustrated in the last division of the table.

As we have noted previously (Section **7c**), saturated carbon forms σ bonds with hybrid orbitals having a 1/4 content of s component, while ethylenic and benzenoid carbon forms single bonds from orbitals with a 1/3 content, and acetylenic carbon from orbitals with a 1/2 content of s component: therefore, relatively to saturated carbon, ethylenic and benzenoid carbon is moderately electronegative, while acetylenic carbon is somewhat strongly electronegative. The inductive effects ($-I$) which these unsaturated atoms thus initiate should

TABLE 57-5.—THERMODYNAMICALLY CORRECTED ACIDITY CONSTANTS OF UNSATURATED ACIDS IN WATER AT 25°.

Acid	Formula	10^5K_a
Acrylic	$CH_2:CH\cdot CO_2H$	5.56
Propionic	$CH_3\cdot CH_2\cdot CO_2H$	1.33
Vinylacetic	$CH_2:CH\cdot CH_2\cdot CO_2H$	4.48
n-Butyric	$CH_3\cdot CH_2\cdot CH_2\cdot CO_2H$	1.50
Allylacetic	$CH_2:CH\cdot CH_2\cdot CH_2\cdot CO_2H$	2.11
n-Valeric	$CH_3\cdot CH_2\cdot CH_2\cdot CH_2\cdot CO_2H$	1.44
Benzoic	$C_6H_5\cdot CO_2H$	6.27
*cyclo*Hexanecarboxylic	$C_6H_{11}\cdot CO_2H$	1.26
Phenylacetic	$C_6H_5\cdot CH_2\cdot CO_2H$	4.88
*cyclo*Hexaneacetic	$C_6H_{11}\cdot CH_2\cdot CO_2H$	1.58
β-Phenylpropionic	$C_6H_5\cdot CH_2\cdot CH_2\cdot CO_2H$	2.19
n-Butyric	$CH_3\cdot CH_2\cdot CH_2\cdot CO_2H$	1.50
trans-Crotonic	$CH_3\cdot CH:CH\cdot CO_2H$	2.03
Tetrolic	$CH_3\cdot C\vdots C\cdot CO_2H$	222.8
β-Phenylpropionic	$C_6H_5\cdot CH_2\cdot CH_2\cdot CO_2H$	2.19
trans-Cinnamic	$C_6H_5\cdot CH:CH\cdot CO_2H$	3.65
cis-Cinnamic	$C_6H_5\cdot CH:CH\cdot CO_2H$	13.2
Phenylpropiolic	$C_6H_5\cdot C\vdots C\cdot CO_2H$	590

be diminished by relay through saturated carbon bonds. The data reflect these conclusions qualitatively; but there are several detailed points requiring notice.

On looking over the figures either for the series of acids, acrylic, vinylacetic, allylacetic, or for the series benzoic, phenylacetic, β-phenylpropionic, one feels that the first interval is not as large, relatively to the second, as corresponds to the usual form of loss of polar effects by relay through single bonds. However, there is an obvious explanation for this. The mesomeric effect must take a hand in settling the acid strengths of acrylic and benzoic acids; and, if it acted alone it would make them weaker than the saturated acids (p. 1121). What we observe is the excess of the inductive effect over a weaker opposing mesomeric effect.

A consideration of the markedly different strengths of *cis*- and *trans*-cinnamic acids confirms this interpretation. To *trans*-cinnamic acid the remarks just made will apply. But in *cis*-cinnamic acid the phenyl and carboxyl groups must be twisted out of the plane of the bonds of the intervening ethylenic group, just as in *cis*-azobenzene the two phenyl groups are twisted from the plane of the bonds of the azo-group (Section **11c**; Fig. 11-2). Thus in *cis*-cinnamic acid there will be no functional conjugation, and no mesomeric effect, or scarcely any; and so we find in this acid a better manifestation than is shown by any of the other $\alpha\beta$-unsaturated acids of what the inductive effect of an ethylenic centre can do.

Along any series of acids of the form, paraffinic, $\alpha\beta$-olefinic, $\alpha\beta$-acetylenic, the acids become stronger, but the second interval is much greater than the first. This is to be correlated with the deduction that the change of $s-p$ composition of the bond-forming carbon orbitals is twice as great across the second interval as across the first. Supposing that we do not here consider *cis*-cinnamic acid or other non-planar *cis*-acids, another factor contributes to the observed large difference in the intervals, namely, that the opposition of the mesomeric effect is expected to occur at a flat-rate, being no greater for the triple than for the double bond, since it is stereochemically possible for only one bond-orbital of the acetylenic π shell to be conjugated with the carboxyl group. Thus one can read into the figures that, if it were not for the mesomeric effect, we should find the strengths of paraffinic, $\alpha\beta$-olefinic, and $\alpha\beta$-acetylenic acids to have orders of magnitude related as those of 1, 10, and 1000, with a doubled logarithmic difference across the second interval, reflecting the doubled change of orbital composition.

When an electronegative atom, such as chlorine, is substituted for hydrogen in a paraffinic acid, the acidity constant is raised. The increase falls sharply with increasing distance between the substituent and the carboxyl group. These points are illustrated in Tables 57-6

TABLE 57-6.—ACIDITY CONSTANTS OF CHLORO-SUBSTITUTED PARAFFINIC ACIDS IN WATER AT 25°.

Acid	10^5K_a				
	Unsub.	α-Cl	β-Cl	γ-Cl	δ-Cl
Acetic	1.75	139			
Propionic	1.33	132	10.1		
n-Butyric	1.50	106	8.9	3.0	
n-Valeric	1.44	—	—	—	1.9
	Unsub.	Monochlor-	Dichlor-	Trichlor-	
Acetic	1.75	139	5,500	222,000	

TABLE 57-7.—ACIDITY CONSTANTS OF SUBSTITUTED ACETIC ACIDS IN WATER AT 25°.

X in $CH_2X \cdot CO_2H$	CH_2Ph	NHPh	OPh	F
10^5K_a	2.2	3.9	68	260
X in $CH_2X \cdot CO_2H$	CH_2Me	NHMe	OMe	F
10^5K_a	1.5	—	33	260
X in $CH_2X \cdot CO_2H$	F	Cl	Br	I
10^5K_a	260	139	128	67

and 57-7. Presumably the results register co-operating inductive ($-I$) and field effects, though we would need better computing methods than are yet available to apportion the total effect between these two mechanisms.

The effect of formally neutral polar groups in modifying the acidity of saturated acids depends on the position of the substituting atom in the Mendeléjeff table, as will be obvious from Table 57-7. The orders illustrated are those of electronegativity, and correspond to series already given (Section **7c**) for the inductive effect ($-I$):

$$CR_3 < NR_2 < OR < F \qquad I < Br < Cl < F$$

The electropositivity of deuterium relative to ordinary hydrogen was discovered through observations on the effect of deuterium substitution on acid strengths.[25] The effects are small but constant in direction: acid strengths are always reduced. Some representative figures are in Table 57-8.[26,27] The effects in formic, acetic, and pivalic

TABLE 57-8.—EFFECTS OF DEUTERIUM SUBSTITUTION ON ACID STRENGTHS IN WATER AT 25°.

Deutero-acid	K_H/K_D	$pK_D - pK_H$	ΔpK per D atom
$D \cdot CO_2H$	1.085	0.035	0.035
$CD_3 \cdot CO_2H$	1.033	0.014	0.005
$(CD_3)_3C \cdot CO_2H$	1.042	0.018	0.002
$C_6D_5 \cdot CO_2H$	1.024	0.010	—
$C_6D_5 \cdot OH$	1.12	0.05	—

[25] E. A. Halevi and M. Nussim, *Bull. Res. Council, Israel*, 1956, **A, 5**, 263; *ibid.*, 1957, **A, 6**, 167, *idem* and A. Ron, *J. Chem. Soc.*, **1963**, 966; E. A. Halevi, *Tetrahedron*, 1957, **1**, 174; *idem*, *Prog. Phys. Org. Chem.*, 1963, **1**, 109.

[26] R. P. Bell and W. T. B. Miller, *Trans. Faraday Soc.*, 1963, **59**, 1147.

[27] A. Streitwieser jr. and H. S. Klein, *J. Am. Chem. Soc.*, 1963, **85**, 2759.

acids must be essentially inductive. Those in benzoic acid and phenol will be propagated partly by a conjugative mechanism.

(57d) Polar Effects Involving Conjugation: The Mesomeric Effect.—When we review the effects of substituents introduced at an unsaturated carbon atom in an olefinic or aromatic acid, we find evidence of mesomeric effects superposed on the field and inductive effects. This much can be gathered from the acidity constants[28] of several series of aromatic acids, as set out in Table 57-9. Values for ortho-substituents are included in the table, but they are for later discussion. The values for the meta- and para-substituents show, in the first place, the already illustrated general effects of polarity: electropositive alkyl groups always weaken the acid; and electronegative hydroxyl, alkoxyl, halogen, and nitro-substituents (apart from the disturbance next to be mentioned) strengthen it, halogens more than hydroxyl or alkoxyl, and the dipolar-bonded nitro-group most of all. There are no qualitative exceptions to this general statement among the meta-substituted compounds; but there are among the para-compounds, and, within the latter class, among those whose substituents have unshared electrons capable of conjugation with the aromatic system. Some of these para-substitutents, in particular, hydroxyl and alkoxyl, actually weaken the acid; and those that do not weaken it, notably the halogens, strengthen it less than do the same substituents acting from meta-positions, although other neutral groups exert their polar effects, of whatever sign, more strongly from para- than from meta-positions.

There is, then, an acid-weakening disturbance associated with para-substituents having unshared electrons adjacent to the benzene ring. This is surely a mesomeric effect[20] ($+M$). It is more prominent with oxygen substituents than with halogens, in accordance with the now familiar sequence for the $+M$ effect (Section **7e**):

$$\text{OR} > \text{Hal}$$

It can be verified from the table that this disturbance is most pronounced in the phenylboronic acid series, and thereafter falls off from series to series in the order,

phenylboronic > benzoic > cinnamic > phenylacetic > β-phenylpropionic

This is wholly consistent with its identification as a mesomeric effect.

[28] They are from the article by J. F. J. Dippy (ref. 23). The measurements of series A–D are by this author and his coworkers, while those of series E are by G. E. K. Branch and his collaborators.

TABLE 57-9.—THERMODYNAMICALLY CORRECTED ACIDITY CONSTANTS OF AROMATIC ACIDS.

(A) Benzoic Acids: 10^5K_a in Water at 25°

	CH_3	H	OH	OMe	F	NO_2
ortho-	12.3	6.27	105	8.06	54.1	671
meta-	5.35	6.27	8.3	8.17	13.6	32.1
para-	4.24	6.27	2.62	3.38	7.22	37.0

(B) Phenylacetic Acids: 10^5K_a in Water at 25°

	CH_3	H		OMe	Cl	NO_2
ortho-	—	4.88		—	8.60	9.90
meta-	—	4.88		—	7.24	10.8
para-	4.27	4.88		4.36	6.45	14.1

(C) β-Phenylpropionic Acids: 10^5K_a in Water at 25°

	CH_3	H		OMe	Cl	NO_2
ortho-	2.17	2.19		1.57	2.65	3.13
meta-	2.10	2.19		2.22	2.60	—
para-	2.07	2.19		2.04	2.47	3.36

(D) *trans*-Cinnamic Acids: 10^5K_a in Water at 25°

	CH_3	H	OH	OMe	Cl	NO_2
ortho-	3.16	3.65	2.44	3.45	5.83	7.07
meta-	3.61	3.65	4.00	4.21	5.08	7.58
para-	2.73	3.65	—	2.89	3.86	8.99

(E) Phenylboronic Acids: $10^{10}K_a$ in 25% aqueous EtOH at 25°

	CH_3	H		OEt	Cl	NO_2
ortho-	0.261	1.97		0.91	14.0	5.6
meta-	1.4	1.97		3.05	13.5	69
para-	1.0	1.97		0.608	6.30	98

There is through-conjugation between the influencing group, the benzene ring, and the acidic centre in the first three series, and it is most compact in the first, and least in the third:

$X—C_6H_4—B(OH)_2$ $X—C_6H_4—C(=O)OH$

$X—C_6H_4—CH=CH—C(=O)OH$

The conjugation is only between the influencing group and the benzene ring in the last two of the five series, and hence its polarising effect will suffer loss by single-bond relay—more loss when two single bonds intervene, as in the fifth series.

The manner of variation of the $+M$ effect with period number in a given Mendeléjeff group, for instance, the halogen group, follows from measurements of acid strengths. The relevant data[29] are in Table 57-10, which assembles acidity constants for the monohalogeno-derivatives of benzoic acids, of phenylboronic acids, and of phenols, and basicity constants for the monohalogeno-anilines. Values for ortho-halogeno-compounds are included, but are not for present discussion. It can be noticed that meta- and para-halogen substituents nearly always strengthen acids and weaken bases, but that they never strengthen the acids or weaken the bases as much when acting from the para-position as when acting from the meta-position. The para-fluorine substituent even slightly weakens phenol as an acid, only slightly strengthens benzoic acid, and barely succeeds in weakening aniline as a base. This is part of the generalisation that the failure of the halogens to act from para-positions as they do from meta-positions is most pronounced in the case of fluorine, and falls progressively through the halogen series towards iodine. In other words, the acid-weakening disturbance, which we have credited to the mesomeric effect, falls in the order already given for the $+M$ effect (Section **7e**):

$$F > Cl > Br > I$$

In detail, the relation of fluorine to the other halogens with respect to the intensity of the mesomeric effect, appears in the data for the benzoic and phenylboronic acids, and the relation of all four halogens is shown by the figures for the phenols and anilines. Historically,

[29] These figures also are from the article by J. F. J. Dippy (ref. 23). The measurements of series A are by him and his coworkers, those of series B by R. Kuhn and A. Wassermann, those of series C by G. E. K. Branch and his collaborators, and those of series D and E by G. M. Bennett, G. L. Brooks, and S. Glasstone.

TABLE 57-10.—THERMODYNAMICALLY CORRECTED ACIDITY AND BASICITY CONSTANTS FOR HALOGEN-SUBSTITUTED AROMATIC ACIDS AND BASES.

Position	H	F	Cl	Br	I
(A) Benzoic Acids: 10^5K_a in Water at 25°					
ortho-........	6.27	54.1	114	140	137
meta-........	6.27	13.6	14.8	15.4	14.1
para-........	6.27	7.22	10.5	10.7	—
(B) Benzoic Acids: 10^5K_a in 50% aqueous MeOH at 18°					
ortho........	0.513	6.61	7.08	7.08	6.6
meta-........	0.513	1.41	1.45	1.35	1.41
para-........	0.513	0.832	1.00	0.933	1.00
(C) Phenylboronic Acids: $10^{10}K_a$ in 25% aqueous EtOH at 25°					
ortho-........	1.97	—	14.0	—	—
meta-........	1.97	11.0	13.5	14.6	—
para-........	1.97	3.66	6.30	7.26	—
(D) Phenols: $10^{10}K_a$ in 30% aqueous EtOH at 25°					
ortho-........	0.32	4.27	10.2	9.78	9.12
meta-........	0.32	1.51	4.90	4.37	3.89
para-........	0.32	0.26	1.32	1.55	2.19
(E) Anilines: $10^{12}K_b$ in 30% aqueous EtOH at 25°					
ortho-........	126	2.95	1.35	1.00	0.36
meta-........	126	10.5	8.51	7.94	7.59
para-........	126	120	28.8	21.9	15.1

this relation was not theoretically foreseen, but was deduced by Branch and his collaborators[30] from the strengths of the phenylboronic acids, by Dippy, Watson, and Williams from the strengths of aromatic carboxylic acids,[31] and by Bennett and Glasstone and their coworkers[32] from measurements on the phenols and anilines. The electronic interpretation was supplied by Remick[33] later (Section 7e).

[30] B. Bettman, G. E. K. Branch, and D. L. Yabroff, *J. Am. Chem. Soc.*, 1934, 56, 1865.

[31] J. F. J. Dippy, H. B. Watson, and F. R. Williams, *J. Chem. Soc.*, 1935, 346; J. F. J. Dippy and R. H. Lewis, *ibid.*, 1936, 644.

[32] G. Baddeley, G. M. Bennett, S. Glasstone, and Brynmor Jones, *J. Chem. Soc.*, 1935, 1827.

[33] A. E. Remick, "Electronic Interpretations of Organic Chemistry," Wiley, New York, 1st Edn., 1943, p. 66.

This interpretation, it will be recalled, is that the overlap of atomic *p*-orbitals, necessary for the increased multiplicity of bonding involved in the $+M$ effect, is restricted by differences of size between the substituent atom and carbon. It follows that the $+M$ effect should fall with increasing atomic number, not only among the halogens, but also in other Mendeléjeff groups. Baker and his coworkers confirmed this for the series oxygen, sulphur, selenium, by a study of the strengths of benzoic acids, meta- and para-substituted by the groups, ·OMe, ·SMe, and ·SeMe. Their results,[34] given in Table 57-11, show that, while the substituents strengthen the acid when acting from meta-positions, they weaken it when acting from para-positions; and that the weakening effect diminishes towards higher atomic numbers. As

TABLE 57-11.—ACIDITY CONSTANTS OF BENZOIC ACIDS: 10^5K_a IN 30% AQUEOUS EtOH AT 20°.

	H	OMe	SMe	SeMe
meta-................	1.57	1.93	1.82	1.84
para-................	1.57	0.78	0.97	1.01

mentioned in Section **54a,** the same investigators derived the same conclusion from a study of the cyanohydrin equilibria of benzaldehydes. Thus, as already noted in Section **7e,** the $+M$ effect of the oxygen family of elements conforms to the sequence.

$$OR > SR > SeR$$

(57e) Steric and Other Short-Range Effects.—Effects of short-range forces on acid strength certainly exist. They are somewhat complicated; but part of their apparent complication arises from a cause for which they themselves are not to blame, namely, that we can observe them only in superposition on the field, inductive, and mesomeric effects, which, although they are not specifically short-range effects, are at their strongest at small distances. Of the specifically short-range effects of substituents, we can distinguish the following: (1) a *primary steric effect,* that is, steric compression exerted in different degrees in the conjugate acid and base; (2) a *secondary steric effect,* that is, a pressure-produced twisting of the acidic or basic group, with a consequent breakdown of conjugation, and therefore a modification of the mesomeric effect on acid strength; (3) chemically specific acts of combination of the substituent with the acidic or basic centre or with its solvation shell, as by hydrogen-bonding or co-ordination. This is not an exhaustive list of all conceivable local effects: for, while

[34] J. W. Baker, G. F. C. Barrett, and W. T. Tweed, *J. Chem. Soc.*, **1952,** 2831.

it refers throughout to exchange forces, it leaves electro-kinetic forces out of account.

All local effects, whether arising from forces which are not necessarily local, or from forces of an essentially local type, must be expected to influence, not only the heat of reaction, but also the entropy change. However, the observations are not yet extensive enough to allow of the isolation of these thermodynamic factors.

Flürscheim first pointed out[35] that all ortho-substituents, even electropositive methyl, increased the strength of a benzoic acid. This is sufficiently illustrated[36] by the acidity constants in the foregoing Tables 57-9 and 57-10 (but salicylic acid is a special case, to be discussed later). Flürscheim's explanation is equivalent to what we have called the primary steric effect: he saw in the observations a holding-off of the hydrogen ion by a volume-filling group. That acid strengths can be increased by such a mechanism was a fruitful idea, as will be illustrated below; but it is doubtful whether the benzoic acids constitute a good example. For the effective size of a carboxylate ion with its solvation shell will be greater than that of the undissociated carboxyl group, and therefore a differential primary steric effect due to a neighbouring substituent should weaken the acid. Thus the acid-strengthening effect of ortho-groups to which Flürscheim drew attention cannot be explained in this way: but it can be explained as a secondary steric effect on the following lines.

A carboxyl group bound to the benzene ring is of $-M$ type, and it exhibits the properties thus summarised more strongly than does the carboxylate-ion group (Section **7e**). The aromatic-to-carboxyl conjugation, then, brings electrons into the carboxyl group, and it brings them into the undissociated group more than into its anionic modification. Therefore aromatic conjugation weakens a benzoic acid. And therefore, if steric pressure twists the carboxyl group out of the

[35] B. Flürscheim, *J. Chem. Soc.*, 1909, **95**, 718.

[36] The case of the electropositive *t*-butyl substituent was subsequently investigated by J. B. Shoesmith and A. Mackie (*J. Chem. Soc.*, **1936**, **300**). Their values (apparently thermodynamically uncorrected) for 10^5K_a in water at 25° are as follows:

$C_6H_5\cdot CO_2H$	6.5	*o*-$Me_3C\cdot C_6H_4\cdot CO_2H$	35
		m-$Me_3C\cdot C_6H_4\cdot CO_2H$	5.2
		p-$Me_3C\cdot C_6H_4\cdot CO_2H$	4.2

By comparison with Table 57-9, one sees that, whereas, in the meta- and para-positions, the *t*-butyl group acts very much like the methyl group, an ortho-*t*-butyl group has a distinctly greater acidifying influence than an ortho-methyl group, in agreement with the suggested incursion of steric factors.

aromatic plane, thus breaking down the conjugation, the acid will be strengthened.

The same interpretation can be used in accounting for differences in strength of the stereoisomeric olefinic acids. Some illustrations are given in Table 57-12. The figures suggest that a stereo-change, which brings the larger of the two β-substituents, whether it be electropositive methyl or electronegative phenyl or chlorine, over from the *trans*- to the *cis*-position with respect to the carboxyl group, strengthens the acid. On account of size only, we should expect a methyl, or a phenyl, or a chlorine substituent, if *cis*-related to the carboxyl group, to cause a twisting of the latter out of the ethylenic plane, and thus to strengthen the acid.

The short-range character of the effect through which ortho-substituents in a benzoic acid, even when electropositive, strengthen the acid, is confirmed by the absence of such a strengthening influence of ortho-methyl groups in the series of β-phenylpropionic acids, and also in the series of cinnamic acids, as illustrated in Table 57-9 (p. 1116).

Flürscheim had a second group of examples, namely, the primary aniline bases, by which he illustrated his steric theory. He pointed out that all ortho-substituents, even electropositive methyl groups, reduce the basic strength of an aniline. He pictured the ortho-substituent as fending off the hydrogen ions, and thus making the base weaker: this is again equivalent to our primary steric effect. Now the aniline bases really might be expected to exhibit this effect. For their conjugate acids are ionic, and thus the acidic centre, being

Table 57-12.—Acidity Constants of Some Stereoisomeric αβ-Olefinic Acids: 10^5K_a in Water

Temp.	Isomer	10^5K_a	Isomer	10^5K_a
18°	$CH_3—C—H$ ‖ $H—C—CO_2H$	1.95	$H—C—CH_3$ ‖ $H—C—CO_2H$	3.9
18°	$CH_3—C—H$ ‖ $CH_3—C—CO_2H$	1.1	$H—C—CH_3$ ‖ $CH_3—C—CO_2H$	5.1
25°	$CH_3—C—H$ ‖ $Cl—C—CO_2H$	72	$H—C—CH_3$ ‖ $Cl—C—CO_2H$	158
25°	$C_6H_5—C—H$ ‖ $H—C—CO_2H$	3.65	$H—C—C_6H_5$ ‖ $H—C—CO_2H$	13.2
18°	$Cl—C—H$ ‖ $H—C—CO_2H$	22.2	$H—C—Cl$ ‖ $H—C—CO_2H$	47.7

strongly solvated, would almost certainly have a larger effective volume than the amino-group in the neutral base. Therefore, differential steric compression should increase the relative thermodynamic stability of the base, that is, it should make the base weaker, or, in other words, its conjugate acid stronger.

These expectations stand in contrast to those which relate to the secondary steric effect. First, we can show that, if the secondary steric effect were operative, it would work in the opposite direction. For now it is the base, and not the acid, which is conjugated with the aromatic ring; and since it is a $+M$ type of conjugation, it withdraws electrons from the basic group. Therefore any destruction of conjugation through twisting will cause electrons to pass back into the basic group, making the base stronger, or, in other words, its conjugate acid weaker. Secondly, we have the evidence of Hampson's work on dipole moments (Section **8f**) that, because of the small size of the primary amino-group, the twisting, on which the secondary steric effect depends, would be either non-existent, or at best very small.

Therefore the generalisation concerning basic strengths noted by Flürscheim can hardly be explained otherwise than as he suggested, that is, by a primary steric effect. Some examples of the effect of ortho-halogen substituents on the strengths of aniline bases are included in Table 57-10; but these substituents are strongly electronegative, and therefore their behaviour, though quantitatively notable, is not qualitatively distinctive. However, the two examples cited in the upper part of Table 57-13 illustrate the influence of ortho-location in a qualitatively clear form.[37] The methyl group, as a $+I$ group, when meta-situated, decreases the acid strength of the anilinium ion slightly, and, when para-situated, decreases it somewhat strongly; but when in the ortho-position, it increases the strength of the acid. The methoxyl group is a $-I+M$ group, the $+M$ character of which can be strongly exerted from an ortho- or para-position: consistently it increases acid strength when meta-, and decreases it when para-, situated; but when ortho-situated it increases acid strength. Evidently, then, ortho-substitution, independently of the polarity of the substituent, has a general acidifying influence on anilinium ions.

A check upon these conclusions can be obtained by turning to the N-substituted aniline bases. Here in contrast, as we see from the

[37] The values in Table 56-12 are cited by J. F. J. Dippy (ref. 23.). Those on the aniline bases are due to N. F. Hall and M. R. Sprinkle (*J. Am. Chem. Soc.*, **1932, 54,** 3469), and those on the dimethylanilines to W. C. Davies and H. W. Addis (*J. Chem. Soc.*, **1937**, 1622).

TABLE 57-13.—ACIDITY CONSTANTS OF THE CONJUGATE ACIDS OF SOME RING-MONOSUBSTITUTED ANILINES AND DIMETHYLANILINES.

X		Me	H	OMe
$C_6H_4X\cdot\overset{+}{N}H_3$: 10^5K_a in water at 25°				
X	ortho-	4.1	2.4	3.2
	meta-	2.05	2.4	6.3
	para-	0.74	2.4	0.51
$C_6H_4X\cdot\overset{+}{N}Me_2H$: 10^5K_a in 50% aqueous EtOH at 20°				
X	ortho-	0.85	6.2	0.32
	para-	1.7	6.2	0.69

lower part of Table 57-13, ortho-substitution by methyl or methoxyl lowers the acidity of NN-dimethyl-anilinium ions.

Now, in the original discovery of the secondary steric effect by Hampson, it was shown by the use of dipole moments (Section **8f**) that the dimethylamino-group is large enough to be twisted out of the aromatic plane by ortho-methyl groups, even though the primary amino-group is too small to be thus disturbed. There is also chemical evidence to this effect. It was discovered many years ago[38] that ortho-substituents, including methyl and ethoxyl groups, strongly depress the para-reactivity of NN-dialkylanilines towards electrophilic reagents, such as diazonium ions, nitrous acid, and formaldehyde, although substituents of the type of those named have no such effect in the absence of the N-alkyl groups. Verkade and Wepster and their collaborators have extended these observations to a number of other reactions, and have done this on quantitative lines. Most definitively, they have studied the electronic absorption spectra of the amines, and have observed the conjugation band of NN-dimethylaniline weaken and disappear as ortho-alkyl substituents are introduced and increased in size or number.[39] Two ortho-methyl groups or one ortho-*t*-butyl group suffice to suppress conjugation between the nitrogen atom and the ring practically completely. When these substituents are intro-

[38] O. Fischer, *Ber.*, 1880, **13**, 807; A. Weinberg, *Ber.*, 1892, **25**, 1610; E. Bamberger and F. Meimberg, *Ber.*, 1895, **28**, 1887; P. Friedländer, *Monatsh.*, 1898, **19**, 627.

[39] J. Burgers, M. A. Hoefnagel, P. E. Verkade, H. Visier, and B. M. Wepster, *Rec. trav. chim.*, 1958, **77**, 491; references are given to eleven earlier papers, 1949–1957, by authors of the same group, where some of the data, brought together in this comprehensive paper, are to be found.

duced into aniline itself, there is no suppression of conjugation. N-methylaniline and N-ethylaniline behave in an intermediate manner.

The same workers have measured the basicity constants of a large number of aniline bases: a sample of their results is in Table 57-14. Making use of the spectral intensities of the conjugation band, they were able to offer the following semi-quantitative analysis of the factors that determine basic strength. From measurements of the basic strength of para- and meta-alkyl derivatives of aniline, N-alkylanilines, and NN-dialkylanilines, it was concluded that any simple alkyl group would, when para-situated, increase basicity to the extent of raising the pK_a of the conjugate acid of the amine by 0.4 pK_a unit; and that if the alkyl group were meta-situated, the increment of pK_a would be 0.15 unit. These effects could be taken as polar, and, for simple alkyl groups, as inductive effects. It was assumed, as indicated in the third column of Table 57-14, that, if the alkyl substituents were ortho-situated, the same polar effect, in the absence of specifically local influences, would provide an increment to pK_a of 0.4 unit. The secondary steric effects of ortho-substituents were now

TABLE 57-14.—ACIDITY CONSTANTS OF THE CONJUGATE ACIDS OF SOME RING-ALKYLATED ANILINES AND NN-DIMETHYLANILINES.

Substituents	pK_a in 50% aq. EtOH	Increments in pK_a for		
		Inductive effect	Secondary steric effect	Primary steric effect
In $C_6H_5NH_2$:				
—	4.26	—	—	—
2-Me	4.09	+0.4	—	−0.6
2-*t*-Bu	3.38	+0.4	—	−1.3
2,6-Me_2	3.49	+0.8	—	−1.5
2,4,6-Me_3	4.00	+1.2	—	−1.5
2,6-Me_2-4-*t*-Bu	3.88	+1.2	—	−1.6
2,4-Me_2-6-*t*-Bu	3.40	+1.2	—	−2.1
2-Me-4,6-*t*-Bu_2	3.35	+1.2	—	−2.1
2,4,6-*t*-Bu_3	2.20	+1.2	—	−3.3
In $C_6H_5 \cdot NMe_2$:				
—	4.39	—	—	—
2-Me	5.15	+0.4	+1.8	−1.4
2-*t*-Bu	4.28	+0.4	+2.9	−3.4
2,6-Me_2	4.81	+0.8	+2.6	−3.0
2,4,6-Me_3	5.19	+1.2	+2.8	−3.2
2,4-Me_2-6-*t*-Bu	2.93	+1.2	+2.8	−5.5
2-Me-4,6-*t*-Bu_2	2.77	+1.2	+2.9	−5.7

allowed for, as shown in the fourth column of the table, by assuming an increment proportional to the decrease in intensity of the conjugation band. The increment corresponding to its complete destruction was 3 pK_a units. The primary steric effects of the ortho-substituents, both in the absence and the presence of N-substituents, were then computed by difference. As shown in the fifth column of the table, these increments in pK_a are all negative, as they should be. They are numerically greater in like derivatives of dimethylaniline, than of aniline, and in either of these series, they increase in magnitude with the number and size of the ortho-alkyl groups, as is to be expected. As an example of how a nett effect is made up, we may compare dimethylaniline with its 2-methyl-4,6-di-*t*-butyl derivative. The alkyl substituents reduce the basicity constant of the trialkyl derivative by 40-fold; but this factor is made up from an increase by a factor of 16 on account of the inductive effect, a decrease by a factor of 500,000 coming from the primary steric effect, and an increase by a factor of 800 from the secondary steric effect.

As stated at the commencement of this Section, we have to expect short-range effects on acid strength, not only on account of the general causes already discussed, the primary and secondary steric effects, but also, in special cases, by reason of specific interactions, such as hydrogen bonding and co-ordination. The data already cited offer some possible examples of these forms of interaction.

It will have been noticed in Table 57-9 that, whereas an ortho-methoxyl substituent increases the strength of benzoic acid by a factor of only 1.3, an ortho-hydroxyl group increases it by a factor of 17. That the smaller of two similarly polar groups in a benzoic acid should be so much more acidifying cannot be explained as a steric effect. It could, however, be attributed to internal hydrogen-bonding, which, partly in an electrostatic manner and partly through covalency change, brings a new positive charge into the carboxyl group, and therefore must have an acid-strengthening influence:

$$\mathrm{C_6H_4(C(OH){=}O\cdots H{-}O)} \rightleftarrows \mathrm{C_6H_4(C(OH){=}O^{+}{-}H\cdots \bar{O})}$$

Another possible example can be seen, though with more associated doubt, among the arylboronic acids, the data for which are in Table 57-9. Most of the figures in division (E) of the table can be understood in qualitatively the same way as the figures in division (A) for the benzoic acids. The exception of salicylic acid has been mentioned. The other main exception is *o*-nitrophenylboronic acid. Among the benzoic acids, strongly electronegative substituents are more strongly acidifying when in the ortho-position than when in other positions. The same is true for the chloro-substituent in the arylboronic acids. But it is not true for the nitro-substituent: the acidifying influence of the ortho nitro-group in this series is remarkably feeble. A plausible explanation of this is ready to hand: for as Branch and his coworkers pointed out,[30] the ortho-nitro-group is suitable, in both its electronic structure and its stereochemical disposition, to enter into an acid-weakening co-ordination with the boron atom:

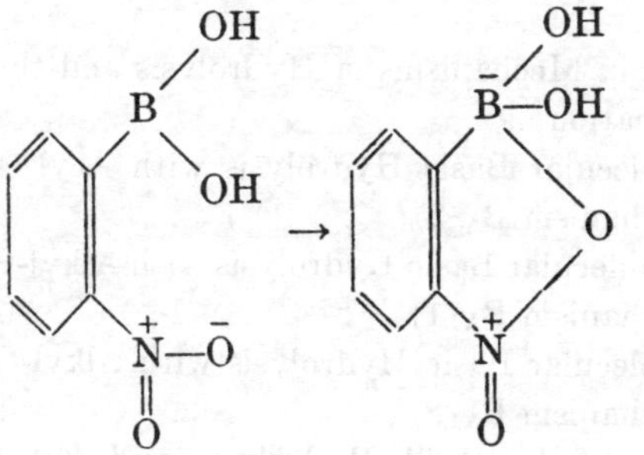

CHAPTER XV

Carboxyl and Phosphate Reactions

THE reactions of the carboxyl group are related both to reversible nucleophilic additions and to nucleophilic substitutions. We shall consider in turn those carboxyl reactions in which the attacking nucleophilic atom is oxygen, nitrogen, and carbon.

(58) HYDROLYSIS OF CARBOXYLIC ESTERS AND CARBOXYL ESTERIFICATION[1]

(58a) The Six Mechanisms of Hydrolysis and the Three of Esterification.[2]—In the reactions of carboxyl esterification and hydrolysis a number of distinct mechanisms may be recognised. They can be classified by reference to three features of these reactions.

The first guide to classification is the nature of the reagent. We know that esters may be hydrolysed by alkalis or by acids, and many circumstances convince us that different mechanisms or groups of mechanisms apply in these two cases. A less well-known form of hydrolysis occurs in neutral solution, and this can be shown to be more than a simple extrapolation of the alkaline and acid reactions. Thus it might appear that there are three main groups of mechanisms; but we shall regard two of these groups as related more closely to each other than to the third. For in both alkaline and neutral hydrolysis, the carboxyl form which undergoes reaction is the neutral ester molecule, $R'\cdot CO_2R$, while in acid hydrolysis it is the ionic conjugate acid, $R'\cdot CO_2HR^+$. The same sub-division is in principle applicable to esterification. Alkaline esterification is precluded by the stability of the carboxylate ion. Neutral esterification is conceivable, but has not been established: if it were realised, the reacting carboxyl form would be $R'\cdot CO_2H$. Acid-catalysed esterification is well known, and the reacting entity is $R'\cdot CO_2H_2^+$. We have to consider hydrolysis and esterification together, since either amounts to a retrogression of the other. We can include the reactions of oxygen exchange between acids and water as a specialisation (R to H) either of hydrolysis or of esterification; and we can include the transesterification of esters with alcohols as a generalisation (H to R) of either hydrolysis or esterifica-

[1] J. N. E. Day and C. K. Ingold, *Trans. Faraday Soc.*, 1941, 37, 686.
[2] S. C. Datta, J. N. E. Day, and C. K. Ingold, *J. Chem. Soc.*, 1939, 838; E. D. Hughes, C. K. Ingold, and S. Masterman, *ibid.*, p. 840.

tion. For all these reactions, we make one main division of mechanisms according to whether or not a preliminary proton uptake by the carboxyl compound is involved.

In order to elaborate the classification, we turn to a second diagnostic feature, namely, the position of rupture of the carboxyl compound. There are several ways of determining this, one general and the others limited, but all so easy to operate that the result need never remain unknown. For hydrolysis the possible modes of rupture, and the names given to them, are as follows:

$R'\cdot CO \mid OR + H \mid OH$	$R'\cdot CO\cdot O \mid R + HO \mid H$
Acyl-oxygen fission	**Alkyl-oxygen fission**

For esterification the corresponding alternatives are as below:

$R'\cdot CO \mid OH + H \mid OR$	$R'\cdot CO\cdot O \mid H + HO \mid R$
Acyl-oxygen fission	**Alkyl-oxygen fission**

Now it is found that, for alkaline hydrolysis, acyl-oxygen fission is usual but not invariable; and that, for neutral hydrolysis, alkyl-oxygen fission is not infrequent. Thus within the main group of mechanisms for which the attacked entity is the neutral molecule, $R'\cdot CO_2R$, there are two sub-groups, distinguished by the position of rupture of the ester group. It has been found also that, in acid-catalysed hydrolysis and esterification, in which the attacked entity is the conjugate-acidic ion, $R'\cdot CO_2HR^+$ or $R'\cdot CO_2H_2^+$, either acyl-oxygen or alkyl-oxygen fission may take place according to the structure and conditions. Thus our original two-fold classification of mechanisms becomes four-fold.

Having assigned a mechanism to its class, basic or acidic, and with acyl-oxygen or alkyl-oxygen fission, the final step must be to elucidate its nature as exactly as possible with the aid of reaction kinetics, supplemented by the study of reaction products where stereochemical or other relevant distinctions can be drawn. The general result of work on these lines has been to show that, within certain of the classes at least, two mechanisms exist, which are related to each other just like the bimolecular and unimolecular mechanisms of nucleophilic substitution or elimination. On account of the analogy we call such mechanisms "bimolecular" and "unimolecular."

The classification described is summarised in Table 58-1. As a convenient notation, we symbolise "basic" mechanisms, including the alkaline and related neutral mechanisms, by B, and "acidic" mechanisms by A; we denote acyl-oxygen and alkyl-oxygen fission by subscripts

TABLE 58-1.—MECHANISMS OF CARBOXYL HYDROLYSIS AND ESTERIFICATION.

Type of mechanism	Form attacked	Known reactions	Fission	
			Acyl-	Alkyl-
Basic	$R'\cdot CO_2R$	Hydrolysis	—	$B_{AL}1$
			$B_{AC}2$	$B_{AL}2$
Acidic	$R'\cdot CO_2HR^+$ or $R'\cdot CO_2H_2^+$	Hydrolysis and esterification	$A_{AC}1$	$A_{AL}1$
			$A_{AC}2$	—

AC and AL, respectively;[3] and we indicate molecularity by 2 or 1 as usual. Our three criteria allow for eight mechanisms, of which, as the table shows, six can claim to have been observed.

Many more than six mechanisms of hydrolysis and esterification have been suggested at various times, but some of the suggestions are elaborations of others. Almost any hypothetical mechanism can be elaborated by the introduction of additional rapid proton movements, and in other ways; but unless such occurrences affect the observable chemistry of the reaction, one has no basis for discussing them: it seems preferable to discuss each mechanism in its simplest conceivable form.

(58b) Bimolecular Basic Hydrolysis with Acyl-Oxygen Fission (Mechanism $B_{AC}2$).—The hydrolysis of carboxylic esters by hydroxide ion in aqueous solution is well known to involve acyl-oxygen fission, and to follow a second-order kinetic law. Theory suggests only one mechanism consistent with these observations, namely, the bimolecular mechanism $B_{AC}2$. We can represent it on the model of carbonyl addition and its retrogression, as follows:

$$\overset{-}{HO} + \underset{R'}{\overset{O}{\overset{\|}{C}}}\text{—OR} \underset{\text{fast}}{\overset{\text{slow}}{\rightleftharpoons}} HO\text{—}\underset{R'}{\overset{O^-}{C}}\text{—OR} \underset{\text{slow}}{\overset{\text{fast}}{\rightleftharpoons}} HO\text{—}\underset{R'}{\overset{O}{\overset{\|}{C}}} + \overset{-}{OR} \qquad (B_{AC}2)$$

$$(R'\cdot CO\cdot OH + OR^- \xrightarrow[\text{fast}]{} R'\cdot CO\cdot O^- + HOR)$$

The process is in principle reversible, but in practice is driven completely to the right by the final proton transfer from the formed carboxylic acid to the alkali present in the solution. We can represent

[3] In the paper by Day and the writer (ref. 1) primes were used instead of these more explanatory subscripts.

the same mechanism in an alternative way by using the model of nucleophilic substitution thus:

$$\bar{H\bar{O}} + \underset{\underset{R'}{|}}{\overset{\overset{O}{\|}}{C}}\text{—OR} \underset{}{\overset{\text{slow}}{\rightleftharpoons}} \left[\overset{\sim\frac{1}{2}-}{H\bar{O}}\cdots\underset{\underset{R'}{|}}{\overset{\overset{O}{\|}}{C}}\cdots\overset{\sim\frac{1}{2}-}{\bar{O}R} \right] \underset{\text{slow}}{\longrightarrow} \text{HO—}\underset{\underset{R'}{|}}{\overset{\overset{O}{\|}}{C}} + \bar{O}R \quad (B_{AC}2)$$

$$(R'\cdot CO\cdot OH + OR^- \underset{\text{fast}}{\longrightarrow} R'CO\cdot O^- + HOR)$$

Here, the intermediate complex is put in brackets, and in the middle of the reaction-indicating arrows, because, if it really possessed the electron distribution exhibited, and had no way of achieving greater stability, it would probably be a transition state, with an energy maximum in the reaction co-ordinate, rather than a molecule, having energy minima in all normal co-ordinates. It is, indeed, more unlikely that none of the anionic charge on the complex ion should be borne by the original carbonyl oxygen atom, than that the whole of it should be so borne, as in the expression based on addition. This expression depicts a more stable complex, one which might be a molecule. The real complex will be more stable still, because it will be mesomeric between the representations based on pure addition and pure substitution. As we shall note below, its status as a molecule has been experimentally established. We shall find it convenient to retain the two representations, recognising that they are extremes, because each signalises useful analogies.

Evidence of the nature of the alkaline hydrolysis of esters was first produced in 1912 by Holmberg. He used a substituted alkyl group R, which was asymmetric at the point of union; and he assumed that, if R were to separate from this point in the course of reaction, then R would not retain its stereochemical configuration. In the example of O-acetylmalic acid, $CH_3\cdot CO_2R$, where $R = \cdot CH(CO_2H)\cdot CH_2\cdot CO_2H$, he showed[4] that the asymmetric group did fully retain its configuration during alkaline hydrolysis. He concluded that R did not separate. The loophole in this argument is one which he was not in a position to see, namely, that if R separated as R^+, then it still might conceivably retain its configuration, owing to an intervention by one of the carboxylate-ion groups (Sections **33e** and **33g**).

Other methods of diagnosis were subsequently devised. Hilda Ingold and the writer considered a form of R which, if liberated as R^+, would be mesomeric, and would therefore yield isomeric alcohols.[5]

[4] B. Holmberg, *Ber.*, 1912, **45**, 2997

[5] C. K. Ingold, and E. H. Ingold, *J. Chem. Soc.*, **1932**, 758.

Crotyl and 1-methylallyl, $\cdot CH_2\cdot CH{:}CHMe$ and $CH_2{:}CH\cdot CHMe\cdot$, are forms of R for which this is true, and Prévost had already shown[6] that acetates containing these radicals R are hydrolysed by alkali without isomerisation.

Norton and Quayle[7] used a similar principle when they let R be the *neo*pentyl radical, $\cdot CH_2\cdot CMe_3$, knowing that, if it were liberated as a cation, it would react in rearranged form, $CH_2Me\cdot CMe_2\cdot$, giving *t*-amyl alcohol. It was observed that *neo*pentyl esters, such as the acetate, undergo alkaline hydrolysis to give unrearranged *neo*pentyl alcohol.

All these methods are limited by the necessity for choosing a special form of R; but the following method, first used in this problem by Polanyi and Szabo,[8] is completely general. They employed solvent water enriched in ^{18}O, and showed, in the example of the alkaline hydrolysis of *n*-amyl acetate, that the oxygen from the medium does not appear in the formed alcohol, and therefore must go into the acid. This result clearly requires acyl-oxygen fission:

$$R'\cdot CO\,\vert\,\cdot OR + H\,\vert\,\overset{*}{O}H \rightarrow R'\cdot CO\cdot\overset{*}{O}H + HOR$$

Long and Friedman[9] have given a similar demonstration for the alkaline hydrolysis of γ-butyrolactone.

The kinetic classification of the alkaline hydrolysis of carboxylic esters as a second-order reaction was established in 1881 by Warder, in the example of the aqueous hydrolysis of ethyl acetate.[10]

The question of whether the most condensed intermediate state is a molecule, having a life which is long in comparison with a collision period, or is only the transition state of a reaction-giving collision, has been settled by Bender.[11]

He employed ethyl, *iso*propyl, and *t*-butyl benzoates, and, as solvent, either water or aqueous dioxan, the water in either case being enriched in ^{18}O; and he compared the rates of exchange of oxygen between the medium and the ester, as determined in ester recovered after different amounts of partial hydrolysis, with the rate of the hydrolysis. He found the rate of exchange to be from 10% to 40%, according to the ester and the medium, of the rate of hydrolysis. This

[6] C. Prévost, *Ann. chim.*, 1928, **10**, 147.
[7] H. M. Norton and O. R. Quayle, *J. Am. Chem. Soc.*, 1940, **62**, 1170.
[8] M. Polanyi and A. L. Szabo, *Trans. Faraday Soc.*, 1934, **30**, 508.
[9] F. A. Long and L. Friedman, *J. Am. Chem. Soc.*, 1950, **72**, 3692.
[10] R. B. Warder, *Ber.*, 1881, **14**, 1361
[11] M. L. Bender, *J. Am. Chem. Soc.*, 1951, **73**, 1626; M. L. Bender, R. D. Ginger, and J. P. Unik, *ibid.*, 1958, **80**, 1044.

shows that the intermediate complex lives long enough to survive the proton shift required to bring its two non-alkylated oxygen atoms into equivalence, so that either might split off to regenerate ester: when the alkylated oxygen splits off, the hydrolysis products are formed. If we use the addition model, the whole of the σ-π electronic readjustment occurs in the formation and destruction of the complex, and none in the proton shift; but, as already noted, this must be a limiting situation:

$$\mathrm{H\overset{*}{\underset{-}{O}}} + \mathrm{R'{-}\overset{\displaystyle O}{\overset{\|}{C}}{-}OR} \rightleftarrows \mathrm{H\overset{*}{O}{-}\underset{\displaystyle R'}{\overset{\displaystyle O^-}{C}}{-}OR} \rightleftarrows \mathrm{R'{\cdot}C\overset{*}{O}_2H} + \mathrm{\overset{-}{O}R}$$

$$\updownarrows$$

$$\mathrm{H\overset{-}{O}} + \mathrm{\overset{*}{O}{=}\underset{\displaystyle R'}{C}{-}OR} \rightleftarrows \mathrm{\overset{*}{\underset{-}{O}}{-}\underset{\displaystyle R'}{\overset{\displaystyle H\overset{*}{O}}{C}}{-}OR} \rightleftarrows \mathrm{R'{\cdot}C\overset{*}{O}_2H} + \mathrm{\overset{-}{O}R}$$

Let us now consider structural effects on rate of hydrolysis by mechanism $B_{AC}2$. The intermediate complex is negatively charged. Therefore we must expect electropositive substituents to retard, and electronegative to accelerate, the hydrolysis of esters by this mechanism. Furthermore, since the rate-controlling process is bimolecular, we must expect steric retardation from substituents close to the reaction centre.

The first quantitative investigation of constitutional effects on the second-order rate of alkaline hydrolysis of carboxylic esters was that of Reicher,[12] who in 1885 and subsequently examined aliphatic esters having unbranched and branched alkyl groups as R and R′ in $R'{\cdot}CO_2R$. His work was extended in the field of aliphatic esters by Olsson,[13] by Skrabal,[14] and by Kindler,[15] whose results,[16] besides confirming the retarding effect of alkyl substituents, show the accelerating influence of the groups Cl, $\cdot CO_2Me$, $\cdot COMe$, $\cdot CH_2{\cdot}COMe$, and $\cdot CH_2{\cdot}OMe$, and the retarding influence of a negative ionic charge, as

[12] L. T. Reicher, *Ann.*, 1885, **228**, 257; 1886, **232**, 103; 1887, **238**, 276.

[13] L. Smith and H. Olsson, *Z. physik. Chem.*, 1922, **102**, 26; 1925, **118**, 99; H. Olsson, *ibid.*, p. 107; *ibid.*, 1927, **125**, 243; 1928, **133**, 233.

[14] A. Skrabal and A. H. Hügetz, *Monatsh.*, 1926, **47**, 17; A. Skrabal and M. Rückert, *ibid.*, 1928, **50**, 369.

[15] K. Kindler, *Ann.*, 1927, **452**, 90; *Ber.*, 1936, **69**, 2792.

[16] They have been summarised and discussed already by L. P. Hammett, "Physical Organic Chemistry," McGraw-Hill, 1940, Chap. 7.

TABLE 58-2.—RELATIVE RATES OF SECOND-ORDER ALKALINE HYDROLYSIS OF ALIPHATIC CARBOXYLIC ESTERS.

		(A) In water at 25°			
$CH_3\cdot CO_2R$	R......	Me	Et	*i*-Pr	*t*-Bu
	rate.....	1	0.601	0.146	0.0084
$R'\cdot CO_2Me$	R'......	$\cdot H$	$\cdot CH_3$	$\cdot CH_2Cl$	$\cdot CHCl_2$
	rate.....	223	1	761	16000
$R'\cdot CO_2Me$	R'......	$\cdot CO_2Me$	CO_2^-	$\cdot CH_2\cdot CO_2Me$	$\cdot CH_2\cdot CO_2^-$
	rate.....	170000	8.4	13.7	0.19
$R'\cdot CO_2Et$	R'......	$\cdot CH_3$	$\cdot CH_2\cdot CH_3$	$\cdot CO\cdot CH_3$	$CH_2\cdot CO\cdot CH_3$
	rate.....	0.601	0.553	10000	2.66
$R'\cdot CO_2Et$	R'......	$\cdot CH_3$	$\cdot CH_2\cdot OMe$	$\cdot CH_2\cdot OEt$	$\cdot CH_2\cdot OH$
	rate.....	0.601	11.9	6.03	6.08
		(B) In 88% aq. EtOH at 30°			
$R'\cdot CO_2Et$	R'......	$\cdot CH_3$	$\cdot CH_2\cdot CH_3$	$\cdot CH(CH_3)_2$	$\cdot C(CH_3)_3$
	rate.....	1	0.470	0.100	0.0105
$R'\cdot CO_2Et$	R'......	$\cdot(CH_2)_2\cdot CH_3$	$\cdot(CH_2)_3CH_3$	$\cdot CH_2\cdot C_6H_5$	$\cdot C_6H_5$
	rate.....	0.274	0.262	1.322	0.102

illustrated in Table 58-2. Clearly polar effects are acting as they should, whatever steric effects may be doing.

The effect of substituents on second-order rates of alkaline hydrolysis of aromatic esters, $R'\cdot CO_2R$, where either R′ or R are phenyl or substituted phenyl groups, was first studied in an extensive way by Kindler,[17] whose work was developed, especially with respect to the temperature coefficient of reaction rate and the resulting Arrhenius parameters, by Nathan and the writer,[18] by Evans, Gordon, and Watson,[19] and by Tommila and Hinshelwood.[20] As to absolute rate, it is found that the substituents, Me, OMe if para-, and NH_2, retard the reaction, while halogen substituents, and the NO_2 group, accelerate it. This is illustrated in Table 58-3. It is to be noted that the NH_2 group retards much more effectively from the para-position in R′, than from the meta-position in R′, or from the para-position in R: the large effect exerted from the para-position in R′ is clearly to be ascribed to conjugation between the amino- and carboxyl groups through the aromatic ring. All these results can be understood on

[17] K. Kindler, *Ann.*, 1926, **450**, 1; 1927, **452**, 90; 1928, **464**, 278; *Ber.*, 1936, **69**, 2792.

[18] C. K. Ingold and W. S. Nathan, *J. Chem. Soc.*, **1936**, 222.

[19] D. P. Evans, J. J. Gordon, and H. B. Watson, *J. Chem. Soc.*, **1937**, 1430.

[20] E. Tommila and C. N. Hinshelwood, *J. Chem. Soc.*, **1938**, 1801; E. Tommila, *Ann. Acad. Sci. Fennicae*, 1941, **A, 57**, No. 3; **A, 59**, Nos. 3, 4, 5, 9, and 10.

TABLE 58-3.—RELATIVE RATES OF SECOND-ORDER ALKALINE HYDROLYSIS OF AROMATIC CARBOXYLIC ESTERS.

(A) $C_6H_4X \cdot CO_2Et$ in "85%" aq. EtOH at 25°

X	NH_2	OMe	Me	H	F	Cl	Br	I	NO_2
p-	0.023	0.209	0.456	1	2.03	4.31	5.25	5.05	110
m-	—	—	0.697	1	—	7.52	—	—	69.0
o-	—	—	0.125	1	3.74	2.24	—	—	8.71

(B) $C_6H_4X \cdot CO_2Et$ in "60%" aq. Me_2CO at 25°

X	NH_2	Me	H	NO_2
p-	0.0293	0.403	1	85.1
m-	0.574	0.596	1	47.7

(C) $CH_3 \cdot CO \cdot OC_6H_4X$ in "60%" aq. Me_2CO at 0°

X	NH_2	Me	H	NO_2
p-	0.510	0.602	1	18.8
m-	—	0.699	1	13.0

the basis that $-I$ or $-M$ effects accelerate, while $+I$ and $+M$ effects retard reaction. It is to be observed also that ortho-substituents, with the exception of fluorine, retard more, or accelerate less, than corresponding para-substituents: presumably a steric retardation is being superposed on the polar effects of all but the smallest of ortho-substituents.

By means of a study of the temperature coefficients of these rates it has been found that the kinetic effect of meta- and para-substituents is exerted almost entirely on the Arrhenius energy of activation E_A, the Arrhenius frequency factor A being unaltered by the substituents. It has also been found that the kinetic effect of ortho-substituents is exerted, not only in the energy of activation, but also in the frequency factor, which is markedly reduced by all ortho-substituents, excepting fluorine. This is illustrated, for the hydrolysis of esters $C_6H_4X \cdot CO_2Et$ in "85%" aqueous ethyl alcohol, by the plot in Fig. 58-1 of E_A against $\log 10^5k_2(25°)$, and particularly by the relation of the points to the straight line of slope $-2.303\boldsymbol{R}T$ (where $T = 298°$) drawn through the point X = H. This line represents an invariant frequency factor, and displacements to the left of the line measure reductions in the frequency factor. The displacements, which are shown only by ortho-substituents (but not by fluorine), are taken to mean that, while the energy of activation can be modified, not only by local effects, but also by transmitted polar effects, the entropy of activation becomes modified only by local interference with the assembly and articulation of the reactants, and of components of the solvation shell of the transition state (Section **6d**).

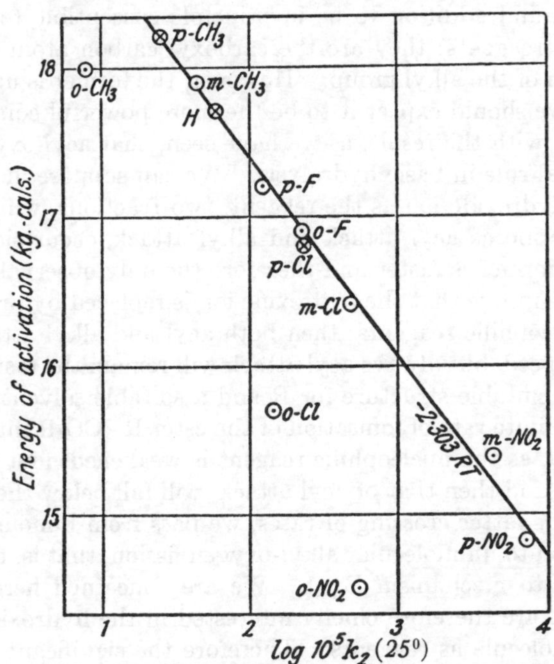

Fig. 58-1.—Alkaline hydrolysis of esters $C_6H_4X \cdot CO_2Et$ in 85% aqueous EtOH: effect of substituents X on the Arrhenius parameters E_A and A. Points on the line represent rates modified through effects on E_A only, A remaining constant. Displacements to the left of the line measure reductions in A. (Reproduced with permission from Evans, Gordon, and Watson, *J. Chem. Soc.*, 1937, 1430.)

Evans, Gordon, and Watson have applied the same kind of analysis to aliphatic esters.[21] In particular, they have measured the temperature coefficients of the rates of alkaline hydrolysis in 85% aqueous ethyl alcohol of normal and branched-chain saturated aliphatic esters $R' \cdot CO_2Et$. Though the rate differences were on the whole smaller in this series than in the above-mentioned aromatic series of esters, the general result was similar. It was that branching in R′, elsewhere than at the **α**-carbon atom, affected only the Arrhenius energy of activation, leaving the frequency factor nearly unaltered, whereas branching at the α-carbon atom reduced the frequency factor.

(58c) Unimolecular Basic Hydrolysis with Alkyl-Oxygen Fission (Mechanism $B_{AL}1$).—The ester molecule, $R' \cdot CO_2R$, contains two carbon atoms which are indicated by our knowledge of nucleophilic

[21] D. P. Evans, J. J. Gordon, and H. B. Watson, *J. Chem. Soc.*, **1938, 1439.**

substitution and addition to be in principle susceptible to attack by nucleophilic reagents: they are the carboxyl carbon atom and the α-carbon atom of the alkyl group. However, the former is unsaturated, and hence we should expect it to be the more powerful competitor for the reagent, with the result, as we have seen, that acyl-oxygen fission is the general rule in basic hydrolysis. We can suppose, nevertheless, that, with hydroxide ion as the reagent, two reactions, which we may shortly describe as acyl attack and alkyl attack, occur side by side, though the former is faster and therefore the only observable process. Let us now suppose that the hydroxide ion is replaced by progressively weaker nucleophilic reagents: then both acyl and alkyl attack will be reduced in speed, but always acyl attack will remain the faster process. Assuming a suitable structure for R and a suitable solvent, there will be a certain finite rate of ionisation of the ester $R' \cdot CO_2R$ into $R' \cdot CO_2^-$ and R^+; and, as the nucleophilic reagent is weakened, first the rate of alkyl attack and then that of acyl attack, will fall below the ionisation rate. At this latter crossing of rates, we pass from bimolecular acyl-oxygen fission to unimolecular alkyl-oxygen fission, that is, from mechanism $B_{AC}2$ to mechanism $B_{AL}1$. We are concerned here with hydrolysis, and are therefore chiefly interested in the hydroxide ion and the water molecule as reagents. Therefore the significant conclusion is that, *if* the described change of mechanism occurs before the nucleophilic reagent has been so far weakened as to become a water molecule, then, although alkaline hydrolysis will pursue mechanism $B_{AC}2$, hydrolysis in neutral solution will proceed by mechanism $B_{AL}1$.

Mechanism $B_{AL}1$ may be formulated as follows:

$$\left.\begin{array}{l} R{-}O \cdot CO \cdot R' \underset{\text{fast}}{\overset{\text{slow}}{\rightleftharpoons}} R^+ + \bar{O} \cdot CO \cdot R' \\ \\ R^+ + OH_2 \underset{\text{slow}}{\overset{\text{fast}}{\rightleftharpoons}} R{-}OH_2^+ \end{array}\right\} \qquad (B_{AL}1)$$

$$(R \cdot \overset{+}{O}H_2 + \bar{O} \cdot CO \cdot R' \xrightarrow[\text{fast}]{} ROH + HO \cdot CO \cdot R')$$

Apart from the final proton transfer, it constitutes a typical unimolecular nucleophilic substitution. It is reversible in principle, but in practice the proton transfer from the alkyloxonium ion to the carboxylate ion will drive it completely in the direction of hydrolysis.

The characteristics by which this mechanism should be recognisable are as follows. First, it is a basic mechanism: it will not require acid, but may proceed in neutral or weakly alkaline solution. Secondly, it will be possible to establish alkyl-oxygen fission by any of the usual methods: if the α-carbon atom of R is asymmetric, an optically active ester will give a racemised alcohol; or, if R is a substituted allyl group, it may become isomerised during hydrolysis; or, if R is of a form liable to Wagner rearrangement, as in camphene esters, it may suffer rearrangement during hydrolysis; and, unconditionally, the ^{18}O method may be applied. Thirdly, the kinetics of hydrolysis should have one of the forms appropriate to unimolecular substitution. Fourthly, as to polar effects on rate, electropositive, and especially $+E$, groups, such as methoxyl, if suitably situated in R, should strongly accelerate reaction; and so also should electronegative groups, such as nitro-groups, if suitably located in R′. Fifthly, the reaction, as a unimolecular process, should not be sensitive to steric retardation. And lastly, the reaction should be much accelerated by an increase in polarity of the solvent.

The first evidence concerning this mechanism employed the criterion of optical activity, and was furnished by Kenyon and his coworkers, who encountered this form of reaction during their experiments on the preparation of optically active alcohols by hydrolysis of resolved hydrogen phthalates. Their original form of R consisted of 1,3-disubstituted allyl groups, which are known to have a considerable tendency to pass into cationic forms R^+. They found that optically active 1,3-dimethylallyl hydrogen phthalate and 1-methyl-3-phenylallyl hydrogen phthalate, on hydrolysis in weakly alkaline aqueous solution, gave racemic alcohols, although, on hydrolysis with concentrated alcoholic alkali, the esters yielded optically active alcohols.[22] The inference was, first, that the reaction with *concentrated alcoholic* alkali involved bimolecular acyl attack, $B_{AC}2$, which could not racemise the alkyl group; and, secondly, that, in *dilute aqueous* alkali, the rate of this second-order process was so far reduced, and the rate of unimolecular alkyl fission, $B_{AL}1$, was so much increased, as to leave the latter mechanism in control, which, since it produced a cationic form R^+ of the alkyl group, led to racemisation. The experiments were subsequently extended outside the series of substituted allyl esters, chiefly to esters of benzhydryl and 1-phenylethyl derivatives, and to some naphthalene analogues. It was found that the different alkyl radicals differed considerably in the tendency of their esters to use the racemising $B_{AL}1$ mechanism of hydrolysis, and that the differences corresponded to the expected stabilities of the relevant carbonium ions R^+. Thus, optically active *p*-methoxybenzhydryl hy-

[22] J. Kenyon, S. M. Partridge, and H. Phillips, *J. Chem. Soc.*, **1936**, 85; W. J. Hills, J. Kenyon, and H. Phillips *ibid.*, p. 576.

drogen phthalate gave a racemic alcohol even with 10*N* aqueous sodium hydroxide,[23] while active *p*-phenoxybenzhydryl and 1-*p*-anisylethyl hydrogen phthalates required quite dilute alkali,[24] and the unsubstituted 1-phenylethyl ester needed an almost neutral solution,[25] in order to do so. This is in agreement with the expected order of ability of the substituents on the carbinol carbon atom to stabilise the corresponding carbonium ion:

$$\text{MeO}-C_6H_4- \;>\; \text{PhO}-C_6H_4- \;>\; C_6H_5- \;>\; \text{Me}-$$

The first of these inequalities arises because the oxygen atom of the phenoxy-group has competing opportunities for conjugation.

Kenyon and his collaborators obtained confirmation of the occurrence of alkyl-oxygen fission of the allyl esters under hydrolysis by dilute aqueous alkali, by observations of occurrence of anionotropic change. They found[26] that 1-phenyl-3-methylallyl hydrogen phthalate, on hydrolysis with concentrated methyl alcoholic alkali, gave only its own alcohol, but that, if the solvent were made more aqueous, and especially if the alkali were made more dilute, the produced alcohol was mainly the isomeric 1-methyl-3-phenylallyl alcohol. The interpretation was that the change of conditions has produced a change of mechanism: with concentrated alkali and a poor ionising solvent mechanism $B_{AC}2$ predominates, while with low alkalinity and a good ionising medium mechanism $B_{AL}1$ assumes control.

The same workers have used the nature of the products to establish alkyl-oxygen fission for most of the same esters in the generalised reactions of ether and ester formation by solvolysis in alcoholic or carboxylic-acid solvents. Thus 1,3-dimethylallyl hydrogen phthalate, on treatment with methyl alcohol, gave (racemic) 1,3-dimethylallyl methyl ether, a reaction which must involve alkyl-oxygen fission of the ester; and the same ester, by treatment with acetic acid, gave (racemic) 1,3-dimethylallyl acetate:[27]

$$\text{MeOH} + \text{R}\cdot\text{O}\cdot\text{CO}\cdot\text{R}' \rightarrow \text{MeO}\cdot\text{R} + \text{HO}\cdot\text{CO}\cdot\text{R}'$$
$$CH_3\cdot CO_2H + \text{R}\cdot\text{O}\cdot\text{CO}\cdot\text{R}' \rightarrow CH_3\cdot CO_2R + \text{HO}\cdot\text{CO}\cdot\text{R}'$$

[23] M. P. Balfe, M. A. Doughty, J. Kenyon, and R. Poplett, *J. Chem. Soc.*, **1942**, 605.

[24] M. P. Balfe, A. A. Evans, J. Kenyon, and K. N. Nandi, *J. Chem. Soc.*, **1946**, 803; M. P. Balfe, J. Kenyon, and R. Wicks, *ibid.*, p. 807.

[25] M. P. Balfe, G. H. Bevan, and J. Kenyon, *J. Chem. Soc.*, **1951**, 376.

[26] J. Kenyon, S. M. Partridge, and H. Phillips, *J. Chem. Soc.*, **1937**, 207.

[27] M. P. Balfe, W. J. Hills, J. Kenyon, H. Phillips, and B. C. Platt, *J. Chem. Soc.*, **1942**, 556.

Similarly, *p*-methoxybenzhydryl hydrogen phthalate and methyl alcohol gave racemic *p*-methoxybenzhydryl methyl ether;[28] 1,1-naphthylethyl hydrogen phthalate and formic acid gave racemic 1,1-naphthylethyl formate;[29] and several esters of 1-phenylethyl and some analogous radicals, including formates, acetates, benzoates, and hydrogen phthalate, gave racemic ethers or esters on solvolysis with methyl or ethyl alcohol or with formic or acetic acid.[30]

It has not been established, in any of the preceding examples of hydrolysis and its generalisations by mechanism $B_{AL}1$, that the kinetics are in fact characteristic of unimolecular reactions, for instance, that the reaction rates of hydrolysis or ether formation are insensitive to alkali. However, this want has been supplied in some other cases. Hammond and Rudesill examined the conversion of triphenylmethyl benzoate, in a solvent of mixed ethyl alcohol and methyl ethyl ketone, into triphenylmethyl ethyl ether and benzoic acid, a reaction which must involve alkyl-oxygen fission:

$$EtOH + Ph_3C{\cdot}O{\cdot}CO{\cdot}C_6H_5 \rightarrow EtO{\cdot}CPh_3 + HO{\cdot}CO{\cdot}C_6H_5$$

They confirmed[31] its unimolecular nature by showing that it had a strict first-order rate, unaccelerated by added sodium ethoxide, apart from a salt effect. A second, closely similar, case is that of the conversion of triphenylmethyl acetate in solvent methyl alcohol into triphenylmethyl methyl ether and acetic acid:

$$MeOH + Ph_3C{\cdot}O{\cdot}CO{\cdot}CH_3 \rightarrow MeO{\cdot}CPh_3 + HO{\cdot}CO{\cdot}CH_3$$

Gomberg and Davies[32] established the nature of the products of this reaction, whilst Bunton and Konasiewicz have shown[33] that it has a first-order rate, unaccelerated by methoxide ions.

Bunton, Comyns, Graham, and Quayle have investigated the hydrolysis under various conditions, including alkaline and neutral conditions, of a number of esters of 2,4,6-triphenylbenzoic acid, in which bimolecular acyl attack is considerably repressed by steric retardation.[34] In spite of this, the methyl, ethyl, *n*-propyl, *iso*butyl, and

28 M. P. Balfe, M. A. Doughty, J. Kenyon, and R. Poplett, *J. Chem. Soc.*, **1942,** 605; C. A. Bunton and T. Hadwick, *ibid.*, **1957,** 3043.

29 M. P. Balfe, E. A. W. Downer, A. A. Evans, J. Kenyon, R. Poplett, C. E. Searle, and A. L. Tárnowey, *J. Chem. Soc.*, **1946,** 797.

30 M. P. Balfe, G. H. Bevan, and J. Kenyon, *J. Chem. Soc.*, **1951,** 376.

31 G. S. Hammond and J. T. Rudesill, *J. Am. Chem. Soc.*, 1950, **72,** 2769.

32 M. Gomberg and G. T. Davies, *Ber.*, 1903, **36,** 3926.

33 C. A. Bunton and Alicja Konasiewicz, *J. Chem. Soc.*, **1955,** 1354.

34 C. A. Bunton, A. E. Comyns, J. Graham, and J. R. Quayle, *J. Chem. Soc.*, **1955,** 3817.

*iso*propyl esters suffer alkaline hydrolysis in aqueous 95% methyl alcohol by mechanism $B_{AC}2$, the second-order rates, all in the region of 10^3 times smaller than those of the corresponding esters of benzoic acid, decreasing slowly along the alkyl series, as is characteristic of this mechanism (Table 58-2). However, the *t*-butyl ester underwent hydrolysis faster than any of the lower esters, and required no alkali, the reaction having a first-order rate, which was not increased by added alkali. It followed that the hydrolysis was unimolecular. That it involved alkyl-oxygen fission was proved by the ^{18}O method:

$$H_2\overset{*}{O} + t\text{-BuO}\cdot CO\cdot C_6H_2Ph_3 \rightarrow t\text{-Bu}\overset{*}{O}H + HO\cdot CO\cdot C_6H_2Ph_3$$

Furthermore, since this reaction is evidently much faster than the corresponding (unrealised) unimolecular reactions of the methyl, ethyl, and *iso*propyl esters, it is exhibiting the expected accelerative action of electropositive alkyl substituents, and also the expected absence of steric retardation. The reaction was shown to be considerably accelerated by making the medium more aqueous. Thus the evidence for mechanism $B_{AL}1$ is in this example as complete as it could be.

(58d) Bimolecular Basic Hydrolysis with Alkyl-Oxygen Fission (Mechanism $B_{AL}2$).—According to the explanation, given above, of the relation between mechanisms $B_{AC}2$ and $B_{AL}1$, the remaining basic mechanism $B_{AL}2$ would appear to be incapable of observation. Actually it has been observed, first, in a special system, and secondly, in an ordinary system, but with special measures to incapacitate the usual masking effect of mechanism $B_{AC}2$.

For hydrolysis, mechanism $B_{AL}2$ may be formulated as follows:

$$H_2O + R{-}O\cdot CO\cdot R' \underset{\text{slow}}{\overset{\text{slow}}{\rightleftharpoons}} H_2\overset{+}{O}R + \overset{-}{O}\cdot CO\cdot R' \qquad (B_{AL}2)$$

$$(R\cdot\overset{+}{O}H_2 + \overset{-}{O}\cdot CO\cdot R' \xrightarrow[\text{fast}]{} ROH + HO\cdot CO\cdot R')$$

The process may be regarded as reversible in principle, although the final proton transfer from the alkyloxonium ion to the carboxylate ion will direct it in practice completely from left to right.

The observable characteristics of this mechanism are, first, that it should require no acid, secondly, that it should involve alkyl-oxygen fission, and thirdly, that it should be bimolecular. The last two points are covered together, when it is shown that a group R, asymmetric at the point of binding, becomes wholly inverted during hydrolysis. Polar and steric effects, and also solvent and salt effects, on rate could be predicted. It should be added that the argument from total inversion is unsafe in principle, because this stereochemical result could be given by a unimolecular ionisation with very efficient screening (Section **33f**). But our experience of the extensive racemisation accompanying mechanism $B_{AC}1$ in a like solvent may provide a reassuring contrast. And a confirmatory test based on products can be applied, as we shall see.

The special system in which this mechanism has been observed is the β-lactone system. It was first recognised[35] in the example of β-malolactonic acid. In alkaline, or in somewhat concentrated acid solution, this internal ester is hydrolysed with retention of configuration at the asymmetric centre, presumably by basic and acidic mechanisms of acyl-oxygen fission. However, over an intermediate *p*H range, it suffers a slower hydrolysis with inversion of configuration, and therefore by a bimolecular mechanism of alkyl-oxygen fission $B_{AL}2$. The diagram ($R=CO_2H$) shows the different positions of splitting: the acid reaction will be discussed later:

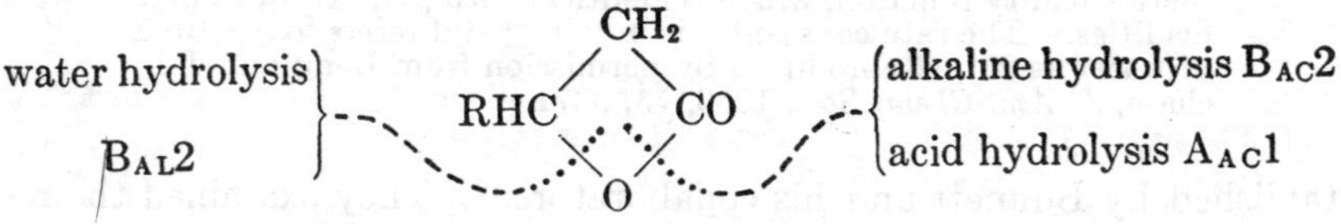

water hydrolysis $B_{AL}2$ — CH_2 / RHC — CO / O — alkaline hydrolysis $B_{AC}2$; acid hydrolysis $A_{AC}1$

Olson and Miller[36] discovered another case in β-butyrolactone ($R=CH_3$), which exhibits all the same phenomena. Olson and Hyde proved by the ^{18}O method that, in neutral hydrolysis, fission is on the alkyl side.[37] Long and Purchase[38] examined the simplest member of the series, β-propiolactone ($R=H$). In this case the stereochemical criterion is not available, but as Fig. 58-2 shows, the kinetic phenomena are so similar to those of the homologous lactone that the same mechanisms must be held to apply. Consistently with this conclusion, Bartlett and Rylander have shown[39] that, whereas the first product of the reaction of β-propiolactone with methoxide ions is the hydroxy-ester $HO\cdot CH_2\cdot CH_2\cdot CO_2Me$, the lactone reacts with initially neutral methyl alcohol to give the methoxy-acid $MeO\cdot CH_2\cdot CH_2\cdot CO_2H$.

The generality of mechanism $B_{AL}2$ in principle, despite its usual eclipse by the faster mechanism $B_{AC}2$ in basic hydrolyses, has been es-

[35] W. A. Cowdrey, E. D. Hughes, C. K. Ingold, S. Masterman, and A. D. Scott, *J. Chem. Soc.*, **1937**, 1264.

[36] A. R. Olson and R. J. Miller, *J. Am. Chem. Soc.*, 1938, **60**, 2690.

[37] A. R. Olson and J. L. Hyde, *J. Am. Chem. Soc.*, 1941, **63**, 2459.

[38] F. A. Long and Mary Purchase, *J. Am. Chem. Soc.*, 1950, **73**, 3267.

[39] P. D. Bartlett and P. N. Rylander, *J. Am. Chem. Soc.*, 1951, **73**, 4273

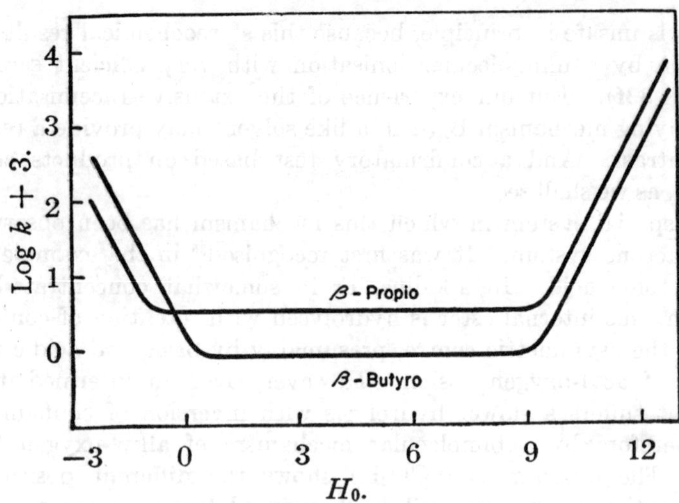

FIG. 58-2.—Rates of hydrolysis of two β-lactones: H_0 is Hammett's acidity function, which is identical with pH, except at high acidities. The rate constant k is in min.$^{-1}$ and refers to reactions in water at 25°. (Reproduced by permission from Long and Purchase, *J. Am. Chem. Soc.*, 1950, **73**, 3271.)

tablished by Bunnett and his collaborators.[40] They examined the reaction of sodium methoxide with methyl benzoate in solvent methyl alcohol. In this system, reaction $B_{AC}2$ is a transesterification, which replaces each original molecule with an identical one: however rapidly this happens, it cannot mask reaction $B_{AL}2$, if the latter process occurs. That it does occur was shown by the isolation in high yield of dimethyl ether:

$$Me\bar{O} + MeO \cdot CO \cdot C_6H_5 \rightarrow MeOMe + \bar{O} \cdot CO \cdot C_6H_5$$

The reaction was qualitatively shown to depend on the methoxide ion, and therefore it must have the mechanism indicated, which is simply a special case of S_N2 substitution. The same method has been used to establish mechanism $B_{AL}2$ in the basic methanolysis of methyl 2,4,6-triphenylbenzoate.[34]

(58e) Unimolecular Acid Hydrolysis and Esterification with Acyl-Oxygen Fission (Mechanism $A_{AC}1$).—The acid hydrolysis of esters and esterification are the reverse of each other. They will, in given circumstances, pursue identical mechanisms in their respective directions, in accordance with the principle of microscopic reversibility.

[40] J. F. Bunnett, M. M. Robison, and F. C. Pennington, *J. Am. Chem. Soc.*, 1950, **72**, 2328.

With acid-catalysed hydrolysis and esterification may be classed, as a specialisation, the acid-promoted oxygen-exchange reaction of acids, and, as a generalisation, acid-catalysed transesterification.

There are two mechanisms of acid-catalysed hydrolysis and esterification with acyl-oxygen fission, the unimolecular mechanism signalised in the title of this Section, and a corresponding bimolecular mechanism. In order to establish that a mechanism is one of these, it has in general to be shown that acyl-oxygen fission is involved, though this is self-evident in the special case of the oxygen-exchange of acids.

Holmberg was the first to provide such an indication for acid hydrolysis.[4] He did this by the method which seeks to detect a configurational change in a group R, which is asymmetric at its point of union in the ester $R'\cdot CO_2R$. He showed that in the acid hydrolysis of O-acetylmalic acid, $CH_3\cdot CO_2R$, where $R=CH(CO_2H)\cdot CH_2\cdot CO_2H$, the asymmetric group retains its configuration.

The method of choosing a form of R, which, if liberated as R^+, would be mesomeric, and would accordingly lead to isomeric, anionotropically related products, was applied by Hilda Ingold and the writer to both acid hydrolysis and esterification in the example of 1-methylallyl and 3-methylallyl (crotyl) acetates: no isomerisation was observed in these reactions.[41]

The ^{18}O method has been applied to establish acyl-oxygen fission in the acid hydrolysis of methyl hydrogen succinate,[42] and in that of benzhydryl formate,[43] and again in that of γ-butyrolactone.[44] It has been employed to prove the same type of fission in the esterification of benzoic acid with methyl alcohol.[45]

The two mechanisms of acid-catalysed hydrolysis and esterification with acyl-oxygen fission both involve pre-equilibrium with an adding proton, but differ in what afterwards happens to the oxonium ion thus formed. In the unimolecular mechanism,[41] $A_{AC}1$, the oxonium ion first undergoes a rate-controlling heterolytic fission, just as a sulphonium ion would in unimolecular nucleophilic substitution. This produces a carbonium ion, more specifically, an acylium ion $R'\cdot CO^+$, which is then attacked rapidly by a hydroxylic molecule, as in the final step of a unimolecular solvolytic substitution. And lastly, a proton, equivalent to that originally taken up, is split off. All proton

[41] C. K. Ingold and E. H. Ingold, *J. Chem. Soc.*, **1932**, 758.

[42] S. C. Datta, J. N. E. Day, and C. K. Ingold, *J. Chem. Soc.*, **1939**, 838.

[43] C. A. Bunton, J. N. E. Day, R. H. Flowers, P. Sheel, and J. L. Wood, *J. Chem. Soc.*, **1957**, 963.

[44] F. A. Long and L. Friedman, *J. Am. Chem. Soc.*, 1950, **72**, 3692.

[45] I. Roberts and H. C. Urey, *J. Am. Chem. Soc.*, 1938, **60**, 2391.

transfers are regarded as effectively instantaneous. As heretofore, the mechanism is formulated in a reversible manner, so that, read forwards, it applies to hydrolysis and, backwards, to esterification. The character (so to say) of the mechanism lies in its middle two stages, and, on account of their correspondence to the two stages of unimolecular substitution, the mechanism is called unimolecular, and labelled $A_{AC}1$:

$$\mathrm{R'{\cdot}CO{\cdot}OR} + \overset{+}{\mathrm{H}} \underset{\text{fast}}{\overset{\text{fast}}{\rightleftharpoons}} \mathrm{R'{\cdot}CO{\cdot}\overset{+}{O}HR}$$

$$\left.\begin{array}{l} \mathrm{R'{\cdot}CO{\cdot}\overset{+}{O}HR} \underset{\text{fast}}{\overset{\text{slow}}{\rightleftharpoons}} \mathrm{R'{\cdot}\overset{+}{C}O} + \mathrm{HOR} \\ \mathrm{R'{\cdot}\overset{+}{C}O} + \mathrm{OH_2} \underset{\text{slow}}{\overset{\text{fast}}{\rightleftharpoons}} \mathrm{R'{\cdot}CO{\cdot}\overset{+}{O}H_2} \end{array}\right\} \quad (A_{AC}1)$$

$$\mathrm{R'{\cdot}CO{\cdot}\overset{+}{O}H_2} \underset{\text{fast}}{\overset{\text{fast}}{\rightleftharpoons}} \mathrm{R'{\cdot}CO{\cdot}OH} + \overset{+}{\mathrm{H}}$$

The bimolecular mechanism,[42,46] $A_{AC}2$, is derived from mechanism $A_{AC}1$ just as bimolecular nucleophilic substitution is derived from unimolecular substitution: the life of the acylium ion is pictured as being reduced to the order of a collision period, so that the two stages, which previously represented the formation and destruction of this ion, become fused into a single bimolecular process. The initial proton uptake, and the final proton loss, are fast reversible processes as before. The characteristic stage of this mechanism is the middle one, and, on account of its analogy with bimolecular substitution, the mechanism is described as bimolecular and labelled $A_{AC}2$:

$$\mathrm{R'{\cdot}CO{\cdot}OR} + \overset{+}{\mathrm{H}} \underset{\text{fast}}{\overset{\text{fast}}{\rightleftharpoons}} \mathrm{R'{\cdot}CO{\cdot}\overset{+}{O}HR}$$

$$\mathrm{R'{\cdot}CO{\cdot}\overset{+}{O}HR} + \mathrm{OH_2} \underset{\text{slow}}{\overset{\text{slow}}{\rightleftharpoons}} \mathrm{R'{\cdot}CO{\cdot}\overset{+}{O}H_2} + \mathrm{HOR} \quad (A_{AC}2)$$

$$\mathrm{R'{\cdot}CO{\cdot}\overset{+}{O}H_2} \underset{\text{fast}}{\overset{\text{fast}}{\rightleftharpoons}} \mathrm{R'{\cdot}CO{\cdot}OH} + \overset{+}{\mathrm{H}}$$

[46] H. B. Watson, "Modern Theories of Organic Chemistry," Oxford Univ. Press, 1937, p. 130.

As with the basic mechanism $B_{AC}2$, the rate-controlling stage of this acidic bimolecular mechanism can be represented with hypothetical detail based either on the model of carbonyl addition and its retrogression,

$$H_2O + \overset{\overset{\displaystyle O}{\|}}{\underset{\underset{\displaystyle R'}{|}}{C}} - \overset{+}{O}HR \underset{\text{fast}}{\overset{\text{slow}}{\rightleftharpoons}} H_2\overset{+}{O} - \overset{\overset{\displaystyle O^-}{|}}{\underset{\underset{\displaystyle R'}{|}}{C}} - \overset{+}{O}HR \underset{\text{slow}}{\overset{\text{fast}}{\rightleftharpoons}} H_2\overset{+}{O} - \overset{\overset{\displaystyle O}{\|}}{\underset{\underset{\displaystyle R'}{|}}{C}} + HOR \qquad (A_{AC}2)$$

or on that of nucleophilic substitution,

$$H_2O + \overset{\overset{\displaystyle O}{\|}}{\underset{\underset{\displaystyle R'}{|}}{C}} - \overset{+}{O}HR \underset{}{\overset{\text{slow}}{\rightleftharpoons}} \left[\overset{\sim\frac{1}{2}+}{H_2O} \cdots \overset{\overset{\displaystyle O}{\|}}{\underset{\underset{\displaystyle R'}{|}}{C}} \cdots \overset{\sim\frac{1}{2}+}{O}HR \right] \underset{\text{slow}}{\rightleftharpoons} H_2\overset{+}{O} - \overset{\overset{\displaystyle O}{\|}}{\underset{\underset{\displaystyle R'}{|}}{C}} + HOR \qquad (A_{AC}2)$$

It is assumed that these are limiting representations, and that the actual intermediate complex has a charge distribution intermediate between those shown, and a stability greater than would be possessed by either of the represented structures, one of which is a molecule and the other a transition state. We shall note later that the intermediate complex is indeed a molecule.

The mechanisms $A_{AC}1$ and $A_{AC}2$ are both kinetically of first order in ester: in either mechanism, the first-order rate-constant in ester, k_1, is a good rate parameter at all acidities. In dilute acids only, both mechanisms are of first order in hydrogen ions. But the mechanisms show drastic differences of acid dependence in concentrated solutions of strong acids. As an introductory approximation, let us consider the older approach to the distinction between these mechanisms. Mechanism $A_{AC}1$ requires the pre-equilibrium formation of the conjugate acid of the ester, which then suffers a slow unimolecular heterolysis. The only concentration of kinetic importance is thus the stationary concentration of the conjugate acid, and this is thermodynamically controlled. Therefore when, on increasing the concentration of the aqueous strong acid, Hammett's equilibrium measure of acidity h_0 begins to diverge from $[H^+]$, the rate is expected to follow more closely the equilibrium measure h_0. Mechanism $A_{AC}2$ also requires pre-equilibrium proton uptake, but then requires the adding of a water molecule *in the rate-controlling step*. Kinetically, this is equivalent to the addition of H_3O^+ in a bimolecular rate-controlling process. Therefore, when $[H_3O^+]$ and h_0 begin to differ appreciably, rate is expected more closely to follow the kinetically more relevant quantity $[H_3O^+]$.

This is a fairly good approximation for moderate acid concentrations; but, in order to follow the distinction of behaviour of the two mechanisms up to the highest acid concentrations, we need a more sophisticated theory of acidity parameters. The way to such a theory was pointed out by Bunnett[47] (cf. Section **52a**). The Hammett function h_0, or, in the convenient logarithmic form, $-H_0 = \log_{10} h_0$, was developed in order to express the equilibrium extent of proton transfers from aqueous acid media to indicator bases, all of which were nitrogen bases. But in principle, every type of base (in strictest principle, every base) requires its own acidity function. The reason is that, when we increase the concentration of an aqueous strong acid, we not only increase the activity of hydrogen ions, but also, beyond a certain point, significantly decrease the activity of water. And whilst the formation of all conjugate acids has, as its uniform requirement, the uptake of a proton, the different types of conjugate acid differ considerably in their requirements of hydration. Thus, a relatively hydrophobic conjugate acid, one in whose formation, at the expense of hydrated hydrogen ion, bound water is released, will be additionally favoured on that account in a more concentrated acid medium in which the water activity has been reduced. According to Bunnett, the steepness with which $-H_0$ rises above the logarithm of the hydrogen-ion concentration measures the amount of bound water released on the formation of the indicator acids employed in the determination of the function H_0. If the conjugate acid of a general substrate is less hydrated than they are, its generalised acidity function $-H_S$ will rise more steeply than $-H_0$; and if the conjugate acid is more hydrated than the indicator acids, then $-H_S$ will rise less steeply than $-H_0$.

The expression of this theory in a quantitative form suitable for the study of mechanism in ester hydrolysis has been given and illustrated by Yates and McClelland.[48] We are concerned now with the method rather than with the results, but it will be convenient to illustrate their method with some of their results, though leaving over for the moment more general description of their results. Their experimental field comprised the hydrolysis of various alkyl and aryl acetates in aqueous sulphuric acid media.

Both the mechanisms $A_{AC}1$ and $A_{AC}2$ start with the pre-equilibrium

[47] J. F. Bunnett, *J. Am. Chem. Soc.*, 1961, **83**, 4056 *et seq.* (four papers).

[48] K. Yates and R. A. McClelland, *J. Am. Chem. Soc.*, 1967, **89**, 2686. The writer is much indebted to Dr. Keith Yates for having allowed him to see this paper in manuscript before its publication.

formation of the conjugate acid of the ester. The first step was therefore to determine the acidity function which expresses the extent of this thermodynamically controlled proton transfer. For all those esters for which spectrometric measurement of pre-equilibria could be made, Yates and McClelland found that the extents of proton transfer were represented by a practically uniform acidity function $-H_S$, which gave a linear plot against $-H_0$ with a slope of 0.62. This less-than-unit slope means only that the esterium ions are more hydrated than are Hammett's indicator ions.

With this acidity function to take quantitative account of the common pre-equilibrium step in the two mechanisms, Yates and McClelland could "isolate" the distinctive, and rate-controlling, second steps. These steps differ in their water requirements, and therefore the exercise was to determine how the rates of these individual steps vary with water activity as acid concentration is increased. The method was to plot the difference $\log k_1 - (-H_S)$ or, what is equivalent, the sum $\log k_1 + mH_0$, where $m = 0.62$, against $\log a_{H_2O}$. Provided that the equilibrium proportion of the conjugate acid of the ester is small, the sum $\log k_1 + mH_0$ is proportional to the free energy of activation of the whole hydrolysis, *less* the free energy of the pre-equilibrium step.

In mechanism $A_{AC}1$, the second step replaces the esterium ion, which is a pure oxonium ion, by an acylium ion, which is in part an oxonium ion and in part a carbonium ion: it is the cation of a pseudo-base. To the extent that it is a carbonium ion, it will be less hydrated than a pure oxonium ion. Actually, what is relevant for rate is, not the acylium ion itself, but the transition state on the way from the esterium ion to the acylium ion. But even this is expected to be somewhat less hydrated than the initial esterium ion. Hence we have to expect that, as a_{H_2O} drops with increasing acid concentration, the sum $\log k_1 + mH_0$ will rise to a small extent; *i.e.*, there will be a small negative correlation. As is shown for three simple aliphatic acetates in Fig. 58-3, in media over the range 85–100% by weight sulphuric acid in which mechanism $A_{AC}1$ prevails, the sum does rise when plotted against falling $\log a_{H_2O}$, with a slope of -0.2. Statistically, 0.2 molecule of bound water is released to the solvent when the esterium ion is converted to the transition state leading to the acylium ion. Phenyl acetate could not be studied in the more concentrated sulphuric acid media, because sulphonation took place; but *p*-nitrophenyl acetate could be so studied. It went over to mechanism $A_{AC}1$ at concentrations above 70% by weight of sulphuric acid; and again the slope of $\log k_1 + mH_0$ plotted against $\log a_{H_2O}$ was -0.2.

In mechanism $A_{AC}2$, the second step consumes a water molecule, which must be fully present in its bimolecular transition state. If this were all, one would expect that, as log a_{H_2O} drops with increasing acid concentration, the sum log k_1+mH_0 would suffer an accompanying drop, with a slope of unity, which could be described as the "kinetic order" in water. Actually, the water-dependence of the mechanism is greater than this, as might have been expected. For our formulae as written above (p. 1146) are oversimplified, in that the water molecules that must initially bring a proton into either acidic mechanism, and must finally take it away again, are not shown. Yet, it is very likely that the water molecule, which will take the proton away in the third step of mechanism $A_{AC}2$, will be hydrogen-bonded at the end of the second step to the proton which it will remove; and it may be present, and helping to distribute positive charge, in the transition state of the second step. If that is so, the slope of the plot of log k_1+mH_0 against log a_{H2O}, that is, the "kinetic order" in water, would be two. As shown for the same three esters in Fig. 58-3, over the range of media 0–80% sulphuric acid in which mechanism $A_{AC}2$ prevails, the slope is 2.0 ± 0.1. The data for ethyl acetate are due to

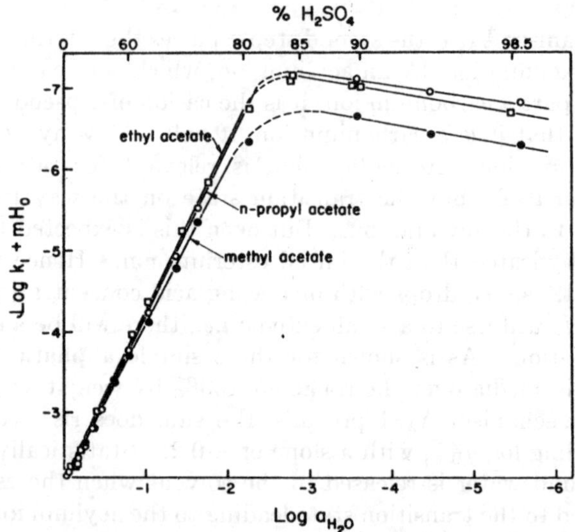

FIG. 58-3.—Rate-acidity dependence for the hydrolysis of alkyl acetates in aqueous sulphuric acid at 25°. Plot of log k_1+mH_0 *versus* log a_{H_2O} for methyl, ethyl, and *n*-propyl acetates (k_1 is the first-order rate-constant in min.$^{-1}$, and $m=0.62$). (Reproduced with permission from Yates and McClelland, *J. Am. Chem. Soc.*, 1967, **89**, 2686.)

Lane.[49] Yates and McClelland found the same slope for secondary alkyl acetates in the range 0–70% sulphuric acid, for benzyl acetate in the range 0–60%, and for phenyl, *p*-chlorophenyl and *p*-nitrophenyl acetates in the range 0–50% sulphuric acid. Thus mechanism $A_{AC}2$ prevails generally throughout the more aqueous end of the range of sulphuric acid media.

The broad qualitative distinction between mechanisms $A_{AC}1$ and $A_{AC}2$ with respect to the dependence of the specific rate k_1 on the concentration of the strong acid therefore amounts to this: in mechanism $A_{AC}1$, the specific rate rises with acid concentration, always somewhat faster than the acidity function, and on an ever-steepening curve, but in mechanism $A_{AC}2$, the rate rises less steeply than the acidity function, and with a diminishing slope, which takes it through a rate maximum, and thereafter with increasing steepness of descent either to zero rate as the water activity reaches zero, or to some low value at which an alternative mechanism takes over. We shall illustrate rate curves of these forms later.

Other observationally possible distinctions between mechanisms $A_{AC}1$ and $A_{AC}2$ can be foreseen. Rates of hydrolysis and esterification by mechanism $A_{AC}1$ should be greatly increased by electropositive substituents in the acyl group, which will not much impede proton addition at the alkyl oxygen atom, but will powerfully assist the rate-controlling heterolysis at the acyl carbon atom; and this effect should be much stronger than any kinetic effect of such substituents on mechanism $A_{AC}2$. Rates by mechanism $A_{AC}1$ should be insensitive to steric retardation: here is another gross distinction from mechanism $A_{AC}2$. Yet other distinctions can be devised. If an ester is hydrolysed by mechanism $A_{AC}1$ in an aqueous acid containing ^{18}O, this isotope cannot get into the ester ahead of the hydrolysis of the latter; but the ^{18}O istotope could so get incorporated, if the mechanism of hydrolysis were $A_{AC}2$. Long's observation (Section **30a**) that unimolecular mechanisms generally have higher (more positive or less negative) entropies of activation than bimolecular, applies to the acid hydrolyses of esters, and so provides another criterion of the molecularity of hydrolysis. Finally, rates by mechanism $A_{AC}1$ should be highly sensitive to the solvent, and indeed the mechanism should work best in solvents, such as sulphuric acid, in which acylium ions are known to be stable (Section **24e**).

The first direct evidence of the occurrence of carboxyl reactions by mechanism $A_{AC}1$ was obtained by Treffers and Hammett,[50] who proved

[49] C. A. Lane, *J. Am. Chem. Soc.*, 1964, **86**, 2521.

[50] H. P. Treffers and L. P. Hammett, *J. Am. Chem. Soc.*, 1937, **59**, 1708.

that mesitoic acid (2, 4, 6-trimethylbenzoic acid) produces a four-fold depression of the freezing-point of solvent sulphuric acid, a result which shows that it is converted into the mesitoylium ion:

$$C_6H_2Me_3 \cdot CO_2H + H_2SO_4 \rightarrow C_6H_2Me_3 \cdot CO_2H_2^+ + HSO_4^-$$

$$C_6H_2Me_3 \cdot CO_2H_2^+ + H_2SO_4 \rightarrow C_6H_2Me_3 \cdot CO^+ + H_3O^+ + HSO_4^-$$

Benzoic acid, on the other hand, gave a two-fold depression, an indication that here the initial proton transfer is complete, but that any further conversion to benzoylium ion is insufficient for cryoscopic detection. The similar behaviour of the esters of these acids, and its significance for hydrolysis, was shown by the observation that a freshly made solution of methyl mesitoate in sulphuric acid, on being poured into water, gave a quantitative precipitation of mesitoic acid, whereas methyl benzoate, on similar treatment, remained almost wholly unhydrolysed. This result forms a striking contrast to the known retarding effects of ortho-substituents, including ortho-methyl substituents, in the acid hydrolysis of benzoic esters in aqueous solvents, and in the esterification of benzoic acids in alcoholic media. The difference is a clear indication of duality of mechanism, and its direction is in harmony with the idea that the reactions have the unimolecular mechanism $A_{AC}1$ in sulphuric acid, but the bimolecular mechanism $A_{AC}2$ in aqueous or alcoholic solvents. Sulphuric acid is one of the best solvents known for producing dehydrated 'onium ions from acids; and we can see in the contrasts illustrated both the anticipated strong polar effect of electropositive methyl substituents, and the absence of steric retardation by ortho-substituents, in the reactions in sulphuric acid.

In the reactions of mesitoic acid and its ester in sulphuric acid, the formation of the acylium ion is rapid and complete; but the production of such an ion need be neither rapid nor complete, in order that it may constitute an intermediate for mechanism $A_{AC}1$. Indeed, in those cases in which kinetics can be examined, acylium-ion production must be slow, because it is rate-determining; and the stationary concentration of acylium ion might be very small. Such is the case in the hydrolysis of methyl benzoate by water in solvent sulphuric acid, which has been kinetically examined by Graham and Hughes.[51] The reaction is slow (half-life 7.7 hours at 20°), and is of first order with respect to ester, but zeroth-order with respect to water in concentrations up to $1M$. Methyl *p*-toluate underwent hydrolysis with similar kinetics,

[51] J. Graham and E. D. Hughes, results personally communicated. (Cf. the first edition of this book.)

the reaction being four times faster. Three of Yates and McClelland's examples of the hydrolysis of simple aliphatic esters by mechanism $A_{AC}1$ in sulphuric acid containing amounts of up to 15% by weight of water have been illustrated in Fig. 58-3. The similar behaviour of *p*-nitrophenyl acetate in media containing up to 30% of water has been mentioned.

When the very concentrated solution of the hydrolysing strong acid, such as sulphuric acid, is gradually diluted, then mesitoic esters, as the substrates being hydrolysed, maintain the use of mechanism $A_{AC}1$ to greater dilutions than do esters of benzoic acids without ortho-substituents, or than esters of simple aliphatic acids, for example, acetates. Bender found that methyl mesitoate used mechanism $A_{AC}1$ in 3*M* aqueous sulphuric acid, as he judged both from the closer correspondence of the rate to h_0 than to $[H^+]$, and from the absence of any uptake of ^{18}O from the medium into the unhydrolysed ester.[52] Long found that methyl and α-glyceryl mesitoates underwent hydrolysis in 4*M* aqueous sulphuric acid, or in 6*M* aqueous perchloric acid, by mechanism $A_{AC}1$, as he deduced from the near correspondence of the rate to h_0, whereas methyl or α-glyceryl esters of benzoic acid, *p*-anisic acid, or 3,4,5-trimethoxybenzoic acid underwent hydrolysis in the same media by mechanism $A_{AC}2$, as he concluded from the better correspondence of the rates with $[H^+]$ than with h_0.[53] Bunton and his coworkers studied the ^{18}O-exchange of mesitoic and benzoic acids with aqueous strong acids.[54] Mesitoic acid in a 60 vol.:40 vol. dioxan-water mixture containing 0.4–3.0*M* perchloric acid exchanged ^{18}O with a rate that followed h_0, and had an entropy of activation of +9 cal./deg./mole: the conclusion was that this exchange was proceeding by mechanism $A_{AC}1$. In contrast, benzoic acid in water containing 0.4–3.0*M* sulphuric acid exchanged ^{18}O at a rate that followed $[H^+]$, and had an entropy of activation of −30 cal./deg./mole; and the conclusion was that this exchange was using mechanism $A_{AC}2$.

(58f) Bimolecular Acid Hydrolysis and Esterification with Acyl-Oxygen Fission (Mechanism $A_{AC}2$).—The theory of mechanism $A_{AC}2$, and of its kinetics, and of the other properties which allow it to be distinguished from mechanism $A_{AC}1$, have been set out in the preceding Section. This was done in order to bring out the many contrasts between the two mechanisms. Of these two acid mechanisms, mechanism $A_{AC}2$ is on the whole the commoner if the acid catalyst is in dilute or only moderately concentrated solution. Most esters

[52] M. Bender, H. Ladenheim, and M. C. Chen, *J. Am. Chem. Soc.*, 1961, **83**, 123.

[53] C. T. Chmiel and F. A. Long, *J. Am. Chem. Soc.*, 1956, **78**, 3326.

[54] C. A. Bunton, D. H. James, and J. B. Senior, *J. Chem. Soc.*, **1960**, 3364.

(excepting some of special classes, such as esters of tertiary alcohols, and aromatic esters with carboxyl groups sterically well shielded on the acyl side) are hydrolysed by the bimolecular mechanism $A_{AC}2$ in dilute or moderately dilute aqueous solutions of strong acids, for instance, dilute hydrochloric or sulphuric acid. Likewise, the acids of these esters are esterified by mechanism $A_{AC}2$ in dilute alcoholic solutions of strong acids, for instance, by the Fischer-Speier method of heating the acid in a dilute alcoholic solution of hydrogen chloride.

This was the mechanism concerned in all the early work on rates of acid hydrolysis and esterification, work which was formative for the subject of reaction kinetics in general, and helped to link it to chemical thermodynamics. In 1862, Berthelot and Péan de Saint Gilles showed[55] how equilibrium in the reversible formation of ethyl acetate changed with the proportions of the reactants; and they deduced that the rates of the opposing reactions vary as the products of the concentrations of the interacting substances. Guldberg and Waage[56] drew largely on this work when generalising the principle of mass-action in relation to kinetics. The kinetic order of the hydrolysis of esters by aqueous acids was shown by Ostwald[57] to correspond to proportionality of the rate to $[H^+][R'\cdot CO_2R]$, and this demonstration was direct as to the dependence of the rate on ester, though indirect with reference to its dependence on hydrogen ion. Concerning the latter point, what was shown was that the specific rates of hydrolysis of methyl acetate by dilute aqueous solutions of identical concentrations of a long series of acids, ranging from strong to weak, were very nearly proportional, over a range of 200:1, to the electrical conductances of the solutions of the acids. This was in 1884: after the promulgation of the theory of electrolytic dissociation three years later, its significance became clear, namely, that rate is proportional to $[H^+]$, and that nearly all the electric current is carried by H^+. The kinetic order of esterification of carboxylic acids under catalysis by strong acids in alcoholic solvents was established in a fully direct way by Goldschmidt,[58] who found rates proportional to $[H^+][R'\cdot CO_2H]$. Since the transition state for esterification, and for the acid hydrolysis of esters, must be the same, this result implies the previously stated kinetic law for acid hydrolysis, the common transition state being composed either from $H^+ + R'\cdot CO_2H + ROH$ or, alternatively, from

[55] P. E. M. Berthelot and L. Péan de Saint Gilles, *Ann. Chim.*, 1862, **65**, 385; 1863, **68**, 225.

[56] C. M. Guldberg and P. Waage, "Etudes sur les affinités chimiques," Brögger and Cristie, Christiania, 1867; *J. prakt. Chem.*, 1879, **19**, 69.

[57] W. Ostwald, *J. prakt. Chem.*, 1884, **30**, 93.

[58] H. Goldschmidt, *Ber.*, 1895, **28**, 3218.

$H^+ + R'\cdot CO_2R + H_2O$. Direct demonstrations of the kinetic law for acid hydrolysis in aqueous solvents appear in a number of later investigations, for example, those of Drushel,[59] and of Palomaa.[60]

The kinetics characteristic of mechanism $A_{AC}2$, over the range of acid concentrations within which it applies, have been described in the preceding Section. We may now note some of the other characteristics of the mechanism.

Bender has shown[61] that the complex, formed by ester, water, and hydrogen ion, in hydrolysis by mechanism $A_{AC}2$, is a molecule, and not merely a transition state. This he did with the aid of water enriched in ^{18}O, as in his corresponding demonstration relating to the basic mechanism $B_{AC}2$. The example taken was the hydrolysis of ethyl benzoate in water with added perchloric acid as the catalyst. It was found that the rate of exchange of oxygen between ester and water, as determined in ester recovered after various amounts of partial hydrolysis, was a considerable fraction, about 20%, of the rate of hydrolysis. This shows that the intermediate complex lives long enough to permit the proton shifts which are required to bring its non-alkylated oxygen atoms into equivalence. The principle may be illustrated, as before, by the use of the addition model, though we recognise that this constitutes only a limiting representation of the involved changes in electron distribution:

$$H_2\overset{*}{O} + \underset{R'}{\overset{O}{\overset{\|}{C}}}-\overset{+}{O}HR \rightleftharpoons H_2\underset{*}{\overset{+}{O}}-\underset{R'}{\overset{O^-}{C}}-\overset{+}{O}HR \rightleftharpoons R'\cdot C\overset{*}{O}_2H_2^+ + HOR$$

$$\updownarrows$$

$$H_2O + \overset{*}{O}=\underset{R'}{C}-\overset{+}{O}HR \rightleftharpoons \underset{*}{\overset{-}{O}}-\underset{R'}{\overset{H_2\overset{+}{O}}{C}}-\overset{+}{O}HR \rightleftharpoons R'\cdot C\overset{*}{O}_2H_2^+ + HOR$$

Strong retarding steric effects on acid-catalysed esterification were established in the last century by the work of Victor Meyer, Sudborough, and Kellas. In Section **34a** reference was made to this work, and in particular to Meyer's demonstration that two ortho-substituents in a benzoic acid, independently of their polar nature, greatly retard

[59] W. A. Drushel, *Am. J. Sci.*, 1912, **34**, 69; 1914, **37**, 514.

[60] M. H. Palomaa, *Ann. Acad. Sci. Fennicae*, 1913, A, **4**, No. 2; 1917, **A, 10**, No. 16.

[61] M. L. Bender, *J. Am. Chem. Soc.*, 1951, **73**, 1626.

esterification, though ortho-substituents have no such effect in a phenylacetic acid. About that time, and early in the present century, this work was developed in a more quantitative manner by Goldschmidt,[62] by Kailan,[63] and by Sudborough,[64] who measured rate-constants of esterification of benzoic acids containing substituents: their data showed small polar effects of meta- and para-substituents, together with a notable retarding effect of ortho-substituents, which seemed to depend more on size than on polarity. In extension of earlier semi-quantitative work by Menshutkin, a systematic study of constitutional influences on the kinetics of esterification of aliphatic acids was made by Sudborough and his coworkers,[64] who noted the retarding effect of chain branching near the reaction site. During the 1920's the acid hydrolysis of aliphatic esters, many of them containing non-hydrocarbon substituents, was kinetically investigated by Skrabal and his collaborators,[65] whose results again demonstrate the smallness of polar effects, and the considerable steric retardations caused by substituents near the carboxyl group. In the 1930's several series of investigations were reported. One was by Palomaa and his coworkers,[66] who dealt with the kinetics of hydrolysis of aliphatic esters containing hydrocarbon and non-hydrocarbon substituents, and also with the kinetics of esterification of similarly constituted acids. Hinshelwood and his collaborators[67] studied the kinetics of both ester hydrolysis and esterification in both the aliphatic and aromatic series, with special reference to the effects of substituents on rate-constants and on Arrhenius parameters. In work which extended into the 1940's, Hartman and his coworkers[68] investigated rates and Arrhenius parameters for the

[62] H. Goldschmidt, *Ber.*, 1895, **28**, 3210; H. Goldschmidt, and O. Udby, *Z. physik. Chem.*, 1907, **60**, 728.

[63] A. Kailan, *Ann.*, 1907, **351**, 186.

[64] J. J. Sudborough and L. L. Lloyd, *J. Chem. Soc.*, 1899, **75**, 467; J. J. Sudborough and J. M. Gittins, *ibid.*, 1908, **93**, 210; J. J. Sudborough and M. K. Turner, *ibid*, 1912, **101**, 237.

[65] A. Skrabal, F. Pfaff, and H. Airoldi, *Monatsh.*, 1924, **45**, 141; A. Skrabal and A. M. Hügetz, *ibid.*, 1926, **47**, 17; A. Skrabal and A. Zahorka, *ibid.*, 1927, **48**, 459; A. Skrabal and M. Rückert, *ibid.*, 1928, **50**, 369.

[66] M. H. Palomaa, E. J. Salmi, J. I. Jansson, and T. Salo, *Ber.*, 1935, **68**, 303; M. H. Palomaa and K. R. Turkimadi, *ibid.*, p. 887; M. H. Palomaa and T. A. Siitonen, *Ber.*, 1936, **69**, 1338.

[67] C. N. Hinshelwood and A. R. Legard, *J. Chem. Soc.*, **1935**, 1588; E. W. T. Turner and C. N. Hinshelwood, *ibid.*, **1938**, 862; E. Tommila and C. N. Hinshelwood, *ibid.*, p. 1001.

[68] R. J. Hartman and A. M. Borders, *J. Am. Chem. Soc.*, 1937, **59**, 2107; R. J. Hartman, L. B. Storms, and A. G. Gassmann, *ibid.*, 1939, **61**, 2167; R. J. Hartman and A. G. Gassmann, *ibid.*, 1940, **62**, 1559; 1941, **63**, 2393; R. J. Hartman, H. M. Hoogsteen, and J. A. Moede, *ibid.*, 1944, **66**, 1714.

esterification of many substituted benzoic acids. Further work on similar lines continues to appear. Only a small proportion of this large body of results has been drawn upon in the construction of Tables 58-4 and 58-5, which will, however, suffice to illustrate the general weakness of polar influences, and the considerable importance of steric retardations.

One sees in the comparisons given how small is the effect, for example, of replacing electropositive CH_3 by strongly electronegative $CO \cdot CH_3$ or CO_2CH_3 on rate in the aliphatic series, and again, how small is the kinetic effect of introducing a *p*-NO_2-group in the aromatic series, quite unlike the effect of such constitutional changes on alkaline hydrolysis, as shown in Tables 58-2 and 58-3 (pp. 1135, 1136). On the other hand, one observes the notable retarding effect of any group of three substituents, whether they be Me_3, or Cl_3, or Ph_3, adjacent to an aliphatic carboxyl carbon atom, and also the marked retarding influence of ortho-substituents in the aromatic series. It is fortunate for the development of organic chemistry that Victor Meyer selected the reaction of esterification for the purpose of demonstrating the principle of steric hindrance: had he chosen the alkaline hydrolysis of carboxylic esters the phenomenon would still have been present, but the results would have been less easy to assign to a single dominating cause.

The reason for the smallness of polar effects in bimolecular acid hydrolysis and esterification is qualitatively obvious: any polar effect acts on this mechanism in two nearly compensating ways. Either it enhances pre-equilibrium protonation but retards rate-controlling attack on the conjugate acid by the water or alcohol, or it represses the protonation but accelerates the nucleophilic attack. In bimolecular basic hydrolysis one has no such compensation: here, the only kinetically significant process is the nucleophilic attack.

(58g) Unimolecular Acid Hydrolysis and Esterification with Alkyl-Oxygen Fission (Mechanism $A_{AL}1$).—As described in Section **58c**, it is possible, with a suitable choice of R, to observe hydrolysis of $R' \cdot CO_2R$ by mechanism $B_{AL}1$, which involves, as its rate-determining step, the following heterolysis of the neutral ester molecule to yield a carbonium ion:

$$R' \cdot CO_2R \rightarrow R' \cdot CO_2^- + R^+$$

This makes it certain that, again with an appropriate choice of R, it will be possible to realise hydrolysis by mechanism $A_{AL}1$, which requires the analogous, but undoubtedly much more facile heterolysis of the ionic conjugate acid of the ester. And since the ionic conjugate acids of some alcohols have the capacity for heterolysis to a carbonium ion, it is equally clear that one may observe esterification by mechanism

TABLE 58-4.—RELATIVE RATES OF ACID-CATALYSED HYDROLYSIS OF ALIPHATIC ESTERS AND OF ESTERIFICATION OF ALIPHATIC ACIDS.

(A) Hydrolysis by HCl in water at 25°

$CH_3\cdot CO_2R$	R.....	Me	Et	*i*-Pr	*t*-Bu
	rate....	1	0.97	0.53	1.15[1]
$CH_3\cdot CO_2R$	R.....	CH_2Ph	$\cdot CH_2\cdot CH_2\cdot OH$	$\cdot CH{:}CH_2$	$\cdot C_6H_5$
	rate....	0.96	0.69	1.20	0.69
$R'\cdot CO_2Me$	R'.....	H	Me	$\cdot CO_2Me$	$\cdot CH_2\cdot CH_2\cdot CO_2Me$
	rate....	21.3	1	1.71	0.35
$R'\cdot CO_2Me$	R'.....	$\cdot CH_3$	$\cdot COMe$	$\cdot CH_2\cdot COMe$	$\cdot CH_2\cdot CH_2\cdot COMe$
	rate....	1	1.20	0.16	0.23

(B) Hydrolysis by $PhSO_3H$ in 60% aq. EtOH at 60°

$R'\cdot CO_2Et$	R'.....	$\cdot CH_3$	$\cdot CH_2Cl$	$\cdot CHCl_2$	$\cdot CCl_3$
	rate....	1	0.91	0.40	0.11

(C) Esterification by HCl in EtOH at 14.5°

$R'\cdot CO_2H$	R'.....	Me	Et	*i*-Pr	*t*-Bu
	rate....	1	0.83	0.27	0.025
$R'\cdot CO_2H$	R'.....	$\cdot CH_3$	$\cdot CH_2Cl$	$\cdot CHCl_2$	$\cdot CCl_3$
	rate....	1	0.83	0.017	0.010
$R'\cdot CO_2H$	R'.....	$\cdot CH_3$	$\cdot CH_2Ph$	$\cdot CHPh_2$	$\cdot CPh_3$
	rate....	1	0.56	0.015	0.000

[1] This figure is probably increased by the incursion of hydrolysis by mechanism $A_{AL}1$ (Section 58g).

TABLE 58-5.—RELATIVE RATES OF ACID-CATALYSED HYDROLYSIS OF AROMATIC ESTERS AND OF ESTERIFICATION OF AROMATIC ACIDS.

(A) Hydrolysis of $C_6H_4X\cdot CO_2Et$ by $PhSO_3H$ in 60% aq. EtOH at 100°

X..................	OMe	Me	H	Br	NO_2
p-..................	0.92	0.97	1	0.98	1.03
m-..................	—	—	1	—	0.99
o-..................	—	—	1	—	0.36

(B) Hydrolysis of $CH_3\cdot CO\cdot O\cdot C_6H_4X$ by $PhSO_3H$ in 60% aq. EtOH at 25°

X..........................	Me	H	CO_2H	NO_2
p-..........................	1.06	1	0.89	—
m-..........................	0.97	1	0.86	0.70

(C) Esterification of $C_6H_4X\cdot CO_2H$ by HCl in MeOH at 25°

X..........................	Me	H	Br	NO_2
p-..........................	1.03	1	0.64	0.45
m-..........................	1.13	1	0.65	0.38
o-..........................	0.33	1	0.29	0.028

$A_{AL}1$. The stages of this mechanism may be set out as follows:

$$R'\cdot CO\cdot OR + \overset{+}{H} \underset{\text{fast}}{\overset{\text{fast}}{\rightleftharpoons}} R'\cdot CO\cdot \overset{+}{O}HR$$

$$\left.\begin{aligned} R'\cdot CO\cdot \overset{+}{O}HR &\underset{\text{fast}}{\overset{\text{slow}}{\rightleftharpoons}} R'\cdot CO\cdot OH + \overset{+}{R} \\ \overset{+}{R} + OH_2 &\underset{\text{slow}}{\overset{\text{fast}}{\rightleftharpoons}} R\cdot \overset{+}{O}H_2 \end{aligned}\right\} \quad (A_{AL}1)$$

$$R\overset{+}{O}H_2 \underset{\text{fast}}{\overset{\text{fast}}{\rightleftharpoons}} R\cdot OH + \overset{+}{H}$$

In either direction the rate-determining step is the unimolecular heterolysis of an oxonium ion.

The expected characteristics of this mechanism are as follows. It should be acid catalysed. It should involve alkyl-oxygen fission, as might be proved, for example, by the ^{18}O method. It should in appropriate cases show the usual signs of the liberation of R^+: thus, if R is asymmetric at the point of its union, it should suffer racemisation, possibly with some excess of inversion; and if R^+ is of such a form that, when liberated, it would decompose to give an olefin, or undergo a Wagner rearrangement, or some other kind of rearrangement, then these effects should be observed to accompany the hydrolysis or esterification. The rate of reaction by this mechanism should show strong polar effects, in particular, strong acceleration under the influence of electron-releasing groups in R. The rate should be insensitive to steric retardation. It should show the entropy effect of a unimolecular reaction. Isotopically labelled oxygen from the medium should not get incorporated into an ester ahead of its hydrolysis.

Tertiary alkyl groups are among the forms of R which should be favourable to this mechanism, and a preliminary indication of its incursion in acid hydrolysis can be seen in some results of Skrabal, which are summarised in the top line of Table 58-4. The rate of acid hydrolysis of *t*-butyl acetate is considerably greater than would be expected from the rates applying to methyl, ethyl, and *iso*propyl acetates. Indeed, the rates for the series go through a minimum, strongly reminiscent of the minimum in the rates of hydrolysis of corresponding alkyl halides, which was part of the originally offered evidence of duality of mechanism in aliphatic substitution (Section

28a). Skrabal's rates can be understood, if it is assumed that methyl, ethyl, and *iso*propyl acetates suffer acid hydrolysis by mechanism $A_{AC}2$, which is being sterically retarded increasingly along the series, but that, in the case of *t*-butyl acetate, the faster mechanism $A_{AL}1$ assumes control, in consequence of the relatively considerable stability of the *t*-butyl group as a carbonium ion.

This rate minimum in the branching homologous series, Me>Et >*i*-Pr ¦ <*t*-Bu, for the rates of hydrolysis of alkyl acetates in dilute aqueous hydrochloric acid marks a switch from mechanism $A_{AC}2$ on the left of the dotted line to mechanism $A_{AC}1$ on the right. Another rate minimum, occurring one step earlier in the same series, Me>Et¦ <*i*-Pr<*t*-Bu, has been observed by Leisten for the hydrolysis of alkyl benzoates in concentrated sulphuric acid.[69] This minimum marks a different mechanistic switch, one between two unimolecular mechanisms: it is, as Leisten recognised, a switch from mechanism $A_{AC}1$ to mechanism $A_{AL}1$ in the concentrated acid medium. Leisten showed that the kinetic effects of polar substituents, such as a *p*-nitro-group in the benzene ring, were qualitatively opposite on the two sides of the mechanistic switch-point, just as the effects of methyl substitutuents in the alkyl part of the molecule are qualitatively opposite.

Some evidence of mechanism $A_{AL}1$ in association with a secondary alkyl group had already been obtained by Hughes, Masterman, and the writer by stereochemical observations on esterification.[70] They observed that optically active 2-octyl alcohol, on esterification with acetic acid in excess of the latter as solvent, and with sulphuric acid as catalyst, gave an extensively racemised ester.

Bunton and Konasiewicz have shown[33] that triphenylmethyl benzoate undergoes acid-catalysed hydrolysis in aqueous dioxan with alkyl-oxygen fission as proved by the ^{18}O-method; and also that it undergoes an analogous acid-catalysed methanolysis, in which one of the products is triphenylmethyl methyl ether:

$$CH_3\cdot CO\cdot O\cdot CPh_3 + H_2\overset{*}{O} \xrightarrow[H^+]{} CH_3\cdot CO\cdot OH + H\overset{*}{O}\cdot CPh_3$$

$$CH_3\cdot O\cdot CO\cdot CPh_3 + MeOH \xrightarrow[H^+]{} CH_3\cdot CO\cdot OH + MeO\cdot CPh_3$$

Even though the proof of mechanism is not kinetically complete, there can be no real doubt that these reactions exemplify mechanism $A_{AL}1$.

[69] J. L. Leisten, J. Chem. Soc., 1956, 1572.

[70] E. D. Hughes, C. K. Ingold, and S. Masterman, *J. Chem. Soc.*, **1939**, 840.

The stereochemical criterion for distinguishing between a unimolecular, and a possible bimolecular, acid-hydrolysis with alkyl-oxygen fission has been applied by Bunton and his colleagues, in the example of an optically active tertiary alkyl acetate.[71] Active methylethyl*iso*hexylcarbinyl acetate was hydrolysed in 70% aqueous dioxan with catalysis by hydrochloric acid. The formed methylethyl*iso*hexylcarbinol was mainly racemic, though it contained about 10% of the optically inverted carbinol:

$$\text{(active) } CH_3\cdot CO\cdot O\cdot CMeEtHex^i \xrightarrow[H^+]{} CH_3\cdot CO_2H + HO\cdot CMeEtHex^i \text{ (DL)}$$

It was shown that, although the carbinol itself suffers racemisation in aqueous dioxan in the presence of an acid catalyst, this reaction takes place too slowly to be made responsible for more than a small fraction of the racemisation observed to accompany hydrolysis of the ester. It was concluded that the aqueous acid hydrolysis of tertiary alkyl acetates takes place by mechanism $A_{AL}1$.

In the investigation by Yates and McClelland[48] of the kinetics of the acid hydrolysis of alkyl and aryl acetates in aqueous sulphuric acid media, a number of examples of this third acid mechanism, $A_{AL}1$, were encountered. This mechanism was kinetically characterised in the following manner.

Mechanism $A_{AL}1$, like the other acidic mechanisms, starts with a pre-equilibrium proton uptake. This preliminary step of the mechanism can therefore be taken into quantitative account by means of the ester acidity function $-H_S$, or its approximation $-mH_0$ with $m=0.62$. The second, and rate-controlling, step of the mechanism can therefore be "isolated" through the function $\log k_1-(-H_S)$, or $\log k_1+mH_0$, which measures its free energy of activation. This step is a unimolecular heterolysis, but it will have a water requirement, in particular, a negative one, because it will release water, and hence will be favoured by a medium of low water activity. In this step, an esterium ion is converted into a pure carbonium ion, which will be much less hydrated. The state which is most directly relevant to the rate is, of course, not the carbonium ion itself, but the transition state through which it is formed; but even this must be very substantially less hydrated than the initial esterium ion. It follows that, when, with increasing acid concentration, the water activity falls, the quantity $\log k_1+mH_0$ should rise substantially. Thus, the transition state

[71] C. A. Bunton, E. D. Hughes, C. K. Ingold, and D. F. Meigh, *Nature*, 1950, **166**, 679.

leading to the alkylium ion of mechanism $A_{AL}1$ requires a fairly large negative dependence of log k_1+mH_0 on log a_{H_2O}, almost certainly a larger dependence than that of the gradient -0.2 which characterised the transition state leading to the acylium ion of mechanism $A_{AC}1$.

When log k_1+mH_0 was plotted against log a_{H_2O} for the secondary aliphatic esters, *iso*propyl acetate and *s*-butyl acetate, bilinear curves were obtained of the same form as those shown for methyl and primary aliphatic esters in Fig. 58-3. The primary aralphyl ester, benzyl acetate, gave another such curve, except that its investigation to high acidities was limited by other reactions. The left-hand members of these bilinear curves had the common slope, $+2.0\pm0.1$, characteristic of mechanism $A_{AC}2$. This slope held up to 70% by weight sulphuric acid for the secondary alkyl acetates, and up to 60% acid for benzyl acetate. The right-hand members of the curves for the secondary acetates had the negative slope, -0.6. The curve for benzyl acetate could be extended far enough only to show that it had a substantial negative slope, but not far enough to allow the slope to be measured. These relatively large negative slopes are taken to be characteristic of mechanism $A_{AL}1$. *t*-Butyl acetate could not be investigated satisfactorily in this solvent system; but data for the rate of its hydrolysis in aqueous hydrochloric acid disclosed a possibly larger negative dependence of rate on water activity, and, moreover, one which is operating already in quite dilute acid solutions, though it is difficult to measure, because the water activity changes so slowly. It would appear that mechanism $A_{AC}2$ has no noticeable range of validity for this tertiary alkyl ester: mechanism $A_{AL}1$ takes charge from the beginning of the acid concentration range.

The qualitative rate pattern characteristic of mechanism $A_{AL}1$ follows from these findings; and it is that, as the acid concentration is increased, the rate rises with ever-increasing steepness. This happens from indefinitely low acid concentrations upwards in the example of *t*-butyl acetate. In the acid hydrolyses of the secondary alkyl acetates and of benzyl acetate, mechanism $A_{AL}1$ takes over from mechanism $A_{AL}2$ at a certain point as the acid concentration is raised. Before this change of mechanism takes place, mechanism $A_{AC}2$ has carried the rate over a maximum; but then, before the rate has fallen to zero, mechanism $A_{AL}1$ assumes charge, and the rate rises again very steeply.

Figure 58-4 is a simplified conspectus of the division of responsibility for rate of hydrolysis between the three acid mechanisms, over the range of ester structure and medium acidity covered in Yates and McClelland's kinetic investigation. The almost co-incident curves for the two secondary acetates are presented by a single curve. So are

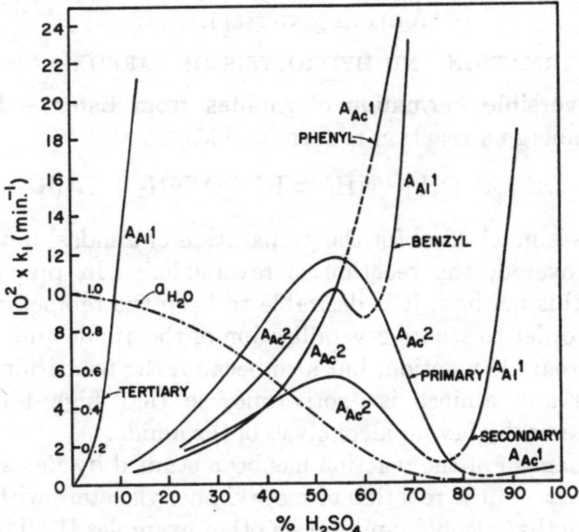

FIG. 58-4.—Hydrolysis of acetates in aqueous sulphuric acid (k_1 in min.$^{-1}$ at 25°). Schematic conspectus of rate-acidity curves for primary, secondary, and tertiary alkyl, benzyl, and phenyl acetates; and the assigned mechanisms. (Reproduced with permission from Yates and McClelland, *J. Am. Chem. Soc.*, 1967, 89, 2686.)

the practically coincident curves for the two aliphatic primary esters. The curve for methyl acetate is not drawn separately: it would follow the shape of the curve for the aliphatic primary esters, but would lie a little higher in the diagram (as can be deduced from Fig. 58-3). A single curve does duty for phenyl acetate and the substituted phenyl acetates.

The already-mentioned rate minima in the series of branching homologous alkyl groups are, so far as acetates are concerned, sections of this diagram, or rather, sections of the more complete diagram of which it is a simplification. If we take a section along any vertical line in the range 0–70% sulphuric acid, we obtain the Skrabal rate minimum:

$$(A_{AC}2)\quad \text{Me} > \text{Et} > i\text{-Pr} \;|\; < t\text{-Bu} \quad (A_{AL}1)$$

If we take the section in the range 90–100% sulphuric acid, we obtain the Leisten minimum, which marks a different mechanistic transition:

$$(A_{AC}1)\quad \text{Me} > \text{Et} \;|\; < i\text{-Pr} < t\text{-Bu} \quad (A_{AL}1)$$

(59) FORMATION AND HYDROLYSIS OF CARBOXYLAMIDES

(59a) Reversible Formation of Amides from Esters.—Esters and ammonia undergo a reaction to form amides:

$$R'\cdot CO\cdot OR + NH_3 \rightleftarrows R'\cdot CO\cdot NH_2 + HOR$$

The process is much used for the preparation of amides; but as Lothar Meyer discovered, the reaction is reversible.[72] In preparations of amides by this method, it is desirable to keep the temperature down, not only in order to secure crystallisation of the amide and thus to defeat the retrograde reaction, but also because the formation of amides from esters and amines is exothermic, so that high temperatures thermodynamically favour alcoholysis of the amide.

The mechanism of the reaction has been studied by Betts and Hammett in the case of the reaction of methyl phenylacetate with ammonia in solvent methyl alcohol, and in two other examples.[73] They showed that the reaction is of the usually assumed second-order form only to a rough approximation, and, in particular, that the order with respect to ammonia lies between 1.0 and 1.5. They interpreted the unit order in ammonia as describing the rate of addition of ammonia to the ester, and the excess over unit order as an effect of a concurrent addition of amide ion, formed with the aid of a second ammonia molecule through the pre-equilibrium

$$2NH_3 \rightleftharpoons NH_4^+ + NH_2^-$$

in a concentration proportional to the square-root of the ammonia concentration. This idea of a specific base catalysis, which implies that the second ammonia molecule contributes nothing to the composition of the transition rate, has been called in question. For Bunnett and Davies[74] have shown that the conversion of ethyl formate with *n*-butylamine into form-*n*-butylamide in ethyl alcohol is general base-catalysed, each catalysing base therefore forming a part of the transition state relevant to its own catalysis. In the case of this amide formation, there was no uncatalysed rate term of order unity in *n*-butylamine. There was a rate term of order 1.5 in *n*-butylamine, which Bunnett and Davies interpreted as due to catalysis by ethoxide ions formed in the pre-equilibrium,

$$n\text{-}C_4H_9\cdot NH_2 + EtOH \rightleftharpoons n\text{-}C_4H_9\cdot NH_3^+ + OEt^-$$

in concentration proportional to the square-root of that of the amine.

[72] L. Meyer, *Ber.*, 1889, **22**, **24**.

[73] R. L. Betts and L. P. Hammett, *J. Am. Chem. Soc.*, 1937, **59**, **1568**.

[74] J. F. Bunnett and G. T. Davies, *J. Am. Chem. Soc.*, 1960, **82**, **665**.

And there was a term of order 2.0 in the amine, representing catalysis by the amine molecule itself.

The uncatalysed reaction of Betts and Hammett implies a reaction of $B_{AC}2$ type: an initial bimolecular reaction between the amine and the ester is the slow step. The reaction can be represented alternatively on the model of carbonyl addition and its reversal, and on that of nucleophilic aliphatic substitution:

$$H_3N + \overset{\overset{O}{\|}}{\underset{\underset{R'}{|}}{C}}\text{—OR} \underset{\text{fast}}{\overset{\text{slow}}{\rightleftharpoons}} H_3\overset{+}{N}\text{—}\overset{\overset{O^-}{|}}{\underset{\underset{R'}{|}}{C}}\text{—OR} \underset{\text{slow}}{\overset{\text{fast}}{\rightleftharpoons}} H_3\overset{+}{N}\text{—}\overset{\overset{O}{\|}}{\underset{\underset{R'}{|}}{C}} + \overset{-}{O}R \quad (B_{AC}2)$$

$$H_3N + \overset{\overset{O}{\|}}{\underset{\underset{R'}{|}}{C}}\text{—OR} \overset{\text{slow}}{\rightleftharpoons} \left[H_3\overset{\delta+}{N}\cdots\overset{\overset{O}{\|}}{\underset{\underset{R'}{|}}{C}}\cdots\overset{\delta-}{O}R \right] \underset{\text{slow}}{\rightleftharpoons} H_3\overset{+}{N}\text{—}\overset{\overset{O}{\|}}{\underset{\underset{R'}{|}}{C}} + \overset{-}{O}R \quad (B_{AC}2)$$

The implication of the double representation is that the electronic distribution in the intermediate complex, whether it is a molecule or a transition state, is intermediate between the expressed distributions. The general base-catalysed mechanism of Bunnett and Davies has to treat the last step, the loss of an alcohol molecule from an addition complex, as the slow step, which the catalysing base assists:

$$R''NH_2 + \overset{\overset{O}{\|}}{\underset{\underset{R'}{|}}{C}}\text{—OR} \overset{\text{fast}}{\rightleftharpoons} R''NH\text{—}\overset{\overset{OH}{|}}{\underset{\underset{R'}{|}}{C}}\text{—OR}$$

$$R''NH\text{—}\overset{\overset{OH\cdots B}{|}}{\underset{\underset{R'}{|}}{C}}\text{—OR} \overset{\text{fast}}{\rightleftharpoons} R''NH\text{—}\overset{\overset{^-O\quad H\text{—}B^+}{|\qquad\ |}}{\underset{\underset{R'}{|}}{C}}\text{—OR}$$

$$\overset{\text{slow}}{\rightleftharpoons} R''NH\text{—}\overset{\overset{O}{\|}}{\underset{\underset{R'}{|}}{C}} + \overset{\overset{H}{|}}{O}R + B$$

The effect of polar substituents on rate of amide formation is qualitatively as expected for the uncatalysed reaction: as far as is known, electron-attracting substituents accelerate and electron-releasing substituents retard reaction, as will be illustrated below. The polar requirements of the general base-catalysed reaction are qualitatively ambiguous, and are therefore not inconsistent *prima facie* with general experience of the effects of substituents. It was pointed out by Hans Meyer that esters of strong acids, such as trichloroacetic acid, form amides rapidly, while those of weak acids, such as trimethylacetic acid, do so slowly.[75] Gorvin showed[76] in a semi-quantitative way that aromatic substituents affect the rates of reaction of ethyl benzoates in accordance with the following sequence:

$$p\text{-NO}_2 > m\text{-NO}_2 > \text{H} > p\text{-Me} > p\text{-MeO} > p\text{-NH}_2 > p\text{-O}^-$$

Gordon, Miller, and Day have studied the rates of reaction of several series of esters with ammonia.[77] They establish certain rate series, for example, the following for alkyl acetates, $CH_3 \cdot CO_2R$,

$$\text{R} = \text{Ph} > \text{CH}_2\text{:CH} > \text{Me} > \text{Et} > i\text{-Pr} > t\text{-Bu}$$

and the following series for methyl esters, $R' \cdot CO_2Me$,

$$\text{R}' = \text{H} > \text{Me} > \text{Et} > i\text{-Pr} > t\text{-Bu}$$

These results probably represent a mixture of polar and steric effects. Certainly steric effects must be expected in a mechanism of $B_{AC}2$ type. Unfortunately we do not know to what extents the reactions for which substituent effects have been observed are uncatalysed and catalysed. The only recorded substituent effects which are definitely associated with kinetic form are those of the para-substituents in Betts and Hammett's reactions of methyl phenylacetate and its ring substitution products with ammonia in solvent methyl alcohol.[73] The rate series,

$$p\text{-NO}_2 > p\text{-Cl} > \text{H}$$

was found with rate ratios 3.2:1.8:1 for the (uncatalysed) reaction of first order in ammonia, and 5.9:2.1:1, for the (catalysed) reaction of order 1.5 in ammonia. The similarity of the pattern of substituent effects is more easily understood in terms of a mechanism, like Betts and Hammett's, which puts rate-control into the first step, alike of the uncatalysed and catalysed reactions, than in terms of a mechanism that would transfer rate-control to the last step of a base-catalysed mechanism. Further clarification of this matter is needed.

[75] H. Meyer, *Monatsh.*, 1906, 27, 31.

[76] J. H. Gorvin, *J. Chem. Soc.*, 1945, 732.

[77] M. Gordon, J. G. Miller, and A. R. Day, *J. Am. Chem. Soc.*, 1948, 70, 1946; 1949, 71, 1245; E. M. Arnett, J. G. Miller, and A. R. Day, *ibid.*, 1950, 72, 5635.

(59b) Basic and Acid Hydrolysis of Amides.—Amides can be hydrolysed either by aqueous alkalis or by aqueous strong acids. Both reactions were studied by Reid.[78] He showed that the alkaline reaction follows a second-order course, with the rate proportional to [amide][OH^-], thereby making it clear that the mechanism is of type $B_{AC}2$. The methods of representation, and the implications of the double representation, are as explained in other examples of $B_{AC}2$ reactions:

$$H\bar{O} + \underset{R'}{\overset{O}{\overset{\|}{C}}}—NH_2 \underset{\text{fast}}{\overset{\text{slow}}{\rightleftharpoons}} HO—\underset{R'}{\overset{O^-}{C}}—NH_2 \underset{\text{slow}}{\overset{\text{fast}}{\rightleftharpoons}} HO—\underset{R'}{\overset{O}{\overset{\|}{C}}} + \bar{N}H_2 \quad (B_{AC}2)$$

$$H\bar{O} + \underset{R'}{\overset{O}{\overset{\|}{C}}}—NH_2 \overset{\text{slow}}{\longleftarrow} \left[\overset{\delta-}{HO} \cdots \underset{R'}{\overset{O}{\overset{\|}{C}}} \cdots \overset{\delta-}{NH_2} \right] \underset{\text{slow}}{\longrightarrow} HO—\underset{R'}{\overset{O}{\overset{\|}{C}}} + \bar{N}H_2 \quad (B_{AC}2)$$

$$(R' \cdot CO_2H + NH_2^- \underset{\text{fast}}{\longrightarrow} R' \cdot CO_2^- + NH_3)$$

Bender has shown[11] that the most condensed intermediate state in the basic hydrolysis of an amide is a molecular rather than a transition state. The evidence is that an amide undergoing alkaline hydrolysis in water containing ^{18}O will incorporate a certain proportion of this isotope before it becomes hydrolysed.

As before, we have to expect that electron-attracting groups will accelerate, and electron-releasing groups retard, the reaction, which will also be sensitive to steric retardation. Reid investigated the effects of aromatic substituents on the rates of hydrolysis of substituted benzamides with aqueous barium hydroxide. Some of his rate-constants are reproduced on a relative scale in Table 59-1. The figures show that electron-attracting meta- and para-substituents do, indeed, accelerate, and electron-releasing substituents retard hydrolysis. They show also that ortho-substituents retard the reaction independently of their polarity, in agreement with the assumption of a strong steric effect.

As to acid hydrolysis, Reid showed that, in not too concentrated aqueous solutions of strong acids, the rate is proportional to [amide][H^+]. Since the conditions are not those in which we should expect the conjugate acid of the amide to undergo heterolysis to an

[78] E. E. Reid, *Am. Chem. J.*, 1899, **21**, 284; 1900, **24**, 397; I. Meloche and K. J. Laidler, *J. Am. Chem. Soc.*, 1951, **73**, 1712.

TABLE 59-1.—RELATIVE RATES OF SECOND-ORDER ALKALINE HYDROLYSIS OF SUBSTITUTED BENZAMIDES IN WATER AT 100° (REID).

Substituent....	O^-	NH_2	OMe	Me	H	I	Br	NO_2
para-........	—	0.20	0.49	0.65	1	1.69	1.91	—
meta-........	0.19	0.93	—	0.83	1	2.60	2.97	5.60
ortho-........	0.064	—	—	0.054	1	0.138	0.254	—

acylium ion, a mechanism of type $A_{AC}2$ is presumed. It may be represented either on the model of carbonyl addition and its retrogression, or on that of nucleophilic substitution, with the significance already noted in other examples:

$$H_2O + \overset{\overset{O}{\|}}{\underset{\underset{R'}{|}}{C}}-\overset{+}{N}H_3 \underset{\text{fast}}{\overset{\text{slow}}{\rightleftharpoons}} H_2\overset{+}{O}-\overset{\overset{O^-}{|}}{\underset{\underset{R'}{|}}{C}}-\overset{+}{N}H_3 \underset{\text{slow}}{\overset{\text{fast}}{\rightleftharpoons}} H_2\overset{+}{O}-\overset{\overset{O}{\|}}{\underset{\underset{R'}{|}}{C}}+NH_3 \qquad (A_{AC}2)$$

$$H_2O + \overset{\overset{O}{\|}}{\underset{\underset{R'}{|}}{C}}-\overset{+}{N}H_3 \overset{\text{slow}}{\rightleftharpoons} \left[\overset{\delta+}{H_2O}\cdots\overset{\overset{O}{\|}}{\underset{\underset{R'}{|}}{C}}\cdots\overset{\delta+}{N}H_3\right] \underset{\text{slow}}{\rightleftharpoons} H_2\overset{+}{O}-\overset{\overset{O}{\|}}{\underset{\underset{R'}{|}}{C}}+NH_3 \qquad (A_{AC}2)$$

$$(R'\cdot CO_2H_2^+ + NH_3 \xrightarrow[\text{fast}]{} R'\cdot CO_2H + NH_4^+)$$

As explained in Section **58f**, mechanism $A_{AC}2$ requires that substituents should exert only weak polar effects, but that, when suitably situated, they should exert strong steric effects. Reid studied the influence of aromatic substituents on the rates of hydrolysis of benzamides in aqueous $N/2$ hydrochloric acid: his figures are reproduced on a relative scale in Table 59-2. They make it clear that meta- and para-substituents, however strongly polar, have little effect on the rate, while ortho-substituents, whatever their polarity, markedly retard the reaction.

The kinetics of the acid-catalysed hydrolysis of amides in water has been studied in another connexion. Since the acid hydrolysis of

TABLE 59-2.—RELATIVE RATES OF HYDROLYSIS OF SUBSTITUTED BENZAMIDES BY N/2 HYDROCHLORIC ACID IN WATER AT 100° (REID).

Substituent....	NH_2	OH	Me	H	I	Br	Cl	NO_2
para-........	0.85	—	0.84	1	—	0.86	0.91	1.13
meta-........	0.81	—	0.87	1	—	0.94	—	0.94
ortho-........	0.085	0.208	0.105	1	0.051	—	0.153	0.026

amides is somewhat slow, it can conveniently be investigated with quite high concentrations of the catalysing acid; and it has been found[79] that, as the concentration of the strong acid is increased, the rate goes through a maximum. In the example of the hydrolysis of formamide with aqueous hydrochloric acid, the maximum occurs at about 6*N* acid, but the figure is somewhat different for aqueous sulphuric acid, and is not the same for different amides.

This is the usual behaviour for an $A_{AC}2$ mechanism in concentrated aqueous acids, as already described for the acid hydrolysis of esters. It can become more complicated in the case of amides by extensive protonation; that is, protonation may be showing signs of impending saturation at the same time as water activity is declining, in the growing concentration of the strong acid. The matter has been studied quantitatively by Yates and his collaborators.[80] The first step was to establish an acidity function H_A for amides, in order to take account of their pre-equilibrium protonation. This allowed the water dependence of the second and rate-controlling step of the mechanism to be studied. The positive dependence of $\log k' + H_A$ on $\log a_{H_2O}$ is greater than for the $A_{AC}2$ hydrolysis of esters, and corresponds to an "order" in water of 3, rather than 2. It would appear that the transition state contains, not only the water which is to substitute as a nucleophile at carbon, and the water molecule which is later to take its proton away, but also another water molecule, perhps one which will help the amino-group to be lost in ammonium form in the acid solution.

There is evidence that another of the three known acid mechanisms of carboxyl hydrolysis is applicable to amides. Lacey has shown[81] that N-*t*-alkyl-substituted amides are hydrolysed, either by boiling 30% sulphuric acid or by cold 98% acid, to give unsubstituted carboxylamides and thereafter the acids, with elimination of the *t*-alkyl group as a tertiary alcohol or the olefins derivable from it. The N-alkyl groups used were *t*-butyl and "*t*-octyl" (1,1,3,3-tetramethylbutyl). The amides were of formic, acetic, and chloroacetic acids, and of benzoic acid and its substitution products containing methoxy-, chloro-, and nitro-groups in the ring. Among the substituted benzamides the rate order was $p\text{-MeO} > \text{H} > p\text{-Cl} > p\text{-NO}_2$.

[79] A. Beurath, *Z. anorg. Chem.*, 1926, **151,** 53; H. v. Euler and A. Ölander, *Z. physik. Chem.*, 1928, **131,** 107; T. W. J. Taylor, *J. Chem. Soc.*, **1930,** 2741; V. K. Krieble and R. A. Holst, *J. Am. Chem. Soc.*, 1938, **60,** 2976. J. T. Edwards and S. C. R. Meacock, *J. Chem. Soc.*, **1957,** 2000.

[80] K. Yates, J. B. Stevens, and A. R. Katritzky, *Can. J. Chem.*, 1964, **42,** 1957; K. Yates and J. B. Stevens, *ibid.*, 1965, **43,** 529; K. Yates and J. C. Riordan, *ibid.*, p. 2328.

[81] R. N. Lacey, *J. Chem. Soc.*, **1960,** 1633.

The products obtained by Lacey are those of alkyl-nitrogen bond fission; and even in the absence of a kinetic investigation, one can feel certain, simply from the type of alkyl group with which this peculiar mode of hydrolysis appears, that mechanism $A_{AL}1$ is under observation. The kinetic effect of ring substituents in benzamides is consistent with this interpretation. For Reid's work showed (see Table 59-2) that the polar effect of ring substituents on amide hydrolysis with acyl-nitrogen bond fission is very small. This means that the effect of polarity in pre-equilibrium protonation is almost balanced by its effect on nucleophilic attack in the acyl group. If we move the position of nucleophilic attack further off, that is, to the alkyl group, as required in mechanism $A_{AL}1$, we expect the polar effect on pre-equilibrium protonation to be left in control. This would produce polar effects such as Lacey observed.

(60) REACTIONS OF CARBOXYLIC ESTERS WITH CARBANIONS

There are in principle two main sides to this subject. They correspond to those of the addition of carbanions to carbonyl compounds: the carbanions either may be produced by extraction of a proton from pseudo-acids, or they may be derived from metal alkyls, for example, Grignard reagents. The addition of pseudo-acids, through their carbanions, to esters has been studied intensively over a long period, though not as yet with the tool of reaction kinetics. This is the *Claisen condensation*. It has a most distinguished history, which will be summarised in this Section. The addition of metal alkyls to esters has been widely employed synthetically, but, so far, has been largely neglected with respect to mechanism; and no account of the detailed position of this subject can profitably be included here.

(60a) The Claisen Condensation.—These reactions consist essentially of condensations between a carboxylic ester unrestricted as to form, and an ester, ketone, or nitrile, containing α-hydrogen, to give a β-ketonic, or, in case a formic ester is the first-mentioned reactant, a β-aldehydic, ester, ketone, or nitrile, with the elimination of a molecule of alcohol. Such condensations have usually been effected by means of sodium, or sodium methoxide or ethoxide either in solid form or in solution in the corresponding alcohol. More powerful condensing agents have been used, such as sodium amide, mesityl magnesium bromide, and sodium triphenylmethide.

The first example of a Claisen condensation was that discovered by Geuther in 1863, namely, the conversion of ethyl acetate by means of sodium into ethyl acetoacetate. The reaction was generalised greatly after 1887, when Claisen began his work on the mechanism and the general chemistry of the procéss. From 1894 Dieckmann developed the use of the reaction to close rings: this type of application is generally known as the *Dieckmann reaction.*

Some examples of Claisen condensations, including some Dieckmann reactions, are formulated below. In all these cases there are enough α-hydrogen atoms in the factors to cause the products to be keto-enolic tautomers. This is not a strict necessity of the reaction, but it does enable it to go forward more easily than it would otherwise, as will be explained later. In the equations given, the keto-enolic products are, for consistency, represented in their ketonic forms, whatever may be the position of equilibrium in the prototropic systems of these substances, as they are ordinarily seen and handled:

$$2\,CH_3\cdot CO_2Et \rightarrow CH_3\cdot CO\cdot CH_2\cdot CO_2Et + EtOH \quad [82]$$

$$(CO_2Et)_2 + CH_3\cdot CO_2Et \rightarrow EtO_2C\cdot CO\cdot CH_2\cdot CO_2Et + EtOH \quad [83]$$

$$HCO_2Et + \begin{array}{l} CH_2\cdot CO_2Et \\ | \\ C_6H_5 \end{array} \rightarrow \begin{array}{l} CHO\cdot CH\cdot CO_2Et \\ \qquad\;\; | \\ \qquad\; C_6H_5 \end{array} + EtOH \quad [84]$$

$$2\begin{array}{l} CH_2\cdot CO_2Et \\ | \\ CH_3 \end{array} \rightarrow \begin{array}{l} CH_2\cdot CO\cdot CH\cdot CO_2Et \\ | \qquad\qquad\; | \\ CH_3 \qquad\quad CH_3 \end{array} + EtOH \quad [85]$$

$$C_6H_5\cdot CO_2Et + CH_3\cdot CO\cdot CH_3 \rightarrow C_6H_5\cdot CO\cdot CH_2\cdot CO\cdot CH_3 + EtOH \quad [86]$$

$$HCO_2Et + \begin{array}{l} CH_2\cdot CO{-}CH_2 \\ | \qquad\qquad\; | \\ CH_2\cdot CH_2\cdot CH_2 \end{array} \rightarrow \begin{array}{l} HCO\cdot CH\cdot CO{-}CH_2 \\ \qquad\;\; | \qquad\qquad | \\ \qquad CH_2\cdot CH_2\cdot CH_2 \end{array} + EtOH \quad [87]$$

$$\begin{array}{l} CH_2\cdot CH_2\cdot CO_2Et \\ | \\ CH_2\cdot CH_2\cdot CO_2Et \end{array} \rightarrow \begin{array}{l} CH_2\cdot CH_2\cdot CO \\ | \qquad\qquad\quad | \\ CH_2{-}{-}{-}CH\cdot CO_2Et \end{array} + EtOH \quad [88]$$

$$2\begin{array}{l} CH_2\cdot CO_2Et \\ | \\ CH_2\cdot CO_2Et \end{array} \rightarrow \begin{array}{l} CH_2\cdot CO\cdot CH\cdot CO_2Et \\ | \qquad\qquad\quad | \\ EtO_2C\cdot CH\cdot CO\cdot CH_2 \end{array} + 2EtOH \quad [89]$$

[82] A. Geuther, *Arch. Pharm.*, 1863, **106**, 97; *Jahresber.*, **1863**, 323.

[83] W. Wisliscenus, *Ann.*, 1888, **246**, 306.

[84] W. Wisliscenus, *Ber.*, 1887, **20**, 2930; *Ann.*, 1896, **291**, 147.

[85] R. Hellon and A. Oppenheim, *Ber.*, 1877, **10**, 699; A. Israel, *Ann.*, 1885, **231**, 187.

[86] L. Claisen, *Ber.*, 1887, **20**, 655.

[87] O. Wallach and A. Steindorff, *Ann.*, 1903, **329**, 109.

[88] W. Dieckmann, *Ber.*, 1894, **27**, 102.

[89] H. v. Fehling, *Ann.*, 1844, **49**, 154; C. Duisberg, *Ber.*, 1883, **16**, 133.

$$\begin{matrix} CO_2Et \\ | \\ CO_2Et \end{matrix} + \begin{matrix} CH_2\cdot CO_2Et \\ CH_2 \\ CH_2\cdot CO_2Et \end{matrix} \rightarrow \begin{matrix} CO\cdot CH\cdot CO_2Et \\ | \quad CH_2 \\ CO\cdot CH\cdot CO_2Et \end{matrix} + 2\,EtOH$$ [90]

As early as 1901 Lapworth appreciated the principle that properties, like those possessed by α-hydrogen "activated" by a neighbouring carboxyl, or other competent group, should be shown by γ-hydrogen if connected with such a group through an intervening $\alpha\beta$-ethylenic bond. He employed the Claisen reaction in order to illustrate this phenomenon, showing, in particular, that ethyl oxalate condenses with the γ-position of ethyl crotonate under the influence of sodium ethoxide:[91]

$$EtO_2C\cdot CO\cdot OEt + CH_3\cdot CH{:}CH\cdot CO_2Et$$
$$\rightarrow EtO_2C\cdot CO\cdot CH_2\cdot CH{:}CH\cdot CO_2Et + EtOH$$

The first serious attempt to propound a mechanism for the Claisen reaction was made in 1887–8 by Claisen and Lowman.[92] They believed that they had observed the addition of sodium alkoxides RONa to esters $R'\cdot CO_2R$, and had isolated addition products of the type $R'\cdot C(OR)_2\cdot ONa$. They suggested that such compounds were intermediates in the condensation, the final stage of which was an elimination of 2ROH by interaction of the addition compound with a molecule containing two α-hydrogen atoms. Thus the formation of ethyl acetoacetate was regarded as proceeding in the following steps:

$$CH_3\cdot CO\cdot OEt + EtONa \rightarrow CH_3\cdot C(ONa)(OEt)_2$$
$$CH_3\cdot C(ONa)(OEt)_2 + CH_3\cdot CO_2Et$$
$$\rightarrow CH_3\cdot C(ONa){:}CH\cdot CO_2Et + 2EtOH$$

This theory implied that the active condensing agent was not sodium, but sodium ethoxide, which was assumed to be formed, at first, from the added sodium and some initial trace of alcohol, and subsequently, in continually increasing quantities, from sodium and the alcohol produced in the reaction. It was pointed out that the reaction starts slowly, indeed, more slowly the more thoroughly the ethyl acetate is freed from alcohol, but gathers speed as it proceeds. There can be no doubt[93] that, in their identification of the condensing agent, Claisen and Lowman were right. It appears that they were not right in

[90] W. Dieckmann, *Ber.*, 1894, 27, 965.

[91] A. Lapworth, *J. Chem. Soc.*, 1901, 79, 1265.

[92] L. Claisen and O. Lowman, *Ber.*, 1887, 20, 651; 1888, 21, 1147.

[93] J. M. Snell and B. M. McElvain, *J. Am. Chem. Soc.*, 1931, 53, 2310.

supposing that they had isolated addition compounds of the type of their assumed intermediates.[94] It has long seemed obvious that they were wrong in assuming such an intermediate, since it cannot help the introduction of an acetic ester residue into a carboxyl group to begin by destroying the unsaturation of the latter.

One of the arguments by which Claisen supported his reaction mechanism was that, unlike ethyl acetate, propionate, and *n*-butyrate, ethyl *iso*butyrate undergoes no self-condensation when treated with sodium or sodium ethoxide. Even ethyl oxalate, which usually participates in Claisen condensations with especial ease, fails thus to react with ethyl *iso*butyrate. Claisen's interpretation was that ethyl *iso*butyrate, having only one α-hydrogen atom, would not permit the double elimination of alcohol, which the second stage of his scheme required. However, a much more satisfying explanation of the matter was given by Dieckmann.[95] In 1900 he discovered the general reversibility of the Claisen condensation, and also the effect of alkyl substituents adjacent to the reaction site in pressing back the equilibrium in the direction of the factors. Ethyl acetoacetate itself is only slightly alcoholised to ethyl acetate by alcoholic sodium ethoxide; but its α-alkyl derivatives are alcoholised extensively enough very appreciably to limit the yield in which a product, such as ethyl α-propiopropionate, could possibly be formed by condensation under like conditions; and the $\alpha\alpha$-dialkyl derivatives of ethyl acetoacetate are practically completely alcoholised in such conditions. Thus Dieckmann made it clear that the non-formation of ethyl α-*iso*butyro*iso*butyrate, in the conditions of his work, was part of a graded series of constitutional thermodynamic effects, and was not due to lack of a piece of the machinery demanded by the actual mechanism of the reaction, which could work perfectly well backwards, if not forwards. These demonstrations of equilibria, and of constitutional effects thereon, corresponded closely to what was established, partly about the same time and partly later, for the aldol and Michael reactions (Section **54a** and **b**). However, Dieckmann's only inference concerning Claisen condensations was that Claisen's scheme must be formulated reversibly, and must be split up into more stages, in order to avoid the requirement of elimination of two alcohol molecules as a condition of carbon-carbon bonding. Dieckmann's modification of Claisen's mechanism may be illustrated as follows:

[94] J. F. Bunnett, M. M. Robison, and F. C. Pennington, *J. Am. Chem. Soc.*, 1950, 72, 2328.

[95] W. Dieckmann, *Ber.*, 1900, 33, 2670.

$$CH_3{\cdot}CO{\cdot}OEt + EtONa \rightleftarrows CH_3{\cdot}C(ONa)(OEt)_2$$

$$CH_3{\cdot}C(ONa)(OEt)_2 + CH_3{\cdot}CO_2Et \rightleftarrows CH_3{\cdot}C(ONa)(OEt){\cdot}CH_2{\cdot}CO_2Et + EtOH$$

$$CH_3{\cdot}C(ONa)(OEt){\cdot}CH_2{\cdot}CO_2Et \rightleftarrows CH_3{\cdot}CO{\cdot}CH_2{\cdot}CO_2Et + EtONa$$

Nef advanced a very different theory of this reaction.[96] Like the Claisen-Dieckmann theory, Nef's theory has a certain element of correctness. Its valuable feature is that, instead of making an ester-alkoxide addition complex the intermediate, Nef cast for this role a metal substitution product of the ester. From here onward he erred, inasmuch as he pictured the metal derivative as the unsaturated accepting molecule, to which the other reactant adds, instead of the opposite way around. His scheme for the formation of ethyl acetoacetate was as follows:[97]

$$CH_2{=}C(ONa)(OEt) + H{-}CH_2{\cdot}CO_2Et \rightarrow H{\cdot}CH_2{-}C(ONa)(OEt){\cdot}CH_2{\cdot}CO_2Et$$

$$CH_3{\cdot}C(ONa)(OEt){\cdot}CH_2{\cdot}CO_2Et \rightarrow CH_3{\cdot}CO{\cdot}CH_2{\cdot}CO_2Et + EtONa$$

It was an evident weakness of this theory that it could not be applied in cases such as the formation of ethyl benzoylacetate.

Michael's ideas were much more nearly correct.[98] He, like Nef, adopted a metal derivative as his intermediate. But Michael gave it its correct function, namely, that of the adding reagent, the carboxyl group of another molecule being the accepting unsaturated system:

$$CH_3{\cdot}\underset{\underset{OEt}{|}}{\overset{\overset{O}{\|}}{C}} + CH_2{:}\underset{\underset{OEt}{|}}{C}{-}\overset{\overset{Na}{|}}{O} \rightarrow CH_3{\cdot}\underset{\underset{OEt}{|}}{\overset{\overset{O-Na}{|}}{C}}{-}CH_2{\cdot}\underset{\underset{OEt}{|}}{C}{=}O$$

$$\rightarrow CH_3{\cdot}CO{\cdot}CH_2{\cdot}CO_2Et + EtONa$$

This scheme can be applied to any Claisen condensation. Michael's theory was, however, incomplete, as is illustrated by the fact that he was led into certain minor errors. For example, he opposed Claisen's assumption that sodium ethoxide, rather than sodium, is the active condensing agent in the formation of ethyl acetoacetate; and for this opinion he offered the bad reason that better yields had been obtained with sodium than with sodium ethoxide as the added reagent. He did

[96] J. U. Nef, *Ann.*, 1897, **298**, 202.

[97] Here, as often elsewhere, Nef wrote the active unsaturated bond as a single bond between atoms each having a free valency.

[98] A. Michael, *Ber.*, 1900, **33**, 3731; 1905, **38**, 1922.

not appreciate (as others subsequently have not) that yields afford no evidence of mechanism, unless they are shown to be determined by the rate of the reaction, and not by the rates of other reactions, or by thermodynamic factors. Probably the real reason why Michael preferred to regard sodium as the reagent was because he felt that best through the free element, by an atom-for-atom replacement of hydrogen, could sodium be introduced into ethyl acetate. He had not the idea of a base reversibly removing a hydrogen ion from ethyl acetate. Although Michael, earlier than most, recognised the importance of electrochemical quality in reactions, he did not go so far as to assume that the special reactivity of his sodium compound depended on the ions it would give.

What was lacking in Michael's theory was made good in Lapworth's, which (except that it was not, of course, expressed in terms of the electronic theory of valency) is identical with what we believe today.[99] This is that a base, for example an alkoxide ion, reversibly removes a proton from the adding ester or ketone or nitrile; that the resulting anion reversibly combines with a carboxyl carbon atom, just as a cyanide ion does with carbonyl carbon in cyanohydrin formation; and that the more complex anion thus produced reversibly loses an alkoxide ion. The following equilibria would be involved in the formation of ethyl acetoacetate:

$$\bar{\text{O}}\text{Et} + \text{CH}_3\cdot\text{CO}_2\text{Et} \rightleftarrows \text{HOEt} + \bar{\text{C}}\text{H}_2\cdot\text{CO}_2\text{Et} \qquad (1)$$

$$(\text{B}_{\text{AC}}2)\begin{cases} \text{EtO}_2\text{C}\cdot\bar{\text{C}}\text{H}_2 + \overset{\displaystyle \text{O}}{\overset{\|}{\underset{\underset{\displaystyle \text{CH}_3}{|}}{\text{C}}}}\text{—OEt} \rightleftarrows \text{EtO}_2\text{C}\cdot\text{CH}_2\text{—}\overset{\displaystyle \text{O}^-}{\overset{|}{\underset{\underset{\displaystyle \text{CH}_3}{|}}{\text{C}}}}\text{—OEt} & (2) \\[2ex] \text{EtO}_2\text{C}\cdot\text{CH}_2\cdot\overset{\displaystyle \text{O}^-}{\overset{|}{\underset{\underset{\displaystyle \text{CH}_3}{|}}{\text{C}}}}\text{—OEt} \rightleftarrows \text{EtO}_2\text{C}\cdot\text{CH}_2\cdot\text{CO}\cdot\text{CH}_3 + \bar{\text{O}}\text{Et} & (3) \end{cases}$$

$$\bar{\text{O}}\text{Et} + \text{CH}_3\cdot\text{CO}\cdot\text{CH}_2\cdot\text{CO}_2\text{Et} \rightleftarrows \text{CH}_3\cdot\text{CO}\cdot\bar{\text{C}}\text{H}\cdot\text{CO}_2\text{Et} + \text{HOEt} \qquad (4)$$

The only modifications which are now made in this theory amount to interpreting it in terms of the electronic theory of valency, and recognising the mesomeric nature of the involved carbanions.[100]

The above equilibrium (4) is not part of the condensation mecha-

[99] A. Lapworth, *J. Chem. Soc.*, 1901, **79**, 1265; A. C. O. Hahn and A. Lapworth, *Proc. Chem. Soc.*, 1903, **19**, 189.

[100] F. Arndt and B. Eistert, *Ber.*, 1936, **69**, 2381.

nism. But it would be involved when, as in the example formulated, the condensation product contains ionising hydrogen; and when involved it would contribute to the overall thermodynamic balance, which determines the possible extent of condensation. Thus, the circumstance that ethyl acetoacetate, as produced in the above sequence of processes, is largely converted into its anion in equilibrium (4), tends to promote the forward reactions of equilibria (1), (2), and (3). An equilibrium of the type of (4) is not available to give this assistance to the forward reaction in the example of the condensation of ethyl *iso*butyrate with itself to give ethyl α-*iso*butyro*iso*butyrate.

The circumstance that an alcohol molecule occurs on the right-hand side of equation (1) is a factor restraining the forward reactions of equilibria (1), (2), and (3). No doubt this is one of the reasons why ethyl acetoacetate is produced in better yield with the aid of sodium than with sodium ethoxide, or, in other words, in the presence of a smaller, rather than a larger amount of ethyl alcohol.

Some independent evidence bearing on the occurrence of equilibrium (1) is available. Kenyon and Young have shown[101] that optically active esters of the form $R_1R_2CH\cdot CO_2Et$ are racemised in the presence of sodium ethoxide. Brown and Eberly have found[102] that esters containing α-hydrogen undergo hydrogen exchange with "heavy alcohol," EtOD, containing sodium ethoxide, and that the rate of exchange parallels the reactivity of the esters with respect to the participation of their α-hydrogen in Claisen condensations.

Equations (2) and (3) together represent a $B_{AC}2$ type of mechanism, as represented on the model of carbonyl addition. The same mechanism might be represented on the model of nucleophilic substitution. Equilibria (2) and (3) would then become replaced by a single equilibrium, attained by way of a transition state identical with the previously written anionic addition complex except with respect to the distribution of charge:

$$EtO_2C\cdot\overset{-}{C}H_2 + \underset{\displaystyle CH_3}{\overset{\displaystyle O}{\overset{\|}{\underset{|}{C}}}}\!-\!OEt \rightleftarrows \left[EtO_2C\cdot\overset{\delta-}{C}H_2\cdots\cdots\underset{\displaystyle CH_3}{\overset{\displaystyle O}{\overset{\|}{\underset{|}{C}}}}\cdots\cdots\overset{\delta-}{O}Et \right] \rightleftarrows$$

$$EtO_2C\cdot CH_2\!-\!\underset{\displaystyle CH_3}{\overset{\displaystyle O}{\overset{\|}{\underset{|}{C}}}} + \overset{-}{O}Et \qquad (B_{AC}2)$$

[101] J. Kenyon and D. P. Young, *J. Chem. Soc.*, 1940, 216.
[102] W. G. Brown and K. Eberly, *J. Am. Chem. Soc.*, 1940, 62, 113.

Theory indicates that the most condensed anionic complex will actually possess an intermediate distribution of charge. Whether the complex has the length of life which would characterise it as a molecule, rather than a transition state, has not yet been determined, though analogy suggests that it is probably a molecule.

The use of stronger bases than ethoxide ions for the purpose of effecting Claisen condensations was at first developed empirically. Claisen himself[103] introduced the employment of sodium amide, showing that it is in many cases a more satisfactory preparative reagent than either sodium or sodium ethoxide.

Spielman and Schmidt[104] recorded a further advance in technique when they initiated the use of mesityl magnesium bromide (2, 4, 6-trimethylphenyl magnesium bromide), showing that it could be used to effect a number of previously unrealised Claisen condensations, including the self-condensation of ethyl *iso*butyrate. Such a reagent might have been expected itself to attack the nucleus of carboxyl carbon, and thus to bring about a Grignard reaction; however, we must assume that the steric effect of the ortho-methyl substituents prevents this, but does not suffice to prevent combination of the mesitide ion with the spatially more exposed, pseudo-acidic proton.

A still better condensing agent was discovered by Hauser and Renfrow,[105] who, guided by the theoretical requirements revealed in the equilibria already illustrated, demonstrated the value of sodium triphenylmethide as a condensing agent. Much of its value derives from the circumstance that the triphenylmethide ion, replacing the ethoxide ion in an equilibrium of type (1), brings it entirely over to the right, thereby driving the succeeding reactions forward in a complete equilibrium. The reagent sometimes has available a second source of power, which is that, when the β-ketonic ester has not an α-hydrogen atom to engage in an equilibrium of type (4), but has a γ-hydrogen atom, then the triphenylmethide ion can do extensively what an alkoxide ion can do only to a minute extent, namely, extract a γ-proton, and thus provide an equilibrium, which, except for the location of the proton transfer, is of the type of (4), and will draw the preceding reactions forward in a complete equilibrium. Probably both these effects contribute to the formation, by Hauser and Renfrow's method, of ethyl α-*iso*butyro*iso*butyrate, which is thus produced in better yield than by the method of Spielman and Schmidt:

[103] L. Claisen, *Ber.*, 1905, **38**, 693.

[104] M. A. Spielman and M. T. Schmidt, *J. Am. Chem. Soc.*, 1937, **59**, 2009.

[105] C. R. Hauser and W. B. Renfrow, jr., *J. Am. Chem. Soc.*, 1937, **59**, 1823; W. B. Renfrow jr. and C. R. Hauser, *ibid.*, 1938, **60**, 463.

$$(CH_3)_2CH\cdot CO\cdot OEt + CH(CH_3)_2\cdot CO_2Et \xrightleftharpoons{Ph_3C^-} (CH_3)_2CH\cdot CO\cdot C(CH_3)_2\cdot CO_2Et + EtOH$$

Only the first factor can be operative in the previously unrealised condensation, which Hauser and Renfrow effected by their method, of ethyl benzoate with ethyl *iso*butyrate to give ethyl α-benzoyl*iso*butyrate:

$$C_6H_5\cdot CO_2Et + CH(CH_3)_2\cdot CO_2Et \xrightleftharpoons{Ph_3C^-} C_6H_5\cdot CO\cdot C(CH_3)_2\cdot CO_2Et + EtOH$$

However, an incursion of the second factor, when enough time is allowed for the probably slow process of γ-proton transfer from formed ethyl α-*iso*butyro*iso*butyrate, would furnish a plausible explanation of the following observation. This is that, whereas a mixture of ethyl benzoate and ethyl *iso*butyrate, when treated for a short time with sodium triphenylmethide, gives ethyl α-benzoyl*iso*butyrate as the main condensation product, on prolonging the treatment, this substance disappears, ethyl benzoate is regenerated, and ethyl α-*iso*butyro*iso*butyrate becomes the chief condensation product.

(61) HYDROLYSIS OF PHOSPHATE ESTERS

To pass in one step from the mechanisms of reactions of esters of the monobasic carboxylic acid group to those of the esters of the tribasic phosphoric acid group seems drastic; but the study of phosphate esters has been pressed ahead of logically intermediate studies, because of the biological importance of organic phosphates. It may be expected that the complete pattern of mechanisms participating in phosphate reactions will be highly elaborate, and that what is known of it now is very far from being the whole. Phosphoric acid can provide as substrates mono-, di-, and tri-alkyl esters, the first two of which can furnish conjugate-base substrates, whilst all three can provide conjugate acid substrates—eight possible types of substrate, not counting second conjugate bases or acids. The identification of a mechanism requires as a minimum three determinations: (1) the operative substrate and the attacking nucleophile, (2) the position of the bond fission in the substrate, (3) the molecularity of that process. After that, further details may require to be filled in. The two positions of bond fission, namely, at the alkyl-oxygen bond and at the acyl-oxygen bond, may now be distinguished as carbon-oxygen and phosphorus-oxygen bond fission.

(61a) Mechanisms of Hydrolysis of Phosphate Mono-esters.—The general character of the variation with *p*H of the rate of hydrolysis of simple alkyl dihydrogen phosphates has been known for a considerable time.[106] It contrasts strongly with the behaviour of carboxylic esters. Hydrolysis of the phosphates in alkaline solution, instead of being fast, is very slow; but the rate rises towards the neutral point and beyond to a maximum at about *p*H 4, near where carboxyl hydrolysis rates would pass through a minimum. On increasing the acidity further, the rate falls from this maximum to a minimum at about *p*H 0.5; and then it rises again in strongly acid solution. Bailly and also Desjobert held that the relatively high rate around *p*H 4 was due to a reaction of the mono-anion with water; and now that we have extensive kinetic data on the reaction, and on related reactions, this idea provides a more plausible chemical picture than the kinetically equivalent alternative of a reaction between the undissociated acid molecule and hydroxide ions.

Butcher and Westheimer showed that optically active 1-methoxy-2-propyl dihydrogen phosphate, on hydrolysis at *p*H 4, gave 1-methoxy-2-propanol with totally retained configuration.[107] This has not the significance, subsequently ascribed to it by others, of proving phosphorus-oxygen bond fission, because the 1-methoxy-2-propyl group has a configuration-holding methoxyl substituent (Section **33e**). But the same workers showed by the ^{18}O-method that phosphorus-oxygen bond fission is here involved.

Bunton, Vernon, and their coworkers determined the rate-*p*H profile, shown in Fig. 61-1, for the aqueous hydrolysis of methyl dihydrogen phosphate. From it, they deduced the presence of three kinetically distinct reactions, for each of which they determined the kinetic form, rate-constant, and the position or positions of the bond fission. It was shown that the three kinetically distinct reactions represent at least four individual reactions. The molecularity with respect to solvent water was estimated in some cases.[108]

[106] J. Chevalier, *Compt. rend.*, 1898, **127,** 60; R. H. A. Plummer and F. H. Scott, *J. Chem. Soc.*, 1908, **93,** 1699; M. C. Bailly, *Bull. soc. chim.* (France), 1942, **9,** 340, 405; P. Fleury, *Compt. rend.*, 1945, **221,** 416; A. Desjobert, *ibid.*, 1947, **224,** 575; *Bull. soc. chim.* (France), 1947, **14,** 809; *Bull. soc. chim. biol.*, 1954, **36,** 475.

[107] W. W. Butcher and F. H. Westheimer, *J. Am. Chem. Soc.*, 1955, **77,** 2420; J. Kumamoto and F. H. Westheimer, *ibid.*, p. 2515.

[108] C. A. Vernon, *Spec. Pubs. Chem. Soc.*, 1957, **8,** 17; C. A. Bunton, D. R. Llewellyn, K. G. Oldham, and C. A. Vernon, *J. Chem. Soc.*, **1958,** 3574; cf. C. A. Bunton, D. Kellermann, K. G. Oldham, and C. A. Vernon, *ibid.*, **1966, B,** 292.

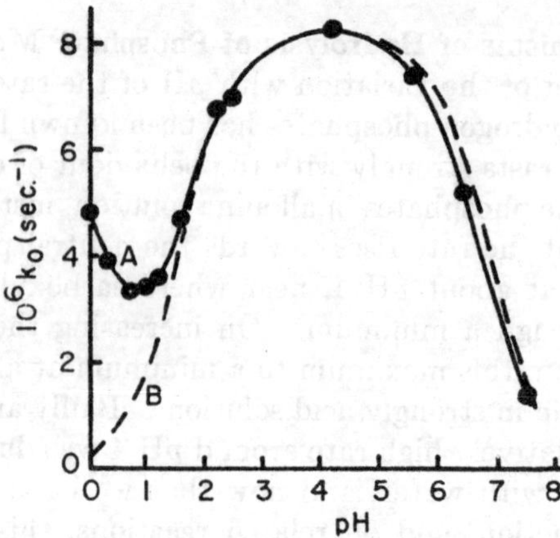

FIG. 61-1.—Rate of hydrolysis of methyl dihydrogen phosphate in water at 100.1°. A: experimental. B: calculated for reaction through the mono-anion. (Reproduced by permission from Bunton, Llewellyn, Oldham, and Vernon, *J. Chem. Soc.*, 1958, 3579.)

The reaction which accounts for practically the whole of the rate from *p*H 2 to *p*H7 is the reaction of the mono-anion in or with water. Its contribution to the rate-*p*H profile, computed from the concentration of the mono-anion, as calculated from the determined first acidity constant of the acid-ester, is given by the broken line in Fig. 61-1. It was shown by the ^{18}O method that this reaction is characterised by exclusive fission at the phosphorus-oxygen bond.

The molecularity of this reaction with respect to water is not known. But it was deduced from the observations (Sections **61b** and **61d**) that the relatively high rate of hydrolysis of the mono-anion of methyl dihydrogen phosphate is repeated in oxygen exchange between water and the mono-anion of ortho-phosphoric acid, and is not repeated in hydrolysis of the anion of dimethyl hydrogen phosphate, that the reaction requires that the phosphoryl phosphorus atom bears *both* of the groups —OH and —O⁻. This structure is what is required for a unimolecular breakdown of the anion to methyl alcohol and a monomeric metaphosphate ion, which would at once hydrate to orthophosphate and might competitively polymerise to stable tri- or other polymeric metaphosphates:

$$\mathrm{Me{-}O{-}\overset{\overset{\displaystyle O}{\|}}{\underset{\underset{\displaystyle H{-}O}{|}}{P}}{-}O^-} \rightarrow \mathrm{MeOH} + \mathrm{\overset{\overset{\displaystyle O}{\|}}{\underset{\underset{\displaystyle O^-}{|}}{P}}{=}O} \qquad (\mathrm{B^-_{AC}1})$$

The formation of trimetaphosphoric acid has been detected. This assumes zero molecularity in water. If unit molecularity in water is assumed, other possibilities arise. Westheimer hypothetically included a water molecule in the cyclic part of the transition state, so converting it from a four-cycle to a six-cycle.[107] Vernon allows for the possibility that attack by a water molecule at the phosphorus atom could provide additional assistance for release of the methoxyl group.[108] Water might act in both these ways simultaneously. Until the molecularity of the process with respect to water is determined, one must remain open-minded as to all these possibilities.

The dominating form of hydrolysis at the more acidic end of the pH range consists in reactions of an ionic conjugate acid of the ester. The conjugate acid is formed in pre-equilibrium: this is indicated by the small positive kinetic effect of replacing H_2O by D_2O in the solvent. The rate-controlling step is thus a substitution in the conjugate acid. The overall rate of acid hydrolysis follows $[H^+]$ more closely than h_0 up to $8N$ perchloric acid. This shows that the transition state of the rate-controlling step is as much hydrated as the initial state consisting of a hydrated hydrogen ion and the acid-ester molecule. Hydrolysis with ^{18}O-enriched water showed that the acid hydrolysis consists of two concurrent reactions of like kinetics: 65% of the total reaction went with carbon-oxygen bond fission, and 35% with phosphorus-oxygen bond fission. The acid-ester also underwent a comparable amount of oxygen exchange ahead of its hydrolysis: this implies phosphorus-oxygen fission with the loss of an unesterified hydroxyl group.[108]

These reactions were plausibly represented as bimolecular nucleophilic substitutions by water molecules, either at carbon, or at quadriligant phosphorus, in one or another of the ionic conjugate acids of the methyl dihydrogen ester. Hydrolysis with carbon-oxygen bond fission was represented as follows:

$$H_2O + MeO\overset{+}{H}\cdot PO(OH)_2 \rightarrow H_2\overset{+}{O}\cdot Me + HO\cdot PO(OH)_2 \qquad (A_{AL}2)$$

and with phosphorus-oxygen fission by the expression:

$$H_2O + PO(OH)_2\cdot\overset{+}{O}HMe \rightarrow H_2\overset{+}{O}\cdot PO(OH)_2 + HOMe \qquad (A_{AC}2)$$

The oxygen exchange prior to hydrolysis was analogously represented as a bimolecular nucleophilic substitution at phosphorus in an isomeric ionic conjugate acid:

$$H_2\overset{*}{O} + PO(OH)(\overset{+}{O}H_2)(OMe) \rightarrow H_2\overset{+*}{O}\cdot PO(OH)(OMe) + H_2O$$

All these bimolecular substitutions by water require a molecularity in water of at least one.

It is not to be expected that bimolecular nucleophilic substitution at carbon in the form just described, *i.e.*, acid hydrolysis by mechanism $A_{AL}2$, will prevail among alkyl phosphates outside the range of methyl and primary alkyl groups. Probably for secondary, and certainly for tertiary alkyl groups, and even for primary alkyl groups which contain a strongly electron-releasing α-substituent, we should find acid hydrolysis by mechanism $A_{AL}1$. The last-mentioned area of expectation of this mechanism is illustrated later.

Between the anionic mechanism and the two conjugate-acid mechanisms, there was found, by analysis of the rate-*p*H profile, a neutral mechanism, that is, a reaction of hydrolysis between the non-ionised acid-ester molecule and a water molecule. It has a strong positive salt effect, as would be expected of a reaction between two neutral species which goes through a polar transition state to make, as it must, a pair of ions. Measurements of ^{18}O-transfer showed that the main position of fission in this reaction is at the carbon-oxygen bond. The occurrence of a kinetically similar reaction with phosphorus-oxygen bond fission is not excluded, because the detection of such is considerably obscured by overlapping by the anion and the conjugate-acid mechanisms.

The molecularity of the neutral reaction with respect to water has not yet been determined. But the hydrolysis with carbon-oxygen bond fission was plausibly assumed to be a bimolecular nucleophilic substitution by water at carbon:

$$H_2O + MeO\cdot PO(OH)_2 \rightarrow H_2\overset{+}{O}Me + \overset{-}{O}\cdot PO(OH)_2 \qquad (B_{AL}2)$$

This assignment of mechanism is consistent with a comparison of the rate with that of a neutral hydrolysis by mechanism $B_{AL}1$ which is mentioned below.

Again, we shall not expect mechanism $B_{AL}2$ to apply generally to the neutral hydrolysis of alkyl dihydrogen phosphates outside the range of methyl and primary alkyl groups. Possibly for secondary alkyl, and certainly for tertiary alkyl dihydrogen phosphates, as well as for the case which we shall illustrate, that of the dihydrogen phosphate of a substituted primary alkyl group with a strongly electron-releasing α-substituent, the expected neutral mechanism is $B_{AL}1$.

Bunton and Vernon's example of an electron-releasing alkyl group was the biologically significant one of a sugar phosphate.[109] The rate-*p*H profile for the aqueous hydrolysis of α-D-glucopyranosyl dihydrogen phosphate rose from very low rates in alkaline solution to a near flat around *p*H 5, when the concentration of the mono-anion was approaching its maximum; but then, instead of falling again as, with increasing acidity, this species became replaced by the non-ionised acid-ester molecule, it rose anew; and this new rise in rate was linear, from *p*H 4 to *p*H 0.5, with the degree of replacement of the mono-anion by the non-ionised molecule. In this case then, the reaction of the molecule with or in water, instead of being slower than the reaction of the anion, as in the hydrolysis of methyl dihydrogen phosphate, was much faster. Concurrently with the change from a reaction of the mono-anion to one of the non-ionised molecule, the position of bond fission, as determined by the ^{18}O-method, changed from the phosphorus-oxygen bond of the mono-anion to the carbon-oxygen bond of the non-ionised molecule.

Although the molecularities of these reactions with respect to water are not established, it seems obvious to assume the same mechanism, $B^{-}_{AC}1$, for the hydrolysis of the mono-anion of α-D-glucopyranosyl dihydrogen phosphate as for hydrolysis of the mono-anion of methyl dihydrogen phosphate. The positions of fission are the same, both phosphorus-oxygen, and the rates are of the same order of magnitude

The positions of fission in the hydrolysis of the non-ionised pyranosyl ester and the non-ionised methyl ester are again the same, both carbon-oxygen; but the great difference between the rates would be very difficult to understand as a constitutional effect on the bimolecular mechanism $B_{AL}2$. The rate for the non-ionised pyranosyl ester is 10^5 times greater than for the non-ionised methyl ester. It is easy to agree that the mechanism has changed from $B_{AL}2$ to $B_{AL}1$, consistently with the known S_N1 mechanism of hydrolysis of pyranosyl halides.[109] The constitutional effect which gives the high rates is, of course, the ether linking, which, just as in the hydrolysis of chloromethyl ethers, conjugates with the breaking bond, so to give a carbonium ion which is in part an oxonium ion, and, as the mesomeric cation of a pseudo-base, has a much enhanced stability. The rate-controlling step of hydrolysis is thus unimolecular, and the mechanism is $B_{AL}1$:

HO·CH$_2$ … O … OH … HO … HO … O–PO(OH)$_2$ —slow step→ HO·CH$_2$ … O$^+$ … OH … HO … HO … CH + $\bar{\text{O}}$·PO(OH)$_2$ ($B_{AL}1$)

In strongly acid solution, for instance in 0.5–3.4 *N* perchloric acid, a conjugate-acid mechanism of hydrolysis supervened, the specific

[109] C. A. Bunton, D. R. Llewellyn, K. G. Oldham, and C. A. Vernon, *J. Chem. Soc.*, 1958, 3588.

rate of which was much greater still. It follows from the above conclusion concerning the unimolecular nature of the reaction of the non-ionised pyranosyl ester that the reaction of its conjugate acid must be unimolecular. For the extra proton would greatly increase rate by this mechanism by creating a more fugitive leaving group. Specific kinetic support for this conclusion was found, inasmuch as the rate rose with acidity approximately as Hammett's h_0, unlike the reaction of the conjugate acid of methyl dihydrogen phosphate, the rate of which rose more nearly as $[H^+]$. This proves that the transition state of hydrolysis of the conjugate acid of the pyranosyl ester has a lower molecularity in water than has the transition state of hydrolysis of the conjugate acid of the methyl ester: the bimolecular substitution by water in the methyl conjugate acid has changed to a unimolecular heterolysis of the pyranosyl conjugate acid.[109] It is consistent that, whereas the reaction of the methyl conjugate acid consists of two reactions, one involving carbon-oxygen and the other phosphorus-oxygen bond fission, the reaction of the pyranosyl conjugate acid leads to carbon-oxygen bond fission only.[109] For every reason, then, the rate-controlling step of the reaction of the pyranosyl conjugate acid must be concluded to be unimolecular, and the mechanism of hydrolysis $A_{AL}1$:

HO·CH₂ ... OH ... HO ... HO ... HO^+ ... $PO(OH)_2$ $\xrightarrow[\text{step}]{\text{slow}}$ HO·CH₂ ... OH ... HO ... OH ... $\overset{+}{C}H$ + $HO{\cdot}PO(OH)_2$ ($A_{AL}1$)

(61b) Mechanisms of Hydrolysis of Phosphate Di-esters.—The hydrolysis of dibenzyl hydrogen phosphate was studied by Westheimer and his coworkers.[110] They did not observe any reaction between the anion and water, but did find a slow reaction of the anion with hydroxide ions. There was an easily observed reaction of the non-ionised acid-ester with water, which proceeded predominantly with carbon-oxygen bond fission. And there was a fairly fast acid-catalysed reaction, presumably a reaction of the conjugate acid in or with water, which proceeded wholly with carbon-oxygen fission.

Bunton and Vernon and their coworkers found analogous reactions in their study of the kinetics and products of hydrolysis of dimethyl

[110] K. Kumamoto, J. R. Cox jr., and F. H. Westheimer, *J. Am. Chem. Soc.*, 1956, **78**, 4858.

hydrogen phosphate.[111] They could set an upper limit to the rate of the unobservably slow reaction of the anion with water. They found that the slow second-order reaction between the anion and hydroxide ions involves predominating carbon-oxygen bond fission. This is presumably a bimolecular nucleophilic substitution at carbon:

$$HO^- + MeO \cdot PO(OMe) \cdot O^- \rightarrow HOMe + O \cdot PO(OMe) \cdot O^- \qquad (B^-_{AL}2)$$

According to Westheimer and his collaborators, some 10% of the second-order reaction involves phosphorus-oxygen bond fission.[110] This will constitute a bimolecular nucleophilic substitution at phosphorus:

$$HO^- + PO(OMe_2) \cdot O^- \rightarrow HO \cdot PO(OMe) \cdot O^- + OMe^- \qquad (B^-_{AC}2)$$

Bunton and Vernon found that the hydrolysis of the non-ionised acid-ester molecule also consisted of two parallel reactions: 78% of the total process went with carbon-oxygen bond fission, and 22% with phosphorus-oxygen bond fission. They assigned both mechanisms as bimolecular substitutions, because of their kinetic evidence that hydrolysis even of the protonated substrate is essentially bimolecular:

$$H_2O + MeO \cdot PO(OMe)(OH) \rightarrow H_2\overset{+}{O}Me + \overset{-}{O} \cdot PO(OMe)(OH) \qquad (B_{AL}2)$$

$$H_2O + PO(OMe_2)(OH) \rightarrow H_2\overset{+}{O} \cdot PO(OMe)(OH) + \overset{-}{O}Me \qquad (B_{AC}2)$$

Hydrolysis through the ionic conjugate acid of the substrate again consisted of two concurrent reactions: 89% of the total process went with carbon-oxygen bond fission and 11% with phosphorus-oxygen bond fission. Between $1N$ and $3N$ perchloric acid, the rate of the overall reaction rose with acidity proportionally to the concentration $[H^+]$, and not at all proportionately to Hammett's h_0. It followed that the transition state carried all the bound water in the initial state, and hence included water as a reagent. These reactions were therefore assigned bimolecular mechanisms:

$$H_2O + Me\overset{+}{O}H \cdot PO(OMe)(OH)$$

$$\rightarrow H_2\overset{+}{O}Me + HO \cdot PO(OMe)(OH) \qquad (A_{AL}2)$$

$$H_2O + PO(OH)(OMe)(\overset{+}{O}HMe)$$

$$\rightarrow H_2\overset{+}{O} \cdot PO(OH)(OMe) + HOMe \qquad (A_{AC}2)$$

[111] C. A. Bunton, M. M. Mhala, K. G. Oldham, and C. A. Vernon, *J. Chem. Soc.*, **1960**, 3233.

To within a power of ten, the rates of these reaction mechanisms were the same as those of the corresponding acid hydrolyses of methyl dihydrogen phosphate (cf. Table 61-1, p. 1190).

A remarkable kinetic effect, apparently of stereochemical origin, on both the alkaline and the acid hydrolysis of phosphate di-esters arises in the cyclic phosphates of 1,2-glycols. This first came to light through an elucidation, due essentially to Brown and Todd, of the depolymerisation of ribonucleic acid in its hydrolysis to nucleotides. Slightly simplified, their scheme amounts to a transesterification, which esterifies the 2-hydroxyl group of the ribose residue at the expense of the inter-monomer ester link, so to give a monomeric di-ester, which is subsequently hydrolysed to mono-esters:[112]

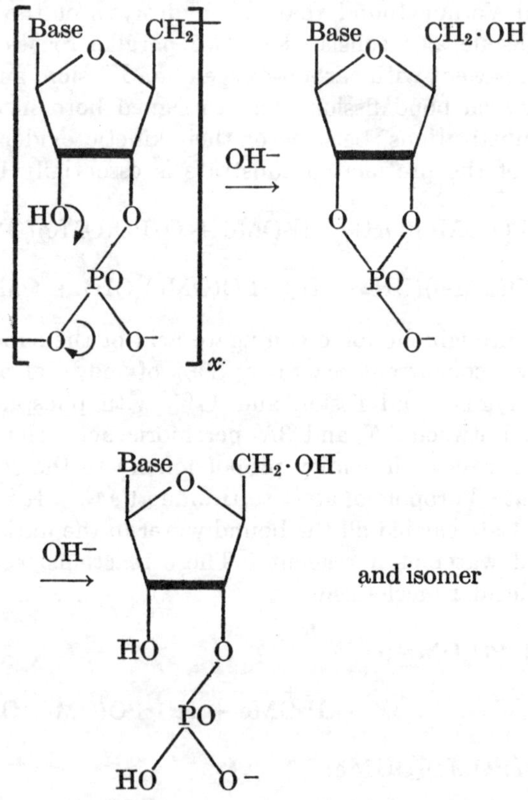

In order to make this theory operative, it was necessary to assume that the cyclic di-ester would undergo hydrolysis much more rapidly than

[112] D. M. Brown and A. R. Todd, *J. Chem. Soc.*, 1952, 52.

simple acyclic esters do. Todd and his coworkers were able to synthesise such cyclic esters and to show that they do indeed have the required property of rapid hydrolysis.[113]

Westheimer and his collaborators have gone to considerable lengths to define the structural requirements for this kinetic effect. They have examined a number of simple model compounds such as ethylene hydrogen phosphate.[110,114] They have found that cyclic phosphates and phosphonates, which contain the diester grouping —O·PO·O— as part of a five-membered ring, are hydrolysed, both in alkaline and in acid solution, some 10^5–10^8 times faster than their open-chain analogues. The high reaction rate conferred by the cyclic ester structure is not restricted to the hydrolytic opening of the ring. In a cyclic di-ester, such as ethylene hydrogen phosphate, it applies to both the ring opening and the concurrent exchange of oxygen between the unesterified hydroxyl group and the solvent, an exchange which does not, of course, open the ring. This sharing of the kinetic effect of the ring between two concurrent reactions, one of which opens the ring whilst the other does not, applies to both the alkaline and acid hydrolysis of the cyclic di-esters, that is, to the second-order reaction of the anion with hydroxide ion, and to hydrolysis through the conjugate acid of the acid-ester. These accelerated reactions go with exclusive phosphorus-oxygen bond fission. Neither alkaline nor acid carbon-bond fission, and no neutral reaction, that is, no reaction of the non-ionised acid-ester molecule, had a rate large enough, in comparison with the accelerated rates, to admit detection.

The interpretation offered by Haake and Westheimer is as follows. The bond angle at phosphorus in the ester group of the five-membered ring approximates to 90° (the other ring angles averaging 112.5°). This geometry can be accommodated only with several kilocalories per mole of strain to the initial state of tetrahedrally hybridised phosphorus in phosphates. On the other hand, in the trigonal bipyramidal configuration assumed for quinqueligant phosphorus in an S_N2-type transition state, such a phosphorus angle can be accommodated without strain to one of the 90°-angles of that model, though not of course to any of the 120°-angles. Its strainless accommodation in the transition state results in a substantial reduction of the activation energy of the nucleophilic substitution. It is a consequence of this group ar-

[113] D. M. Brown, D. I. Magrath, and A. R. Todd, *J. Chem. Soc.*, **1952,** **2708.**

[114] P. C. Haake and F. H. Westheimer, *J. Am. Chem. Soc.*, 1961, **83,** 1102; E. T. Kaiser, M. Pamar, and F. H. Westheimer, *ibid.*, 1963, **85,** 602; F. Covitz and F. H. Westheimer, *ibid.*, p. 1773; A. Eberhard and F. H. Westheimer, *ibid.*, 1965, **87,** 253; E. A. Dennis and F. H. Westheimer, *ibid.*, 1966, **88,** 3431, 3432.

rangement in the transition state that the usual angle of about 180° between the lines of approach and recession of the exchanging groups must be reduced to approximately 120°; and that therefore the line of approach of the entering ligand makes approximately equal angles with the lines of recession of two alternative leaving ligands. The loss of one of these would involve the opening of the phosphate-ester ring, whilst the departure of the other, which is the unesterified hydroxyl group, would lead to oxygen exchange. Both these processes therefore share the kinetic benefit resulting from the loss of strain on activation. This is illustrated for acid hydrolysis below:

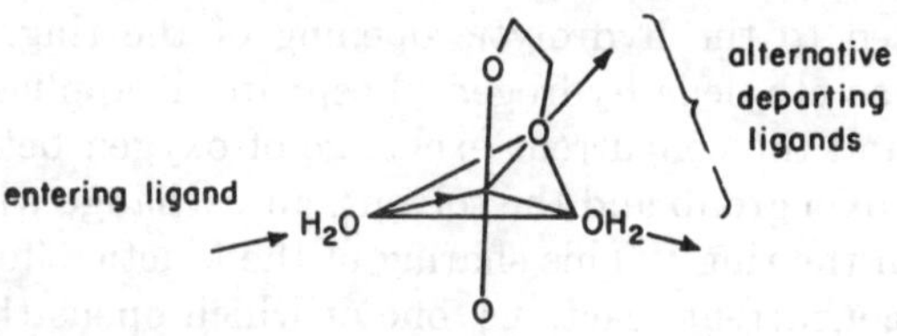

alternative departing ligands

entering ligand H_2O OH_2

(61c) Mechanisms of Hydrolysis of Phosphate Tri-esters.—As Blumenthal and Herbert first showed, the hydrolysis of trimethyl phosphate in alkaline ^{18}O-enriched water proceeds with fission of the phosphorus-oxygen bond.[115] Bunton, Vernon, and their coworkers showed that this is the exclusive mode of fission both of trimethyl phosphate and triphenyl phosphate in alkaline solution.[116] In the reaction of triphenyl phosphate a careful search for ^{18}O uptake into the ester prior to its hydrolysis, uptake such as would have indicated preliminary reversible addition, failed to reveal any. These reactions were therefore regarded as bimolecular nucleophilic substitutions at phosphorus:

$$H\bar{O} + PO(OR)_3 \rightarrow HO\cdot PO(OR)_2 + \bar{O}R \qquad (B_{AC}2)$$

Bunton and Vernon have extended their studies to include hydrolyses in neutral and acid solution.[116] Trimethyl phosphate underwent a first-order hydrolysis in water. Experiments with ^{18}O-enriched water showed that this reaction is characterised by carbon-oxygen bond fission. The reaction was assigned a bimolecular mechanism:

$$H_2O + MeO\cdot PO(OMe)_2 \rightarrow H_2\overset{+}{O}Me + \bar{O}\cdot PO(OMe)_2 \qquad (B_{AL}2)$$

[115] E. Blumenthal and J. B. M. Herbert, *Trans. Faraday Soc.*, 1945, 41, 611.

[116] P. W. C. Barnard, C. A. Bunton, D. R. Llewellyn, C. A. Vernon, and V. A. Welch, *J. Chem. Soc.*, 1961, 2670; P. W. C. Barnard, C. A. Bunton, D. Kellermann, M. M. Mhala, B. Silver, C. A. Vernon, and V. A. Welch, *ibid.*, 1966, 227.

The rates of hydrolysis of mono-, di- and trimethyl phosphates by mechanism $B_{AL}2$ form a monatonic series. At 100°, the rates are in the approximate ratios, 1:7:70.

The rate for trimethyl phosphate is high enough to allow it to be made responsible for the difficulty in observing the acid-catalysed reaction in solutions of up to $3N$ of perchloric acid in water.[117] On the other hand, acid catalysis can be observed, as Thain has shown, in aqueous dioxan, in which the rate of the neutral reaction is relatively much reduced.[118]

Westheimer's stereochemical phenomenon reappears among tri-esters.[114] Esters, such as methyl ethylene phosphate, which contain the divalent ester grouping —O·PO·O— in a five-membered ring, show both abnormally fast bimolecular hydrolyses with hydroxide ions, $B_{AC}2$, and abnormally fast acid-catalysed hydrolyses, which probably proceed by mechanism $A_{AC}2$. Both types of reaction are associated exclusively with phosphorus-oxygen bond fission. Reactions of either type comprise two concurrent reactions, in one of which the five-membered ring is opened whilst in the other, the acyclic alkoxyl group is lost, the ring being preserved. The second of these reactions corresponds to the oxygen-exchange reaction of cyclic di-ester hydrogen phosphates. In the alkaline and acid hydrolyses of the tri-esters, therefore, both the ring-opening and the reaction involving the acyclic oxy-group share the accelerating effect of the presence of the ring. All this fits in with Westheimer's theory, as explained already in the example of di-ester hydrogen phosphates. In the cyclic tri-esters, as in the cyclic di-ester hydrogen phosphates, a neutral reaction was not observed.

Triphenyl phosphate displays acid catalysis in aqueous dioxan solvents.[116] Experiments with ^{18}O-water showed that this reaction proceeds with extensive phosphorus-oxygen bond fission. The rate passed through a maximum in moderately concentrated acid, for instance, at about $1.7N$ perchloric acid in "60%" aqueous dioxan, the exact value depending on the dioxan:water ratio and on added salts if any. This

[117] It seems possible also that tri-esters are less easily protonated than acid esters, in that internal hydrogen bonding in the latter would facilitate proton uptake:

$$H^+ + \underset{\diagdown \ \ \diagup}{\overset{\ \ H}{O\diagup \ \ \diagdown OR}}\ \underset{PO(OR)}{} \rightarrow \underset{\diagdown\ \ \diagup}{HO\quad \overset{+}{O}HR}\ \underset{PO(OR)}{}$$

[118] E. M. Thain, *J. Chem. Soc.*, **1957**, 4694. These observations were made with tri-ethyl phosphate.

indicates that the reaction is quite water-demanding, so that its rate will drop to zero as the thermodynamic activity of the solvent water drops to zero. It is assigned the mechanism $A_{AC}2$, with the following rate-controlling step:

$$H_2O + PO(OPh)_2(\overset{+}{O}HPh) \rightarrow H_2\overset{+}{O}\cdot PO(OPh)_2 + HOPh \qquad (A_{AC}2)$$

(61d) Summary of Mechanisms of Hydrolysis and Oxygen Exchange.—Table 61-1 contains a summary of rate constants and mechanisms given by Bunton, Vernon, and their coworkers for the hydrolysis of mono-, di-, and trimethyl phosphate and mono-α-glucopyranosyl phosphate in water under various conditions of alkalinity and acidity.

TABLE 61-1.—RATE-CONSTANTS AT 100° AND MECHANISMS OF HYDROLYSIS OF PHOSPHATE ESTERS (BUNTON AND VERNON).

Form of substrate.......	Mono-anion[a]		Molecule[a]		Conj. Acid[b]	
Bond fission............	C—O	O—P	C—O	O—P	C—O	O—P
Mechanisms............	$B^-_{AL}2$	$B^-_{AC}1$	$B_{AL}2$	$B_{AC}2$	$A_{AL}2$	$A_{AC}2$
Ester and reagent						
$(HO)_3PO + H_2O$		4.03		1.3		0.55
$(MeO)(HO)_2PO + H_2O$		8.23	0.05		2.00	1.08
$(MeO)_2(HO)PO + H_2O$		<0.001	3.3	0.9	0.91	0.11
$(MeO)_3PO + H_2O$			36.5			
			$B_{AL}1$		$A_{AL}1$	
$(Glu)(HO)_2PO$[c] $+ H_2O$		13.0	30,300		32 (25°)[d]	
		$B^-_{AC}2$				
$(MeO)_2(HO)PO + OH^-$	slow	v. slow				
$(MeO)_3PO + OH^-$				~40,000[e]		

[a] Rate-constants as $10^6 k_1$, with k_1 in sec.$^{-1}$ at 100° with $\mu = 0$.

[b] Rate-constants as $10^6 k_2$ with k_2 in sec.$^{-1}$ mole^{-1} l. at 100°, $\mu = 0$.

[c] Glu = α-D-glucopyranosyl.

[d] The rate-constant at 25° from rate with $[HClO_4] = 0.5M$. At higher concentrations of acid the rate follows h_0 more closely than $[H^+]$.

[e] This figure is $10^6 k_2$ in sec.$^{-1}$ mole^{-1} l., extrapolated to 100° from rates at lower temperatures.

Oxygen exchange between a phosphate group and solvent water is a specialisation of hydrolysis, and we have noticed several times that the hydrolysis of an acid-ester is accompanied by oxygen exchange with an unesterified hydroxyl group of the phosphate residue. Oxygen exchange in the phosphate group requires phosphorus-oxygen bond fission. The best-studied example of such oxygen exchange is that of phosphoric acid itself, and the rate constants for the three observed mechanisms of exchange are in Table 61-1.

Bunton, Llewellyn, Vernon, and Welch measured the rate of oxygen exchange between orthophosphoric acid and water for *p*H 8 to 8*N* perchloric acid.[119] The rate-*p*H profile from *p*H 8 to *p*H 0 is so closely similar to that shown in Fig. 61-1 for the hydrolysis of metbyl dihydrogen phosphate that, if the numbers were taken away from the axes oi that diagram, one could hardly tell to which of the two reactions it referred. In the curve for the exchange, the absolute rates are about half as big as for the hydrolyses, the rate maximum is at *p*H 5 instead of 4, and the minimum is at *p*H 1 instead of 0.5. Analysis shows that the reaction between *p*H 3 and *p*H 8 is again one of the mono-anion. Its rate, as can be seen from Table 61-1, is of the same order of magnitude as that of hydrolysis of those acid-esters which, in this *p*H range, contain one ionised and one non-ionised hydroxyl group. The rate of exchange of the conjugate acid is similarly related to the rates of hydrolysis of esters through their conjugate acids with phosphorus-oxygen bond fission. The rate of exchange through the non-ionised molecule is relatively prominent, but again may be comparable with those non-ionic acyl hydrolyses that are not too much overshadowed by alkyl hydrolyses to be measured.

[119] C. A. Bunton, D. R. Llewellyn, C. A. Vernon, and V. A. Welch, *J. Chem. Soc.*, 1961, 1636.

CHAPTER XVI

Polar Energy

(62) ADDITIVE AND PROPORTIONAL POLAR ENERGIES

(62a) The Expectation of Additivity and Proportionality.—Any general and exact theory of polar effects on reaction equilibria or on reaction rates is far out of reach at the present time. However, we have noticed in previous Chapters several approximately quantitative theoretical treatments, which imply that the polar effects of certain types of substituents on the free energy of reaction, or on the free energy of activation for certain types of reaction may be additive or proportional to an approximation. Let us recall two examples.

The first will be Bjerrum's theory of the field effect of an ionic substituent on an ionisation equilibrium (Section **57b**). The theory is that the electrostatic potential field of the substituent will have a calculable value V_1 at the point to which the counter-ionic reagent of charge q_1 must come in the final state of the reaction. The consequential energy increment is V_1q_1, and this, after a statistical correction which is part of an entropy term, Bjerrum treats as an addition to the free-energy change of the reaction. It is here implied that, if the ionic substituent were different, in the sense of having a different charge or effective charge, or being differently situated, so that it produced a potential V_2 at the same point as before, then the addition to the polar energy would be V_2q_1. Further, if the first-mentioned substituent and the second-mentioned were present together, though spaced sufficiently to allow them to act in independence, then the addition to the free energy would be $(V_1+V_2)q_1$. This is simple additivity. It is likewise implied that, if, instead of considering, with Bjerrum, the uptake of a proton, we should consider the uptake of some other ion, such as a mercuric ion, of charge q_2, then the free-energy contributions due to the first substituent, to the second, and to both together, would be V_1q_2, V_2q_2, and $(V_1+V_2)q_2$, respectively. This is simple proportionality.

The additivity and proportionality depend vitally on the constitution of the polar energy terms. Each term is a product of two factors, one of which represents a single physical magnitude of one reactant whilst the other represents a single physical magnitude of the other. What is vital is that each factor measures only one electrostatic quantity. The two reactants must collectively provide the two quantities, but not necessarily on the one-to-one basis here described. Obviously, if we had to take account of comparable energies derived by multiplying a charge into a potential and a (point) dipole moment into a potential gradient, and so reckon with a two-term expression such as $qV + \mu$ grad V, proportionality could not be expected.

The conditions for additivity and proportionality in polar effects on reaction equilibria have a complete parallel in the conditions for these properties in polar effects on reaction rate. In accordance with transition-state theory, we replace the point in the final state, at which a charge is raised to a potential, by a corresponding point in the transition state. The additivity and proportionality now refer to the free energy of activation.

The other example which it is convenient here to recall is a theory of inductive effects of ionic substituents such as ammonium poles on rates of olefin-forming elimination by the bimolecular mechanism E2 (Section **39b**). Here, we calculate the charge q_1 conferred inductively by the substituent on the β-hydrogen atom. Then we compute the potential V_1 at the point occupied by that atom in the potential field of the basic reagent when in its transition-state position. The resulting energy term is q_1V_1— as before, but with the factors from interchanged sources. Obviously, we can consider variations in the polar substituent, leading to changes in q, and variations in the basic reagent, leading to changes in V, and so deduce additivity and proportionality in the energy terms, as before. The conditions for additivity and proportionality will be the same as before. This example has to do with reaction rates, but examples could be devised in which an analogous discussion would have to do with equilibria.

One can see the possibility of extending the additivity or proportionality of the thermodynamic or kinetic energy parameters of reactions more widely than is directly represented in these two examples. The relation between any pair of reactants is reciprocal—either reactant may be regarded as the substrate and the other as the reagent. Substitutions may be successive and cumulative, so leading overall to drastic changes of chemical structure. Hence it is conceivable that some markedly different reactions could be brought into the kinds of correlation illustrated.

If we are concerned with the thermodynamic properties of reactions, then, in the present context, a reaction is different, if its stoicheiometry is different, or if the physical state in which it occurs is different, in particular, if the solvent is different. If we are dealing with kinetic properties, then a reaction is different, if either its initial state or transition state is different, that is, if either its stoicheiometry, or its mechanism, or the rate-controlling stage of its mechanism, is different; and again the reaction is different, if the physical state in which it occurs is different.

According to these principles, the field for trial comparisons with experiment is wide, but the conditions for the demonstration of simple additivity and proportionality of energy effects are restricted. Steric effects and ponderal effects must be inappreciable. (Ponderal effects are always small.) The polar effects of simultaneous substituents must be independent. And every polar effect must be expressible as an energy which is the simple product of the same two physical quantities over the whole range of the comparison. As we shall see later, this range of application can be widened at the cost of employing additional parameters of reaction, the need for which is, however, already indicated by the theory of organic chemistry (Section 7).

If the chemical reaction, which is being influenced by the polar effect of a substituent with respect to its equilibrium, were being conducted adiabatically, the polar effect, considered as an electrostatic work term, would appear thermodynamically as a change in the internal energy ΔU. If, however, the reaction is conducted in the normal way in a thermostat, and at sensibly constant volume, there will be an equivalent heat change ΔH. There will accordingly be an entropy change ΔS. The free-energy change ΔG will be composed from both the enthalpy change ΔH and the entropy change ΔS. Similar statements will apply if the reaction is being influenced by the polar effect with respect to its rate. Supposing the reaction to be conducted isothermally and at constant volume, the polar effect will modify both the activation parameters $\Delta H^{\neq}$ and $\Delta S^{\neq}$. And through both it will modify the free energy of activation $\Delta G^{\neq}$.

In their comprehensive discussion of relations between the free-energy changes of reaction, or of activation of different reactions, Leffler and Grunwald considered effects arising from the dependence of free energy on temperature, as expressed in the equation $\Delta G = \Delta H - T\Delta S$.[1] They first consider a temperature range such that ΔH may be taken as constant, ΔC_p being assumed to be zero. They also consider the more relaxed condition in which ΔC_p is treated as constant, though not necessarily zero, over the temperature range. For both cases they show that, if the contributions $\delta\Delta G$ of a series of substituents to the free-energy change ΔG are observed to be accurately proportional for two reactions, and if such proportionality holds over the temperature range, then the contributions $\delta\Delta H$ of the substituents to

[1] J. E. Leffler and E. Grunwald, "Rates and Equilibria of Organic Reactions," Wiley, New York and London, 1963, Chaps. 6 and 9.

the enthalpy change ΔH of either reaction will be proportional to their contributions $\delta\Delta S$ to the entropy change ΔS of that reaction. Hence either of these contributions $\delta\Delta H$ or $\delta\Delta S$ will be proportional to the contributions $\delta\Delta G$ to the free-energy change ΔG of that reaction. And all this will be true for either reaction, at any one temperature within the temperature range. Thus, distinguishing the two reactions by subscripts 1 and 2, the originally observed proportionality between $\delta\Delta G_1$ and $\delta\Delta G_2$ becomes part of the six-fold proportionality,

$$\delta\Delta G_1 \propto \delta\Delta H_1 \propto \delta\Delta S_1 \propto \delta\Delta G_2 \propto \delta\Delta H_2 \propto \delta\Delta S_2$$

Thus, the observed proportionality between the contributions $\delta\Delta G$, made by the substituents to the free-energy changes ΔG of the two reactions, will entail a like proportionality between their contributions $\delta\Delta H$ to the enthalpy ΔH, and one between their contributions $\delta\Delta S$ to the entropy changes ΔS of the reactions.

It will be understood that this thermodynamic theorem does not in itself justify the expectation of any of these proportionalities. It says only that, *if* one of them exists, the others will. As we have already seen, proportionalities are expected only if polar energies can be expressed as single products of two factors, and if steric and ponderal effects are absent. An experimentally demonstrated proportionality between $\delta\Delta H$ and $\delta\Delta S$ is illustrated in Fig. 57-1 (p. 1110). Here the conditions are well fulfilled. The reaction is the ionisation equilibrium of methaemoglobins, influenced by ionic substituents large distances, such as 30 *A*, away in a rigid structure. Nothing but a coulombic field could span the distances; the local environment is constant; and even the mass is sensibly constant.

Leffler and Grunwald extended their proposition to include kinetic comparisons. If an exact proportionality between the substituent contributions $\delta\Delta G^{\neq}$ to the kinetic parameter $\Delta G^{\neq}$ for two reactions is found to hold over a range of temperature, then the analogous six-fold proportionality will follow, and, in particular, the substituent contributions $\delta\Delta H^{\neq}$ will be proportional for the two reactions, and so will be the substituent contributions $\delta\Delta S^{\neq}$. The conditions for these proportionalities are the same as before: polar energy terms must be constituted as single binary products, and the substituents must introduce no steric or ponderal effects.

(62b) Proportionality of Energies in Acid-Base Catalysis.—The first discovery of proportionality in structural contributions to free-energy changes in reactions was made by Brönsted and Pedersen in 1924. In that year they discovered[2] general-base catalysis. The re-

[2] J. N. Brönsted and K. Pedersen, *Z. physik. Chem.*, 1924, **108**, 185.

action catalysed was the decomposition of nitramide. And in the course of this work they noticed an approximately regular relation between the catalytic rate-constants given by different bases and their basic strengths. On going from one base to a stronger one, the increment in the logarithm of the catalytic rate-constants was a constant fraction of the increment in the logarithm of the basicity constants of the bases.[2] In the immediately following years other reactions were investigated with like results, for instance, the mutarotation of glucose, and the iodination of acetone. In this work, general-acid catalysis was discovered, and with it a similarly linear relation between the logarithms of the catalytic rate-constants and the logarithms of the acidity constants of the catalysing acids.[3] Of course, the basicity constants of bases can be expressed as acidity constants of their conjugate acids, and so the two linear relations can be expressed in a common form, which is known as *Brönsted's relation.* It may be written,

$$\delta \log k = B\delta \log K_a$$

where k is a catalytic rate-constant, K_a is the acidity constant of the acid catalyst, or of the conjugate acid of the basic catalyst, and the operator δ refers to differences made by a change of catalyst.[4] Since, quite generally (Sections **6c** and **6d**),

$$\log K = -\frac{\Delta G}{2.303\,RT} \quad \text{and} \quad \log k = -\frac{\Delta G^{\neq}}{2.303\,RT} + \log\frac{kT}{h}$$

Brönsted's relation can be rewritten as a proportionality between structural contributions to the free energy of activation of the catalysed reaction, and to the free energy of the acid-base equilibria of the catalysts:

$$\delta\Delta G^{\neq} = B\delta\Delta G_a$$

At the time of its promulgation, there was no theory of the Brönsted relation. Indeed, in the 1920's, before the advent of transition-state theory, it was a surprise to everyone that there could be a simple relation between the thermodynamics of one reaction and the kinetics of another.

[3] J. N. Brönsted and H. C. Duus, *Z. physik. Chem.*, 1925, **117,** 299; H. M. Dawson and J. S. Carter, *J. Chem. Soc.*, **1926,** 2282; H. M. Dawson and N. C. Dean, *ibid.*, p. 2872; H. M. Dawson and C. M. Hoskins, *ibid.*, p. 3166; J. N. Brönsted and E. A. Guggenheim, *J. Am. Chem. Soc.*, 1927, **49,** 2554; J. N. Brönsted, *Chem. Revs.*, 1928, **5,** 322; cf. R. P. Bell, "Acid-base Catalysis," Clarendon Press, Oxford, 1941.

[4] The constants should be statistically corrected for the number of equivalent protons, or places for protons, in the reactants.

One of the most thorough studies of general-acid catalysis is that by Bell and Higginson on the dehydration of acetaldehyde hydrate in "92%" aqueous acetone:[5]

$$CH_3 \cdot CH(OH)_2 \xrightarrow{HA} CH_3CHO + H_2O$$

The logarithms of the rates of the reaction catalysed in this solvent at 25° by a series of aliphatic and aromatic carboxylic acids and of phenols are plotted in Fig. 62-1 against the acidity constants of the catalysts in water at 25°. The correlation runs over five orders of magnitude in rate and ten in acid strength.

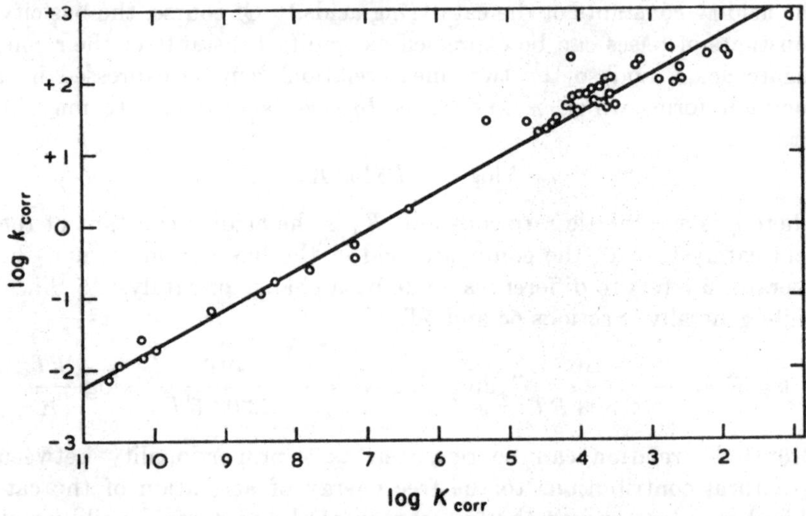

FIG. 62-1.—Bell and Higginson's data for general-acid catalysis by uncharged carboxylic acids and phenols of the dehydration of acetaldehyde hydrate in 92% aqueous acetone at 25°. (A statistical correction is made to K and to k, when reactants contain equivalent protons or sites for protons.)

The correlation is, however, not exact. Bearing in mind that logarithms are somewhat insensitive functions of their arguments, some of the deviations appear quite large among the uncharged carboxylic and phenolic acid catalysts illustrated. Considerably larger deviations would appear, if we would include the many measured acids of other types, such as oximes, enols of β-diketones, *aci*-forms of nitroalkanes, or charged acids. This can mean either that structural effects other than polar effects are present, or that the conditions for proportionality in polar energy terms are unfulfilled.

It is apparent in the detailed data that steric effects are an im-

[5] R. P. Bell and W. C. E. Higginson, *Proc. Roy. Soc.*, 1949, **A, 147**, 141.

portant source of deviations. Steric effects weaken uncharged acids, largely by reducing the solvation of their anions; and they reduce reaction rates, largely by reason of the greater material congestion in bimolecular transition states than in initial states. But these two effects, measured in terms of energy differences, do not, of course, have to be proportional, and certainly not with the proportionality constant, B, of the slope of the line in Fig. 62-1. In formic, acetic, and pivalic acids, the steric effects of successive methyl substitution bear more heavily on the acid strengths than on the reaction rates, with the result that the point for formic acid lies to the right and that for pivalic acid to the left of a line of the slope illustrated through the point for acetic acid. In substituted benzoic acids, the steric effects of ortho-substituents affect the reaction rates relatively more strongly, wherefore a line of the same slope, drawn to give the best fit to points for meta- and para-substituted benzoic acids, would leave on its right the points for ortho-substituted benzoic acids.

The other general cause of deviations is, as already foreshadowed, that it is an idealisation to represent the electrical energy of a polar effect as a single product, which leads to proportionality relations just because it is single. Polar energy must in principle be constituted as a sum of products, because account has to be taken of the independent properties of polarisation and polarisability. It can be seen in the data for this and other acid- or base-catalysed reactions that marked deviations arise when a conjugated system extends between the site of the structural change and that of the reaction. These are the circumstances in which we can expect substantial polarisability effects, which will add new product terms.

(62c) Additivity of Energies in Electrophilic Aromatic Substitution.—The recognition of additivity in polar energies, under certain restrictions of structure and reaction, also goes back to the 1920's. The original discovery was made by Bradfield and Brynmor Jones[6] in 1928. Their reaction was the chlorination of aryl alkyl ethers by chlorine in "99%" acetic acid at 20°. The ethers were of the forms,

RO–C₆H₄–X (para)   RO–C₆H₄–X (ortho)   RO–C₆H₃X–X

where R and X were variable, so that there were three points in the molecule at which changes of structure could be made simultaneously. The alkyl group could be a benzyl group, and then could itself contain aromatic substituents. It was found that, if the aromatic substituents

[6] A. E. Bradfield and B. Jones, *J. Chem. Soc.*, **1928**, 1006, 3073; **1931**, 2903.

TABLE 62-1.—RELATIVE RATES OF CHLORINATION OF ARYL ALKYL ETHERS $RO \cdot C_6H_4X$ AND $RO \cdot C_6H_3X_2$: EFFECTS OF VARIATION IN R (BRADFIELD AND JONES).

R..........	Me	Et	*n*-Pr	*i*-Pr	*n*-Bu	Benzyl and substituted benzyl			
						H	*p*-Cl	*m*-NO_2	*p*-NO_2
X or X_2									
p-CO_2H	100	198	215	444	221	70	—	—	—
p-NO_2	100	200	221	—	—	—	—	—	—
p-Cl	100	199	225	439	222	67	394	16.0	14.2
o-Cl	100	199	—	—	—	—	—	—	14.4
p-Br	100	200	227	438	—	68	—	16.0	14.1
o-Br	100	—	—	—	—	—	—	—	13.8
2,4-Cl_2	—	199	—	—	—	68	—	—	—
2,4-Br_2	100	200	—	—	—	64	—	—	—

TABLE 62.2.—RELATIVE RATES OF CHLORINATION OF ARYL ALKYL ETHERS $RO \cdot C_6H_4X$: EFFECTS OF VARIATIONS IN X (BRADFIELD AND JONES).

X...........	*p*-CO_2H	*p*-NO_2	*p*-Cl	*o*-Cl	*p*-Br
R					
Me	100	0.674	276	916	281
Et	100	0.682	278	925	284
n-Pr	100	0.691	288	—	294
i-Pr	100	—	272	—	279
n-Bu	100	—	283	—	—
$PhCH_2$	100	—	269	899	273

X were held the same, whilst the alkyl group R was varied, the rates bore to one another ratios which were independent of the nature and position of the substituents X, as illustrated in Table 62-1; and reciprocally that, if the group R was kept the same, and the substituent X, or the two substituents X, were changed, then the rates bore ratios that were independent of R, as shown in Table 62-2.

This reciprocal proportionality of the rate when simultaneously present substituents are varied clearly implies additivity in the contributions made by the several substituents to the free energy of activation. Denoting the substituents by i, we can write the symbolic expression of this finding thus:

$$\delta\Delta G^{\neq} = \sum_i \delta\Delta G_i^{\neq}$$

This *Bradfield-Jones relation* has, as we know, widespread application in electrophilic aromatic substitution; and it is often used for the approximate computation of partial rate factors for substitutions in the presence of simultaneously present substituents, when the partial rate factors applying to the singly present substituents are known. However, the additive relationship is not often so accurately fulfilled as it was in the original work of Bradfield and Brynmor Jones, whose results, here expressed as relative rates, would appear even more regular, if re-expressed as logarithms of rates.

A reason for the very close fulfilment of additivity in this particular family of reactions is easy to see. The groups X are inductively electronegative, and are meta-situated with respect to the site or sites of the electrophilic substitution. They will act mainly by inductive polarisation $-I$, and the associated field effect. On the contrary, the groups RO are conjugatively electropositive, and are ortho- or para-situated with respect to the site or sites of electrophilic substitution. These groups will activate almost entirely by the conjugative effect $+K$, and therefore essentially by polarisability effects $+E$ (Section **21c**). This sharp difference in the modes of electron displacement by which the two kinds of groups contribute to the overall activation will help to keep their contributions independent, and, in terms of polar energies, additive.

(62d) Proportionality of Energy Effects of Aromatic meta- and para-Substituents.—In 1935, Hammett[7] and Burkhardt[8] independently discovered that the differences made by *m*- or *p*-substituents to the logarithms of equilibrium or rate-constants of reactions in an aromatic side-chain are proportional for any two of a variety of such reactions. Both investigators recognised the limitation of the relation to *m*- and *p*-substituents in benzene derivatives, and, in particular, that *o*-substituents do not conform. Both emphasized the empirical character of the relation. Both, it so happens, chose the aqueous ionisation equilibria of benzoic acids as the standard process to whose substituent increments of free energy those of other processes within the scope of the relation could be shown to be proportional, and therefore proportional to one another.

If δ_σ, as an operator, indicates a difference due to a substituent, and if k_ρ is a rate or equilibrium constant for a reaction, and K is an equilibrium constant of ionisation of a benzoic acid, then the relation described may be symbolised

[7] L. P. Hammett, *Chem. Revs.*, 1935, **17**, 225; "Physical Organic Chemistry," McGraw-Hill Co., New York and London, 1940, Chap. 7.

[8] G. N. Burkhardt, *Nature*, 1935, **136**, 684; G. N. Burkhardt, W. G. K. Ford, and E. Singleton, *J. Chem. Soc.*, **1936**, 17.

$$\delta_\sigma \log k_\rho = \rho\delta_\sigma \log K$$

where ρ is a constant depending only on the reaction.

Figure 62-2 reproduces one of Burkhardt's graphical representations,[8] in which the effects of *m*- and *p*-substituents on the logarithms of the rate-constants of several side-chain reactions (his own or from the literature), are shown to be linearly correlated with the logarithms

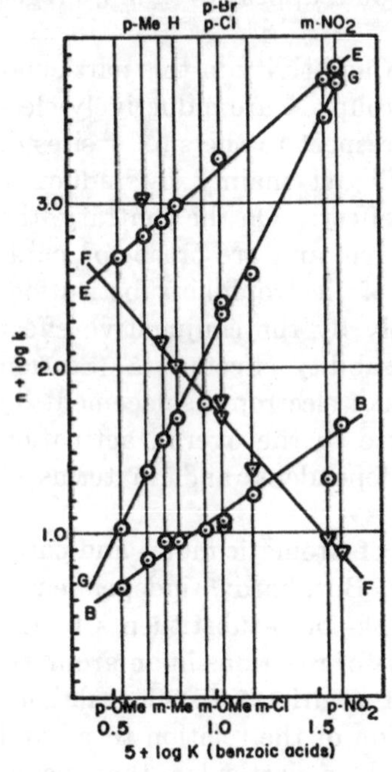

B = Aqueous acid hydrolysis (49°) of substituted phenyl bisulphates (Burkhardt).
E = Aqueous alkaline hydrolysis (100°) of substituted benzamides (Reid).
F = Solvolysis in aqueous ethanol of substituted benzyl chlorides (Olivier).
G = Alkaline hydrolysis in aqueous ethanol of substituted ethyl benzoates (Kindler).

The ordinates for each reaction contain an arbitrary constant *n*. (Reproduced by permission from Burkhardt, Ford, and Singleton, *J. Chem. Soc.*, **1936**, 22.)

FIG. 62.2.—Differences due to *m*- and *p*-substituents in the logarithms of rate-constants of the following reactions (ordinates) versus such differences for the acidity constants of benzoic acids in water at 25° (abscissae).

of the acidity constants of correspondingly substituted benzoic acids. In the above notation the slopes of the straight lines are ρ values.

It is not clear that Burkhardt then understood (though a discussion had just been published that could have suggested a reason[9]) why one of his points for the solvolysis of benzyl chlorides lies nowhere near the linear curve. The solvolysis of benzyl chloride itself proceeds by mechanism S_N2 in aqueous organic solvents if not too highly aqueous, and in any event is near the S_N2-S_N1 mechanistic border (Section **28b**). The aberrant point indicates that, in the

[9] E. D. Hughes and C. K. Ingold, *J. Chem. Soc.*, 1935, 244.

presence of the electron-releasing *p*-methyl substituent, the mechanism has shifted from S_N2 so far towards S_N1, that the "bad" point may be the first point on a new and much steeper line that could be realised by extending the diagram to the left.[10]

At the time of its promulgation, there was no *explicit* theory of the Hammett-Burkhardt relation.[11] Hammett has consistently maintained (and indeed extolled) its empiricism.[12] However, it has a theoretical interpretation, as set down in Section **62a**, above. And in a sense it has always had one, because, as there explained, the interpretation with respect to equilibria has been implicit in organic chemical theory since the mid-1920's, and with respect to rates since the advent of transition-state theory in 1932–35. The interpretation is that, if all effects on equilibrium and rate except polar effects can be neglected (as they cannot in the presence of ortho-substituents), and if the polar energies can be represented each as a single product of the same two electrical quantities (as may be excluded by strong polarisabilities), then we must find proportionality between such single products and one of their factors, when the other factor is kept constant.

In 1940, Hammett[7] restated his and Burkhardt's relation in a form which has been generally used ever since. The differences δ_σ are taken as between a general substituent and its specialisation to hydrogen (subscript zero):

$$\log k - \log k_0 = \rho(\log K - \log K_0)$$

The factor log (K/K_0) is dependent only on the substituent, and is written σ, whilst ρ depends only on the reaction:

$$\log \frac{k}{k_0} = \rho\sigma$$

[10] The change from the straight line to the steeper line may not be sharp; for we expect a change of mechanism not to be absolutely sharp (Section **28a**). Rounded plots covering several substituents have occasionally been observed in S_N2 reactions mechanistically near the S_N2–S_N1 border. A good example is that of the exchange reaction of substituted benzhydryl thiocyanates with thiocyanate ion, which in polar organic solvents proceeds by concurrent S_N2 and S_N1 mechanisms (both near the border), of which the former gives a markedly rounded plot, and the latter a steep plot (A. Ceccon, I. Papa, and A. Fava, *J. Am. Chem. Soc.*, 1966, **88**, 4643).

[11] This relation (= equation) is nearly always signalised under Hammett's name alone (not by Hammett, than whom none could be more generous); but it was discovered by both investigators, though the $\rho\sigma$ notation was (later) introduced by Hammett. (An "equation" can, of course, be stated in words, as well as in symbols.)

[12] L. P. Hammett, *J. Chem. Ed.*, 1966, **43**, 464.

There is another field besides that of aromatic side-chain reactions for which differences due to *m*- and *p*-substituents in free energy of activation are approximately proportional for two reactions. This is the field of electrophilic aromatic substitutions. Its discovery, and the main demonstrations of its extension, are the work of H. C. Brown and his collatorators.[13] Again, *o*-substituents do not conform. If we assume such proportionality in free-energy differences in, for example, nitration, and consider rates of nitration of C_6H_5R in the position to which the variable substituent R is para, then we could set up the equation,

$$\log \frac{k_{p-\mathrm{R}}^{\mathrm{nitr.}}}{k_{p-\mathrm{H}}^{\mathrm{nitr.}}} = \log f_p^{\mathrm{nitr.}} = \sigma_p \rho^{\mathrm{nitr.}}$$

where use has been made of the definition (Section **21b**) of partial rate factors, *f*. We could write a similar equation for the rates of nitration of C_6H_5R in a position to which the substituent R is meta. And then by division of one equation by the other, we would obtain the equation below, from which the dependence on nitration has disappeared from the right-hand side, because $\rho^{\mathrm{nitr.}}$ has cancelled. This "quotient equation," as we shall call it,

$$\frac{\log f_p}{\log f_m} = \frac{\sigma_p}{\sigma_m}$$

depends on the substituent but not on the reaction. For a given substituent, the left-hand side will therefore be the same for nitrations, halogenations, mercurations, Friedel-Crafts alkylations, and so on. This equation can be put in another form. By subtracting the reciprocal of each side from unity, and replacing the function $\sigma_p/(\sigma_p-\sigma_m)$ of benzoic ionisation constants by a single constant b_{R}, we obtain

$$\log f_p = b_{\mathrm{R}} \log \frac{f_p}{f_m}$$

This is known as *Brown's selectivity relation.* A subscript R has been added to the proportionality constant *b*, as a reminder that it depends on the chemical nature (not the position) of the substituent. But for a given substituent, the equation as a whole is independent of the reaction. Qualitatively, it says that the more strongly a reaction re-

[13] H. C. Brown and K. L. Nelson, *J. Am. Chem. Soc.*, 1953, **75**, 6292; H. C. Brown and C. W. McGary, *ibid.*, 1955, **77**, 2300. For a comprehensive account, see L. M. Stock and H. C. Brown, "Advances in Physical Organic Chemistry," Editor V. Gold, Academic Press, London and New York, Vol. 1, 1963, p. 35.

sponds in changed rates to a substituent, the more strongly it will respond in changed ratios of rates of meta- and para-substitution, or, in in other words, in changed product ratios.

As to the quantitative value of the relation, the data for toluene (R = Me), which has been kinetically investigated with respect to about 50 substitutions (in this context, the same stoicheiometric substitution in a different medium is a different substitution), are as internally consistent as any one can find. The selectivity constant b_{Me} has the mean value 1.31 ± 0.10. The standard deviation, $\pm 8\%$, is larger than warranted by the experimental uncertainties. If we compute b as $\sigma_p/(\sigma_p - \sigma_m)$, the value obtained is 1.68. This is 27% larger than is required for best fit to the data. Transformation of the quotient equation to Brown's form reduced the errors. On using the quotient equation directly, one finds that $\log f_p/\log f_m$, which should be constant, has a mean value 4.0 ± 0.5. The standard deviation is now 12.5%. If one computes the constant as σ_p/σ_m, the value is 2.6, in poor agreement with the empirical value 4.0.

It is easy to suggest a reason why the data for effects of *m*- and *p*-substituents on aromatic side-chain reactions and on electrophilic aromatic substitutions disagree so strongly when ensconced together under the same too small umbrella. Generally and in principle, the polar energy contribution of a substituent towards the free energy of a reaction, or of its activation, consists, not of one two-factor product, but of several, which differ in that the factors of each product depend in different ways on the substituent and on the reaction. The simplest situation arises when one such product, due, for example, to the operation of the inductive effect and any associated field effect, is so dominating that other polar effects may be neglected, or at least subsumed by suitably "cooking" the constants that should describe only the effect of the dominating product. Very many aromatic side-chain reactions do approximately conform to this situation, though many conspicuously do not, as we shall see. But among electrophilic aromatic substitutions, especially those influenced by *p*-substituents, marked deviations are widespread. The reason for the difference is that conjugation between the substituent and the reaction site can be more direct in nuclear substitution than in side-chain reactions. The significance of conjugation in this connexion resides mainly in the powerful part played by the conjugative polarisability effect ($+E$) in electrophilic aromatic substitution (Section **21c**). And, to follow the matter through, a polarisability effect will provide, at simplest, another energy term, one composed differently from the first one, and therefore with a different dependence on the substituent and the reaction. The sum of two differently constituted energy terms of comparable magnitudes cannot be represented by a single energy term determined by two constants.

Historically, what was done in face of these and other like troubles was to invent many alternative sets of σ constants (more than will be discussed in this Chapter), each for use in some specialised situation; and to choose new ρ constants to suit each set. These procedures can be criticised as designed to prolong the forcing of data into a formulation shown by long-accepted theory to be too narrow. On the other side it can fairly be said, (a) that they were first-aid measures, and (b) that they did act as a stepping stone towards a broader formulation, one more in line with theory.

(62e) Deviations from Proportionality in the Energy Effects of Aromatic meta- and para-Substituents.—Table 62-3 shows a sample of some substituent constants that are quoted for *m*- and *p*-aromatic substituents.[14] For the moment let us consider only the unmodified σ constants, in the top lines of the first and second sections of the table. And let us start by recapitulating the significance of these constants. On being multiplied by the ρ constant for a particular reaction, a set of such σ constants describes, for that reaction, the logarithmic spread of its equilibrium or rate constants which is caused by a series of substituents. The constant ρ measures the spread for that reaction, relative to the spread similarly caused in the ionisation constants of benzoic acids, the standard reaction for which ρ is taken as unity. Electronegative substituents increase the acidity of benzoic acids, and hence algebraically positive σ constants express electronegativity, and algebraically negative σ constants electropositivity, except for some substituents of the $-I+K$ class (and the $+I-K$ class, not exemplified), which have an ambiguous polarity. We may note that the $-I+K$ substituent, methoxyl, has a positive (*i.e.*, electronegative) σ in the *m*-position, from which its conjugation does not extend quite closely to the reaction site, and a negative (electropositive) σ in the *p*-position, from which its conjugation does lead closely to, if not right into, the reaction site. Evidently conjugation plays a minor role in the former case, but a major role in the latter. The effect of position is less marked in the $-I+K$ halogen substituents. Here, inductive electronegativity determines the positive sign of σ in both

[14] The constants of Table 62-3 and the associated reaction constants of Table 62-4 are nearly all from compilations by the following: H. H. Jaffé, *Chem. Revs.*, 1953, **53,** 191; Y. Okamoto and H. C. Brown, *J. Org. Chem.*, 1957, **22,** 485; *idem*, *J. Am. Chem. Soc.*, 1958, **80,** 4979; D. H. McDaniels and H. C. Brown, *J. Org. Chem.*, 1958, **23,** 420.

TABLE 62-3.—SOME SUBSTITUTED CONSTANTS OF AROMATIC *m*- AND *p*-SUBSTITUENTS.

	Me_2N	MeO	F	Cl	Me	*t*-Bu	CF_3	CO_2Et	COMe	CN	SO_2Me	NO_2	N_2^+
						Meta							
σ	—	0.11	0.34	0.37	−0.07	−0.10	0.43	0.37	0.38	0.56	0.52	0.71	1.76
σ^+	—	0.05	0.33	0.40	−0.07	−0.06	0.52	0.37	—	0.56	—	0.67	—
						Para							
σ	−0.83	−0.27	0.06	0.23	−0.17	−0.20	0.54	0.45	0.50	0.66	0.49	0.78	1.91
σ^+	−1.7	−0.78	−0.07	0.11	−0.31	−0.26	0.61	0.48	—	0.65	—	0.79	—
σ^-	—	—	—	—	—	—	—	0.67	0.87	1.00	1.05	1.27	3.2
						Para Differences							
σ-σ^+	0.9	0.51	0.13	0.12	0.14	0.06	−0.07	—	—	—	—	—	—
σ^--σ	—	—	—	—	—	—	—	0.22	0.37	0.34	0.56	0.49	1.3

locations, but the increased effect of conjugation in the *p*-position reduces the positive magnitude of σ. We must, however, not treat para-meta differences of σ generally as measuring conjugation: the difference of position from which inductive and field effects extend would in any case create differences in σ.

In order to complete this sketch of applications of the Hammett-Burkhardt relation, let us consider next the figures in the top section of Table 62-4. The table contains[14] a sample of the reaction constants of reactions subject to influences from *m*- and *p*-substituents. The sample is only a small one, because so many reaction constants have been quoted: the same reaction done in a different solvent needs a different constant. The top section of the table contains values of ρ primarily intended for use with the unmodified substituent constants σ. The first entry refers to the fiducial reaction, the equilibrium ionisation of benzoic acids. Because ρ is here set equal to unity, other reactions which are promoted by electronegative substituents will have positive

Table 62-4.—Some Reaction Constants for Use with Substituent Constants of Aromatic *m*- and *p*-Substitution. (E = equilibrium, R = rate.)

		Values of ρ for use with σ	
$ArCO_2H$	E	Deprotonation, water, 25°	(1.00)
ArO^-	R	Reaction with EtI (S_N2), ethanol, 42°	− 0.99
$ArCH_2Cl$	R	Reaction with I^- (S_N2), acetone, 20°	0.78
$ArNH_2$	R	Reaction with PhCOCl (S_N2), benzene, 25°	− 2.78
ArCOCl	R	Reaction with $PhNH_2$ (S_N2), benzene, 25°	1.22
$ArCO_2Et$	R	Alk. hydrol. ($B_{AC}2$), "85%" ethanol, 35°	2.46
$ArCO_2H$	R	Esterification ($A_{AC}2$), ethanol, 25°	− 0.47
ArOCOMe	R	Acid hydrol. ($A_{AC}2$), "60%" acetone, 25°	− 0.20
$ArCONH_2$	R	Alk. hydrol. ($B_{AC}2$), "60%" ethanol, 53°	1.36
$ArCONH_2$	R	Acid hydrol. ($A_{AC}2$), "60%" ethanol, 52°	− 0.48
		Values of ρ for use with σ^+	
$ArCMe_2Cl$	R	Solvolysis (S_N1), "90%" acetone, 25°	− 4.52
Ar_3COH	E	Ionisation through conjugate acid, water, 25°	− 3.64
$ArPh_2CCl$	R	Solvolysis (S_N1), 40% EtOH + 60% Et_2O, 0°	− 2.34
$ArCH:CH \cdot CO_2H$	R	Addition Cl_2, acetic acid, 24°	− 4.01
ArH	R	Nitration, HNO_3, $MeNO_2$ or Ac_2O, 0° or 25°	− 6.22
ArH	R	Bromination, HOBr + H^+, "50%" dioxan, 25°	− 5.78
ArH	R	Chlorination, Cl_2, acetic acid, 25°	− 8.06
ArH	R	Bromination, Br_2, acetic acid, 25°	−12.14
		Values of ρ for use with σ^-	
ArOH	E	Deprotonation, water, 25°	2.01
$ArNH_3^+$	E	Deprotonation, water, 25°	2.77
$ArCH_2 \cdot CH_2Br$	R	Reaction with OEt^- ethanol, 30°	2.15
o-$C_6H_3NO_2Cl$	R	Reaction with OMe^- (S_N2), methanol, 25°	3.90

ρ values, whilst those promoted by electropositive substituents will have negative ones. The broad features of the figures are then easily understood, for instance, why the sign of ρ changes when the substituent-bearing aryl group is changed from one reactant to the other in the S_N2-type substitutions, and why the positive ρ values characteristic of the $B_{AC}2$ mechanisms of hydrolysis of carboxylic esters and amides give place to negative values (in principle, less positive or negative) in corresponding $A_{AC}2$ mechanisms.

Okamoto and Brown[14] recognised two large classes of reactions whose equilibria or rates are influenced by *m*- and *p*-aromatic substituents to extents which show large and systematic deviations from those calculated as $\rho\sigma$ products. One class comprised aromatic side-chain reactions, which in equilibria produced an α-carbonium ionic centre, or else whose rates were controlled by the formation of an α-carbonium ionic centre. The examples included equilibria in the formation of triarylmethyl carbonium ions, rates of solvolyses by the S_N1 mechanism of benzyl, benzhydryl, and triarylmethyl compounds, and the addition in polar solvents of molecular chlorine to cinnamic acid and styryl ketones. The other class of reactions consisted of electrophilic aromatic substitutions. In the rate-controlling step of these reactions, the substituting agent is taken up in such a way that the ring itself bears a carbonium ionic charge. The pattern of the deviations was shown to be the same in both groups of examples. *m*-Substituents and non-conjugated *p*-substituents produced no significant deviations; neither did electronegatively conjugated *p*-substituents (*e.g.*, NO_2). But electropositively conjugated *p*-substituents (*e.g.*, MeO) produced deviations which apparently increased with the power of the substituent to conjugate. The deviations were always in the same direction, *viz.*, that the reaction went further, or went faster, than the Hammett-Burkhardt relation would predict.

It was clear to Okamoto and Brown that the deviations arose from conjugation between the *p*-substituents and the formed or forming carbonium ion: the conjugation added a negative term to the free energy of reaction, or of its activation. Okamoto and Brown proposed to cover the deviations in a new formulation, patterned on the $\rho\sigma$ formulation, but specific for aromatic α-carbonium-ion reactions and aromatic electrophilic substitutions. This formulation was not necessarily to be tied to any reactions outside its own sphere, and could therefore employ an internal standard reaction, rather than the standard of benzoic acid ionisations, as a reaction for defining substituent constants. It will be recalled that Brown's selectivity constants are poorly correlated with σ values based on benzoic acid ionisations. With new substituent constants, based on an internal standard, the correlation could be foreseen to be, as, indeed, it is, much better.

The internal standard chosen was of the first of the reactions listed in the middle section of Table 62-4, *viz.*, the hydrolysis in specified conditions of cumyl ($\alpha\alpha$-dimethylbenzyl) chloride. Its reaction constant was, however, taken, not as $+1$, but as -4.52, because that made the substituent constants, called σ^+, derived from the effect of substituents on its rate, minimally different from σ for *m*-substituents, as is illustrated in the top section of Table 62-3 (p .1207). For *p*-substituents, as shown in the middle section of this table, there is also substantial agreement between σ^+ and σ, except for electropositively conjugated $(+K)$ substituents. Among these, one finds differences which are large for amino- and oxy-groups, small for the halogens, and for methyl (and primary and secondary alkyl) groups, and smaller to negligibility otherwise. Differences between σ^+ and σ are listed in the bottom section of the table. They may be taken to measure the strength of conjugation of the substituents.

With the aid of these σ^+ values, ρ values for use with them were determined for other α-carbonium ion reactions of aromatic side-chains, and for electrophilic aromatic substitutions, as exemplified in the middle section of Table 62-4. All these reactions, in common with the fiducial reaction of the hydrolysis of cumyl chloride, are facilitated by electron supply to the reaction centre, *i.e.*, by electropositively acting substituents, and hence all these ρ values are negative. In magnitude, they are particularly large for the aromatic substitutions. And in this field one can see the operation of de la Mare's principle (Section **22c**) that electromeric effects $+E$ from substituents in *p*-positions are exerted more powerfully in electrophilic substitutions by uncharged carriers than by cationic carriers of the same entering substituent.

The upper of the two diagrams in Fig. 62-3 illustrates the need for some change in formulation, if the deviations from linearity associated with electropositively conjugated para-substituents in Hammett-Burkhardt's plots are to be avoided. The lower diagram illustrates how well the replacement of σ values by σ^+ values can straighten out the deviations. But let it be admitted at once that the reaction taken for illustration was selected: σ^+ plots do not always behave in such an exemplary way, as we shall see.

There is another, less thoroughly investigated, but similarly large area of reactions, which exhibit systematic deviations from $\rho\sigma$ linearity. These failures occur at the other end of a $\rho\sigma$ plot, the end containing the electron-absorbing $(-I-K)$ substituents. But again the anom-

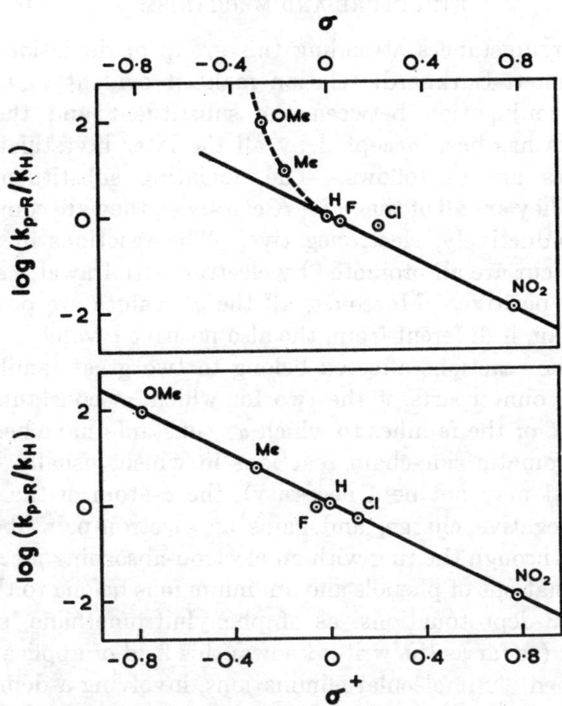

FIG. 62-3.—Plots of log (k_{p-R}/k_H) against σ and against σ^+ for *p*-substituents. The rates are for the ethanolysis of *p*-monosubstituted triphenylmethyl chlorides in 40% EtOH/60% Et_2O at 0°, as measured by A. C. Nixon and G. E. K. Branch, *J. Am. Chem. Soc.*, 1936, **58**, 492.

alies are associated only with *p*-substituents, and again their direction is to make certain substituents act more strongly than the $\rho\sigma$ product would allow. Hammett first noticed this type of deviation in the behaviour of the nitro-group; and he suspected then (1940) that it would be found more widely, as, indeed, it subsequently was found by Roberts, Bordwell, and others.[15] The matter was formalised by compiling yet another series of substituent constants for employment where the deviations occurred or were serious. Some of these constants, as compiled by Jaffé,[14] are listed under the designation σ^- in the second section of Table 62-3. The values are for *p*-substituents: where no entries appear, σ^- may be taken as identical with σ; and for all *m*-substituents, σ^- may be set equal to σ.

[15] J. D. Roberts and E. A. McElhill, *J. Am. Chem. Soc.*, 1950, **72**, 628; F. G. Bordwell and G. D. Cooper, *ibid.*, 1952, **74**, 1058.

All the circumstances attending this group of deviations from the simple Hammett-Burkhardt relation make it evident that they also arise from conjugation between the substituent and the reaction centre. This has been accepted by all the later investigators. The circumstances are as follows. The deviating substituents are *p*-situated. They are all of the $-I-K$ class; *i.e.*, they are conjugatively, as well as inductively, electronegative. The reactions in which the deviations occur are all promoted by electron withdrawal; *i.e.*, all their ρ values are positive. Moreover, all the σ^- values are positive, and are larger than, if different from, the also positive σ values. Most significantly, the reactions affected belong to two great families, which are obvious counterparts of the two for which σ^+ constants were invented. One of the families to which σ^- constants have been applied comprises aromatic side-chain reactions in which, usually by proton loss (but that may not be a necessity), the α-atom of the side-chain receives a negative charge, and gains an electron-pair liberated for conjugation through the ring with an electron-absorbing *p*-substituent. The deprotonations of phenols and anilinium ions belong to this family. Prototropic α-deprotonations, as of phenylnitromethane, should belong, though (as far as the writer knows) this field of application is not yet exemplified. Bimolecular eliminations, involving α-deprotonation and leading to styrenes, have been shown by Saunders and Williams to belong to the same family of side-chain reactions.[16] The other great family consists in the bimolecular reactions of nucleophilic aromatic substitution. Their inclusion in the same system of deviations has been demonstrated by Bunnett and his collaborators.[17] Examples of reactions belonging to the two families are given in the third section of Table 62-4.

It is generally agreed, then, that these deviations from $\rho\sigma$ linearity are connected with conjugatively electronegative effects of *p*-substituents. The differences $\sigma^- - \sigma$ listed in the last line of Table 62-3 may accordingly be taken as measures of the conjugating power of the $-K$-type substituents. Figure 62-4 illustrates a case in which failure of the $\rho\sigma$ relation is largely rectified by the use of σ^- in place of σ.

(62f) Energy of Polar Effects of Aromatic meta- and para-Substituents as a Sum of Products.—We now consider further the two major groups of deviations from proportionality in free energy effects, and first those shown by conjugatively electropositive *p*-substituents. These deviations show strongly near the electropositive ends of $\rho\sigma$

[16] W. H. Saunders jr. and R. A. Williams, *J. Am. Chem. Soc.*, 1957, **79**, 3712.

[17] J. F. Bunnett, F. Draper jr., P. R. Ryason, P. Noble jr., R. G. Tonkyn, and R. F. Zahler, *J. Am. Chem. Soc.*, 1953, **75**, 642.

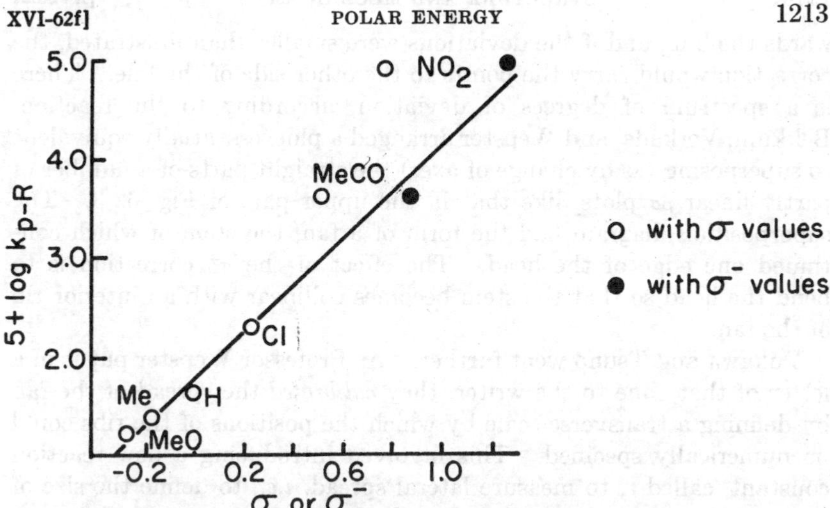

FIG. 62-4.—Plots of log k_{p-R} against σ and σ^- for para-substituents. The rate-constants k_{p-R} are for bimolecular olefin-forming eliminations from *p*-substituted 2-phenylethyl bromides by reaction with ethoxide ions in ethanol at 30°. (Reproduced with permission from Saunders and Williams, *J. Am. Chem. Soc.*, 1957, **79**, 3714.)

plots, as the upper diagram of Fig. 62-3 illustrates (p. 1211). They are the deviations to which Okamoto and Brown's σ^+ constants have been applied. We have been illustrating with Okamoto and Brown's σ^+ constants largely because they are more extensively documented than anyone else's σ^+ constants. But quite a number of alternative sets of σ^+ values, each with its own set of ρ values, have been proposed by other workers. The mere fact that several alternatives exist shows that Okamoto and Brown's constants should not be taken as fixed numbers for general application.

This lack of general applicability was pointed out in 1959 by van Bekkum, Verkade, and Wepster,[18] and also by Yukawa and Tsuno.[19] Both groups showed that if, near the electropositive end of a $\rho\sigma$ plot one finds positive deviations by conjugatively electropositive *p*-substituents, as illustrated in the upper diagram of Fig. 62-3, then to replace σ by Okamoto and Brown's σ^+ may bring the aberrant points onto the line, as it does in that illustration; or it may not, and more often does not. In a case in which the deviations are larger than illustrated, the σ^+ correction would bring the points only part way to-

[18] H. van Bekkum, P. E. Verkade, and B. M. Wepster, *Rec. trav. chim.*, 1959, **78**, 85.

[19] Y. Tsumo, T. Ibata, and Y. Yukawa, *Bull. Chem. Soc. Japan*, 1959, **32**, 960; Y. Yukawa and Y. Tsumo, *ibid.*, 965, 971.

wards the line; and if the deviations were smaller than illustrated, the correction would carry the points to the other side of the line. There is a spectrum of degrees of deviation, according to the reaction. Bekkum, Verkade, and Wepster arranged a plot, essentially equivalent to superposing (as by change of axes) the straight parts of a number of partly linear $\rho\sigma$ plots, like that in the upper part of Fig. 62-3. The superposition diagram had the form of a fan, the stem of which continued one edge of the head. The effect of the σ^+ correction is to bend the head so that the stem becomes collinear with an interior rib of the fan.

Yukawa and Tsuno went further. As Professor Wepster put it in a letter of that time to the writer, they *calibrated* the spread of the fan by defining a transverse scale by which the positions of the ribs could be numerically specified. This involved introducing a new reaction constant, called r, to measure lateral spread, *i.e.*, to define the size of those deviations from $\rho\sigma$ linearity which are characteristic of a reaction. The unit of r was taken as its value when the replacement of σ by Okamoto and Brown's σ^+ exactly corrected the deviations. Thus r was made unity for Okamoto and Brown's standard reaction, the hydrolysis of cumyl chloride under their conditions. In this case, one can say that the correction needed to σ is $\sigma^+ - \sigma$. In the general case, the needed correction is $r(\sigma^+ - \sigma)$. The constant r can be less than or greater than unity. Values have been determined which range from 0.2 to more than 2. In these terms, the *Yukawa-Tsuno equation* is

$$\log \frac{k}{k_0} = \rho\{\sigma + r(\sigma^+ - \sigma)\}$$

Some values of the reaction constant r are given in Table 62-5. They are, of course, significant only in the presence of p-substituents, since for m-substituents σ^+ is taken as equal to σ, wherefore r becomes indeterminate.

As an instrument for the representation of kinetic and thermodynamic effects of m- and p-substituents, but not o-substituents, this equation is highly successful. Yukawa and Tsuno examined some thirty-five reactions in their first papers on the equation. They all gave good linear plots of $\log k$ or $\log K$ against $\sigma + r(\sigma^+ - \sigma)$ — plots as good as the lower plot of Fig. 62-3, which is good, because r for the reaction represented happens to be close to unity. But r can vary widely, as Table 62-5 shows. Other investigators, notably Eaborn,[20]

[20] R. W. Bott and C. Eaborn, *J. Chem. Soc.*, **1963**, 2139; R. Baker, R. W. Bott, and C. Eaborn, *ibid.*, **1964**, 627; R. W. Bott, C. Eaborn, and D. R. M. Walton, *ibid.*, **1965**, 384.

TABLE 62-5.—SOME REACTION CONSTANTS FOR USE IN THE YUKAWA-TSUNO EQUATION.

(E = equilibrium, R = rate)

			ρ	r
$ArCMe_2Cl$	R	Hydrolysis, "90%" acetone, 25°	−4.52	(1.00)
$ArB(OH)_2$	R	Brominolysis, "20%," acetic acid, 25°	−3.84	2.29
Ar_2CHCl	R	Methanolysis, methanol, 25°	−4.02	1.23
ArH	R	Bromination, $HOBr+H^+$, "50%" dioxan, 25°	−5.28	1.14
ArH	R	Nitration, HNO_3, $MeNO_2$, or HOAc, 25°	−6.38	0.90
$ArCPh_2Cl$	R	Ethanolysis, "40%" EtOH + "60%" Et_2O, 0°	−2.52	0.88
ArN:NPh	E	Basicity, "20%" EtOH, 25°	−2.29	0.85
$ArCOCHN_2$	R	Acid decomposition, acetic acid, 40°	−0.82	0.56
ArCMe:NOH	R	Beckmann rearr., "94%" H_2SO_4, 51°	−1.98	0.43
ArCH(OH)·CH:CH(Me)	R	Anionotropy, "60%" dioxan, 30°	−4.06	0.40
Ar_2CN_2	R	Decomposition by HOBz, toluene, 25°	−1.57	0.19

have used the Yukawa-Tsuno equation with much success. It can be said that the equation ought to do well, because it has four constants. However, they have not all to be determined simultaneously, but can be found, as they have been, σ and ρ together, and then σ^+, and then r, severally, from non-overlapping data designed *ad hoc* to fix the quantities individually.

Table 62-5 also shows that Okamoto and Brown's definition of the family of reactions requiring the sort of treatment towards which their use of the σ^+ constant was a first step was too narrow. It is not necessary that the final state in an equilibrium, or the transition state in a rate process, should have a carbonium ionic centre either in the benzene ring or on an atom directly bound to the ring. The losses of nitrogen from aromatic derivatives of diazomethane are believed to depend on a carbene rather than a carbonium-ion intermediate. The real need is only that the final or transition states shall contain an electron-absorbing centre of any kind that is strong enough effectively to excite the active conjugation of an electropositively conjugated para-substituent.

But the special interest of the Yukawa-Tsuno equation is that it is the first equation to be proposed for polar substituent effects on reactions which is consistent with the pattern of organic chemical theory, as developed in and since the mid-1920's.

It has been recognised by all who have concerned themselves with deviations from simple $\rho\sigma$ products that the main deviations are associated with conjugation. As to how the conjugation acts, two theoretical considerations, both going back to 1927, may be recalled.

The first is that a polar effect in general comprises both polarisation and polarisability. In a polarisation, the substituent creates a potential field in which the reagent, and hence the reacting system, undergoes a change of energy. This energy term can in the simplest approximation be represented by the product of a constant for the polar potential at the ultimate or critical location of the reagent (according as one is dealing with equilibria or rates), and a constant for the effective charge which at that location represents the spatial distribution of charges carried by the reagent. (Point multipoles are an inappropriate concept in such intimate situations.) Polarisability will add another energy term quite differently constituted. The substituent factor will be different, because it now involves a polarisability. The reaction factor will also be different, because the effective charge in the reagent will act on the polarisability to produce an extra potential; and then it, and so the reacting system, will undergo an energy change in the extra polar potential so created. Taking polarisability in this approximation as a field-independent symmetric tensor expressing harmonic electron displacements, the required equation will have a two-term four-constant form, and could be symbolised,

$$\log \frac{K}{K_0} \quad \text{or} \quad \log \frac{k}{k_0} = \rho_0\sigma_0 + \rho_+\sigma_+$$

This is the Yukawa-Tsuno equation in other symbols.

The second long-established consideration that we have to recall is that of the connexion between the principle of polar duplexity and conjugation. Why cannot conjugation be "lumped in" with induction? Why does it take conjugation to enforce the recognition of polar duplexity? The reason is simply that conjugation, by giving new mobility to the most loosely bound electrons in a molecule, and hence in a reacting system of molecules, much enhances polarisability. In quantal terms, it reduces excitation energies. As polarisability is a sum of terms each inversely proportional to an excitation energy, even one small excitation energy will provide a large, often outstanding, contribution to the polarisability (Section **7g**). Therefore, as was experimentally demonstrated in 1927 for polar effects in electrophilic aromatic substitution, a substituent which secures that conjugation will be increased in the course of reaction will enlarge, usually much enlarge, the contribution of polarisability to the reaction. It follows that Yukawa and Tsuno's second work term, even if negligible, or empirically subsumable, in the absence of a substituent having this property of enhancing conjugation in reaction, is unlikely to be negligible or subsumable in the presence of such a substituent (cf. Section **7a** and **21c**).

It would not be correct to define the family of reactions which show the electronegative deviations to which σ^--type corrections have been or could be applied as those reactions in whose final or transition states carbanionic or other fully-formed basic centres arise either in the benzene ring or on an atom directly bound to it. For example, the formation of styrenes listed in the last section of Table 62-4 is an E2 reaction, not an E1cB reaction; that is, it does not proceed by way of an intermediate carbanion. The real condition for the deviations is that the final or transition state should contain an electron-supplying centre of any kind that is sufficiently active effectively to excite functional conjugation in an electronegatively conjugated para-substituent.

Finally, and mainly in order to look forward, let us look back at the deviations from $\rho\sigma$ linearity which are shown in a large class of reactions by conjugatively electronegative *p*-substituents, and are shown especially strongly by those substituents (*e.g.*, NO_2) of this class which figure near the electronegative ends of $\rho\sigma$ plots. They are the deviations which Jaffé proposed[14] to cover by the substituent constant here called σ^-. We may assume that it was an accident of history that caused the electropositive group of deviations, those which σ^+ constants were invented to correct, to be the first group to be sufficiently carefully investigated to disclose dispersion of the deviations previously thought uniform enough to be covered by fixed σ^+-type corrections. This discovery produced the Yukawa-Tsuno equation. Therefore we should expect that a similarly careful study of the electronegative deviations, of reactions such as those to which σ^- constants have been applied, would reveal an analogous dispersion.[21] Such a discovery would provide the empirical basis for a broadened Yukawa-Tsuno equation:

$$\log \frac{K}{K_0} \quad \text{or} \quad \log \frac{k}{k_0} = \rho\{\sigma + r^+(\sigma^+ - \sigma) + r^-(\sigma^- - \sigma)\}$$
$$= \rho\{\sigma + r(\sigma^+ + \sigma^- - 2\sigma)\}$$

[21] Such a study has been begun: the rates of basic hydrolysis of phenyl esters having $-K$-type *p*-substituents need σ-factors of the form $\sigma + r^-(\sigma^- - \sigma)$ with $r^- = 0.2$–0.3 (J. J. Ryan and A. A. Humffray, *J. Chem. Soc.*, **1966, B**, 842; **1967, B**, 468.) The significant conjugation here is of the same type as that concerned with the acidity of phenols.

the simplified second form arising if r^+ and r^- can be taken as a single set of constants r.

A broadened equation of this type is expected theoretically. For the short-range polarisability relevant to reaction is far from being the field-independent tensor of homogeneous polarisability: the electron displacement may be highly anharmonic. We have known since 1927 that polarisability effects have sense bias (Sections **7** and **21c**). Hence we cannot imagine being able for general purposes to represent the polarisability of a substituent in reactions by less than two constants, corresponding to the two electropolar senses. So, by extension of the previous argument we come to the three-term equation,

$$\log \frac{K}{K_0} \quad \text{or} \quad \log \frac{k}{k_0} = \rho_0\sigma_0 + \rho_+\sigma_+ + \rho_-\sigma_-$$

$$= \rho_0\sigma_0 + \rho_\pm(\sigma_+ + \sigma_-)$$

its five-constant form arising if ρ_+ and ρ_- need not be differentiated.[22] This equation is the same as that written above in Yukawa-Tsuno-type notation. It suggests the type of extension to which we can look forward.

(62g) Proportionality of Energy Effects of Spatially Remote Aliphatic Substituents.—The three immediately preceding Sections are limited to effects on reactions of aromatic *m*- and *p*-substituents, substituents remote enough not to involve interference from primary steric effects. Owing to the usual conformational flexibility in the aliphatic series, it is more difficult there to organise a like degree of fixed remoteness. But this has been done, by Roberts and Moreland, by the use of bridge-heads for the sites of the influencing substituent and the reaction-carrying side-group.[23] Their system comprised 4-substituted *dicyclo*(2.2.2)octane-1-carboxylic acids or other 1-carboxylic derivatives, $4\text{-RC}(CH_2 \cdot CH_2)_3C \cdot CO_2H$, and so on.

The substituent constants, called σ', were defined by reference to substituent effects on the acidity constants of the acids in "50%" aqueous ethanol at 25°. The reaction constant, ρ', for this reaction was taken as 1.464, the value of ρ found for the ionisation of benzoic acids in that solvent, in terms of the value, unity, for ionisation in water. The formal definition of σ' is therefore

[22] The writer had this "theoretical" equation (in other symbols) in the manuscript of the first edition of this book, but then took out the section containing it (one on polar energies), having decided that it was better at that date to leave empirical development to find its own way forward, as it brilliantly has done.

[23] J. D. Roberts and W. T. Moreland jr., *J. Am. Chem. Soc.*, 1953, **75**, 2167.

$$1.464\sigma' = \log\left(\frac{K}{K_0}\right)$$

But, of course, the comparison of σ' with aromatic σ values will make sense only if the solvent effect at 25°, as between water and "50%" aqueous ethanol, on the ionisation of *dicyclo*(2.2.2)octane-1-carboxylic acid is the same as on that of benzoic acid. It may not be exactly the same.

The four σ' values, determined by Roberts and Moreland, are in the upper portion of Table 62-6. They are compared in the table with aromatic σ_{meta} and σ_{para} values.

In aromatic systems, polar transmission is aided by the conductivity of the benzene ring. A polar effect reaching the benzene ring, even at a meta-position to the reaction site, is in part conjugatively transferred to ring positions nearer to the reaction site. If the polar effect reaches the ring at the para-position, it will in part be thus conjugatively transferred to the ring position which either is the reaction site or bears the side-group containing the reaction site. All such effects of aromatic conjugation are cut away in Roberts and Moreland's system: that was their object. Provided that ponderal effects can be neglected, as they usually can, their 4-substituents can influence reaction only by inductive and field effects, the latter probably having the greater importance.

We may note some expected consequences. The substituents OH and Br, which as aromatic substituents are of $-I+K$ type, will, in

TABLE 62-6.—SUBSTITUENT CONSTANTS σ' AND REACTION CONSTANTS ρ', FOR REACTIONS OF 4-SUBSTITUTED *dicyclo*(2.2.2)OCTANE-1-CARBOXYLIC COMPOUNDS. COMPARISON OF σ' WITH AROMATIC σ_{meta} AND σ_{para} CONSTANTS (ROBERTS AND MORELAND).

R	σ'	σ_{meta}	σ_{para}
OH	0.28	0.12	−0.27
Br	0.43	0.39	0.23
CO_2Et	0.30	0.37	0.45
CN	0.58	0.56	0.66

		E = equilibrium, R = Rate	ρ'
$RC(CH_2\cdot CH_2)_3C\cdot CO_2H$	E	Ionisation, "50%" EtOH, 25°	(1.464)
	R	Reaction with Ph_2CN_2, EtOH, 30°	0.70
$RC(CH_2\cdot CH_2)_3C\cdot CO_2Et$	R	Alk. hydr., "87.8%" EtOH, 30°	2.24

the *dicyclo*-octane system, show only $-I$ character. So they will give positive σ' constants, of magnitudes in the inductive order OH < Br. The lost aromatic conjugation being electropositive, these σ' constants will be algebraically more positive even than the aromatic σ_{meta} constants, and much more positive than the σ_{para} values. All these expectations are illustrated in Table 62-6. The substituents CO_2Et and CN, which as aromatic substituents are of $-I-K$ type, will, in the bridged aliphatic system, again show only $-I$ character, and so will give positive σ' constants. But now the lost aromatic conjugation is electronegative, and hence the σ' values should be somewhat less positive than aromatic σ_{meta} constants, and considerably less positive than σ_{para} values. The signs of the σ' values, and of three of the four differences, and the greater magnitude of the differences from σ_{para} than from σ_{meta} constants, can be seen in the table to be as expected. One difference, $\sigma_{\text{meta}}-\sigma'$ for CN, has the "wrong" sign; but it is so small that a change of 5% in σ' could invert the sign. The experimental measurements are likely to be in error by less than this discrepancy, but it can be doubted whether the assumed identity of solvent effects on the ionisation of the *dicyclo*-octane acid and of benzoic acid, as implied by the factor 1.464 put into the definition of σ', can be guaranteed to within such a small margin.

When the values of log k for the two reaction series investigated with respect to rate were plotted against the determined substituent constants σ', in accordance with the assumed equation

$$\log \frac{k}{k_0} = \sigma'\rho'$$

good straight lines were obtained, as illustrated in Fig. 62-5. The slopes of such lines give the ρ' values set down in the lower part of Table 62-6.

(62h) Elimination of Some Steric Effects: Additivity and Proportionality in Residual Polar Energies.—Substituents in open-chain aliphatic reactions, and ortho-substituents in reactions of aromatic compounds, usually introduce polar and appreciable steric effects together. We have no general method of analysis of the resulting thermodynamic or kinetic data which will extract the separate polar and steric contributions to these composite structural effects. Nevertheless, an early suggestion[24] as to a rough method, limited in application to the hydrolysis of carboxylic esters—in principle, to reactions having two mechanisms which differ only in the number of protons in

[24] C. K. Ingold, *J. Chem. Soc.*, **1930**, 1032.

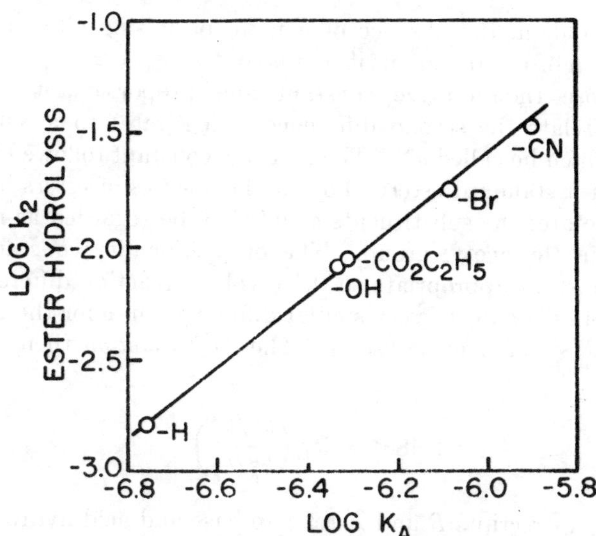

FIG. 62-5.—Plot of the logarithms of the second-order rate-constants of saponification of the *dicyclo*-octane carboxylic ethyl esters against the logarithm of the acidity constants of the corresponding acids, in the respective conditions specified for these reactions in Table 62-6. The values log K_A plotted as abscissae are equivalent to σ' values, apart from a zero-adjustment and a scale-factor. (Reproduced by permission from Roberts and Moreland, *J. Am. Chem. Soc.*, 1953, **75**, 2167.)

their transition states—has been made the starting point of fruitful development by Taft.[25]

The suggestion was that steric effects would approximately cancel in the ratio of the rates of bimolecular acid and basic hydrolysis of an ester, and that therefore polar effects would be measured by changes in that ratio from one ester to another. Of course, this assumption cannot be exactly true. It is true that the two transition states for ester hydrolysis are iso-electronic, and differ only by two protons. But an extra proton is expected to shrink an electronic system, and if such contraction were not the same after a change of substituent, *i.e.*, if size had a finite *second* difference, steric effects would be incompletely eliminated.[26] However, the elimination might be complete enough to

[25] R. W. Taft jr., *J. Am. Chem. Soc.*, 1952, **74**, 2729, 3120; 1953, **75**, 4231; "Steric Effects in Organic Chemistry," Editor M. S. Newman, Wiley, New York, 1956, Chap. 13.

[26] It has been suggested that first differences of solvation energy may spoil the procedure, but that is not so. Only second differences have to be assumed negligible.

be useful, and, in the absence of a more promising alternative, one must try it in order to find out if that is so.

Taft chose the additive constant and proportionality constant needed to relate the second difference of log (rate) to a substituent constant which he called σ^*. The additive constant followed from the selection of a standard ester. For one long series of esters his choice was the acetate: the substituents could then be regarded as replacing hydrogen in the acetyl group. The proportionality constant was a reaction constant appropriate to the involved reaction difference, and was an average (2.48) of very similar differences in ρ for the basic and acid hydrolysis of benzoic esters. The *Taft equation* then takes the form

$$2.48\sigma^* = \log\left(\frac{k^B/k^A}{k_0^B/k_0^A}\right)$$

where the superscripts B and A refer to base and acid hydrolysis, and the subscripts zero indicate rections of the standard ester, *e.g.*, acetate.

Table 62-7 contains some σ^* constants derived by Taft from ester hydrolysis rates. This particular table is limited to substituted acetates having only one substituent replacing a hydrogen atom of the acetyl group. Each value of σ^* is determined with the alcoholic radical and the physical conditions kept constant.

One can see at a glance that the σ^* values display polar regularity; but several more detailed points are worth noting. The first is that

TABLE 62-7.—TAFT'S σ^* SUBSTITUENT CONSTANTS FROM ESTER HYDROLYSIS RATES: ACETATES CONTAINING A SINGLE SUBSTITUENT IN THE ACETYL GROUP.

Substituent in $\cdot CO\cdot CH_3$	σ^* rel. to acetate	$2.2\sigma'$	Substituent in $\cdot CO\cdot CH_3$	σ^* rel. to acetate	$2.2\sigma'$
$\cdot NMe_3^+$	1.90	—	$\cdot CN$	1.30	1.27
$\cdot SO_2\cdot Me$	1.52	—	$\cdot CO\cdot CH_3$	0.60	—
$\cdot F$	1.10	—	$\cdot CH_2\cdot NO_2$	0.50	—
{ $\cdot Cl$	1.05	—	$\cdot CH{:}CHMe$	0.13	—
{ $\cdot CH_2Cl$	0.385	—	{ $\cdot Ph$	0.215	—
$\cdot Br$	1.00	1.00	{ $\cdot CH_2Ph$	0.08	—
$\cdot I$	0.85	—	{ $\cdot CH_2\cdot CH_2Ph$	0.02	—
$\cdot OPh$	0.85	—	$\cdot Me$	−0.10	—
$\cdot OH$	0.56	0.62	$\cdot Et$	−0.115	—
$\cdot OMe$	0.52	—	$\cdot$Pr-*i*	−0.125	—
{ $\cdot CF_3$	0.72	—	$\cdot$Bu-*t*	−0.165	—
{ $\cdot CH_2\cdot CF_3$	0.32	—	$\cdot CH(CH_2)_5$	−0.06	—
{ $\cdot CH_2\cdot CH_2\cdot CF_3$	0.12	—	$\cdot SiMe_3$	−0.26	—

these values, which by their derivation should represent almost pure polar effects, are proportional, where comparison can be made, with Roberts and Moreland's σ' values, which for a different reason also measure almost pure polar effects. The constant of proportionality is $\sigma^*/\sigma' = 2.2$.

Next, as we can see from any of the sets of homologous groups linked by a brace in Table 62-7, the factor of attenuation by transmission through one CC bond of the polar effects measured by σ^* is around 2.7–2.8. This agrees with the figure 2.8 deduced by Branch and Calvin from a consideration of strengths of aliphatic acids.[27] The existence of such a factor, even though it is only approximate, implies bond-by-bond transmission, *i.e.*, that the main polar effect being measured by σ^* is the inductive effect. If this were true in Roberts and Moreland's dicyclic system, the ratio σ^*/σ' would be about 7 (allowing for transmission by three paths through three bonds). The fact that this ratio is only 2.2 is consistent with our intuitive expectation that the main polar effect measured by σ' is the field effect.

The most interesting property of the σ^* values for single substituents in Table 62-7 is their additivity. This again shows their almost complete freedom from steric effects, inasmuch as the latter, because of the character of the non-bonding force law (Section **5c**), are very far from additive. We have noted this with reference to the methyl substituents in the *neo*pentyl group and the *neo*hexyl group (Sections **34b** and **39b**): in the bimolecular reactions affected (S_N2 and E2, respectively) the third methyl substituents in these groups are much more inhibitory than the first two. Taft has determined σ^* values for esters having two and three substituents in the acetyl group. His values are compared in Table 62-8 with the figures obtained by the addition of single substituent values from Table 62-7.

Table 62-8.—Taft's σ^* Constants for Acetates Containing Two and Three Substituents in the Acetyl Group.

Substituents in $\cdot CO \cdot CH_3$	σ^* exptl.	σ^* by addn.	Substituents in $\cdot CO \cdot CH_3$	σ^* exptl.	σ^* by addn.
F, F	2.05	2.20	Me, *t*-Bu	−0.28	−0.265
Cl, Cl	1.94	2.10	Me, Ph	0.11	0.115
Me, Me	−0.19	−0.20	Et, Ph	0.04	0.10
Ph, Ph	0.405	0.43	Cl, Cl, Cl	2.65	3.15
Ph, OH	0.765	0.775	Me, Me, Me	−0.30	−0.30

[27] G. E. K. Branch and M. Calvin, "The Theory of Organic Chemistry," Prentice-Hall, Englewood Cliffs, N. J., 1941, Chap. 6.

The one large discrepancy is in the figures for trichloroacetates. This might arise, as Taft suggests, from an experimental inaccuracy. But it might arise from a real failure in additivity. Such failure should occur when cumulative polar substitution has effected a proportionally substantial approach towards the electrical saturation of induction.

Table 62-9 refers to other esters which Taft has investigated. On the left are given some σ^* values relative to formates. The entries here are of known or possible parents for the treatment of substituent effects. Thus the first entry refers to the parent acetates, the effects of substitution in which have just been discussed. The acetates are here shown to be related to formates by the σ^* difference, acetates-minus-formates, −0.49. The second entry refers to parent acrylates, whose σ^* difference, acrylates-minus-formates, is 0.16. The σ^* constants of some *trans*-β-monosubstituted acrylates are given, relative to acrylates, on the right of the table. Both sets of figures show obvious polar series. One might be momentarily surprised that styryl in the left-hand column of figures, and phenyl in the right-hand column, are given algebraically negative, *i.e.*, electropositive, values. However, this reminds us that the "test-piece" in all these molecules is a carbalkoxyl group, which is itself electronegative. Because of its polarising action, all groups, especially those conjugated with it, will have σ^* values which are less positive, even when they are not actually negative as these two values are, than they would have been if the substituents could have been attached to a non-polar test group.

Table 62-9.—Taft's σ^* Constants for Substituents in the Acyl Residues of Formates and Acrylates.

Substituent in $\cdot CO \cdot H$	σ^* rel. to formates	*trans*-β-Substituent in $\cdot CO \cdot CH:CH_2$	σ^* rel. to acrylates
$\cdot CH_3$	−0.49	$\cdot NO_2$	1.05
$\cdot CH:CH_2$	0.16	$\cdot Cl$	0.25
$\cdot C_6H_5$	0.11	$\cdot CCl_3$	0.54
$\cdot CH:CHPh$	−0.08	$\cdot CHCl_2$	0.23
$\cdot C \vdots CPh$	0.86	$\cdot Ph$	−0.24
$\cdot CO \cdot CH_3$	1.16	$\cdot Me$	−0.29
$\cdot CO \cdot OCH_3$	1.51		

The other important series of esters examined by Taft is that of benzoic esters containing one ortho-substituent. The relation of the parent benzoic esters to other esters is given by the third entry on the left in Table 62-9: the benzoate-minus-formate difference is 0.11. The σ^* values for the ortho-substituted benzoic esters relative to benzoic esters are set out in Table 62-10. They are believed to be purely polar values, and hence one would like to compare them with meta- or para- σ values, which are also purely polar for a different reason. In the benzene ring, we have the complication of interior conjugation, and so Taft makes comparison primarily with para- σ values, in the belief that the conjugative contributions to the conveyance of polarity from the substituent to the test group are more nearly comparable as between *o*- and *p*-, than as between *o*- and *m*-substituents. The ortho-para comparisons are in Table 62-10.

Supposing steric effects to have been completely eliminated, we still do not expect the two sets of constants to be identical. For, first, the field effect will be differently weighted in the two positions; and second, the polar paths, though analogously composed of conjugation and induction, are by no means identical. But we should expect purely

TABLE 62-10.—TAFT'S σ^* CONSTANTS FOR ORTHO-SUBSTITUENTS IN BENZOATES.

Substituent X in ·CO·Ph	σ^* for ortho-X rel. to benzoates	σ for para-X
OMe	−0.39	−0.27
Me	−0.17	−0.17
F	0.24	0.06
Cl	0.20	0.23
Br	0.21	0.23
I	0.21	0.18
NO_2	0.78	0.78

polar substituent constants to follow similar trends in the two positions. And this is approximately what Table 62-10 shows.

Taft proposed that the changes induced by substituents in log k or log K in reactions other than those of ester hydrolysis (for which substituent constants σ^* can be determined) will be found proportional to the σ^* values of the substituents as given by ester hydrolysis. This proposition may be written,

$$\log (K/K_0) \quad \text{or} \quad \log (k/k_0) = \rho^*\sigma^*$$

where ρ^* is an empirically determined proportionality constant for the reaction. In graphical terms, this means that log k or log K, plotted against σ^*, should give a straight line of slope ρ^*.

This relation is not characterised by the accuracy to which we were introduced in a restricted field by the Roberts-Moreland equation, or the equal and much more widespread accuracy to which the Yukawa-Tsuno relation has accustomed us. When Taft's relation was promulgated, our standards had not thus been raised. Some reactions fit well, but some fit indifferently. This relation cannot have general accuracy extending over reactions in which steric effects are important, because it compares log K or log k, which in principle are dependent on both polar and steric factors, with σ^*, which is designed to be dependent on polar effects only. One cannot get a straight line, or any other sort of line, by plotting a function of two independent variables of comparable importance, which are both allowed to vary, against a function of one of those variables only.

This takes us back to the historical beginnings of linear free-energy relations. For the theoretical position is quite similar to that of the Brönsted relation. Here, one compares catalytic log k with acidic log K, two quantities which are in principle dependent on both polar and steric effects, but with different relative weightings. The fact that, by leaving out the worst-fitting groups of cases, one can achieve the mediocre linearity illustrated in Fig. 62-1 (p. 1198) means only that, for these reactions, polar effects are much more important than steric, so that variations in the relative weighting of the factors have no more than a small absolute effect. In a plot like that illustrated, one is seeing the line consequent on a dominating polar effect through a cloud of small or medium-sized steric disturbances. Brönsted plots are to do with protolytic processes, and in such, steric effects are of somewhat small general importance, just as they are in olefin eliminations (cf. Section **39**); and the reason is the same, namely that, in both types of reaction, protons are transferred from relatively exposed situations.

For many classes of reaction, besides those of general-acid catalysis, polar effects dominate over steric. And as long as the steric contribution remains minor, we can expect to be able approximately to correlate a measured quantity dependent in principle on polar and steric effects, but in practice mainly on polar effects, with a quantity designed to measure polar effects only. Many of the reactions to which the Brönsted relation has been applied with some success appear again in the lists of reactions which have been offered by Taft in support of his proportionality relation. So do many other reactions in which again only relatively unimportant steric effects would be expected. However, though it is limited in application and precision, Taft's $\rho^*\sigma^*$ relation does extend the range of reactions for which the general truth can be numerically demonstrated that polar effects are ubiquitous in organic chemistry, showing widespread domination, and that small steric effects are also widespread, but that strong steric effects require special structural circumstances for their development.

CHAPTER XVII

Stable Radicals

AN EXPLANATION is needed of the word "stable" in the title of this Chapter. In Chapter V we surveyed the general methods of production of radicals. In Chapters VI, VII, and XIII we considered the main classes of reactions in which radicals engage with aromatic, aliphatic, and olefinic compounds. In these studies the point of view throughout was kinetic. The thermodynamic matter of the stability of radicals was therefore left untouched. Most kinetically important radicals are quite unstable relative to their factors and products. Any quantitative knowledge that we can obtain as to the thermodynamic stability of radicals must come from measurements of the proportions in which the radicals arise in homolysis-colligation equilibria. Such knowledge is therefore restricted to radicals that do arise in measurable equilibrium proportions. It is restricted to radicals which are much more stable than most of the kinetically important radicals, and are, indeed, among the most stable organic radicals known.

(63) ARYLMETHYL, ARYLAMINYL, AROXYL, AND RELATED RADICALS

(63a) The Triphenylmethyl Radical.—In 1900 Gomberg,[1] in attempting to prepare hexaphenylethane from triphenylmethyl chloride by reaction with silver, obtained a colourless solid substance, whose yellow solution in benzene showed great reactivity. Oxygen was immediately absorbed to give a peroxide, $Ph_3C \cdot O \cdot O \cdot CPh_3$. So was nitric oxide to give the nitroso-compound $Ph_3C \cdot NO$. And so was iodine to form triphenyliodomethane, Ph_3CI. For these and similar reasons, Gomberg regarded his substance as the radical, triphenylmethyl, Ph_3C. Its molecular weight, as given by the depression of the freezing point of benzene, was, however, very much nearer that of hexaphenylethane, Ph_6C_2, than that of triphenylmethyl, Ph_3C.

Gomberg was more impressed by the colour and the reactivity than by the molecular weight. However, Heintschel[2] and also Jacobson[3] made attempts to reconcile the colour and chemical properties with the molecular weight, by devising for Gomberg's substance quinonoid structures of the molecular weight of hexaphenylethane, but of such

[1] M. Gomberg, *J. Am. Chem. Soc.*, 1900, **22,** 757; *Ber.*, 1900, **33,** 3150.
[2] K. Heintschel, *Ber.*, 1903, **36,** 320, 579.
[3] P. Jacobson, *Ber.*, 1905, **38,** 196.

unknown types that they could at that time be assumed to have the necessary colour and reactivity. In this period appraisal of the evidence was made the more difficult by some further observations to which we shall come; but there were some, notably Baeyer,[4] Flurscheim,[5] and Werner,[6] who, despite these complexities, could see the picture of a dissociative equilibrium involving a densely coloured, highly reactive radical, in a proportion too small for measurement by the cryoscopic method. Then, in 1908, this picture was completely exposed by Schmidlin,[7] who discovered the rate difference between the dissociation which produced triphenylmethyl and the reactions of that substance with reagents such as Gomberg had used. Schmidlin employed that difference to demonstrate the distinct and successive character of these processes:

$$\underset{\text{colourless}}{Ph_3C\cdot CPh_3} \underset{\text{slow}}{\overset{\text{benzene}}{\rightleftharpoons}} \underset{\text{yellow}}{2Ph_3C\cdot} \underset{\text{fast}}{\overset{O_2}{\longrightarrow}} \underset{\text{precipitated}}{Ph_3C\cdot O\cdot O\cdot CPh_3}$$

When the yellow solution in benzene was shaken with air, the colour was immediately discharged, and the peroxide was precipitated in an amount which accounted for only a small proportion (some units %) of the original hexa-arylethane. But, oxygen being excluded, the colour returned in a matter of minutes, and then, by admitting oxygen, it could again be immediately discharged, with the precipitation of a further similarly small proportion of peroxide. This cycle could then be repeated a number of times.

One factor which complicated the early judgments arose as a consequence of Walden's observation of 1903 that hexaphenylethane gave highly electrically conducting, deep yellow solutions in sulphur dioxide.[8] A different dissociative process was here under observation:

$$Ph_3C\cdot CPH_3 \overset{SO_2}{\rightleftharpoons} Ph_3C^+ + Ph_3C^-$$

The cation was that of solutions, well known to Walden, of triphenylmethyl chloride in sulphur dioxide. The anion was that of triphenyl methyl-sodium in basic solvents such as ammonia. So, one had to reckon with "three triphenylmethyls," the cation, the radical, and the anion, Ph_3C^+, $PH_3C\cdot$, and PH_3C^-; and it was at first not always easy

[4] A. v. Baeyer and V. Villiger, *Ber.*, 1902, **35**, 1189.

[5] B. Flurscheim, *J. prak. Chem.*, 1905, **71**, 505.

[6] A. Werner, *Ber.*, 1906, **39**, 1278.

[7] J. Schmidlin, *Ber.*, 1908, **41**, 2471.

[8] P. Walden, *Z. physik. Chem.*, 1903, **43**, 386.

to remember that they are very different entities, and that observations or conclusions relating to any one of them could not automatically be carried into the chemistry of the others.

The other main factor of complication consisted in the mesomerism of all the "triarylmethyls," in particular the radical and the cation. In 1907 Gomberg convinced himself that the radical had a quinonoid constitution[9] (which in part it has). His evidence was that the bromine atom in *p*-bromophenyl-diphenylmethyl could be extracted with metallic silver, as though the carbon atom which carried it lacked benzenoid character (which in part it did). This type of *p*-halogen lability was reproduced in other examples, and new evidence was adduced which actually applied to the cation, rather than the radical.[10] This was that tri-(*p*-bromophenyl)methyl chloride, though it undergoes no change in solvent benzene, comes into equilibrium with *p*-chlorophenyl-di-(*p*-bromophenyl)methyl bromide in solution in sulphur dioxide. This shows that the originally dissociating chloride ion can return to a *p*-carbon atom (as the mesomeric structure of the carbonium ion would allow) so to give a quinonoid molecule,

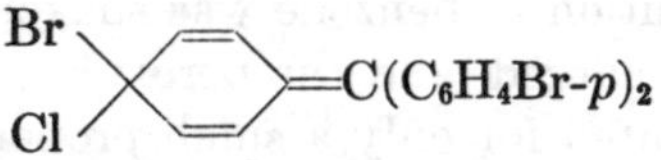

$$\text{(Br)(Cl)}C_6H_4{=}C(C_6H_4Br\text{-}p)_2$$

from which either chloride ion or bromide ion can dissociate, finally to recombine at the central carbon atom producing the isomers found.

(63b) Rate and Extent of Formation of Triphenylmethyl.—There are three methods in general of measuring the compositions in dissociation equilibria in which radicals are more or less extensively produced. The most widely used in the triarylmethyl series is by cryoscopic determination of mean molecular weight. But this is unsuitable for measuring the dissociation of hexaphenylethane, because the error of the method, a few units percent, is of the same order of magnitude as the degree of dissociation in the usual cryoscopic solvents, such as benzene, at the concentrations convenient for cryoscopic measurements.

The second method is by colorimetric estimation of the concentration of the radical. This is suitable to the case of hexaphenylethane, because one can work at much higher dilutions, thereby increasing the degree of dissociation. It is, indeed, a necessity of the method that one can go to high degrees of dissociation, since for calibration purposes one has to know the extinction coefficient of the radical. In

[9] M. Gomberg, *Ber.*, 1907, **40,** 1851.

[10] M. Gomberg and H. Cone, *Ann.*, 1910, **376,** 183; M. Gomberg and D. D. van Slyke, *J. Am. Chem. Soc.*, 1911, **33,** 531.

other words, one must be able to match the deviations from Beer's law to Ostwald's dilution law.

The third method is by measurement of the magnetic property of the unpaired electron in the radical. The older approach to this, *viz.*, by measurement of the paramagnetic susceptibility of the radical as a whole, is not satisfactory, because it is at present impossible sufficiently reliably to compute the magnetic-orbit diamagnetism of the radical, on which the paramagnetism of the unpaired electron is superposed. However, measurement by means of the electron-spin magnetic-resonance spectrum is reliable, because it is a direct measurement of the spin inversions of unpaired spins in the externally applied magnetic field, and is thus independent of the magnetic properties of the orbital motion of the electrons as a whole. The position of the line in the magnetic-resonance spectrum gives the energy difference due to spin inversion in the magnetic field, and the suitably calibrated line intensity gives the density of unpaired spins, and hence the concentration of radicals. Very low concentrations of radicals, $10^{-7}M$ or less, can be detected in this way, and larger concentrations can be measured. Additional information is frequently forthcoming. Magnetic interaction between the unpaired electron and not-too-distant atomic nuclei with spin, particularly the protons of bound hydrogen atoms, appears as a hyperfine splitting of the electron-spin resonance line. This helps to locate the unpaired electron in the radical. Distribution of the unpaired electron by mesomerism among several atoms may lead to several electron-spin resonance lines, each with its characteristic hyperfine splitting. From the relative intensities one may deduce the quantitative distribution of the unpaired electron among its possible positions. In accordance with the uncertainty principle, short-lived radicals have diffuse energy levels, and hence give broad electron-spin lines. Radical half-lives in the range 10^{-10}–10^{-6} second can be estimated by line-width in the electron-spin magnetic-resonance spectrum.

It was shown in 1911 by Piccard[11] that the colour of solutions of hexaphenylethane gave evidence of its dependence on dissociation by its deviations from Beer's law, *i.e.*, by the increase of total colour on dilution. On this basis, Ziegler and Ewald in 1929 developed a calibrated method for measurement of equilibrium compositions, and hence for the determination of equilibrium constants.[12] Thus, for solutions of hexaphenylethane in benzene at 20°, the relation between the percentage dissociation, 100α, and the dilution, $v=[Ph_6C_2]^{-1}$, ran

[11] J. Piccard, *Ann.*, 1911, **381,** 347.
[12] K. Ziegler and L. Ewald, *Ann.*, 1929, **473,** 163.

as follows:

v (M^{-1})...........	12.5	98	885	25,700	76,000
100α.............	3.6	9.6	25.8	77.5	90

These figures lead to the equilibrium constant,

$$K = [Ph_3C]^2/[Ph_6C_2] = 4.1 \times 10^{-4} \text{ mole/l.}$$

The temperature coefficient of the equilibrium constant gave the increment of enthalpy as 11.3 kcal./mole, and the increment of entropy as 23.1 cal./mole/deg. The increase in free energy was only 4.54 kcal./mole; and so, as always, entropy is an important factor promoting dissociation. We shall refer in Section **63d** to Ziegler and Ewald's work on solvent effects on these quantities.

Ziegler, Ewald, and Orth showed that the reaction of hexaphenylethane with iodine is a first-order process, the rate of which is independent of the concentration of iodine.[13] Evidently the iodination was an S_H1 reaction, rate-controlled by a slow preliminary homolysis:

$$\left.\begin{aligned} Ph_3C\cdot CPh_3 &\xrightleftharpoons{\text{slow}} Ph_3C\cdot + Ph_3C\cdot \\ Ph_3C\cdot + I_2 &\xrightarrow{\text{fast}} Ph_3C\cdot I + I\cdot \end{aligned}\right\} \quad (S_H1)$$

Although the preliminary homolysis would be considerably reversed in the absence of a trap for the formed radicals, it goes forward to completion in the presence of such a fast-acting trap as iodine is. Thus, by following the uptake of iodine kinetically, one has a method of measuring the rate of dissociation of hexaphenylethane.

Ziegler, Orth, and Weber established similar kinetics for the uptake of nitric oxide.[14] Provided that this is above a certain minimum pressure, it is sufficiently fast-acting as a trap for triphenylmethyl radicals to furnish a first-order reaction, with a rate independent of the pressure of nitric oxide. Here, then, is another S_H1 process:

$$\left.\begin{aligned} Ph_3C\cdot CPh_3 &\xrightleftharpoons{\text{slow}} Ph_3C\cdot + Ph_3C\cdot \\ Ph_3C\cdot + NO &\xrightarrow{\text{fast}} Ph_3C\cdot NO \end{aligned}\right\} \quad (S_H1)$$

Again the measured rate was that of the preliminary homolysis. It was essentially identical with the rate of uptake of iodine in the same solvent and at the same temperature.

Ziegler, Ewald, Seib, and Luttringhaus showed that the uptake of

[13] K. Ziegler, L. Ewald, and P. Orth, *Ann.*, 1930, **479**, 277.
[14] K. Ziegler, P. Orth, and K. Weber, *Ann.*, 1933, **504**, 131.

oxygen by hexaphenylethane went faster than the uptake of nitric oxide.[15] They traced the discrepancy to the incursion, in autoxidation, of a chain reaction initiated by formed triphenylmethylperoxy radicals, which to an appreciable extent attack undissociated hexaphenylethane molecules. They overcame this complication by adding a known trap for the peroxy radicals, *viz.*, pyrogallol, which hydrogenated them to give, as the final product, triphenylmethyl hydroperoxide:

$$\left.\begin{array}{r}
Ph_3C\cdot CPh_3 \underset{}{\overset{\text{slow}}{\rightleftharpoons}} Ph_3C\cdot + Ph_3C\cdot \\
Ph_3C\cdot + O_2 \xrightarrow{\text{fast}} Ph_3C\cdot O\cdot O\cdot \\
Ph_3C\cdot O\cdot O\cdot + H \xrightarrow{\text{fast}} Ph_3C\cdot O\cdot OH
\end{array}\right\} \qquad (S_H1)$$

The rate of uptake of oxygen was now of first order, and was independent of the oxygen pressure. Being controlled by the same preliminary homolysis, it was identical with the rate of uptake of nitric oxide in like conditions.

On grounds of mutual consistency, Ziegler regarded the rates of chain-quenched autoxidation, and of nitric oxide uptake, as the most accurate measures of the rate of dissociation. The rates measured by the iodine method tended to run somewhat high, probably because of some uneliminated side-reaction. For the rate of dissociation of hexaphenylethane in toluene at 0°, he and his collaborators found $k_1 = 0.0025$ sec.$^{-1}$. From the temperature coefficient of the rate, they obtained the Arrhenius frequency factor, 0.5×10^{-13} sec.$^{-1}$, a normal figure for a unimolecular reaction. The Arrhenius energy of activation was 19.0 ± 1.0 kcal./mole. They also studied the effect of solvent variation on these kinetic parameters, with results which will be noted in Section **63d**.[14,15,16]

Taking the endothermicity of dissociation of hexaphenylethane as having an average value of 11.5 kcal./mole in the usual solvents, and the activation energy of homolysis as 19 kcal./mole, it follows that the activation energy of radical colligation is 7.5 kcal./mole. Thus the radicals do not just fall together, but have to be pressed together before they can colligate. Two reasons for this can be suggested. One is that the radical centre is distributed by mesomerism in the three phenyl groups, and must be concentrated at the exo-cyclic carbon atom to permit colligation. The other is that the central bonds of the free

[15] K. Ziegler, L. Ewald, and A. Seib, *Ann.*, 1933, **504**, 162, 182; K. Ziegler and A. Luttringhaus, *ibid.*, p. 189.

[16] K. Ziegler, A. Seib, K. Knoevenagel, P. Herte, and F. Andreas, *Ann.*, 1942, **551**, 150.

radical are coplanar, and must be bent towards a pyramidal configuration in order to allow colligation. Energy must be supplied for the inception of these processes, before much becomes returned by the resulting colligation.

(63c) Effects of Structure on the Stability of Triarylmethyls.—Throughout the first decade of this century, the difficulty of detecting in a cryoscopic molecular weight the dissociation of hexaphenylethane, or of any of its simple substitution products that were investigated in that period, had remained a source of unease. It was therefore an important event when, in 1910, Schlenk and his coworkers reported triarylmethyls whose equilibrium degrees of formation by dissociation of the hexa-arylethanes were large, and in one case total. The systems examined were those obtained by replacing one, then two, and then all three phenyl groups of triphenylmethyl by *p*-biphenylyl groups, *p*-$C_6H_5 \cdot C_6H_4$—. The result was that, in benzene at 5°, and in the concentrations 2–3% convenient for cryoscopic measurement, the percentage of dissociation into radicals increased from below the limits of measurement by that method in triphenylmethyl, to 15%, to 80%, and to 100%, as the three phenyl groups were successively replaced. The radicals were, of course, all deeply coloured. On evaporation of the benzene solutions, the radical with one biphenylyl group recolligated to give back the colourless hexa-arylethane. So did the radical with two biphenylyl groups, despite the great extent of its formation in solution. But the radical with three biphenylyl groups refused to recolligate, and on evaporation was recovered as a black solid—the first crystalline triarylmethyl radical.

This pioneering investigation showed clearly that one could increase the equilibrium degree of dissociation of a hexa-arylethane by expanding the aryl groups to polynuclear forms. It was later shown that this could also be done by the use of naphthyl groups, phenyl-substituted vinyl groups, and other polynuclear groups. Examples are shown in the upper part of Table 63-1.

The simple alkyl and halogen substitution products of hexaphenylethane show small degrees of dissociation, comparable with those of hexaphenylethane itself. But these substitution products have been less accurately investigated, with the result that most of the reported figures are not reliable enough to quote, and provide no differences of any value for the purpose of defining the effect of the substituent on the homolytic equilibria. The known strong effects of polar substituents in hexaphenylethane on these equilibria come mainly from the *o*- and *p*-methoxyl and the *p*-nitro-substituents; and data relating to

TABLE 63-1.—APPROXIMATE PERCENTAGES OF HOMOLYTIC DISSOCIATION OF HEXA-ARYLETHANES IN BENZENE AT 5° AND IN CONCENTRATIONS 2–3% BY WEIGHT.

Hexa-arylethane[a]	% Dissoc.	Ref.	Hexa-arylethane[a]	% Dissoc	Ref.
$\{Ph_3C—\}_2$	~5	*b*	$\{\beta$-$NaphPh_2C—\}_2$	33	18
$\{p$-$BiphPh_2C—\}_2$	15	17	$\{\alpha$-$NaphPh_2C—\}_2$	60	18
$\{p$-$Biph_2PhC—\}_2$	80	17	$\{Ph_2C{:}CH\cdot CPh_2—\}_2$	80	19
$\{p$-$Biph_3C—\}_2$	~100	17	$\left\{\begin{matrix}PhC{:}CPh \\ \vert \\ PhC{:}CPh\end{matrix} > CPh—\right\}_2$	100	20
$\{o$-$MeOC_6H_4\cdot CPh_2—\}_2$	26	21	$\{(m$-$MeOC_6H_4)_3C—\}_2$	13	22
$\{(o$-$MeOC_6H_4)_2CPh—\}_2$	40	22	$\{p$-$MeOC_6H_4\cdot CPh_2—\}_2$	23	24
$\{(o$-$MeOC_6H_4)_3C—\}_2$	80—100	23	$\{(p$-$NO_2C_6H_4)_3C—\}_2$	100	25

[a] *p*-Biph = *p*-biphenylyl; Naph = Naphthyl.
[b] Calculated from the enthalpy and entropy (Section **62b**)

these groups are in the lower part of Table 63-1. Methoxyl is strongly electropositively conjugating, and nitroxyl strongly electronegatively conjugating: both cause marked increases in the extent of radical formation.

The data of Table 63-1 were discussed by Burton and the writer in 1929, on lines that have remained essentially unchanged.[26] The latter discussion, part of which applied to the theory of organic chemistry as a whole, was the first which related mesomerism to the uncertainty principle, so taking the driving force of conjugative electron redistribution to be of quantal origin. Effects of polar conjugation on carbonium ions and carbanions were discussed. A conjugated $+M$-type

[17] W. Schlenk, T. Weinkal, and A. Herzenstein, *Ann.*, 1910, **372,** 1; W. Schlenk and A. Herzenstein, *Ber.*, 1910, **43,** 1753.

[18] M. Gomberg and C. S. Schoepfle, *J. Am. Chem. Soc.*, 1917, **39,** 1652; M. Gomberg and F. W. Sullivan, *ibid.*, 1922, **44,** 1810.

[19] K. Ziegler, *Ann.*, 1923, **434,** 34.

[20] K. Ziegler and B. Schnell, *Ann.*, 1925, **445,** 266.

[21] M. Gomberg and D. Nishida, *J. Am. Chem. Soc.*, 1923, **45,** 190.

[22] S. T. Bowden, *J. Chem. Soc.*, **1957,** 4235.

[23] H. Lund, *J. Am. Chem. Soc.*, 1927, **49,** 1346.

[24] M. Gomberg and O. C. Buckler, *J. Am. Chem. Soc.*, 1923, **45,** 207.

[25] K. Ziegler and E. Boye, *Ann.*, 1927, **458,** 248.

[26] C. K. Ingold, *Ann. Reports on Progress Chem.* (Chem. Soc. London), 1928, **25,** 164; H. Burton and C. K. Ingold, *Proc. Leeds Phil. Soc.*, Sci. Sect., 1929, **1,** 421.

substituent would stabilise a carbonium ion by spreading the electron deficiency so that no valency orbital remained wholly unoccupied, *e.g.*, MeÖ—C⁺. A conjugated $-M$-type substituent would stabilise a carbanion by spreading its unshared electrons, so allowing all conjugated electrons some shared character, *e.g.*, O_2N—C⁻. The main point of the more specialised part of the discussion was that a carbon radical, with its one-electron deficiency and its one unshared electron, needed both those spreading processes to give it stability. The special property of aryl and conjugated arylvinyl substituents was that they were ambipolar, that is, $\pm M$-substituents. This was the key to their singular effectiveness for the building of stable carbon radicals:

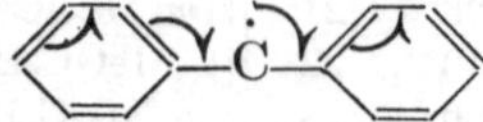

The more the conjugation, that is, the more the spreading of both the kinds described, as in polynuclear aryl groups, the better for radical stability, as illustrated in the upper portion of Table 63-1. Today we think the same, though we would add that steric effects play a certain part. But the more general cause must be polar. Steric effects could not, for example, be held responsible for the great increase in dissociation which occurs when phenyl substituents are replaced by *p*-biphenylyl substituents.

Carbon is an element whose cation and anion, when charges are localised, are both too unstable, relatively to reaction products, to allow the ions any permanent existence in solution. Even in the triphenyl-substituted ions Ph_3C^+ and Ph_3C^-, which by reason of their spread charges can exist in solution, there is plenty of room for further stabilisation by appropriate polar substituents in the phenyl groups. A $+M$ substituent, such as *o*- or *p*-methoxyl, will thus stabilise the cation, and a $-M$ substituent, such as *o*- or *p*-nitroxyl, will stabilise the anion. It could be deduced[26] that such strong improvements in ion stability would be reflected in the effect of the polar substituents on radical stability. For *o*- and *p*-methoxyl and for *p*-nitroxyl we have the data to show that this is so, as illustrated in the lower portion of Table 63-1.

When one phenyl group of each trio in hexaphenylethane is replaced by an alkyl group (not more bulky than phenyl), no measurable or even visible amount of a diphenylalkyl radical is formed in equilibrium at, or anywhere near, room temperature, though such radicals are formed as kinetic intermediates at rates which can be measured by Ziegler's methods. However, when the group replacing phenyl is not alkyl, but is a group of the $-M$ class, such as an acyl or cyano-group, then, as Löwenbein and his collaborators have shown,[27] discernible equilibrium homolysis may arise. Though these $-M$ groups, supplementing two phenyl groups, have a distinct effect in promoting homolytic dissociation, they are not as good for that purpose as a third $\pm M$ phenyl group would be. Thus, diphenylbenzoylmethyl is formed in equilibrium from its dimer to just about the same extent in boiling toluene as triphenylmethyl is from its dimer in freezing benzene. The following is a sample of equilibrium constants governing the homolytic formation of diarylacylmethyls in toluene at 110°:

	Ph—Ċ(Me)—Ph	Ph—Ċ(CO·Ph)—Ph
10^4K....	0.0	4.3

(benzene ring)—ĊPh—CO—O (lactone)	(naphthalene ring)—ĊPh—CO—O (lactone)
6.6	88

The effect of cyano-groups in promoting dissociation, though discernible by reversible colour development on heating in solvents, is smaller than that of acyl groups.

When a phenyl group in each trio in hexaphenylethane is replaced by a bulky aliphatic substituent, dissociation to radicals may be increased. This was strikingly shown by Schlenk and Mark,[28] who used triphenylmethyl as the replacing group. It is, of course, an aliphatic group (aralphyl), having no direct conjugation with the seat of dissociation. Presumably it acts by building up non-bonding pressure: models show that, unlike hexaphenylethane, it would do so in all conformations. Supplementing two phenyl groups in the stabilisation of a carbon radical, it is highly effective—much more effective than a third phenyl group. In benzene at the freezing point decaphenyl-*n*-

[27] A. Löwenbein, *Ber.*, 1925, **50**, 601; *idem* and R. F. Gargarin, *ibid.*, p. 2643; A. Löwenbein and H. Schmidt, *Ber.*, 1927, **60**, 1851; A. Löwenbein and L. Schuster, *Ann.*, 1930, **481**, 106.

[28] W. Schlenk and E. Mark, *Ber.*, 1922, **55**, 2285, 2299.

butane is wholly dissociated into pentaphenylethyl. Conant and his coworkers examined the effect of *t*-butyl as a replacing group.[29] It also assists two phenyl groups in stabilising a carbon radical, but not as well as a phenyl group would. The formation of diphenyl*neo*pentyl radical from its ethane dimer is only a trace conversion, indicated by a faint colour in solvents at temperatures up to 50°. (Above that temperature the substance decomposes with loss of colour.) When the phenyl group in Schlenk's phenyldi-*p*-biphenylylethyl is replaced by *t*-butyl, the resulting radical, di-*p*-biphenylyl*neo*pentyl, is only a little less extensively formed. These examples are set out below, with figures which can be compared with those of related examples in Table 63-1.

	$Ph—\dot{C}(CPh_3)—Ph$	$Ph—\dot{C}(CMe_3)—Ph$	$p\text{-}PhC_6H_4—\dot{C}(CMe_3)—C_6H_4Ph\text{-}p$
% Dissociation in cold solvents....	100%	~0%	60%, 0.06M, C_6H_6, 5°

(63d) Solvent Effects on the Rate and Extent of Formation of Triphenylmethyl.—Some of the rate and equilibrium constants determined by Ziegler and his collaborators for the homolysis of hexaphenylethane in a variety of solvents are assembled in Table 63-2. The rate figures [14,15,16] are first-order constants at 0°. The equilibrium constants[12] are for 20°. The same solvents were not usually taken for

TABLE 63-2.—RATE AND EQUILIBRIUM CONSTANTS FOR THE HOMOLYSIS OF HEXAPHENYLETHANE IN VARIOUS SOLVENTS (ZIEGLER).

Rate: k_1 in sec.$^{-1}$ at 0°		*Equilibrium:* K in mole/l. at 20°	
Solvent	10^3k_1	Solvent	10_4K
Acetonitrile	1.1	Propionitrile	1.2
Ethyl cyanoacetate	1.8	Ethyl benzoate	1.7
Mesityl oxide	2.1	Acetophenone	1.7
Pyridine	2.2	Dioxan	2.5
Toluene	2.5	Bromobenzene	3.7
Ethyl alcohol	2.8	—	—
Ethylene bromide	3.3	Ethylene bromide	3.9
—	—	Benzene	4.1
Carbon tetrachloride	3.9	Chloroform	6.9
Carbon disulphide	4.2	Carbon disulphide	19.2

[29] J. B. Conant and N. M. Bigelow, *J. Am. Chem. Soc.*, 1928, **50**, 2041; J. B. Conant and R. F. Schultz, *ibid.*, 1933, **55**, 2098.

the two types of measurement, but they are matched as far as possible in two columns of the table, each of which follows the order of the figures.

The run of the rate figures is very different from any applying to heterolytic reactions. The high-dielectric solvent, acetonitrile, which gives relatively high rates in all heterolytic reactions of uncharged reactants, is the slowest of the solvents for the homolysis. The fastest solvents are the non-polar carbon tetrachloride and carbon disulphide. The hydroxylic solvent, ethyl alcohol, has no special position. The whole series of rates is comprised within a factor of 4. The equilibrium figures follow a roughly similar series. The equilibrium extent of formation of the radical is smallest in the aliphatic nitrile, and greatest in carbon disulphide. These figures show a generally wider spread than the others, and carbon disulphide provides a salient figure, with the result that the whole range covers a factor of 16.

It would seem that solvation differences widen from the transition state of homolysis to the final state, and that therefore the main factor controlling the solvent effects is solvation of the forming, or better, the fully formed, radical. The figures suggest a general relation with polarisability, and show that carbon disulphide, which, it may be recalled, is quite special in its power of destroying the spectroscopic symmetry of dissolved benzene (Section **14a**), and is thought to have a relatively high affinity for chlorine atoms (Section **37b**), is also able to solvate the carbon radical particularly well. This may be because sulphur in carbon disulphide is an unsaturated second-row element, possessing, and conferring on that molecule, both a low ionisation potential, and a low electron affinity arising from low-lying empty orbitals. Bearing in mind the presumed duplex nature of the internal processes of stabilisation of a carbon radical (Section **63c**), this capacity of carbon disulphide to offer easy interaction with both its electrons and its empty orbitals might be the key to its apparent affinity for the triphenylmethyl radical.

(63e) Diarylaminyls.[30]—Tetraphenylhydrazine was first prepared by Wieland in 1911. He obtained it by the oxidation of diphenylamine with potassium permanganate in acetone. It was a colourless substance, which gave solutions that were colourless at room temperature, but reversibly developed a green colour at temperatures near 100°. The coloured solutions did not obey Beer's law: the variation of colour intensity with dilution showed that the coloured material

[30] H. Wieland, *Ann.*, 1911, **381**, 200; H. Wieland and H. Lecher, *Ber.*, 1912, **45**, 2600; H. Wieland, *Ber.*, 1915, **48**, 1078.

was being produced by dissociation. Tetraphenylhydrazine took up nitric oxide to give diphenylnitrosamine, $Ph_2N \cdot NO$, and triphenylmethyl to produce pentaphenylmethylamine, $Ph_2N \cdot CPh_3$. Wieland ascribed the colour and reactions to the reversible formation of the diphenylaminyl radical:

$$Ph_2N \cdot NPh_2 \rightleftharpoons 2Ph_2N \cdot$$

The degree of dissociation was obviously small and was not measured in this example. However, Cain and Wiselogle subsequently employed the reaction with nitric oxide to measure the rate of dissociation of tetraphenylhydrazine.[31] The reaction is of first order, with a rate independent of the pressure of nitric oxide above a certain threshold pressure. It is another S_H1 reaction, and hence can be used to measure dissociation rate:

$$\left.\begin{array}{l} Ph_2N \cdot NPh_2 \xrightleftharpoons{\text{slow}} Ph_2N \cdot + Ph_2N \cdot \\ Ph_2N \cdot + NO \xrightarrow{\text{fast}} Ph_2N \cdot NO \end{array}\right\} \quad (S_H1)$$

The measurements were made in solvent *o*-dichlorobenzene at 75–100°. At 100° the rate-constant was 0.0037 sec.$^{-1}$. The set of rate data gave an Arrhenius frequency factor of about 10^{15} sec.$^{-1}$ and an activation energy of about 30 kcal./mole. Even though great accuracy is not claimed, the activation energy must be considerably greater than the endothermicity.

In the absence of a reagent, the system tetraphenylhydrazine-diphenylaminyl is susceptible, as Wieland showed,[30] to the disproportionation,

$$2\ Ph_2N \cdot NPh_2 \rightarrow 2Ph_2NH + \text{[dihydrophenazine ring structure with two NPh groups]}$$

Wieland studied the effect of polar substituents in the phenyl groups of tetraphenylhydrazine on the extent of its homolytic dissociation.[30] Tetraphenylhydrazine itself shows reversible colour development in boiling toluene (110°), but not in boiling benzene (80°). Tetra-*p*-tolylhydrazine shows such an effect in boiling benzene. Thus the *p*-methyl group seems to have a small promoting effect on the dissocia-

[31] C. K. Cain and F. Y. Wiselogle, *J. Am. Chem. Soc.*, 1940, **62**, 1163.

tion. But the strong effects came from $+M$ substituents electropositively conjugated with the seat of dissociation. Tetra-*p*-anisylhydrazine formed deep green solutions at room temperature and below. Its degree of dissociation was probably some units percent at cryoscopic concentrations, but not quite large enough to be measured at the freezing point of benzene or nitrobenzene (5–6°). However, tetra-*p*-dimethylaminophenyl-hydrazine forms strongly yellow solutions, in which it is dissociated to the extent of 10% in benzene and 20% in nitrobenzene at the freezing points of these solvents. The order of extent to which the substituents promote dissociation was therefore *p*-Me_2N > *p*-MeO > *p*-Me. At the other extreme, the $-M$ group *p*-NO_2 inhibited dissociation. Wieland commented on the way in which these effects follow those of the substituents on electrophilic aromatic substitution, and deviate from the pattern of substituent effects on the dissociations leading to triarylmethyls.

Burton and the writer discussed these phenomena.[26] They called attention to the polar dissymmetry of the aminyl radical, by pointing in parallel to the corresponding cation and anion. Unlike the tercligant carbon cation and anion, which apart from charge delocalisation can have no permanent existence in solution, the biligant nitrogen cation alone is unstable to that degree, whilst the anion is relatively stable. The main reason is, of course, that the nuclear charge of nitrogen is greater. Hence the chief requirement for the structural stabilisation of a biligant nitrogen radical is, as for the biligant cation, to spread, and thus partly to repair on nitrogen, the electron deficiency of the radical centre. The spreading of the unshared electrons matters much less. The argument is the same as that by which we concluded, by comparing related cations and anions, that, for example, the bromine atom should be, as it is known to be, an electrophilic radical (Section **55a**). The biligant nitrogen radical should likewise be an electrophilic radical. Hence we can understand the series of *p*-substituents found by Wieland for the promotion of thermodynamic stability in aminyl radicals: Me_2N > MeO > Me > H > NO_2.

(63f) Aroxyls.—The radicals we have to discuss here have relations to two familiar fields of chemistry. First, they belong to the general class of oxy-radicals RO·, formed by homolysis of peroxides, which are very well known as chain-initiating species. Their kinetic importance in this matter derives from the fact that they are unstable in the environments in which they are produced. Secondly, everyone is familiar with one group of comparatively stable aroxyl radicals, namely, the quinhydrones. There can be little doubt that they are made as stable as they are by their $+M$-type *o*- or *p*-hydroxyl substituents. However, their chemistry is complicated by their ionisation: they form reactive radical-anions with great ease.

In 1922, Goldschmidt[32] found that guaiacol (*o*-methoxyphenol), on oxidation by lead peroxide, forms a green solution, instantly decolorised by quinol or by triphenylmethyl. He suggested that the aroxyl radical was formed, and was only partly associated to its dimer, which, not unnaturally, but incorrectly, he took to be the diaryl peroxide. But neither the radical nor its dimer could be isolated. However, by working with dibenzoguaiacol, *i.e.*, 9-methoxy-10-phenanthrol, and using alkaline ferricyanide as the oxidising agent, he was able to obtain a colourless solid, and show that it was the dimer of the radical. The solutions of this substance were initially colourless; but they developed, over some hours at room temperature, a deepening yellow-green colour. Cryoscopic determinations of molecular weight showed that dissociation was occurring, to a limit, in the conditions used, of 37%. At any time, the colour could be instantly discharged by a reducing agent, such as quinol, or alternatively by triphenylmethyl. The product of reduction was the guaiacol, and the product of the reaction with triphenylmethyl, on hydrolysis, gave triphenylcarbinol.

Goldschmidt assumed that his homolytic equilibrium was between an aroxyl radical and a diaryl peroxide, $2\mathrm{ArO}\cdot \rightleftharpoons \mathrm{ArO}\cdot\mathrm{OAr}$. But, in common with all other reputed diaryl peroxides, this one has been shown not to exist as such, at least at ordinary temperatures. It appears that, in contrast to dialkyl and diacyl peroxides, the central bond of diaryl peroxides is weakened to destruction, presumably by the lateral aryl-oxygen conjugation. The isolable dimers of aroxyl radicals are got by ortho- or para-, O—C or C—C coupling of the radicals, not by O—O coupling. When a substituent is at the coupling position, O—C coupling to give an aryloxy*cyclo*hexadienone (which has the conjugation of an ester vinylogue) is preferred. Of course, when the substituent is a hydrogen atom, it migrates to give the phenolic tautomer, and the aromatisation becomes a factor in determining relative stability. In Goldschmidt's example, the coupling is necessarily ortho and involves O—C coupling. Hence the correct formulation of his equilibrium is as follows:[33]

[32] S. Goldschmidt, *Ber.*, 1922, **55**, 3194; *idem* and W. Schmidt, *ibid.*, p. 3197; S. Goldschmidt and C. Steigerwald, *Ann.*, 1924, **438**, 202; S. Goldschmidt, A. Vogt, and M. A. Bredig, *Ann.*, 1925, **445**, 123.

[33] E. Müller, K. Schurr, and K. Scheffler, *Ann.*, 1959, **627**, 132.

$$2\ (\text{OMe-substituted phenanthroxyl radical}) \rightleftharpoons \text{dimer}$$

OMe

2 ⇌

O

OMe

O

O

MeO

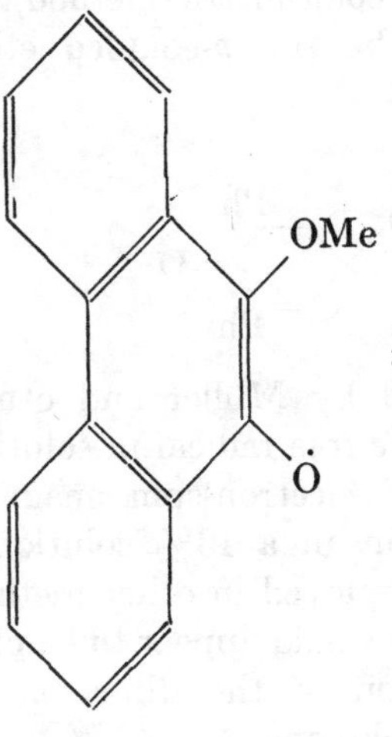

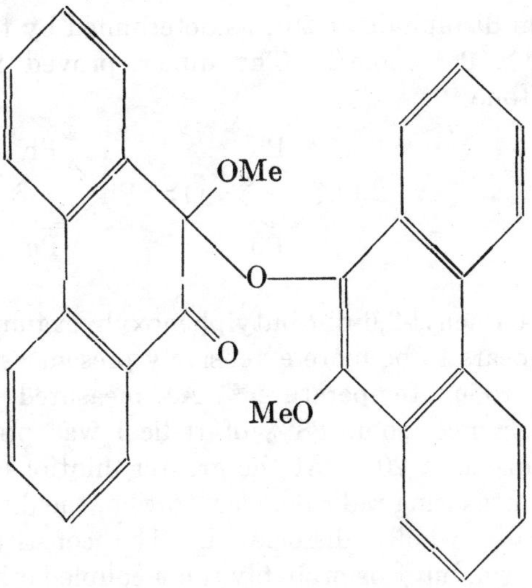

Thermodynamically, the aroxyl radicals which have been obtained in solution or as solids must be enormously more stable than their peroxide dimers, because their stability is comparable with or greater than that of the most stable of the ring-coupled isomers of the peroxides.

For the reasons explained in Section **63c**, aroxyl radicals, like diarylaminyl radicals, are expected to be electronegative, and therefore to be stabilised by *o*- or *p*-substituents of $+M$-type, such as methoxyl, or by $\pm M$ substituents, such as phenyl or the benzo-group, whose properties include the $+M$-property. Both types of stabilising groups are present in Goldschmidt's examples. Generalising, aroxyls 2,4,6-trisubstituted with phenyl, alkoxyl, and *t*-butyl groups are among the most stable radicals known. They are all obtained by Goldschmidt's methods of oxidising the related phenols with metal oxides or alkaline ferricyanide. The effectiveness of the *t*-butyl group is unexpected, but, as it appears to be required that such groups occupy ortho-positions, the development of steric pressures may be an important contributory cause.

2,4,6-Triphenylphenoxyl, studied by Dimroth and his coworkers, is obtainable in the solid state only as its dimer, with which, however, the radical comes into measurable equilibrium in solution at and near room temperature.[34] For example, the equilibrium constant in car-

[34] K. Dimroth, F. Kalk, and G. Neubauer, *Chem. Ber.*, 1957, **90**, 2098; K. Dimroth and G. Neubauer, *Angew. Chem.*, 1957, **69**, 95.

bon disulphide at 20°, as determined by the colorimetric method, was 2.4×10^{-5} mole/l. The dimer proved to be the *p*-coupled ether-ketone:[35]

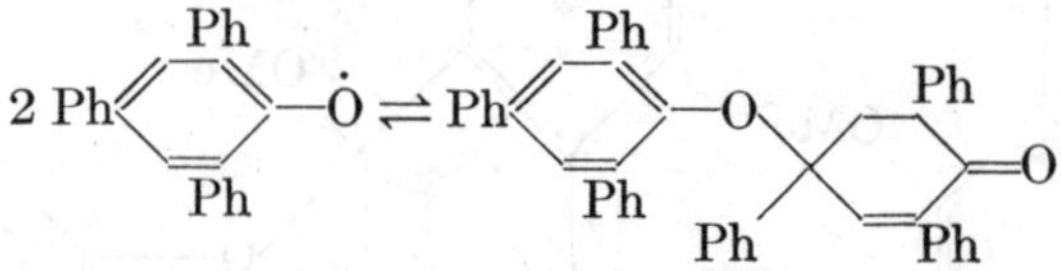

Ph Ph
2 Ph—⟨ring⟩—Ȯ ⇌ Ph—⟨ring⟩—O—⟨ring⟩=O
Ph Ph Ph Ph Ph Ph

4-Phenyl-2,6-di-*t*-butylphenoxyl, examined by Müller and others, appears to be more extensively present as the free radical in solutions at room temperature.[36] As measured by electron-spin magnetic resonance, some 88% of radical was present in a 10% solution in benzene at 20°. At the greater dilutions employed in other methods of measuring radical concentration, the dimer would appear to be practically wholly dissociated. The constitution of the dimer is not known, but it is probably the *p*-coupled ether-ketone.

2-Methoxy-4,6-di-*t*-butylphenoxyl, investigated by Petranek and his coworkers, and by Howgill and Middleton,[37] is a blue radical, which comes to measurable equilibrium in solution with its dimer. The dimer is shown by its proton-magnetic-resonance spectrum almost certainly to be the 4-coupled ether-ketone:

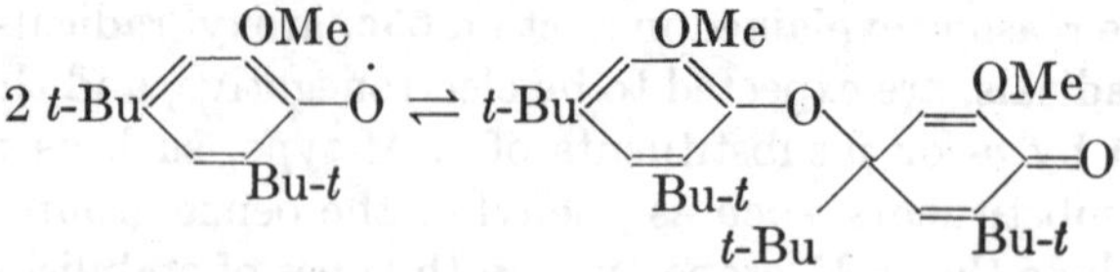

OMe OMe OMe
2 *t*-Bu—⟨ring⟩—Ȯ ⇌ *t*-Bu—⟨ring⟩—O—⟨ring⟩=O
Bu-*t* Bu-*t* *t*-Bu Bu-*t*

The two best-known aroxyl radicals which are fully stable in the solid state were both discovered contemporaneously by Cook and by Müller and their respective collaborators. They are 4-methoxy-2,6-di-*t*-butylphenoxyl[38] and 2,4,6-tri-*t*-butylphenoxyl.[39] They are both black solids, the former giving a red and the latter a blue solution. The formation of dimers has not been detected:

[35] K. Dimroth, F. Kalk, R. Sell, and K. Schlömer, *Ann.*, 1959, **624,** 51; K. Dimroth and A. Berudt, *Angew. Chem. internat. Edit.*, 1964, **3,** 385.

[36] E. Müller, A. Schick, and K. Scheffler, *Chem. Ber.*, 1959, **92,** 474.

[37] J. Petranek, J. Plieř, D. Doskočilova, *Tetrahedron Letters*, **1967,** 1979; F. R. Hewgill and B. S. Middleton, *J. Chem. Soc.*, **1967, C,** 2316.

[38] E. Müller and K. Ley, *Chem. Ber.*, 1955, **88,** 601; C. D. Cook, *J. Am. Chem. Soc.*, 1956, **78,** 2002.

[39] C. D. Cook, *J. Org. Chem.*, 1953, **18,** 291; C. D. Cook and R. C. Woodworth, *J. Am. Chem. Soc.*, 1953, **75,** 6242; E. Müller and K. Ley, *Chem. Ber.*, 1954, **87,** 922; *idem* and W. Kiedaisch, ibid., p. 1605.

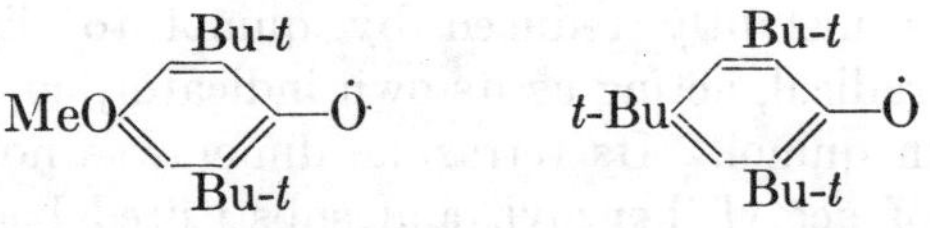

$$\text{MeO}\text{-C}_6\text{H}_2(\text{Bu-}t)_2\text{-}\dot{\text{O}} \qquad t\text{-Bu-C}_6\text{H}_2(\text{Bu-}t)_2\text{-}\dot{\text{O}}$$

Stable aroxyl radicals

(63g) Triaryl- and Diarylacyl-hydrazyls.[40]—In 1920, Goldschmidt discovered that the hexa-aryltetrazanes are more extensively dissociable to triarylhydrazyls than Wieland's tetra-arylhydrazines were to diarylaminyls. When triphenylhydrazine was shaken with lead peroxide in diethyl ether at room temperature, a deep blue solution was obtained, which contained much of the triphenylhydrazyl radical. When the experiment was repeated at $-60°$ in dimethyl ether, the hexaphenyltetrazane was isolated as a very pale green solid. Its blue solutions displayed the Beer's-law deviations indicative of a partial dissociation:

$$\text{Ph}_2\text{N}\cdot\text{NPh}\cdot\text{NPh}\cdot\text{NPh}_2 \rightleftharpoons 2\,\text{Ph}_2\text{N}\cdot\text{NPh}\cdot$$

The blue solution reacted instantly with quinol to give triphenylhydrazine, and instantly also with nitric oxide to give N-nitroso-triphenylhydrazine; and it reacted more slowly with triphenylmethyl. Left to itself, it decomposed to diphenylamine and quinone bis-diphenylhydrazone, $\text{Ph}_2\text{N}\cdot\text{N}{=}\text{C}_6\text{H}_4{=}\text{N}\cdot\text{NPh}_2$.

One other triarylhydrazyl may be particularly described, because of its remarkable stability, and because it is a link with the diarylacyl-hydrazyl series, to which we shall come. This is diphenylpicryl-hydrazyl, which Goldschmidt and Renn[40] prepared by condensing *as*-diphenylhydrazine with picryl chloride, and oxidising the formed diphenylpicrylhydrazine with lead peroxide in ether. They obtained the radical as a violet-black solid, looking like potassium permanganate. It was subsequently shown[41] to be paramagnetic, with a susceptibility consistent with that estimated for one unpaired electron-spin per molecule. Its electron-spin magnetic-resonance spectrum has been studied in detail.[42] The violet solution has a light absorption which obeyed Beer's law, and was not reduced in intensity on cooling to $-80°$. The molecular weight of the substance in solution was normal for the fully dissociated hydrazyl. It did not absorb nitric

[40] S. Goldschmidt, *Ber.*, 1920, **53**, 44; *idem* and K. Euler, *Ber.*, 1922, **55**, 616; S. Goldschmidt and K. Renn, *ibid.*, p. 628; S. Goldschmidt, *Ann.*, 1924, **437**, 194; *idem* and J. Bader, *Ann.*, 1929, **473**, 137.

[41] E. Müller, I. Müller-Rodloff, and N. Bunge, *Ann.*, 1935, **520**, 235.

[42] A. L. Buchachenko, "Stable Radicals," trans. C. N. Turton and T. I. Turton, Consultants Bureau, New York, 1965, Chap. 4.

oxide, but was instantly reduced by quinol to diphenylpicrylhydrazine. The radical, acting as its own indicator, could conveniently be titrated with quinol. Its tetrazane dimer was not obtained.

By the use of acetyl, benzoyl, and substituted benzoyl groups as the acyl substituents, Goldschmidt and his coworkers[40] prepared various diarylacylhydrazines of the type $Ar_2N \cdot NAcH$ and $ArAcN \cdot NArH$. By oxidation they converted these hydrazines into tetraaryldiacyltetrazanes and/or their homolysis products, diarylacylhydrazyls, of the types (A) and (B) below, which are respectively named $\alpha\alpha$-diaryl-β-acyl-β-hydrazyls and $\alpha\beta$-diaryl-α-acyl-β-hydrazyls:

$$Ar_2N \cdot NAc \cdot NAc \cdot NAr_2 \rightleftharpoons 2\ Ar_2N \cdot \dot{N}Ac \qquad \text{(A)}$$

$$ArAcN \cdot NAr \cdot NAr \cdot NArAc \rightleftharpoons 2\ ArAcN \cdot \dot{N}Ar \qquad \text{(B)}$$

Nearly all these radicals are stable in the sense of undergoing no self-decomposition, apart from their reversible colligation to the tetrazanes. Therefore they allowed this process to be studied in some detail. All the tetrazanes were at least partly dissociated in solution to hydrazyls; and some were totally dissociated. After dissolution of the tetrazanes, the equilibria were established observably slowly (often in a matter of minutes) at room temperature; and, when established, the equilibria could be "frozen" by cooling to low temperatures. As to reactions, most of the radicals combined more or less slowly with nitric oxide, and with triphenylmethyl; but all of them were instantly reduced, even at low temperatures, by quinol or by hydrazobenzene, to form the diarylacylhydrazines. On this distinction of rate between the slow formation and fast reduction of the radicals, Goldschmidt based a titrimetric method of measuring equilibrium degrees of dissociation. The solution was allowed to attain equilibrium at the required temperature. Then it was quickly cooled to a low temperature, and titrated to destruction of the colour by the reducing agent at that temperature.

Goldschmidt and his coworkers determined a large number of equilibrium constants for the dissociation of their tetrazanes in various solvents at various temperatures. The sample of their results contained in Table 63-3 refers to the formation of $\alpha\alpha$-diaryl-β-acyl-β-hydrazyls, and indicates the contrasting effects of polar structural changes in the "acyl" (we include picryl) and aryl groups.

The meaning of Table 13-3 is clearly that the greater the electron absorption into the acyl group, *and* the greater the electron release from the aryl groups, the more stable the radicals will be. In 1929 the observations were summarised in this way, and interpreted on the lines applied to other types of radicals,[26] as described in Sections

TABLE 63-3.—EQUILIBRIUM CONSTANTS (K IN MOLE/L.) FOR THE REACTIONS $Ar_2N \cdot NAc \cdot NAc \cdot NAr_2 \rightleftharpoons 2Ar_2N \cdot \dot{N}Ac$ (GOLDSCHMIDT).

Acyl in Radicals $Ph_2N \cdot \dot{N}Acyl$	Solvent	Temp.	Found 10^4K	Found or estimated for solvent toluene at −18°
Acetyl	Toluene	−18°	small	small
Benzoyl	Toluene	−18°	1.14	1.14
p-Nitrobenzoyl	Toluene	−18°	5.3	5.3
Picryl	Toluene	−18°	100% dissoc.	100% dissoc.
R, R in Radicals $(p\text{-}RC_6H_4)_2N \cdot \dot{N}(COPh)$				
NO_2, NO_2	Chloroform	0°	0.006	*ca.* 0.00014
NO_2, H	Chloroform	−18°	0.83	*ca.* 0.04
Br, Br	Toluene	−18°	0.145	0.145
Br, H	Toluene	−18°	0.33	0.33
H, H	Toluene	−18°	1.14	1.14
Me, H	Toluene	−18°	4.3	4.3
Me, Me	Toluene	−18°	17	17
MeO, H	Acetone	−18°	35	*ca.* 25
MeO, MeO	Acetone	−50°	100% dissoc.	100% dissoc.

63c–63f. The present application is conveniently approached by comparing the hydrazyls with the aminyls. Biligant aminyl radicals are electronegative, as was deduced from the much greater stability of the biligant nitrogen anion than of the biligant nitrogen cation. The hydrazyl radicals will be very much less electronegative, for whilst the related anion is in the same case as before, the corresponding cation, being now partly quadriligant, will be made more stable:

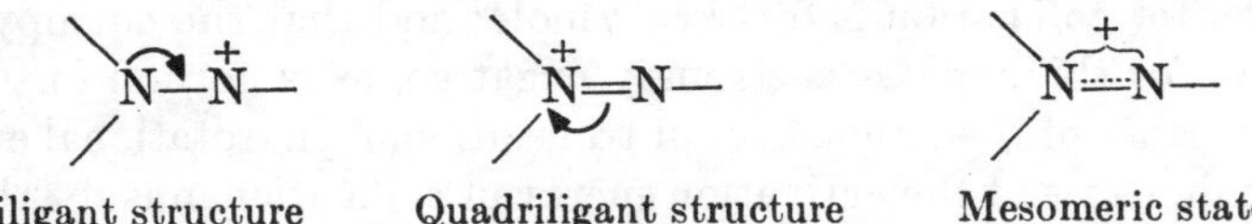

Biligant structure Quadriligant structure Mesomeric state

From the electronegativity of aminyl radicals, it was deduced that they will be stabilised by electropositive substituents, because it was much more important to spread (as for the related cation) the electron deficiency than to spread (as for the anion) the excess of unshared electrons. By an analogous argument, hydrazyl radicals will be stabilised both by electropositive and by electronegative substituents, because a similar importance now attaches to the spreading both of the electron deficiency and of the excess of unshared electrons:

$$\begin{array}{c} \diagdown \\ N{-}\dot{N}{-} \\ \diagup \end{array}$$

The principal canonical structures are the non-dipolar and dipolar structures,

$$\begin{array}{c}\diagdown\\ N{-}\dot{N}{-}\\ \diagup\end{array} \quad \text{and} \quad \begin{array}{c}\diagdown\\ \overset{\cdot+}{N}{-}\overset{-}{N}{-}\\ \diagup\end{array}$$

and it is the second of these, the dipolar structure, which is mainly responsible for the stabilising effects of polar substituents. Goldschmidt showed that both polar kinds of substitution do improve the stability of hydrazyls, and that both kinds of stabilisation can be made effective simultaneously. It has been shown[42] that, in diphenylpicrylhydrazyl, 62% of the unpaired spin is on the picryl-bearing nitrogen atom, as in the non-dipolar structure, whilst the remainder is on the other nitrogen atom, as in the dipolar structure, with a minor amount of dispersal into the phenyl rings.

Wilmarth and Schwartz have determined a series of both equilibrium-constants and rate-constants for the formation, from tetrazanes, of *p*-substituted $\alpha\alpha$-diphenyl-β-benzoyl-β-hydrazyls in solvent acetone, over such temperature ranges that energies and entropies of reaction, and of activation, can be calculated.[43] Some of their results are in Table 63-4. The homolyses are endothermic by 7–11 kcal./mole, and involve, as dissociation should, a large entropy increase. The energies of activation for homolysis are higher, about 15–17 kcal./mole; and the entropies of activation for homolysis are mildly negative, though this means little, because of the conventional omission from entropies of activation of entropy in the reaction coordinate (Section **6d**). By difference one finds that the energy of activation for colligation is 6–8 kcal./mole; and that the entropy of activation for this process is strongly negative, as is normal for associations because of the large losses of translational and rotational entropy. The main cause of the activation energy of colligation must be the need to effect some preliminary concentration of unpaired spin on the colligating nitrogen atoms, from the other nitrogen atom, and from the substituents.

The solvent effect[40] on these equilibria is considerably stronger than that applying to the equilibrium for homolysis of hexaphenylethane to triphenylmethyl (Section **63d**). Over the four solvents noted in Table 63-5, the equilibrium constants for homolysis to $\alpha\alpha$-diphenyl-β-

[43] W. K. Wilmarth and M. Schwartz, *J. Am. Chem. Soc.*, 1955, **77**, 4543.

TABLE 63-4.—ENERGIES (IN KCAL./MOLE) AND ENTROPIES (IN CAL./MOLE/DEG.) OF REACTION AND OF ACTIVATION OF THE REACTIONS $(p\text{-}RC_6H_4)_2N\cdot N(COPh)\cdot N(COPh)\cdot N(C_6H_4R\text{-}p)_2 \rightleftharpoons 2\ (p\text{-}RC_6H_4)_2N\cdot \dot{N}(COPh)$ IN SOLVENT ACETONE (WILMARTH AND SCHWARTZ).

R, R	Equilibrium		Homolysis		Colligation	
	ΔH	ΔS	$\Delta H^{\neq}$	$\Delta S^{\neq}$	$\Delta H^{\neq}$	$\Delta S^{\neq}$
Br, Br	11.2	25.1	17.2	−2.7	6.0	−27.8
Br, H	10.9	23.2	16.6	−6.6	5.7	−29.8
H, H	9.2	23.9	16.6	−7.6	7.4	−31.3
Me, H	7.9	19.6	15.8	−8.0	8.0	−27.6
Me, Me	6.7	18.0	15.0	−10.3	8.3	−28.3

benzoyl-β-hydrazyl at −18° cover an 80-fold range. Whereas the heat of the dissociation to triphenylmethyl is comparatively insensitive to changes of solvent, that of the dissociation to αα-diphenyl-β-benzoyl-β-hydrazyl varies considerably with changes of solvent, always in company with a variation of like direction in the entropy.

TABLE 63-5.—SOLVENT EFFECTS ON THE EQUILIBRIUM CONSTANT, AND ON THE HEAT AND ENTROPY OF DISSOCIATION TO αα-DIPHENYL-β-BENZOYL HYDRAZYL (GOLDSCHMIDT).

Solvent	Ether	Toluene	Acetone	Chloroform
10^4K, −18° (K in mole/l.)	0.27	1.14	1.48	23.6
ΔH (kcal./mole)	9.6	10.3	8.0	5.5
ΔS (cal./mole/deg.)	16.9	22.4	13.7	5.7

A complicated situation is disclosed here, as is not unexpected. For whereas in the hydrocarbon dissociation, solvation will be generally slight, and concentrated mainly on one constitutional feature, that of radical unsaturation in the radical, in the nitrogen-chain dissociation, all nitrogen atoms in the factor and in the product will be strongly solvated, so that thermodynamic parameters record only small differences between large quantities.

(h) Diaryl- and Dialkyl-aminoxyls.—Most of these radicals are stable in the solid state, and are fully monomeric in solution, even at low temperatures. Some of the radicals are known and are stable in the pure liquid and gaseous states. The radicals may be called aminoxyls, as above, or alternatively aminyl-oxides; for study of their electron-spin magnetic-resonance spectra has shown that their unpaired spin is practically equally divided between the oxygen and nitrogen atoms. The principal canonical structures of the radicals are quite analogous to those of the hydrazyls. We may call them the non-dipolar and dipolar structures,

$$\gt\dot{N}\text{—}O \quad \text{and} \quad \gt\overset{+}{\dot{N}}\text{—}\overset{-}{O}$$

In the mesomeric state, there is a slightly greater concentration of electrons on oxygen, than on the picryl-bearing nitrogen atom of diphenylpicrylhydrazyl, and hence a greater concentration of unpaired spin on the nitrogen atom of aminoxyls than on the disubstituted nitrogen atom of the hydrazyl. None of the possible dimers of the aminoxyls

$$R_2N\cdot O\cdot O\cdot NR_2, \quad R_2N\cdot O\cdot \overset{+}{N}R_2\cdot \overset{-}{O}, \quad \text{or} \quad \overset{-}{O}\text{—}\overset{+}{N}R_2\cdot \overset{+}{N}R_2\cdot \overset{-}{O}$$

is known in solution.

Diphenylaminoxyl, Ph_2NO, was prepared by Wieland and Offenbächer in 1914.[44] They obtained it by oxidation of diphenylhydroxylamine with silver oxide in ether. A red solution resulted from which the radical crystallised in dark red needles, m.p. 62°. A second method of obtaining it, due to Thomas,[45] is by peroxidation of diphenylamine: *t*-butylperoxy radicals, from *t*-butylhydroperoxide and ceric ions, oxidise the diphenylamine in a chain reaction as follows:

$$t\text{-BuO}_2\text{H} + \text{Ce}^{4+} \rightarrow t\text{-Bu}\dot{\text{O}}_2 + \text{H}^+ + \text{Ce}^{3+}$$

$$\left.\begin{array}{l} \text{Ph}_2\text{NH} + t\text{-Bu}\dot{\text{O}} \rightarrow \text{Ph}_2\dot{\text{N}} + t\text{-BuOH} \\ \text{Ph}_2\dot{\text{N}} + t\text{-Bu}\dot{\text{O}}_2 \rightarrow \text{Ph}_2\text{N}\dot{\text{O}} + t\text{-Bu}\dot{\text{O}} \end{array}\right\} \text{chain}$$

The radical can be grown in large crystals, isomorphous with benzophenone, with which it forms mixed crystals. On attempting to keep it at room temperature, it undergoes deep-seated decomposition, though it can be kept for a considerable time below −15°. All methods of molecular-weight determination show that it is monomeric, even at low temperatures. It is instantly reduced by a variety of reducing agents; and it combines at once with nitric oxide and with triphenylmethyl, though the immediate products of addition of these radicals undergo complex decompositions.

Most of the known substituted diphenylaminoxyls are generally similar to diphenylaminoxyl: they are not very stable substances. There are, however, some exceptional members of the series, which are very much more stable. The simplest of these are di-*p*-anisylaminoxyl,

[44] H. Wieland and M. Offenbächer, *Ber.*, 1914, **47**, 2111.

[45] J. R. Thomas, *J. Am. Chem. Soc.*, 1960, **82**, 5955.

discovered in 1919 by Kurt Meyer and Billroth,[46] and di-*p*-nitrophenylaminoxyl, prepared in 1920 by Wieland and Roth.[47] The former crystallises in copper-coloured plates, melting with decomposition at 120–150°, and the latter as dark red crystals, m.p. 109°. These radicals, like the products of their further substitution, can be kept indefinitely at ordinary temperature. They are strictly monomeric in all investigated conditions, and have one unit of electron spin, and the expected type of electron-magnetic-resonance spectrum.[48,49]

If these qualitative indications of stabilisation by conjugating methoxy and nitro-groups can be accepted, even though they lack the documentation of measured equilibrium constants, an analogy with hydrazyls is apparent; for hydrazyls, as we have seen, are stabilised by both $+M$ and $-M$ substituents. The analogy is not perfect, because the possible positions for substituents are more limited in aminoxyls than in hydrazyls. But still a conjugating $+M$-group such as methoxyl, and a conjugating $-M$ group such as nitroxyl, can both fill up octets and/or increase bonding, as illustrated with respect to the dipolar radical structures below:

$$(MeO-C_6H_4-)_2\dot{N}^{+}-O^{-} \qquad (O_2N-C_6H_4-)_2\dot{N}^{+}-O^{-}$$

A most interesting feature of aminoxyl radicals is that one can obtain stable aliphatic aminoxyls without formal conjugation. For the very few examples known, it would seem that $+I$ and $-I$ substituents favour stability, and can do so sufficiently to create very stable radicals.[50]

The first of these radicals to be described was di-*t*-butylaminoxyl, *t*-Bu_2NO. It was prepared in 1961 by Hoffmann and Henderson by the action of sodium on 2-nitro*iso*butane.[51] The sodium may be replaced by other very strong bases such as metal alkyls, and even Grignard reagents.[52] Di-*t*-butylaminoxyl is a red liquid of b.p. 75°/35 mm. When heated it undergoes no change up to 120°. It is stable in air and water. It is stable to dilute aqueous alkali. Its electron spin magnetic-resonance spectrum shows that its one unpaired

[46] K. H. Meyer, and H. G. Billroth, *Ber.*, 1919, **52**, 1476.

[47] H. Wieland and K. Roth, *Ber.*, 1920, **53**, 210.

[48] L. Cambio, *Gazz. chim. ital.*, 1933, **63**, 579.

[49] A. L. Buchachenko, *Optika i Spektroskopiya*, 1962, **13**, 795.

[50] E. G. Rozantsev, *Russian Chemical Reviews* (*Uspecki Khimii*), 1966, **35**, 658.

[51] A. K. Hoffmann and A. T. Henderson, *J. Am. Chem. Soc.*, 1961, **83**, 4671; A. K. Hoffmann, A. M. Fieldman, E. Gelblum, and W. G. Hodgson, *ibid.*, 1964, **86**, 639.

[52] R. Brière and A. Rassat, *Bull. soc. chim* (France), 1965, 378.

spin is divided, just as in aromatic aminoxyls, equally between its nitrogen and oxygen atoms.[42,51]

We can qualitatively understand this stability on the basis that the electropositive effect, $+I$, of the two tertiary alkyl groups would both increase the electron occupancy of the incomplete valency shell of the radical and increase its internal bonding. The non-dipolar and dipolar structures of the radical are shown below:

t-Bu
$\dot{\text{N}}$—$\dot{\text{O}}$
t-Bu

t-Bu
$\overset{\cdot +}{\text{N}}$—$\text{O}^-$
t-Bu

F_3C
N—$\dot{\text{O}}$
F_3C

F_3C
$\overset{\cdot +}{\text{N}}$—$\text{O}^-$
F_3C

The formulae above include the illustrations of the complementary case of radical stabilisation by the electronegative inductive effect, $-I$, of the trifluoromethyl group in bistrifluoromethylaminoxyl. This radical was prepared contemporaneously by Blackley[53] and by Makarov[54] and their respective collaborators in 1965. It is obtained by the action of oxidising agents ($KMnO_4$, Ag_2O, F_2) on bistrifluoromethylhydroxylamine, $(CF_3)_2N\cdot OH$, which is itself prepared from trifluoronitrosomethane, $CF_3\cdot NO$, by the action of ammonia, or by hydrolysis of its photo-dimer. The radical, $(CF_3)_2NO$, appears as a purple gas, which is stable in air and water, and in aqueous alkali. It combines with nitric oxide to give $(CF_3)_2NO\cdot NO$, which is, in fact, the photo-dimer of trifluoronitrosomethane. At lower temperatures the gaseous radical condenses to a deep purple liquid, b.p. $-25°$ At still lower temperatures, the liquid turns brown, and freezes to a yellow solid, m.p. $-70°$. A study of the electron-magnetic-resonance spectrum at various temperatures shows that the gas at 25° consists entirely of the radical, with one unpaired spin per molecule, but that the liquid at low temperatures is partly associated, and that the solid is wholly associated to what is assumed to be the diamagnetic dimer.

[53] W. D. Blackley and R. R. Reinhard, *J. Am. Chem. Soc.*, 1965, **87**, 802.

[54] S. P. Makarov, A. Yo. Yakubovich, S. S. Dubov, and A. N. Medvedev, *Dokl. Akad. Nauk S.S.S.R.*, 1965, **160**, 2139; cf. I. V. Miroshnichenko, G. M. Levin, S. P. Makarov, and A. F. Videiko, *Zhur. Strukt. Khim.*, 1965, **6**, 776.

The heat of dissociation of the dimer to the radical has been estimated as 2.5 kcal./mole.

Again we may suppose that a polar effect, now an electronegative inductive effect, $-I$, increases bonding as illustrated above, though it must decrease the total electron content of the NO group. The effect of polar substitution on bonding in both di-*t*-butylaminoxyl and bistrifluoromethylaminoxyl can be expressed in molecular orbital terms in a common statement. It is that, in either radical, one electron of the NO group must be alone in an antibonding orbital. If a polar effect of either sign should concentrate this electron on one atom or the other, then its antibonding effect, which depends on its being on both, will be reduced, with a resultant increase in overall bonding.

INDEX

Note: Where continuous or repeated references to a subject extend over no more than three consecutive pages, only the first such page is recorded below, but where over longer passages, the length is indicated.